AF518647

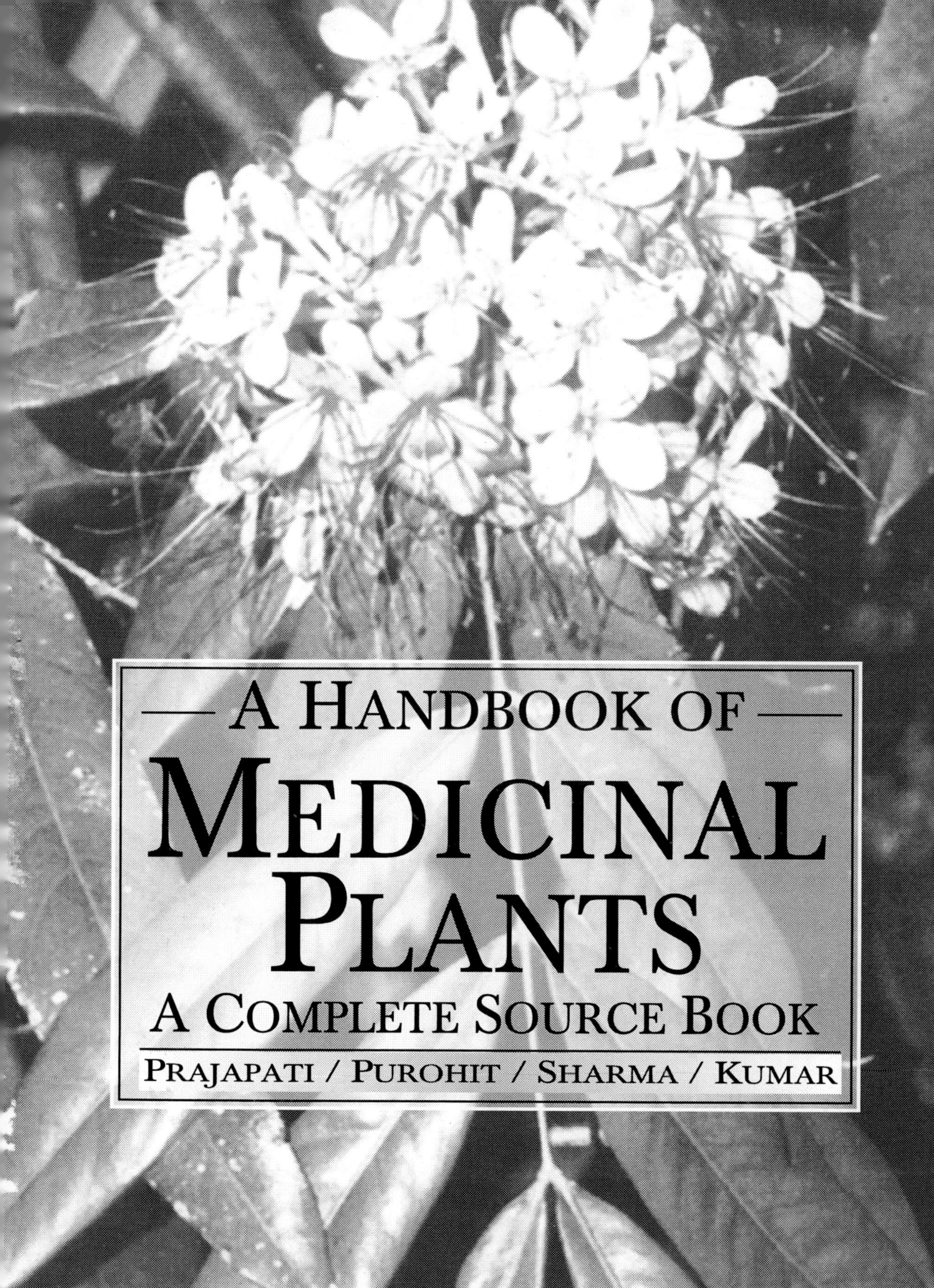
A HANDBOOK OF
MEDICINAL
PLANTS
A COMPLETE SOURCE BOOK
PRAJAPATI / PUROHIT / SHARMA / KUMAR

— A HANDBOOK OF —

MEDICINAL PLANTS

A COMPLETE SOURCE BOOK

Narayan Das Prajapati
S. S. Purohit
Arun K. Sharma
Tarun Kumar

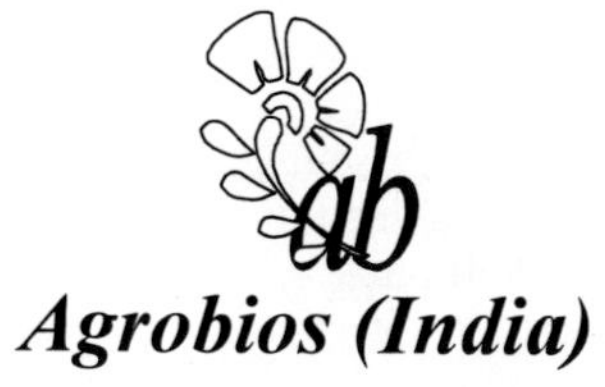

Agrobios (India)

Narayan Das Prajapati
Member, National Medicinal Plants Board
Department of Indian System of Medicine & Homeopathy
Ministry of Health and Family Welfare, Government of India, New Delhi

Dr. S. S. Purohit
Ex-Head, Department of Botany, Dungar College, Bikaner

Arun K. Sharma
Scientist (Agronomy), Central Arid Zone Research Institute, Jodhpur

Tarun Kumar
M.Sc. (Medicinal Plants)
Gujarat Ayurved University, Jamnagar

Published by:

Agrobios (India)
Agro House, Behind Nasrani Cinema
Chopasani Road, Jodhpur 342 003
Phone: 91-0291-2643993, 2642319
E. Mail: agrobiosindia@gmail.com

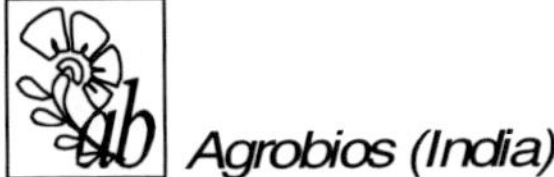

First Published, 2003
Print:2018

ISBN: 978-81-7754-134-2

Published by: Dr. Updesh Purohit for Agrobios (India), Jodhpur
Lasertypeset at: Yashee Computers, Jodhpur
Cover and Plates Design by: Shyam
Printed at: AGROBIOS DIGITALS, Jodhpur

PREFACE

Medicinal plants are the local heritage with global importance. World is endowed with a rich wealth of medicinal plants. The variety and sheer number of plants with therapeutic properties is quite astonishing. It is estimated that around 70,000 plant specie, from lichens to towering trees, have been used at one time or another for medicinal purposes. The herbs provide the starting material for the isolation or synthesis of conventional drugs. In India, medicinal plants have made a good contribution to the development of ancient Indian *Material Medica*. During the past one century there has been a rapid extension of the allopathic system of medical treatment in India. It generated commercial demand for pharmacopoeial drugs and their products in India. Efforts have been made to introduce many of these drug plants to farmers. Several research institutes have undertaken studies on the cultivation practices of medicinal plants, which were found suitable and remunerative for commercial cultivation.

Medicinal plants have curative properties due to the presence of various complex chemical substances of different composition, which are found as secondary plant metabolites in one or more parts of these plants. These plant metabolities, according to their composition, are grouped as alkaloids, glycosides, corticosteroids, essential oils, etc.

During the past decade, a dramatic increase in exports of medicinal plants attests to worldwide interest in these products as well as in traditional health systems. In the last 10 years, for example, India's exports of medicinal plants have trebled. But with most of these plants being taken from the wild, hundreds of species are now threatened with extinction because of overharvesting, destructive collection techniques, and conversion of habitats to crop-based agriculture. For instance, the small coniferous Himalayan yew (*Taxus baccata*) has recently become a heavily traded species. Similarly, *senna* is being grown extensively in arid region of India.

The pharmaceutical industries have made massive investment on pharmacological, clinical and chemical researches all over the world in past five decades. Efforts have been made to discover still more potent plant drugs. In fact, a few new drug plants have successfully been passed the tests of commercial screening. The benefits of these efforts would reach to the masses in future if farmers initiates commercial cultivation of medicinal plants. In fact, agricultural studies on medicinal plants, by its very nature, demand an equally large investment and higher priority. India, in particular, has a big scope for the development of pharmaceutical and phytochemical industry.

The Indian Pharmacopoeia (1966) recognized eighty five drug plants whose ingredients are used in various pharmaceutical preparations. We have however, confine our text to a few important commercially grown medicinal plants whose cultivation deserves priority in out national economy.

This book is divided in four sections: **Section – I:** Medicinal Plants : An overview, **Section II:** Medicinal Plants: A to Z, **Section III:** Colour Atlas, and **Section IV:** Medicinal Plants: Resources. The book will be useful for farmers, nursery men, growers, pharmaceutical and ayurvedic herbal companies, extractors, exporters, importers, large and small-scale organic cultivaters, seed production companies, scientists of various research institutes, consultants, planters associations, herbal hospitals, etc.

We acknowledge our thanks to various sources from where the text material, photographs, economic-data and resources have been used.

We also thank to Dr. Updesh Purohit of Agrobios (India) for quality production in record time.

Authors

CONTENTS

Section I: Medicinal Plants: An Overview

***Section II**: Medicinal Plants- A to Z*

Section III: *Medicinal Plants- Colour Atlas*

PLATE : 34

194 *Celosia argentea*
195 *Celosia cristata*
196 *Celtis australis*
197 *Centaurea centaurium*
198 *Centaurea cyanus*
199 *Centaurea jacea*
200 *Centella asiatica*

PLATE : 35

201 *Cephalonploa segetum*
202 *Ceratonia siliqua*
203 *Cerbera manghas*
204 *Ceterach officinarum*
205 *Chaenomeles sinensis*
206 *Chaenomeles speciosa*

PLATE : 36

207 *Chamomilla recutita*
208 *Cheiranthus cheiri*
209 *Chelidonium majus*
210 *Chenopodium bonus-henricus*
211 *Chloranthus joponicus*
212 *Chlorophytum borivilianum*

PLATE : 37

213 *Chrysanthemum cinerariifolium*
214 *Chrysanthemum coronarium*
215 *Chrysanthemum leucanthemum*
216 *Chrysanthemum morifolium*
217 *Chrysanthemum parthenium*
218 *Cichorium intybus*
219 *Cichoriun intybus*

PLATE : 38

220 *Cichorum endivia*
221 *Cicjorium intybus*
222 *Cimicifuga foetida*
223 *Cimicifuga heracleifolia*
224 *Cimicifuga racemosa*
225 *Cinchona officinalis*
226 *Cinnamomum cassia*

PLATE : 39

227 *Cinnamomum tamala*
228 *Cinnamomum verum*
229 *Cirsium japonicum*
230 *Cissampelos pareira*
231 *Cissus quadrangularis*

PLATE : 40

232 *Cistanche tubulosa*
233 *Citrullus colocynthis*
234 *Citrullus lanatus*
235 *Citrus aurantium*
236 *Citrus aurantium*
237 *Citrus limon*
238 *Citrus medica Linn*

PLATE : 41

239 *Citrus reticulata*
240 *Citrus sinensis*
241 *Citrus unshiu*
242 *Clematis hexapetala*
243 *Clematis mandschurica*
244 *Clematis vitalba*

PLATE : 42

245 *Cleome gynandra*
246 *Clerodendrum serratum*
247 *Clitoria ternatea*
248 *Cnicus benedictus*

PLATE : 43

249 *Cnidium officinale*
250 *Coccinia grandis*
251 *Cocos nucifera*
252 *Codiaeum variegatum*
253 *Codonopsis pilosula*
254 *Coffea arabica*

PLATE : 44

255 *Coix lacryma-jobi*
256 *Colchicum autumnale*
257 *Coleus barbatus*
258 *Coleus forskohlii*
259 *Colocasia esculenta*
260 *Commelina diffusa*

PLATE : 45

261 *Commersonia bartramia*
262 *Commiphora wightii*
263 *Conium maculatum*
264 *Convallaria majalis*
265 *Convolvulus arvensis*
266 *Convolvulus microphyllus*

PLATE : 46

267 *Copsicum frutescens*
268 *Coptis chinensis*
269 *Corchonus dipresces*
270 *Cordia subcordata*
271 *Cordyline fruticosa*
272 *Cornus mas*

PLATE : 47

273 *Cornus officinalis*

274 *Cornus sanguinea*
275 *Corydalis ternata*
276 *Corydalis yanhusuo*
277 *Corylus avellana*
278 *Costus speciosus*
279 *Countium kusnezoffii*

PLATE : 48

280 *Crataegus monogyna*
281 *Crataegus pinnatifida*
282 *Crataeva nurvala*
283 *Crinum asiaticum*
284 *Crithmum maritimum*
285 *Crocus sativus*

PLATE : 49

286 *Croton tiglium*
287 *Cucumis citrullus*
288 *Cucumis sativus*
289 *Cucurbita maxima*
290 *Cuminum cyminum*
291 *Cupressus sempervirens*
292 *Curcuma aromatica*
293 *Curcuma longa*

PLATE : 50

294 *Cuscuta chinensis*
295 *Cuscuta epithymum*
296 *Cuscuta reflexa*
297 *Cycas circinalis*
298 *Cydonia oblonga*
299 *Cynanchum ascyrifolium*

PLATE : 51

300 *Cynanchum atratum*
301 *Cynanchum wilfordii*
302 *Cynara scolymus*
303 *Cynodon dactylon*
304 *Cynoglossum officinale*
305 *Daphne mezereum*
306 *Datura innoxia*
307 *Datura Metal*
308 *Datura stramonium*

PLATE : 52

309 *Datura suaveolens*
310 *Daucus carota*
311 *Davallia fijiensis*
312 *Decaspermum fructicosum*
313 *Dendrobium nobile*
314 *Dendrocalamus giganteus*
315 *Dendrocnide harveyi*
316 *Dianthus chinensis*

PLATE : 53

317 *Dianthus superbus*
318 *Dichroa febrifuga*
319 *Dictamnus albus*
320 *Dictamnus albus*
321 *Dictamnus dasycarpus*
322 *Digitalis lutea*
323 *Digitalis purpurea*

PLATE : 54

324 *Dioscorea bulbifera*
325 *Dioscorea opposita*
326 *Diosorea batatas*
327 *Diospyros kaki*
328 *Dipsacus fullonum*
329 *Dolichos lablab*
330 *Drosera rotundifolia*

PLATE : 55

331 *Dryopteris crassirhizoma*
332 *Dryopteris filix-mas*
333 *Ecballium elaterium*
334 *Echinops latifolius*
335 *Echinops setifer*
336 *Echium vulgare*
337 *Eclipata prostrata*

PLATE : 56

338 *Elettaria cardamomum*
339 *Eleutherococcus sessiliflorus*
340 *Elsholtzia ciliata*
341 *Elsholtzia splendens*
342 *Elytraria acholis*
343 *Embelia ribes*

PLATE : 57

344 *Emblica offcinalis*
345 *Enicostema hysopefolium*
346 *Ephedra gerardiana*
347 *Ephedra sinica*
348 *Epilobium angustifolium*

PLATE : 58

349 *Epimedium koreanum*
350 *Epimedium sagittatum*
351 *Equisetum arvense*
352 *Equisetum hyemale*
353 *Erigeron canadensis*
354 *Eriobotrya japonica*
355 *Eryngium campestre*
356 *Erythrina variegata*

PLATE : 59

357 *Eucalyptus citriodora*
358 *Eucalyptus globulus*
359 *Eucommia ulmoides*
360 *Eugenia aromatic*
361 *Eugenia caryophyllata*
362 *Euodia hortensis*

PLATE : 60

363 *Euodia officinalis*
364 *Euonymus alatus*
365 *Eupatorium cannabinum*
366 *Euphorbia caducifolia*
367 *Euphorbia fidjiana*
368 *Euphorbia hirta*
369 *Euphorbia lathyrus*

PLATE : 61

370 *Euphorbia caducifolia*
371 *Euphorbia neriifolia*
372 *Euphorbia pekinensis*
373 *Euphorbia royleana*
374 *Euphrasia officinalis*
375 *Euryale ferox*
376 *Evodia rutaecarpa*
377 *Evolvulus alsinoides*

PLATE : 62

378 *Fagonia cretica*
379 *Fagus aylvatica*
380 *Farsetia hamiltonii*
381 *Ferula asafoetida*
382 *Ficus bengalensis*
383 *Ficus benjamina*
384 *Ficus carica*
385 *Ficus glomerata*

PLATE : 63

386 *Ficus religiosa*
387 *Foeniculum vulgare*
388 *Forsythia suspensa*
389 *Forsythia viridissima*
390 *Fragaria vesca*
391 *Frainus rhynchophylla*
392 *Fraxinus excelsior*

PLATE : 64

393 *Fucus vesciculosus*
394 *Fyllinga brevifolia*
395 *Galega officinalis*
396 *Galium aparine*
397 *Galium verum*
398 *Garcinia sessilis*
399 *Gardenia jasminoides*
400 *Gardinia gummifera*

PLATE : 65

401 *Gardenia taitensis*
402 *Gastrodia elata*
403 *Geniostoma rupestre*
404 *Gentiana acaulis*
405 *Gentiana litea*
406 *Gentiana scabra*

PLATE : 66

407 *Geranium robertianum*
408 *Ginkgo biloba*
409 *Glechoma hederacea*
410 *Gleditsia japonica*
411 *Glehnia littoralis*
412 *Globularia vulgaris*
413 *Gloriosa superba*
414 *Glossonema varians*

PLATE : 67

415 *Glycine max*
416 *Glycyrrhiza glabra*
417 *Glycyrrhiza uralensis*
418 *Gossypium herbaceum*
419 *Grewia tenax*
420 *Grindelia robusta*

PLATE : 68

421 *Guettarda speciosa*
422 *Gymnema sylvestre*
423 *Gyrocarpus americanus*
424 *Hamamelis virginiana*
425 *Hedera helix*
426 *Helianthus annuus*
427 *Helicteres isora*

PLATE : 69

428 *Heliotropium curasavicum*
429 *Hemerocallis fulva*
430 *Hemidionius indicus*
431 *Heracleum sphondylium*
432 *Hernandia nymphaeifolia*
433 *Hibiscus rosa-sinensis*
434 *Hibiscus syriacus*
435 *Hibiscus tiliaceus*

PLATE : 70

436 *Hieracium pilosella*
437 *Hipophae rhamnoides*
438 *Holarrhena antldysenterica*
439 *Holoptarlia intragifolia*

440 *Hordeum vulgare*
441 *Houttuynia cordata*

PLATE : 71
442 *Hoya australis*
443 *Humulus lupulus*
444 *Hyatis pectinata*
445 *Hyoscyamus niger*
446 *Hypericum perforatum*
447 *Hyssopus officinalis*
448 *Ilex aquifolium*

PLATE : 72
449 *Impatiens balsamina*
450 *Inocarpus fagifer*
451 *Inula helenium*
452 *Inula japonica*
453 *Inula racemosa*
454 *Ipomoea digitata*

PLATE : 73
455 *Ipomoea indica*
456 *Ipomoea nil*
457 *Iris germanica*
458 *Iris pseudacorus*
459 *Jasminum grandiflorum*
460 *Jatropha curcas*
461 *Juglans regia*

PLATE : 74
462 *Juglans sinensis*
463 *Juncus effusus*
464 *Juniperus communis*
465 *Juniperus sabina*
466 *Justicia sendarusse*
467 *Kalopanax pictus*
468 *Kochia scoparia*
469 *Kyllinga nemoralis*

PLATE : 75
470 *Lactuca sativa*
471 *Lactuca virosa*
472 *Lamium album*
473 *Lantana camara*
474 *Larix decidua*
475 *Laurus nobilis*
476 *Lavandula angustifolia*

PLATE : 76
477 *Lawsonia inermis*
478 *Leontopodium alpinum*
479 *Leonurus cardiaca*
480 *Leonurus japonicus*
481 *Leonurus sibiricus*
482 *Leptadenia pyrotechnica*

PLATE : 77
483 *Leptadenia reticulata*
484 *Leucas cephalotes*
485 *Levisticum officinale*
486 *Ligusticum chuanxiong*
487 *Ligustrum lucidum*
488 *Ligustrum vulgare*
489 *Lilium candidum*

PLATE : 78
490 *Lilium lancifolium*
491 *Linaria cymbalaria*
492 *Linaria vulgaris*
493 *Lindera strychnifolia*
494 *Linum usitatissimum*
495 *Lippia citridora*
496 *Liquidambar formosana*

PLATE : 79
497 *Liriope platyphylla*
498 *Litchi chinensis*
499 *Lobelia chinensis*
500 *Lobelia inflata*
501 *Lonicera caprifolium*
502 *Lonicera Japonica*
503 *Lophatherum gracile*

PLATE : 80
504 *Lotus corniculatus*
505 *Luffa cylindrica*
506 *Lupinus albus*
507 *Lycium barbarum*
508 *Lycium chinense*
509 *Lycoperdon bovista*
510 *Lycopersicon esculentum*
511 *Lycopodium clavatum*

PLATE : 81
512 *Lycopus lucidus*
513 *Lygodium japonicum*
514 *Lythrum salicaria*
515 *Magnolia denudata*
516 *Magnolia officinalis*
517 *Malus sylvestris*

PLATE : 82
518 *Malva sylvestris*
519 *Malva verticillata*
520 *Manihot esculenta*
521 *Marrubium vulgare*

604 *Petasites albus*
605 *Petroselinum crispum*

PLATE : 95

606 *Peucedanum decursivum*
607 *Peucedanum japonicum*
608 *Peucedanum ostruthium*
609 *Pharbitis nil*
610 *Phaseolus vulgaris*
611 *Phellodendron amurense*
612 *Phlomis umbrosa*

PLATE : 96

613 *Phragmites communis*
614 *Phyllanthus niruri*
615 *Phymatosorus scolopendeia*
616 *Physalis alkekengi*
617 *Physalis angulata*
618 *Physalis minima*

PLATE : 97

619 *Phytolaca esculenta*
620 *Phytolacca acinosa*
621 *Phytolacca americana*
622 *Phytolacca dioica*
623 *Picea abies*
624 *Picrasma quassioides*
625 *Pimpinella saxifraga*
626 *Pinellia pedatisecta*

PLATE : 98

627 *Pinellia ternata*
628 *Pinguicula vulgaris*
629 *Pinus koraiensis*
630 *Pinus mugo*
631 *Pinus sylvestris*
632 *Piper longum*
633 *Piper methysticum*

PLATE : 99

634 *Piper nigrum*
635 *Piper purberulum*
636 *Pistacia lentiscus*
637 *Pisum sativum*
638 *Plantago asiatica*
639 *Plantago depressa*
640 *Plantago lanceolata*

PLATE : 100

641 *Plantago major*
642 *Plantago media*
643 *Plantago ovata Forsk*
644 *Plantago psyllium*
645 *Plantanus orientalis*
646 *Plantycladus arientalis*

PLATE : 101

647 *Platycodon grandiflorum*
648 *Pluchea lanceolata*
649 *Plumbago zeylanica*
650 *Plumeria rubra*
651 *Polygonatum kingianum*

PLATE : 102

652 *Polygonatum odoratum*
653 *Polygonum aviculare*
654 *Polygonum bistorta*
655 *Polygonum dichrotomum*
656 *Polygonum multiflorum*
657 *Polygonum tinctorium*

PLATE : 103

658 *Polypodium vulgare*
659 *Polyscias fruticosa*
660 *Pometia pinnata*
661 *Poncirus trifoliata*
662 *Pongamia pinnata*
663 *Portulaca oleracea*

PLATE : 104

664 *Portulaca quadrifida*
665 *Posostemon cablin*
666 *Potentilla anserina*
667 *Potentilla chinensis*
668 *Potentilla reptans*
669 *Potentilla tormentilla*

PLATE : 105

670 *Premna serratifolia*
671 *Primula veris*
672 *Prunella vulgaris*
673 *Prunus armeniaca*
674 *Prunus avium*
675 *Prunus domestica*

PLATE : 106

676 *Prunus japonica*
677 *Prunus laurocerasus*
678 *Prunus mume*
679 *Prunus persica*
680 *Prunus spinosa*
681 *Psidium guajava*

PLATE : 107

682 *Psilotum nudum*
683 *Psoralea corylifolia*
684 *Psychotria insularum*

685 *Pueraria lobata*
686 *Pulmonaria officinalis*
687 *Pulsatilla chinensis*
688 *Pulsatilla koreana*

PLATE : 108

689 *Punica granatum*
690 *Putranjiva roxburghii*
691 *Pyrrosia lingua*
692 *Quercus robur*
693 *Quisquqlis indica*

PLATE : 109

694 *Ranunculus ficaria*
695 *Rauwolfia serpentina Benth*
696 *Rauwolfia tetrafela*
697 *Rehmannia glutinosa*
698 *Rheum palmatum*
699 *Rheum undulatum*

PLATE : 110

700 *Rhododendron ferrugineum*
701 *Rhus chinensis*
702 *Ribes grossularia*
703 *Ribes rubrum*
704 *Ricinus communis*

PLATE : 111

705 *Rivea hypocrateriformis*
706 *Robinia pseudacacia*
707 *Rorippa sarmentosa*
708 *Rosa canina*
709 *Rosa laevigata*
710 *Rosa multiflora*
711 *Rosa rugosa*

PLATE : 112

712 *Rosmarinus officinalis*
713 *Rubia akane*
714 *Rubia cordifolia*
715 *Rubia tinctorum*
716 *Rubus coreanus*
717 *Rubus fruticosus*
718 *Rubus idaeus*
719 *Rumex acetosella*
720 *Ruscus actuleatus*

PLATE : 113

721 *Ruta graveolens*
722 *Saccharum officinarum*
723 *Salix alba*
724 *Salvadora persica*
725 *Salvia miltiorrhiza*
726 *Salvia officinalis*
727 *Sambucus ebulus*
728 *Sambucus nigra*
729 *Sambucus racemosa*

PLATE : 114

730 *Sanguisorba officinalis*
731 *Sanicula europaea*
732 *Sansevieria trifasciata*
733 *Santalum album*
734 *Santolina chamaecyparissus*
735 *Saponaria officinalis*
736 *Saposhnikovia divaricata*

PLATE : 115

737 *Saraca asoka*
738 *Satureja hortensis*
739 *Scabiosa succisa*
740 *Scaevola taccada*
741 *Schisandra chinensis*

PLATE : 116

742 *Schizonepeta tenuifolia*
743 *Scolopendrium officinale*
744 *Scopolia japonica*
745 *Scrophularia buergeriana*
746 *Scrophularia ningpoensis*

PLATE : 117

747 *Scutellaria baicalensis*
748 *Scutellaria barbata*
749 *Sedum acre*
750 *Seetzenia lanata*
751 *Semecarpus anacardium*
752 *Sempervivum arachnoideum*
753 *Senecio vulgaris*

PLATE : 118

754 *Sesbania grandiflora*
755 *Siberian ginseng*
756 *Sida cordifolia*
757 *Siegesbeckia orientalis*
758 *Simmondsia chinensis*
759 *Sinapis alba*
760 *Sisal sislana*
761 *Sisymbrium officinale*

PLATE : 119

762 *Smilax aspera*
763 *Smilex china*
764 *Solanum dulcamara*
765 *Solanum indicum*
766 *Solanum melongena*

767 *Solanum nigrum*
768 *Solanum tuberosum*
769 *Solanum viride*

PLATE : 120

770 *Solanum xanthocarpum*
771 *Soldanella alpina*
772 *Solidago virgaurea*
773 *Sophora flavescens*
774 *Sophora japonica*
775 *Sorbus aucuparia*
776 *Sorghum bicolor*
777 *Spartium junceum*

PLATE : 121

778 *Spathoglottis pacifica*
779 *Spondias dulcis*
780 *Stachys officinalis*
781 *Stellaria dichotoma*
782 *Stellaria media*
783 *Striga gesnerioides*
784 *Swertia chirata*

PLATE : 122

785 *Symplocarpus foetidus*
786 *Syzygium cornocarpum*
787 *Syzygium cumini*
788 *Syzygium malaccense*
789 *Tacca lentopetaloides*

PLATE : 123

790 *Tamarindus indica*
791 *Tamarix gallica*
792 *Tamus communis*
793 *Tanacetum vulgare*
794 *Taraxacum mongolicum*
795 *Taraxacum officinale*
796 *Tarenna sambucina*
797 *Taxus baccata*

PLATE : 124

798 *Tecomella undulata*
799 *Tectona grandis*
800 *Tephrosea purpurea*
801 *Terminalia arjuna*
802 *Terminalia bellirica*

PLATE : 125

803 *Terminalia catappa*
804 *Terminalia chebula*
805 *Tetrapanax papyrifer*
806 *Teucrium chamaedrys*
807 *Theobroma cacao*
808 *Thespesia populnea*
809 *Thevetia peruviana*

PLATE : 126

810 *Thuja occidentalis*
811 *Thuja orientalis*
812 *Thymus serpyllum*
813 *Thymus vulgaris*
814 *Tilia platyphyllos*
815 *Tinospora Cordifolia*
816 *Torilis japonica*
817 *Torreya nucifera*

PLATE : 127

818 *Tragopogon pratensis*
819 *Trianthema portulacastrum*
820 *Tribulus terrestris*
821 *Trichodesma indicum*
822 *Trifolium arvense*
823 *Trigonella foenum-graecum*
824 *Trollius europaeus*
825 *Tropaeolum majus*

PLATE : 128

826 *Tussilago farfara*
827 *Tylophora indica*
828 *Typha orientalis*
829 *Ulmus macrocarpa*
830 *Ulmus procera*
831 *Umbilicus rupestris*
832 *Urtica urens*
833 *Utricularia vulgaris*

PLATE : 129

834 *Vaccinium myrtillus*
835 *Vaccinium vitis-idaea*
836 *Valeriana fauriei*
837 *Valeriana officinalis*
838 *Valeriana wallichii*
839 *Vanilla planifolia*

PLATE : 130

840 *Veratrum album*
841 *Veratrum maackii*
842 *Verbascum thapsus*
843 *Verbena officinalis*
844 *Vernonia cinerea*
845 *Veronicastrum sibiricum*
846 *Vicia faba*

PLATE : 131

847 *Vigna marina*
848 *Vinca minor*

Section IV: Medicinal Plants- Resources

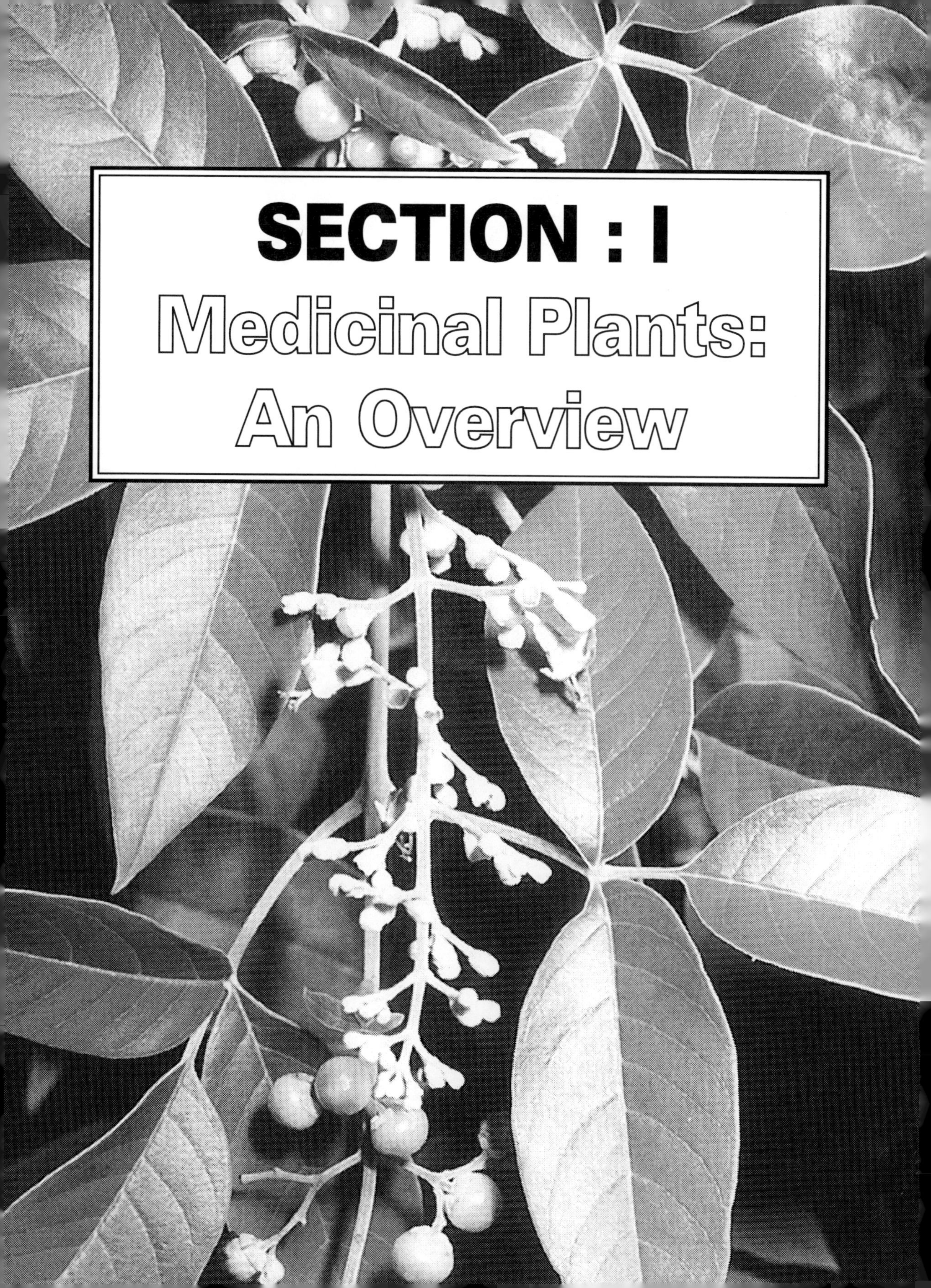

SECTION : I

Medicinal Plants: An Overview

1 MEDICINAL PLANTS: AN OVERVIEW

Medicinal plants are the local heritage with global importance. World is endowed with a rich wealth of medicinal plants. Herbs have always been the principal form of medicine in India and presently they are becoming popular throughout the developed world, as people strive to stay healthy in the face of chronic stress and pollution, and to treat illness with medicines that work in concert with the body's own defences. People in Europe, North America and Australia are consulting trained herbal professionals and are using the plant medicines. Medicinal plants also play an important role in the lives of rural people, particularly in remote parts of developing countries with few health facilities.

The variety and sheer number of plants with therapeutic properties is quite astonishing. It is estimated that around 70,000 plant specie, from lichens to towering trees, have been used at one time or another for medicinal purposes. The herbs provide the starting material for the isolation or synthesis of conventional drugs. In Ayurveda about 2,000 plant species are considered to have medicinal value, while the Chinese *Pharmacopoeia* lists over 5,700 traditional medicines, most of which are of plant origin. About 500 herbs are still employed within conventional medicine, although whole plants are rarely used.

In India, medicinal plants have made a good contribution to the development of ancient Indian *Material Medica*. One of the earliest treatises on Indian medicine, the *Charak Samhita* (1000 B.C.), records the use of over 340 drugs of vegetable origin. Most of these continue to be gathered from wild plants to meet the demand of the medical profession. Thus, despite the rich heritage of knowledge on the use of plant drugs, little attention had been paid to grow them as field crops in the country till the latter part of the nineteenth century.

During the past one century there has been a rapid extension of the allopathic system of medical treatment in India. It generated commercial demand for pharmacopoeial drugs and their products in India. Efforts have been made to introduce many of these drug plants to farmers. Several research institutes have undertaken studies on the cultivation practices of medicinal plants, which were found suitable and remunerative for commercial cultivation. The agronomic practices for growing poppy, *isabgol, senna,* cinchona, ipecac, belladonna, ergot and few others have been developed and there is now localized cultivation of these medicinal plants commercially.

Medicinal plants have curative properties due to the presence of various complex chemical substances of different composition, which are found as secondary plant metabolites in one or more parts of these plants. These plant metabolities, according to their composition, are grouped as alkaloids, glycosides, corticosteroids, essential oils, etc. The alkaloids form the largest group, which includes morphine and *codein* (poppy), strychnine and *brucine* (nux vomica), *quinine* (cinchona), ergotamine (ergot), *hyocyamine* (belladonna) scolapomine (*datura*), emetine (ipecac), cocaine (coco), ephedrine (*Ephedra*), reserpine (*Rauwolfia*), caffeine (tea dust), aconitine (aconite), vascine (vasaca) santonin (*Artemisia*), lobelin (Lobelia) and a large number of others. Glycosides form another important group represented by digoxin (foxglove), stropanthin (*Strophanthus*), glycyrrhizin (liquorice), barbolin (aloe), sannocides (senna), etc. Corticosteroids have come into sennocides (senna), etc. Corticosteroids have come into prominence recently and diosgenin (*Dioscorea*), solasodin (*Solanum* sp.), etc. now command a large world demand. Some essential oils such as those of valerian *kutch* and peppermint also possess medicating properties and are used in the pharmaceutical industry. However, it should be stated in all fairness that our knowledge of the genetic and physiological make–up of most of the medicinal plants is poor and we know still less about the biosynthetic pathways leading to the formation of active constituents for which these crops are valued.

Medicinal and aromatic plants are found in forest areas throughout South Asia, from the plains to the high Himalayas, with the greatest concentration in the tropical and subtropical belts and arid region of Thar desert. India recognizes more than 2,500 plant species as having medicinal value, Sri Lanka about 1,400, and Nepal around 700. Some of these, found at high altitudes in particularly stressful environments, grow very slowly and cannot live elsewhere. Others are more broadly distributed and adapt more easily to different ecological conditions.

During the past decade, a dramatic increase in exports of medicinal plants attests to worldwide interest in these products as well as in traditional health systems. In the last 10 years, for example, India's exports of medicinal plants have trebled. But with most of these plants being taken from the wild, hundreds of species are now threatened with extinction because of overharvesting, destructive collection techniques, and conversion of habitats to crop–based agriculture. For instance, the small coniferous Himalayan yew (*Taxus baccata*) has recently become a heavily traded species. Similarly, *senna* is being grown extensively in arid region of India.

The pharmaceutical industries have made massive investment on pharmacological, clinical and chemical researches all over the world in past five decades. Efforts have been made to discover still more potent plant drugs. In fact, a few new drug plants have successfully been passed the tests of commercial screening. The benefits of these efforts would reach to the masses in future if farmers initiates commercial cultivation of medicinal plants. In fact, agricultural studies on medicinal plants, by its very nature, demand an equally large investment and higher priority. India, in particular, has a big scope for the development of pharmaceutical and phytochemical industry.

The Indian Pharmacopoeia (1966) recognized eighty five drug plants whose ingredients are used in various pharmaceutical preparations. We have however, confine our text to a few important commercially grown medicinal plants whose cultivation deserves priority in out national economy.

FUTURE STRATEGY FOR MEDICINAL PLANTS

World bank group have several project to support the cultivation of medicinal plants through various lending and nonlending initiatives, the World Bank is assisting the countries of South Asia to address these needs. Some of these efforts are, The Kerala Forestry Project, The Sri Lanka Medicinal Plants Project, Ritigala Community Based Development and Environment Management Foundation, The India Capacity Building for Food and Drugs Quality Control Project, etc. There is a need to launch number of projects for arid region of India.

Although the Bank has supported some pioneering work in the South Asia region related to medicinal plants and, more generally, natural resource management, much remains to be done. In the future, it will be important to mainstream medicinal plants and other nontimber forest products into natural resource management and development programs. To boost the quality of plant resource management and increase supplies of these resources:

1. Agricultural support agencies should strengthen extension efforts to farmers.
2. Research institutions need to improve basic knowledge about cultivation practices and dissemination of plant species.

3. Conservation agencies and NGOs should promote conservation of vulnerable species at the grass–roots level.

4. Community organizations need to adopt sustainable collection and management practices on public lands.

5. Profitable private enterprises for processing, transporting, and marketing must be developed.

6. Government institutions need to be strengthened to regulate these important resources and, at the same time, foster their sustainable development and conservation.

7. Future initiatives should also link the management and conservation of medicinal plants (and other non–timber forest products) with the commercial development of these resources. In this spirit, every new forestry project should be designed to have a significant effect on the sustained use of non–timber forest products. Management and conservation must be integrated with programs in other sectors: in health, to foster better use of plant materials; in education, to build awareness of the need for protection and judicious development; and in agriculture, to strengthen farmer extension methods for plant cultivation.

8. The Bank's new lending instruments–learning and innovation loans and adaptable program loans–are well suited to these efforts. They can allow for project design flexibility to incorporate lessons learned, encourage institutional reforms, and, where appropriate, foster pilot exercises to test new approaches. With the commitment of governments, local communities, and NGOs, coupled with international support, the medicinal plant resources of South Asia have a chance of surviving, thriving, and continuing to aid billions of people.

9. The Global Environment Facility (GEF) provides grant and concessional funds to developing countries and those with economies in transition for projects and activities that address four aspects of the global environment: biological diversity, climate change, international waters, and the ozone layer. Activities related to land degradation, primarily those addressing deforestation and desertification as they relate to the focal areas, are also eligible for funding. Along with the United Nations Development Programme and the United Nations Environment Programme, the World Bank is an implementing agency for the GEF.

2 HISTORY OF MEDICINAL PLANTS: A WORLD SCENARIO

To trace the history of herbalism one must go back to the history of pharmacology, for until the last century medicinal plants were still being processed for general use. The discovery of the curative properties in plants must have sprung from some human instinct. Primitive man used plants for both food and medicine. He would have learnt, after perhaps many unfortunate experiences, that some plants contained certain properties, and was able to identify them by the results they induced. He would also have observed, which plants animals utilized when they were sick. After seeing an injured deer rubbing itself against the geum, he might have discovered, for instance, that this plant would hel his own wounds; and realized that dog tooth grass would act as an emetic, as it did with the cat. Many remarkable examples of animals intuitively knowing how to treat themselves with appropriate plants are quoted by numerous writers. Cicero, for example, mentions the hartwort being used by young does to ease parturition, while Plutarch refers to bears using the wild arum (lords–and–ladies). Cases of accidental poisoning must have been common occurrences before the beginning; curative herbs had been distinguished from the poisonous ones. The German botanist Mollisch made an interesting observation concerning six plants containing caffeine–namely coffee, cola, mate, tea, cocaa and guarana; among innumerable plant species man was able to pick out these six with great precision, even though they lack particular features, which enable them to be easily distinguished for their medical properties.

EARLY ORIGINS: THE 19TH CENTURY

Medicinal plants have been crucial in sustaining the health and the well being of mankind. People were knowing the importance of Linseed (*Linum usitatissimum*) oil as nutritious cooking oil, fuel, a cosmetic balm for the skin, in treatmnent of bronchitis, respiratory catarrh, boils, digestive disorders, and fibre to make fibric. A 60,000–year–old burial site excavated in Iraq, for instance, was found to contain eight different medicinal plants, including ephedra (*Ephedra sinica*). The inclusion of the plants in the tomb suggests they had supernatural significance as well as medicinal value. In many civilizations plants were considered to have souls. Even Aristotle, the 4th–century BC Greek philosopher, thought that plants had a *psyche*, albeit of a lesser order than the human soul. In medieval Europe, the Doctrine of Signatures stated there was a connection between how a plant looked–*God's signature*–and how it might be used medicinally. For example, the mottled leaves of lungwort (*Pulmonaria officinalis*), were thought to resemble lung tissue, and the plant is still used to treat ailments of the respiratory tract. Similarly, in Western cultures, it is a belief that plant spirits linger. In Bratin people do not cut down elder trees (*Sambucus nigra*) for fear of arousing the anger of the Elder Mother, the spirit who lived in and protected the tree. In Hind culture, plants are sacred to specific divinities. For example, the bael tree (*Aegle marmelos*) is said to shelter Lord Shiva, the god of health, beneath its branches. Andes in South America believe that the coca plant (*Erythroxylum coca*) is protected by Mama Coca, a spirit who must be respected and placated if the leaves are to be harvested and used.

In many traditional societies illness is thought to stem from malignant forces or possession by spirits. If a member of the tribe falls ill, the shaman (the *medicine* man or woman) is expected to intercede with the spirit world to bring about a cure. Shamans often enter the spiritual realm with the aid of hallucinogenic plants or fungi, such as ayahuasca (*Banisteriopsis caapi*), taken by Amazonian shamans, or fly agaric (*Amanita muscaria*), taken by traditional healers of the Siberian steppes.

It is generally recognized that by our ancestors that a wide range of medicinal plants have healing powers. Until the 20th century, every village and rural community had a wealth of herbal folklore. They have tried and tested local plants for a range of common health problems. Thye were using herbal plants as teas and lotions or even mixed with lard and rubbed in as an ointment. People were aware of good and bad effect of herbal plants. For example, eating of a particular root, leaf or berry by watching animal behaviour after they have eaten or rubbed against certain plant. These observations have also added to medicinal values of the forest plants. For example, if one watches sheep or cattle, they almost unerringly steer a path past poisonous plant such as ragwort (*Senecio jacobaea*), or oleander (*Nerium oleander*). Such close observations helped to know the people about poisonous or medicinal value of the plants.

In Egypt, the Middle East, India and China civilizations grew from 3000 BC on wards, therefore, the use of herbs became more sophisticated. They made first written accounts of medicinal plants. They listed dozens of medicinal plants, their uses and related spells and incantations. They indicated the medicinal value of herbs like myrrh (*Commiphora molmol*), castor oil (*Ricinus communis*), and garlic (*Allium sativum*).

In India, the *Vedas* are the, epic poems written *c.* 1500 BC. These volumes contain rich material on the herbal lore of that time. The *Vedas* were followed in about 700 BC by the *Charaka Samhita*, written by the physician Charaka. He is know as is known father of medicine in India. This medical treatise includes details of around 350 herbal medicines. Amongst them are visnaga (*Ammi visnaga*), a herb of Middle Eastern origin that has of Middle Eastern origin that has recently proven effective in the treatment of asthma, and gotu kola (*Centella asiatica*), which has long been used to treat leprosy.

By about 500 BC in developed cultures, medicine began to separate from the magical and spiritual world. Hippocrates (460–377 BC), the Greek is known father of medicine. He considered illness to be a natural rather than a supernatural phenomenon. He also felt that medicine shold be given without ritual ceremonies or magic.

The book, *Yellow Emperor's Classic of Internal Medicine* is the earliest Chinese medical text written in the 1st century BC. It includes text about rational medicine and treating illness before examination of the entire context, symptoms, observations of the emotions and attitudes. If one insists on the presence of ghosts and spirits one cannot speak of therapeutics.

Foundation of Major Herbal Tradition 300 BC–AD 600

In second century BC trade of many medicinal and culinary herbs between Europe, the Middle East, India, and Asia was established. Cloves (*Eugenia caryophyllata*), for example, native to the Philippines and the Molucca Islands near New Guinea, were imported into China in the 3rd century BC, and first arrived in Egypt around AD 176. As the centuries passed, cloves' popularity grew and by the 8th century AD, their strong aromatic flavour and powerfully antiseptic and analgesic properties were familiar throughout most of Europe.

As trade and interest in herbal medicines and spices flourished. These plants were known for their various known medicinal value and properties. In China, the *Divine Husbandman's Classic (Shen' nong Bencaojing)*, written in the 1st century AD, has 364 entries, of which 252 are herbal medicines, including bupleurum (*Bupleurum chinense*), coltsfoot (*Tussilago farfara*), and *gan cao* (*Glycyrrhiza uralensis*). Such literature laid the foundations for the continuos development and refinement of Chinese herbal medicine.

In Europe, Dioscorides the, a Greek physician wrote the first European herbal book *De Materia Medica* in a 1st–century AD. He presented accurate and authoritative work on herbal medicines. He indicated the medicinal importance of many plants like juniper (*Juniperus communis*), elm (*Ulmus carpinifolia*), peony (*Paeonia officinalis*), and burdock (*Arctium lappa*). He listed about 600 herbs in all. The text had an astonishing influence on Western medicine and was used as a principal reference in Europe until the 17th century and translated into Anglo–Saxon, Persian and Hebrew languages. In AD 512, *De Materia Medica* became the first herbal to feature pictures of the plants discussed. Made for Juliana Arnicia, the daughter of the Roman emperor Flavius Avicius Olybrius, it contained nearly 400 full–page colour illustrations.

Galen (AD 131–200), physician to the Roman emperor Marcus Aurelius, had an equally profound influence on the development of herbal medicine. Galen drew inspiration from Hippocrates and based his theories on the *theory of the four humours*. His ideas shaped and, some would say, distorted medical practice for the next 1,400 years.

In India and in China, elaborate medical systems somewhat resembling the theory of the four humors developed that have endured to the present day.

Though European, Indian and Chinese system differ widely, they all consider that imbalance within the constituent elements of the body is the cause of illness, and that the aim of the healer is to restore balance, often with the aid of herbal remedies.

Traditional Folk Healing in Middle Ages

The theories of *Galenic, Ayurvedic* (Indian) and Chinese traditional medicine were used for treatment of mankind, which are still being used by some indigenous peoples who have little access to conventional medicines. One should not underestimate the medical skills of apparently undeveloped communities–particularly during the so–called Dark Ages in medical Europe. Though many people had a surprisingly sophisticated understanding of plant medicine.

In 11th–century, Monastic hospital in Scotland, monks were using exotic herbs such as opium poppy (*Papaver somniferum*), and marijuana (*Cannabis sativa*), as painkillers and anaesthetics. Similarly, the herbalists in Myddfai (a village in South Wales) were aware of Hippocrates' writings in the 16th century AD and used a wide variety of medicinal plants. The major text indicated the following aspects of treatment:

To strengthen the sight	Take Eyebright and Red Fennel, a handful of each, and half a handful of Rue, distil, and wash your eye daily therewith.
To destroy a worm in the tooth	Take the root of the ear, bruise, and apply to the patient's tooth for three nights, and it will kill the worm.

Indian and Islamic Medicine AD 500–1500

The Arabic culture in AD 500–1300 gained the classical Greek and Roman ideas for medicinal plants. They preserved and elaborated them. The spread of Islamic culture along North Africa and into present–day Italy, Spain and Portugal led to the founding of renowned medical schools, notably at Cordoba in Spain. The Arabs were expert pharmacists, blending and mixing herbs to improve their medicinal effect and their taste. Their contacts with both Indian and Chinese medical traditions meant that they had a remarkable range of medical and herbal knowledge to draw on and develop. Avicenna (AD 980–1037), author of *Canon of Medicine,* was the most famous physician of the day, but perhaps the most unusual herbal connection was made a century before his time by Ibn Cordoba, an intrepid Arab seafarer, who brought ginseng root (*Panax ginseng*), from China to Europe. This valuable tonic herb was to be regularly imported into Europe from the 16th century onwards.

India had golden age of medicine in 7th century. Thousands of students studied *Ayurveda* at Indian university, especially at Nalanda. There, scholars recorded the medical achievements of the time, with advance such as the development of hospitals, maternity homes and the planting of medicinal herb gardens.

Central and South American Cures

On the other side of the world, the ancient civilizations of Central and South and South America–Maya, Aztec and Inca–all had herbal traditions with profound understanding of local medicinal plants. One account tells of Incas taking local herbalists from what is now Bolivia back to their capital Cuzco in Peru because of the herbalists' great capabilities, which reputedly included growing penicillin on green banana skins.

At the same time, medicine and religion were still closely interwoven in these cultures, possibly even more so than in Europe. One gruesome account tells of Aztec sufferers of skin diseases who sought to appease the god Xipe Totec by wearing the flayed skins of sacrificial victims. Fortunately, a supernatural appeal to the gods was not the sole means to relieve this and other afflictions. Many herbs were available as alternative treatments, including sarsaparilla (*Smilax* spp), a tonic and cleaning herb that was used in treatments for a variety of skin complaints including eczema and psoriasis.

Use of Medicinal Plants in European Countries (AD 1000–1400)

European scholars were influenced by Arabic medical learning in the early Middle Ages.

The classical Greek, Roman and Egyptian literature were preserved in the libraries of Constantinople (later Istanbul) which filtered back to Europe. This encouraged European scholars to establish hospitals, medical schools and universities. The medical school at Salerno on the west coast of Italy is one of the prime institutes. It not only allowed students from all faiths–Christian, Moslem and Jewish–to study medicine, but it also allowed women to train as physicians.

Herbs were, of course, central to the healing process. An adage from the Salerno school on sage (*Salvia officinalis*), went as follows: *Salvia salvatrix, natura conciliatrix* (sage, the savoiour; nature, the conciliator).

By the 12th century, trade with Asia and Africa was expanding and new herbs spices were being regularly imported into Europe. Hildegard of Bingen (1098–1179) the famous German mystic and herbal authority, considered galangal (*Alpinia officinarum*),–used in Asia as a warming and nourishing spice for the digestive system–to be the "spice of life", given by God to provide health and to product against illness.

Development in Asia

Marco Polo's travels to China in the 14th century coincided with the unification of the whole of Asia from the Yellow Sea in China to the Black Sea in south–eastern Europe by Genghis Khan and his grandson Kublai Khan, whose capital was in China, not far from Beijing. Neither the Chinese nor Ayurvedic medical traditions were directly threatened by this conquest. The rulers of Mongol tried to stop use of a few toxic plants like aconite (*Aconitum napellus*). The people were using aconite as alternative of arrow poison–one that could have been used against the ruling powers. Mongols have tried to make unification between the two medical disciplines. In other parts of Asia, such as

Vietnam and Japan, Chinese culture and medicine exerted the primary influence. While *kampoh*–the traditional herbal medicine of Japan–is distinctive to that country, its roots stem from Chinese practices.

Trade Promotion of Medicinal Plant (AD 1400–1700)

In Middle ages Trade routes had expanded. People used to bring exotic new herbs in their wake. From the 15th century onwards, an explosion in trade led to a cornucopia of new herbs becoming readily available in Europe. They included plants such as ginger (*Zingiber officinale*), cardamom (*Eletteria cardamomum*), nutmeg (*Myristica fragrans*), turmeric (*Curcuma longa*), cinnamon (*Cinnamomum verum*), and senna (*Cassia senna*). The trade in herbs was not entirely one way. The European herb sage, for example, came into use in China, where it was considered to be a valuable *yin* tonic.

In 1942, ships of Columbus arrived in the Caribbean, which was followed in the rapid conquest and colonization of Central and South America by the Spanish and Portuguese. Along with their booty of plundered gold, the conquistadors returned to the Old World with previously unheard–of medicinal plants. Various herbs from the Americas had highly potent medicinal actions. They soon became available in the apothecaries of the major European cities. Plants such as lignum vitae (*Guaiacum officinale*), and cinchona (*Cinchona*) were used for treatment of fever, malaria, syphilis, smallpox and other serious illnesses.

The rural communities tried to grow foreign plants for medicinal and food value. Garlic offers one of the earliest and clearest examples. These plants were originated in central Asia which were grown in Egypt around 4500 BC.

Similarly, in later centuries potatoes (*Solanum tuberosum*), and maize (*Zea maize*), (both native to South America) become common foods for all. These plants have clear medicinal as well as nutritional benefits. Potato juice is a valuable remedy for the treatment of arthritis, while corn–silk makes an effective decoction for urinary problems such as cystitis.

Vale of Medicinal Plants for Health and Hygiene (AD1400–1700)

From 12th and 18th centuries, the influx of exotic medicinal plants added large number of useful European herbs. Conceivably, an overall improvement of health in Europe might have resulted. After all, not only were new medicinal plants available, but Europeans had the opportunity to observe the different medical practices of people in South America, China, Japan and especially in India, where trade was well established. From the mid–14th century onwards, plague killed millions, in some cases close to 50 per cent of the population. No medical treatment–herbal or mineral–was able to alter its fatal course. Epidemics continued to determine the cities of Europe and Asia well into the 18th century. A recent outbreak in India in 1994 reawakened the terror inspired simply at the mention of the wood plague. Syphilis was another disease spread by seafarers. It was reputedly brought back from the Caribbean to Naples by Columbus' crew in the 1490s, spreading quickly throughout Europe and to the rest of the World, reaching China in 1550. European doctors had little success in combating diseases as devastating as plague. The medicine they practiced was based on the blind acceptance of Galen's humoral principles. Perhaps if, as in Chinese and Indian medicine, European medicine had continued to evolve, revising ancient medical texts and reinterpreting them in the light of new discoveries, it would have had grater success.

Impact of Paracelsus Views

Paracelsus (1493–1541) was one of the key European figures of the 16th century. He was an influential force in the future development of chemistry, conventional medicine herbal medicine and homeopathy. Though he is known as the concerned itself with the transmutation of base materials to gold, and the search for immortal life. Paracelsus also observed interest in the Doctrine of Signatures–the ancient theory that held that a plant's appearance indicated the ailments it would treat–and affirmed the value of locally grown medicinal herbs over expensive, improved specimens.

Culpeper was wounded during the English Civil War while fighting for the Commonwealth. He felt the needs of the ordinary poor people who unable to afford neither the services of a doctor nor the expensive imported herbs. The Arabian physicians and Paracelsus, Culpeper developed a medical system that blended astrology and vast personal experience of the therapeutic uses of local plants. The details were published in n North America (1700) the form of a book–*Herbal.* It became an instant bestseller and was published in several subsequent editions.

Paracelsus was a well known figure in the field of new chemical medicine by the end of the 16th century. He was also of the opinion that metallic poisons like mercury, antimony and arsenic should be used with caution.

Modern medicine proved as important *vital force* for mankind, however the importance of the vital force was diminished in the West by the philosophy of René Descartes (1596–1650). He was a French mathematician who divided the world into body and mind, nature and ideas. His philosophy ordained that the intangible vital force that maintains life and governs good health was the province of religion rather than of the newly self–aware "science" of medicine. To the new medical establishment, inching it way forward towards scientifically sound medical practices, *supernatural* concepts such as the vital force were a reminder of the ignorance and superstition that were part and parcel of older healing practices.

In traditional Chinese medicine, *qi* is the primal energy that maintains life and health. In Ayurveda, it is *prana,* and in the Western tradition. Hippocrates writes about "*vis medicatrix naturae*" or the healing power of nature, while modern Western medical herbalists and homeopaths use the term "vital force".

Scientific Approach in Using Medicinal Plants

There was a gap in proper understanding of medicinal plants for mankind in past because traditional medicine generally lacked scientific explanation. In *American Indian Medicine* (University of Oklahoma Press, 1970), Virgil Vogel provided a good example of *ignorant* folk medicine outstripping scientific understanding in therapeutic applications. The discovery of the medicinal value of foxglove (*Digitalis purpurea*) is another case where traditional herbal knowledge led to a major advance in medicine. Dr. William Withering (1741–1799), a conventionally trained doctor with a long interest in medicinal plants. Started to investigate foxglove after encountering a family recipe for curing dropsy (water retention). He found that in some regions of England, foxglove was traditionally used to treat this condition, which is often of the indications of a failing heart. In 1785, he published *Account of the Foxglove,* documenting dozens of carefully recorded case histories, and showing how foxglove's powerful (and potentially dangerous) active constituents, now known as cardiac glycosides, made it a valuable plant medicine for dropsy. Cardiac glycosides remain in common use to the present day. Yet despite this clear–cut example of the possibilities inherent in a marriage of herbal medicine and scientific method, conventional medicine was to take another path in the 19th century.

New Frontiers and New Herbal Medicines

Wherever Europeans settled during the great migrations of the 18th and 19th centuries–North America, South America, southern Africa or Australia–much of the European medicine familiar from home was either unavailable or prohibitively expensive. Settlers cam to learn that native peoples were a wellspring of information about the medicinal virtues of indigenous plants. For example, European settlers in southern Africa learned about the diuretic properties of buchu (*Barosma betulina*), from native peoples; and Australian settlers came to understand the remarkable antiseptic properties of tea tree (*Melaleuca alternifolia*), from observing the medicine as it exists today is a blend of Aztec, Mayan and Spanish herbs and practices.

In North America, native herbalists were particularly adept at healing external wounds and bites–being superior in many respects to their European counterparts in the area respects to their European counterparts in this area of medicine. This is not surprising, given the range of highly effective medicinal plants Native Americans had discovered–including well-known herbs such as Echinacea (*Echinacea angustifolia*), goldenseal (*Hydrastis Canadensis*) and lobelia (*Lobelia inflata*).

European settlers learned much from observing native practices. Over the course of the 19th and early 20th centuries, as pioneers moved west across the frontier territory, new plants were constantly being added to the official three species mentioned above, about 170 native plants were listed in *The Pharmacopoeia of the United States.*

Western Impact on Asian Medicine

In Chinese medicine, there has always been a debate as to what degree illness arises from cold, and to what degree it arises from heat. The *Shanghanlun* (*On Cold–Induced Maladies*), written in the 2nd century AD, and revised and reinterpreted in commentarie sover the last 1,800 years, recommends the herb cinnamon (*Cinnamomum verum*), asa principal remedy when the patient "shivers with fever, breathers heavily and feels nauseous". In the 14th century illness and febrile illness, and treated them in different ways, and this distinction was elaborated in greater and greater detail by different Chinese herbalists right up to the 19th century.

Western biomedicine had impact on traditional practices of China and India during the early 19th century. This was certainly beneficial in many respects. The judicious incorporation of scientific principles and methods into traditional herbal healing offers the possibility of greatly refining the effectiveness of treatment.

However, in India, during British rule, Western medicine, eventually become the only alternative of *Ayurveda.* Western practice was introduced not as a complement to traditional medicine, but rather as a means to supplant it. Before 1835, the Western physicians and their Indian counterparts were exchanging knowledge; thereafter only Western medicine was recognized as legitimate and the Eastern systems were actively discouraged.

THE HISTORY OF AYURVEDA

Gradually accumulated practical and systematic medical knowledge in India is called **Ayurveda**. Medicinal knowledge gained over trial and error over the thousands of years in India and neighbouring regions of central Asia/ south East Asia has been systematized some four thousand years ago in a system of medicine called Ayurveda.

Ayurveda (pronounced *I–your–vay–da*), the science of life, prevention and longevity is the oldest and most holistic or comprehensive medical system available. It was placed in written form over 2,000 years ago in India, it is said to be a world medicine. Before the advent of writing, the ancient wisdom of healing, prevention and longevity was a part of the spiritual tradition of a universal religion. Medical knowledge from all areas of the world gathered in India, and the famous sage Vyasa, put into writing the complete knowledge of Ayurveda, along with the more directly spiritual insights of ethics, virtue and Self–realization.

In Ayurveda the methods used to acquire this knowledge of the uses of herbs, foods, aromas, gems, colors, yoga, mantras, lifestyle and surgery. The sage–physician/surgeons of the time were the same sages or seers, deeply devoted holy people, who saw health as an integral part of spiritual life. It is said that they received their training of Ayurveda through direct cognition during meditation. In other words, the knowledge of the use of the various methods of healing, prevention, longevity and surgery came through Divine revelation; there was no guessing or testing and harming animals. These revelations were transcribed from the oral tradition into book form, interspersed with the other aspects of life and spirituality.

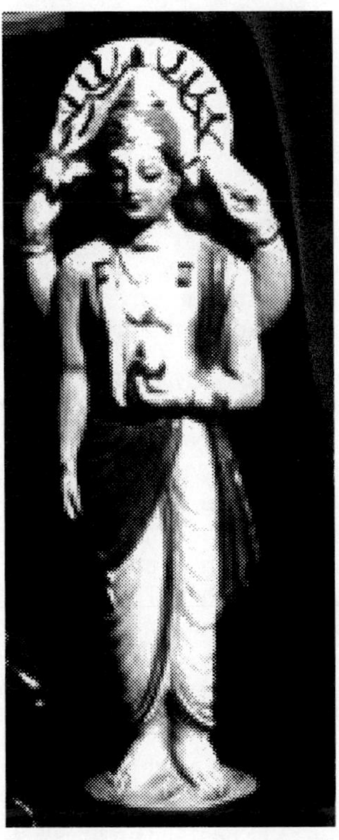

Fig. 1.1: Dhanvantari Lord of Ayurvedic Healing. According to the *Puranas* this incarnation of Vishnu was a ruler of Benares whooriginated a universally effective system of traditional herbalmedicine. He holds a golden leech (symbolic of blood purification) and a medicinal plant (*Tinospora cordifolia*, "Amrita") in his right hands, and the conch of wisdom and pot of rejuvenating nectar in his left. The tulsi–beed mala around his neck, plant–wreath halo, and his sometimes blue–tinted skin emphasizehis connection to Vishnu the Preserver.

The Vedas; *Rik, Sama, Yajur and Atharva.* Ayurveda was used in conjunction with Vedic astrology (Jyotish–inner light). At later dates, Ayurveda was organized into its own compact system of health and considered an auxiliary branch of the Vedas, called an ***Upaveda*** (limb of the Veda), because it dealt with the healing aspects of spirituality, and not directly discussing spiritual development). These authors took the passages related to Ayurveda from the various Vedas and made separate books, dealing only with Ayurveda. Among the Rik Veda's 10,572 hymns, are found discussions of the three doshas, *Vayu, Pitta and Kapha;* organ transplants, and artificial limbs, the use of herbs to heal the diseases of the mind and body and to foster longevity. Within the Atharva Veda's 5,977 hymns, are discussions of anatomy, physiology and surgery.

Around 1500 B.C., Ayurveda was delineated into eight specific branches of medicine. There were two main schools of Ayurveda at that time, Atreya– the school of physicians; and *Dhanvantari*– the school of surgeons.

These two schools made Ayurveda a more scientifically verifiable and classifiable medical system. Through research and testing, they dispelled the doubts of the more practical and scientific minded, removing the aura of mystery that surrounded the concept of Divine revelation. Consequently Ayurveda grew into a respected and widely used system of healing in India. People from numerous countries came to Indian Ayurvedic schools to learn about this world medicine– in its completeness. Chinese, Tibetans, Greeks, Romans, Egyptians, Afghanistanis, Persians, and more travelled to learn the complete wisdom and bring it back to their own countries.

There are two main re–organizers of Ayurveda whose works are still existing in tact today– Charak and Sushrut. The third major treatise is called the Ashtanga Hridaya which is a concise version of the works of Charak and Sushrut. Thus the three main ancient Ayurvedic texts that are still used today are, the *Charak Samhita* (compilation), *Sushrut Samhita* and the *Ashtangha Hridaya Samhita*. These books are believed to be over 1,200 years old. It is because these texts still contain the original and complete knowledge of this Ayurvedic world medicine, that Ayurveda is known today as the only complete medical system still in existence. Other forms of medicine from various cultures, although parallel, are missing parts of the original information.

Charak represented the Atreya school of physicians, discussing physiology, anatomy, etiology, pathogenesis, symptoms and signs of disease; methodology of diagnosis, treatment and prescription of patients; prevention and longevity. Included were internal and external causes of illness. Charak states that the first cause of illness is the loss of faith in the Divine. In other words, when a person does not have the experience that God is inside us, and, outside– in all things, this separation of vision creates a gap in which longing or suffering for oneness of vision occurs. This suffering is the beginning of spiritual, mental and physical disease. External causes of health included time of day, seasons, diet and lifestyle. There is a whole section discussing the medicinal aspects of herbs, diet, and reversing of the aging process. For the skeptical modern person, who wonders if this ancient wisdom can be believed, one only need to read Charak's month–by–month description of the development of the fetus in the womb to see its exact parallels to what we know today from using modern technical machinery.

Sushruta comes from the Dhanvantari school of surgeons. In America, there is a society of surgeons who named themselves the Sushruta Society. In this text, there are detailed and sophisticated discussions of surgical equipment; the classification of abscesses, burns, fractures, wounds, amputation, plastic surgery, anal/rectal surgery, which are validated by modern medicines technical equipment and research. There is a complete discussion of the human anatomy; the bones, joints, nerves, heart, blood vessels, circulatory system etc., again, corroborated by todays methods of mechanical investigation. From the Sushrut Samhita, we learn of the first science of massage, using marma points or vital body points, which parallel Chinese acupuncture. Even the popular Polarity Massage Therapy in America, was developed by a man after studying massage in India.

Antiquity of System

There is a refreshing lack of mumbo–jumbo mystery mongering, and in many cases modern techniques confirms the genuineness of the claims of Ayurvedic doctors. Unfortunately fakes and quacks out to make a fast buck distort the teachings.

Origins

The origins of this system of course are lost in time. In legend it is said to have been taught by the creator, Brahma, to the Prajapati Daksha. (One of the lords of the animals) who taught it in turn to the divine twins called the Asvins. These Aswins are the heavenly healers. They taught Indra, the chief of the shining ones. The personages mentioned were deities of early Vedic times.

When mankind started suffering from various diseases the wise men like Bharadvaja learnt from Indra the knowledge of medicine. Gradually the huge amount of knowledge accumulated was divided systematically into 8 branches.

THE BRANCHES OF AYURVEDA

Branch	Meaning
Kaya chikitsa	Internal medicine
Baala	Pediatrics
Graha	Treatment of diseases arising from possession by pathogens, evil spirits, etc. Mainly diseases of a mental nature.
Urdhvanga	Dealing with the eyes, ear, nose, throat and dentistry
Salya	Surgery including plastic surgery
Danstra	Insect bites, poisons (Toxicology)
Rasayana	Diseases of advancing age
Prasuti	Gynecology and obstetrics

BASIC CONCEPTS OF AYURVEDA

Vyaadhi, or disease in Ayurveda is due to an imbalance of three fundamental elements of the body. These are VATA, PITTA and KAPHA. The entire universe is made of five *Maha bhootas,* or great *elements.* (that are not material in the usual sense of the term, and are types of energy.) For identifying them they are called:

1. *Akaasa* (roughly, space)
2. *Vaayu* (air)
3. *Tejas* (light)
4. *Ap* (water)
5. *Prithvi* (earth)

Vaata	Human bodies are mainly made of Akasa, Vaayu with a little of Teja, Ap and Prithvi. Vaata is what allows one to interact with the environment. Briefly, vaata tramsmits sense impressions to the mind and responses to various places of the body, maintains the integrity of the body and proper functioning of its various constituent elements, the sensory organs of touch and sound depend on vaata: the Dhaatus and Malas (tissue material and waste matter) are transported by vaata. It stimulates Agni and produces joy. It forms the embryo in the womb into particular shapes It is the evidence of life.
Pitta	Is the primary constituent of the living body whose structure is Tejas ("luminous light"). Its function is balncing and transformative. Its functions in particular are — vision, digestion, production of heat, Hunger, thirst, softness and suppleness of body, lustre, cheerfullness and intelligence.
Kapha	Is one of the primary constituents of body, having "water" and "earth" as elements. Function of pitta is conserving and stabilising . It organises the tissues (into their microscopic and macroscopic form)

Disease in Ayurveda

Disease is called ***Vyaadhi*** in ayurveda. It is the state of body and mind in which they are subjected to discomfort, pain and injury. The fundamental cause is imbalance of the three Vaata, Pitta and kapha. Fairly elaborate classification of diseases is done in Ayurveda. It is according to the trauma (abhigaata).

Adhyatmika	physical and psychic type, constitutional
Adhibhautika	caused by environment
Aadhidaivika	caused by gods or spirits

More practical classification for treatment

Aadi– bala pravritta	Genetically predisposed
Janma– bala	Congenital
Dosha –bala	caused by imbalances in Vaata, Pitta, Kapha.
Sanghata–bala	Traumatic
Kaala–bala	Seasonal, time linked
Daiva –bala	Gods or demons
Svabhaava –bala	natural changes

Ayurvedic Treatment Differs from Modern Medicine

Ayurvedic treatment differs from modern medicine in the way the disease is viewed. Usually ayurvedic practitioners say antibiotics may have their uses, especially in surgery, but that antibiotics basically attack the germs which are considered to cause disease.

The ayurvedic doctors prefer that the balance of the body be restored. The causative factors, which allow the germs to grow has to be removed, not just quickly attacking the germs they say.

Drugs

The drugs used in Ayurveda are made by several processess from vegetable and mineral raw materials. It appears mostly plant alkaloids are the active ingredients. Obviously barring some chemical changes it is mostly natural derivates (modern medicines are also based upon these but proportion of synthetic derivate is more.).

However the plants growing in particular soils, with pattern of weather, sunlight, time of harvesting, method of preparation of medicine all are very important. The identical species of plant growing in rain forest and city backyard may not have the same medicinal value.

EUROPE

Each of the world's Major herbal traditions has developed its own framework for making sense of illness. In Europe, the model for understanding and explaining illness was the", which persisted well into the 17th century it was laid down by Galen (AD 131–201), physician to the Roman emperor Mercus Aerelius. Galen was born in Pergamum and part of his medical practice involved caring for the gladiators of the city, which gave him the opportunity to learn about anatomy and the remedies best suited to healing wounds. He wrote literally hundred of books and his influence on European conventional and herbal medicine has been immense. To this day, plant medicines are sometimes called Galenicals to distinguish them from synthesized drugs.

The Theory of the Four Humours

Galen developed his ideas from the texts of Hippocrates (460–*c.* 377 BC) and Aristotle (384–322 BC), who in turn had been influenced by Egyptian and Indian ideas. Hippocrates, expanding on the early belief that the world was made up of the elements fire, air, earth and water, classified herbs as having hot, dry, cold and most properties. Aristotle developed and endorsed the theory of the four humours. According to the theory, four principal fluids–or humours–exist within the body; blood, choler (yellow bile), melancholy (black bile) and phlegm. The *ideal* person bore all four in equal proportion. However, in most people, one or more humours predominate, giving rise to particular temperatures or characters. For instance, excess choler produced a choleric–type person, who was likely to be short–tempered, sallow, ambitious and vengeful. Galen also believed that *pneuma* (spirit) was taken in with each breath, and processed in the body to form the "vital spirit". Vitality and health depended upon the proper balance between the four humours and the four elements and the correct mix with the inspired *pneuma.*

Influence of Classical Herbalists

Two other classical writers strongly influenced the European herbal tradition. Dioscorides (AD 40–90), a Greek–born Roman army on herbal medicines, *De Materia Medica,* based on observations of nearly 600 plants. Pliny the Elder (AD 23–79) drew together writings from over 400 authors in his *Natural History,* recording, amongst other things, herbal lore of the time. Much traditional European knowledge of medicinal herbs comes from Dioscorides and Pliny. One of the most interesting herbs mentioned by both is mandrake (*Mandragora officinarum*). With a forked root that resembles the human shape, mandrake was credited with great magical and healing powers. It was recommended by Dioscorides for many ailments, including sleeplessnessand inflammation of the eyes.

With the collapse of the Roman empire in the 4th century AD, the debate about how illness arose and how it should be treated shifted to the East. By the 9th century, Islamic physicians had translated much of Galen's work into Arabic, and his ideas affected the development of Arabic medicine into the Middle Age, influencing Avicenna (980–1037). Later in the Middle Age, Galen's writings were translated back into Latin from the Arabic and, for 400 years, his ideas sway and were diligently applied in European medical practice. Even in the 16th and 17th centuries, students in university medical schools were given an academic training in the principles of the humoural system, as established by Galen. They learnt how to diagnose an imbalance of the humours, and the methods of restoring equilibrium, primarily bloodletting and purging.

Printing and Herbal Medicine

The invention of printing in the 15th century changed the face of herbal medicine in Europe. Before that time, European folk medicine had been handed down from generation to generation. While some early herbals were written in Anglo–Saxon, Icelandic and Welsh, for example, for the most part the tradition was orally based.

During the following centuries, herbals were published throughout Europe in different languages, making standardized catalogues of herbs and their applications accessible to the general public, not just to those who understood Latin. As literacy rates rose, women in particular used the advice in the herbals to treat their families.

In some cases, the printed herbals were written by physicians, and largely reflected the writings of classical authors such as Dioscorides. In other instances, they were based directly on first–hand experience–the English herbals of John Gerard (1597) and Nicholas Culpeper (1652) being good examples.

John Gerard's *The Herball* is clearly the work of horticulturist, rather than of a herbal practitioner, but is nonetheless a mine of information. The book includes many plans that had been recently brought back to Europe by explorers and traders.

Culpeper's *The English Physitian* has been widely used as a practical reference book every since its publication. It is a rich blend of personal and practical experience, traditional European medicine and astrological thought. Each herb is assigned a "temperature European medicine and astrological thought. Each herb is assigned a "temperature", a use within the humoural system, and a ruling planet and star. Like Dioscorides' *De Materia Medica* it has the merit of being based on close observation and extensive experience in the use of herbal medicines.

Foreign Herbs and Synthesized Drugs

The growing use of foreign herbs in the 17th prompted heated debate about the relative value of indigenous European herbs, but for the majority of the population this was irrelevant as the imported herbs were well out of their price range. In the end, it created a rift in herbal medicine. Poor and rural peoples used locally available herbs, while affluent city–dewellers and aristocrats purchased plants of foreign origin, prescribed by university–trained physicians. By the beginning of the 18th century, approximately 70 per cent of plant medicines stocked by European apothecaries were imported. Over time, this city–based herbalism evolved into conventional scientific medicine, which in turn rejected its herbal roots and regarded plant medicines as inferior.

Once conventional medicine established its monopoly of practice–in most European countries by the end of the 19th century–it became (and in many cases still remains) illegal to practice herbalism without medical certification. In Greece, traditional herbalists, known as *komboyannites,* were persecuted, and the word itself became an insult meaning 'trickster' or "quick". In France and Italy, experienced traditional herbalists were imprisoned for providing treatment to their patients. The renaissance in herbal medicine that has occurred in the last 25 years offers hope that official censure will change.

Modern Practitioners

The pattern of herbal medicine across Europe today is remarkably varied, but a common thread runs through the different traditions and practices. Most European herbalists use orthodox methods of diagnosis, looking for signs of infection and inflammation, for example. However, most also try to establish a broad, holistic picture, placing the illness in the context of the patient's life as a whole. Herbalists then choose plant medicines and recommend suitable dietary and lifestyle changes that will allow the body's self–regenerating powers–the modern equivalent of the "vital spirit"–to establish good health once again. Recovery may take longer than it would if treated with conventional medicine, but relief is generally enduring and free from side effects.

A patient with a stomach ulcer, for example, may be treated with a variety of herbs such as meadowsweet (*Filipendula ulmaria*), German chamomile (*Chamomilla recutita*), marshmallow (*Althaea officinalis*), and deadly nightshade (*Atropa belladonna*), to soothe inflammation, astringe and protect the inner lining of the stomach, and reduce excess acid production. In addition, herbal practitioners also address poor dietary habits, bad posture and stress–which are all conditions that may have undermined the body's healing ability. Problems such as these are reversed with herbs to relieve stress, a diet rich in non–acidic vegetables and fruits, and exercise.

Popular Herbs

In European herbal medicine, native herbs are still highly popular. Alpine plants such s arnica (*Arnica Montana*), and pasque flower (*Anemone pulsatilla*), are much used in Swiss, German, Italian and French herbal medicine, while comfrey (*Symphytum officinale*), is particulary well liked in Britain. These has also been a surge in demand for exotic herbs. The Chinese ginkgo tree (*Ginkgo biloba*), which improves circulation of blood to the head and helps the memory, is now cultivated in vast plantations in France, and became the bestselling medicine of all in Germany in 1992.

European Traditions and the Future

Sales of over–the–counter medicines in Europe are increasing at a dramatic rate. In the UK between 1990 and 1995, sales clamed by 25 per cent. Herbal medicine or *phytotherapy* is so esteemed in Germany that conventionally trained doctors routinely prescribes herbs along with orthodox drugs. In contrast, herbalism in the UK was practiced by those who have trained in herbal rather than conventional medical schools; providing treatment that is complementary to conventional medicine. The picture is again different in Spain. Some doctors prescribe herbal medicines, but traditional herbalists, *curanderos*, still practice. They learn by apprenticeship, gathering herbs from the wild and preparing their own medicines.

How the European Union will mango to legislate the safe practice of each of these three types of herbalism remains to be seen, but each has a significant contribution to make in a future in which people are free to free choose the treatment that accords with their ideas and wishes.

INDIA

The Name Ayurveda Deriver from two Indian words: *ayur*, meaning life and *veda*, meaning knowledge or science. Ayurvedic medicine is more than a system of healing. It is way of life encompassing science, religion and philosophy that enhances well–being, increase longevity and ultimately brings self–realization. It aims to bring about a union of physical, emotional and spiritual health, known as *swathya*. This state enables the individual to enter into a harmonious relationship with cosmic consciousness.

Early Origins

Ayurveda evolved over 5,000 years ago in the far reaches of the Himalaya from the deep wisdom of spiritually enlightened prophets, of *rishis*. Their wisdom was transmitted orally from teacher to disciple, and eventually set down in Sanskrit poetry known as the *Vedas*. These writing, during to approximately 1500 BC, distilled the prevailing historical, religious, philosophical and medical knowledge.

The Influence of Ayurveda

Other systems of medicine such as the Chines, Tibetan and Islamic (Unani Tibb) traditions have their roots in Ayurveda. For example, the Buddha (born *c.* 550 BC) was a follower of Ayurveda, and the spread of Buddhism into Tibet during the following centuries was accompanied by increased practice of Ayurveda.

The ancient civilizations were linked to one another by trade routes, campaigns and wars. Arab traders spread knowledge of Indian plants and Ayurvedic medicine was studied by Arab physicians, who included Indian plants in their *Material Medica*. This knowledge was passed on to the ancient Greeks and Romans, whose practices were eventually from the basis of European medicine.

The Five Elements

Ayurveda is a unique holistic system, based on the interaction of body, mind and spirit. In Ayurveda, the origin of all aspects of existence is pure intellect or consciousness. Energy and matter are one. Energy is manifested in five elements–ether, air, fire, water and earth–which together form the basis of all matter. In the body, ether is present in the cavities of the mouth, abdomen, digestive tract, thorax and lungs. Air is manifested in the movements of the heart, expansion and contraction of the lungs, and the workings of the digestive tract and the nervous system. Fire is manifested in the digestive system, metabolism body temperature, vision and intelligence. Water is present in the digestive juices, salivary glands, mucous membranes, blood and cytoplasm. Earth exists in the nails, skin and hair, as well as in the elements that hold the body together: bones, cartilage, muscles and tendons.

The five elements manifest in the functioning of the five senses, and they are closely related to our ability to perceive and interact with the environment in which we live. In Ayurveda, ether, air, fire, water and earth correspond to hearing, touch, vision and taste small respectively.

The *Doshas* and Health

The five elements combine to form three basic forces, known as the *tridoshas*, which exist in everything in the universe, and influence all mental and physical processes. From ether and air, the principle *vata* is created; fire and water yield the fire principle *pitta*; and earth and water produce the water principle *kapha*. The principles correspond closely to the three humors of Tibetan medicine and somewhat resemble Galen's theory of the four humours.

According to Ayurveda, we are all born with a particular balance of *doshas*. The proportions are largely determined by the balance of *doshas* in our parents at the time of our conception. Our body type, temperament, and susceptibility to illnesses are largely governed by the predominant *dosha*. In this way we inherit our basic constitution, called the ***prakruti***, which remains unaltered throughout our lives. The first requirement for health in Ayurveda is a proper balance of the *doshas*. If the balance is upset, illness, *ryadhi*, results. The disruption may be manifested in physical discomfort and pain, or in mental and emotional suffering, including jealousy, anger, fear and sorrow. While our balance of *doshas* influences vulnerability to certain kinds of illness, the principle do not work in a vacuum. The effect our lifestyle has on our *prakruti–vakruti*–has a strong effect upon overall health, and it may easily disrupt *dosha* balance.

Illness may also result if the flow of energy, *prana*, around the body is interrupted. The flow is relayed via the seven *charkas* (psychic energy centers), which are situated at various points along the spinal column, from the crown of the head to the tailbone. If the energy flowing between these centers is blocked, the likelihood of ill health increases.

An Aurvedic practitioner first carefully assesses *prakruti* and *vakruti*–constitution and lifestyle. This involves taking a detailed case history and carefully examining the body, paying attention to the build, the lines in the face and hands, and skin and hair type–all of which point to more profound aspects of the patient's condition. However, the main foundation on which diagnosis rests re the appearance of the tongue, and the pulse rate. In these respects, Ayurvedic has much in common with Chinese and Tibetan medicine, in which these two indicators are also of the greatest importance. A very complex technique for taking the patient's pulse has been developed by Ayurvedic practitioners, requiring many years' experience.

When a *dosha* imbalance has been diagnosed, medical treatment and lifestyle advice are provided. The first step is eliminating toxins and the main cleansing and rejuvenation programme, known as *panchakarma*, includes therapeutic vomiting, purging, enemas, nasal administration of medication and purification of the blood.

Categories of Treatments

Usually, treatments fall into following main categories:

1. Medicines from natural sources
2. Dietary regimes
3. Behavioural modifications

Medicines, foods and lifestyle activities are all classified according to their effect on the three *doshas*. For instance, a health problem associated with an excess of *kapha*, the water principle, is characterized by catarrh, excess weight, fluid retention and lethargy. The practitioner would prescribe the consumption of warm, dry, light foods, because the quality of *kapha* is cool and damp. Avoidance of cold damp foods (such as wheat, sugar and milk products), which increase *kapha*, would also be advised. Herbal remedies would include warming species such as ginger (*Zingiber officinale*), cinnamon (*Cinnamomum verum*), and cayenne (*Capsicum frutescensi)*, as well as biters such as turmeric (*Curcuma longa*), and aloe vera (*Aloc vera*).

Herbal Quality or Energy

In Ayurveda system, the specific choice of herbal remedy depends on its *quality* or energy, which is determined according to twenty attributes (*vimshati guna*) such as hot, cold, wet, dry, heavy or light. Ayurveda also classifies remedies according to six tastes–sweet, sour, salty, bitter pungent and astringent. Sweet, sour and salty substances increase water (*kapha*) and decrease air (*vata*); bitter, pungent and astringent remedies increase air and decrease water; and sour, salty and pungent herbs increase fire (*pitta*).

Preparations and Treatments

In addition to plant extracts, Ayurvedic medicines include honey and dairy produce, and sometimes–minute doses of minerals such as salt are added. Remedies take the form of pills, powers, balms and infusions, and most contain several different ingredients, all carefully balanced to individual needs. Treatments might include washes and enemas or the application of poultices as well as massage with warm herbal oil, burning incense, the use of precious stones and metals, and ritual purification for imbalanced mind and emotions. The chanting of mantras (incantation based on sacred texts), breathing and mediation exercise may be advised, due to the power of sound and the effect of vibration and meditation on the body, mind and spirit.

Importance of Ayurvedic Medicine

The importance of Ayurveda is proved in part by its timelessness, since it has existed as an unbroken tradition for thousands of years. Ayurveda's value lies in the fact that it is not a medical science that deals solely with treatment of disease. Instead, it offers practical guidelines for living, which are applicable to every facet of daily existence. It also seeks to reconcile health and lifestyle with the universal aspects of existence, and thus it enhances the well–being, longevity and harmony of all those who practice it. For these reasons, traditional Western practices.

CHINA

Traditional Chinese Medicine and the herbal tradition that is part of a developed separately from Chinese folk medicine. It arose from ideas recorded between 200 BC and AD 100 in the *Yellow Emperor's Classic of Internal Medicine (Huang Di Nei Jung)*. This text is based on detailed observations of nature and a deep understanding of the way that all life is subject to natural laws. It contains concepts that are fundamental to TCM, including *yin* and *yang*, the five elements (*wu* *xing*); and the theory of the effect of nature upon health. In Traditional Chinese Medicine, living in harmony with these principles is the key to good health and longevity. According to the *Yellow Emperor's Classic*, members of previous generations lived for a hundred years, and had constitution so strong that illness was cured by incantations alone. Only later, as human vitality, or *qi*, declined and people became *overactive.... going against the joy the life*, did herbal medicine, acupuncture and other branches of Traditional Chinese Medicine become necessary.

Basic Theories

Unlike other herbal traditions that have a unified theory for making sense of illness and disease (for example, the European theory of the four humours), Traditional Chinese Medicine has two quite different systems–the *yin* and *yang* theory and the five elements, similar to Indian tradition. They developed quite separately in China and the five elements system was only accepted and fully incorporated into Chinese medicine during the Song dynasty (AD 960–1279). To this day, differences between these theories are reflected in practitioners' approaches to diagnosis and treatment. According to Traditional Chinese Medicine everything in the universe is composed of *yin* and *yang*–words that were first used to denote the dark and light side of a valley. Everything has *yin* and *yang* aspects, or complementary opposites–such as day and night, up and down, wet and dry. Every *yin* or *yang* category can itself also be subdivided–so that while the front of the body is *yin* relative to the back, which is *yang*, the abdomen is *yin* relative to the chest, which is *yang*. The five elements theory associates constituents of the natural world–wood, fire, earth, metal and water–with other fundamentals such as seasons, emotions and parts of the body. Each element gives rise to the next in a perpetual fashion. For this reason, the system might be more accurately described as the five phases, representing the processes of continual movement in life. The five elements have a central role in Chinese herbal medicine, in the grouping of taste of herbs and parts of the body.

Diagnosis and Treatment

In Traditional Chinese Medicine causes of illness depends on the patterns of disharmony, which are expression of imbalance between *yini* and *yang*. Particular attention is given to reading the pulse and tongue, both of which are very important for an accurate diagnosis. The health results depends from a deficiency or excess of either *yin* or *yang*.

For example, cold, is not just the result of a virus (though this clearly is a cause), but a sign that the body is not adapting to external factors such as wind–heart, wind–cold or summer–heat. Similarly, a high temperature indicates too much *yang* and shivering is the result of an excess of *yin*. Therefore, the Chinese herbal practitioner is to restore harmony between *yin* and *yang* both within the patient's body and between the patient and the world at large.

Uses of Chinese Herbs

In *Encyclopedia of Traditional Chinese Medicinal Substances* which has about 5,757 and most of them are herbs. The Communist Revolution in 1949 helped swell the number of plants used in Traditional Chinese Medicine, because herbs that had previously only been employed in folk medicine were incorporated into the tradition.

The herbal tradition of Traditional Chinese Medicine has developed the taste and other characteristics of herbs. They became closely linked with their therapeutic uses. *The Divine Husbandman's Classic (Shen'nong Bencaojing*, 1st century AD) lists about 252 herbal medicines and indicated their tastes and temperatures. In present time, Chinese herbalists still directly relate the taste and temperatures of a herb directly to its therapeutic use. Sweet–tasting herbs such as ginseng (*Panax ginseng*) are prescribed to tone, harmonize and moisten, while bitter–tasting herbs such as *dan shen* (*Salvia miltiorrhiza*) are employed to drain and dry excess dampness. Similarly, hot–testing herbs are used for treating cold conditions and vice versa. A taste of the herbs and temperature are linked to their specific types of illness. For example, Baical skullcap (*Scutellaria baicalensis*), which is bitter–tasting and cold is a drying, cooling herb for conditions such as fever and irritability, brought on by patterns of excess heat.

The Traditional Chinese Medicine mainly depends set mixtures of herbs. Such mixtures have proven effectiveness as tonics or remedies for specific illnesses. Many are available over the counter and are used by millions of people every day in China and around the world. Chinese herbalists often take a formula as a starting point and then add other herbs to the mixture. There are hundreds of formulate, one of the most famous being *Four Things Soup*, a tonic given to regulate the menstrual cycle and tone the reproductive system. It consists of Chinese angelica (*Angelica sinensis*), rehamannia (*Rehmannia glutinosa*), *chuang xiong* (*Ligusticum wallachii*) and white peony (*Paeonia lactiflora*). Traditional Chinese Medicine uses tinctures or alcoholic extracts of herbs, but only infrequently. Generally, patients are given mixtures of roots and bark to take as decoctions two or three times a day.

Influence of Traditional Chinese Medicine in Japan and Korea

Japan and Korea have been strongly influenced by ideas of Traditional Chinese Medicine practices. *Kampoh*, traditional Japanese medicine, traces its origins back to the 5th century AD, when Buddhist monks from Korea introduced their healing arts, largely derived from Chinese medicine, into Japan. In the following century, the Empress Suiko (AD 592–628) sent envoys to China to study that country's culture and medicine. Direct Chinese influence on Japanese medicine, which was practiced for the most part by the monks, continued for 1,000 years.

In the 16th century, In Japan, *kampoh* has developed its own cultural identity and characteristic traits. However, certain Chinese concepts of *yin, yang* and *ki* (*qi*) continued to have their central roles. The concept of *kampoh* in Japan was passed on to the younger generations to keep the tradition alive. In the last 20 years the number of practitioners has greatly increased. The concept of *kampoh* is currently taught at Toyama University in Honsu.

Korean herbal medicine is very similar to Traditional Chinese Medicine, and almost all the Chinese herbs are used in Korea. Ginseng (*Panax ginseng*) has been cultivated in Korea for home use and export since 1300.

Importance of Chinese Herbal Medicine

Even today, Traditional Chinese Medicine is the valid medical system in China and available to the Chinese on an equal footing with conventional Western medicine. Herbs are used mainly for chronic conditions, while Western medicine is more frequently employed, for serious acute illness. Several Chinese universities have included Traditional Chinese Medicine in their syllabi. Teaching and research on herbal medicine, their development and massive input of plant resources will help to revitalize herbalism worldwide.

Worldwide many governments have officially recognized Chinese herbal medicine. In 1995, the French government signed an agreement with the Chinese to establish a hospital in Pairs, offering acupuncture and traditional Chinese herbal medicine. In the same way that ephedra (*Ephedra sinica*), was discovered to be such an excellent medicine for allergies and asthma, so increasing numbers of Chinese herbs will be found to have major health benefits, and there is little doubt that over the next few decades Chinese herbal medicine will continue to grow in popularity around the world.

AFRICA

The Therapeutic Use of medicinal plant Africa dates back to the earliest times. Ancient Egyptian writings confirm that herbal medicines have been valued in North Africa for millennia. The Ebers papyrus (*c.* 1500 BC), one of the oldest surviving medical texts, includes over 870 prescriptions and formulae, 700 medicinal herbs–including gentian (*Gentiana lutea*), aloe (*Aloe vera*), and opium poppy (*Papaver somniferum*)–and covers conditions ranging from chest complaints to crocodile bite. The medicinal arts put forward in this and other Egyptian texts formed the intellectual foundation of African medicine.

In the more remote areas of Africa, nomadic peoples, such as the Berber of Morocco and the Topnaar of Namibia, have herbal traditions that remain largely unaffected by changes in medicine in the world at large. For these peoples, healing is linked to a magical world in which spirits influence illness and death. In Berber culture, possession by a *djinn* (spirit) is a major cause of sickness, and herbs with *magical* properties are given to restore health. If the patient fails to recover, their condition is likely to be attributed to a curse or to the "evil eye".

The Topnaar formerly depended completely on their environment for medicines, using the few medicinal plants that grow in such harsh and arid conditions. Although they are now heavily influenced by the Western way of life and have lost much of their plant lore, they continue to employ many indigenous plants medicinally. The stem of the seaweed *Ecklonia maxima,* for example, is roasted, mixed with petroleum jelly and rubbed into wounds and burns, while *Hoodia currori,* a low–lying cactus, is stripped of its thorns and outer skin and eaten raw to treat coughs and colds.

Throughout Africa, thousands of different wild and locally grown medicinal plants are sold in the markets. Some are prescribed as medicines for home use. Others, such s kanna (*Membryanthemum* spp.) and iboga (*Tabernanthe iboga*), are chewed to combat fatigue, and are taken intoxicants in religious ceremonies. According to local accounts in the Congo and Gabon, iboga's stimulant effect was discovered when observers saw wild boars and gorillas dig up and eat the roots, and subsequently become frenzied.

Traditional and Conventional Care in Africa

Though conventional Western medicine is well established throughout Africa, however, in rural areas, far from medical and hospital services, traditional medicine remains the only areas conventional health care services can be limited and in this situation, traditional provides of care such as spiritualists, herbaists and midwives are the main source of treatment available for the majority of the population. The World Health Organization aims to help African countries pioneered in providing training of traditional medicines. In one center in Ghana, conventionally trained medical staff–work hand–in–hand with traditional herbal practitioners.

The Discovery of New Herbal Cures

Along with encouraging the safer use of herbal medicines, medical centers are researching their use in detail. For example, Pygeum (*Pygeum africanum*) grows in Angola, Mozambique, Cameroon and South Africa was traditionally used in central and southern Africa to treat urinary problems. Today, pygeum is regularly prescribed in conventional French and Italian medicine for prostate problems. Of the plants currently under investigation in Africa, two shrubs *Bridelia ferruginea* (found in eastern and western grasslands) and *Indigofera arrecta* (found in tropical areas), show promise in the treatment of diabetes.

AUSTRALIA

Australia is also considered as one of the homes of an ancient herbal tradition. The **Aborigines**, believed to have settled in Australia over 60,000 years ago, developed a sophisticated empirical understanding of indigenous plants, many of which, such as eucalyptus (*Eucalyptus globules*), are unique to Australia, While much of this knowledge has vanished with its keepers, there is currently a high level of interest in native herbal traditions. The Aborigines probably had a more robust health than the early European settlers who displaced them. They had very different ideas of health, disease and illness, in which the influence of the spirit world played a major role. In common with other hunter–gatherer societies, the Aborigines devoted much time to ritual, which reinforced the sense of place and purpose in the lives of each individual. They used sense plants and the laying on of hands in a complex weave of culture and medicine.

The influx of Europeans in the 18th century was disastrous for the Aborigines. Nevertheless, a little is known of Aboriginal medicine. Aromatic herbs, such as eucalyptus, were often crushed and inhaled to treat many common illnesses, including respiratory disease such as flu. Without metal technology, water could not be boiled, but decoctions were made by heating water with hot stones. These were drunk or applied externally. It is known that skin eruptions, such as boils and scabies, were common and that they were treated with acacia (*Acacia* spp), while acute diarrhea was used to treat fevers.

Several native Australian plants are popular around the world. Research into fever bark resulted in the discovery of the alkaloid reserpine, which markedly lowers blood pressure. The substance is now prescribed by herbalists and conventional practitioners alike. Eucalyptus and tea tree (*Melaleuca alternifolia*) yield essential oils that are employed worldwide as antiseptics. Other native Australian plants are now used in Australian herbalism because of their medicinal use elsewhere, for example gotu kola (*Centella asiatica*) and visnaga (*Ammi visnaga*), which have a long history of medicinal use in India and the Middle East.

In Australia, early British settlers imported European medicinal plants, such as vervain (*Verbena officinalis*), hawthorn (*Crataegus* spp.), mullein (*Verbascum thapsus*), and dandelion (*Taraxacum officinale*), which have now all become naturalized. Native American plants have also found their way to Australia, including prickly pear (*Opuntia ficus–indica*) and Canadian fleabane (*Erigeron Canadensis*). As Australian herbalists generally follow the Anglo–American herbal tradition, these plants are often employed in local practice.

In Australia, Traditional Chinese medicine has its substantial influence. Chinese immigrants in the 19th century spread the knowledge of herbal formula and gained a reputation for their effectiveness. During the 1980s, a renaissance in all branches of herbal medicine began, and today Australia has three colleges of traditional Chinese medicine. Chinese herbs are also quite frequently used by Australian herbalists, and Chinese patent medicines are widely available in health food shops.

Australia is the considered as one of the important centers of growing Indonesian, New Zealand and Ayurvedic medicines. The potential of many native herbs is also being explored–the most notable example being the Moreton Bay chestnut tree (*Castonospermum australe*), one of the many plant medicines with potential in treating AIDS. Commercial cultivation of medicinal plants is expanding with herbs such as tea tree opium poppy (*Papaver somniferum*) becoming major crops. In Tasmania, trails are now under way to try to grow ginseng (*Panax ginseng*) and goldenseal (*Hydrastis Canadensis,*), two plants that are very difficult to cultivate.

NORTH AMERICA

Stretching, From the Arctic Wilds of Canada and Alaska to the tropical regions of Panama, North and Central America covers diverse geographical regions and harbours an immense variety of medicinal plants. Most of them are indigenous, but others–such as nutmeg, ginger and tamarind–were introduced from the Old World from the 16th century onwards. Likewise, native American medicinal plants–such as corn, cocoa, cayenne and sunflower–were introduced to Europe, Asia and Africa. This trade of species was an important part of the interplay between the Old and New World's herbal traditions.

CENTRAL AMERICA

Herbal medicines are usually practiced in rural areas of Central America (in Guatemala and Mexico). In the Mexican tradition, loss of "balance" between hot and cold elements within the body is thought to be the underlying cause of illness, and the healer's art is restore balance and vitality. Mexican herbal medicine is not a static tradition, but has evolved from a shafting blend of Aztec, Mayan and Spanish influences. The *Badianus Manuscript*, the first American herbal listed the medicinal uses of 251 Mexican species. They include damiana (*Turnera diffusa*), taken by the Maya as an aphrodisiac, and mesquite (*Prosopis juliflora*) used by the Aztecs as an eye lotion. Both species are still used medicinally, alongside European herbs such pennyroyal (*Mentha pulegium*) and thyme (*Thymus vulgaris*). It is thought that approximately 65 per cent of the plants used by traditional Mexican herbalists originated in Europe. Projects in the Dominican Republic and Nicaraua, for example, are teaching women how to use local herbs within their communities, while in Cuba doctors increasingly prescribe medicinal herbs to make up for the scarcity of conventional medicines.

Caribbean Herbal Medicine

Throughout the Caribbean, domestic herbal medicine remains popular. Some of the widely used herbs include fever grass or lemon grass (*Cymbopogon citrates*), which, is its name suggests, is used to treat fevers, and cerasee (*Momordica charantia*), a creeping vine that is prized as a *cure–all* on many of the islands. Cerasee has been shown to have an ability to lower blood sugar levels and may help to slow down the onset of diabetes, a relatively common illness among Afro–Caribbeans. The medical and religious customs on each Caribbean island vary, but on many they reflect the African traditions of transported slaves, especially of the Yoruba people shipped from West Africa, who carried on the practices of their homelands. Tobacco (*Nicotiana tabacum*), for example, is used for divination in many American cultures, including in Santeria and Voodoo religious rituals, as are other herbs, including garlic (*Allium sativum*) and cayenne (*Capsicum frutescens*).

Shamanism

Moving north, Native American herbal medicine in what is now the United States was and is primarily shamanistic in nature, involving herbal lore, ritual and magic. Shamanistic societies from Siberia to the Amazon believe that, in serious illness, the soul of the sick person has been take over by malign forces. The shaman's role is to heal both the physical *and* the spiritual dimension of the illness. The patient cannot be truly cured until his or her soul has been freed from evil spirits. Shamanistic ceremonies and rites to heal the sick person's spirit include dancing, chanting, drumming, playing games, and the stirring of ashes or sprinkling of water. By taking hallucinogens such as peyote (*Lophophora williamsii*), the shaman is able to reach out to the spirit world and heal both the individual and the community as a whole.

In all Native American cultures from Canada to Chile, herbs are thought to have spiritual energy and many of them are invested with great magical power. The Iroquosis believe that cardinal lobelia (*Lobelia cardinalis, L. inflata*), and morning glory (*Ipomoea pandurata*) have the ability to heal or harm, and should be picked, stored and used with great care. Morning glory is considered so powerful that even touching it could cause harm. The Iroquois use the plant as a remedy for coughs, tuberculosis and other ailments, and also take it as a decoction with sunflower seeds (*Heliantus annus*) as a sacrament in spring and autumn rituals.

The first European settlers in North America, arriving in the early 17th century, trended to dismiss Native American medical practices as nothing more than primitive savagery. The settlers relied largely on imported herbal medicines, or on European plants hardy enough to grow in eastern North America.

As time went by, however, the settlers increased contact with indigenous peoples in the frontier regions fostered a healthy respect for their healing skills. Sometimes settlers adopted not just the plants but the harvesting and therapeutic methods as well as Joseph Doddridge, in *Notes on the Settlement and Indian Wars* (1876), relates that butternut bark (*Juglans cinerea*) was peeled downwards if it was to be used as a purgative (acting "downwards" by purging the bowels), and upwards for use as an emetic (acting "upwards" by providing vomiting).

Using many herbs, these practitioners sought to harmonize "the organic tissues with the vital force", with the aim of restoring equilibrium within the body. Believing the stomach was the source of disease; Physiomedicalists used herbs that induced vomiting, such as poke root (*Phytolacca decandra*), to cleanse the organ. Other herbs such as echinacea (*Echinacea* spp), now recognized as an excellent immune–stimulant, and goldenseal (*Hydrastis Canadensis*) a tonic and anti–inflammatory were then prescribed to aid recovery.

The second half of the 19th century was an extraordinary time for American natural medicine. In addition to engendering osteopathy and chiropractic at the turn of the century, it also re–investigated herbal medicine in Britian to such a degree that Physiomedicalism became an Anglo–American herbal tradition. To this day, British herbalists still use a far wider variety of North American medicinal herbs than do their European counterparts.

In the US, herbal medicine went into steep decline after 1907 because of the government's decision to limit financial support for medical training to conventional medical schools. Since that time, herbal medicine in both the US and Canada has existed only on the fringes of conventional health care. In much of the US, it is illegal to practice herbal medicine without medical qualifications, but courses in herbalism are not offered at medical schools.

Herbal Medicine in South America conjures up images of shamanistic rituals and a collection of thousands of as yet unclassified plants under the thick canopy of the rainforest. But these are only two facets of the continent's herbal tradition–those of the Amazon and Orinoco regions. Distinctly different plants and practices are found in other areas, for example on the Bolivian Andes plateau, on the humid plains of Paraguay and in cities such as Rio de Janeiro.

Ever since the Spanish conquest in the early 16th century, European writers have remarked on the huge variety of plant medicines used by native peoples. The important plants are as follows:

Anise (*Pimpinella anisum*)	A digestive remedy for colic and griping that originally came from the Mediterranean, is sold alongside unusual native medicines.
Arquitects (*Culcitium reflexum*)	A diuretic and detoxifying herb traditionally used to treat toxicity and infections, including syphilis.
Ayahuasca (*Banisteriopsis caapi*)	It is a powerful medicine enables the shaman (priest) to communicate with the spirit world and cure the patient's ill health.
Cinchona (*Cinchona* spp.)	A traditional Andean fever remedy, which the Spaniards first discovered around 1630.
Coca (*Erythroxylum coca*)	An important medicine in South America for nausea and vomiting, toothache and asthma. It is also completely interwoven into the culture of indigenous Amazonian and Andean peoples and serves as a precise example of the unique relationships that traditional peoples have with plant world.

Ipecacuanha (*Cephaelis ipecacuanha*)	Commonly found in over–the–counter cough preparations–was taken by Brazilian native peoples to treat amoebic dysentery.
Maté (*Ilex paraguariensis*)	It grows in western regions of the continent, makes a stimulating beverage that is prepared and drunk like tea. Maté has become so popular it is now cultivated in Spain and Portugal as well as in South America.
Pareira (*Chondrodendron tomentosum*)	A climbing vine of the rainforest, for example, yields the poison curare used in hunting, and is taken medicinally to treat retention, bruising and insanity. Sadly, however, the herbal medicine of many indigenous groups is now under threat as the rainforests disappear.
Potato (*Solanum tuberosum*)	Cultivated in over 60 different varieties by the Inca. Its use are wide–ranging, but it is particularly effective as a poultice for skin conditions.

TYPES OF THERAPY

Homoeopathy

Although homoeopathy has only been systematized for about two centuries, it roots go back much further. As a method of treatment, it is quite different from any other and wholly unconventional in concept. The term was first introduced into England in 1827 and derives form the Greek words *homoios* meaning similar, and *pathos*meaning pain. This literal meaning, however, of 'similar to the pain', fails to give any practical clue as to how an illness can be cured by means of the same illness.

The Hippocratic concept that *like can be treated with like* makes it clearer and it is on this concept that homoeopathy is based. Accustomed as we are today to an almost constant stream of new discoveries emerging in various scientific areas, it is difficult for us to grasp the full significance of this Hippocratic statement and its fortunate rediscovery by the German physician, Christian Friedrich Samuel Hahnemann (1755–1843).

With this Hippocratic concept in mind, Hahnemann regulated the methods of diagnosis and the homoeopathic procedure that is still practiced today. By the age of twenty he was already a qualified doctor and, like all eighteenth–century physicians, was prescribing preparations and procedures (including traditional blood–letting) consistent with contemporary pharmaceutical knowledge and methods. Being keenly observant, however, he came to doubt the efficacy of these centuries–hallowed treatments.

He remarked, too, that medicines often prescribed in good faith only tended to aggravate the illness. He began, therefore, to criticize openly many of the common practices of contemporary medicine pointing out that the use of certain medicines was not always founded on sound scientific reason.

In his main work, Organon (1810) wrote as follows: *Allopathich treatment* (a term created by Hahnemann to high the contrast between the current school of thought and his own; it derives from the Greek *allos* meaning different and *pathos* meaning pain, and indicates how illnesses are cured by a different derivative action] without ever being able to remove and cure the original (dissimilar) chronic disease, only develops new artificial diseases beside it. As daily experience shows, this practice renders the patient much worse and more incurable than before. It would be described as criminal treason against the principles of cure of mix the two systems of medicine according to the pleasure of the patient. The ordinary physician imagines the can get over the difficulties of antipathic treatment by giving a stronger dose of the remedy at each renewed aggravation of the illness. By this method and equally transient suppression of disease is affected and then there is still greater necessity for giving ever–increasing quantities of the palliative. There ensure either another more serious disease or, frequently, danger to life, and then death itself.

Hahnemann's mission in life was to discover ways of curing the sick in a natural way, with simple medicines. His determined research led him to read a treatise by a nineteenth–century Edinburgh doctor, William Cullen, on the properties o quinine and on certain 'strangenesses' that became apparent in people who habitually took it. Spurred on by scientific curiosity, he began to experiment on himself, and thus began to formulate the basic o homoeopathy. He observed, in fact, that concentrated doses of quinine produced a fever similar to that of malaria, although it was well known that quinine was used to combat the disease.

In this connection Hahnemann said, *All the morbid symptoms and alterations in health that each medicine is especially capable of developing in the healthy individual must first be observed as far as possible, before the physician can hope to find among them, and to select, the suitable homoeopathich remedies for most of the natural diseases.*

This was an affirmation of 'like treating like', and it wsas from this point that the salient features of the homoeopathic doctrine were drawn:

1. Determination of the symptoms created in a healthy person by the use of various substances;
2. Comparisons of these symptoms with those relative to known illnesses;
3. The use of tested substances, appropriately prepared, in the treatment of a particular illness.

Returning to the concepts of his basic text, Hahnemann says:' Whichever medicine contains, in the symptoms observed from its use, the greatest similarity to the totality of symptoms of a given case of natural disease, this medicine will be the most certain homoeopathic remedy for the illness. A medicine selected in this manner produces its own artificial disease on those very parts and points of the organism now suffering from the natural disease. The instinctive automatic vital force is from that time forward no longer affected by the natural disease, but solely by the stronger similar medicinal disease. Because the moderate medicinal disease is produced by a small dose of the medicine, it is overcome by the increased energy of the vital force and soon spontaneously disappears, leaving the body free from all disease.'

This statement not only encapsulates the certainty the he felt in having found a new path, and, in his view, the only one to be taken in dealing with all diseases, but also introduces the new concept of dynamization, here translated from the German by the phrase 'the vital force'. It is important to ponder a little on this term, as it is the cornerstone of homoeopathic preparations.

The experiments on healthy persons with a wide variety of animal, vegetable and preparing earliest remedies, and thus laying the foundations for the first written descriptions of homoeopathy. Once he and established that a particular substance had a specific effect on a disease, Hahnemann went on to the dynamization process. Starting with the mother tincture of the substance, the next step was to dilute one drop of the tincture with 99 drops of alcohol. After being shaken bigorously, one drop of this dilution was then diluted with another 99 drops of alcohol, and so on for as many times as was necessary to achieve the required degree of dilution. This method produced solutions in hundredths but, of course, this could be altered to tenths of fiftieths or whatever strength was required merely by varying the number of drops of alcohol. Each solution obtained would thus have a different degree of dynamization of the product.

To dynamize, therefore, does not mean to dissolve or fraction the initial product as much as possible; dynamizing enables the substance initial product as much as possible. Dynamizing enables the substance–by dilution and the shaking given to each dilution–to release its properties, with an emphasis on quantity.

The same method is still used for homoeopathic products, although obviously many more aspects are taken into account today than could possibly have been conceived in Hahnemann's lifetime.

It is easy to imagine the dust that would normally have been found in a laboratory as well as the spores and fungi present in poorly washed test–tubes, which would have become part of the homoeopathic product and would have been quite different from that being sought or, at least, would have considerably reduced the efficacy of the preparation.

Such dangers are avoided nowadays by preparing the products in totally sterile surrounding, with constant levels of temperature and humidity, using tinctures extracted from medicinal plants specially grown in unpolluted soil without fertilizers or other chemical products. Thus both doctor and patient can be completely confident of the purity of the curative product whose action will be based exclusively on the transformed original element.

From a diagnostic point of view, the practice of homoeopathy is not restricted simply to the study of the actual disease but also takes into account the patient's state of mind, treating the person as a whole. Rather than investigating the illness or disease as something contracted by the person in question, it studies the actual patient. The diagnosis of a homoeopathic doctor is based on information that is quite outside the usual area of interest, and questions are put to the patient about his psychological condition, which to anyone not familiar with the basic philosophy of homoeopathy might appear irrelevant. In this way, a pattern of symptoms is built up, which enables the practitioner to prescribe the appropriately dynamized homoeopathic medicine, which, in a healthy person, would produce the same symptoms as have been diagnosed in the patient.

Thus there is no standard remedy for all patients suffering from a particular disease but a wide variety of medicines, which have to be selected carefully for each individual.

This is a remarkable innovative approach that is not always accepted by those practicing allopathic medicine. Hahnemann introduced a detailed code of practices for all homoeopathic doctors to follow when examining a patient, who is best summarized in the following paragraph from the Organon. *The examination of each individual case of disease demands of the physician nothing but sound senses and freedom from prejudice, attention in observing and fidelity in tracing the picture of the disease.*

He also stressed that mass–produced prescriptions should be avoided and that it was not possible to affect a proper cure without treating each case in 'a rigorous manner and on a personal level'. This is known as 'individualization'.

The opposition that has been mounted by the conventional medical profession against homoeopathy ever since its discovery, and which continues to this day, is motivated by two developments: the increase in the number of homoeopathic schools, and the high dynamization of the preparations.

After Hahnemann's death, many homoeopathic schools were established because of the novelty of the subject. With a view to giving it greater scientific validity, and in a quest for new knowledge, some detached themselves, to a greater or lesser extent, from the basic methodology created by its originator. The schools, therefore, became divided between 'purists' and 'non–purists'.

The purists adhered scrupulously to the rules laid down in the Organon in which Hahnemann had described how every disease could be overcome by a single medicine, by a single substance, used in different dynamizations for different degrees of illness. The non–purists, on the other hand, used a greater variety of drugs, which were often linked with non–homoeopathic remedies.

The dissension, apart from causing considerable confusion, was to bring discredit on homoeopathic methodology as a whole; this discredit was increased further by the second development mentioned above; the high dynamization of the products.

Although the remarkable effects of vaccines had already been proved, the medicinal action of highly diluted and dynamized homoeopathic products has not been widely accepted. Even today, the fact that homoeopathy has not made greater strides, or won more general recognition, is due to the use of these preparations.

Homoeopathic schools and hospitals have long been established in many European countries, and new ones are being set up all the time. Many members of the medicinal profession as well as the general public are showing increasing interest in homoeopathic theories and practices. Whatever the various reasons for this, they surely stem from a fundamental desire to return, as far as possible, to natural healing methods.

The large majorities of homoeopathic preparations contain a plant base, which, even if derived from plants containing toxic principles, yield many curative properties, and may be administered with complete safety. Homoeopathy, along with aromatherapy, is firmly establishing itself as a reality, furnishing phtotherapy with a serious scientific basis in a manner that, only a short while ago, would have been deemed impossible.

Aromatherapy

Aromatherapy is regarded as specialized branch of phytotherapy, concerns the use of essential oils for their healing properties. We have already seen how difficult is to extract essences, how expensive they are to produce and how extensively they have been used in a variety of ways.

Our ancestors used essential oils to embalm their dead, to render putrefied substances more tolerable, and as food preservatives. These examples not only confirm the fact that essences have always had other uses apart from the making of perfume but emphasize what is often a fundamental characteristic–their anti–bacterial qualities. It is obvious that any treatment in which essential oils are used either internally or externally requires a high standard of purity, which is not always maintained in essences produced for the perfume manufactures. For this reason, all essences that are extracted for medicinal purposes should be obtained from plants grown under controlled conditions in which no chemical products of any kind have been used.

All essences can be divided into three categories:

1. Terpenic
2. Oxygenated
3. Sulphurized

The most important element of a given essence determines the category to which it belongs.

The quintessence, known in modern terms as the active principle, has been sought since the time of Paracelsus as the sole element in the entire plant possessing curative properties. Experiments of guineapigs and humans have now established that when only a small–albeit the most important–part of the total essence is used, the medicinal effect on a particular illness often differs from the anticipated result. It is evident, therefore, that an essential oil should be used in its entirety, rather than broken down into its various components, in order to achieve a more vigorous, total synergic action.

Despite the fact that aromatic drugs are recognized as having a valuable antiseptic quality, they are still not sufficiently utilized, even though the results obtained have extremely successful. Almost any bacterial attack is treated nowadays with antibiotics or other similar–acting drugs. Consequently, although the infection is suppressed, the body becomes debilitated and has difficulty in restoring its natural defense mechanism.

Another factor to be considered is that the action of pharmaceutical drugs does not remain constant over a period of time, as germs become resistant to ever–increasing doses. This makes it necessary, therefore, to create new and stronger drugs, which, unfortunately, still have the same harmful side effects on the whole system.

In contrast to this, the results of recent research now show that essences perform a specific antibiotic action and produce no secondary effects whatsoever on the organic functioning of the body. For example, essence of thyme has greater antiseptic power than hydrogen peroxide and guaiacol, due to its thymol antiseptic power that hydrogen peroxide and guaiacol, due to its thymol content. A water solution of essence of thyme kills the typhus bacillus in two minutes, streptococcus in four minutes and the tuberculosis bacillus in one hour. Similarly, essence of lemon kills the meningitis bacillus in a quarter of an hour, and staphylococcus and pneumococcus in one hour.

It is interesting to recall that in olden days people sprinkled themselves with the essences of rosemary, thyme, sage and other fragrant plants as a protection against contagious diseases during epidemics. The good sense of this practice it today fully endorsed, as is proved by over own current use of atomized sprays comprising a mixture of essences with a phenolic (carbolic acid) content, which can easily sterilize a room full of bacilli. Were such a procedure to be adopted in hospitals and operating theatres, almost total asepsis could be achieved.

Furthermore, germs do not become resistant to the action of the essences, so that the latter's effect on them does not diminish during their active life. This is the determining factor in differentiating between essential oils and antibiotics. Although essences do not act directly on germs, they have an unfavourable effect on their habitat, causing them to disappear as a result of the unsuitable environment thus produced. This is the manner in which conditions such as festering sores and the early stages of necroses have been healed when treated with solutions of essential oils.

It has been suggested that the fragrance of the solution merely masks the foul smell of the sore, but this is not so. The essence suppresses the sore by blending with the products of deterioration of yield non–toxic compounds. In addition, may people have, at some time, suffered from a form of skin inflammation, which, when treated with an appropriate solution, has healed quite quickly without the tissues being in any way affected. A great many tests have, in fact, been carried out on both superficial and deep burns, in all instances with positive results.

A further important factor, absent in other types of medication designed for the same purpose, is the speed of absorption, which makes essences particularly suitable of the comprehensive treatment of a wide variety of infections. This rate can actually be measured in many different essences and is an invaluable quality in cases requiring the fastest possible curative action.

It is only right to mention that many women have had unhappy experiences of this rapidity of action. After using a new perfume, they have noticed allergic reactions or other phenomena almost immediately on a part of all the skin, which is entirely use to absorption of the essential oils. A simple test can be carried out by spreading some garlic essence on the sole of one foot; after only a few minutes, the breath will have the characteristic garlicky odour. The essence has been absorbed by osmosis and has quickly entered the bloodstream. This is clearly a vital factor in cases when speedy action is necessary, and oral or parenteral (otherwise than through the digestive system) administration of the medicament through osmosis.

Essences, however, are not only effective because of their bactericidal action. There is much evidence to show that their healing effect is, in fact, obtained by means of a range of activities. Essences can be categorized according to these activities: antispasmodic or spasmolytic, stimulatory, cicatrizant, antifermentative and hormonal. In this connection, it is remarkable how the traditional use of certain plants has now been justified by qualitative analyses.

It has been proved that many plants, for example, produce substances with hormonal qualities similar to the female ovarian hormones and, therefore, behave in the same way. Sage, hops, willow and liquorice have long been popular remedies to increase the milk–flow of a nursing mother or to correct and stabilize the menstrual flow, and science has now confirmed their efficacy and revealed the reasons for it. There are probably many other types of plant that produce such hormones, or others that are akin to them. It is important, therefore, that these valuable natural resources should be discovered, classified and used, under strict medical control, to avoid dependence on ill–tolerated synthetic preparations.

Many people have personal experience of the antiputrefactive and antifermentative uses of certain essential oil–producing plants such as fennel, anise and coriander, which are especially effective remedies against such complaints as gastritis and colitis.

Why do essences posses such curative powers? How can their action be explained? Science still has to find the definitive answers to questions such as these, although there is no shortage to theories. One important hypothesis, propounded by the Russian surgeon, V.P.F. attempts to prolong its life by producing special substances known as biostimulants.

In current pharmacology these substances are obtained from the female placenta, which produces them in considerable quantities. When used on sick organisms, biostimulants excite the organic defense mechanisms and thus encourage the healing process. It is deduced, therefore, that essences, too, when separated by the distillation process from the plant that has produced them, must themselves create stimulants, since they possess the healing action just described. This theory is supported simply by our sense of smell, as it is most unusual for the fragrance of a living plant to be the same as that of the essence extracted from it. This necessarily suggests that some kind of modification must take place during the extraction process.

Georges Lakhovsky explained it on rate of vibration. According to this theory, every organ has an established wavelength and any variation in its frequency could cause a specific disease. The essence would be able to reverse the variation, restoring the frequency to normal, and thus affecting a cure.

However, it very difficult to decide about any theory without further examinations. The fact emerges that essential oils act quickly and safely; so there seems to be a valid argument in favour of restoring them to a prime position in the pharmacopoeia.

Several oils are used in the cosmetic and perfume industries, which disregard their medicinal action unless that action is an obvious one. In such cases, a thorough check of the cosmetic preparation, in which the essential oils is contained, must be made because there may be a hidden secondary action, which may prove harmful. The cosmetic expert, therefore, must work closely with someone who has a sound knowledge of aromatherapy. This will ensure that the product is not only suitable for its purpose, but that any potentially harmful side effects can be recongnized and eliminated.

3 MEDICINAL PLANTS AND HUMAN SYSTEM

THE STATUS

Plant remedies are harmless, provided they are selected carefully and taken under medical guidance. This type of treatment never has to be brought to a sudden half because of any adverse effect on the patient, although in some cases it may have to be concluded because it is too mild or is taking too long.

It should be noted that not all illnesses are suitable for herbal treatment. Obviously, it cannot be the answer for patients in need of more radical attention such as surgical operations and bone setting, or for those whose life depends on quick–acting treatment.

People were making use of plant, having discovered their beneficial and curative effects, long before scientific explanations were advanced. They soon came to separate edible species from poisonous ones and gradually learned how to select the most useful parts of such plants. This wealth of acquired knowledge was passed on verbally and, as so often happens when information depends on word on mouth, facts became distorted and all kinds of imaginary powers were attributed to certain plant. Although a certain mystique still surrounds herbs and their medicinal usage today, progress in scientific research has greatly clarified the subject. Officinal plants now have accepted botanical names, whilst attempts have been made to analyze them chemically and distinguish at least some of the many components and active principles.

Such analyses have recently led to the production of similar compounds by synthetic means. These are not only more convenient to take but are also easier to store. On the face of it, the two types of product would seem to be analogous. Experiments have shown, however, that from a curative point of view substances extracted from medicinal plants and the equivalent substances produced synthetically behave differently. There is variation in the absorption capacity, and the natural product has a milder effect on the system than the man–made one. Other tests have shown that synthetic drugs afford a faster rate of recovery, but that plant substances have a much more positive and lasting effect.

These, however, are not the only reasons for the present return to treatment with 'simples', as medicinal herbs were once known. Some of the interest springs, firstly, form the fact that many people are already familiar with herbs. Who, for instance, has not heard of camomile, mint or basil? Secondly, fragrant herbalist shops are themselves and attraction, exuding an atmosphere of charm and confidence.

MODERN HERBALISM OR PHYTOTHERAPY

The study of modern herbalism (phytotherapy) is rapidly evolving throughout the world. New commercial organizations are emerging to study hitherto unknown medicinal plants, adding to the information about those already classified and selecting new seeds from cultures, in order to obtain qualitative and quantitative optimal yields, and to elaborate new, scientifically tested recipes for the more effective treatment of specific illnesses. This is not campaign against synthetic drugs, for that would be a serious mistake–some complaints respond well to herbal remedies while others react better to synthetic ones. The sole objective, of both types of medicine, is to restore the patient to good health. It is desirable, therefore, that research in both fields should continue without conflict.

Phytotherapy is once again being recognized for the healing qualities it can offer mankind, though this time on a much wider scale and supported by all the facilities of modern science. The links with past superstitions are not entirely broken, however, for although some old legends cannot be upheld against the evidence of microscopes and electronic calculators, research scientists never cease to be amazed, even perplexed, when an active principle, which ahs already been defined and classified, behaves in a way that is at variance with the experimentally tested results. Such behaviour certainly explains the bewilderment of ancient scholars who could only hold supernatural powers responsible for the active properties of such plants.

We now know that these unexpected results are due to the synergetic action of the various components of a plant and not merely of the active principle on which interest is usually focused.

Te phenomenon of synergism is extensively used in modern therapies at all levels. Briefly, it involves the association of two or more drugs whose interaction may produce the following results:

1. By equal action (synergism by addition), each of the various drugs performs the same function on the substrata of the organism;
2. By different action (synergism by potentiation), the various drugs exert collateral action on different substrata of the organism;
3. By antagonistic action (synergism by degradation), the drugs, which individually have their own action, when combined, produce a result, which is different from the predicted one.

It is obvious that exhaustive research into plants containing such a large number of active principles must offer a vast range of possibilities. Unfortunately, large–scale experimental treatment cannot be considered for hospital patients. It would take too long and would also be uneconomic, as in most countries patients are kept in hospital for as short a period as possible. Apart from a few particular cases, experiments have generally been carried out exceptional circum–synthetic drugs was precarious or non–existent.

Another useful contribution to the better understanding of phytotherapeutic treatments is being provided by countries, which, though they have a low level of technology, are the largest exporters of officinal plants. It is, therefore, in these countries that phytotherapy is most widely used, even in hospitals, although unfortunately their research facilities are limited. Information concerning the result achieved is, nevertheless, highly important, as the data is then studied and examined in depth in more developed countries where research teams are better equipped to carry out the necessary work.

HOW MEDICINAL PLANTS WORK

In current age, modern medicine offers an unparalleled opportunity to relieve disease symptoms and save lives. Modern surgical techniques, such as keyhole surgery and plastic surgery, and the whole range of diagnostic and life–support machinery now available can all be used to improve the chances of recovery from serious illness of injury.

Since ancient time, orthodox pharmaceutical medicines were the only solution to sustain life and counter infections. Despite of the dramatic advances and advantages of conventional medicine, or biomedicine it has been established that herbal medicine has offered a great solution to cure diseases of human being. From last fifty years or so, men have relied almost entirely on plants to treat all manner of illnesses, from minor problems such as coughs and colds to life–threatening diseases such as tuberculosis and malaria. Today, herbal remedies are coming back into prominence because the efficacy of conventional medicines such as antibiotics, which once had near–universal effectiveness against serous infections, is on the wane. Over the years, infections organisms have developed resistance to synthesized drugs, and the herb *qing hao* (*Artemisia annua*), and its active consistent artemisin, for example, are now being used to treat malaria in areas of the world where the protozoa causing the infection no longer respond to conventional treatment.

Herbal medicine offers conventional treatments, providing safe, well–tolerated remedies for chronic illnesses. It is experiencing a dramatic renaissance in Western countries, partly because no effective conventional treatment as yet exists for many chronic illnesses, such as asthma, arthritis and irritable bowel syndrome. In addition, concern over the side effects of biomedicine is encouraging people to look for more gentle forms of treatment. It is estimated that 10–20% of hospital patients in the West are there due to the side effects of conventional medical treatment.

Herbal medicin should be used wisely. Most commonly used herbs are extremely safe to use. But some plants can produce side effects and, like all medicines, herbal remedies must be treated with respect. It is necessary to take or use certain plants only under the guidance of a well–trained practitioner, to avoid adverse consequences. It has been observed that Ephedra (*Ephedra sinica*), can be extremely toxic at the wrong dosage, and comfrey (*Symphytum officinale*), a very popular herb in the past, is thought to cause severe or even fatal liver damage in rare circumstances. Therefore, herbal medicine should be used correctly, however, the chances of developing a serious side–effect are remote.

WHY HERBAL MEDICINE IS USED?

Herbal medicines have the ability of a to affect body systems. The effects are dependent on the chemical constituents present in the plant used. Scientists first started extracting and isolating chemicals from plants in the 18th century, and since that time we have grown accustomed to looking at herbs and their effects in terms of the active constituents they contain. This *Encyclopedia* is no exception, providing details of all the main active constituents of the medicinal herbs featured and explaining their actions.

Pure and isolated plant constituents are of great importance because they have given various world's most useful drugs. For example, tubocurarine, the most powerful muscle relaxant in existence, is derived from curare (*Chondrodendron tomentosum*), and the strongest painkiller of all, morphine, comes from opium poppy (*Papaver somniferum*). Many anaesthetics are also derived from plants, for example cocaine, which comes from coca (*Erythroxylum coca*). It is hard to think of a world deprived of the antimalarial properties of quinine (derived from *Cinchona*); or the heart remedy digoxin (from *Digitalis*) or the cough–relieving properties of ephedrine (from *Ephedra sinica*), which is present in many prescription and over –the–counter cold remedies. These and many other conventional medicines are all derived from isolated plant constituents. These are most effective of all conventional drugs.

Value of Whole Plants

Biomedicines are literally god/goddess gift, rather than developed in a laboratory. Though it is difficult to understand the actions of individual active constituents of the herbal medicine. In fact, biomedicine is ultimately about the use and actions of whole plants. Therefore, it is essential to identify the key parts of the plants. The whole herb is worth more than the sum of its parts and scientific research is increasingly showing that the active constituents of many herbs, for example those in ginkgo (*Ginkgo biloba*), interact in complex ways to produce the therapeutic effect of the remedy as whole. Plants contain hundreds, if not thousands, of different constituent chemical chemicals that interact in complex ways. Frequently, we simply do not know in detail how a particular herb works–even though its medicinal benefit is well established. The pharmacological approach to understanding how whole herbs work is like working on a jigsaw where only some of the pieces have been provided. Furthermore, although it is very useful to know that a plant contains certain active constituents, such information can be misleading on its own. For example, tea (*Camellia sinensis*) and coffee (*Coffea arabica*), contain approximately the same levels of caffeine. Tea, however, contains a much greater quantity of tannins (which give tea its sour, astringent taste).

These constituents reduce the amount of nutrients and drugs that are absorbed from the intestines into the blood–stream, and consequently less caffeine is absorbed. As a result, and true to most people's experience, tea is less stimulating than coffee. This example reveals a couple of fundamental truths about herbal medicine. Firstly, the experience of the herbal practitioner and of the patient often provide the most reliable guide to the medicinal effect of individual herbs. Secondly the value of a medicinal herb cannot be reduced simply to a list of its active constituents.

Plants Serve as Foods and Medicines

A plant is an immediate source of medicine, which can be extracted, titrated and preserved. A great many natural drugs, which cannot be synthetically duplicated, may, therefore, be selected for possible use. In view of the large number of active principles produced by plants, we can only wonder at the incredibly vast reservoir nature has to offer, in which unlimited reserves of medicinal ingredients are still largely untapped. What is more, these ingredients are not presented to use in the form of pills a potions but as flowers, fruit, leaves and seeds.

It can be argued that during the last few decades, there has been a progressive decline in the relationship between man and his surroundings. We live in a society orientated to the production of consumer goods that are designed to make our lives as easy as possible but which, all too often, become quickly obsolete. The cost, even if economically acceptable, is, from the ecological viewpoint, enormously damaging.

One of the main consequences of this artificially forced lifestyle is the increasing number of younger people who are falling victim to fatal illnesses, which were at one time found almost exclusively in the elderly. The health problems that plague modern society are well–know in the medical world, but the rapid strides being made in current pharmacology are barely able to keep pace with them, and even the vast range of drugs available is often far from satisfactory. Underlying the praises heaped upon such products for their efficacy is a more cautious note of warning. This propaganda, voiced in a low key, invites the consumer to turn to more natural alternative medicines, many of which were once widely used, but have long since been abandoned in favour of 'progress'.

As a result of this new trend, a large number of people who are perhaps skeptical or apprehensive about 'conventional' drugs have now turned to alternative treatments, and in particular treatments that make use of medicinal plants. They are quite willing to place their trust in the competence of herbalists, amateurs or professionals, who often have no formal medical background whatsoever. In their attempt to achieve good health by 'natural' means, they are tempted by expensive little packets of attractively wrapped and cleverly advertised herbs claiming to cure every type of complaint.

There is no official guarantee as to the purity of these products and certainly non as regards their effectiveness. The possibility always remains that the uncontrolled administration of unsuitable and toxic remains that the uncontrolled administration of unsuitable and toxic herbs may produce effects, which are as harmful as the indiscriminate use of synthetic products. Furthermore, phytotherapeutic treatment (i.e. treatment by means of vegetable drugs) is often ineffective when it involves the use of dried plants such as those sold in health shops. Since the majority of these dried plants are imported and will inevitably have been gathered some time previously, the active principles contained I them will almost certainly be considerably reduced and, in many cases, will be non–existent. The failure of a treatment involving the use of medicinal or 'officinal' herbs (as they are some times called) is often due to the age of the plants; as with traditional medicines, their active properties expire after a given period. The main difference, however, is that natural products that have lost their active qualities are not harmful to the system.

One of the main advantages is undoubtedly the opportunity to use a wide range of essential elements, provided by ka living organism of plant origin, for the human organism. This natural affinity allows total assimilation of all those elements, developed by the growth organs of the plant that are indispensable to human life. This natural affinity allows total assimilation of all hose elements, developed by the growth organs of the plant that are indispensable to human life. This is borne out by some doctors who prefer to recommend the inclusion of large amounts of cereals, vegetables or fruit in the daily diet rather than prescribe pharmaceutical products, especially in the treatment of deficient ailments in the young.

The human body is much better suited to treatment with herbal remedies than with isolated chemical medicines. The digestive systems and physiology of human have evolved side–by–side utility of plants over tens of thousands of years. Men have generated digesting and utilizing capacity of plant–based foods, which also have medicinal values. The demarcation line between *foods* and *medicines* may not always be clear. For example, lemons, papayas onions and oats sevre as foods and medicines both. Lemon (*Citrus limon*) improves resistance to infection; papaya (*Carica papaya*), is taken in some parts of the world to expel worms; onion (*Allium capa*) relieves bronchial infections; and oats (*Avena sativa*) support convalescence. Indeed, herbal medicine comes into its own when the distinctions between foods and medicines are removed.

Plants increase stamina, help the nervous system to function correctly, provide a good supply of B vitamins, and maintain regular bowel function.

The strategies of herbal treatments adopted by herbal practitioners to prevent illness or restore health in their patients may be different in varied herbal traditions across the world, but the effects that herbal medicines within the body of human always improve health. There are many thousands of medicinal plants in the use throughout the world, with a tremendous range of actions and degrees of potency. Most have a specific action on particular body systems and are known to be suitable for treating certain types of ailments for specific actions.

Plants are being used for improving the quality of the diet and sustaining or regulating good health. The saying *You are what you eat* is by and large true, though herbalists prefer to quality it, saying *You are what you absorb from what you eat*. Herbal medicines not only provide nutrients, but when needed they also strengthen and support the action of the digestive systems, speeding up the rate of proceeding food and improving the absorption of nutrients.

Oxygen is needed by human body for respiration. It is another kind of nutrient for functioning of lungs and respiratory system. It can be helped with herbs that relax the bronchial muscles and stimulate respiration. Once taken in by the body, nutrients and medicines are carried to the body's estimated three trillion cells. The circulatory system has a remarkable ability to adapt to an endlessly shifting pattern of demand. At rest, the flow of blood is mainly towards the centre of the body, while when active the muscles in the limbs make huge demands. Herbal medicines work to encourage the circulation in particular ways, for example, they encourage blood to flow to the surface of the body; others stimulate the heart to pump more efficiently, while others relax the muscles of the arteries, lowering blood pressure.

Human physiology acts in such a way that nutrients are circulated in body cells and waste matters are removed. All too often in our polluted world, high levels of toxicity in the body are an underlying cause of ill health, and herbalists use a wide range of cleansing herbs that improve the body's ability to remove toxins. Perhaps the finest example of a detoxifying herb is burdock (*Arctium lappa*), which is used extensively in both Western and Chinese medicine. Once herbs such as this reduce the toxic *load* the body is ableto invest greater resources repairing and strengthening damaged tissue and weakened organs.

The skin also plays an important role in good health. Antiseptic plants fight infection, while vulnerary (wound–healing) herbs such as comfrey (*Symphytum officinale,*) encourage blood clotting and help speed the healing wounds.

It is a common observation that good health is dependent on on a healthy balanced nervous system. In order to ensure long–term good health of the nervous systems, it is important to adapt well to life's daily demands to avoid excessive anxiety, worry or depression, and to take sufficient rest and exercise. Human Nervous system does not work in isolation. It is complemented by the endocrine system, which controls the release of a whole symphony of hormones, including the sex hormones, which control fertility and often affect vitality and mood. The nervous system is also intimately linked with the immune system, which controls the ability to resist infection and to recover from illness and injury. Nervous system is a very complex and is a part of electrical, chemical and mechanical functions andf all the parts should work harmoniously for good health. Human body has has infinite capacity of its controlling this systems under environmental adjustments and change to external pressures. This ability to adapt to the external world while the body's internal workings remain constant is known as *homeostasis*. Several herbs work with the immune, nervous and endocrine systems to help the body adapt more effectively to stresses and strains of all kinds–physical, mental emotional and even spiritual. They are effective because they work in tune with the body's processes.

Certain herbs are *adaptogenic,* meaning that they have in ability to help people to adapt, either by supporting the nervous system and easing nervous and emotional tension, or by working directly with the body's own physiological processes to maintain health. The prime example of an adaptogenic herb is ginseng (*Panax ginseng*), which is an effective remedy at times of great mental or physical stress, but in certain cases can also be taken when a relaxing effect is required, for example to relieve headaches, or to ensure a good night's sleep.

COMPLEX NATURAL MEDICINES

A herb is not serve as a *magic bullet because it has* complex natural medicinal effect because it is composed of several active constituents which work on different human body systems. By combining scientific research into active constituents with clinical observation and traditional knowledge of the whole plant, we can develop a rounded picture of each herb's range of medicinal uses.

The medicinal plants are classified and identify on the basis of their actions, for example whether they are sedative, antiseptic or diuretic, and the degree to which affect different body systems. Herbs often have a pronounced action on a particular body system, for example a plant that is strongly antiseptic in the digestive tract may be less so in the respiratory tract. Examples of how herbs work on the body are given below.

Disease	Name of plant(s)	Used in
Skin		
Antiseptics	Tea tree (*Melaleuca alternifolia,*),	Disinfects the skin.
Emollients	Marigold (*Calendula officinalis*),	Deduces itchiness, redness and soreness
Astringents	Witch hazel (*Hamamelis virginiana,*)	Tighten the skin
Depuratives	Burdock (*Arctium lappa)*	Encourages removal of waste products
Healing and vulneary herbs	Self–heal (*Prunella vulgaris*) and comfrey (*Symphytum officinale*)	Aids the healing of cuts, wounds and abrasions.
Immune System		
Immune stimulants	Echinacea (*Echinacea* spp) and lapacho (*Tabebuia* spp)	Encourages the immune system of ward off infection
Respiratory System		
Antiseptics and antibiotics	Garlic (*Allium sativum*)	Helps the lungs resist infection
Expectorants	Elecampane *(Inula helenium*)	Stimulates the coughing up of mucus
Demulcents	Marshmallow (*Althaea officinalis*)	Smooth irriated membranes
Spasmolytics	Visnaga (*Ammi visnaga*)	Relax bronchial muscles
Endocrine Glands		
Adaptogens	Ginseng (*Panax ginseng,*)	Help the body adjust to external pressures and stress
Hormonally active herbs	Agnus castus (*Vitex agnus–castus*)	Stimulates production of sex and other hormones
Emmenagogues	Black cohosh (*Cimicifuga racemosa*)	Encourages or regulate menstruation
Urinary System		
Antiseptics	Buchu (*Barosma betulina*)	Disinfect the urinary tubules
Astringents	Horsetail (*Equisetum arvense*)	Tighten and protect the urinary tubules
Diuretics	Cornsilk (*Zea mays*) stimulate the flow of urine	
Musculo–Skeletal System		
Analgesics	Yellow jasmine (*Gelsemium sempervirens*)	Relieve joint and nerve pain
Anti–inflammatories	White willow (*Salix alba*)	Reduce swelling and pain in joints
Antispasmodics	Cinchona (*Cinchona* spp.)	Relax tense and cramped muscles.
Nervous System		
Nervine	Rosemary (*Rosmarinus officinalis*)	Support and strengthen the nervous system
Relaxants	Lemon balm (*Melissa officinalis*)	Relax the nervous system
Sedatives	Mistletoe (*Viscum album*)	Reduce nervous activity
Stimulants	Kola nut (*Cola acuminata*)	Increase nervous activity
Tonics	Oats (*Avena sativa*)	Improve nerve function and tone, and help to restore the nervous system as a whole
Circulation and Heart		
Cardiotonics	Ddan shen *(Salvia miltiorrhiza*)	Vary in action. Some slow heart beat

Disease	Name of plant(s)	Used in
		rate, while others increase it. Some improve the regularity and strength of the heart's contractions.
Circulatory stimulants	Cayenne (*Capsicum frutescens*)	Improves the circulation of blood to the extremities
Diaphoretics	Juhua (*Chrysanthemum* x *morifolium*)	Encourages blood flow to the surface to the body, promote sweating and lower blood pressure
Spasmolytics	Cramp bark (Viburnum opulus)	Relax the muscles, helping to lower blood pressure
Digestive Organs		
Antiseptics	Ginger (*Zingiber officinalis*)	Protects against infection
Astringents	Bistort (*Polygonum bistorta*)	Tighten up the inner lining of the intestines and create a protective coating over them
Bitters	Wormwood (*Artemisia absinthum*)	Stimulate secretion of digestive juices by the stomach and intestines
Carminaties	Sweet flag (*Acorus calamus*)	Relieve wind and griping pain
Cholagogues	Fringe tree (*Chionanthus virginicus*)	Improves the flow of bile into the intestines
Choleretics	Artichoke (*Cynara scolymus*)	Stimulates secretion of bile by the liver
Demulcents	Psyllium (*Plantago* spp.)	Soothes the digestive system and protect against acidity and irritation
Hepatics	Bupleurum (*Bupleurum chinense*)	Prevents liver damage
Laxatives	Senna (*Cassia senna*)	Stimulate bowel movements
Stomachis	Cardamom (*Eletteria cardamomum*)	Protect and support and stomach

4 CLASSIFICATION, IDENTIFICATION AND NAMING OF MEDICINAL PLANTS

OVERVIEW

Nature is characterized by diversity. No two individuals are exactly alike. Some individuals have identical genomes (arrays of genes). However, in appearance, even *clonal populations* or identical twins exhibit differences. Every culture has a system for grouping individuals for a variety of practical purpose; names are attached to the groups and the component types of which they are comprised. As long as a culture remained closed to the outside world there was no problem with the culture–based nomenclature. However, as cultures merged with each other and plant materials were moved across cultural and geographic lines, it became necessary, for effective cross–cultural communication, to have a universal system of naming plants. This system ensured that corn, even though called maize in another culture, would have a neutral name and mean the same crop to all people.

Some superficial differences automatically place organisms into distinct classes. For example, there are plants and there are animals. In plants, some bear flowers, others do not some have broad leaves, others have narrow leaves; some bear fleshy fruits, others bear grains; and so on. These *natural systems* of classification are arbitrary and reflect the used human cultures have for plants. Other forms of nomenclature are based on scientific principles that have universal application. This chapter explores the origin and nature of these difference systems for grouping and naming plants.

SCIENTIFIC AND BOTANICAL SYSTEMS OF CLASSIFICATION

Scientific systems of classification go beyond the superficial or natural system by employing a number of criteria that include morphological, anatomical, ultrastructural, physiological, phytochemical, cytological, and evolutionary (phylogenetical) criteria. Pyrame de Candole is credited with the introduction of the term *taxonomy* as the science of classifying and naming plants. Taxonomy is sometimes used synonymously with *systematics.* The latter, however, is a field of biology involved with the study of diversity among organisms to establish their natural (evolutionary) relationship, making taxonomy a discipline of systematics.

In plant identification, individuals are assigned to descending series of related plants, based on their known common characteristics. For example, a marigold plant is first placed in a more distant group with plants that have seed, then among seed plants with flowers, and eventually in the most closely associated groups of varieties of marigold. In terms of *botanical nomenclature* (naming plants), Carolus Linnaeus is credited with developing the current Latin–based system called the binomial nomenclature (because an individual is given two names, as opposed to the polynomial system, which was more descriptive). The international body that sets the rules for naming plants by this system publishes the *International Code of Botanical Nomenclature (ICBN)* to provide guidelines for standardizing the naming of plants. These rules are revised as new scientific evidence becomes available.

TAXONOMIC GROUPS

Seven general classification categories have been defined in plants. These classification can be arranged in order from the most inclusive group (*kingdom*) to the least inclusive group (*species*). Each of these groups constitutes a taxon (plural: *taxa*). In addition to these basic groups, subcategories are used in certain cases. These include such as *subdivision, subclass, suborder, subspecies,* and *variety* (or *cultivar*). An example of plant classification is presented in table 1–1.

According to the binomial nomenclature, each individual has two–part name; the first part is called the genus (plural: *genera*) and second part is called a *specific epithet* or *species.* This system is equivalent to surnames and first names in the naming of people.

Kingdoms

Placing organisms into groups is a work in progress. Traditionally, living organisms are recognized as belonging to one of two categories or kingdom: the *plant kingdom* or the *animal kingdom.* However, as science advances and knowledge increases, this scheme periodically comes under review. From the two–kingdom scheme evolved the three–, four–, and five–kingdom classifications of organisms. Even the five–kingdom scheme is deemed inadequate by

Table 4.1. An Example of Scientific Classification of Plants

Taxon	Example	Common Name
Kingdom	Plantae	Plant
Division	Magnoliophyta	Flowering plant
Class	Liliopsida	Monocot
Order	Liliales	Lily order
Family	Liliaceae	Lily order
Genus	*Allium*	
Species	*Allium cepa*	Onion

R. H. Whittaker (1969) proposed the five–kingdom classification. The criteria for the classification are cellular structure (complexity) and forms of nutrition (photosynthesis, ingestion, or absorption of food in solution).

Even though horticulture focuses on organisms in Kingdom Plantae, other kingdoms are directly or indirectly important to the field. Horticulture exists because of humans (Kingdom Animalia). The field was developed by humans. Organisms in the Kingdom Monera, Protoctista, and Fungi include those that are pathogen of horticultural plants, namely, bacteria, fungi, and viruses.

1. **Kingdom Monera.** Monera is a kingdom of unicellular (one–called) organisms (2.11). They are called prokaryotes and have no nuclear membrane or compartmentalization into distinct organelles. They re produce primarily by cell division and are mostly heterotrophic (cannot make organic compounds and thus feed on material made by others). Bacteria are classified under this kingdom.

2. **Kingdom production.** The Kingdom Production includes algae (green, brown, and red), slime molds, and eukaryotes (cells with a nuclear membrane and compartmentalization).

3. **Kingdom Fungi.** Fungi are filamentous eukaryotes that lack plastids and the photosynthetic pigment (chlorophyll). Thus, they feed on dead or living organisms. Most plant diseases are caused by fungi.

4. **Kingdom Animalia.** Kingdom Animalia consists of multicellular organisms that are eukaryotes but without cell walls, plastids, and capacity for photosynthesis (processing of food production from the sun by plants). Animals generally ingest their food and reproduce primarily by sexual means. Animals have the highest level of organization and tissue differentiation of any organism in any kingdom. They have complex sensory and neuromotor systems.

5. **Kingdom Plantae.** Organisms in the Kingdom Plantae are photosynthetic (make food from inorganic materials; few plants are heterotrophic, that is, feeding on organic material from other sources). They are multicellular, have cell walls, and live on land.

Table 4.2. The Five Kingdoms of Organisms as Described by Whittaker

Monera (Have Prokaryotic Cells)
Bacteria
Protoctista (Have Eukaryotic Cells)
Algae
Slime molds
Flagellate fungi
Protozoa
Sponges
Fungi (Absorb Food in Solution)
True fungi
Plantae (Produce Own Food by the Process of Photosynthesis)
Bryophytes
Vascular plants
Animalia (Ingest Their Food)
Multicellular animals

Divisions of Kingdom Plantae

Several divisions are recognized in the Kingdom Plantae. These divisions can be divided into two major categories: *bryophytes* (nonvascular plants–the mosses, hornworts, and liverworts) and vascular plants. Vascular plants are large bodied and have three primary vegetative organs, stem, leaves, and roots, and also conducting tissues (vascular tissue). Vascular plants may produce seeds or be seedless. Most plants of horticultural interest are vascular plants.

In terms of relative abundance, more than 80 per cent of all species in the plant kingdom are flowering plants. Even though gymnosperms (seed plants whose seeds are not enclosed within an ovary during development) make up only 0.2 per cent of species in the plant kingdom, conifers (e.g., pines) occur on about one–third of forested lands of the world.

Variety Versus Cultivar

The lowest and least–inclusive taxon is the species, as already indicated. Species may be subdivided into specific categories. A botanical variety is a naturally occurring variant of the species that is significantly different from the general species originally described. Botanical varieties may differ in subtle or more visible ways, such as in color, shape, size, chemical quality, or some other traits. Instead of two names, as expected in the binomial nomenclature, a variety requires the use of a third name after the introduction of the abdreviation var. (for *variety*). For example, broccoli is called *Brassica oleraceae* var. *botrytis.*

Through plant breeding, humans sometimes create new variants that are maintained under human supervision (as opposed to being naturally maintained, as is the case in varieties). The product of plant breeding is called a *cultivar,* a contraction of two terms–*cultivated* and *variety.*

Table 4.3. The Divisions of the Kingdom Plantae

	Divisions	Common Name
Bryophytes	Hepaticophyta	Liverworts
	Anthocerotophyta	Hornworts
	Bryophyta	Mosses
Vascular plants	Psilotophyta	Whisk ferns
Seedless	Lycophyta	Club mosses
	Sphenophyta	Horsetails
	Pterophyta	Ferns
Seeded	Pinophyta	Gynosperms
	Subdivision: Cycadicae	Cycads
	Subdivision: Pinicae	
	Class: Ginkgoatae	Ginkgo
	Class: Pinatae	Conifers
	Subdivision: Gneticae	Gnetum
	Magnoliophyta	Flowering plants
	Class: Liliopsida	Monocots
	Class: Mangoliopsida	Dicots

Cultivars are maintained as clones in vegetatively propagated (increasing the number of plants by using plant parts other than seed) species and as lines in species propagated by seed under specific conditions. Many flowers and vegetables have cultivars that are propagated by seed, whereas others are *hybrids* (F_1 seed from a cross of two different parents).

Rules in Classification

In plant taxonomy, the ending of a name is often characteristic of the taxon. Classes often end in –*opsida* (e.g., Magnoliopsida). Names ending in –*ae* are subclasses of class names (depending on the classification system). Exceptions include several families such as Compositae (now called Asteraceae). Plant orders end in –*ales* (e.g., Rosales [roses]) while family names end in –aceae (e.g., Rosaceae).

These higher–order taxa are not routinely encountered, unless one is conducting taxonomic studies. The binomial names (genus and species) are the most frequently encountered. When you walk through a botanical garden, or even a college campus where there is good horticulture program or a good grounds and gardens department, you may find that some plants in the landscape are labeled with the correct binomial name or scientific name, as well as the common name. The family name is quite frequently indicated.

For writing names following rules have been framed at the binomial level:

1. All the binary name must be underlined or written in italics.
2. The genus name starts with an uppercase letter, and the species name is written in lowercase throughout. The term *species* is both singular and plural. It may be shortened to spp., for the plural species.

3. In technical writing, an initial L. may follow the species, indicating that Linnaeus first named the plant. Other abbreviations may be encountered in the literature. An example of a full binary name for corn, for example, *Zea mays* L. The genus may be abbreviated (e.g., *Z. mays* L.). Some plants may have a subspecies and hence a third name added to the binary name. In such a case, the third name is also underlined or italicized.
4. Whereas the generic name can be written alone to refer to individuals in the group, the specific epithet cannot be used by itself (i.e., *Zea* but not *mays*).
5. At the bottom of the taxa hierarchy is variety, which is the naturally occurring and very closely related variant. As previously indicated, the binomial name is followed by the abbreviation var. and then the variety name. Cultivar names are not underlined or italicized (e.g., *Lycopersicon esculentum* Mill. Cultivar 'Big Red' or L. *esculentum* cv. 'Big Red').

Specific epithets are adjectival in nature. Many genera can have the same specific epithet. Some of them indicate color, such as *alba* (white), *variegata* (variegated), *rubrum* (red), and *aureum* (golden). Example are, *vulgaris* (common), *esculentus* (edible), *sativus* (cultivated), *tuberosum* (bearing tubers), and *officinalis* (medcinal).

In developing new horticultural cultivars, plant breeders employ a variety of techniques. The conventional techniques involve crossing or hybridizing plant that differ in desirable characteristics. In terms of taxonomic hierarchy, hybridization can be routinely performed at the base of the hierarchy (i.e., among varieties or cultivars of the same species). Crossing at other levels such as among species (*interspecies hybridization* leads to genetic complications. Such a cross is problematic and has limited success, requiring the use of additional technique, such as *embryo rescue*, in some cases.

Other Classification Systems (Operational)

A number of operational classification systems are employed simultaneously in the field of horticulture. The following are some of the major systems.

Seasonal Growth Cycle

Plants may be classified into three general groups based on growth cycle. Growth cycle refers to the period from first establishment (e.g., by seed) to when the plant dies. The three categories are as follows:

Annuals

An annual plant lives through only one growing season, completing its life cycle (seed, seedling, flowering, fruiting, and death) in that period. This group includes many weeds, garden flowers, vegetables, and wild flowers. The duration of a life cycle is variable and may be a few weeks to several months, depending on the species. Annuals are the basis of a major horticultural production group called annual bedding plants. These plants are produced largely for use in the landscape and also the vegetable garden. Popular annual flowers are geranium (*Geranium* spp.), zommoa (*Zinnia elegans*), marigold (*Tagetes* spp.), and pansy (*Viola tricolor*). In cultivation, certain vegetables such as tomato (*Lycopersicon esculentum*) are produced an annual cycle.

Biennials

A biennial is a plant that completes its life cycle in two growing seasons. In the first season, it produces only basal leaves; it grows a stem, produces flowers and fruits, and dies in the second season. The plant usually requires some special environmental condition or treatment such as exposure to a cold temperature (*vernalization* to be induced to enter the reproductive phase. Examples of biennials are sugar beet (*Beta vulgaris*) and onion (*Allium cepa*). Even though annuals and biennials rarely become woody in temperature regions, these plants may sometimes produce secondary growth in their stems and roots.

Perennials

Perennials may be herbaceous of woody. They persist year–round through the adverse weather of the non–growing seasons (winter or drought) and then flower and fruit after a variable number of years of vegetative growth beyond the second year. Herbaceous perennials survive the unfavorable season as dormant underground structures (e.g., roots, rhizomes, bulbs, and tubers that are modified primary vegetative parts of the part of the plant. Examples of herbaceous perennials are turfgrasses such as bermudagrass (*Cynodon dactylon*) and flowers such as daylilies (*Lilium* spp.) and irises (*Iris* spp.)

Woody perennials may be vines, shrubs, or trees. These plants do not die back in adverse seasons but usually suspend active growth. Although some perennials may flower in the first year of planting, woody perennials flower only when they become adult plants. This stage may be attained within a few years or even after 100 years. Woody perennials may be categorized into two types:

Evergreen

Evergreen perennials maintain green leaves year–round. Some leaves may be lost, but not all at one time. Example of evergreen perennials are citrus (*Citrus* spp.) and pine (*Pinus* spp.).

Deciduous

Deciduous plants shed their leaves at the same time during one of the seasons of the year (dry cold). New leaves are developed from dormant buds upon the return of favorable growing conditions. Examples of deciduous perennials are oak (*Quercus* spp.) and elm (*Ulmus* spp.). It should be mentioned that intermediate conditions occur in which some plants do not lose all of their leaves (*semideciduous*).

Kinds of Stems

There are three general classes of horticultural plants based on stem type. However, intermediates do occur between these classes.

Herbs

Herbs are plants with soft, nonwoody stems. They have primary vegetative parts. Example include corn (*Zea mays*), many potted plants, many annual bedding plants, and many vegetables. In another usage, the term *herbs* is associated with spices (plants that are aromatic or fragrant and used to flavor foods or beverages).

Shrubs

A shrub has no main trunk. Branches arise from the ground level on a shrub. It is woody and has secondary tissue. Shrubs are perennials and usually smaller than trees. Examples of shrubs are dogwood (*Cornus* spp.), kalmia (*Kalmia* spp.) and azalea (*Rhododnedron* spp.).

Trees

Trees are large plants characterized by one main trunk. They branch on the upper pert of the plant, are woody, and have secondary tissue. Examples include pine (*Pinus* spp.), oak (*Quercus* spp.), cedar (*Cedrus* spp.), and orange (*Citrus sinesis*).

Common Stem Growth Forms

The criterion for classification is how the stem stands in relation to the ground. There are several types of stem growth forms, the most common ones including the following.

Erect

A stem is erect if, without artificial support, it stands upright (stands at a 90–degree angle to the ground level). Because of the effect of strong winds and other environmental factors, an erect plant may incline slightly. Trees have erect stems. To adapt crop plants to mechanized harvesting, plant breeders have developed what are called "bush" cultivars. These plants have strong stems and stiff branches.

Decumbent

The stems of decumbent plants are extremely inclined, with the tips raised. An example is peanut (*Arachis hypogaea*).

Creeping (or repent)

A plant is described as creeping when it crawls on the ground, producing adventitious roots at specific points on the stem. Stems that grow horizontally in this fashion are called *stolons.* The strawberry plant (*Fragaria* spp.) has creeping stems.

Climbing

Climbers are vines that, without additional support, will creep on the ground. There are three general modes of the climbing. *Twiners* are climbing plants that simply wrap their stringy stems around their support, as occurs in sweet potato (*Ipomea batatas*). Another group of climbers develop cylindrical structures called tendrils that are used to coil around the support on physical contact. An example of a plant that climbs by this method is the garden pea (*Pisum sativum*). The third mode of climbing is by adventitious roots formed on aerial parts of the plants, as found in the English ivy (*Hedera helix*) and *Philodendron.*

CLASSIFICATION OF FRUITS

Fruits can be classified on a botanical basis and for several operational purposes.

Botanical Classification

Fruits exhibit a variety of apparent differences that may be used for classification. Some fruits are borne on herbaceous plants and others on woody plants. A very common operational way of classifying fruits is according to fruit succulence and texture on maturity and ripening. On this basis there are two basic kinds of fruits–*fleshy fruits* and *dry fruits.* However, anatomically, fruits are distinguished by the arrangement of the carpels from which they developed. A carpel is sometimes called the *pistil* (consisting of a stigma, style, and ovary), the female reproductive structure.

A fruit is mature ovary. The ovary may have one or more carpels. Even though the fruit is a mature ovary, some fruits include other parts of the flower and are called *accessory fruits.* Combining carpel number, succulence characteristics, and anatomical features, fruits may be classified into three kinds, *simple, multiple,* or *aggregate.*

Simple fruits develop from a single carpel or sometimes from the fusing together of several carpels. This group of fruits is very diverse. When mature and ripe, the fruit may be soft and fleshy, dry and woody, or have a papery texture. There are three types of fleshy fruits.

Fleshy fruits

Drupe

A drupe may comprise one to several carpels. Usually, each carpel contains one seed. The endocarp (inner layer) of the fruit is hard and stony and is usually highly attached to the seed. Examples are cherry (*Prunus* spp.), olive, coconut (*Cocos nucifera*), peach (*Prunus persica*), and plum (*Prunus domestica*).

Berry

A berry is a fruit characterized by an inner pulp that contains a few to several seeds but not pits. It is formed from one or several carpels. Examples are tomato (*Lycopersicon esculentum*), grape (*Vitis* spp.), and pepper (*Capsicum anuum*). If the exocarp (skin) is leathery and contains oils, as in the citrus fruits (e.g., orange [*Citrus sinensis*], lemon [*Citurs lemon*], and grapefruit [Citrus paradisi]), the berry is called a hesperidium. Some berries have a rind, as in watermelon (*Citrullus vulgaris*), cucumber (*Cucumis sativus*), and pumpkin (*Cucurbita pepo*). This type of a berry is called a *pepo.*

Pome

A pome is a pitted fruit with a stony interior. The pit usually contains one seed chamber and one seed. This very specialized fruit type develops from the ovary, with most of the fleshy part formed from the receptacle tissue (the enlarged base of the perianth). Pomes are characteristic of one subfamily of the family Rosaceae (rose family). Examples of pomes are apple (*Pyrus malus*), pear (*Pyrus communis*), and quince (*Cydonia oblonga*).

Dry fruits. Dry fruits are not juicy or succulent when mature and ripe. When dry, they may split open and discharge their seeds (called *dehiscent fruits*) or retain their seeds (called *indehiscent fruits*).

Dehiscent Fruits. A fruit developed from a single carpel may split from only one side at maturity to discharge its seeds. Such a fruit is called a follicle. Examples are columbine (*Aquilegia* spp.), milkweed (*Asclepias* spp.), larkspur (*Delphinium* spp.), and magnolia (Magnolia spp.). Sometimes, the splitting of the ovary occurs along two seams, with seeds borne on only one of the halves of the spilt ovary. Such a fruit is called a legume, example being pea (*Pisum sativum*), bean (*Phaseolus vulgaris*), and peanut (*Arachis hypogaea*). In a third type of dehiscent fruit, called *silique* or *silicle*, seeds are attached to central structure, as occurs in radish (*Raphanus sativus*) and mustard (*Brassica campestris*). The most common dehiscent simple seeds are discharged when the capsule splits longitudinally. In some species, seeds are discharged when the capsule splits longitudinally. In others, seeds exit through holes near the top of the capsule, such as in lily (*Lilum* spp.), iris (*Iris* spp.), and poppy (*Papaver* spp.).

Indehiscent Fruits. Some indehjiscent fruits may have a hard *pericarp* (exocarp + mesocarp + endocarp). This stony fruit wall is cracked in order to reach the seed. Such fruits are called nuts, as found in chestnut (*Castanea* spp.) and hazelnut (*Corylus* spp.). Nuts develop from a compound ovary. Sometimes the pericarp of the fruit is thin and the ovaries occur in pairs, as found in dill (*Anethum graveolens*) and carrot (*Daucus carota*). This fruit type is called a schizocarp. In maple (*Acer* spp.), ash (*Fraxinus* spp.), elm (*Ulmus* spp.), and other species, the pericarp has a wing and is called a samara. Where the pericarp is not winged but the single seed is attached to the pericarp only at its base, the fruit is called an *achene.* Achenes are the most common indehiscent fruits. Example are the buttercup family (Ranuculaceae) and sunflower. In cereal grains (Poaceae or grass family), the seed, unlike in an achene, is fully fused to the pericarp. This fruit type is called a *caryopsis* or grain.

Other Operational Classifications

Fruits may also be classified according to other operational uses.

Temperate fruits or tropical fruits

Temperature fruits are fruits from plants adapted to cool climates, and tropical fruits are produced on plants adapted to warm climates. For example, apple (*Pyrus malus*), peach (*Prunus domestica*) are temperate fruits, whereas mango (*Mangifera indica*) and coconut (*Cocosnucifera*) are tropical fruits.

Fruit trees

Tree fruits are fruits borne on trees, such as apple (*Pyrus malus*) and mango (*Mangifera indica*).

Small fruits

Small fruits are predominantly woody, perennial, dicot angiosperms. They are usually vegetatively propagated and bear small– to moderate–sized fruits on herbs, vines, or shrubs. Examples are grape (*Vitis* spp.), strawberry (*Fragaria* spp.), and blackberry (*Rubus* spp.). Small fruits require training and pruning (removal of parts of the shoot) to control growth and remove old canes (branches) to obtain desired plant shape and high productivity.

Bramble fruits

Bramble fruits are nontree fruits that usually require physical support (such as a trellis) during cultivation. Examples are raspberry (*Rubus* spp.), blackberry (*Rubus* spp.), and boysenberry) (*Rubus* spp.). Bramble fruits also require training and pruning in cultivation.

Classification of Vegetables

Vegetables may be classified on the basis of life cycle, edible or economic parts of the plant (use), adaptation, and botanical features.

Life cycle

Based on life cycle, vegetables may be classified as annuals, biennials, or perennials.

Annual

Most vegetable garden crops are true annuals, such as corn (*Zea mays*), or are cultivated as annuals, such as tomato (*Lycopersicon esculentum*). These plants are selected for either fall or summer cultivation. They require a few weeks to several months to maturity, depending on the cultivar.

Biennial

Few popular vegetable garden crops are biennials, and, even then, they are frequently cultivated as annuals and replanted each season. Examples are sugar beet (*Beta vulgaris*) and carrot (*Daucus carota*).

Perennial

Whenever perennial vegetable garden crops are cultivated, they must be strategically located so as not to interfere with seasonal land preparation activities needed for planting annual crops. These plants may be pruned to control growth or to remove dead tissue. Examples are asparagus (*Asparagus officinalis*) and horseradish (*Rorippa armoracia*).

Edible or Economic Parts

Vegetables may be operationally classified according to the parts of the plant harvested for food or other uses.

Pods

Pods are legumes that are harvested prematurely, cooked, and eaten with the seeds inside. When harvesting is delayed, pods develop fiber and become stringy and undesirable for fresh use. Examples are green bean and okra.

Roots

Sometimes primary plant parts (stem root, and leaf) may become modified as storage organs for food. Roots may become enlarged as a result of the accumulation of stored food. The roots are dug and eaten baked, boiled, or fried. An example is the sweet potato.

Bulbs

Like roots, bulbs are modified stems and leaves, as found in onions. The stem is highly compressed to form what is called a basal plate, while the leaves are storage organs.

Tubers

Tubers look like modified roots. The difference between them is that tubers are swollen stems, whereas roots are swollen roots.

Greens

Greens are vegetable crops whose leaves are usually picked at tender stages to be used for food. The leaves are generally cooked before being eaten.

Adaptation

Just like fruits, certain vegetable species prefer cool temperatures during production, and others prefer warm temperatures. Based on seasons in which they grow best, vegetables may be classified into two groupings.

Cool season

Cool–season crops require monthly temperatures of 15–18°C (60–65°F). Examples are sugar beet (*Beta vulgaris*) and cabbage (*Brassica oleracea*).

Warm season

Warm–season crops prefer monthly temperatures of 18–27°C. Examples are okra (*Hibiscus esculentus*), eggplant ((*Solanum melongena*), corn (*Zea mays*), and shallot (*Allium cepa*).

It should be mentioned that plant breeders have developed cultivars with wide adaptation for many crop species. For example, popular garden crops including corn, tomato, and pepper are grown over a wide range of climates. Even though cultivars with cold or heat tolerance may have been bred for different crops, commercial large–scale production occurs n regions of best adaptation of these crops, unless production is under a controlled environment (greenhouse).

Botanical Features

Vegetables may be classified according to specific botanical characteristics they share in common.

Vines

Vines are plants with stems that need physical support; without it they creep on the ground or climb onto other nearby plants in cultivation. Examples are squash, pumpkin, and cucumber.

Solanaceous plants

Solanaceous plants belong to the family Solanaceae. Examples are eggplant, tomato, and pepper.

Cole crops

Cole plants belong to the Brassica family. Example are cabbage, cauliflower, and broccoli (*Brassica oleracea* var *botrytis*).

Classification of Ornamental Plants

Ornamental plants may also be classified based on stem type, growth cycle, leaf form, use, and other characteristics.

Herbaceous Ornamental Plants

Herbaceous plants are non–woody. Many horticultural plants, especially those grown indoors, are non–woody. They have a wide variety of uses in landscapes as well. They may be classified in various ways.

Growth cycle

Annuals

Annual ornamentals are planted each season. Flowering annuals are prominent in the landscape in favorable seasons, providing most of the color. Versatile landscape plants can be used to fill in gaps, provide color in bulb beds after the bulbs have bloomed, and create colorful flower beds, hanging baskets (flowers grown in containers and hung), and cut flowers (flowers grown and cut for use). Examples include petunia (*Petunia* spp.), zinnia (*Zinnia elegans*), and marigold (*Tagetes* spp.).

Biennials

Biennial ornamentals are vegetative in their first year of growth and bloom in the next season. Examples are foxglove (*Digitalis* spp.) and hollyhock.

Perennials

Since perennials live for a long time in the landscape, locating them requires a great deal of thought and planning. Perennials may be flowering or non–flowering.

Flowering

Flowering perennials may be planted in flower beds in the fall season to provide early blooms, after which annuals may be planted. Examples are geranium (*Geranium* spp.), lily (*Lilium* spp.), and tulip (*Tulipa* spp.).

Foliage. Foliage, or nonflowering, perennials are popular for indoor use in houses and offices as potted plants. Examples are coleus (*Coleus blumei*), sansevieria (*Sansevieria* spp.), and dumbcane (*Dieffenbachia*).

Other Operational Classifications

Herbaceous plants may be used in a variety of other ways, both indoors and outdoors.

Bedding plants

Bedding plants are annual plants raised for planting outdoors in flower beds. They are usually started from seed indoors in the off–season and transplanted later in the growing seasons. Examples include petunia (*Petunia* spp.), zinnia (*Zinnia elegans*), pansy (*Viola tricolor*), and marigold (*Tagetes* spp.).

Hanging plants

Hanging basket plants are plants, annual or perennial, flowering or foliage, that are grown in decorative containers and hung by equally elegant ropes from the ceiling in the patio, in the doorway area, or from decorative plant poles. Examples are geranium (*Geranium* spp.) and spider plant (*Chlorophytum comosum*).

Houseplants

Indoor plants or house plants, are plants adapted to indoor conditions. They are grown in containers, are usually slow growing, and may be flowering or foliage plants. Examples are sansevieria (*Sansevieria* spp.) and Indian rubber plant (*Ficus elastica*).

Woody Medicinal Plants

Woody ornamentals differ in size and growth pattern. Some shed their leaves and are called *deciduous*, whereas others maintain fresh leaves year–round and are called *evergreen*. Some are shrubs, and others are trees. Woody ornamentals may be grown in a perennial garden along with herbaceous perennials. When choosing these plants, attention should be paid to growth habit, color, texture, shape, and adaptation.

Shrubs

As previously described, a shrub is a perennial woody plant of relatively low stature and usually produces multiple stems that arise from the ground or very close to it. Shrubs, which may be sued as hedge plants or ground cover, can be classified as deciduous or evergreen.

Deciduous shrubs

Deciduous shrubs shed their leaves at some point in the year. Example are lilac (*Sylinga vulgaris*), honeysuckle (*Lonicera japonica*), and barberry (*Berberis* spp.).

Evergrren shrubs

Evergreen shrubs may be further divide into two groups according to leaf size.

Narrow leaf. Narrow leaf shrubs have need–like leaves, as in pine (*Pinus* spp.) and juniper (*Juniperus* spp.).

Broadleaf

Broadleaf shrubs have large leaf lamina, as in gardenia (*Gardenia* spp.) and rhododendron.

Trees

Trees are the largest plant materials in the landscape and thus should be located with care. They can overwhelm a house in the adult stage if inappropriate trees species are planted. Trees can also modify the local climate (e.g., as shade trees or wind breaks).

Deciduous trees

Examples of deciduous trees birch (*Betula papyrifera*), elm (*Ulmus* spp.), and willow (*Salix* spp.)

Evergreen trees

Narrow leaf. Examples of narrow leaf evergreen trees are spruce (*Picea* spp.) and red cedar (*Juniperus viginiana*).

Broadleaf. Examples of broadleaf evergreen trees are holy (*Ilex opaca*) and citrus (*Citrus* spp.).

Vines

Vines are climbers and can be manipulated to create a variety of structures and for various functions in the landscape. Like trees and shrubs, vines can be deciduous or evergreen.

Deciduous vines. An example of a deciduous vine is clematis (Clematis recta).

Evergreen vines. An example of an evergreen vine is English ivy (Hedera helix).

Classification Based on Hardiness (Adaptation)

Plants can be classified according to their hardiness or adaptation to local climate. Certain trees are able to thrive under cold temperature, whereas others prefer warm or tropical conditions. The U.S. Department of Agriculture (USDA) Plant Hardiness Zone map divides the United States into 10 zones. Zones 1 is the coldest, and zone 10 is the warmest. Plants' adaptive ranges may be narrow or broad. For example, a shrub such as cinquefoil (*Potentilla fruticosa*) is adaptable to zones 2 through 7, and lantana (*Lantana camara* 'Nivea' L.). is adapted to zones 9 and 10. All plants may be placed into one or more of these hardiness zones.

5 CULTIVATION OF MEDICINAL PLANTS: AN ECO–FRIENDLY APPROACH

ECO–FRIENDLY FARMING

World needs eco–friendly farming systems for sustainable agriculture. This is the need of the present day. There is an urgent need to develop farming techniques, which are sustainable from environmental, production, and socioeconomic points of view. The means to guarantee sufficient food production in the next decades and beyond is critical because modern agriculture production throughout the world does not appear to be sustainable in the long–term. The agricultural community is thus setting it hopes on *sustainable agriculture,* which will maintain the cycles of input–output and ecosystem balance. Definition form FAO (1988), seems appropriate in this contest

> *Sustainable rural development is the management and conservation of the natural resource base, and the orientation of technological and institutional change in such a manner as to assure the attainment and continued satisfaction of human needs for the present and future generations. Such sustainable development, in the agriculture, forestry and fishers sectors, conserves land, water, plant and animal genetic resources, is environmentally non–degrading, technically appropriate, economically viable and socially acceptable.*

Evolution of Sustainable Agriculture

In the 1960s and 1970s, a growing environmental agriculture movement evolved in response to increasing soil erosion, pesticide use, and groundwater contamination. Simultaneously, economic conditions for farmers were becoming more stressful and the number of family farms declined.

In 1980s, Wes Jackson of The Land Institute in Salina, K. S., began using the term *sustainable agriculture* to describe an alternative system of agriculture based upon resource conservation and quality of rural life.

While sustainable agriculture has become the umbrella under which, many of the above–mentioned alternatives farming systems fall, it is important to note that sustainable agriculture is really a long–term goal, not a specific set of farming practices. In temperate zones sustainable agriculture was defined as such:

> *Sustainable agriculture is a philosophy based on human goals and on understanding the long–term impact of our activities on the environment and on other species. Use of this philosophy guides our application of prior experience and the latest scientific advances to create integrated, resource–conserving, equitable farming systems. These systems reduce environmental degradation, maintain agricultural productivity, promote economic viability in both the short and long term and maintain stable rural communities and quality of life.*

In this context, sustainable agriculture embraces all agricultural systems, striving to meet these criteria. Many aspects of modern conventional agriculture are included in sustainable agriculture, just as are many aspects of alternative farming systems.

One aspect of modern agriculture receiving a lot of attention in the sustainable agriculture discussion is the use of chemical inputs to supply fertility and pest control. White agriculture chemicals will continue to play an important role in American agriculture. Many farmers are looking at alternatives due to environmental, economical, or regulatory reasons. In a transition to farming systems more reliant on biological methods of production, low–input farming serves as in intermediary step.

Sustainable agriculture emphasizes the conservation of its own resources. For a farm to be sustainable, it must produce adequate amounts of high–quality foods, be environmentally safe, and where appropriate, be profitable. Sustainable farms minimize their purchased inputs (fertilizers, energy and equipment) and rely, as much as possible on the renewable resources of the farm itself. This is especially important in the 90 per cent of farms that exist in the third world, where these inputs are often not available or affordable.

Agricultural ecosystems, unlike the natural ecosystems, are human manipulated ecosystems and regular and sometimes intense disturbances are a major part of economically viable agriculture management systems.

Sustainable agriculture is a complex issue associated with producing food while maintaining our biophysical resources including soil, water and bita with no adverse impacts on the wider environment. It should:

1. Maintain or improve the production of 'clean' food
2. Maintain or improve the quality of landscapes, which includes soils, water, biota and aesthetics.
3. Have minimal impact on the wide environment.
4. Be economically viable
5. Be acceptable to society.

There are different concepts of sustainable agriculture, but none is generally accepted. It embraces several forms of non–conventional agriculture that are often called organic, alternative, ecological or low input. However, from economic and ecological perspectives, two basic criteria must be met if agriculture is to be sustainable in the long term. These are:

Sustainable farming uses some form of integrated pest management for pest control, and this can include the use of chemical pesticides that are not used by organic farmers. Thus, sustainable agriculture does not mean a return to the farming methods of the late 1800's. Rather, it combines traditional techniques that stress conservation with modern technologies, such as improved seed, modern equipment for low–tillage practices, integrated pest management that relies heavily on biological control principles, and weed control that depends on crop rotations. Sustainable farms try to use wind or solar energy instead of purchased energy, and use organic animal manure and nitrogen–fixing legumes as green manure to maintain soil fertility, as much as possible, thereby minimizing the need to purchase inputs from outside the farm. The use of genetically engineered crop strains is certainly not excluded by sustainable farming. The emphasis is on maintaining the environment, not on rules about what can or cannot be done. Profits from sustainable farms can exceed those of conventional farms.

Innovative farmers have developed many alternative farming methods and systems. These systems consist of a wide variety of integrated practices and methods suited to the specific needs, limitations, resource bases and economic conditions of different farms. To make wider adoption possible, however, farmers need to receive information and technical assistance in developing new management skills.

There are several established approaches to ecofriendly farming systems. A common thread in all schools is an emphasis on biological systems to supply fertility and pest control rather than chemical inputs.

ORGANIC FARMING

The most widely recognized alternative farming system. Modern organic farming evolved as an alternative to chemical agriculture in the 1940s, largely in response to the publications of J.I. Rodale in the U.S., Lady Eve Balfour in England, and Sir Albert Howard in India.

In 1980, U.S.D.A. released a landmark report on organic farming. The report defined organic farming as:

> *Organic farming is a production system, which avoids or largely excludes the use of synthetically compounded fertilizers, pesticides, growth regulators, and livestock feed additives. To the maximum extent feasible, organic farming systems rely upon crop rotations, crop residues, animal manures, legumes, green manures, off–farm organic wastes, mechanical cultivation, mineral–bearing rocks, and aspects of biological pest control to maintain soil productivity and tilth, to supply plant nutrients, and to control insects, weeds, and other pests.*

BIOLOGICAL FARMING

Biological farming has become synonymous with farmers using the Reams fertility system as the basis for crop production. *Eco–agriculture* is the term used to describe this system by the monthly Acres, U.S.A. The Reams system is based on the LaMotte–Morgan soil test and the use or rock phosphate, calcium carbonate, and compost to achieve nutrient ratios of 7:1 calcium to magnesium, 2:1 phosphorus to potassium, and so on. Biological farming allows the use of selected chemical fertilizers (avoiding disruptive materials such as anhydrous ammonia and potassium chloride) and adopts low–inputs approaches to use of herbicides and insecticides.

Diagnostic instruments to monitor plant and soil conditions are frequently used in biological farming. These include refractometers to monitor sugar content (Brix) in plant tissue sap; electrical conductivity meters to monitor ERGS (or energy released per gram of soil); ORPS meters (or oxygen reduction potential of soil); and radionics. Based on data gathered, foliar sprays containing biostimulatns and soluble nutrients are applied. The Pandol Brothers, a large commercial fruit and vegetable operation in California, reduced their annual pesticide bill from US $500,000 to US $50,000 per year after adopting a Biological Fertility Program.

NATURE FARMING

Nature Farming was developed in Japan in the 1930s by Mokichi Okada, who later formed the Mokichi Okada Association (MOA). Nature Farming parallels organic farming in many ways but includes special emphasis on soil health through composts rather than organic fertilizer, when possible. Kyusei Nature Farming, a branch group, emphasizes use of microbial preparations in addition to traditional Nature Farming is most active in the Pacific rim, California and Hawaii.

In addition to these methods–based approaches to sustainable farming, regenerative agriculture and permaculture are widely recognized. However, these latter systems, like sustainable agriculture, are more conceptually oriented than methods–based.

REGENERATIVE AGRICULTURE

In regenerative agriculture bunds on nature's own inherent capacity to cope with pests, enhance soil fertility, and increase productivity. It implies a continuing ability to re–create the resources that the system requires. In practice, regenerative agriculture uses low–input and organic farming systems as a framework to achieve these goals.

PERMACULTURE

Permaculture is a contraction of *permanent agriculture.* The term was coined by Bill Mollison, an Australian forest ecologist, in 1978. Permaculture is concerned with designing ecological human habitats and food production systems, and follows specific guidelines and principles in the design of these systems. To the extent that permaculture is not a production system, per se, but rather a land use planning philosophy, it is not limited to a specific method of production. Thus, practically any site–specific ecological farming system is amenable to permaculture.

Some of the Eco–friendly farming systems are described here in detail:

ALTERNATE AGRICULTURE

Plant growth and crop production are complex processes that depend on many interactions between organisms. The trend of modern agriculture has been:

1. To substitute monoculture and continuous culture for crop rotation and diversified agriculture
2. To use genetically more uniform plants, that have a narrow genetic base
3. To use inorganic fertilizers, rather than the more difficult–to–use organic manures, in combination with green manures
4. To use herbicides and pesticides to combat weeds and pests, rather than more complex biological control mechanisms
5. To make bigger fields by eliminating all vegetation between them

Recently, there has been a resurgence of interest in alternative agriculture, organic farming and sustainable agriculture. In 1989, the Board on Agriculture of the National Research Council of the United States lent credence to this movement with the publication of a major study called *Alternative Agriculture.* Alternative agriculture is not a single system of organic, low input, regenerative, or sustainable farming. All these systems share an emphasis on management practices and on biological relationships between organisms.

Alternative agriculture recognizes that a piece of land on which crop plants are grown is first and foremost an ecosystem, and not a factory. An ecosystem has many interacting organisms that must remain in balance. Many natural processes occur in such an ecosystem and farmers should take advantage of these natural processes, rather than try to circumvent them or destroy them with chemicals. Alternative agriculture rejects certain practices (such as heavy use of inorganic fertilizers), but most important are the practices it favours:

1. Tillage that minimizes soil erosion even if it is more expensive
2. Reliance on animal manures and green manures with minimal input of inorganic fertilizers
3. Integrated pest management for pest control
4. Management systems, such as crop rotations, that help control weeds and disease organisms
5. These techniques are not new of course, although some of them have been refined in recent years.

> *Organic farming is defined as production system, which avoids or largely excludes the use of synthetically compounded fertilizers, pesticides, growth regulators, and livestock feed additives. To the maximum extent feasible, organic farming systems rely upon crop rotations, crop residues, animal manures, legumes, green manures, off–farm organic wastes, mechanical cultivation mineral–bearing rocks, and aspects of biological pest control to maintain soil productivity and to supply plant nutrients, and to control insects, weeds and other pests (USDA, 1980).*

The above definition of organic farming seems to be more appropriate as it considers the important aspects like sustainability of natural resources and environment. Organic farming is a production system which favours maximum use of organic material (crop residues, animal excreta, legumes, on and off farm organic wastes, growth regulators, bio–pesticides etc.) and discourages use of synthetically produced agro–inputs, for maintaining soil productivity and fertility and pest management under conditions of sustainable natural resources and healthy environment.

ECOLOGICAL AGRICULTURE

The growing concern about environmental degradation, dwindling natural resources and urgency to meet the food needs of the increasing population are compelling farm scientists and policy makers to seriously examine alternatives to chemical agriculture. A sustainable agriculture backed–up by *green technologies* in an integrated farming system has been considered a promising and potential pathway. The twin problems confronting agricultural production are all pervasive erosion of natural resources such as land, water and biodiversity, fast declining soil fertility and use efficiency of inputs such as water, fertilizer and energy. Demographic pressures accelerate the first and agronomic deficiencies the second.

The gravity of the environmental degradation, arising from faulty practices, has set several experts in the field to focus attention on ecologically sound, viable and sustainable farming systems. Though there has been a series of scientific and policy conferences on this issue, the sustainable farming methods are yet to get the approval of most agricultural scientists.

There are no serious attempts to develop a package of practices for large–scale adoption of sustainable agriculture in India. Only a few enterprising farmers and private institutions stand testimony to the utility of safe and highly productive natural farming methods.

The adverse effect of pesticides on the environment has been well documented, and their residues in the food chain have endangered the whole life sustaining systems in many regions. Chemical fertilizers have also jeopardized the environment through nitrate poisoning and exterminating the beneficial soil microflora and micro–fauna by adversely altering the chemical and physical structures of the soil.

ECOLOGICAL FARMING SYSTEMS

The shift from chemical to ecological agriculture should, however, be gradual. A sudden switchover can spell disaster and discourage farmers from taking to this course. At least two to three seasons will be needed for the transition, and during the interim years the farmers could build up a sufficient organic base to fertilize the fields and improve the productivity of the soil. Once a state of ecological balance is attained and there are a good number of beneficial organisms to check the explosion of pests and pathogens, crop yields of a high order can be ensured. The cost of cultivation can be brought down substantially as many farm–grown inputs can be integrated efficiently in the farming system.

Ecological farming can be sustainable and profitable too. It is a self–reliant method and has to be an integrated system. Since it is a knowledge–intensive practice, one has to keep pace with the dynamics of nature to increase the biological productivity of the soil.

Since eco–farming uses several farm grown inputs, and less dependent on market purchased inputs, it is economically attractive to the growers. Case studies show that when a chemical far incurred about Rs. 11,250 towards the cost of cultivation per hectare of rice, an organic farm spent Rs. 10,590. Alternatively, if the biofertilizers and organic nutrient supplements such as neem cake are subsidized to extent the same monetary advantage as chemical fertilizers, the cost of ecological farming will come down significantly.

It has been observed that in chemical farming, fertilizers and plant protection chemicals accounted for nearly 30 per cent of the total cost. The cost of market purchased inputs in ecological farming was far less, and bulk of it went towards the purchase of neem cake.

In both the cases, the yield remained almost the same at 5,625 kg paddy per hectare. The straw yield was eight tonnes. The net returns from the ecological farming system at the current cost of Rs. 3. 34 per kg paddy is Rs. 8,197. 50. The chemical farming, the net profit is Rs. 7,500. If one gets a premium price for the poison–free, organically grown rice, the economic returns from the ecological returns from the ecological farming system will be highly encouraging. While the modern system of farming expended nearly 31,000 MJ of energy, the ecological farming method accounted for only 23,400 MJ. High energy inputs such as fertilizer, plant protection chemicals, herbicides and high speed diesel are substituted with biological inputs and low–energy human and cattle power. The output/input ratio in the case of modern farming is 3. 76, while in the case of ecological farming it is more than 4. 95.

Objectives of Ecological Farming

Bringing to match the crop, soil and climate of a region the ecology and farming and gaining from the economy and efficiency of inputs are the objectives of eco–farming. According to Sankaram (1996), this technology may be grouped into four categories.

1. Those that reduce the environmental burden of green house gases (CO_2 and CH_4), global warming, ozone depletion. All attention to promote renewable sources of energy (draught animal power), electrical energy from garbage disposal and biogas from organic wastes.
2. Those that reduce the demand on land, water and biodiversity without adverse effect on agricultural production and nutritive value of food. Nurse the soil back to health, change cropping patterns to maximize ecological productive efficiency, improve, water use efficiency–through conjunctive use of rain, tank, underground, well and river waters; reduce conveyance losses; phase out subsidies.
3. Those that continue to improve crop productivity, under shrinking land resources. (genetic and agronomic) hybrid vigour, gene pyramiding; multiple cropping patterns, integrated nutrient management and integrated pest management.
4. Reduce hunger and poverty, adopt, cost effective farming to bring equity of food price and wage, encourage job promoted growth right in the village to arrest migration as ecological refugees.

For each specific location, eco–farming involves the search for the optimum rather than the maximum in cohesiveness and functional diversity. The fairly general nature of these properties, makes it clear that the designation *ecological* cannot be applied in an absolute sense nor can it be expressed in quantitative terms. It relates, rather, to a development process in which changes in the ecosystem must be continuously assessed to determine whether or not specific measures are of value. This means that farming techniques are not good or bad per se; their value depends on their applicability within a particular system; e.g. whereas minimum tillage may be recommendable in one case, ploughing may be necessary in another. There are scarcely any objective and generally valid criteria for assessing the extent to which a technique is environmentally appropriate for a given farm situation.

Prospects

In contrast, eco–farming systems and techniques have been developed on the basis of a holistic view of man within the biosphere and the awareness of man's dependence on scarce natural resources. In some cases, recognition may have been reached that the use of certain external production inputs is undesirable from the ecological point of view or is, under certain circumstances, even unprofitable. In other cases, as in some developing countries, the inputs may not be available on account of supply constraints where this level of consciousness of these economic conditions prevail. Intensification of farming is sought through more productive use of available resources such as soil nutrients, rain water and local energy, together with the knowledge, labour and initiative of the people.

The term *eco–farming* implies that farming regions and individual farms must be treated as ecological systems. Ecology is a science, which deals with the relationships between organisms and their environment. But in this context the environment is not confined to the natural conditions (e.g. soil, climate); it encompasses the entire complex of physical, economic, social and cultural conditions which affect the growth and development of an organism or organic system.

Eco–farming can be sub–stainable and profitable too. It is a self–reliant method and has to be an integrated system. Since it is a knowledge–intensive practice, one has to keep pace with the dynamics of nature to increase the biological productivity of the soil.

Since eco–farming uses several farm grown inputs, and is less dependent on market purchased inputs, it is economically attractive to the growers. When a chemical farm incurred about Rs. 11,250 towards the cost of cultivation per hectare of rice, an organic farm spent Rs. 10,590. Alternatively, if the biofertilizers and organic nutrient supplements such as *neem* cake are subsidized to extent the same monetary advantage as chemical fertilizers, the cost of ecological farming will come down significantly. It has been observed that in chemical farming, fertilizers and plant protection chemicals accounted for nearly 30 per cent of the total cost. The cost of market purchased inputs in ecological farming was far less.

In both the cases, the yield remained almost the same at 5,625 kg paddy per hectare. The straw yield was eight tonnes. The net returns from the ecological farming system at the current cost of Rs. 3.34 per kg paddy is Rs. 8,197.50. In chemical farming, the net profit is Rs. 7,500. If one gets a premium price for the poison–free, organically grown rice, the economic returns from the ecological returns from the ecological farming system will be highly encouraging.

While the modern system of farming expended nearly 31,000 MJ of energy, the ecological farming method accounted for only 23,400 MJ. High energy inputs such as fertilizer, plant protection chemicals, herbicides and high speed diesel are substituted with biological inputs and low–energy human and cattle power. The output/input ratio in the case of modern farming is 3.76, while in the case of ecological farming it is more than 4.95.

Ecological farming is more labour intensive, and several of its components such as vermicompositing, vermiwash, and generation of botanical pesticides and rearing beneficial insects such as *Trichogramma* parasites, ladybird beetles, and spiders for release in the field as bio–control agents offer scope for unemployed and landless youth.

Group and community endeavour holds the key for successful implementation of ecological farming over larger areas. Community participation in pest control and rodent eradication will be rewarding. Even in the case of developing biofertilizers, such as blue green algae and *Azolla*, group action will pay rich dividends.

> *Instead of giving the labeled* ecological *or* unecological approach*, it would be more correct to refer to the degree of appropriateness of a farming techniques for a specific site and time.*

Integrated Intensive Farming System (IIFS)

The Integrated Intensive Farming Systems (IIFS) methodology provides the pathway to achieving an evergreen revolution in agriculture. According to Prof. M. S. Swaminathan, Chairman, M. S. Swaminathan Research Foundation (MSSRF), Madras, the IFS involves agricultural intensification, diversification and value–addition. It helps improve physical and economic access to food, there by fostering sustainable food security at the level of each individual in a house hold. Emphasis on food security at the individual level is important in view of the growing feminisation of poverty, according to him.

As the name indicates, IIFS involves intensive use of farm resources. To be ecologically sustainable, such intensification should be based on techniques which are knowledge–intensive rather than capital–intensive, and which replace, to the extent possible, market–purchased chemical inputs with farm–grown biological inputs.

Such a shift in the nature of inputs used is brought about through integrated farming involving animal husbandry, fishery and agroforestry. Such integrated farming practices which constitute the second element of the IIFS strategy provide scope for organic recycling. The third element of the strategy is value–addition to every part of the plant and animal biomass through the establishment of bio–refineries. On–farm and off–farm employment can then be linked in a symbiotic manner. In the case of farm–women, who are invariably over worked because of their multiple roles in a household, IIFS aims to reduce the number of hours of work and add economic value to each hour of their work, according to Dr. Swaminathan.

With an ever–expanding urban population, the demand for a side range of processed and pre–cooked foods will expand, as urbanisation leads to diversification of foods habits. The IIFS with its emphasis on crop–live–stock–fish integration responds to this challenge. Also, the emphasis placed on post–harvest technology in IIFS helps both producers and consumers. To sum up, IIFS involves a pro–nature, pro–employment, pro–women and pro–poor orientation to technology and dissemination. It leads to labour diversification and not displacement. It leads to resource–based, in contrast to the widely prevalent commodity–based, agricultural development planning, according to him.

Dr. Swaminathan has prescribed *seven pillars of IFFS* for successful implementation of such systems. Soil health care is fundamental to sustainable intensification. In addition, vermiculture constitutes an essential component of IIFS. IFFS farmers should maintain a *soul health card* to monitor the impact of farming systems on the physical, chemical and microbiological components of the soil.

Water harvesting and management is the next crucial component. Crop and pest management including integrated nutrient supply (INS) and integrated pest management (IPM) systems form important components as well. Energy management and post–harvest component, choice of crops, other components of farming system and information technology are also important. These will help to ensure economic viability, environmental sustainability, social and gender equity in IIFS villages.

It should be emphasized that IIFS will succeed only it is a human–centered rather than a mere technology–drive programmer. It essence is the symbiotic partnership between farming families and their natural resource endoments of land, water forests, flora, fauna and sunlight. Without appropriate public policy support in areas such as, land reform, security of tenure, rural infrastructure. Input and output pricing and marketing small farming will find it difficult to adopt IIFS according to him. The eco–technologies and public policy measures needed to make IIFS a mass movement should receive concurrent attention. The programme will fail if it is based solely on a technological quick–fix approach.

On the other hand, it can trigger an evergreen revolution, if mutually reinforcing packages of technology, training. techo–infrastructure and trade are introduced, according to Dr. Swaminathan.

Ecological agriculture that effectively combines use efficiency of Input and economic yield maximization will begin to prevent the abuse of natural resources. On its progress depends the achievement of food security and sustainability of farming systems. Ecological agriculture will reactivate the fatigued green revolution to move forward through promotion of soil health, package of agronomic practices with each component a blend of tradition and modernity, and a policy to value each input based on its intrinsic worth free from subsidies.

There is the need to recapture local knowledge about framing systems. A synthesis of traditional wisdom and ecological prudence of topical agriculture with modern advances in technology will help higher use efficiency of inputs and sustainable crop yield maximization.

This symbolic of low input sustainable agriculture of (LISA) and sustainable agricultural research and education programme (SAREP) widely promoted in the U. S.

Low External Input Supply Agriculture (LEISA)

Low–Input Agriculture

The term low–input agriculture has been defined as a production activity that uses synthetic fertilizers or pesticides below rates commonly recommended by the Extension Service. It does not mean elimination of these materials. Yields are maintained through greater emphasis on cultural practices, IPM, and utilization of on–farm resources and management.

The LEISA concept seeks to optimize the use of locally available resources by maximizing the complementary and synergistic effects of different components of the farming systems. External inputs are used in a complementary way.

Although, the term *low–input farming* has often been used to describe any system of alternative agriculture, if can be seen that it is distinctly different from organic farming etc. Nevertheless, any system that reduces purchased chemical inputs can be called low–input farming, some examples are:

1. Poultry litter can replace nitrogen fertilizers in the production of watermelons.
2. Legume cover crops can supply the total nitrogen requirements of pecan trees.
3. Compost amended potting mixes produce superior vegetable transplants than traditional soilless mixes.
4. No–till vegetable systems are feasible using reduced herbicide rates to kill cover crops.
5. Subterranean clover living mulches supply nitrogen and weed control in peach orchards.

Integrated pest management is probably the oldest and most widely recognized Extension Service program devoted to low–input agriculture. However, only recently have the *non–chemical* approaches–such as cultural, mechanical, and biological–within the IPM framework been emphasized over the chemical component. Some programs, in fact, are now termed *biologically–intensive IPM.*

The intentions of the LEISA concept are obvious, but in practice the way it differs from integrated agriculture (understood to be a gradual minimization of external inputs) is not too clear. Defining what constitutes *low* inputs will always be difficult, therefore, LEISA remains an ambiguous concept.

Important characteristics of LEISA systems are that thy are based on a preventive approach whereby the problem is tackled at its roots, as opposed to the more symptom–curing nature of *modern agriculture.* Ecological and biological principles are the basis of the farm system. Nature works for the farmer, the farmer does not have to work against it. They are often based on local knowledge and production systems adapted to modern requirements and much less on external expertise. They are generally more labor–intensive compared to the mechanization–and petrochemical–intensive character of the agriculture envisioned by the Green Revolution and what it has become.

Criteria for LEISA

Ecological criteria

1. Balanced use of nutrients and organic matter
2. Efficient use of water resources
3. Diversity of genetic resources
4. Efficient of genetic resources
5. Efficient use of energy sources
6. Minimal negative environmental effects
7. Minimal use of external inputs

Economic criteria

1. Sustained farmer livelihood systems

2. Competitiveness
3. Efficient use of production factors
4. Low relative value of external inputs

Social criteria

1. Wide–spread and equitable adoption potential, especially among small farmers
2. Reduced dependency on external institutions
3. Enhanced food security at the family and national level
4. Respecting and building on indigenous knowledge, beliefs and value systems
5. Contribution to employment generation

BIODYNAMIC AGRICULTURE

Biodynamic farming means biological dynamics. It is a method of organic agriculture, which considers farm as a living system and where one activity affects the other

Biodynamic farming evolved in Europe in the 1920s following lectures on agriculture by the Austrian anthroposophist Rudolf Steiner. Biodynamic farming parallels organic farming in many ways but places greater emphasis on the integration of animals to create a closed nutrient cycle, effect of crop planting dates in relation to the calendar, and awareness of spiritual forces in nature. A unique feature of this system is the use of eight specific preparation derived from cow manure, silica, and herbal extracts to treat compost piles, soils, and crops.

Demeter (tm) is a certification program for and feed produced by strictly biodynamic farming methods. The Community Supported Agriculture (CSA) marketing programs, gathering popularity as an innovative method of subscription farming, were largely introduced into the U.S. by the biodynamic movement. An article on soil quality and financial performance of biodynamic and conventional farms in New Zealand in the April 16, 1993 issue of Science. In a comparison of 16 adjacent farms, the biodynamic farms exhibited superior soil physical, biological and chemical properties and were just as financially viable as their counterparts.

Organic Farming v/s. Biodynamic Farming

The biodynamic farming is more than just another organic method. It stands for a truly scientific way of producing humus. It does not involve in the application of organic matter in a more or less decomposed form but the use of completely digested from of crude organic matter known as stabilized and stable humus. In this aim, the method differs from organic farming. IN the case of biodynamic farming the organic material to be used as basis for compost is transformed either by means of the biodynamic compost preparations or by means of the biodynamic compost starter.

Principles of Biodynamic Farming

1. Biodynamic farming aims to restore humus status of the soil ecosystem to hold its fertility and productivity.
2. Also it helps to restore the soil for a balanced funtioning of flora and fauna. Because soil is a living system wherein the microbes can be fully established and maintained.
3. The biodynamic farming does not deny the role and importance of mineral nutrients of the soil like nitrogen, phosphate, potash, calcium, magnesium etc., and it considers the skilful use of organic matter as the factor for soil life.

4. It involves skilful application of all the factors contributing to soil life and health. Because a plant grows under the influence of abiotic factors like temperature, oxygen, CO_2 light, water etc. And these energies are transformed in the plant system into chemically active energies by way of photosynthesis.
5. Biodynamic farming considers a plant as living entity whih consists not only of mineral elements (like N, P, K, Ca, Mg, Mn, Cl, Fe, etc.,) but also of organic matter such as protein, carbohydrates, cellulose, starch.
6. Biodynamic farming gives importance to enzymes and growth substances.
7. To restore the soil fertility, biodynamic farming gives priority to proper crop rotation Soil exhausiting crops should be cultivated alternatively with fertility restoring crops.
8. It also provides recognition to green manuring and cover cropping.
9. To restore the soil environmental conditions, forests, wind protection and water regulation are important.
10. Biodynamic farming also gives importance to maintain the soil structure (physical characters like bulk density, pore space, water holding capacity and texture).

Rules for using Biodynamic Agriculture

1. Use of biodynamic sprays to stimulate and retain soil fertility
2. Following crop rotation to combat pests and disease and to increase the beneficial micro flora
3. Recycling on farm wastes
4. Following prevention strategies against pest and disease by strengthening plant and animals in the farm.

The produce of this farming is guaranteed by presence of international certification trademark Demeter™ this assures for a buyer that produce is biodynamically grown. The Demeter™ appeared first in Germany around 1928. It is certification trademark of biodynamic farming.

ORGANIC AGRICULTURE SYSTEM

Practicing organic agriculture is managing the agro–ecosystem as an autonomous system, based on the primary production capacity of the soil under the local conditions.

Although there are some differences between these approaches, the common understanding is that practicing organic agriculture is managing the agro–ecosystem as an autonomous system, based on the primary production capacity of the soil under local climatic conditions. Agro–ecosystem management implies treating the system, on any scale, as a living organism supporting its own vital potential for biomass and animal production, along with biological mechanisms for mineral balancing, soil improvement, and pest control. Instead of the tendency towards mechanical thinking characteristic of industrial agriculture, agro–ecosystem management requires a nursing, cultivating attitude, a professional feeling for the organism Farmers, their families, and rural communities, are an integral part of this agro–ecosystem. Both sexes are involved on equal terms.

We thought it an advantage to present a drastic alternative to modern high–tech farming, one totally without synthetic chemicals and fertilizers (nitrogen!!). In this way the reader must think in a different way, and not just adapt to a trend of *using a little bit less*, which is what many so–called sustainable agriculture systems are based on. We advocate the development of consistent sustainable agriculture systems by starting from perhaps a drastic alternative, determine its impossibilities, and develop feasible systems from there.

A hypothetical *High External Input Farmer* (HEIF), who wants (has) to become more *environmentally friendly* will reduce inputs. This is what many would call *integrated agriculture*. There are different grades, usually starting with *Integrated Pest Management* (IPM), adding *Integrated Nutrient Management* (INM), and making a real change when the farm becomes an *Integrated Farm System* (IFS). Continuing the quest to become more environmentally friendly and more sustainable, the farmer will move forward to LEISA when optimizing the IFS. The farmer will end up with an Organic Agriculture System.

The Major Aims of Organic Farming

Many outsiders perceive organic agriculture as a craze, not a method, in which all agrochemicals are dogmatically banned because of private and environmental health concerns. Others believe that yields are much lower in organic agriculture, or that the cost of labor is much higher. In short, it is not an option to solve the world's agricultural problems.

In reality, organic agriculture is a consistent systems approach based on the perception that tomorrow's ecology is more important then today's economy. Its aim is to stop degradation and reestablish natural balances. The economy must readjust to the primary production factors, and not the other way around. Without ecology, there is no economy. If conventional agriculture had been made to pay for the degradation and environmental damage it is causing, the move towards organic farming system would have been made long ago.

Besides this other possible aims of organic agriculture are:

1. To work as much as possible within a closed system and draw upon local resources
2. To maintain the long term fertility of the soil
3. To avoid all forms of pollution caused by agricultural techniques
4. To provide a foodstuff of high nutritional quality in sufficient quantity
5. To reduce the use of fossil energy in agricultural practices to the minimum tending of zero
6. To give to all livestock the conditions of life that conform to their physiological needs
7. To make it possible for agricultural families to earn a living through their work and develop their potentialities as human beings
8. To maintain the rural environment and also preserve non agricultural ecological habitats

Organic agriculture recognizes that *everything effect everything else*, and that one component cannot be taken out of the system, without positively or negatively affecting other things.

Concept of Organic Farming

Organic refers to the agricultural systems used to produce food and fiber. Organic farming systems do not use toxic chemical pesticides or fertilizers. Instead, they are based on the development of biological diversity and the maintenance and replenishment of soil fertility. Organic foods are minimally processed to maintain the integrity of the food without artificial ingredients, preservatives, or irradiation. Organic farming describes two major aspects of alternative agriculture:

1. The substitution of manures and other organic matter for inorganic fertilizers.
2. The use of biological pest control instead of chemical pest control.
3. Approaching organic agriculture from the vantage point of a scientist trained in conventional farming techniques, Harwood (1984) outlines the following assumptions:
4. Organic agriculture is a reversion to the agriculture of the 1940's.

5. Organic agriculture is merely conventional agriculture without the use of chemicals. This assumption often leads to the use of a no–treatment check plot in a conventional experiment as an organic treatment.

6. Organic agriculture is relevant only to backyard gardens.

Organic agriculture is based on the assumption of a difference between chemicals produced by biological organisms and the same chemicals, which have been synthesized in an industrial process.

Difference Between Organic and Conventional Farming

Organic and conventional agriculture belonged to two different paradigms. The fundamental difference between the two competing agricultural paradigms as follows:

Conventional	**Organic**
Centralization	Decentralization
Dependence	Independence
Competition	Community
Domination of nature	Harmony with nature
Specialization	Diversity
Exploitation	Restraint

In contrast, several agro–ecologically based researchers stress more the fluid transition between conventional, integrated and organic farming, as an outcome of different assessments of economic, ecological and social goals. Consequently, technical strategies such as integrated pest management of balanced nutrient supply might improve conventional agriculture to such an extent that it may appear unnecessary to strictly ban pesticides and mineral fertilizers as required by organic standards.

However, there is scientific evidence that organic agriculture differs from conventional agriculture not only gradually but fundamentally. Implementing organic methods consequently seems to provide a new quality in how the agro–ecosystem works. This functioning cannot be explained by summing up single ecological measures. Organic farming seems to improve soil fertility in a way and to an extent, which cannot be achieved by conventional farming even if the later consistently respects some ecologically principles.

Organic agriculture is one of several to sustainable agriculture and many of the techniques used (e.g., inter–cropping, rotation of crops, double–digging, mulching, integration of crops and livestock) are practiced under various agricultural systems. What makes organic agriculture unique, as regulated under various laws and certification programmes, is that: (1) almost all synthetic inputs are prohibited. and (2) *soil building* crop rotations are mandated.

The basic rules of organic production are that natural inputs are approved and synthetic inputs are prohibited, but there are exceptions in both cases. Certain natural inputs determined by the various certification programmes to be harmful to human health or the environment are prohibited (e.g. arsenic). As well, certain synthetic inputs determined to be essential and consistent with organic farming philosophy, are allowed (e.g. insect pheromones). Lists of specific approved synthetic inputs and prohibited natural inputs are maintained by all certification programmes and such a list is under negotiation in Codex. Many certification programmes require additional environmental protection measures in adoption to these two requirements. While many farmers in the developing world do not use synthetic inputs, this alone is not sufficient to classify their operations as organic.

History of Organic Farming

Organic Agriculture Systems are not a repudiation of the assets of modern agricultural technology, neither are they defined by the simple elimination of synthetic fertilizers or pesticides. Methods in organic agriculture are less intensive in terms of synthetic and other external inputs compared with conventional farming methods, but are much more intensive from a biological point of view.

The term *organic farming* was first used by Lord Northbourne in the book, *Look to the Land* Lord Northbourne, who embraced the teachings of Rudolph Steiner and biodynamic farming, had a vision of the farm as a sustainable, ecologically stable, self–contained unit, biologically complete and balanced–a dynamic living organic whole. The term thus did not refer solely to the use of living materials (organic manures, etc) in agriculture although obviously it included them, but with its emphasis on *wholeness* is encompassed best by the definition' of, pertaining to, or characterized by systematic connection or coordination of part of the one whole.'

As defined by a USDA Study Team on Organic Farming, Organic farming is a production system which avoids or largely excludes the use of synthetically compounded fertilizers, pesticides, growth regulators, and livestock feed additives. To the maximum extent feasible, organic farming systems rely upon crop rotations, crop residues, animal manures, legumes, green manures, off–farm organic wastes, mechanical cultivation, mineral–bearing rocks, and aspects of biological pest control to maintain soil productivity and tilth, to supply plant nutrients, and to control insects, weeds and other pests.

> According to the produced Codex definition (FAO), *Organic agriculture is production management system which promotes and enhances agro–ecosystem health, including biodiversity, biological cycles, and soil biological activity. It emphasizes the use of management practices in preference to the use of off–farm inputs, taking into account that regional conditions require locally adapted systems. This is accomplished by using, where possible, agronomic, biological, and mechanical methods, as opposed to using synthetic materials, to fulfill any specific function within the system.*

Organic agriculture systems include approaches and methods like organic/UK), biodynamic/D Rusch–Muller/CH, Lemaire–Boucher/F, regenerative/USA, nature farming/JPN (Fukuoka 1985) and permaculture/AUS (Mollison 1990). These were all developed during this century, most of them the last 50 years.

In the Western world, organic agriculture is fairly well developed. There is a growing market for these products (including imports from developing countries) based on consumers' willingness to pay a substantial premium for reliably labeled, organically grown foods. Various types and methods of organic agriculture have been developed in the Northern Hemisphere, such as the biological–organic and biodynamic method

Needs of Organic Farming

Needs for Organic Inputs

Organic farming is the pathway that leads us to live in harmony with nature. Organic agriculture is the key to a sound development and a sustainable environment. It minimise environment environmental pollution and the use of non–renewable natural resources. It conserves soil fertility and soil erosion through implementation of appropriate conservation principles.

Several reasons have been emphasised for the need of organic agriculture, like limited land holdings, poor socio–economic conditions of farmers, rise in input cost etc. The broadest view shows two major reasons viz., population and environment, emphasised the ultimate need for eco–friendly technologies. FAO estimates that by the year 2000 the global population will be 25% higher than in the mid 1980s and that 90% of this population increase will be in the developing countries like India. It will be necessary to increase the supply of food and other agricultural products to meet their needs. At the moment, many of the methods being used to increase production are damaging to natural resources and the environment and farmers are supposed to invest heavily into inputs to improve yields and productivity. Further, the produce from organic farming has become inevitable. The food containing pesticides and other chemicals are increasingly made obvious by many research studies revealing the presence of pesticide residues in eatables. About one million people suffered from pesticides poisoning and 20,000 die every year due to the toxic effects of these chemicals worldwide but the crop loss due to pest is still 15,000 crores, apart from killing a portion of the human population by the same pesticide use. This perspective is also one of the needs for organic approach to farming. In order to avoid the deleterious effects of synthetic chemical fertilizers and pesticides, organic agriculture is needed as an alternative to provide ecologically safe methods of farming.

Although the concept of organic agriculture has received much elaboration at different levels, the description offered by has been found to be the most comprehensive covering all essential factors.

Organic agriculture is a production system, which avoids or largely excludes the use of inorganic fertilizers, pesticides, growth regulators and livestock feed–additives. To the maximum extent feasible, organic farming system rely on crop rotations, crop residues, animal manures, legumes, green manures, off farm organic wastes and aspects of biological pest control to maintain soil productivity and tilth, to supply plant nutrients and to control insects, weeds and other pests.

Sustainable agriculture, by definition, is that form of farming which produces sufficient food to meet the needs of present generation without eroding ecological assets and productivity of life supporting system of the future generation. The key characterization of organic farming in relation to sustainable soil fertility and organic farming include:

1. Protecting the long–term fertility of soil by maintaining organic matter levels, fostering soil biological activity and careful mechanical intervention.
2. Providing crop nutrients indirectly by using relatively insoluble nutrient sources which are made available to the plants by the action of soil microorganisms.
3. Nitrogen self–sufficiency through use of legumes and biological nitrogen fixation as well as effective recycling of organic materials, including crop residues and livestock wastes.
4. Weed, disease and pest control relying primarily on crop rotations, natural predators, diversity, organic maturing resistant varieties and limited thermal, biological and chemical intervention.
5. The extensive management of livestock, paying full regard to their evolutionary adaptations, behavioural needs and animal welfare issues with respect to nutrition, housing health, breeding and rearing.
6. Careful attention to the impact of farming system on the wider environment and the conservation of wild life and natural habitats.

Organic agriculture is viable alternative to conventional agriculture. It protects the soil from erosion, strengthens natural resources base and sustains biological production at levels commensurate with the carrying capacity of managed agroecosystem because of reduced dependence of fertilizers and plant protection chemicals; problems of environmental pollution are greatly reduced if not totally avoided. The practice leads to regeneration of ecosystem. There is now a demand worldwide for organically grown foods, which command a premium in export markets. The demand for such safe foods is increasing annually and this opportunity needs to be exploited.

Organic agriculture is often associated with low yields. The demands for products of organic agriculture are growing in India. The European Union (EU) and the International Federation of Organic Agriculture Movement (IFOAM) have defined rules for organic agriculture producers. India too needs to establish its own certification scheme to facilitate exports of organic agriculture products and an accreditation agency to certify the produce of the farm. The essential elements of an organic quality assurance scheme are as follows:

1. Development of standards
2. Inspection and verification
3. Certification
4. Accreditation

As low yields are expected, the market's ability to pay a price premium is a key determinant of sustainable growth of organic agriculture. The European Union is currently world's leading market for organic products with various countries within the EU having deficits of fresh organic products. The legislation on organic agriculture varies across countries. At present certification is compulsory for the organic foods exported from India. To encourage mass production and consumption of organic products, there should be clear–cut policies and incentives to promote organic agriculture and necessary infrastructure and market.

National level efforts are needed to facilitate the successful adoption of organic agricultural by the farmers. The approach shall be farmer centered and programmes developed shall create conditions for the conservation and efficient use of locally available resources as inputs in agriculture. Research has also to play to the extent of developing apropriate agro–techniques in conformity with the basic principles of organic agriculture.

In Partnership with Nature

In Organic Agriculture Systems, the interactions described here can be used to develop and manage a holistic farming system which is an autonomous organic agro–ecosystem based on a partnership with nature. Such a system is not static; it should be adapted continuously to changing conditions using practical experience and new knowledge. There is no quick and easy recipe. Redirecting agriculture away from the unsustainable situation of the present requires more than just another set of technologies. It requires an attitude, which emphasizes human and ecosystem capacities, and cultivates them in a structurally sustainable way.

Mobilizing indigenous knowledge and inspiring farmers to grow their crops autonomously in the local agroecosystem places the farmers in the center of farming activities. This is a prerequisite for human resource development of farmers.

The principles mentioned above provide a basis for the development of agricultural methods which fit well in the concept of SARD.

BASIC STANDARDS AND GENERAL PRINCIPLES FOR ORGANIC AGRICULTURE

Organic farming system is based on the dynamic interaction between the soil, the plants, animals, humans, the ecosystem and the environment. The system is directed towards enhancing natural life cycles rather than suppressing nature. It relies largely on locally available resources. Organic farmers have proven to the world that their farming system is distinguishable from other agricultural systems, and above all, is competitive and able to provide agricultural products of good quality while minimising negative side–effects.

Crop and Soil Management

Organic farming systems encourage the use of rotations and manures to maintain soil fertility. Carefully managed soils with a high proportion of humus offer essential advantages with respect to water retention, ion exchange, soil erosion, and animal life in the soil. A high proportion of humus in the soil gives uniform distribution of nutrients and also promotes plant hygiene.

Green manuring and intercropping of legumes is another important aspect for biological farming systems not only in regard to weed control, but also in reducing the leaching of nutrients and in reducing soil erosion. A green cover throughout most of the year is one of the main goals of such farming methods. Depending on the green manure mixture or the legumes used for undersowing, there may be an increase in soil organic matter and soil N as well as in other nutrients.

Choice of Crops and Varieties

1. All seeds and plant material should be certified organic.
2. Species and varieties cultivated should, as far as possible, be adapted to the soil and climatic conditions and be resistant to pests and diseases.
3. A moratorium on all transgenic food and agricultural applications should be imposed.
4. In the choice of varieties genetic diversity should be taken into consideration.

Crop Rotations

Rotations should be as varied as possible and aim to :

1. maintain soil fertility,
2. reduce nitrate leaching,
3. reduce weed, pest and disease problems.

It is recommended that specific rotations including legumes are insisted upon by the certification programmes.

Nutrient Management

Increasing prices of chemical fertilizers have enabled organic wastes to regain an important role in the fertilizer practices on the farm. Good manure management means improved fertilizer value of manure and slurry and less nutrient losses. Composting of all organic waste in general, and of farm yard manure or feedlot manure in particular, is important in organic farming with the following guidelines:

1. Sufficient quantities of organic material should be returned to the soil to increase or at least maintain its humus content on a long term basis.
2. Accumulation of heavy metals and other pollutants should be limited.
3. Organic material produced on organic farms should form the basis of the manurial programme.
4. Management and handling of manure and compost should minimise nutrient losses.
5. Soil pH–values, which are appropriate to the soil type and the crops cultivated, should be maintained.

Use of human faeces is restricted. Consideration should be paid to the absence of pollutants. Steps should be taken to prevent the transmission of pests, parasites and other infectious agents e. g. by high temperature compostsing.

Non synthetic mineral fertilizers and brought in fertilizers of biological origin should be regarded as supplementary and not a replacement for nutrient recycling.

Minimizing the downward movement of nutrients in the soil profile:

(i) The rotation with deep–rooted crops,

(ii) The avoidance of high–solubility nutrient sources,

(iii) The avoidance of mould board ploughing in favour of chisel ploughing,

(iv) The insertion of nutrients into the rotation onto a sod crop, if possible, to maximise uptake, and

(v) The seasonal use of cover crops in and around the major cash crops.

There are differences in nutrient profile with depth between organic and conventional systems, if the assumption is correct and if any of the above practices have a major effect in vertical nutrient movement.

Management of Pests, Diseases and Weeds

Organic farmers' primary strategy in controlling pests and diseases is the prevention. Organic farmers build healthy soils––fertilizing and building soil organic matter through the use of cover crops, compost, and biologically based soil amendments. This produces healthy plants, which are better able to resist disease and insect predation. Organic farmers also rely on a diverse population of soil organisms, insects, birds, and other organisms to keep pest problems in check. When pest populations get out of balance, growers will implement a variety of strategies such as the use of insect predators, mating disruption, traps, and barriers. As a last resort, botanical or other non–toxic pesticides may be applied under restricted conditions. Weeds are controlled through increased cultivation, as well as through cover crops, mulches, flame weeding, crop rotation and similar management methods.

1. Organic farming systems should be carried out in a way which ensures that losses from pests, diseases and weeds are minimised. Emphasis is placed on the use of varieties well–adapted to the environment, a balanced manurial programme, fertile soils of high biological activity, correct rotations, companion planting, green manures, etc.
2. The natural enemies of pests and diseases should be protected and, through proper habitat management, encouraged such as hedges, nesting sites, etc.
3. Weeds are controlled by a number of preventive cultural techniques limiting their development, e. g. suitable rotations, green manures, a balanced manurial programme, early seedbed preparations and predrilling, mulching and by mechanical control. Physical and thermic methods are permitted. Growth Regulations, etc.

Wild Products

The collection should positively contribute to the maintenance of natural areas.

Pollution Control

1. All relevant measures should be taken to minimize pesticide contamination, from outside and within the farm by wind drift, drainage and irrigation. This includes a clearly defined demarcation between conventionally and organically farmed fields.
2. In case of risk or reasonable suspicion of risk of pollution, the certification programme shall set limits for the maximum yearly addition of heavy metals and other pollutants.
3. Accumulation of heavy metals and other pollutants should be limited.

Soil and Water Conservation

The collection should positively contribute to the maintenance of natural areas.

Landscape

1. The certification programmes should, where necessary, set standards for a minimum percentage of the farm area to facilitate biodiversity. These areas should be managed properly and be linked.
2. Areas which might be included in this percentage are:
   - extensive grassland such as moorlands, reed land or dry land
   - in general all areas which are not under rotation and are not heavily manured:
   - extensive pastures, meadows, extensive grassland, extensive orchards, hedges, hedgerows, groups of trees and/or bushes and forest lines
   - ecologically rich fallow land arable land (with no inputs),
   - ecologically diversified (extensive) field margins,
   - waterways, pools, springs, ditches, wetlands, swamps and other water rich areas which are not used for intensive agriculture or aqua production
   - areas with ruderal flora.

PRINCIPLE REQUIREMENTS AND PRE–CONDITIONS

The Organic Agricultural Movement has adopted certain techniques that respect natural ecological balances to avoid products and methods, which are contrary to the principle aims.

The basis for crop production in gardening, farming and forestry is the consideration for the structure and fertility of the soil and surrounding ecosystem, as well providing a diversity of species. This is achieved by a combination of:

1. A versatile crop rotation
2. The recycling of organic material, and includes
3. A wide range of methods for the control of pests, diseases and weeds which avoiding the use of synthetic fertilizers, pesticides and herbicides.
4. The basis for animal husbandry is the respect for physiological and ethiological needs of the animals. This is achieved by a combination of:
5. Providing sufficient amounts of good quality organic fodder
6. Providing husbandry systems appropriate to behavioural needs
7. Proper veterinary treatment
8. Animals are an important part of organic farming system because:
9. They contribute to closing the nutrient cycles,
10. Animals convert organic matter and are thus major contributors to soil fertility
11. Some animal species can utilise agricultural areas which cannot otherwise be used
12. Growing forage crops improves the crop rotation, the diversification and balance of the farming system

13. They may be for draught purposes
14. They can utilise by–products from agricultural production
15. They contribute to higher yields

The basis for natural ecological balances in livestock production is a harmonious relationship between the crop production and animal husbandry. This is achieved by a combination of:

Establishing as much self self–sufficiency of manure and animal feed on the farm unit as possible through specifying maximum stocking rates.

Converting plant protein and energy into animal protein and energy brings about losses during the metabolic process. For this reason crop, production for human nutrition and that for animal nutrition should generally be balanced. The basis of processing organic products is that its vital qualities are maintained through out each step of the process. This is achieved by a combination of:

1. Choosing and developing methods, which are adequate to the specifics of the ingredients.
2. Developing standards, which emphasize careful processing methods, limited refining, energy saving technologies, minimal use of additives and processing aids etc.
3. The production and handling of organic products should seek to minimize the environmental degradation.

CONVERSION FROM CONVENTIONAL TO ORGANIC FARMING

The approach is to fit an organic system into any given local situation. It will thus be clear that organic farming systems cannot be introduced in one day. The period needed to develop an organic agriculture system is called the conversion period.

Conversion Requirements

1. When traditional agricultural methods fulfill the principles of these standards no conversion period is required. When claiming virgin land for organic agriculture, no conversion period is required.
2. The whole farm, including livestock, should be converted according to the standards over a period of time. This time is defined by the certification programme.
3. If a farm is not converted all at once, it should be done on a field by field basis, whereby the full standards are followed from the start of conversion on the relevant fields. The area of landing being managed to the full standards will therefore progressively increase.
4. The composition of a farm unit can vary widely according to geographical conditions, ownership structure, time span, etc.

Farms with Plant Production and Livestock

The entire operation should be seen as a whole. It is not recommended to separate the conversion of individual fields or individual livestock productions, unless this is on the basis of imposed public restrictions or can be justified according to local conditions.

Farming with plant production/livestock and using remote areas (outlaying fields, alpine pastures, etc). When organic farmland and remote areas are operated under the same management, the remote areas in general should be included in the conversion plan as well. Areas which:

1. Requires disproportionately long transportation of farmyard manure,

2. Have very different climatic conditions,
3. In any other way have difficult access in relation to the other operations,
4. May, with restrictions, be operated conventionally, provided that the associated prohibited aids are not kept within the operation area for which certification is applied.
5. Operation of individual, separate farms. If a farmer of farming community operates two or more farms within a local area, all the farms should be converted according to the organic standards.
6. The time taken for conversion of the whole farm should not exceed one complete rotation.

Farmers will probably experience some loss in yields when converting their operation to organic production. There is period of time between the discarding of synthetic inputs and sufficient biological insect populations, nitrogen fixation from legumes) during which pest suppression and fertility problems are typical. The degree of yield loss varies, however, and depends on factors such as the inherent biological attributes of the farm, farmer expertise, and the extent to which synthetic inputs were used under the previous management system. Where soil fertility is low and biological processes have been seriously disrupted, it may take years to restore the ecosystem to the point where organic production is possible. In such cases other sustainable approaches, which allow judicious use of synthetic chemicals, may be more suitable start–up solutions. One strategy to survive the difficult transition period involves converting farms to organic production in partial installments so that the entire operation is not at risk.This is the period in which organic methods are introduced and the organic system is developed. Techniques have to be learned and labor reorganized. Experience shows that such a period takes from three to five years, depending on the situation. Often, a conversion plan is made, but the conversion can be a difficult time for farmers. Banks often deny credit to farmers who convert to a system where they might have lower yields. It might take a few years before pest predators are at full strength again. Farmers have to learn to observe more than they used to. After conversion, the system should be flexible enough to adapt itself from within to any changes in circumstances. From this point of view, it should be an autonomous system.

Limitations

Although this concept fully fits in the goals and criteria of organic agriculture systems are not proposed as a miracle solution for all the problems. One should not set high hopes on a single concept, especially after experience with the Green Revolution and biotechnology, which were understood by many as miracle solutions.

These are assumptions throughout the organic literature of differences between organic and conventional systems with respect to their effects on soil physical properties, soil insect fauna, nutrient flow within the soil, crop health, and nutritional value of the harvested crop. One finds many principles commonly held by organic farmers such as feed the soil and not the crop, and the need to rotate with deep rooted crops to bring nutrients from deep in the soil profile. There are other perplexing observations such as the decline in yields during the process of conversion from conventional to organic practices. These assumptions, principles and observations cover virtually every aspect of crop and animal management in organic systems. Some are readily understandable, but many deal with physical and biological interactions which have not been researched and are little understood.

Initiating Organic Farming

Drylands are the potential place where organic farming can be started first because in drylands–

1. Less effect of high input agriculture thus least residue of pesticide and less time required for conversion

2. Organic manure improve the fertility and water retention capacity of poor soils of drylands
3. Economic conditions of dryland's farmers are also comparatively poor and they are not able to purchase high cost input on the other side they can do the labour intensive operations and both are requirements of organic farming.

Medicinal plants–the First Crops for Organic Farming

Organic farming in drylands can be started with medicinal plants because

1. The forest resource of medicinal plants is decreasing but demand is increasing thus cultivation is the only solution to fill this gap.
2. Medicinal plants are for the curing of disease and any residue of pesticide can convert it into poison. Hence medicinal plants should only be cultivated in organic farming
3. Use of high dose of inputs like fertilizers, irrigation etc may change the composition and quality of medicinal plants. Growing near to natural conditions is the best way to maintain the quality, which is possible in the organic farming.

CONCLUSION

The fast development of technology for increasing production without given due importance to the agro–ecosystem balance resulted in disturbed *natural cycles* of carbon, nutrient and food chain of flora and fauna. The results are visible in terms of decreasing yield and increasing unsustainability in agro–ecosystem. The need is to revive natural balance with sustainable farming concept. There are several approaches has been recommended by various scientist, farmers, and forums. Organic farming is one such approach which emphasis on maintaining the cycle of input–output with ecofriendly methods, is becoming widely recognised by researchers and farmers and gaining popularity in the international market.Organic farming has one distinguish feature of certification as compared to the other sustainable production systems .For certification certain rules and standards has to be followed Although it need both time and money but ultimately get due recognition by the *mother nature* and in the market.

IMPORTANT TIPS FOR CULTIVATION OF MEDICINAL PLANTS

India is endowed with a rich wealth of medicinal plants, which ranked our country in the list of top producers of herbal medicines. This is alarming that the total forest area is reducing which has reduced the total cultivation/collection of medicinal plants in India. If this kind of damage continues, we may lose the wealth of medicinal plants, which will affect the growth of our economy. Therefore, it is essential to cultivate at large scale and to conserve heritage of medicinal plants.

It was an old interest of the farmers to cultivate medicinal plant, and unlimited research efforts have been made to improve the varieties of medicinal plants, however, we are still at the developing stage with regard to cultivation of medicinal plants because there is no standard organization/agency for the certification of these plants in India. Therefore, in such situation it is essential to know the tips and follow them carefully for cultivation of medicinal plants:

1. Try to collect the available literature on medicinal plant which you can able to collect. Read it carefully for many times. The literature is available in the forms of books, magazines, research papers, films, etc. You may develop habit to participate in seminars/conferences or training programmes, etc.

2. Try to visit the farms of those farmers who are cultivating medicinal plants successfully and listen their experiences with special reference to their techniques for growing these plants, storage and packing practices, procedure of their sale, etc.
3. You have to evaluate your own capacity honestly in following ways:
   - You will cultivate the plants at your own.
   - The plants will be cultivated by others on your farm.
   - How much of land you owned?
   - How much time you will spare for cultivation?
   - The land value.
   - It is a ownership/rental land.
   - Type of land and soil quality.
   - Irrigation facilities and climatic condition of your land. Rain fall, wind velocity etc.
4. If you have selected say 'X' plant for cultivation, find out its sale potential and market position. You should know the names of buyer/company, exporters. The plant name should be discussed with these buyers very carefully. When you are satisfied with the capacity and requirements of the buyer along with his terms and condition, then and then proceed with the cultivation. You may know this potential by meeting with the person(s)/ through Internet etc. This is called market survey.
5. You should know that which part of the plant has demand in the market e.g., root, fruit, leaves, flower.
6. You should know various parameters of the standard as required by buyer. This needs market survey.
7. You should know the climatic, edaphic and other requirement of the plant, which you are proposed to cultivate.
8. After extensive survey of the plant, select only 4 or 5 plants for cultivation purpose.
9. Unfortunately, not much new varieties of medicinal plants have been developed, however, a few new varieties have been developed. Therefore, the grower should carefully purchase seeds/planting material from institution/farmer directly. Do not depend on agents etc.
10. Never use fertilizers for cultivation. As far as possible, use organic manure only.
11. Most of the medicinal plants are not infected with diseases, however. If they are infected, try to cure them using indegenous practices or biopesticides. Try to avoid use of chemical pesticides/herbicides.
12. The cultivation of medicinal plants may be a new field for you. Therefore, at initial stage, try to cultivate at small scale to know the characters/properties of the particular plant.
13. When you have started cultivation of medicinal plant, do not advertise much among your fellow–farmers. As and when you get success and launch commercial cultivation, let you propogate your success to others, if you are failed, you may be depressed.
14. After getting success in your venture, let other farmers should know your success and people will join you. This will result into reorganization of your village/place as a prime growing area of a particular medicinal plant.

15. Your success and cultivated area should come in record of local/State Government, specially for those plants which can not be exported.
16. After getting success, try to conduct experimentation on the cultivated plant, this will help you to improve/understand the nature, properties of the plant in detail.
17. For this purpose, it is necessary to read magazines, research papers or to contact research institutions. This will encourage you to develop proper skill for cultivation.
18. Cultivate those medicinal plants, which are banned from export point of view. This will pay you more.

The above guidelines help you to become a successful grower of medicinal plants.

MULTI TIER AGRICULTURE SYSTEM FOR CULTIVATION OF MEDICINAL PLANTS

Earlier, medicinal plants were obtained from the forests. At that time in the forests they were in abundance and the consumption was in milligrams or grams. But now, the situation has reversed due to deforestation, uprooting of the plants for fulfilling the requirements and the craze for herbal globalization. So all the medicinal plants, which require shade and base for climbing, have become endangered. Therefore, the rates have also increased and are unable to fulfill the requirement of the genuine material in the world.

At present time the cultivation of medicinal plants is the only way by which one can fulfill the world's requirement along with quality. Shade loving plants are now some where growing in the open field and the climbers are grown by giving artificial support. So, the rates are too high and quality is not good. Everyone is facing problems. The farmers are unable to cultivate medicinal plants in large scale due to too much expense. The pharmaceutical companies are unable to maintain the quality in their medicines due to variation in raw materials. Exporters and importers also face the same problem.

In this alarming situation MTAS is the only way, which can be helpful for farmers, pharmaceutical companies and the world to get/produce good quality of genuine material in abundance.

Benefits of Multi–Tier Agriculture System (MTAS)

1.	One time ploughing in a life.	Save–expenditure of round the year ploughing
2.	Needs very less water for irrigation.	Save–80% of the expenditure.
3.	One time in a life to purchase the seeds.	Save–expenditure to purchase hybrid seeds every year.
4.	No need of chemical fertilizer, pesticides and weedicides.	Save–100% saving

So, by this waorest area will increase and small–scale cultivator will also be benefited by this system. The produced will be 100% organic. In this time, organically cultivated produce has very good demand in international market so the rates are four times more.

Model of Multi–Tier Agriculture System (MTAS)

Selection of the base plant–For this purpose *Jatropha curcus* is the ideal plant to give shade to shade loving plants and provide a base for the climbers.

Income Generated from One Hectare Land by MTAS

SN	Crop's sowing season	Income per hectare				
1.	*Jatropha curcus* (July 2002)	Octoer–03 10,000	Octor–04 20,000	October–05 30,000	October–06 40,000	
		After that every year Rs. 40,000–50,000 income				
2.	Sonamukhi (*Cassia augustifolia*) (August–2002)	November–02 5,000	March–03 5,000	May–04 5,000	End of crop	
3.	Kounch *Mucuna prurita* July–2003)	December–03 Seed 40,000 Root 5,000	Dec.–04 Seed 40,000 Root 5,000	Dec.–05 Seed 40,000 Root 5,000	Dec.–06 Seed 40,000 Root 5,000	
4.	Kalihari *Gloriosa superba* (Jun–July)	October–2003 Seed 90,000	October–04 Seed 90,000	October–05 Seed 90,000	October–06 Seed 90,000	
5.	Karela *Momordica charantia* 2003–three time in a year			Every year 70,000–80,000		
6.	Pippali *Piper longum* (July–2003)	Nov.–03 60,000	Nov.–04 60,000	Nov.–05 60,000	Nov.–06 60,000	Nov.–07 60,000
7.	Sweth Musli *Chlorophytum boriviliamum* (June–2003)			9 months crop 4 lacs rupees every year per hectare		
8.	Ashwagandha *Withania somnifera* (August–2003)			6 months crop 25,000 per year per hectare		
9.	Sarpagandha *Rauwolfia serpentina* (July–2003)			18 months crop 2 lacs rupees every year		
10.	Haldi *Curcuma longa* (July–2003)			6 months crop 60,000 every year		
11.	Adrak *Zingiber officinales* (July–2003)			6 months crop 60,000 every year		

Note: Crop No. 7–11, total five crops cover 0.75 hectare are and remaining 0.25 hectare area covered by Jatropha.

Selection of climbers: Selection of the climber is done according to the climatic condition of the regions. Mainly, the following climbers are common for every/region:

- Kounch–*Mucuna prurita*
- Kalihari–*Gloriosa superba*
- Pippali–*Piper longum*
- Karela–*Momordica charantia*

Selection of shade Crops

- Sweth musli–*Chlorophytum boriviliamum*

- Sarpagandha–*Rauwolfia serprntina*
- Haridra–*Curcuma longa*
- Adrak–*Zingiber officinales*
- Ashwagandha–*Withania somnifera*

Irrigation

In first year, water should be supplied only to the rows of *Jatropha curcus.* In second year rain gun system is best for M.T.A.S. By this system we can save manpower, electricity and soil erosion. In this system, water will first fall on the leaves of Jatropha, then drop by drop it will fall in the soil. So 100% water will be absorbed by the soil.

Disease and protection

- The neem oil in March–April should paint every year main stem of Jatropha
- Spray the neem oil on the crop.
- Cow urine can also be sprayed.
- Make a paste of neem leaves, dhatura leaves and ark leaves, dissolve it in water and then spray.
- Guggul smoke also helps to protect the crop against viruses.
- Hang a bell in the field and ring the bell daily at the time of sun set. The sound waves from the bell will kill the viruses.

Benefits for farmers & the world

- Good quality and genuine material will always be available.
- From the farmers, pharmaceutical industries can buy–back, so they will get similar quality of raw material. No variation will come in medicine which comes due to crude material.

In this way we can solve this problem along with conservation of medicinal plants.

6 DISEASES OF MEDICINAL PLANTS

Along with the earliest records of cultivated plants there are references to diseases of plants, but for ages these maladies were ascribed to mysterious causes, such as *visitations, acts of God, works of the devil,* and so on. Plant diseases have been known to all since the times immemorial, but they have not been precisely defined by anyone. Literally the word disease means disease, which scientifically hardly carries any meaning. Disease is not the cause but is the result; and that it is not the condition. Disease in plants may be caused by living or non–living agencies like fungi, bacteria, viruses, algae, nematodes, phanerogamic parasites and unfavourable environmental factors. Infected plants do recover in some cases. Seedlings of many crops mildly suffering from damping–off or blights might recover with age, corn lines may quickly sensor newer roots to compensate for the roots rotted by fungi. In these cases, we can call the infected plants or plant parts diseased, till complete recovery takes place. The plant becomes diseased, however, if large number of spots develop on the leaves to affect its growth or reproduction. Whetzel (1929) coined the word suscept for a diseased plant. According to Stakman and Harrar (1957) *the plant disease is physiological disorder or structural abnormality that is harmful to the plant or to any of its parts or products or that reduces their economic value.*

CAUTION

Though we are presenting the various methods and use of fungicides for control of plant diseases, which are in use by various growers and scientists, however, authors are not recommending them. The authors believe in organic farming only and recommend that the cultivators should use organically produced fungicides.

WHAT IS A PLANT DISEASE?

Plant diseases in a general sense is used to indicate those disturbance of the structure and functions of the plant which threaten its existence as a useful or desirable object from the cultivator's point of view. Plant disease, a condition where the normal functions are disturbed and harmed; may be divided into infectious, i.e., caused by a pathogen, and non–infectious, caused by other factors. The former be called **diseases** and the latter **disorders**. A plant infected by a pathogen may not show any symptoms, i.e., it is not obviously diseased; but since such a plant may be a source of inoculum it is probably best described as diseased. The word disease is often incorrectly used i.e., as a synonym for a pathogen; disease means host + pathogen.

- **Host:** A cell or organism that acts as the habitat for the growth of another organism; the cell or organism upon or in which parasitic organisms live.

- **Pathogen:** An organism, often a microorganism, a virus or viroid, which causes disease. It can be applied to a species, race, strain, or isolate. A pathogen may be a virulent and a host may be tolerant of a pathogen.
- **Pathogenesis:** Pathogenesis is the sequence of processes from host and pathogen contact to the complete syndrome.
- **Pathogenic:** Pathogenic is having the characteristics of a pathogen.
- **Pathogenicity:** Pathogenicity having the characteristics to cause disease. Virulence should not be considered as synonymous with pathogenicity.
- **Symptom:** Symptom is a visible or otherwise detectable abnormality arising from a disease or a disorder; symptomatology, a displeasing word, is the study of symptoms. Symptom may be acute, chronic, local, masked, mild, primary, secondary, systemic etc.
- **Pathology:** Pathology is the study of the nature of disease through the study of its cause, processes, and effects, along with the associated alternations of structure and function.

Recently Dr. H. H. Whetzel of Cornell University defined plant disease as: *A plant disease is a continuous harmful process that is usually caused by a microorganism and is manifested by visible morphological changes called symptoms.* Whatever is happening to the plant is generally a step–by–step process or a series of process or a series of processes rather than a single isolated event.

A HEALTHY PLANT

1. A plant is healthy when it can carry out its basic physiological functions, including:
2. Normal cell division, differentiation, and developments;
3. Absorption of water and minerals from the soil and translocation of these nutrients throughout the plant;
4. Photosynthesis and translocation of the photosynthetic products to areas of utilization or storage;
5. Metabolism of synthesized compounds;
6. Reproduction; and
7. Storage of food supplies for overwintering or reproduction. Plants become diseased whenever any of these functions are significantly disrupted.

PLANT AND PATHOGEN RELATIONSHIPS

The plant pathogen like Bacteria, Fungi, Mycoplasmas, Nematodes, Rickettsia–like Bacteria, Spiroplasmas, Viruses and Viroids cause various types of diseases by establishing a close relationship with the host plant. Plant pathogens weaken or destroys cells and tissue, reducing or eliminating the ability to perform their normal physiological functions and resulting in disease symptoms and reduced plant growth or death. Pathogens may infect various plant parts like root, leaf, xylem vessels fruits, reproductive structure etc. The action of a pathogen on plant part(s) is presented in Fig. 4.1. They are as follows:

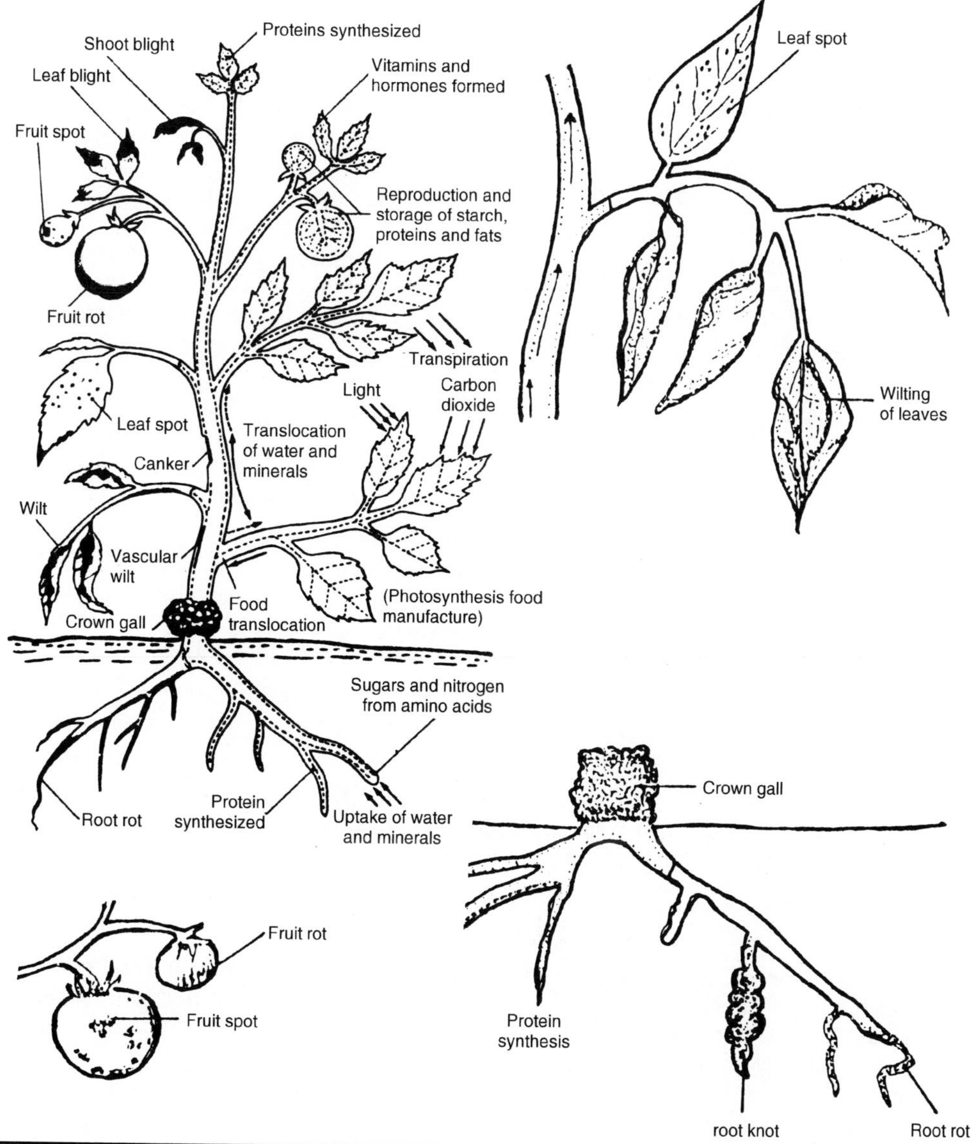

Fig. 6.1: Basic plant functions can be interfered with by common types of plant diseases.

1. When a pathogen infects the root, as occurs in root rot, it interferes with absorption of water and nutrients from the soil;
2. When a pathogen infects the xylem vessels, as occurs in vascular wilts and certain cankers, interferes with translocation of water and minerals to the crown of the plant;
3. When a pathogen infects the foilage, as occurs in leaf spots, blights, and mosaics, interferes with photosynthesis;

4. When a pathogen infects the cortex, as occurs in cortical canker and viral infections of phloem, interferes with the downward translocation of photosynthetic products;
5. When a pathogen infects reproductive structures, as occur in bacterial and fungal blights and microbial infections of flowers, interfere with reproduction; and when a pathogen infects fruit, as occur in fruit rots, interfere with reproduction and/or storage of reserve foods for the new plant.

Infected plants can develop a variety of morphological abnormalities. Pathogens that penetrate plants directly often elicit a morphological response from the plant that may result in the formation of abscission or gum layers. The cell walls of infected plant tissues are often modified, resulting in swelling or other distortions of the cell due to the production of enzymes by the pathogenic microorganisms that degrade cell–wall components and may disrupt cell permeability, leading to leakage and death of the plant cells.

STEPS IN DISEASE DEVELOPMENT

A disease generally can be considered to develop in a step–by–step progression. However, the progression may be modified depending upon the particular pathogen and circumstances of inoculum type, placement, dissemination, or other factors.

- **Inoculum is placed in position:** The microorganism is disseminated and somehow reaches the surface of a host plant. This occurs by wind, water, insects or some other means capable of transporting or disseminating a part of the pathogen. Often, usually in the case of fungi, the pathogen may grow a relatively short distance through the soil to the host.
- **Spore Germination:** This applies only to fungus spores and is somewhat analogous to seed germination in higher plants. Moisture is generally necessary for spores or other propagules to produce a germ tube or infective mycellium.
- **Ingress:** This is the entrance of the microorganism into the plant and can be accomplished in one of several ways such as the direct penetration through the plant epidermis by a germ tube or entrance through a natural opening or a wound.
- **Infection:** This is the establishment of the pathogen within the host and may not be accompanied by outward or visible symptoms.
- **Disease Induction:** This is the response on the part of invaded plant cells and is evident by visible disease symptoms. Each plant disease has its own symptoms that are unique to that particular host–pathogen relationship. However, a microorganism that can cause disease on a large number of plant species may cause similar symptoms on each species.

Proof of Pathogenicity

How is a particular microorganism proven to be the cause of a plant disease ? Robert Koch, a German, who investigated diseases in animals and people formulated a series of criteria or rules that should be observed in any attempt to prove that a particular organism is the cause of a certain disease. These rules, now commonly referred to as Koch's Postulates, are followed as closely as possible to prove any organism is the cause of a plant disease. The essential features of the rules of proof are as follows:

1. The suspected organism must be found in every observed case of the disease.
2. It must be isolated and grown in pure culture on various media so that its identity can be established.
3. Healthy plants must be inoculated from pure cultures.

4. Typical symptoms of the disease in question must develop in those inoculated plants.
5. The organism must be re isolated from the plant part showing typical symptoms and again grown in pure culture until it is proven to be the same as that originally isolated and used in the inoculations.
6. Nevertheless, Koch's Postulates are still followed as closely as possible in proving an agent is the cause of a disease.

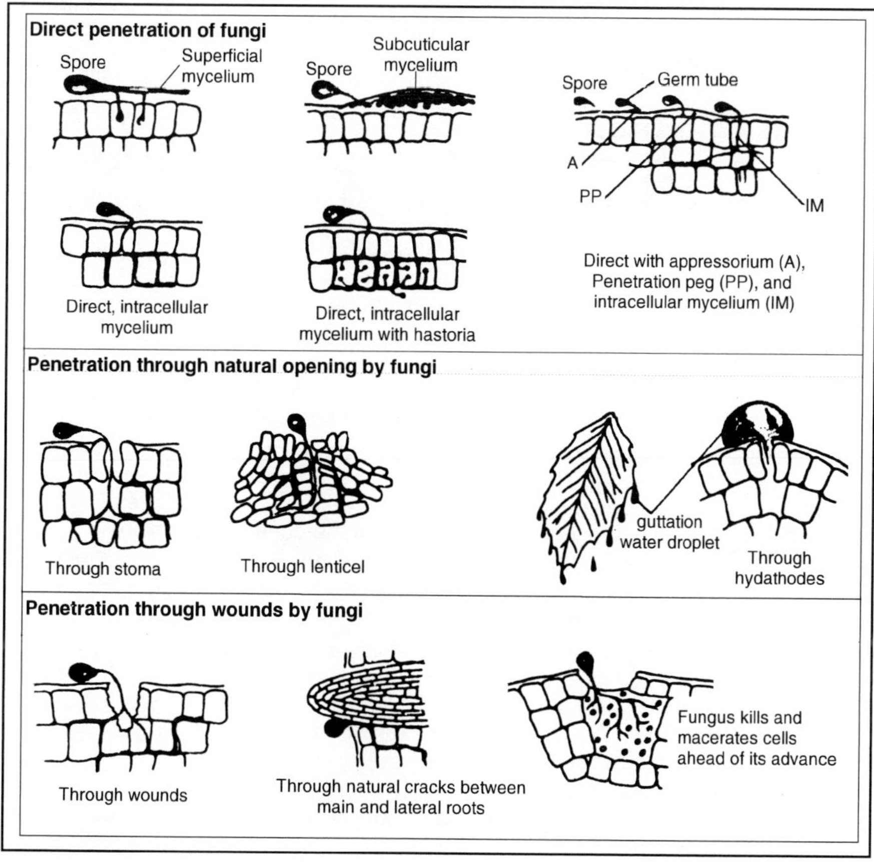

Fig. 6.2: Illustration of entry of plant pathogen in host.

NATURE AND CLASSIFICATION OF PLANT DISEASES

Disease is not a living organism, it, therefore, cannot grow or reproduce. Every disease is certainly due to a cause, which is never absent in case of any disease. The infectious plant diseases differ from the non–infectious ones in the sense that the former can be induced in a healthy plant by transferring the cause. Plant diseases manifest themselves in the form of symptoms. The expressions of diseases condition are known as symptoms which are more dependable in certain cases e.g., presence of mycelial mat or sclerotia or reproductive bodies of the microorganism in the infected region constitute signs, which have great diagnostic value. The typical symptoms observed in plant diseases are started below.

The different types of external and internal symptoms have been grouped into three categories, which are

Hyperplasia: It is the over–development of tissue due to stimulation of cells. The increase in size is due to abnormal enlargement of component cells, is called hypertrophy. The example of hyperplasia are crown gall of apple, club root of crucifers, white rust of crucifers, cedar rust and nematode galls on various crops, etc.

Necrosis: It is the decay or rotting of tissues due to derangement of cells. The death of cells, tissues or organs forms the different necrotic symptoms in different plant diseases. Following are the example of diseases of necrosis:

Types of Necrosis Occur in Plants

Rot	This type of necrosis is not localized and parenchyma, collenchyma and pith tissues all are infected. Depending upon the organ of plant attacked, colour and condition of tissues various types of rots have been described. On the basis of plant organ involved, the different rots have been called as root rots, foot rots, collar rots, neck rots, bud rots and fruit rots. On the basis of colour, white, red, black and brown rots have been recognized. On the basis of firmness of tissues, soft rots (tissues become soft), dry rots (tissues maintain firmness) and wet rots (tissue start decaying or putrefying) have been designated. While root rot and stem rot affect the plants after they are established, the soft rot affects fishy parts of the plants (mainly fruits and vegetables).
Cankers	It is the corky necrosis and results in the destruction of woody tissues and is deep seated. Cankerous growth occurs due to the hypertrophy of cambium tissues. Cankers are usually slow rots but can also spread rapidly. Cankers of mango, citrus and woody plants are the common examples.
Blights	These are characterized by very rapid and extensive necrosis of the whole plant or plant parts. On the basis of infected plant parts, names like leaf blight, twig blight, shoot blight, blossom blight and collar blight have described.
Spots	The necrosis may be local. Spots may develop on leaf, stem and fruit. The locally water–soaked or swollen (blotch) or chlorotic or killed tissues get coloured. In many diseases, the leaf spots are very characteristic. In some diseases, the infected tissues of the spot fall out leaving a hole behind, which is called the shot hole.
Damping–off	Seedlings of various crops suffer from this type of necrosis. Tissues in the basal portion of the stem or in the crown region are attacked. Infected tissues become too weak to support the stand to plants which ultimately topple down.
Wilts	In wilts, vascular tissues may be affected. Pathogenic wilts incited by fungi and bacteria are well. In cabbage yellows, the vascular tissues become from yellow to dark brown. In black rot of crucifers, the vascular tissues become black or brown, and do not turn yellow.
Scab	Necrosis is usually superficial and restricted mainly to the epidermal region. The scab may be induced by living or non–living agencies (mechanical injury).

Hypoplasia: It is the underdevelopment of tissues due to subnormal multiplication of cells. This causes reduction in size of the whole plant or plant parts or reduction in chlorophyll may occur. Hypoplasia can be expressed in the forms of stunting (stung of maize), smelling of leaves (little leaf of brinjal) or colour changes in leaves (yellowing or mosaics). These symptoms can be induced by living or non–living agencies. A condition in which plant parts remain arrested in their growth or entirely suppressed is called atrophy.

CLASSIFICATION OF PLANT DISEASES

Classification of plant diseases depends on the purpose. To designate the perpetuation, categories like soil–borne diseases and seed–borne diseases are commonly used. Plant diseases are often referred to by the type of symptoms like wilts, blights and rots etc. Some diseases occur only in the fields, while others occur in the storage or show up in the markets and accordingly they are called field diseases, storage diseases and market disease, respectively. Plant diseases are also grouped on the basis of host plants, e.g. diseases of pulse crops, diseases of forage crops, diseases of cereals etc. The two classification based on the casual agent and prevalence and periodicity are mentioned below:

Classification on the Basis of Main Casual Agent

A. **Diseases due to animate causes (living causes).**

1. Due to animals: Nematodes, Insects, Mites, Higher animals
2. Due to plants: Fungi, Slime moulds, Bacteria, Algae, Phanerogamic parasites

B. **Diseases due to inanimate (non–living) causes.**

1. Due to unfavourable soil conditions: (a) Physical composition–soil structure, soil moisture, soil aeration etc., (b) Chemical composition–excess of deficiency of elements. pH, presence of harmful salts etc.
2. Due to unfavourable climatic conditions: Temperature, Relative humidity, rains and snow, Wind and hail, Light and lightening
3. Diseases due to unfavourable practice. Chemical and mechanical injury.
4. Diseases due to fumes, gases and smoke.
5. Diseases due to plant metabolic products in transit and storage.

C. **Diseases due to viruses.**

Classification on the Basis of Prevalence and Periodicity

Sporadic diseases: Occurring at irregular locations and intervals, e.g., angular leaf sport of cucumber and blotch diseases of cucumber.

Endemic diseases: Occurring more or less constantly in moderate to severe form, e.g., onion smut and cabbage yellows.

Epiphytotic (epidemic) diseases: Occurring widely and periodically, e.g., cereal rusts and powdery mildew of grapes.

Pandemic diseases: Occurring throughout the continents or subcontinents and resulting in mass mortality, e.g., late blight of potato.

THE DISEASES OF MEDICINAL PLANTS

Belladonna

Belladonna (*Atropa belladonna* L. and *Atropa acuminata* Royle ex Lendle) is a perennial herb. The drug belladonna is obtained from the flowering tops and roots.

Leaf Spots

The leaves of Belladonna ate affected by leaf spot diseases, leaf necrosis. **Causal organism:** It is caused by fungous *Ascochyta atropae* Bres. Pycnidia found on the spots are globose to oval, immersed in necrotic tissue, light brown, ostiolate, without a beak. A leaf spot disease is also caused by *Cercospora atropae* Kuashmina. The conidiophores are produced on the spots in tufts. They are olive brown in colour. Conidia are clavate, cylindrical, broadly rounded at the base and tapered towards the apex. **Symptoms:** Consisted of greyish, white irregular spots with slight depression on the upper surface of the leaves. Later these spots coalesced and became necrotic resulting in defoliation and finally leading to the death of the plants. Pycnidia containing pycniospores have often been found on necrotic spots. The disease caused heavy loss to the yield and foliage production. The spots are mainly confined to the upper surface of the leaves. Severe infection resulted in drying and death of leaves. **Control:** Studies have shown that six sprays of Blitox–50 (Copper oxychloride) might be able to control the disease. The best control was reported by the application of Blitox–50 followed by Bavistin and Dithane Z–78.

Roots–Rots

Various fungi cause root–rot diseases of belladonna. Root–rot has been reported to be one of the serious diseases of this crop. The disease is found epiphytotic in commercial plantations in Jammu and Kashmir. The disease appeared in the beginning of summer when day temperature started increasing beyond 30°C and the disease remained prevalent upto the end of September. Nearly 16–20% plants were observed to be affected. Both youngnursery plants and older plants were affected. *Pythium.*

Roots–Rot Caused by *Phythium*: Causal organisms: *Phythium butleri* Subramaniam. **Symptoms:** The symptoms were sudden wilting of the aerial portions leading to drying and death of plants. The basal portion of the stem and roots showed browning and extensive disintegration of cortical tissues. **Control:** Drenching of seedlings in nursery with Dithane Z–78, Dexon or Benlate was found to control the disease. Fumigation of the soil with methyl bromide and treatment of seeds with Captan are also recommended for the control. Cultural practices such as avoiding excessive irrigation and crop rotation were useful to check the incidence of the disease.

Root–rot caused by *Fusarium:* It was observed as serious threat in the commercial plantations in Jammu and Kashmir. Nearly 40% of the plants were affected by the disease. **Causal organism:** *Fusarium solani* (Mart) Sacc. Optimum temperature for growth and conidia formation in culture is 28°C. **Symptoms:** The symptoms consisted of yellowing of the leaves followed by wilting dehydration and death of plants. Root stem region of infected plants showed extensive disintegration of cortical tissue. Mature and full grown plants before or after flowering were more susceptible for infection. **Control:** Treatment with Dithane Z–78 or Benlate has been reported to control the disease. Crop rotation is also recommended to be beneficial to check the disease.

Root–rot caused *Phytophthora nicotianae* Bide Haan ***nicotianae:*** It is reported from Kashmir valley. **Symptoms:** The visible symptoms appeared first on the aerial parts. Drooping of young leaves and branches, yellowing of older leaves and drying of whole apical portion of the plants or partial drying of leaves of some branches were typical symptoms of the diseases. The infection developed initially in the collar region and then on root and stem. The infected stems were yellowish brown in colour and root were dirty brown.

Root–rot caused *Phytophthora erythroseptica* Pethybr: It was reported to cause pink rot of belladonna in England. The disease was severe in Scotland during summer months. **Control:** Application of chloropicrin, Bordeaux mixture (2:2:50) or any offer copper fungicide were found effective to control the disease. Raising of the nursery on raised beds and avoidance of excess irrigation and crop rotation were found useful as preventive measures. Seed treatment with Captan or Agrosan GN was also found to be effective to minimize the disease incidence.

Collar Rot

Causal organism: *Rhizoctonia solani* Kuhn. **Symptoms:** The disease mainly affected the seedling. The infection normally starts at collar region as elongated water soaked lesions which girdle entire stem ultimately resulting in toppling of the plants. The decay of roots is followed by wilting and drooping of foliage. Severely infected plants invariably died.

Belladonna Mosaic

Smith (1943) described a new virus disease on *A. belladonna.* The virus is sap transmissible to tobacco and other solanaceous plants. The virus is inactivated at temperatures between 75–80°C. Sap extracted from infected plants remained active for 6–11 days. **Causal organism:** It is caused by Belladonna mosaic virus. **Symptoms:** Belladonna plants showing similar symptoms of belladonna mosaic virus has also been reported.

Belladonna Mottle

Belladonna mottle caused by a virus was first reported from Europe. **Causal organism:** Belladonna mottle virus (BML). Belladonna mottle virus is a RNA–containing virus. The virus is strongly immunogenic. The virus apparently has a structure similar to that of turnip yellow mosaic virus. **Symptoms:** The virus caused mild mottling and sometimes deformation in *A. belladonna.* The naturally infected plants were often found in the plant community. The infected plants showed severe mosaic, mottling and vein banding symptoms. The virus is readily transmitted by sap inoculation and by beetle and insect species. When tested by sap inoculation most of the solanaceous plants were infected systemically. Symptom expression in all hosts is variable.

Cinchona

Cinchona species are shrubs or trees upto 30 m tall.

Seedling Blight

Seedling blight of *Cinchona* caused by *Phytophthora* species have plagued growers in many parts of Asia and Africa. A similar disease was found economically important in establishing *Cinchona* plantations in South America. **Causal organism:** *Phytophthora palmivora* Butl. **Symptoms:** The disease was found to be destructive to the seedlings in the nursery. A discoloured area is evident in the collar region of the seedlings during the onset of the disease. The discolouration gradually extends until it reaches the cotyledons, which became flaccid and turned downwards. The leaves gradually became yellow, lost their turgidity and many fell down in extreme cases. Discoloured area soon showed rotting, which proceeded from the bark to the vascular region and the seedlings gradually drooped downwards and eventually died. Under moist conditions, copious mycelial growth was observed on the rotted tissue. **Control:** In Peru control was apparently obtained by eradicating wilted seedling from the beds. Regular application of copper fungicides along with good sticker could be able to control *Phytophthora.* Selection of resistant high alkaloid containing clones would be the most suitable method of control. Attempts have been made to control the disease by soil fumigation or soil sterilization. In Indonesia effective control was obtained by weekly application of fungicides. Application of chloropicrin or DD mixture at a rate of 336 kg/ha., or by injecting 2 ml of the chemical at 20 days intervals at 10–12 cm depth or sprinkling dilute formalin or (iv) drenching with carbamate fungicide. Spraying of the foliage and the base of the stem and drenching the soil with 10% Bordeaux mixture or any other copper fungicide is practiced for the control of the disease.

Die–back

Symptoms: Cinchona hybrids were found to be affected by tip blight disease or die–back. Causal organisms: *Phytophthora parasitica* Dast. The pathogen was isolated from leaf blade, petiole and stem material. **Control:** Destruction of dead plants and spraying of Bordeaux mixture have been found useful to control the disease.

Pink–disease

The disease was first reported from Darjeeling (McRae, 1930). The disease was found to be present for a long time in West India. **Causal organism:** *Corticium salmonicolor* Berk & Br (Syn: *Pellicularia salmonicolor* (Berk & Br) Dastur. **Symptoms:** The disease usually affected small twigs and branches. The leaves were found to lose their colour, gradually turned yellow. The branches also withered rapidly. The affected part is often covered with rose or white crust and somewhat cracked on the underside of the infected branches. The spread of the disease was influenced by moisture. **Control:** Only some cultural practices and prophylatic treatment might be useful for reducing the losses caused by the disease. Less favourable condition for the establishment of the disease can be created by providing less humid atmosphere. Free circulation of air, reduction of shade, thin planting and good drainage. Cutting of disease affected branches and their destruction by burning might also help to reduce disease incidence. Prophylatic spray of 1% Bordeaux mixture has been recommended for the pink disease of rubber.

Canker

Two distinct bark disease of Cinchona, called stripe canker and girdle canker have been reported to cause serious losses to plantings in Guatemala.

Stripe canker: It is found in the rootstock and scion of practically all clones **Causal organism:** *Phytophthora cinnamomi* Rands. **Symptoms:** Infection apparently originated in the roots and advanced upward through the union and into the stem of the tree. The disease is characterized by vertical, linear, slightly sunken stripes of dead and dying inner bark. The stripe varied in width and length and reached to the full length of the tree in later stages. There might be several infection courts in roots giving rise to several stripes on the stem.

Girdle canker: Girdle canker appeared to be localized just above the union in the scion of some selections and hybrids The girdle canker girdles the tree. **Causal organism:** *Phytophthora parasitica* Dastur. **Symptoms:** The bark of the scion above the graft union is killed and became sunken in a horizontal band. The sunken appearance is accentuated by inrolling of callus tissue above and below the dead area. The canker may spread upto the stem of the scion and no true infection was found to be below and graft union into the root stock. Leaves turned yellow and there was a gradual die–back of twigs and branches, culminating eventually in the death of entire tree. **Control:** Destruction of diseased plants and spraying the plants with fungicides as a prophylatic measure are the only control measures for both the canker diseases.

Damping–off

Damping–off of *Cinchona* seedlings and wilting of sprouts of vegetatively propagated nurseries have been reported from South India (Ramakrishnan, 1949). **Causal organism:** *Phythium vexans* de Bary. Hyphae without septa. **Symptoms:** Roots of infected seedlings or sprouts showed rotting and water soaked lesions appeared at the base below soil level. One to three year old plants were also affected. The infected plants showed reddening of leaves which drooped down and ultimately defoliated. Large number of roots of such plants were blackened and died. The cortex of the roots easily sloughed off. Hyphae were present in the cortex and sometimes in xylem vessels. **Control:** Some of the control measures used against diseases caused by *Pythium* species can be adopted. However, no specific control measure for this disease has been recommended.

Brown Root–rot

The extend of damage si not known although the disease is wide spread. **Causal organism:** *Fomes lamaoensis* (Murr) Sacc & Trott. **Control:** Removal of diseased bushes and old stumps would be useful to restrict the spread of the disease. Application of quick–lime near the decaying bushes or stumps are practiced to destroy all remnants of affected roots. This practice might minimize the chances of spread of the disease.

Minor Diseases

Damping–off: Damping–off of seedlings was commonly observed in over crowded nurseries particularly at the lower elevation. **Causal Organism:** The disease was caused by *Macrophomina phaseoli* (Mauld) Ashby (Winters, 1950). **Control:** Removal of affected plants and excess of shade, restricting watering and application of copper fungicide was recommended for control. Treating the seed–beds with chloropcrin before sowing and covering the soil with sphagenum moss is helpful in preventing the disease.

Root and Collar–rot: Seedling in the nursery were found to be affected by root–rot and collar–rot. Colar–rot was also observed in young trees. The disease was reported to be caused be *Sclerotium rolfsii* Sacc. Destruction of dead plants and earthing up the trees were found to help in reducing the spread of the disease.

Coleus

Coleus forskohlii (Wild) Birq. is an Indian medicinal plant. It is a perennial aromatic herb growing wild from Simla eastwards to Nepal, in the hills of Bihar, Gujarat and Peninsular India. The is cultivated in Maharashtra and Gujarat for edible roots which are often used as pickles.

Leaf Blight

Severe leaf infection of *C. forskohlii* cultivated in the experimental plantations has been reported during cool, cloudy and rainy weather. **Causal organism:** *Rhizoctonia solani* Kuhn. **Symptoms:** Symptoms consisted of water soaked leaf spots that increased rapidily in size and became light and then turned to brown in colour. The spots coalesced resulting in blight symptoms. Severe infection caused defoliation and death of the plants.

Root–knot

Coleus forskohlii is reported to be affected by root–gall or root–knot disease. Nematode infected plants though stunted appear as luxuriant as the normal plants. The disease was found to affect the plants in the third month after planting. **Causal organism:** *Meloidogyne incognita* (Kofoid & White) Chitwood. **Symptoms:** The symptoms consist of stunting, wilting of leaves and the basal part of the stem turned brownish–black. The diseased roots are totally damaged. The infection caused yellow patches in the plantations. **Control:** Attempts have been made to control the disease by biological control methods. However, crop rotation and use of suitable nematocides would be beneficial to minimize the loss of yield.

Datura

Datura species are annual bushy herbs. It is rarely cultivated on large scale. The only species which is still used in crude form is *D. stramonium* and is cultivated in Europe and South America. Major constituents of *Datura* are hyoscyamine and hyoscine.

Leaf Spot

The disease was found on leaves of *Datura stramonium, D. metel* and *D. innoxia.* A large number of plants growing in the experimental plantations were found to suffer by the disease. **Causal organism:** *Alternaria tenuissima* (Fr) Wiltshire. **Symptoms:** The infection caused severe defoliation causing considerable economic loss. Spots are characteristically dark–brown, round to oval or slightly irregular, coalescing and forming large necrotic area.

Leaf Blight

Datura innoxia growing in experimental and commercial plantations was found to suffer from a leaf blight disease. **Causal organism:** *Alternaria alternata* (Fr) Keissler. **Symptoms:** Early infection of the disease appeared as water soaked circular spots on the leaves. In later stages the spots coalesced, became dull yellow and turned light brown due to the death of infected tissue. Concentric rings appeared on the dead tissue of old spots. A single spot on a leaf caused curling of the entire leaf in advance stage of infection. Wilting of the entire branch occurred when two or three leaves of a branch were affected. **Control:** No control measure for the disease is reported. However, fungicidal spray using dithiocarbamates, such as Dithane Z–78 or Dithane M–45 would be useful to control the disease.

Leaf Blight and Fruit–rot

Datura metel and *D. stramonium* growing in the experimental plots were found affected by this disease. Leaf blight and pod blight were reported on *D. metel* from Israel (Halfon–Meiri, 1973). Similar disease was found on *D. stramonium* in Lucknow, India. **Causal organisms:** *Alternaria crassa* (Sacc) Rands. **Symptoms:** The infection was first observed on leaves as small necrotic spots. The infection was later spread to the fruits resulting in fruit blight and rot. The mycelium penetrated beneth the seed–coat in most infected seeds. **Control:** Excellent control of the fungus was achieved by disinfection with Thiram suspension. Seed treatment with organo–mercurial dust did not give efficient control of the fungus.

Root–rot

Causal organisms: *Sclerotium rolfsii* Sacc. and *Corticium solanii* (Perill & Delacr) Bourd & Glaz. **Symptoms:** Infected plants showed yellowing, gradual wilting resulting in the death of plants. Root and foot–rot diseases show almost similar symptoms was observed in the experimental plantations. The disease affected plants of all ages, more destructive on young plants. Seedlings showed damping–off and were killed within weeks. In matured plants older leaves showed yellowing. As the disease advanced, severe rotting occurred leading to death and disintegration of plants. **Control:** Usual control measures include disinfection of planting materials, adjustment of soil pH and fertilizer regime. Cultural methods, such as deep burial of infected crop residue and crop rotation are often beneficial. Use of soil fumigants suchas formalin, methylbromide are also beneficial. Pentachlobenzene is considered to be useful to control the fungus.

Distortion Mosaic

The virus caused severe systemic mosaic with puckering and leaf distortion in *Datura stramonium*. The disease was reported to be caused by a strain of cucumber mosaic virus This disease was also reported on *D. innoxia*. The main symptoms were yellowing of veins followed by slight inward rolling and distortion of leaves.

Virus Wilt

Early symptoms of the disease on *D. stramonium, D. innoxia* and *D. metel* were vein clearing followed by necrosis which spread over conducting elements of leaf stalk and stem, resulting in wilting of leaves and whole plants. The virus was transmitted non–persistently by *Myzus persicae*. The causeal virus is not yet identified.

Little leaf

The infected plants showed retarded growth. The leaves became smaller and pale in colour. Infected plants flowered rarely and leaves were small crowded at internodes and apex of the branches. The infection was observed on *D. metel*. The virus was graft transmissible to *D. innoxia* and *D. stramonium* apart from other plants.

Mosaic

A number of mosaic diseases have been reported on *Datura* species. **Symptoms: A**lternatively dark and light green patches, varying in size and shape on leaf lamina and growth was retarded. The symptoms were similar to Tobacco mosaic virus (TMV). Electron microscopic studies showed straight, rod–like particles similar to TMV. A virus disease producing symptoms of vein clearing, mosaic, leaf puckering, distortion and filiform leaves on *D. metel* growing in waste land was reported from Andhra Pradesh, India. A potyvirus was also isolated from *D. stramonium* in Yemen. A mosaic disease of *D. metel* causing stunted growth, reduction in leaf size and light and dark green areas on leaf blade with blighter like patches was reported from India. The mosaic infected plants showed retarded growth and produced lesser number of flowers and fruits compared to healthy plants.

Digitalis

Digitalis was used in folk medicine in England as early as tenth century. The plant is a native of British Island and Western Europe.

Anthracnose

This disease has been reported from USA, UK, Japan, Czechoslovakia and other European countries and Asia. Causal organism: *Colletotrichum fuscum* Laub. **Symptoms:** They are consisted of purplish–brown, circular or angular spots, 1 to 4 μm in diameter on the leaf surfaces; small, sunken, fusiform lesions occur on veins and petioles. Numerous dark brown setae are produced in the black, pulvirate acervuli. The pathogen is known to be seed borne and it easily spread in the seed beds. The disease caused considerable damage the *D. lanata* in commercial plantings. All five species namely, *D. sibirica* Lindl., *D. purpurea, D. ambigua* Murr., *D. ferruginea* L. and *D. lanata* tested were susceptible to the disease, among them *D. ferruginea* and *D. lanata* were the most susceptible. **Control:** The anthracnose disease could be avoided by using disease free seeds. The use of noninfested seeds gave complete freedom from disease. Hot water treatment at 55°C for 15 min. was found to control the organism. Marked reduction in germination usually resulted from treatments longer than 15 min. Seed treatment with a number of fungicides were found to be injurious. Spraying of the crops with 0.5% Bordeaux mixture was found beneficial. Crop rotation and field sanitation also found useful to check the disease.

Leaf–spot

Digitalis purpurea and *D. lanata* were reported to be affected by a number of leaf spot diseases. However, two of them were considered economically important. **Causal organism:** *Septoria digitalis* Pass. **Symptoms:** The disease appeared on leaves as circular spots with purple margin and later the spots became irregular and necrotic with numerous pycnidia in stroma. The fungus has been reported to cause more damage at the cotyledonery stage of the seedlings as also on young plants. perpetuation of the disease has been known through pycnidia, stroma and partly as mycelium in the necrotic issue. The disease is externally seed borne. **Control:** Tilt (propiconazole) at 0.5 lit/ha gave the best protection against the disease.

Viral Diseases

A number of viruses have been reported to infect *Digitalis.* Tobacco mosaic virus (TMV) cucumber mosaic virus (CMV) Tobacco ring spot virus (TRSV) have been reported on *Digitalis* species. Occurrence of beet curly top (BCTV) and broad been wild virus (BWV) have also been occasionally reported.

Dioscorea

Rhizomes of *Dioscorea* species are the source of steroidal sapogenin, diosgenin. Diosgenin itself is not a medicinal product, but it is one of the most important raw materials used for the synthesis of steroidal drugs which include corticosteriods, sex hormones, oral contraceptives and anabolic steroids. Medicinal *Dioscorea* species namely *D. deltoidea, D. floribunda* and *D. composita* are cultivated in many parts of the world.

Rust

Causal organism: *Puccinia dioscorea* Kom. **Symptoms:** The rust infection is observed during the months of October–November on *D. deltoidae.* The symptoms consisted of minute scattered pustules of the fungus on the leaf surface. Both uredal and telial stages of the fungus were observed on infected plants.

Leaf Spots

Causal organism: *Cercospora dioscorea* Ellis & Mart. **Symptoms:** The fungus produced circular spots which are surrounded by dark border. The spots enlarged into irregular size. Abundant spores are produced on the infected leaves. Under humid conditions the disease was found to spread through mycelia (Koch, 1964). This resulted in severe disease incidence.

Leaf Blight

Causal organism: *Glomerella cingulata* (Ston) Spauld. **Symptoms:** The disease symptoms appeared as light brown, small circular spot on the upper surface of the leaves. The spots increased in size in later stage and coalesced forming reddish or dark brown to black patches of blight symptoms. **Control:** Leaf blight of *Dioscorea* species can be controlled by spraying with Dithane Z–78 or Copper fungicides.

Tuber Rot

Tuber rot of *D. floribunda* in nursery beds, fields, storage or transport is a common problem. **Causal organism:** *Aspergillus niger* van Tieghlm. **Symptoms:** Initial symptoms of the disease was purplish brown necrosis of tissue. rotted tissues of the tuber were soft and wet. Decay was associated with fungal infection with black masses of spores. Under humid conditions black masses on the tubers developed rapidly. **Control:** The tuber rot in nursery beds, field and in storage can be prevented by dipping tuber piece in 300 μg solution of benlate or dusting with 0.3 per cent powder.

Ginseng

Ginseng has been recognized for centuries as an important plant used in oriental medicine. What is known as ginseng, is the roots of *Panax ginseng* C.A. Meyers often referred as Korean ginseng or *P. quinquefolium* L. known as American ginseng. Ginseng has been used in Chinese medicine for more than 4000 years. Chinese name of the plant was translated in the Western world as 'Man–shaped Root' or 'Man Essence'. It contains number of saponins in the root termed as 'ginsenosides' or 'panaxosides'. In Chinese medicine ginseng is prescribed as a tonic, stimulant and aphrodisiac. The drug is considered to be an adaptogen and health tonic.

Anthracnose

Anthracnose is an uncommon, but potentially devastating disease of cultivated ginseng. **Causal organism:** Species of *Colletotrichum* (*C. dematium, C. coccodes* and *C. panacicola*) are found to cause anthracnose disease of cultivated species of ginseng. **Symptoms:** The first symptom of injury was seen when one leaflet after another turned brown, afterwards the disease spread down the petiole to the main stalk. Leaflets wilt in wet climates. The leaf spots are sharply delineated. Concentric rings developed within leaf spots, the spots subsequently increased and crumbled, leaving holes in leaflets. Petioles and stems also developed spots and fruiting bodies. **Control:** The disease can be controlled by spraying of Mancozeb, Polyoxin or Iprodione.

Powdery Mildew

A powdery mildew disease was observed on American ginseng (*Panax quinquefolium*) plants in British Columbia, Canada. The disease was found where three year old plants were growing on raised beds under artificial shades. **Causal organism:** *Erysiphe panax* Bai & Wang. **Symptoms:** The upper surface of 5 to 10 leaflets of the plants was covered with colonies of extensive white, superficial mycelium. The leaves became yellow and fell prematurely. No infection of berries or stems were observed. The fungus was identified as a species of *Erysiphe*. The disease is believed to cause severe damage to seed production, root weight and winter hardiness of ginseng plants.

Leaf Blight

Causal organism: *Alternaria panax* Whetzel. **Symptoms:** Infected leaves showed circular brown lesions on the leaf blades. The lesions coalesced resulting in blight symptoms, conidia of the pathogen are produced n the lesions. The pathogen also attacked the stem and produced linear, dark brown and velvety lesions. The stem lesions enlarged with age encircling the entire stem causing death of plant. The flowers and seed stalks were also attacked by the pathogen **Control:** The prevention and control of the disease could be achieved by early fungicidal sprays of Dithane M–45 or Kocide 101 mixed with spreader and sticker in the spring. Use of proper cultural practices for lowering the humidity and wide spacing for air circulation in the plantation is recommended for the prevention of the disease. However, the disease could be controlled by regular spraying of Dithane Z–78, Maneb or Bordeaux mixture.

Root–rot

One of the most serious threats to ginseng cultivation is the root–rot diseases caused by a number of fungi.

1. **Phytophthora root–rot: Causal organism:** *Phytophthora cactorum* (Lebert and Cohn) Schroter. **Symptoms:** The infected roots became discoloured, spongy and watery before they disintegrated. The roots show–scattered black areas which later got rotted. The infected plants showed wilt symptoms. Infected roots changed their colour and turned into soft pulp with pungent odour. The infected roots also showed disintegration. **Control:** Fumigation of soil with fumigants such as Verlox, Mylore, Vapam, etc. showed very effective control of roots–rots caused by *P. cactorum* in large scale forest nurseries. In Japan, Korea and China, cultural practices such as deep furrows between the beds for sufficient drainage were found useful to prevent the disease. Regular spray of protectant fungicides and also the application of systemic fungicides are recommended for the control of the disease. For the control of the leaf blight, foliar spray application of systemic fungicides are recommended.

2. **Fusarium root-rot: Causal organism:** *Fusarium solani* (Mart) Sacc. No reports are available on the control of *Fusarium* root-rot of ginseng. However, usual practice of fungicidal treatment of soil borne diseases would be effective to control the disease. **Control:** Attempts have been made to identify sources of resistance against root-rot pathogen. Some breeding lines have recently been identified to show resistance of *F. solani.*

3. **Cylindrocarpon root-rot: Causal organism:** *Cylindrocarpon destructans* (Zinssm) Scholten. Confusion still exists as to the cause of *Cylindrocarpon* root-rot of ginseng. Another root-rot causing fungus, *Fusarium* is often found associated with *Cylindrocarpon* in this disease.

Root-knot of Nematode

Causal Organism: The disease is caused by *Meloidogyne* spp. The root-knot nematodes are present in various soil types. **Symptoms:** The affected plants show discolourization, stunting and wilting with roots showing characteristic nodule-like swellings called galls. The nematodes attack ginseng roots as soon as they are hatched from the eggs. **Control:** The infected roots produced numerous galls. Suggested control measures are selection of disease-free planting areas, sanitation of farm implements and fumigation of soils with nematicide.

Damping-off Seedling

Post and pre emergence damping-off are common in ginseng seedlings. **Causal Organism:** Soil borne pathogens such as *Pythium* sp. *Rhizoctonia solani* and *Phytophthora* sp. **Symptoms:** Pathogens causing discolourization and root-rot. *Rhizoctonia solani.* Lesions are produced on the succulent stem. Use of fresh straw on the seed-beds is recommended to minimize the disease incidence.

Black Root-rot

Causal Organism: *Sclerotinia panacis.* **Symptoms:** Infected roots showed spongy and watery with black colour. The fungus produced numerous sclerotia. The diseases developed usually in spring. One of the control measures recommend is sanitation by avoiding exchange of soil or infected roots between healthy and diseased areas.

Glycyrrhiza

Dried rhizomes and roots of *Glycyrrhiza glabra* Linn. in known as Liquorice in commerce. The word glycyrrhiza is of Greek origin meaning sweet. Liquorice has been used in medicine more than 4000 years.

Leaf Spot

Causal organism: *Cercospora cavarae* P. & D. Sacc. **Symptoms:** The infection produced dark brown spots on lower surface of the leaves. The spots coalesced and became dark brown lesions. The infected leaves dried and ultimately shed. The infection caused heavy defoliation. **Control:** Fungicidal spray with Dithane Z-78 or Dithane M-45 (0.2%) is recommended for the control of the disease. Bavistin (0.1%) followed by Deltan (0.3%) is also reported to be effective to control the infection.

Leaf Blight

The disease was first observed in Himachal Pradesh, India. Leaf blight is another severe diseases affecting the foliage of liquorice. **Causal organism:** *Phyllosticta glycyrrhizae* (Hollos) Comb. nov. Pycnida were submerged to erumpent, globose, dark and measured. **Symptoms:** Initial symptoms consist of pin–head size dark brown spots. The spots later developed into circular to irregular shapes of 2–3 mm size on both surfaces of leaves. The lesions were dark brown in the centre and surrounded by light brown margins. **Control:** Spraying of the infected plants with Cuperox or Blitox (0.2%) 3–4 times at an interval of six days after the appearance of symptoms is found to control the disease.

Alternaria Leaf Spot

Causal organism: *Alternaria alternata* (Fr.) Keissler. **Symptoms:** Symptoms consist of light brown to black spots on the leaves and stem in the late stage of the season. The spots coalesced resulting in blight symptoms. **Control:** Spraying with Cuperox or Blitox (0.2%) 3–4 times at an interval of 6–7 days is found to control the disease.

Rust

Causal organism: *Uromyces glycyrrhizae* (Rab) Magn. **Symptoms:** Severe systemic and localized rust infection was reported on many wild and cultivated liquorice plants (*G. glabra*) in Southern Italy. The fungus grows systemically in the shoots, mainly in the bark and phloem and in the parts of roots nearest to the crown, mainly in the xylem where it overwinters. Besides, the typical foliar pustules, the fungus induces elongation, resetting, defoliation, browing of the pith and formation of many buds in the crown region. From these buds infected tillers grow in spring which constitute the source of primary infection.

Root–rot, Collar–rot and Wilt

Causal organisms: This disease is reported to be caused by a complex group of fungi which were identified as *Sclerotium* spp. and *Fusarium* spp. in addition to *Rhizoctonia bataticola.* **Symptoms:** The disease started from the planting time. In case of serious infection, complete rotting of the roots was observed, eventually death and decay of whole plant occurred. Infection often spread to the stem and branches of the plants. Dark brown spots were found in the collar region. The collar portion of the infected plants occasionally girdled with the fungus. **Control:** Soil treatment with Bavistin or Benlate is recommended before planting. In case of collar–rot, removal and destruction of aerial portion above the collar region is recommended. Carbendazin (0.05%) is reported to provide control of the disease to a limited extent.

Hyoscyamus

Hyoscyamus species are sources of tropane alkaloids. *Hyoscyamus niger* and *H. muticus* are reported to be affected by a number of diseases caused by fungi, bacteria and viruses.

Leaf Spot

The disease prevalent in Jammu and Kashmir on *H. niger* especially in the shady localities.**Causal organism:** *Ascochyta kashmiriana* Padwick & Merh. **Symptoms:** The disease appeared as orbicular zonate, buff to woody brown spots no the leaf lamina. The spots gradually enlarged and coalesced. In young plants death of leaves due to severe spotting is common.

Leaf Blight

Leaf blight diseases of *H. niger* and *H. muticus* have been reported from India. The disease has a wide spread occurrence. **Causal organism:** *Alternaria alternata* (Fr.) Keissler. **Symptoms:** Initial symptoms in *H. niger* were tiny necrotic spots on matured leaves. The spots enlarged and coalesced which resulted in blight symptoms. The occurrence of the disease was more prevalent on older leaves. In case of *H. muticus* the initial symptoms were scattered, irregular chlorotic spots. The spots later enlarged and coalesced. Severe infection resulted in defoliation.

Seedling Blight

This disease was prevalent in *H. muticus* during the early stages of growth and causes extensive damage. **Causal organism:** *Pythium butleri* Subramaniam. **Symptoms:** Initial symptoms appear as yellowish water soaked lesions on the hypocotyl region. The infection then moved to both stem and root regions. Infected portions became pulpy and dark brown showing soft–rot symptoms. **Control:** Eventhough no control measures are reported, treatment of the infected seedlings with Dithane Z–78 or Dithane M–45 would be useful to check the disease to some extent.

Stem–rot

Both *H. muticus* and *H. niger* were severely affected by stem–rot disease. The disease incidence was severe during the months of December and January in Northern India. **Causal organism:** *Sclerotinia sclerotiorum* (Lib.) de Bary. **Symptoms:** The initial symptoms develop in the form of water soaked lesions on the above ground portion of the plants. The infection rapidly spread upwards resulting in stem–rot and decay of infected plants.

Root–rot

This disease is found in *H. niger.* **Causal organism:** *Thielavia basicola* Zopf. **Symptoms:** The affected plants were stunted in growth with crinkled leaves which became pale yellow. **Control:** Reduction in aerial growth led to bushy appearance. Infected underground portion exhibited rotting of cortical tissue. The spread of the disease has been suggested through endoconidia.

Bacterial Blight

The bacterial blight disease of *H. muticus* was observed in India. **Causal organism:** *Pseudomonas cichorii* (Swingle) Stapp. **Symptoms:** The disease was characterised by the appearance of water soaked lesions on the main stem. The infection gradually expanded to the branches. Infection invariably resulted in wilting and death of affected plants. Pale yellow liquid oozed from the cut ends of infected stem.

Root–knot

Casual organism: *Meloidogyne incognita* (Kofoid & White) Chitwood and *M. javanica* (Treub) Chitwood. The former was more prevalent. **Symptoms:** plants in field were affect by this nematode causing chlorosis and stunting. The infected plants showed root–galls of varying size on the root systems. **Control:** Soil amendments with neem cake was found to be useful for the management of the disease. Inoculation of seedlings with the VAM fungus, *Glomus aggregatum* was found to be beneficial to reduce the multiplication and disease development.

Opium Poppy

Opium poppy (*Papaver somniferum* L.) is one of the most important medicinal plants used by ancient man. The oldest reference of this drug plant is found in Mesopotamia. It is mentioned in Assyrian herbals, 4000 years ago. Various phytopathogenic fungi, bacteria and viruses are known to infect opium poppy causing severe damage to the crop. Majority of the diseases are caused by fungi. Some of the diseases affecting this crop are seedling blight, leaf spot, leaf blight, downy mildew, powdery mildew, wilt, root–rot, capsule–rot, bacterial soft–rot and mosaic diseases. Among these downy mildew, powdery mildew, leaf blight and bacterial soft–rot are major diseases.

Seedlings Blight and Damping–off

Commercial cultivation of opium poppy in Uttar Pradesh (India) were recently found to be affected by a damping–off disease. **Causal organism:** *Pythium ultimum* Trow, *Pythium mamillatum* Meurs. and *Pythium dissotocum* Drechsler. **Symptoms:** The symptoms consisted of rotting of roots and collar region leading to death of seedlings. **Control:** Treatment of seeds with Ridomil MZ–72 WP at 0.12 g/100 g seeds is reported to control the disease. Seed treatment with Captan (0.3%) or soil drenching propamocarb hydrochloride (0.3%) also gave satisfactory control of the disease. The damping–off disease of opium poppy could be effectively managed by macozeb treatment.

Leaf Spots

Causal organism: *Entyloma fuscum* Schorter. **Symptoms:** The symptoms are characterised by cholortic and necrotic areas on the foliage. The infection was often accompanied by curling. Sori in the leaves formed round yellow, later grey or brownish spots.

Causal Organism: *Cercospora papaveri, C. purpurea* and *Alternaria brassicae.* However, all the leaf spot diseases observed till now on this crop are of minor importance, though there is a distinct correlation between leaf–spot infection and morphine, codeine and thebaine contents.

Leaf Blights

A new leaf blight disease of opium poppy was observed in an epidemic form in the poppy plantations in Uttar Pradesh (India). Its causal organism is *Alternaria phragmospora* Van Emden. The disease was prevalent during the winter months. The initial symptoms consisted of small greyish brown spots scattered on the leaves.

Causal organism: *Helminthosporium papaveris* Saw. (Perfect state: *Pleospora papaveraceae* (de Not.) Sacc.). **Symptoms:** Symptoms of the disease appeared as diffused yellow spots, followed by premature drying of the infected leaves. The mycelium from infected leaves advanced to the stem, on which the pathogen produced the perithecia. **Control:** Early sowing was observed to reduce infection caused by *H. papaveris.* Seed disinfection and spraying of seed beds with Bordeaux mixture or other copper fungicides also controlled the disease. Incorporation of lime appreciably reduced the loss. Fungicidal spraying with Systax before flowering reduced infection and increased the yield. Seed disinfection with Organol (0.5 or 1 lg/100 kg seed) significantly reduced the infection (Mraz 1963). Soil treatment with borate and manganese superphosphate (30 kg/ha) reduced the infection significantly. Spraying with Germisan (1%), and dusting with Thiram, Gramisan or Agrosan were found to be the most effective control measure of the disease. Seed dressing with Zaprawa and Nasienna–T and spraying with Synkotox and Dithane M–45 were also effective prophylacetic measures against *H. papaveris.*

In later stages, spots enlarged and coalesced resulting in severe blighting of the leaves. Infection often resulted in yellowing of leaves. Infected peduncle became pink to brown in colour. Severe infection by the pathogen was observed both at the seedling and flowering stages.

Downy Mildew

This is one of the serious and widespread diseases of opium poppy. Downy mildew now occurs in most regions in India (Rajasthan, Madhya Pradesh and Uttar Pradesh). Downy mildew caused 20–30% loss of yield of opium latex. **Causal organism:** *Peronospora arborescens* (Berk) de Bary. **Symptoms:** The infection spread upwards from lower leaves. The entire leaf surface was covered by downy mildew coating, composed of conidiophores and conidia of the pathogen. The stem, branches and even capsules were also attacked resulting in the premature death of the plants. The infection started from the moment the seed germinated and remained during the whole period of growth. The pathogen often causes abnormal development in opium poppy. The pathogen also caused hypertrophy and curvature of stem and flower stalks. The infection was often systemic. The leaves of infected plants remained small, chlorotic and curled downwards. Heavy sporulation occurred on entire lower surface of diseased leaves. The capsule, if formed got shrinken, wringled and dried. Severely infected plants showed extreme stunting. The infected area on the leaf first became chlorotic and then necrotic with large spots. The disease caused extensive damage to the crop cultivated in most sites. **Control:** Crop rotation, wide spacing and avoidance of low lying site for growing poppy reduce incidence of downy mildew. Seed disinfection and spraying seed beds with 0.5% Bordeaux mixture or other copper fungicides was recommended for the control of the disease. Dithane Z-78, Ferban or bisdithane gave 50% are also used for control. Ridomil treatment is the most effective method for the control of downy mildew disease of opium poppy. Higher dozes of phosphorus application to the crop was found to decrease severity of downy mildew while nitrogen increased the disease index. Captan treatment is not recommended as this fungicide inhibited seed germination of opium poppy.

Powdery Mildew

The powdery mildew disease of opium poppy was observed in Pakistan (Zaman and Khan, 1969). The disease has been found in the severe from in many parts of India namely, Rajasthan, Madhya Pradesh and Uttar Pradesh. Poppy cultivation suffer heavy losses on account of this disease. In Rajasthan powdery mildew causes severe damage to the crop. **Causal organism:** *Erysiphe polygoni* DC. **Symptoms:** Powdery mildew disease was observed on 14–16 weeks old poppy plants. The first appearance of the disease in India is in February or early March. The base of the stem is attacked first, where it appeared as small circular patches. Several new colonies of the pathogen continue to appear covering large part of stem. Blackening develops in the affected pats; often the stem appeared black interspersed with green patches. The mycelia spread all over the leaves. The luxurious growth of the fungus is found on the leaf surface in case of severe infection. The entire leaf surface is covered by white powdery masses of mycelium. The age of host is a strong factor influencing the disease development. The disease is never found on plants less than 80 days old. The environmental (mainly temperature) factors also affect the disease development. **Control:** The disease can be effectively controlled by spraying 0.5% wettable sulphur at the time of the appearance of the disease or when the crop attains the age of 80 days. Other fungicides commonly used to control powdery mildew of various crops are also effective for controlling poppy powdery mildew. One spray of Spersul (0.5%) for the control of powdery mildew caused by *E. polygoni* is suggested.

Capsule Infection

A large number of fungi are found to infect opium poppy capsule. **Causal organisms:** *Macrosporium papaveris, Alternaria papaveris* (Bers) Ellis, *Alternaria alternata* (Fr.) Keissler, *Fusarium scirpi* var. *caudatum* Lam and Raw, *Dendryphion penicillatum* (Corda) Fr. **Symptoms:** *Alternaria alternata* infection significantly reduced the morphine content. Similar observation by indicated significant decrease in codeine and thebaine content in opium poppy capsule infected by *A. alternata.* Capsule rot caused by *Dendryphion penicillatum* is prevalent in Rajasthan (India). Most of the capsule infection of opium poppy can be controlled by periodic spray of fungicidal formulations belonging to the group of bisdithiocarbamates. Four to six applications of 200–500 g/ha Bavistin will be a prophylatic measure for maintaining a healthy crop.

Apart from above mentioned diseases poppy is also infected with other diseases like, Bacterial Soft-rots, Cabbage Ring Spot Virus, Beet Yellow Virus, Bean Yellow Virus, Turnip Mosaic Virus, Poppy Mosaic, and Mycoplasma Disease.

Periwinkle

Tropical Periwinkle (*Catharanthus roseus.* L.) G. Don. is known for important medicinal value in folklore of a number of countries, for a long period. The medicinal value of this plant was known even in 50 B.C. (Husain, 1993). However, the importance of this plant in modern medicine was realized by an accidental discovery of the anticancer properties of its leaf alkaloids. Tropical periwinkle was previously known as *Vinca rosea* (L) as well as *Lochnera rosea* (L) Reich.

Die–back

Causal organism: *Colletotrichum dematium* (Pers *ex* Fr.) Grove. **Symptoms:** Die–back is one of the most serious diseases of *C. roseus.* Initial symptoms of the disease consist of withering of the terminal buds of young branches followed by wilting and drying of the young leaves. In later stages infection spreads downwards causing withering of entire branch along with the leaves. In case of severe infection majority of the branches of a plant were found withered and dried.

Another die–back of *C. roseus* was observed in different parts of West Bengal during the monsoon season. **Causal organism:** *Pythium butleri* Subramaniam. **Symptoms:** The symptoms consisted of water soaked spots on the bark, 4–6 inches below the tip, which gradually increased in size and encircled the young stem. Rotting and shredding of the bark resulted in wilting of the tip. The disease became severe during rainy season. The seedlings were also susceptible to the disease.

It is one more die–back disease of *C. roseus.* Causal organism: *Pythium debaryanum* Hesse. **Symptoms:** The symptoms are similar to the disease caused by *P. butleri.* The disease often became severe during rainy season. The plants are partially or completely killed depending upon their age, because younger plants were more susceptible than older ones.

Causal organism: *Pythium aphanidermatum* (Eds) Fitzp.

Control: Die–back disease of *C. roseus* can successfully be controlled by fungicides. It could be effectively controlled by the application of Captafol (Foltaf 80 WP). However, Bavistin 50 WP was not effective. The fungicidal application not only controlled the disease but also gave better yield. Soil solarization can significantly reduce mortality of plants. Integration of host resistance with fungicide treatment is also more effective for the control of die–back.

Stem–rot

Symptoms

This is a new disease of *C. roseus* recently reported. **Causal organism:** *Rhizopus stolonifer* (Ehren) Lind. **Symptoms:** The disease causes serious damage to the crops in commercial plantations. The disease appeared as pale green water soaked lesions on the stem either below the flower head or at the collar region of the plant. infected plants produced slimy wet rot of the cortical tissue due to which affected twigs bend downwards. The infection usually advanced both upwards and downwards resulting in slimy wet rot. In advance stage of infection slimy wet rot turned to pale, then yellowish brown and ultimately dried. Severe infection resulted in premature death of the plants.

Leaf–spot

Rhizoctonia solani is primarily considered as soil fungus. **Causal organism:** *Rhizoctonia solani* Kuhn. (*Thamatephorus cucumeris* (Frank) Donk.). **Symptoms:** The disease first appeared on the lower leaves as water soaked area by the side of midrib near the leaf base which gradually developed to both the sides of the midrib extending towards the tip of the leaves. The affected leaves usually rotted, dried up and appeared black. Drying gradually proceeded towards the tip affecting the branches. **Control:** However, extensive aerial growth is possible under favourable conditions. Hence, chemical treatment of the soil and propogative materials are the most commonly used control methods. Organo–mercury compounds and pentachloronitro benzene are effective in many crops. Cultural practices such as crop rotation, shallow planting, early harvest, etc. also reduced disease incidence. Use of some microorganisms acting as antagonists against this fungus are also reported to be useful to control the disease incidence.

Leaf Blight

Severe leaf blight of *C. roseus* was found to occur in Lucknow. The severity of the disease increased in the rainy season. **Causal organism:** *Alternaria alternata* (Fr.) Keissler. **Symptoms:** The disease appeared as small light brown spots involving almost whole of the surface of the leaf. The lesions later became necrotic with concentric rings.

Target–spot

Causal organism: *Corynespora cassiicola* (Berk and M.A. Curtis) Wei. **Symptoms:** Leaf spots first appeared as small (1–2 mm) necrotic leasions most often associated with margins of leaves of all ages. As spots enlarged, they turned brown, became round to oblong (6.45 × 2 cm) and assumed target like appearance. Eventually entire affected leaves turned yellow and dropped prematurally. Numerous spots were observed on leaves resulting in severe defoliation.

Leaf Blight

Causal organism: *Phytophthora nicotianae* Breda de Haan. **Symptoms:** A leaf blight disease of *C. roseus* was reported from Cochella Valley of California. Initial symptoms were water soaked spots on the leaves. The spots enlarged and turned necrotic, resulting in typical blight symptoms.

Foot–rot

This disease was observed in West Bengal **Causal organism:** *Sclerotium rolfsii* Sacc. (*Corticium rolfsii* Curzi). **Symptoms:** The first symptom of the disease is yellowing and drying of the leaf tips. Young plants wilt and collapsed rapidly. The bark at the collar region is found to be rotted and white mycelial growth is found on the infected area.

Root and Collar–rot

Symptoms

Causal organism: *Pythium aphanidermatum* (Eds.) Fitz. **Symptoms:** Initial symptoms of the disease was the appearance of chlorosis on the plants. The plants later wilted gradually. The wilted plants later collapsed. The wilted plants when uprooted, severe rotting on the root and collar regions was observed. The tissues of cortical regions were severely affected by disintegration. **Control:** Appreciable good control of the disease could be achieved by the application of fungicides. However, introduction of disease resistant cultivars would be useful. Tetraploid lines were reported to show certain amount of resistance to the disease. A combination of resistant varieties and use of appropriate fungicides would be the most effective method for the control of the disease.

Damping–off

Pre–emergence damping–off of *C. roseus* has been reported to cause serious damage to the seedlings. This was reported to be caused by *Phytophthora parasitica* Dastur. Attempt was made to control the disease by aluminium sulphate drenching in the soil.

Flower Blight

Causal organism: *Choanephora cucurbitarium* (Berk. & Rav) Taxter. **Symptoms:** Initial symptoms of the disease were the production of dark grey spots on the petals. The spots often coalesced leading to blight symptoms. The disease caused severe damage under high humid conditions.

Viral Diseases

Three viruses causing different types of mosaic diseases like, Mosaic disease and Tomato Spotted Wilt Virus.

Phyllody

The occurrence of phyllody or little leaf disease of *C. roseus* has been reported by several workers from India. **Causal organism:** The causal organism was identified as mycoplasma or mycoplasma like organism (MLO). **Symptoms:** Typical symptoms of the disease were reduction in the size of leaves, shortening of internodes, extensive branching and stunting with greening of flowers. When the disease intensified the plants turned vegetative with complete loss of flowering and fruiting. The diseased plants often looked like small bushes with stunted growth. Excessive branching was observed the leaves turned chlorotic with pointed tips. There is a complete transformation of the appearance of the diseased plants beyond recognition from the normal plant. The disease caused considerable reduction in the alkaloid content of the plant. **Control:** Tetracycline treatment proved highly successful in limiting the disease symptoms. Treatment with oxytetracycline at 500 μg caused remission of the symptoms. The treatment resulted in amelioration of the disease symptoms. Treated plants were found to produce normal leaves and flowers. Tetracycline and gibberellic acid therapy was more effective.

Plantago

Ripe seeds of *Plantago psyllium* Linn. is known in commerce as Spanish or French psyllium and that of *Plantago ovata* Forsk. is referred as Indian psyllium.

Downy Mildew

Downy mildew is the major and serious disease of *P. ovata.* It causes enormous quantitative and qualitative loss and often becomes a limiting factor in the successful cultivation of the crop. Usually the disease appears at the time of spike initiation. **Causal organism:** The disease is reported to be caused by two pathogens (1) *Peronospora alta* Fuckel (2) *Peronospora plantaginis.* **Symptoms:** Initial symptoms consist of small pale yellow patches on the leaves which progressively spread, completely destroying the leaves. The chlorotic areas develop in the upper surface of the leaves and ash white frost like mycelial growth develops on the lower surface of the leaves. Subsequently, infected leaves become chlorotic and brownish in colour, followed by curling, crinkling and drying of plants. Occasionally, chlorotic streaks, extending along with the midrib of leaves are observed. In such cases profuse downy growth is observed on the lower surface of the leaves. Ultimately, the whole leaf turns necrotic and in severe cases the entire plants appeared blighted. **Control:** It is difficult to keep the disease under control once it has affected the crop extensively. The disease is seed as well as soil borne.

Damping–off

Plantago ovata suffers from both pre–emergence and post–emergence damping–off. Older plants are less susceptible than the young seedlings. **Causal organism:** Damping–off of *Plantago* has been reported to be caused by a number of pathogens (1) *Pythium ultimum* Trow. (Chastagner *et al.,* 1979), (2) *Rhizoctonia solani* Kuh. (Anon, 1980) (3) *Fusarium oxysporum* (Schl) Syn & Hans.

Symptoms: In pre–emergence damping–off young seedlings wither they reach the surface of the soil. While in case of post–emergence damping–off the plantlets are affected first. Initial infection appeared as darkened, water–soaked spot on collar region of the seedlings. The infection extends rapidily leading to the death of seedlings. The disease normally occurred at high temperature and humidity at the time of sowing. **Control:** Seed treatment with metalaxyl or fenaminosulf (5 g/kg) protected the seedlings to a great extent.

Wilt

The disease was found either as damping–off or as late season wilting when the plants started to produce seeds. **Causal organism:** A number of pathogens have been reported to be responsible for the disease (1) *Pythium ultimum* Trow. (Chastagner *et al.,* 1979) (2) *Fusarium oxysporum* (Schl) Syn & Hans (Russell, 1975). (3) *Fusarium solani* Ell & Mart. **Symptoms:** Initial symptoms consist of change in colour of outer leaves from green to silver. Wilting symptoms onset rapidily. The leaves became postrate. Discolourization occurs on the tap root which is accompanied by accumulation of large amount of hyphae in the xylem vessels. Vascular discolourization and cortical root–rot were also observed. **Control:** Seed treatment with a systemic fungicide, such as bavistin or benlate (2.5 g/kg) has been reported to protect the seedlings for a month.

Powdery Mildew

The disease is of minor importance. The disease appeared at the time of flowering. **Causal organism:** *Erysiphe cichoracearum* D. C. **Symptoms:** Small white or greyish spots appeared on the leaves which gradually enlarged and eventually covered the entire plant surface with white powdery mass. **Control:** The disease can be controlled by spraying Karathane W.D. (0.2%) or wettable sulphur compounds immediately after the appearance of the disease.

Leaf Blight

The disease was reported in experimental plantations of *Plantago ovata.* **Causal organism:** *Alternaria alternata* (Fr.) Keissler. **Symptoms:** Symptoms consisted of dull–green yellowish colour on the leaf tip. The older and matured leaves were more severely affected. More than fifty per cent leaf area showed irregular necrotic spots, which enlarged rapidly. In the advance stage, the leaves blackened due to blight symptoms. This was followed by death and drying of the leaves. Severe infection often caused shriveling and blackening of seeds.

Viral Diseases

Eight viruses were observed to infect *Plantago.* Two of them were identified as previously described viruses: Ribgrass Mosaic Virus and Plantain Virus A. However, 6 viruses are believed to be new records. They are tentatively classified as a Potex Virus, a Caulimo Virus, a Poty Virus, a Carla Virus and two isometric viruses with properties similar to the Tobacco Necrosis Virus group and Tombus viruses. Different virus types are known to infect *Plantago* species indicate that the plants have a broad range of susceptibility to plant viruses and may act as a reservoir of viruses which are able to infect other crops.

Podophyllum

The drug Podophyllum is obtained from rhizomes and roots of *Podophyllum peltatum* L. or *P. emodi* Wall (Syn. *Podophyllum hexandrum* Royle). The drug has been used by American Indians as emetic, purgative, etc. *Podophyllum peltatum* is a herb with perennial creeping, fibrous branched rhizomes.

Rust

Mayapple (*Podophyllum peltatum*) is attacked by a non–specific rust fungus. The pathogen is potentially damaging to its host (Sohn and Plicansky, 1977). Host infection occurs via contact with spore–contaminated soil during shoot emergence in early spring (Whetzel *et al.,* 1925).

Causal organism: *Puccinia podophylli* Schw. **Symptoms:** Orange lesions (aecia) develop on leaves within two weeks after infection. Aeciospores shed and immediately reinfect leaves, causing scattered black lesions (telia) from which over wintering teliospores develop. The first generation of the pathogen appears to be most–harmful, since plants are damaged early in their seasonal growth cycle. Heavy aecial infection is associated with a significantly reduced plant growth. Disease impact appears to be much less during the second pathogen generation, since telial development occurs in late spring, just prior to normal leaf senescence.

Rauvolfia

The genus *Rauvolfia* was named in honour of a sixteenth century German Physician and botanist Leonard Rauvolfia. *Rauvolfia serpentina* Benth. is indigenous to India and the neighbouring countries. A number of species of *Rauvolfia* are reported to contain medicinally important alkaloids, only two species of *Rauvolfia* namely *Rauvolfia serpentina* Benth ex Kurz and *Rauvolfia vomitoria* Atz are commercially important and used for the production of therapeutically important alkaloids. Most of the supply of this plant is from wild sources. The plant is cultivated only in small scale in India and Bangladesh. *Rauvolfia serpentina* is susceptible to several diseases caused by fungi and viruses.

Wilt

The wild disease of *R. serpentina* was first observed in Jammu. Since, its first appearance the disease became more and more important, because it caused considerable damage to the crop.

Causal organism: *Fusarium oxysporum* f. sp. *rauvolfii* (Schlecht) **Symptoms:** Initial symptoms of the disease consist of wilting of branches followed by wilting the entire plant. In advance stages, collar region and the root portion below the ground level turned into dark colour. Two year old plants were affected mostly. The distintegration of root cortex was more prominent in the seedling and young plant. The foliage symptoms are characterized by dropping of leaves followed by upward curling. As the disease symptoms advanced, the entire plant was affected resulting in drying of the leaves and death of the plant.

Powdery Mildew

The disease was found prevalent on *R. serpentina* in the plantations in India. **Causal organism:** *Leveillula taurica* (Lev) Atz. **Symptoms:** The characteristic symptom of the disease was rolling of infected leaves enclosing the lower surface of the leaves which is covered with whitish growth of the fungus in patches, consisting of conidia and conidiophores. **Control:** The disease can be controlled by one application of any wettable sulphur preparation (0.3%) or Karathane WD 0.05% at the time of first appearance of the disease.

Leaf Blight and Bud Rot

A leaf blight and bud rot of *R. serpentina* was frequently observed in the experimental plants. **Causal organism:** *Alternaria tenuis* Nees. (Syn: *Alternaria alternata* (Fr) Keissler). **Symptoms:** Initially small brownish circular spots with yellowish margin on the ventral surface of the tender leaves appeared. These spots then enlarged forming large dark brownish circular lesions. The spots covered the entire leaf, resulting in blight symptoms and subsequently leaves died and dropped. In certain cases young and tender portions of the tip of the branches are also infected leading to death of auxiliary buds. The portion of stem just below the affected leaf bud turned purplish black. Young flower buds and even the fruits are also affected. **Control:** The disease can be controlled by spraying the infected plants with Dithane M–45 (0.3%) or by using seed treatment with fungicides also reduced the infection to a great extent.

Leaf Spots

1. **Causal organism:** *Cercospora rauvolfiae* Chupp & Muller. **Symptoms:** The disease appeared as minute yellow spots which gradually increased in size and became dark brown patches. First purple coloured blotches appeared on the ventral surface of the leaves. In about a week's time the infected portions became dark brown in colour. The affected leaves dried and fell off.
2. **Causal organism:** *Rhizoctonia solani* Khun. **Symptoms:** Third leaf blight disease of *R. serpentina* was observed in 4 year old plantations in Madhya Pradesh (India). **Symptoms:** The pathogen attacked the leaves usually at the apex and occasionally at margins. Lower leaves were attacked first and the disease progressed upward.

Target Spot

Rauvolfia serpentina was reported to suffer heavily due to target spot disease The disease caused premature defoliation. **Causal organism:** *Corynespora cassiicola* (Berk & Curt) Wei. **Symptoms:** The leaves are attacked on both surfaces. The infection resulted in the appearance of small brownish spots which gradually enlarged in to circular spots, 2–20 μm diameter with concentric zones due to which the disease is called as 'target spots'. The spots were dark brown on the upper and yellowish brown on the lower surface and are usually surrounded by a pale yellow margin. The lower leaves are infected first, the disease then progressed to upwards. Defoliation of infected plants occurred leaving behind only a few top tender leaves. **Control:** Attempts were made to control the disease. Among the four fungicides tested in the field, application of 0.25% Captan at monthly intervals for six months effectively controlled the disease.

Anthracnose

Causal organism: *Colletotrichum gleosporioides* (Penz) Sacc. **Symptoms:** The symptoms consist of numerous spots and the acervulli scattered all over the leaf. Infection is mainly confined to upper surface of the leaves. The spots enlarged into large circular patches and invaded the surrounding tissues. severely infected leaves dried resulting in defoliation. **Control:** The disease is reported to be controlled by removing infected shoots and avoiding excess watering. Spraying with fermate, Dithane Z–78 and Terlate is also recommended for the control.

Die–back

Rauvolfia serpentina has been reported to be affected by a die–back disease. **Causal organism:** *Colletotrichum dematium*: (Pers) Grove. **Symptoms:** The disease affected the twigs and flowers. Numerous tiny spots found on leaves and stem. Acervuli are scattered all over the surface. Smaller lesions coalesced to form large and circular necrotic patches. Severe infection resulted in drying, defoliation and decapitation. **Control:** The disease is reported to be controlled by spraying the infected plants with Dithane Z–78 (0.2%). In the advance stage of infection pruning of infected parts is recommended. A leaf spot disease and premature defoliation of *R. serpentina* was observed on cultivated plants in Gujarat (India). The symptoms consisted of severe leaf spots and defoliation.

Mosaic

A sap transmissible virus causing mosaic disease of *R. serpentina* has been reported. The virus produced local necrotic lesions on primary leaves of *Phaseolus vulgaris, Nicotiana glutinosa, Datura metel* and *D. innoxia.* The virus was identified as a strain of tobacco mosaic virus. The virus infection was found to affect the alkaloid contents of the roots.

Phyllody

In *R. serpentina* bunchy top disease is common. He suggested the overwintering of the disease in *Catharanthus roseus, Nicotiana tabacum, Solanum melongena* and *Capsicum annum* in Gujarat (India). **Symptoms:** Characteristic symptoms of the disease were retarded growth, shortened internodes, phyllody of flowers. The leaves became small and pale in colour; the floral parts of the infected plants are modified to leaf like structures resulting into a cluster of small leaves in place of inflorescence and leading to complete sterility. The disease was found to appear on all branches or any one flowering branch of the plant. The disease adversely affected the alkaloid content of the plant. The disease is probably caused by a virus resembling Aster yellow virus.

Yellow Vein Mosaic

A yellow vein disease of *R. serpentina* caused by a graft transmissible and whitefly (*Bemisia tabaci*) transmitted virus, was observed in the experimental plantations in Jammu. **Symptoms:** The symptoms consisted of yellowing of young leaves and formation of yellow network in the back ground of green surface. A minor retardation of growth of infected plants was also observed. Reduction in root biomass and total alkaloid contents of roots occurred due to the disease.

Ring Spot

A graft transmissible ring spot disease of *R. serpentina* was observed in the experimental plantations in Jammu. **Symptoms:** Leaves of infected plants showed characteristic concentric yellow rings of different sizes scattered all over the surface of the leaves. The rings gradually enlarged, coalesced and became gradually necrotic. In later stages, the entire infected leaves became necrotic resulting in defoliation. Infection adversely affected the quality of roots and their alkaloid contents.

Green Mosaic

Rauvolfia serpentina was reported to be affected by a severe green mosaic virus. The diseased plants showed severe stunting and the leaves narrowed. Mosaic mottling symptoms were more pronounced in young leaves. **Causal organism:** The virus was identified as a strain of cucumber mosaic virus (CMV). The virus was isometric, 27 nm in diameter and was transmitted by aphid (*Myzus persica*) but not by seeds or soil. Mode of transmission, host range, biophysical properties and serological relationship showed that the virus is an isolate of Cucumber mosaic virus (CMV).

Senna

Dried leaves and pods of *Cassia angustifolia* Vahl is known in commerce as Indian senna and that of *Cassia acutifolia* Delile as Alexandrian senna. Senna was used by Arab physicians as early as 900 A.D. Senna (*Cassia angustifolia* and *Cassia acutifolia*) are affected by a number of diseases. Damping–off, leaf spots and leaf blights are the major diseases of this crop.

Damping–off

Damping–off affecting the seedlings is the most devastating disease of this crop. The disease is common on most of the soils in North–west India where this crop is cultivated. The disease spreads fast, if the drainage is insufficient. **Causal organism:** *Macrophomina phaseolina* (Tassi) Goid (*Syn: Rhizoctonia bataticola* (Taub) Butler). **Symptoms:** The infected plants showed blackening on the collar region extending upwards leading to death of seedlings. Infection caused death of plants in patches in the field. **Control:** Treating the seeds with Thiran or Captan (2.5 g/kg) protects the growing seedlings from the disease. Drenching the field with Bavistin (0.1%) Brassicol (0.2%) or Rhizoctol (0.1–0.5%) is beneficial to delimit the disease or partially control the infection. It is advisable not to grow senna again in the same field where infection was observed earlier.

Leaf Blight

Leaf blight disease has been reported to cause serious damage to senna crop. **Causal organism:** *Alternaria alternata* (Fr.) Keissler. **Symptoms:** Initial symptoms are minute, dark brown circular spots on the laminae especially at the tip and margins of the leaflets. The spots enlarged to 3–8 μm turned brown to black in colour and became irregular. Chlorotic areas from the tip and margins were found to spread over the entire leaf blade leading to drying and premature leaf fall. Older leaves were more susceptible to infection than young ones. *Cassia acutifolia* was less susceptible compared to *C. angustifolia.* The disease was found to affect the quality and quantity of the produce. Chemical analysis of the leaves of infected plants revealed that sennoside, the active principle, content was inversely proportional to leaf blight intensity. **Control:** Spraying of Dithane M–45 (0.15%) thrice at an interval of 15 days for a period of 5–6 weeks is recommended for the control of the disease.

Leaf Spots

A new leaf spot disease of *C. angustifolia* was reported from the experimental plantations in Lucknow (India). **Causal organism:** *Colletotrichum gloeosporioides* (Penz) Sacc. (perfect state: *Glomerella cingulata* (Stonem) Spauld). **Symptoms:** Initial symptoms appeared as small pinhead brown to dark brown spots on the leaf lamina. The spots enlarged towards the margins resulting to death and defoliation.

Withania

Withania somnifera Dunal is an erect, evergreen shrub distributed throughout the drier parts of India and also in the Mediterranean regions. It is cultivated on commercial scales in the central part of India. The commercial drug consists of the dried roots. Several alkaloidal and non alkaloidal compounds were isolated from *W. somnifera.* The important compounds isolated from different parts of the plant are steroidal lactones called Withanolids.

Damping–off and Seedling–rot

Causal organism: *Alternaria alternata* (Fr.) Keissler. **Symptoms:** Damping–off and seedling–rot mortality caused serious damage to the crop. The plant population is drastically reduced which resulted in reduced root yield. The infected plants turned yellowish and finally dried up. In case of damping–off, the leaves of affected plants showed mottling followed by necrotic lesions, curlingand burnt margins. In severe cases of infection whole plant was burnt and died. **Control:** Use of fungicidal treatment of seeds for the control of seedling diseases. Deltan, Dithane M45, Brassicol and Bavistin could protect the seedlings.

Leaf Blight and Die–back

Die–back and leaf blight disease caused significant damage to Ashwagandha crop. **Causal organism:** *Alternaria alternata* (Fr.) Keissler. **Symptoms:** The characteristic symptoms of the disease are the appearance of small light brown spots on leaves and flowers which enlarged, coalesced resulting in blight symptoms. In case of die–back, the disease caused necrosis of tender twigs from the tip backwards. The entire branch or the top of the plant withered. The dead twigs were greyish brown or straw coloured in the advanced stage of infection. **Control:** Use of seeds from disease–free plants, spraying of the crop with fungicides, such as Dithane M–45 (0.3%) or Rovaral (0.2%) have been found to check the spread of the disease. Seed dressings by suitable fungicides has also been found to control the disease to a large extent during the early stage.

Leaf Spot

The disease was reported from Jaipur, India. The disease appeared during the rainy season. **Causal organism:** *Myrothecium roridum* Tode ex Fies. **Symptoms:** Symptoms were small dirty yellow to brown coloured, water soaked spots with a violet periphery and chlorotic halo on the leaves. The spots enlarged coalesced and became brittle. Sporodochia of the fungus were observed in the lower surface of the infected leaves.

Root–knot

Among the phytonematodes, the root–knot nematodes has the widest distribution. Root–knot nematodes are reported to be responsible for the significant reduction in plant growth and yields. **Causal organism:** *Meloidogyne javanica* (Treuk) Chitwood. **Symptoms:** A severe root–knot infection was observed on *W. somnifera*. Infected plants showed yellowing and stunting. Roots of infected plants showed formation of galls, swellings or knots.

Leaf Curl

It is reported in *W. somnifera*. **Causal organism:** Tobacco leaf curl virus. **Symptoms:** The important symptoms of the disease are vein clearing, curling, puckering and occasionally rolling. The surface of infected leaves was wrinkled. Some leaves were malformed.

Witches' Broom

A witches broom disease of *W. somnifera* was reported from Lucknow, India. The disease first appeared in the experimental plantations. The disease then spread to commercial fields causing considerable damage. **Causal organism:** Phytoplasma (Mycoplasma–like organism). **Symptoms:** Typical symptoms of the disease were small leaves, shortening of internodes, excessive branching resulting in witches broom appearance, premature drying and death of infected twigs and leaves. Infected plants remained stunted. **Control:** Treatment of infected plants with tetracycline gave temporary recovery from typical symptoms of the disease after 15–20 days of treatment. Spray with tetracyclines has been recommended for the control of the disease. The recovery of the disease symptoms is often temporary.

It is beyond the scope of the book to describe all the diseases of medicinal plants.

7 PESTS AND PEST MANAGEMENT IN MEDICINAL PLANTS

CAUTION

Though we are presenting the various methods and use of pesticides for control of pests, which are in use by various growers and scientists, however, authors are not recommending them. The authors believe in organic farming only and recommend that the cultivators should use organically produced pesticides.

A HEALTHY PLANT

A plant is healthy when it can carry out its basic physiological functions, including:

Normal cell division, differentiation, and developments;

Absorption of water and minerals from the soil and translocation of these nutrients throughout the plant;

Photosynthesis and translocation of the photosynthetic products to areas of utilization or storage;

Metabolism of synthesized compounds;

Reproduction; and

Storage of food supplies for overwintering or reproduction. Plants become diseased whenever any of these functions are significantly disrupted.

What is Pest?

Any insect that affects the profit of a farmer by harming his or her crops or livestock is called Pest. It may be noted that all insects are not Pests. In other words, there are some useful insects; such as butterfly, honeybee and some parasites on pests.

Control of Pests

There are different methods of Pest control such physical, mechanical, agronomic, biological and chemical. However, farmers usually prefer to apply chemical method in order to avoid loss to crops. But the disadvantage of the chemical method is that, it creates environmental pollution, health hazards, kills the beneficial insects and is very costly system.

Hence one should not depend on a single predominant method, but should utilize all the five methods i.e. physical, mechanical, agronomic, biological and chemical in a safe manner, is an Integrated Pest Management (**IPM**).

For effective and safe measure of pest control, farmers are advised to apply Integrated Pest Management (**IPM**) methods as indicated below;

1. **Physical method:** The pests attack in particular crop at a particular temperature, humidity, sunshine, rainfall and velocity of wind. If farmers are aware of the weather conditions and the life cycle of the their time of growth, they can take care of preventive measures by altering the planting or sowing time of the crop.
2. **Mechanical method:** Carefully collects the pests, their eggs and larvae, and destroys them at regular interval.
3. **Agronomic method**

- Select crops having pest and disease resistant variety.
- Use proper crop rotations.
- Alter sowing / planting time of crops.
- Use the recommended number of ploughing and inter culturing practices.
- Keep the field clean and weed free.
- Use the fertilizer at proper time and in recommended doses.
- Provide timely and light irrigation.

4. **Biological method:**

- Allow the birds to eat the pests and eggs during ploughing and crop growing time.
- Identify the useful parasites and predators on harmful pests.
- Use organic pesticides like neem, tobacco etc. and their products.
- Use repellant like onion, garlic, marigold and tulsi, etc.

ECOLOGICAL PEST MANAGEMENT

Organic and Natural farming, which aim at 'cooperating rather than' confronting with the nature has been hailed as the only answer to bring sustainability to agriculture. In organic farming systems pest control strategies are largely preventative, rather than reactive. Organic farming is not a single method but rather a variety of techniques which are aimed at reducing costs, preserving the environment and protecting human health by eliminating the use of toxic farm chemicals. Masonobu Fukuoka of Japan, considered as the father of Organic farming, has been consistently recording yields of many crops which are comparable to the best yields obtained in Japan, by not using HYVs, chemical fertilizers or pesticides. Use of pesticides and chemical fertilizers does not necessarily lead to better farming than using natural agricultural methods

In the conventional agriculture pests are often controlled with man made chemicals which have following harmful effects:

1. Chemicals kill useful insects which eat pests
2. Chemicals can be very bad for the health of people who use them and people who eat food with small amounts of these chemicals still attached.

3. These chemical can stay in the environment and in the bodies of animals causing problems for many years.
4. They are very simple chemicals and insect pests very quickly, over a few breeding cycles, become unaffected by them.
5. Many farmers in developing countries cannot afford to buy man made chemicals.

Pests–insects, disease causing pathogens, weeds and nematodes are estimated to cause an annual loss of about 33–35 per cent of the potential food production world–wide. In India, according to very conservative estimate, the annual crop losses due to these pests amount to a staggering Rs 25,000 crores. In order to increase agricultural production, many changes have been adopted in the recent past such as use of dwarf high yielding cultivars, higher fertilizer use, increased irrigation sources, intensive cropping, large areas under single crop, extension of new crops in non–conventional areas, large scale movement of seeds etc. All these changes have often led to serious pest problems. The new high yielding cultivars in use today are often more susceptible to pests than the old varieties were. Abundant irrigation and nutrient supply has enabled crops to be grown throughout the year–providing ideal conditions for the pests to multiply. Abandoning many time to planting etc. has further aggravated the problem. With the result, not only the infestation of known major pests has increased, but also hitherto unimportant or unknown pests have emerged as major pests.

The current pest control technology relies heavily on pesticides. The pesticide consumption world–wide which was 148,000 metric tonnes in 1966 has increased to over 302,000 metric tonnes in 1976, the most significant increase being for herbicides which increased from 51,000 to 181,000 metric tonnes. In India, it was nearly 200 metric tonnes in 1955 and about 75,000 tonnes in 1985 and may reach 100,000 tonnes in 1990 and 200,000 tonnes in 2000 AD. Pesticide residues in agricultural commodities are the issue of major concern besides their harmful effects on wild life, and other desirable flora and fauna. Equally worrying thing is about development of resistance in pests to pesticides. There are innumerable instances of insect pests, fungi and weed species showing resistance to pesticide for which they were previously susceptible. Outbreak of American bollworm *Heliothis armigera* in cotton crop in Andhra Pradesh in areas where synthetic pyrethroides were liberally used is indicative of things to come in the future. Such developments have negative impact as it makes room for using higher rate of encourages people to look for chemicals which are more toxic than the ones used previously.

Due to the dangers of using chemical pesticides, there has been a considerable resurgence of interest amongst the scientists to look for alternative methods of pest control. Slowly but steadily there has been growing appreciation about the role of pest resistant cultivars, biological control agents and cultural methods in pest control. These non–chemical or 'bio–environmental' methods are the major components in the integrated management of pests.

The non–chemical methods of pest management certainly form the major components of Organic farming. Management for integration of non–chemical methods of controlling insect pests, disease, weeds and nematodes, is essential for successful organic farming.

Cultural Control

Cultural control is the deliberate manipulation of the environment to make it less favourable for pests by disrupting their reproductive cycles, eliminating their food or making it more favourable for their natural enemies. The following are just a few examples of the diverse ways in which the method can be used.

Sanitation

Sanitation includes the removal or destruction of breeding refuges and over–wintering sites of pests. Removing diseased plants (rouging) or pruning infested parts is important in disease management. To prevent introduction of inoculum, all means of carrying the pathogen should be looked into e.g., seeds or propagating material, water, plant debris, farm–yard manure, implements etc. Collection and destruction of egg masses could be very useful practice in insect management in orchards. Care need to be taken to use well composted manure, as high composting temperature, is expected to damage disease inoculum, weed seeds etc.

The government laws or quarantine play a great role in preventing the introduction of pests by propagating material. The seed certification programmes adopted by the various countries have proved immensely useful in containing the spread of pests.

While it is difficult of check the spread of diseases through irrigation water, systematic weed control along irrigation canals will help in stopping the spread of weed seeds. Similarly, machinery used in an infested field, unless cleaned properly, will aid in spread of disease pathogens and weed seeds. Disinfestation of smaller tools and movement of farm vehicles from less diseased to severely infected fields are general methods of preventing spread of diseases by man and machinery.

Pest population may often be effectively suppressed by destruction of their alternate plant hosts, many may in fact be weeds.

The parasitic weed *Striga* will continue to thrive on sorghum stubbles even after harvest. Unless pulled out, this may be a potential source of infestation in the coming years. Destruction of infested young shoots of sugarcane and the stubbles after harvest helps a great deal in keeping the incidence of sugarcane borer at a very low level.

Tillage

In many developing and under–developed countries, tillage still is the only known method of controlling weeds. The practice however is rapidly being replaced in much of the developed countries with herbicides.

Frequent shallow ploughings given before planting are very effective in controlling annual weeds. This techniques of sowing crop seed in the relatively weed–free soil is termed as 'state seed bed' techniques which is being very widely used in many crops. Being less expensive, this can form an important component of integrated weed management system in many places. However, it may bring back the buried weed seeds on to the surface. Alternatively, a very low dose of a contact herbicide may take care of weeds without disturbing the soil further. Deep ploughing particularly in summer months is very effective against deep rooted perennial weeds as it would expose the underground vegetative parts to hot weather.

With soil tillage, other pests are also killed mainly due to exposure or debris destruction. For example, the wheat sawfly in North Dakota has been reduced by as much as 75 per cent by cultivation .Summer tillage of wheat destroys wheat streak virus reservoirs and viruse's vector the wheat curl mite. Tillage, however, need to be timed to coincide with the susceptible stages of the insects.

Depth of ploughing is also an important factor as burial to atleast 8 cm is necessary to control *Cephalosporium* stripe of wheat, to atleast 15 cm for the bent grass nematode and to atleast 25–30 cm for sorghum downy–mildew . Although the long term effects of reduced tillage have not been studied adequately, some adverse effects are known For example, army worms and corn stalk borers often increase in crops grown under reduced tillage and surface accumulation of crop residues under reduced tillage conditions increases the infestations of termites, slugs, some nematodes and diseases.

Application of Manures and Soil Amendments

Application of soil amendments would change the rhizosphere environment by affecting porosity, aeration, temperature, water holding capacity etc. Healthy crop plants have a greater chance of fighting with pests than under–nourished plants. Besides, soil amendments as such or their decomposition products may have a direct effect. More than thirty disease mainly root rots have been reported to be significantly controlled by application of organic amendments

Incorporation of various kinds of organic amendments to soil also holds promise in long–term control of nematodes. Use of chopped shoots, straw, saw dust, animal manure, cakes etc. have resulted in significant reduction in nematodes population. In India, oil cakes of linseed, mustard, peanut, castor bean, *mahuva, (Madhuca indica)* and neem (*Azadirachta indica*) have proved very effective for nematode control in a variety of crops .

All plant feeding insects have specific nutrient requirements. The incidence of corn leaf hopper (*Dalbulis maidis*) which transmit corn stunt pathogen was reduced at low N levels and at high planting densities .Poor nutrition to crops is also known to affect the reproductive ability of some insects feeding on them .

Increased application of plant nutrients, although, increase the growth of both weeds and crop plants, it benefits crop more. However, increased application of nitrogen is known to reduce *Striga* incidence in cereals. However, other methods of weed control must accompany increased supply of nutrients as weeds are known to deplete large quantities of nutrients from soil, thereby depriving the crop plants of the precious and costly input .

Habitat Diversification

Cropping patterns have undergone drastic changes over the years. Provision of irrigation, development of short duration, photo–insensitive, high yielding varieties of crops have resulted in growing of more number of crops in a year. Consideration of potential pest problems while choosing crops/crop sequences would go a long way in pest management. Following are some of the examples.

Crop rotation

Good crop rotation with non–host plants would result in reduction of pest population either directly by toxic action of the non–host crops or indirectly by depriving them of the food the host plant would have offered had it been grown continuously. Several soil borne diseases of cereal crops are successfully controlled by a crop rotation period of 2–3 years . Soil pathogens that can be controlled by a 3 to 4 year rotation with non–host crops include organisms causing cabbage black rot, bacterial leaf blight of bean and cabbage black leg. Gartic, onion, beet root and Lucerne are suggested as good rotational crops in controlling *Fusarium* wilt of melons and cucumber .Crop rotation is one of the most important measures for controlling plant parasitic nematodes and frequently it appears to be the only economical method for controlling this pest. Effective rotation is widely practised for control of the golden nematode of potatoes, the soybean cyst nematode and the root rust nematode.

Each crop has its own characteristic weeds and they thrive well when the same crop is grown successively. Monoculture of the cereals and use of hormone herbicides have led to serious problems of grass weeds in many parts of the world. In a 3–year study, high populations of *Xanthium pensylvanicum* were associated with soybean than with corn regardless of weed control measures. *Scirups maritamus* a difficult–to–control weed in a continuously flooded low land field was effectively controlled when the rice was rotated with an upland crop.

Rotation is most effective against soil pests (e.g. white grubs, wire worms etc.), which take several years to reach maturity. Until synthetic organic insecticides became available, rotating corn with such crops as oats, clover and soybean was a standard procedure for controlling corn rootworms in mid western United States. In white ant infested areas crops like sugarcane, wheat and chillies should be avoided; instead tobacco or onions maybe grown.

Chief obstacles to success of crop rotations are the pronounced longevity of inoculum/weed seed in soil and frequently wide host ranges of pests. Often populations of a pest other than the target pest may increase on the alternative crop. Some crops used in rotation may often be of very low economic values.

Trap cropping

The practice of attracting pests to small plantings of crops, which are then destroyed or sprayed with a toxicant has been quite successful against some plant nematodes, parasitic weeds and insect pests.

A susceptible crop such as sorghum or sudan grass may be grown before the main crop season to induce germination of *Striga* seeds before it is destroyed. Crops such as groundnut, linseed, cowpea, cotton, sunflower etc. form good rotational crops as they induce germination but are not parasitized by *Striga*.

Some nematodes may also be controlled by trap crops. Highly susceptible crops are allowed to grow in infested fields until the second stage larvae enter the roots and begin to develop. The crop will be destroyed before nematodes mature.

In all these, the plant destruction must properly be timed and implemented, lest the population of pest may increase many–fold.

Intercropping

Inter row space is a potential place for weeds which can be put to better use by intercropping. Intercropping in broad spaced crops such as pigeonpea, sugarcane, cotton, maize, sorghum with fast canopy forming plants, reduce the weed emergence and competition substantially

Lower incidence of insect pests were found on legumes intercropped with maize. Intercrops of clover, spinach, beans and tomato reduced the incidences of *Brevicoryne brassicae* and *Plutella xylostella* in cabbage substantially. Incidence of *Heliothis armigera* reduced in chickpea when grown in association with barley, mustard or whet.

Strip farming

Intervening strip of non–suitable crop prevent movement of insect pests from one strip of a crop to another. Also adjacent strips share unspecialized natural enemies which would move when insect pests build up on the neighbouring strips. The abandonment of strip farming in Peru some years back has been given as the reason for boll worm outbreak on cotton there and certainly re–diversifying the cotton agro–ecosystem has now greatly reduced the incidence of the pest.

Time of Planting

Pest outbreaks occur at particular soil and climatic conditions and planting can be so adjusted that such outbreaks do not coincide with the susceptible stage of the crop.

With diseases, it is reported that the incidences of chickpea wilt and root rot of pea were considerably reduced when the planting was delayed. There are also reports of early sown wheat escaping rust damage and pearl millet sown before 15th July recording less incidence of ergot in North India .

Maize sown late suffers little from damage by maize borer as by then the egg parasite *Trichogramma* is able to keep down the population of the pest. Maize grown in winter is free from borer attack as this pest hibernates during winter. Rice is reported to suffer less from borer attack if transplanted early (before middle of June). Early Maturing cotton varieties (*Bikaneri norma,* H–777 and F–414) have become popular in Punjab and Haryana as they escape pink bollworm attack.

Late sown crop in winter is expected to have less problems with nematodes as they are inactive during this period.

Late planting of wheat reduces infestations of important weeds such as *Chenopedium album,* wild oats (*Avena spp*) and *Phalaris minor.* However, the limitation is, altered planting time may not always be the best one for obtained higher yields.

Water Management

The scab of potato is suppressed by irrigating potato at the time of tuber formation . Wet weather diseases such as halo–blight and anthracnose of beans, early blight and charcoal rot of potatoes can be checked by furrow rather than sprinkler irrigation. Diseases which are favoured by high moisture at the soil surface like damping off or collar rot can be minimized by planting crops in ridges or raised beds. Irrigation often makes it possible to avoid a pest by allowing the crop to be grown out–of–season.

It is a well–known fact that transplanted rice faces very less weed problem compared to other methods, which is mainly due to pudding and impounding of water. Flooding upto 10 to 20 cm early in the season reduced the infestation of many weeds including *Echnochloa crus–galli* but may increase problems with other weeds such as blue green algae. Under irrigated conditions, planting crop–seed in the moisture zone in an otherwise dry seed bed and delaying the first irrigation reduces the weed infestations quite substantially.

Drip irrigation, by virtue of providing water at the base of the plant, results in far lesser weed problem than would be expected from other methods of irrigation. Similarly, overhead sprinkler irrigation in potato effectively controlled potato moth .

Crop Competition

Weeds and crop seeds germinate almost simultaneously and they start competing with each other for water, nutrients and space. Selection of vigorous growing crop cultivar, closer row spacing, higher crop seed rate, proper time and method of fertilizer application etc. are some of the husbandry practices which are likely to play a vital role in weed management. There is much meaning in the saying that *good crop is the best weed killer.*

Among winter cereals, barley is reported to be more competitive than wheat or oat .Maize is having the highest weed suppressing ability (92%) followed by pearl millet (88%), sorghum (81%) and *Setaria* (73%). Amongst non–cereals, cowpea (88%) is more competitive than groundnut (62%), castor (51%) and pigeonpea (54%). Similarly, *Cyperus rotundus* infests lower yield loss in maize and sorghum as compared to groundnut, soybean, and grain legumes .

The high yielding dwarf cultivars of wheat and rice are more vulnerable to weeds and more time is spent in weed removal than in traditional cultivars.

Higher plant population of the crop can put pressure on availability of space for weed growth from relatively early stages of crop growth. Narrow row spacing, higher seed rate and cross sowing all have suppressing effect on weeds.

Close planting tend to produce microenvironment ideal for some fungal diseases, while with others, the same environment may prevent diseases by discouraging an insect vector from feeding. Dense seeding of many crops reduces the losses in yield caused by pathogens and insect pests by providing more plants per hectare.

PHYSICAL AND MECHANICAL CONTROL

Manual Control

Despite major advances in chemical control, hand removal of weeds still remains to be the most practical method of weed control in many developing countries of the world for a variety of reasons. Although back–breaking and laborious hand weeding is quite effective if employed at the right time.

Such manual destruction of other pests is not practicable although, it could be followed to some extent in controlling of some insect pests in orchards, like collecting and destructing the egg masses, mechanical exclusion of insects by placing impenetrable barriers around the host plant etc.

Burning

Flaming with propane burners of infested plants or weeds was practiced widely in western countries before the introduction of chemical pesticides. Burning rice straw has been reported to result in reduced incidence of stem rot of rice caused by *Sclerotium oryzae* . Burning crop residues under direct seeding and reduced tillage conditions has shown to reduce infestation of several pests including weeds.

Flooding

The classical example of use of flooding is for the control of banana wilt. Chlamydospores of *Fusarium* are killed by restricted supply of oxygen in the water stagnated fields. Other fungi showing significant control by flooding are *Verticillium dahliae* in cotton, *Sclerotinia sclerotiorum* in cauliflower and fungus causing black tobacco and bacterial blight of cotton Flooding also effectively controls many arable weeds and that is the reason for reduced weed infestation in transplanted rice as compared to direct seeded rice, as has been discussed earlier.

Many plant parasitic nematodes are reported to be susceptible to flooding .However, a flooding period of 4–8 months is required for effective control of root knot nematodes, which is naturally a limiting factor.

BIOLOGICAL CONTROL

Although still grossly underused, biological control is gaining world recognition as a primary and often essential component of successful integrated pest management.

Classical biological control involves deliberate introduction and establishment of natural enemies in areas where they did not previously occur. The approach is used largely against pests of foreign origin.

In addition to deliberate introduction of biocontrol agents, proper attention needs to be given for conservation and augmentation of natural enemies, that already exist in an area. This need to be treated as an important element in pest management for many insect parasites are much more susceptible to insecticides than the pests they attack.

Biological control agents for insect pests are available in nature abundantly. Several pathogens including viruses such as nuclear polyhedrosis viruses (NPV) and granulosis viruses (GV), bacteria like *Bacillus thuringensis,* fungi like *Metarhizium, Beauveria* and *Verticillium* and protoza like *Schizogregarine* cause diseases in insects and destroy them. Similarly, several insect–parasitoids (parasities thriving on insects) are also known in nature. *Trichogramma* is an egg parasitoid of several pests, particularly of sugarcane internode borer. *Goniozus, Elasmus, Eriborus, Bracon, Trichospilus, Tetrastichus* and *Chelonus* are some of the other parasitoids attacking insect pests. Insect predators such as *Chiloconus, Pharoscymnus, Cryptolaemus, Scymnus* and *Menochilus* feed on mealy bugs, coccids, scales and mites on citrus, grapevine and guava. The mirid predator *Cyrtorhinus* attack brown plant hopper of rice. The green lace wing *Chrysopa,* another most effective insect predator feeds on aphids, mealy bug and young caterpillars.

In biological control of weeds, there is always a fear of biological control agents attacking the crop plants and also a plant considered a weed in one place may not be so in another area. Because of this specificity, the attempts have been primarily against controlling weeds in range lands, forest areas, aquatic environment and parasitic weeds.

Some promising examples include: control of *Eupatorium odorata* by leaf eating caterpillar *Parenchaetus pseudoinsulata;* lantana by *Telenomia scrupulosa; Salvania molesta* (aquatic weed) by *Paulinia acuiminata* (grass hopper); water hyacinth by *Neochetina eichhorniae* and *N. bruchi; Parthenium* by Zogogramula bicolorata *and Smicronyx lutulentus* .Good control of a variety of aquatic weeds by Chinese grass carp (*Ctenopharyangdon idella*) has received world–wide attention. In Japan, there is limited use of tadpole shrimp (*Triopus* spp) to control weeds in flooded rice fields. At the IRRI, the cover effect of *Azolla* spp. is being evaluated as a means of weed control in rice.

In aquatic weed control, biological control holds great potential, as use of chemicals need to be limited because of multifacet uses of water, and mechanical or manual methods are cost prohibitive, and requires frequent treatments.

Increasing the Effectiveness of Bio–control

Artificial structures: Suitable nesting boxes are kept for predatory birds and wasps (*Polistes* spp.) and burlap traps are placed around citrus trees for attracting coccinellid predatory (*Cryptolaemus montrouzieri*) of mealybug.

Food and shelter: Pollen–and nectar–bearing flowering plants are planted on the bunds to provide supplementary food to predatory like chrysopids, coccinellids, predatory mites, syrphid flies and parasitoids.

Controlling ants: Ants interfere with the activities of predators and parasitoids. Control and physical exclusion of ants by putting a band of some botanical around the trunk in citrus orchards increases the efficiency of coccinellid predatory (*Cryptolaemus montrouzieri*) and several parasitoids.

Cultural practices: Avoiding of trash burning in sugarcane protects the parasitoid *Tetrastichus pyrillae* of sugarcane pyrilla. Strip–cutting in alfalfa helps in shifting of the predators to nearby cotton corp. Regular removal of fallen fruits of apple and their destruction reduces the overall population of codling moth. The egg parasitoids released in such orchards are much more effective.

There are a number of examples wherein cultural lowering of the pest population gives more opportunity for the natural enemies to be effective. Thus, if the water shoots in citrus are removed, the populations of leaf–miner, scale–insects, citrus psylla and mealy–bug are reduced.

Trap crops: This is a strategy by which biological control could be made more effective and economic. The target host is attracted to the border rows of a trap crop which is much more preferred than the main crop. The attracted pest on trap crop is more amenable to be economically tackled through biological control in a restricted area. Planting of castor around tobacco nurseries and marigold around main crop for attracting *Spodoptera* and *Helicoverpa* (*Heliothis*) respectively, and releasing egg parasitoids or spraying nuclear polyhedrosis virus could give effective suppression.

Conditions for effectiveness: The time and period of release should be suitable for the natural enemy. It should synchronize with the availability of suitable stage of the pest the release of Trichogrammatid egg parasitoid would be more effective if the release is based on information collected through pheromone traps. Using suitable strain (through artificial selection) adopted to a particular crop ecosystem and pest–management practices increases the success of biological control.

The searching efficacy of parasitoids is increased by applying certain chemicals called fairomones, which are originally isolated from their host species (an example is Trichogrammatid egg parasitoids). Phago–stimulants are applied to the plants to increase the ingestion of leaves sprayed with microbial agents.

For discouraging the activity of hyperparasites, parasitoids should be released at a time when the activity of hyperparasitoids is the least.

Legislation: The Government of India banned the export of frogs, because 90% of the food of frogs is agricultural pests. It has been estimated that catching frogs for export led to the survival of 200,000 tonnes of pests, thereby requiring farmers to spend more on pest control. Legislation is required to ban all such actions which directly or indirectly kill beneficial insects.

Conservation of Biodiversity

Biodiversity should be documented and properly inventoried, so that it can be utilized better. Otherwise, several species facing the threat of extinction will be wiped out before they are studied and named. It will also helps as plan conservation measures.

Conservation of Natural Enemies

Several ways of conservation of natural enemies have been attempted in the past. The use of relatively safer pesticides, and their selective use could conserve the biotic agents. Several other methods of enrichment and conservation of natural enemies include providing artificial structures (nesting boxes for wasps and predatory birds, burlap traps for C. montrouzieri), planting or retaining food and shelter plants of biotic agents on the bunds (retaining pollen and nectar bearing flowering plants Euphorbia, wild clover, etc. to provide supplementary food to parasitoids and predatory; rice gall midges and plant hoppers and their natural enemies survive on weeds like, *Cyperus* during off season and later shift to rice crop providing early suppression of the pests), placing bundles of rice straw for attracting spiders, retention of crop stubble, grass weed heaps for maintaining predator population, collecting egg masses of borers and putting them in a bamboo cage cum percher (which permits escape of egg parasitoids and allow the predatory birds to perch, and trap and kill the hatching larvae) are effective. In addition to nest boxes, nesting material, perching sites and water pans, retaining bushes (*Acalypha, Hibiscus*, crotons, etc.) helps retention or predatory birds in the desired area. Controlling ants (which interfere with the activity of biotic agents), avoiding complete trash burning (to conserve sugarcane pyrilla parasitoids), regular removal of fallen fruits (to increase the effectiveness of egg parasitoids due to overall lowering of population of the pests), strip cutting of alfalfa (to increase biotic agents in the adjoining crops), use of trap crops (planting castor around tobacco attracts *S. litura* to deposit the egg masses which are either collected or T. remus in released), use of semiochemicals or kairomones (to increase the searching ability and retention of the parasitoids, of gall midge, lafhopper and other pests from wild hosts to rice), use of organic manures instead of chemical fertilizers (to conserve predaceous arthropods such as carabid beetles and enhance the efficiency of plant disease antagonists), synchronizing the release of parasitoid with the availability of appropriate stage of the host and enacting suitable legislation (to prevent indiscriminate killing of beneficial organisms) have been suggested from time to time. Per cent parasitism of yellow stem borer (*Scirpophaga incertulas*) egg masses is significantly more in transplanted rice than direct seeding, which indicates the importance of the method of planting in attracting natural enemies.

Biopesticides

The natural occurrence of diseases caused by microorganism is common in both insect and weed populations and is a major natural mortality factor in many situations. For many practical reasons however, use of microorganisms for pest control involve their culture in artificial media and later introduction of comparatively large amounts of inoculum into the field at an appropriate time and place. The technique is possible only with those microorganisms that can be readily cultured in artificial media and moreover than can be induced to produce spores or other suitable resting stages which permit storage and application. Many fungi and bacteria can be handled in this way but insect viruses have the limitation that they have to be raised in living insects. This is unfortunate as insect viruses probably have greater potential for pest control than any other group of microorganisms because of their virulence and selectivity.

As these biocontrol agents (microbial pathogens) are applied on the targeted pests in much the same way as chemical pesticides, they are often termed as *biopesticides* or *natural pesticides*. Microbial phytotoxins, allelochemicals and other biocides of plant origin are also discussed here.

Bacillus thuringensis a bacterial pathogen infecting a wide range of insect pests is the most common microbial insecticide in use today. The disease agent is marketed by several companies and is registered for use against the insect caterpillar pests that attack a wide variety of vegetables, flower and ornamental crops. Unlike most chemical insecticides, it can be used on edible products upto the time of harvest. It is selective in action and does not harm parasites or predators of pests of any extent.

Another bacterium *B. popilale* is also commercially available for insect control which is effective against the white grubs *Popillae japonica* and *Hototrichia* spp.

Amongst insect pathogenic fungi, commercial preparations of *Verticillium lecanii* are now available for control of aphids, thrips and whitefly under glass house conditions Effectiveness out of doors is unlikely to be reliable because of the requirement for high humidity for infection to take place.

Several mycoherbicides have been registered in the USA for commercial use of weed control. One such is the formulation of soil–borne fungus *Phytophthora palmivora* for selective control of strangler (milk weed) vine *Morrenia odorata* in citrus groves. Marketed under the trade name 'De vine', it causes lethal root rots of its host plant and persists saprophytically in the soil for extended periods of time.

Extensive research during the last two decades has demonstrated that several plant secondary metabolities (allelochemicals) as well as fungal and microbial foxins posses good pesticidal activity. *Biolophos* isa natural phytotoxin isolated from the fermentation broth of *Streptomyces hygroscopicus* and *S. viridochromogenes* and exhibits strong herbicidal activity against a wide range of grass and broad leaf weeds following application to their foliage. It is currently being marketed in Japan under the trade name *Herbiaceae*. Neem has long been known to have insecticidal properties and applications of neem extracts have been recommended for deterring insect attack, particularly locuss. Vikwood Ltd., USA has formulated a neem seed extract 'Margosan O'. The National Chemical Laboratories, Pune in India has also been successful in developing neem formulations with antifeedant/insecticidal properties.

The allelochemical from marigold–*terthicyl* was found to be highly nematicidal. Another compound *cucurbitacins* has also bee found to be equally effective in controlling nematode populations.

Botanicals Some useful weeds like Lantana, Notchi, Tulsi, Adathoda etc; act as natural repellent to many pests. The indigenous trees like pungam, wood apple, anona and their byproducts have excellent insecticidal value in controlling diamond black moth, heliothis, white files, leafhopper and aphid infestation. The fish oil resin soap (FOS) is a safe, non–posionous natural product used for the control of developed whitefiles, mealybug, wooly aphid etc. A wider range of bio extracts are proved to be more effective in controlling many insect pests and diseases.

Farmers in their traditional wisdom have identified and used a variety of plant products and extracts for pest control, especially in storage. As many as 2121 plant species are reported to possess pest management properties, 1005 species of plants exhibiting insecticidal properties, 384 with antifeedant properties, 297 with repellent properties, 27 with attractant properties and 31 with growth inhibiting properties have been identified. The most–commonly used botanicals are neem (Azadirachta indica), pongamia (Pongamia glabra) and manhua (Madhuca indica). Neem seed kernel extract (2 to 5%) has been found effective against several pests including rice cutworm, diamond backmoth, rice brown plant hopper, rice green leafhoppers, tobacco caterpillar, several species of aphids and mites. Mahua seed kernel extract (5%) is effective against sawfly (Athalia lugens proxima)and others.

The efficacy of vegetable oils in preventing infestation of stored product pests such as bruchids (Callosorbuchus spp.), rice and maize weevils (Sitophitus spp.) has been well documented. Root extracts of Tagetes or Asparagus work as a nematicide for plant parasitic nematodes. Similarly, leaf extracts of many higher plants can inhibit a number of fungal pathogens. A number of plants like *Chenopodium, Bougainvillea,* etc. have also been reported to be sources of antiviral principle.

SOME PREPARATIONS FROM BOTANICALS

Pongam (*Deris indica*)

Pongam extracts serve as natural pesticides. They can be used for controlling a variety of pests. In this section information regarding preparation of various extracts is given.

Pongam Leaf Extract

For 5 litres of water, 1 kilogram Pongam leaf is required. The leaves are soaked overnight in water. The next day the leaves are ground and the extract is filtered. To the extract, an emulsifier is added at the rate of 1 ml/litre. Khadi Soap solution is used as an emulsifier. Khadi soap is soaked overnight in water and the solution is used. The emulsifier helps the extract to stick well to the leaf surface. This extract is beneficial against the leaf eating caterpillars.

Pongam Kernel Extract

50 gms of Pongam kernel powder is required for use in 1 litre of water. The Pongam kernel is pounded gently. It should be pounded in such a way that no oil comes out. The outer coat is removed before pounding. This is used as a manure. The pounded kernel powder is gathered in a muslin pouch and this is soaked overnight in water. The pouch is squeezed and the extract is filtered. To the filtrate, an emulsifier like khadi soap solution is added. One ml of emulsifier is added to one litre of water. 5 kg of Pongam kernel powder is required for preparation of 100 litres of seed kernel extract which can be used for one acre.

Pongam Cake Extract

100 gm of Pongam cake is required for use in 1 litre of water. The Pongam cake is powdered well and tied in a muslin pouch and soaked overnight in water. The next morning the pouch is squeezed

and the extract is taken out. The extract is then filtered and emulsifier is added at the rate of 1 ml for 1 litre of water. It is now ready for spraying. 10 kg of Pongam cake is required for preparation of 100 litres of spray, which can be used for one acre.

Pongam Oil Spray

30 ml of Pongam oil is required for 1 litre of water. The oil is added to the emulsifier (1 ml/1 litre) and stirred well. It is very essential to add the emulsifier and mix properly. This enables the oil to mix with water well. To this, add 1 litre of water and stir well. It should be used immediately. Otherwise, oil droplets start floating. 3 litres of Pongam oil is required for preparation of 100 litres of oil spray, which can be used for one acre.

Pongam–Neem Oil Extract

Pongam oil and Neem oil should be mixed in the ratio of 1:4. Mix 10 ml Pongam oil and 40 ml Neem oil with the emulsifier (1 ml/1 litre). It should be mixed well to enable the water to mix with the oil properly. To this add one litre of water. Shake it well and spray the mixture immediately.

Pongam, Aloe and Neem Extract

1 kg of pounded Pongam cake, 1 kg of pounded Neem cake and 250 gms of pounded Poisonnut tree seeds are taken in a muslim pouch. This is soaked overnight in water. In the morning the pouch is squeezed and the extract is taken out. This is mixed with 1/2 litre of Aloe vera leaf juice. To this 15 litres of water is added. This is again mixed with 2–3 litres of cow's urine. Before spraying 1 litre of this mixture is diluted with 10 litres of water. For an acre 60–100 litres of spray is used. This controls pests of cotton and crossandra effectively.

*Tulsi or Basil (*Oscimum *spp)*

Use of Tulasi for pest control has a long history. It has been traditionally used in Phillipines to repel mosquitoes. It has both repellent and herbicidal properties. Various extracts can be prepared from dried and powdered leaves, flowers and entire plants but their effectiveness appears to vary. Whole plants can be dried and used a san effective insect repellent. In this section information regarding preparation of various extracts is given.

Preparation of Tulasi leaf extract

100 gms of Tulasi leaves are needed to prepara 1 litre extract. The leaves should be soaked in water overnight. The next day the leaves are ground and the extract is filtered. To this 1 ml of khadi soap solution is added and stirred properly. This can be sprayed in the morning hours for effective control of pests.

Aloe *spp.*

Aloe has anti fungal and anti bacterial properties. It also has an attractant property when mixed with castor cake. *Aloe* in combination with other plant products also control a variety of pests efficiently. In this section we can see how various *Aloe* extracts can be prepared.

Aloe–Notchi Extract

For preparation of 50 litres of this extract we require 2 litres of *Aloe* leaf juice. For extracting *Aloe* juice the outer part of the leaves are removed and the mucilaginous part is taken and ground. 5 kg of Notchi leaves (*Vitex negundo*) are taken and immersed in water (enough water to soak the leaves). These leaves are boiled for half an hour and the extract is filtered. The *Aloe* juice and the Notchi extract are mixed together. This can be diluted in 50 litres of water and sprayed.

Melia azadircta

The leaves, bark and fruits are accredited with insect repellant properties. Leaves are placed inside books and folds of woolen garments to protect them from ancient times. The active principle is reported to be an alkaloid, soluble in hot water. A caretenoid, meliatin present in the aqueous extract of leaves acts as a repellant to grasshoppers. The preparation of different *Melia* extracts are described.

Preparation of Melia Extracts

Leaf Extract

For 5 litres of water, 500 grams of green *Melia* leaf is required. Since the quantity of leaves required for preparation of this extract is quite high, (nearly 40 kilograms are required for 1 hectare) this can be used for nursery and kitchen gardens. The leaves are soaked overnight in water. The next day, the leaves are ground and the extract is filtered. To the extract, an emulsifier like khadi soap is added. The emulsifier helps the extract to stick well to the leaf surface.

Kernel Extract

25 gms of *Melia* kernel is required for use in 1 litre of water. The *Melia* kernel is pounded gently. It should be pounded in such a way that no oil comes out. The outer coat is removed before pounding. This is used as a manure. If pounded with seed coat, one and half times seeds are required. The pounded kernel powder is gathered in a muslin pouch and this is soaked overnight in the water. The pouch is squeezed and the extract is filtered. To the filtrate, an emulsifier like soap oil or khadi soap is added. One ml of emulsifier is added to one litre of water.

Cake Extract

50 gms of *Melia* cake is required for 1 litre of water. The *Melia* cake is put in a muslin pouch and soaked in water. It is soaked overnight before use in the morning. It is then filtered and emulsifier is added at the rate of 1 ml for 1 litre of water. It is now ready for spraying.

Oil Spray

15 ml Melia oil is added to the emulsifer (1 ml/litre). It is very essential to add the emulsifier and mix properly. To this, add 1 litre of water and stir well. Only then will the oil and water mix well. It should be used immediately. Otherwise oil droplets start floating.

Custard apple (Annona spp)

The seeds of custard apple possess insecticidal and anti–feedant properties. The powdered seeds are used to destroy worms. Seeds are reported to be contact poison to flies, aphids and several beetles. The combined seed extract of neem and custard apple is toxic to housefly. It is also used as a nematicide. Different alkaloids namely annonine, municine, artabotrine etc. are reported to be found in custard apple. In this section, we shall see how various extract can be prepared.

Custard Apple Leaf Extract

Take 500 grams of custard apple leaves and boil it in 1–2 litres of water. Allow to boil till it becomes $1/4^{th}$ of its original volume. Mix it with 10–15 litres of water and spray over the crop. For an acre, 2–3 kg of leaves are required.

Custard Apple, Calotropis, Tobacco Extract

Take 500 grams of custard apple leaves and boil it in 1–2 litres of water. Allow to boil till it becomes thick. Filter the solution to get the decoction. Take 250 to 300 ml of calotropis extract. Take 500 grams of tobacco leaves and boil it in 1 to 2 litres of water for 45 minutes. Then filter the extract. Take 250 ml of biogas waste (whitish fluid which deposits in the biogas digester) and 100 grams of copper sulphate. Mix the above ingredients with 60 litres of water and spray it over the crop. The above quantity is recommended for an acre.

Custard Apple, Neem, Chilli Extract

Take 2 kg of custard apple leaves and grind it well. Add 500 ml of water and stir it well. Filter to get the extract. The filtrate is kept aside. Take 500 grams of dry fruits of chilli and soak it in water overnight. Next day, grind it and filter the solution to get the extract. Take 1 kg of crushed neem fruits and soak it in 2 litres of water overnight. Filter the extract. Mix all the 3 filtrates with 50–60 litres of water. Filter it again and spray over the crops.

Note: For all the above extracts, add 250 ml of khadi soap solution as an emulsifier before spraying.

Vitex nirgundo

The leaves of vitex are reported to possess insecticidal properties. They are used in storage godowns to ward off insects. Extracts of the leaves and twigs show anti bacterial activities. Vitex in combination with other plant extracts proves to be successful in controlling certain pests. In this section, we shall see how various extracts can be prepared.

Vitex Leaf Extract

Take 2 kg of vitex leaves and soak it in 5 litres of water over night. The next day boil the leaves for 30 minutes and filter and extract. Mix the extract with 10 litres of water and spray. To the extract, add an emulsifier at the rate of 1 ml per litre before spraying. Khadi soap solution is used as an emulsifier. The emulsifier helps the extract to stick well to the leaf surface. For an acre, 6 kg of leaves are required.

Vitex, Aloe Extract

Take 5 kg of vitex leaves and immerse it in 10 litres of water. Boil the leaves for 1/2 an hour and filter the extract. Take 2 kg of aloe leaves and remove the outer part of the leaves. Take the mucilaginous part and ground well with water to get the extract. Mix the above 2 extract with 50–60 litres of water before spraying. To this, add emulsifier at the rate of 1 ml per litre. The above quantity is recommended for an acre.

Vitex, Pongam, Castor, Calatropis Extract

Take 7 kg each of vitex, pongam and castor leaves and 4 kg of small calatropsis leaves. Grind the above ingredients into powder. Mix it with 20 litres of water and boil it for half–an hour. Keep it overnight and filter the extract the next day. Dilute the filtrate with 100 litres of water and spray it over the crops.

Sweet Flag in Pest Control

The powdered rhizome is used as an insecticide for the destruction of fleas, bed bugs, moths, lice etc. It is effective in killing insect pests of stored grains and is considered to be better than chemicals which pose the problem of residual toxicity. The ether extract of the rhizome exhibits ovicidal and insecticidal properties with no residual toxicity. The alcoholic extract inhibits the growth of certain fungi.

Rhizome Extract

Dry the rhizomes in the sun and powder it well. Take 100 gms of rhizome powder and mix it with 4 litres of water. Leaves the solution as such for a day. To this solution, add emulsifier at the rate of 4 ml / litre. The emulsifier could be Khadi soap. It helps the extract to stick well to the leaf surface. 500 gms of rhizome powder is needed to spray for an acre.

Seed Treatment with Rhizome Powder and Cow's Urine

Boil 10 litres of water and cool it the previous day itself. Next morning, add 4 litres of Cow's urine and 200 gm of rhizome powder to the cooled water. Stir it well. Then add seeds, which are to be sown to this solution and mix it well. Remove the damaged seeds, which float on the surface of the solution. Allow the remaining seeds in the same solution for 15 minutes. Filter the solution and separate the seeds. These seeds can be sown directly in the field. This gives protection and resistance against pathogens and pests. 1 litre of cow's urine and 50 gm of rhizome powder is required for treating 1 kg of seed.

Poison nut, Agave, Neem, Pongam Extract

Take leaves of agave, poison nut, neem and pongam in equal quantities. Pound the leaves and soak it in the required quantity of cow's urine overnight. Then filter the solution and dilute it with 50–60 litres of water. Spray this mixture over the crops such as cotton and kanagambaram (*Balenia sp.*). This controls diseases and pests of the crops. For one acre, 2 kg of the above ingredients each and 10–20 litres of cow's urine is required.

Garlic

Garlic is a safe pesticide. It causes no adverse effects on man, animals and environment. One has to take care not to use mineral fertilizers in garlic cultivation since this reduces the concentration of effective substances. The effectiveness of garlic as a pesticide is due to an acrid volatile oil which contains diallyl disulphide, diallyl trisulphide and sulphoxides derived from allicin contained in it.

Various extracts of garlic can be used for pest control. The whole plant, bulbs, leaves and flowers may be used either fresh or dried. Preparation of different Garlic extracts are given in this section.

The preparations/extracts should be used as soon as it is prepared due to the volatile nature of the oil. It remains effective for 4–13 days after application.

Preparation of Garlic Extracts

Bulb Extract

Add 85 grams of chopped garlic to 50 ml of mineral oil (Kerosene). Allow this to stand for 24 hours. Then mix it with 450 ml of water to which 10 ml of soap solution has been added. Shake this mixture well and filter it through a fine cloth. Store this in a container. For application, dilute one part of the emulsion with nineteen parts of clear water. For example, 50 ml of emulsion is mixed with 950 ml of water. The best time to spray it is in the morning. Shake well before application.

Oil Emulsion

Take 50 ml of garlic oil and mix it with an emulsifier, (1 ml/litre of extract). The emulsifier could be soap oil or khadi soap solution. Emulsifier helps the extract to stick well to the leaf surface. Mix the emulsifier properly. To this, add 950 ml of clear water. Stir this well. Only then will the oil and water mix well. This extract should be used immediately. Otherwise oil droplets will start floating. A knapsack sprayer is better for oil emulsion spraying in preference to a hand sprayer.

Garlic–Neem spray

Take 1/2 a handful of neem seeds, 1 kg of garlic, 10 kg neem leaf (tender branches included) and 0.5 kg stem and root bark of Neem. Crush these and reduce it to pulp. To this, add 12 litres of water. Boil this in copper or clay vessel on slow fire till it is reduced to half. If Neem seeds are not available, add 50 g of Neem oil to the finished preparation or boil the mixture to increase viscosity of preparation. After boiling, allow the mixture to cool. Pass this preparation through a sieve and collect the filtered liquid. The material left over in sieve is fibrous. Grind this well and mix it with a light application of neem oil and a small quantity of turmeric boiled in water. Pack it in cellophane bags. This can be spread on ground before cultivation and on plants. This will prevent disease bearing insects and flies from resting on plants. It can be used in addition to the liquid spray, if necessary. Allow the boiled liquid preparation that has been filtered to settle for 4–5 weeks in a sealed jar. At the end of the period, filter it again so that it can be used in a sprayer. For maximum effect, use it at regular intervals of 3 days, and increase it from 3 to 7 days as plants grow. In wet weather, reduce the intervals and apply the undiluted preparation.

Green Chilli–Garlic Extract

Take Green Chilli and Garlic in equal quantities. Grind it together and prepare an extract. Mix it with water in the proportion of 1:200 and sprinkle over crops. This is very effective against aphids and jassids.

Garlic with other Plant Extracts in Cow's Urine

The extracts of Garlic, Chilli, Ginger, Neem oil, Tobacco, Asafoetida are dissolved in 72 hours old Cow's urine and dissolved. Before spraying, an emulsifier is added. For spraying in cotton 30–40 ml of this spray is used with 15 ml of water and 70 ml per 15 ml water is used for spraying in pigeonpea.

Garlic–Pepper Extract

Take two finely grated Garlic bulbs and two teaspoon pepper. Sitr into four litres of hot water. Add a nut sized piece of soap and spray. This is very effective in controlling caterpillars on fruit trees.

*Sweetflag (*Acorus calamus*) for general disease resistance and increasing germination*

Paddy seeds required for sowing in 1 acre of land should be taken. This would be roughly 35 kilos. These seeds should be soaked for two days in water and it should have sprouted. In fact, it should be ready for sowing in the nursery.

Quarter kilo of sweet flat (*Acorus calamus*) should be powdered and soaked in 3 litres of water. This should be soaked overnight. Filter the extract next day. Take 1 litre of this extract and dilute it in 5 litres of water. Soak the sprouted paddy seeds in this extract for half an hour. Dry it in shade for 10 minutes before sowing. By this treatment the germinating capacity increases and also the plant becomes resistance to a wide variety of diseases.

Use of Mint in seed treatment for increasing crop growth and yield

The following is a recipe for increasing crop growth and yield. 200 grams of mint (*Mentha arvensis*) leaves should be mixed with water and ground well. To this 5 litres of water should be added. The sprouted paddy seeds should be soaked in this for half an hour. It should then be shade dried. After this it could be sown. This helps in increasing the crop growth and yield.

Use of Neem for Pest Management

The neem tree (*Azadirachta indica*) is native to tropical South East Asia. It is fast growing, can survive drought and poor soil keeps its leaves all year round. It is a tall tree, up to 30 metres high, with leafy spreading branches. Many white flowers, which smell of honey appear for the first time when the tree is 2 to 3 years old, and the tree bears fruit at 3 to 4 years. The ripe fruit are about 2 cm long and oval shaped. Inside the fruit there is a light–coloured seed about 1.5 cm long.

Although thousand–year–old Sanskrit medical writings mention neem's usefulness, the tree's exciting potential for controlling insects has only recently become clear.

First report about Neem's ability to repeal insects was is in the scientific literature in 1928 and 1929. Two Indian scientists, R.N. Chopra and M.A. Husain, used a 0.001–percent aqueous suspension of ground neem kernels to repel desert locusts. Not until 1962, however, was the real significance demonstrated. That year in field tests in New Delhi, S. Pradhan ground up neem kernels in water and sprayed the resulting suspension over different crops. He found that, although locusts landed on the plants, they refused to eat anything, sometimes for up to 3 weeks after the treatment. Furthermore, she noted that neem kernels were even more potent than the conventional insecticides then available and that neem's repellency was as important as its toxicity. In neighboring insecticide–treated fields, for instance, the insects also died, but not before consuming the crops.

Neem based pesticides are suitable for use in developing countries because the useful chemicals can be easily removed from the neem without the use of expensive and complicated equipment.

Uses of Neem

Almost every part of the tree is used.

1. The wood of the neem tree is strong and resistant to termite damage. It is also good for firewood and making charcoal.
2. The neem tree is good for shade and is often planted for shade on roadsides.
3. Neem extracts are used to treat many health problems. People bathe in neem water to relieve heat rashes and boils. Neem oil is used against stomach ulcers and rheumatism Neem bark contains a strong antiseptic and neem is used to make soap and toothpaste. Neem twigs are used to clean teeth.
4. Neem leaves can be used to make soil less acid.
5. Extracts from the neem tree are also used as mosquito repellents, fertilizers, diabetic food and animal feed.
6. Neem cake, which is left over when oil has been removed from seeds, and leaves, can improve the soil and add plant food and acts as nitrification inhibitor.

Although it has many used, the most important use for neem products is to fight against crop pests and diseases.

Worldwide approximately one third of crops in the field and store are lost to pests each year. The worst affected are maize and rice in Africa and Asia.

Neem for Pest Control

Different parts of the neem tree can affect more than 200 insect species and some nematodes, fungi, bacteria and viruses. Neem contains several active chemicals, which work in different ways; as a result of this, pests are unlikely to become resistant to neem. The most well known chemical in neem is **azadirachtin**. Neem is easy to prepare and use, and is environmentally safe and not harmful to man and animals.

Neem protects itself from the multitude of pests with a multitude of pesticidal ingredients. Its main chemical broadside is a mixture of 3 or 4 related compounds, and it backs these up with 20 or so others that are minor but nonetheless active in one way or another. In the main, these compounds belong to a general class of natural products called *triterpenes*; more specifically, *limonoids*.

Methods of Application

Neem extracts can be applied in many ways, including some of the most sophisticated. For example, they may be employed as sprays, powders, drenches, or diluents in irrigation water–even through trickle– or subsurface–irrigation systems. In addition, they can be applied to plants through injection or topical applications, either as dusts or sprays. Moreover, they can be added to baits that attract insects (a process used, for instance, with cockroaches). They are even burned. For example, neem leaves and seeds and dry neem cake are ingredients in some mosquito coils

No new or unusual technology is required for any of the processing. It can be done using either simple village–scale technology or high–technology methods and industrialized facilities. The most common procedures are summarized below.

Water Extraction

The simplest technique (and the most widely employed today) is to crush or grind the kernels and extract them with water. They may, for example be steeped overnight in a cloth bag suspended in a barrel of water. For reasons not yet understood, this process is less effective than pouring the water into the bag and collecting the extract as it emerges. The resulting crude suspension can be used in the field without further modification. It can also be filtered and employed as a spray–able emulsion.

Water extracts of ground neem leaves are also very useful. Because neem is an evergreen, they are obtainable throughout the year.

Hexane Extraction

If the kernels are grated and steeped in the solvent hexane, only the oil is removed. The oil is not considered an active pesticide. However, new results show that it is an especially interesting material,, which in certain cases can be used to kill the eggs of many types of insect, the larvae of mosquitoes, and various stages of certain pests (such as leafhoppers) that are often hard to control by other means.

The residue left after hexane extraction still contains the main active limonoid ingredients, and subsequent extractions with water or alcohol produce them in large amounts, clean and uncontaminated by oil.

Formulations

As noted, the simplest neem pesticide is a crude extract. However, for more sophisticated use, modifications can be made. These advanced formulations may convert neem extracts into the form of granules, dust, wettable powders, or emulsifiable concentrates. Aqueous extracts can also be formulated with soap for ease of application against skin disease.

Other formulations may involve the addition of chemicals or even the chemical modification of the neem ingredients themselves. These changes may be made to increase shelf stability and reproducibility, and for ease of handling or of scaling up the process. They may also reduce phytotoxicity, the damage to sensitive plants.

One particularly valuable class of additives are those that inhibit ultraviolet degradation. These include sesame oil, lecithin, and *para*–aminobenzoic acid (PABA).

When neem products are exposed to light they begin to lose their ability to control pests. For this reason the commercial neem based insecticide, Margosan–O, that is sold in the USA, contains a sunscreen.

Additives

Mixing neem extracts with other materials can boost their power 10–20–fold. Among these so–called "promoters" are sesame oil, phrethrins (a type of insecticide mostly extracted from chrysanthemum flowers), and piperonyl butoxide. They are used to produce a quicker kill.

Combinations with synthetic pesticides also can work well–they add rapid "knockdown" to neem's ability to suppress the subsequent rebound in the pest population. The effectiveness of neem extracts can even be boosted with the insect–killing bacterium *Bacillus thuringensis* (Bt) to provide a multifaceted pesticide.

Practical methods for preparations

Control of Stored Grain Pest

Dried Neem leaves are mixed with storage grains . When neem is used in this way pests can be kept from the grain for a whole year; but if the grain is already infected with pests the protection will not work.

Method 1

- A ½ cm (1/2 inch) layer of fresh neem leaves, is placed in the bottom of a storage container.
- A layer of sun dried grain (up to 30 cm) is placed on top of this followed by another layer of neem leaves
- These layers can be repeated until the container is full, finishing with a good layer of leaves.
- Neem leaves for grain storage

Method 2

- Dry neem leaves in the sun so that the leaves stay green. Grind them into a powder. Mix the powder with clay and water. Plaster the inside walls of the storage container with the mixture and allow to dry
- Place a layer of neem leaves,, which have been dried in the shade, on the bottom of the container.
- Fill the container with grain
- Place a layer of dried neem leaves on top and close the storage container.

Method 3

If grain is being stored in sacks, neem leaf powder can be mixed directly with the grain, (1 or 2 kilos of powder to 100 kilos of grain).

Uses of Neem Extract

There are many different ways to apply neem extracts. Some of the most common methods are described in this section.

Preparing crushed neem seed

1. The ripe fruit pulp should be removed from the seed as soon possible after harvest, otherwise the seeds may become covered in mould. In some areas birds or fruits bats eat the pulp leaving the seed on the ground.
2. The seeds should then be laid out in a thin layer in the sun to dry out for a few days. The dried seeds should be stored in containers with plenty of air to stop mould growing.
3. The shells have to be removed using stones or a big mortar. The shells can then be removed by winnowing in the same way as with cereals.
4. The kernels are then ground in a mill or in a mortar.

Neem to control stem borers on young plants

1. A small amount of crushed neem seed powder should be mixed with the same amount of dry amount of dry clay or sawdust.
2. The mixture is placed in the funnel of young maize of sorghum plants.
3. Rain will gradually dissolve the active chemicals in the neem seed.
4. This treatment may need to be repeated every 8 to 10 days until the plants flower.

Extracting Neem oil

To press neem oil by hand the kernels of the neem seed should be crushed as described in the previous section

- Add a small amount of water until the mixture forms a firm paste that can be kneaded.
- Knead the paste until oil drops form on the surface.
- Press firmly to extract the oil.
- The kneading and pressing should be continued in turn until the maximum amount of oil is removed. (The oil content of the seed kernel is about 45%).

In some areas there are traditional ways of removing oil from other seeds such as sesame or groundnut. It is a good idea to try these methods with neem.

If the oil is heated in the process, its ability to control insects will not be affected.

Controlling bruchid beetles in stored beans

Neem oil is used to control Bruchid beetles, which are small beetles whose larvae eat into stored beans and other legumes.

- Mix a small quantity of neem seed oil with the beans or seeds before storing.

The oil has a bitter taste but is not reported to change the taste of stored beans for humans to eat

Control of soil–borne pests

The neem cake, which is left after the oil is extracted from the seed, is also useful for controlling several pests, which live in the soil, particularly nematodes.

Neem water extract for plant protection

- Prepare 500g of crushed neem seed kernels as described previously. Mix crushed neem seed with 10 litres of water. It is necessary to use a lot of water because the active ingredients do not dissolve easily. Stir the mixture well and leave to stand for at least 5 hours.
- Spray the neem water directly on vegetables using a sprayer or straw brush.
- The effect lasts for 3 to 6 days. If kept in the dark neem water will be effective for 3 to 6 days.
- It has been estimated that 20–30 kg neem seed (an average yield from 2 trees), can normally treat one hectare.
- If crops have to be watered, water should go directly on the soil because water running over the leaves of sprayed plants may wash off the extract.
- If alcohol is available, 50 times more azadirachtin can be dissolved and extracted.

Water based neem spray to control cutworms

Water based neem spray is most effective against pests such as Cutworms. During the day the caterpillars stay on the ground and fed on plant roots. At night they eat young stems.

Plants most affected include many vegetables and other affected plants include maize. Tobacco and coffee.

VRIKSH AYRVEDA AND ITS USE IN PANT DISORDERS AND THEIR MANAGEMENT

Treating disorders in plants is dealt with in the extensive work *Brihatsamhitha* of Varahamihira as well as in *Agni purana*. There are a number of other works suchas *Vrkshayurveda* of Surapala and *Lokopakaram*, which have a great wealth of information on treatment of plant disorders. To quote Gunaratna: "Just as the human body is subject to health problems, plants too suffer from similar problems such as displacement or dislocation of flower, fruit, leaves, bark and by application of appropriate remedies prescribed in *vrkshayurveda* unnatural growth, deterioration, wounds, fractures etc., can be cured in plants".

Texts of *vrkshayurveda* classify disorders in plants into two types–exogenous and endogenous. The endogenous disorders are caused by the disturbance of the three *doshas*, namely *vaatha*, *pitta* and *kapha*. The exogenous disorders are caused by factors such as pests, cold, hail, lighting, etc. According to *vrkshayurveda*, plants are also understood as having *vaatha*, *pitta* and *kapha* characteristics, like human beings. We should have an overview of this concept to understand disorders in plants.

Prakrithi or Constitution of Plants

Plants can be classified into three types based on their constitution. The broad classification is the same as the classification for human beings, namely *vaatha*, *pitta* and *kapha* constitution. The general characteristics of plants of each of these types are listed below.

Characteristics of Plants with Vaatha *Constitution*

1. Slender and tall
2. Light in weight
3. Have a rough surface

4. Their leaves with or drop away with the slightest heat of the sun.

Characteristics of Plants with Pitta *Constitution*

1. Are able to withstand bright light.
2. Have weak branches which break away easily.
3. Have abundant leaves and flowers.
4. Bear fruits during off season.
5. Are of medium size and height.

Characteristics of Plants with Kapha *Constitution*

1. Possess stout and bulky stems and branches.
2. Plenty of thick leaves.
3. Bear abundant flowers and fruits.
4. House many creepers and climbers around them.

Rationale of Plant Prakrithi: A Comparison with the Human Constitution

According to *ayurveda, vaatha prakrithi* individuals possess a slender and tall body, are light in weight, have rough and dry skin with prominent (bony) joints and present an emaciated look. *Pitta prakrithi* individuals possess a medium–sized body with medium strength, have a tendency to early bladness and graying of the hair, possess yellow or copper coloured skin and have plenty of pimples and freckles on the skin. *Kapha prakrithi* individuals possess a short and bulky body with good strength and withstand stress better than the other two types of constitution. They adjust well with all types of people.

As in the case of humans, it is also true in the case of plants that single prakrithi type is very rare and what one normally encounters are combinations (eg.) *vaata–pitta type, pitta–kapha type, vaata–kapha* etc.

Endogenous Disorders

Vaathaja Problems

Causes: Feeding plants excessively with substances that are dry and astringent vitiates *vaatha*. *Vaatha* is also vitiated during summer as a result of loss of moisture in the soil.

Note: For details regarding Ayurvedic properties (guna) of drugs refer Appendix–II.

Symptoms: Plants affected by *Vaathaja* diseases are lean, deformed, full of knots and globules on the leaves, rough, have low water content and exhibit a loss of sweetness.

Treatment

1. Irrigation with flesh, flat, tallow and ghee could be done.
2. Fumigation with neem, cow's horn, horse's hair, ghee, atis root and oil (*Aconitum heterophyllum*), pig's fat, wild asparagus (*Asparagus racemosus*) and deodar (*Cedrus deodara*) could be attampled.

3. The tumours and protuberances which develop on the sides of the trees due to *vaathaja* disorders could be plastered with cowdung, marking nut (*Semicarpus anacardium*) and fat and watered with carrion both.
4. An infusion of greater galangal (*Alpinia galanga*), winter cherry (*Withania somnifera*), mesua (*Mesua nagassarium*) and long pepper (*Piper longum*) is used to water the plants.
5. If conditions are acute, the tree is watered with an infusion of fennel (*Foeniculum vulgare*), and dill (*Anethum graveolens*) seeds.
6. Fumigation with the leaves of five–leaved chaste tree (*Vitex negundo*), Indian bdellium tree (*Commiphora mukul*), ghee and seeds of karumarudu (*Terminalia tomentosa*) is also done.
7. Dressing of the roots with goat's excreta and oil cake is also beneficial.

Rationale

Therapy is done with ghee, fat, marrow, flesh, etc. for *vaathaja* disorders in human beings. The drugs administered should have the properties associated with them in *ayurveda,* i.e. be sweet, sour and salty in taste, hot in potency, etc. Infusion and poultices are also used to reduce the pain which is characteristic of *vaatha* dosha. The therapeutics is predominantly what is known as "bulk promoting". Drugs such as winter cherry (*Withania somnifera*), greater galangal (*Alpinia galanga*), marking nut tree (*Semicarpus anacardium*), fennel (*Foeniculum vulgare*) and five–leaved chaste tree (*Vitex negundo*), possess these qualities. Fennel (*Foeniculum vulgare*), deodar (*Cedrus deodara*), winter cherry (*Withania somnifera*), are also mentioned in Charaka for treatment of *vaathaja* disorders.

Pittaja Problems

If plants are irrigated with substances that are pungent, sour and saline it vitiates *pitta.* Plants are also prone to *pittaja* diseases in summer and autumn.

Symptoms

Yellowish discolouration of leaves, premature fruiting, oozing in fruits, emaciation due to excess activities of *pitta* and subsequent burning up of body elements, languor of leaves and flowers and fruits bearing a worn–out appearance, are the symptoms of *pittaja* diseases.

Treatment

The plants should be irrigated with substances that are cooling and predominantly sweet in taste. Decoction of sweet liquorice (*Glycyrrhiza glabra*), mahua tree (*Madhuca indica*) and milk mixed with honey is used for irrigation.

Decoction of triphala (*Terminalia bellerica, Terminalia chebula, Phyllanthus emblica*) mixed with ghee and honey is also recommended. The plants could be nurtured with cold and perfumed rose water in which sugar and embelia (*Embelia ribes*) has been dissolved.

Fumigation with sugar, honey and ghee is also suggested.

Treatment is also given with khas–khas grass (*Vettivera zizanioides*), nut grass (*Cyperus rotundus*), honey, milk and ghee.

Rationale

For *pittaja* disorders the line of treatment is the use of drugs which are predominantly sweet, bitter and astringent in taste, cooling and those which are soft and viscous. Substances such as ghee, milk and butter are used extensively. Application of fumes from aromatic substances such as sandal (*Santalum album*), khas–khas grass (*Vettivera zizanioides*) etc. is also beneficial. All that is soft and cold in nature is recommended.

Kaphaja Problems

Causes

Irrigating plants excessively with substances that are sweet, unctuous, sour and cold, can cause *kapha* diseases. Plants are more susceptible to *kaphaja* diseases in winter and spring.

Symptoms

Deformity of leaves, slow maturing of fruits and less taste in fruits are the general symptoms of *kaphaja* diseases.

Treatment

Kaphaja diseases must be pacified with decoctions that are pungent and hot in nature.

A paste of sugar and mustard is applied at the root and then the plant is irrigated with water mixed with the ashes of *sesamum* sp.

The mud and soil around the plant affected by *kaphaja* diseases is removed and replaced with dry and hard soil.

Affected tree could be nurtured with tepid water.

An infusion prepared from barks of parisah (*Ficus arnottiana*), pilklan, country fig (*Ficus racemosa*) and devil tree or biton bark (*Alstonia scholaris*), neem (*Azadirachta indica*), sweet flat (*Acorus calamus*), nut grass (*Cyperus rotundus*) and rohitaka tree (*Aphanamixis polystachya*) is prescribed.

Watering for seven days with decoction of yellow berried nightshade (*Solanum surratense*), sahacara (*Barleria prionitis*), neem (*Azadiracthta indica*), sweet flag (*Acorus calamus*), cutch tree (*Acacia catechu*), black catechu and rosha grass / rusa grass (*Cymbopogon martini*) is recommended.

The roots of affected trees should be dressed with oil cake of white mustard (*Brassica juncea*) and irrigated with water in which sesamum and ashes are dissolved.

Rationale

For treatment of *kaphaja* disorders substances possessing pungent, bitter and astringent taste are used. *Panchamoola* possesses these qualities and is specifically used in *kapha* and *vaatha* disorders [*Panchamoola* is a combination of five plants. They are the bael tree (*Aegle marmelos*), Indian trumpet tree (*Oroxylum indicum*), comb teak (*Gmelina aroborea*), trumpet flower tree (*Stereospermum colais*) and *agnimandam*]. Neem (*Azadirachta indica*) and devil tree (*Alstonia scholaris*) are mentioned in Sushrutha for treatment of *kaphaja* diseases.

Exogenous Disorders

Vrkshayurveda also discusses the treatment of a large number of exogenous disorders and their management. These disorders are of several kinds, such as those caused due to worm infestation, insect attack, trees affected by fire, hail, storm, cold winds, dried trees, cut and broken branches, trees struck by lightning etc.

Cow's Urine in Pest Management

Cow's urine for resistance to Leaf spot disease in paddy

Symptoms of the disease: The leaves show round to oval or irregular brown spots which may coalesce to cause withering of tissues. A velvetty growth may be seen on the glumes. Sometimes browning or greyish browning may be seen at the neck region. The grains show reddish brown discolouration. These spots are like sesamum seeds. Hence this is also called as sesamum leaf spot disease.

Treatment: Paddy seeds required for sowing in 1 acre of land should be taken. This would be roughly 34 kilos. These seeds should be soaked for two days in water and it should have sprouted. In fact, it should be ready for sowing in the nursery.

Take 1 litre of cow's urine and mix it with 5 litres of water. The cow's urine should be collected two days earlier. The paddy seeds which have already been soaked in water and sprouted should be soaked in the mixture of cow's urine and water. It should be soaked for half an hour. After this it should be taken out and shade dried for 15 minutes. It should then be sown in the nursery. This provides resistance to the crop from leaf spot disease.

Caution: Do not increase the quantity of cow's urine. This could decrease the germinating capacity.

Cow's urine for increasing yield

For spraying in one acre 6 litres of cow's urine is required. This cow's urine should be collected two days earlier. It should be mixed with 60 litres of water and sprayed. When this is sprayed during the vegetative stage the growth rate is increased and the crop also becomes resistant to disease.

Use of Milk for resistance to Tungro virus

Symptoms of Tungro virus attack

Older leaves turn yellow orange starting from the tip and margin. Young leaves are mottled with pale green to whitish spots. Root development is poor and grains are usually covered with dark brown blotch. Plants become stunted and bear poor panicles with empty glumes. This disease is transmitted by green leaf hopper (*Nephotettix virescens*).

Treatment

Paddy seeds required for sowing in 1 acre of land should be taken. This would be roughly 35 kilos. These seeds should be soaked for two days in water and it should have sprouted. In fact, it should be ready for sowing in the nursery.

1 litre of milk should be mixed with 5 litres of water. It is better to use cow's milk. The paddy seeds soaked in water and sprouted should be soaked in this mixture of milk and water for half an hour. After this the seeds should be dried and then sown in the nursery.

Note: In Andhra Pradesh tobacco farmers dip their hands in milk before transplanting the seedlings of tobacco. It is an indigenous practice. This prevents the tobacco mosaic virus from attacking the tobacco seedlings.

Growth Regulator or Kunapajala for Yield Increase

Materials required :

Goat's meat	–	1 kg
Sesame	–	¼ kg
Black gram	–	¼ kg
Cow's milk	–	1 litre

The goat's meat should be washed properly and put in 5 litres of water and boiled till it reduces to half the quantity. After this the flesh should be removed and the extract alone should be filtered. Black gram and seasame should be properly powdered. The mixture of these powders should be mixed with the meat extract after it is cooled. After mixing this it should again be boiled. After boiling the mixture is cooled and then milk should be added. This should now be transferred to a mud pot. The mouth of the mud pot should be tied with a cloth. The pot should be buried under the ground or under the compost pit. The extract should be mixed well at least once a day.

After 10 days the extract should be removed and properly filtered. It should be transferred to another pot and closed. Fermentation takes place during this period.

This extract (*kunapajala*) can be applied near the roots or used as a spray. For application near the root zone 3 litres of growth regulator is required. This should be applied near the irrigation channel so as to mix with the water.

500 ml of extract should be mixed with 10 litres of water for use as a foliar spray. This is sprayed twice during the vegetative stage. By using this there is an increase in the number of grains per ear head and also a general increase in the yield. The weight of the grains also increase.

After irrigating the field in which the seedlings are transplanted the growth regulator can also be applied using a hand sprayer on the surface of the water.

Use of Panchagavya for Paddy

Panchagavya is a combination of 5 products obtained from the cow which is used in traditional medicine extensively. These are cowdung, cow's urine, cow's milk, curd and ghee. This is also mentioned in *vrkshayurveda* texts and it has been experimented by us and other farmers. It has a significant role in providing resistance to disease, pests and increasing the overall yield.

Note: The *panchagavya* preparations mentioned here are slightly different from what has been mentioned in the *vrkshayurveda* texts. These modified versions have been standardized by experimental trials.

Materials required

Cowdung mixed with water	–	500 ml.
Cow's urine	–	300 ml.
Cow's milk	–	200 ml.
Curd	–	200 ml.
Ghee	–	100 ml.
Yellow plantain	–	2 nos.
Coconut water	–	300 ml.
Total		1500 ml.

Preparation

All the products mentioned above should be put in a mud pot, mixed properly and kept open for 10 days. It should be mixed every day. It is ready for use in 10 days time. This preparation is based on the method followed by Dr. K. Natarjan of Kodumudi.

The methods of use of *panchagavya* for specific conditions are described in the next few pages.

Panchagavya for Leaf blight treatment

Symptoms of Bacterial leaf blight disease

It is characterized by the appearance of yellow colour water soaked lesions on both the edges of the leaves. Later they coalesce and the entire surface turns into straw colour. The affected leaves roll completely, droop and ultimately the tillers wither away. These symptoms usually appear 4 to 6 weeks after transplanting. Affected plants produce chaffy grains.

Treatment

A 5% panchakavya extract is sprayed on the paddy crop when bacterial leaf blight symptoms are noted. Within 1 week the bacterial leaf blight symptoms disappear completely. For preparation of 5% extract one should use 50 ml. of the panchavkaya prepared for 1 litre of water.

Use of Panchakavya in other crops

When a 3% panchakavya was sprayed on chilli crop within 10 days of spraying it became dark green. In the case of lemon a 3% panchakavya was sprayed during the vegetative stage and the flowering stage. This gave increased yield.

HOST RESISTANCE

The use of plant varieties tolerant of or resistant to pest attack is a proven, effective, economical and safe method of pest control. Plants have diverse means to avoid, tolerate or recover from attack of other organisms. This trait is particularly important in low value crops.

In weed control, the phenomenon of allelopathy– the inhibition of growth of weedy plants by chemicals released by the crop plants–has not been extensively explored but may have a great potential. Superior weed suppressing types have been reported from searches of cucumber (*Cucumis sativus*), oat, sunflower and soybean collections .Some crops have superior ability to complete with weeds for critical growth factors such as moisture, nutrients and light. Cultivars specially bred for more vigorous canopies or root system should provide atleast partial degree of weed control. This along with allelopathy may provide a new valuable approach to weed management.

Occasionally, a variety developed to resist one pest may be more susceptible to another that had not caused much economic damage. Further, insects and diseases are continuously evolving strains that may adopt to formerly resistant plant varieties. The breakdown of plant resistance has become a greater problem with diseases as compared to insect pests, where it is fortunately much less common. Thus every effort should be made to use genes for general resistance and tolerance obtained from diverse sources and to add them to the genes for specific resistance.

Autocidal Control

Autocidal control involves rearing and release of insects that are sterile or are altered genetically in order to suppress members of their own species that are causing pest problems. Although a novel method, not much headway has been made in this direction because of difficulties with the high costs of rearing, sterilizing and liberating the insects

Bheavioural Control

Pheromones

Pheromones are ectohormones secreted by an organism, which elicit behavioral responses from the other members/sex of its own species. These are of different types–sex pheromones (attracting individuals of opposite sex), trail pheromones (helping the other individuals to follow the trial left by others), aggression pheromones (invoking aggression behaviour), etc. Pheromones are extremely selective, non–toxic, highly biodegradable and effective at very low application rates. Synthetic sex pheromones are commercially available and are used for surveillance, monitoring, and control of many lepidopterous pests such as old world bollworm, tobacco caterpillar, spotted bollworm, coding moth, potato tuber moth, diamond back moth, leaf folder, etc. Mass trapping has been attempted against rice stem borer, sweet potato weevil (*Cylas formicarius*) and red palm weevil (*Rhynchophorus ferrugineus*). Mating disruption or disruption of the insect communication system to prevent mating has been attempted against pink bollworm, codling moth, shoot borer and gypsy moth, etc. Pheromone components of *S. incertulas* impregnated in PVC resins and applied by hand at 40 g/ha are reported to be effective in causing up to 94 per cent reduction in the pheromone mediated communication compared to conventional methods.

Fairomones

Fairomones are volatile compounds that evoke behavioural responses adaptively favourable to the receiver. Fairomones are released either by the host plant or by the host insects. While the former issued by the pest and natural enemies to locate their habitats, the latter is used for prey finding and parasitisation/preying. Fairomones from host plant can be effectively used to mass trap the pest species as well as for monitoring. Tremendous strides have been made in identification, formulation and practical application. Use of Fairomonal compounds to increase the efficacy of the predator C. carnea and the egg parasitoid *T. chilonis* has been successfully demonstrated.

SUCCESS RATE OF ECOLOGICAL MANAGEMENT

In developing countries,

1. The rate of adoption is slow.
2. The majority of those programmes focus on pests within categories (insects, pathogens, nematodes or weeds) with little consideration of multiple pest interaction.

OTHER RELATED APPROACHS

There are several other approaches for pest control yet two most popular approach i.e. IPM and BIPM is described here in brief. Both are having all above component and use of pesticide at minimum required level but not complete restriction on use of pesticide. Thus these are not acceptable to organic farming but need to be practsied during transitional phase i.e. shift form conventional to organic farming.

Integrated Pest Management

Integrated Pest Management (IPM) is a component of sustainable agriculture with a sound ecological foundation. Although the concept of IPM had its origins nearly three decades back, the use of pesticides has not declined appreciably. The essence of the IPM concept, lies in the harmonious integration of compatible multiple methods, used singly or in combination against pests including insects, pathogens and weeds. It ensures economic benefits to the farmers and the society at large. The use of economic injury levels (EILs) and scouting for the assessment of pest populations have been the main criteria of IPM.

Biologically Intensive Pest Control (BIPM)

Relies on host–plant resistance, biological control and cultural control and use of biorational pesticides can be integrated. The Previous term IPM has historically aimed at developing systems based as much as possible on biological and other non–chemical methods. The BIPM also allows the selective use of pesticides after maximizing effectiveness of natural controls. BIPM, a more feasible and economical method of pest management has become popular, particularly among small and marginal farmers.

8 HARVEST TECHNOLOGY AND VALUE ADDITION OF MEDICINAL PLANTS

HARVESTING

Harvesting from the Wild

Harvesting medical herbs requires careful planning to ensure the parts are processed in peak condition and fast enough to retain their active ingredients.Wild plants offer a free and natural source of herbal remedies and give the satisfaction of colleting herbs in the traditional way. Furthermore, active constituents are often more highly concentrated in wild plants as the herb is generally likely to be growing in its preferred environment.

Identification

Proper identification of wild plants is essential. Use a field or wild flower guide to help you, as many plants look similar. If in double, do not pick the plant, as poisoning can result from misidentification.

Collect material from healthy plant that are free from disease, insect damage and, in the case of wild plants, pollution. It is important to discard any damaged plants as they can lead to disease or decay in dried plant material. Do not mix cut plant material to avoid mistakes in identification.

Time of Harvest

Harvesting should be done in dry weather, preferably on a sunny morning after the dew has evaporated. Picking in the right weather conditions, when the plant is at its peak of maturity, ensures that it will have a high concentration of active constituents. Unless otherwise stated in the individual plant entries on leaves are best collected as they open during the spring or summer months, flowers as they start to bloom, fruit and berries just as they become ripe, and roots in the autumn once the plant has drawn its vitality back beneath ground. Bark must be gathered with great are if the shrub or tee is to survive–in most cases harvest it in spring or autumn.

Harvesting Correct Useful Parts

In many cases, different parts of the same plant for example the leaves and seeds, can have quite different actions and uses. Make sure that you harvest the correct medicinal part of the plant for your purposes.

PROCESSING

In order to make use of its latent medicinal qualities, a plant must be treated and modified in such a way that its specific curative substances can be extracted. Such transformations form part of what is known as the 'galenic' branch of pharmacy. The active principles contained in every medicinal plant consist of a number of compounds, which, individually or in groups, can have a specific action on the organs or our bodies. Different methods have, therefore, been devised to extracts these substances, either singly or collectively, depending on the result required. Some forms of extraction, being particularly complex, are beyond the skills of laymen and are exclusively the province of the pharmaceutical chemist or similar specialists. Others, of a more simple nature, can be carried out by anyone. There are four basic, simple preparation techniques: decoction, maceration, infusion and juice extraction. Although these are very straightforward methods, they are just as effective as the more elaborate systems involving considerably more complicated processes. These four methods will be discussed separately, with instructions as to the exact procedures for extracting the active principles and the circumstances in which each should be adopted.

Decoction

Decoction is the method normally used for those medicinal herbs whose active principles are difficult to extract because they are contained in woody parts of the plant, or which require prolonged heating in order to pass into solution. The procedures dealt with here only involve water extraction, as more complex forms requiring various solvents are too technical for a book of this nature.

Extraction by decoction involves boiling the whole plant or a part of it in water for a given time and then allowing it to macerate for a further period before filtering. A slight variation of this method is to soak the plant beforehand in cold water for a specific time, depending on the drugs required, in order to soften the leathery part and thus make extraction easier at the decoction stage. This method is reserved for certain plants such as those with a high mucilaginous content.

Decoction is, understandably, quite a drastic method of extraction and one, which is capable of modifying some of the plant compounds. It is important to ensure that the main active principle to be extracted is not affected by other harmful compounds induced by the heat. The boiling process during, which water is added, nearly always destroys the volatile active principles, that is to say, those with a low boiling point. This means, therefore, that the resulting decoction will never possess all the original principles of the drug.

Filtering Operation

The filtering operation is equally important, as it serves to strain off not only the leathery residues of the plant but also the mucilage or deposits of amphorous substances that are carried in solution during the boiling. The liquid obtained is, therefore, always left to clear before the next stage when it is filtered through paper of finely woven linen.

Extraction

Extraction is much more suitable method for obtaining the active principles when the parts of the plant being used are soft and fragile, such as leaves bud or flowers. It is preferable, except in certain cases, to use herbs that have been slightly dried, as the reduction of water content will concentrate the principal constituents. Unlike decoction, this method allows retention of many of the volatile principles, which would otherwise be lost, but does not permit extraction of those requiring a continuously high temperature. An expert, with extensive knowledge of medicinal plants and their medical compounds, can decide, which of these two methods is more suitable for obtaining the active principles required.

Infusion

Infusion entails pouring boiling water over that part of the plant known to contain the required drug. The container should be made of pottery of glass to avoid the formation of tannate of iron, which due to the presence of tannin in almost all plants, would occur it metal were used. As soon a s the water ahs been poured over the plants, the container should be covered, thereby allowing the steam, rich in volatile compounds, to condense. After a given time, which varies for each plant used, the liquid is filtered before being used.

Maceration

The third simple method, known as maceration, is used for medicinal plants whose active principles are soluble in cold water for several hours during, which time all the principles that do not need heat to release them (i.e. that are not thermolabile) will be released into the solution. The yield of mucilage from certain plants, such as the mallow (*Malva*) and marsh mallow (*Althaea officinalis*), is in fact greater when extraction is carried out by means of cold maceration rather than by infusion.

The method of maceration described above is hardly ever used nowadays in the pharmaceutical industry. Instead, tinctures are prepared by diluting a certain amount of fluidextract of the requisite drug with alcohol of a predetermined strength. When, as is sometimes done, a sugar solution is added to spirit solutions, the resulting preparation is known as an *elixir* or *ratafia*. These preparations are, in fact, genuine liqueurs and have been almost abolished in pharmaceutical practice.

If the vehicle of maceration were to be a mixture of alcohol and ether, andethereal tincture' or, more scientifically, an ethereal spirit solution would be obtained. Many varieties of such preparations could once be found in all the pharmacopoeias, but are now little used. The best known is ethereal tincture of valerian.

Extraction

It is a straightforward method used for the extraction of juices. In this case the plants, which contain the required medicinal ingredients must be fresh and have high water content. The Juice, which can be extracted by various methods, contains the mineral salts and vitamins of the plant, together with all the other substances that can be obtained through pressure. Again, the juice will not contain all the active principles of the plant but, on the other hand, cold extraction does not modify the structure of those compounds, which as we have seen, can be altered by heat. In the home, juices can be produced by first parboiling the fresh plants very briefly and then applying pressure with an appropriate utensil such as a small press. Because of the additional heat used for parboiling, however, this method will modify some of the constituents.

Better still, of course, is the modern electric blender, which extracts almost the entire juice content of the plant.

All the methods described above have a time limit; hence they are considered short–term procedures. In fact, the decoction, the influsion, the maceration and the juice all contain biological compounds that immediately undergo processes of oxidization and fermentation that denaturalize the medicinal substance, often making the liquid taste repugnant and, therefore, unusable. To avoid this, it is possible to add preservatives but this, of course, would be quite contrary to the whole concept of non–adulteration, which is the aim of the methods described here. Additions of sugar and alcohol admittedly also enable juices to be kept for a slightly longer period and, if vacuum–bottled with sugars, their properties and the freshness of their components will remain unaltered; unfortunately, this kind of preservation is almost impossible in the average household because the apparatus required is often expensive.

The Problem

The problem of conserving medicinal principles, once extracted, is of the utmost importance. The pharmaceutical industry has, therefore, done much work in this field, producing further preservation techniques so that active principles can be used at any time and in any dosage. The difficulty of tracking down exotic or rare drugs, combined with the relatively short harvesting period of healing herbs, has necessitated the development and regulation of highly advanced methods of extraction and preservation.

Forms of Preparations

Such preparations are known as extracts. They are divided into semi–solid, dry and fluid types; another means of classifying them is by their vehicle of evaporation: water, water and alcohol, or ether. Strictly speaking, an extract is the concentration of all the substances and salts diluted in the juice obtained from it. This concentration is achieved by the use of two fundamental processes: the first is based on freezing and the other on evaporation. The latter, more generally used, consists of putting the juice into an evaporating dish from, which the water content is evaporated at a low heat. Obviously, depending on the length of the evaporation process, different concentrations of the juice will be obtained. Concentrations will thus range from those still possessing a high water content to concentrates in which water is no longer present. The extract obtained is termed soft extracts have a semi–solid honey–like consistency, while dry ones are often composed of solid masses that can be reduced to powder. A classic example of a dry extract is that of aloes, which has the appearance of black, solid lumps, almost vitrified, but which are friable and easily pulverized; an even better known instance is liquorice, which can be reduced to a powder or to liquorice sticks.

Water content of juice

The water content of juice is not, however, always the vehicle of evaporation used in obtaining an extract. Instead, to facilitate concentration through evaporation, a solution of water and alcohol is often used. Alternatively, ether may be used and then recovered through distillation. The addition of these substances to the water enables compounds to dissolve, which are hardly soluble at all in water alone, but which become very soluble in a combination of the two liquids.

The Solvants

Extracts in which ether is used are described as ethereal and those in which alcohol are used as hydroalcoholic. Certainly the most important type of extract is the fluidextract, which has only relatively recently been formulated and accepted in pharmaceutical practice. In comparison with the type of extract previously described it has one property, which makes it extremely useful: one gramme of fluidextract is equivalent to one gramme of the original plant material. In other words, all the active principles contained in a precise quantity of plant matter to be treated are present in the same quantity of fluidextract obtained. The fluid extract makes it possible to have any drug available at any given time (it does not deteriorate quickly and fluid extract obtained. The fluid extract makes it possible to have any drug available at any given time (it does not deteriorate quickly and is not modified, except very slowly, by external agents); it is of a purify and accuracy of tiration that would be impossible to achieve in drugs fresh from the plant.

Alcohol–soluble substances

When, for particular purposes, it is necessary to extract only the alcohol–soluble substances such as alkaloids, bitter principles, and organic acids and colouring substances, another specific method of preparation is used. This is generally known as an alcoholic tincture or, more correctly, spirit solution. Apart from the reason already given, these tinctures are produced because their high alcohol content makes them easy to preserve. A spirit solution can be prepared either by maceration, in which a measured amount of the medicinal plant is immersed in alcohol of a suitable strength for a predetermined length of time and subsequently filtered, or by digestion, passing it through a still. This apparatus is equipped with a cooling flask, which causes the alcohol that ahs been condensed in it to fall back into the receiver flask in which the drugs to be digested have been placed. Because tinctures are very sensitive to light they are always kept in bottles made of dark glass. The alcohol in which the plants have been macerated develops varying degrees of strength, depending on the drug being used and the ease with which it releases its essential constituents, but it is usually not less than 60% vol. Although these are alcoholic preparations they cannot.

The alcohol content is sufficient to obtain an extraction of the soluble compounds if the medicinal plants are allowed to macerate in the wine for the length of time appropriate to each type. Unfortunately, medicated wines are subject to acetic fermentation (that is, they go vinegary) and form sediment just like any other wine. It is, therefore, important to prepare only small quantities and to keep the wine completely airtight and away form the light.

Fixed Solvents

Essential oils are soluble in solvents that are described as fixed if they do not evaporate at a normal temperature, and as volatile if the reverse is the case. Fixed solvents consist of solid or liquid odouless fats such as lard, tallow or refined olive oil. These solvents enable essence to be extracted by means of a method known as *hot enfleurage*. The essence-producing plants are placed in copper containers and left to macerate in fat, which is brought up to a temperature of about 104° F. (40° C.), with more plants being added until the fat is saturated. The fat is then separated from the essence to give a good yield.

Volatile solvents

Extraction with volatile solvents, while presenting much greater difficulties in obtaining the essential oil, has the advantage of making it possible to extract essences from plants that have only very low percentage of the fragrant principle. The volatile solvents normally used are benzene and petroleum ether, which carry both the essence in solution and other products, making it necessary to carry our further, rather laborious tasks in order to obtain a pure products. The first phase of extraction by this method is the soaking of the flowers in an apparatus known as a *digester*. The solution obtained from this is distilled, during, which process the solvent is recovered. The essence' because of the traces of extraneous material contained in it. In order to purify the concrete essence, it is treated with pure alcohol, which takes up the essence, leaving many undissolved impurities. The alcohol is then brought to a low temperature, which enables the remaining impurities to become concentrate. As this stage, the alcohol can be called an extract. To complete the process, the extract is distilled to give the resulting essence a high degree of purity.

Uses of Extracts

These extracts can be used either by themselves or as the basic ingredient of various medicinal compounds, both of which are guaranteed as a homogenous product. Although the method of preparation varies according to the drug, it can be summarized as follows: 1,000 parts of the finely chopped dried plant are left to macerate for several hours in alcohol of the appropriate strength. This alcohol is then strained off and discarded. A similar amount of fresh alcohol is then poured over the same plant matter and a part of it strained off a day later. This alcohol, the weight of which is in direct relation to the type of herb used, is held in reserve. New alcohol is added until the dried plant material is exhausted of all the soluble extracts. The next stage is to distil this second liquid, recovering the alcohol and allowing the rest to evaporate until an extract is obtained, which, when mixed with the part held in reserve, will be of exactly the same weight as the original herb material. Some experts maintain that the solvent action of the alcohol can be improved by the addition of certain substances such as inorganic or organic acids, salts and ammonia. The various pharmacopoeias certainly use one or other these additives. The fluidextract will remain unaltered for a long time If kept in dark glass bottles, which are firmly stoppered.

The above explanation demonstrates the superiority of this method of extraction over the other methods described, and accounts for are almost unreserved use throughout the world.

Unlike fluidextracts, be preserved indefinitely. They react quickly to light and air, which cause flocculation and acetic fermentation.

Looking at the field of galenical preparations (those deriving from plant of natural origins) as a whole, there is one particular preparation reassessed by modern phytotherapy, both because of its successful results and its ease of preparation. It can even be made at home. This is medicinal wine. As long ago as the thirteenth century, Arnold of Villanova wrote his *Incipit* Tractatus de Vinis, the earliest published book on wines, which dealt particularly with 'methods of making preparations with wine basis'. Such wines are made by simply macerating plant drugs in wine, preferably white, with a high alcohol content, such as a fortified wine.

Examination of galenic products

These are examined are the *alcoholates* or *spirits*, produced by the distillation of spirit solutions. The difference between spirits and spirit solutions is that the former, through distillation, contain only the volatile principles of the drug and not the fixed principle, as do the latter. For the distillation, 70–80% vol. alcohols are generally used, after appropriate maceration. Only a certain part of the distillate is retained, so as not to change its characteristics with substances of low volatility, which remain in the flask, following the concentration of the watery part. Some of the best known spirit solutions still used today are aqua vitae of lemon balm and Hungary water, or spirit of rosemary, the former being used as a digestive antispasmodic and the latter as a perfume component. Spirits have excellent preservation qualities due to their high alcohol content.

Syrups Preparation

Instead of using alcohol as a preservative for garden herbs, sugar can be sued in a concentrated form. By adopting this alternative, sugary solutions can be made, which contain medicinal substances; they are known as *syrups*. Syrups also serve to disguise the unpleasant taste of many medicines.

Ordinary syrup is made by dissolving a certain quantity of sugar in water, at a low heat; the mixture needs to be stirred frequently and allowed to evaporate sufficiently to obtain the concentration necessary to achieve the characteristic density f syrup. The curative substances are then dissolved in it and it is these that determine the particular qualities of each type of syrup. If the resulting liquid is cloudy, it can be clarified. Syrups should be stored in hermetically sealed bottles and kept in a cool dry place, preferably away from the light. Despite such precautions, syrup is prone to alteration, especially when the additives are organic. In such cases, the syrup will have to be re–boiled in order to increase its density and, therefore, its preservation potential. Instead of sugar, honey can be substituted using the same procedure. Such preparations are called *mellitus* or honeyed syrups. For instance, 'melrosette' or 'honey of roses', which is still made for children, belongs to this category.

Electuaries of Conserves

Nowadays there is a growing demand for plants and vegetables that have not been contaminated with insecticides or fungicides, to be used in a natural form as natural form as possible. The interest in macrobiotics ash even brought back a number of preparations, which, due to their short shelf life, had become neglected. These confections are known as *electuaries* of *conserves* and are in the form of paste made by mixing the pulp of fruits, which have special nutritive of medicinal properties, with certain powders, honey of syrups. Some of these are sold commercially but, because of the high percentage of organic substances in them, preservatives have to be added. The macrobiotic diet makes use of several types of electuaries in this double role of supplementary food and medicine.

Use of Oil as solvent

When medicinal substances are dissolved in oil rather than the usual solvents, the preparations can be made either by dissolving one part of an oily fluid extract of a particular plant in a given quantity of refined olive oil or, alternatively, by boiling the plant itself in the oil and then filtering the as rheumatism, in which an oily preparation is required to facilitate localized massages.

Closely related to the medicated oils are the ointments, also known as *salves* or *unguents*, the base of which is usually a semi–solid, fatty or greasy substance such as lard or wool–fat (lanolin). They may be prepared simply by mixing powdered vegetal drugs into the fat, or the fat these ointments are all intended for external use.

At one time simple ointments such as these were very well known and widely used, but nowadays they have been largely replaced by commercial products containing chemical additives. The creams and liniments found on the market today tend to have quite different bases. Sometimes, however, we are reminded of remedies, which must have been familiar to our ancestors, when we see an old apothecary jar bearing a name such as unguent of polar or unguent of lily root. In Britain there is, increasingly, a tendency towards these simple creams containing no chemical additives.

Distillation Process

Distillation process is of fundamental importance for obtaining those ubiquitous ingredients of so many medicines and cosmetics known as essential oils or essences. These are not only used for their aromatic qualities, and s the main ingredients in perfumery, but also as the main medicinal ingredients in modern aromatherapy. The rest of this section, therefore, is devoted to a fairly detailed description of various processes necessary for the production of these oils.

Essences

Essences are complex substances, which are often fragrant and, although not oily, when placed on paper will produce a translucent effect. It is now possible to reproduce a great many essential oils chemically, and although this might suggest that distillation is an outdated method, that is not the case.

The essences derived from plants do not merely consist of open or more compounds, which it is possible to reproduce, but of a whole combination of substances, which are often undefined. It is not difficult to differentiate between the natural and the synthetic essences, because the natural perfume is altogether more delicate. There are also cases were chemistry has to make use of natural raw materials in order to reproduce some of the compounds synthetically produced.

The reasons why plants manufacture essential oils are still being investigated. A Few of the many theories formulated have some credibility, but what is certain, in any event, is that essences are beneficial to the economy of a plant, enabling it to manufacture other products. Some authorities maintain they are either waste materials, which have not yet been eliminated or that they are a means of protection against excessive sunshine. It is, in fact, true to say that nearly all–alpine plants are scented and the perfume that surrounds them serves as a filter through, which the solar rays must penetrate.

Essences are quite easily altered, and the least change in temperature or humidity is enough to allow the enzymes present to become activated. Another factor to be borne in mind when gathering herbs is the effect of light on the amount of essential oil contained in plants at different times of day. Experienced collectors, knowing just when the healing properties of each type of plant are at their peak, can decide exactly when to harvest it in order to derive the most benefit. Thus in some plants, the amount of essence will be reduced by light, whereas in others it will be concentrated. The composition of the soil may also affect the size of the yield.

Having made these points, it has to be said that the most satisfactory extraction is obtained when there is the least possible alteration to the characteristics of the essence itself. This type of extraction, which is described as *cold*, entails no change in the composition of the oil because no heat is involved. Unfortunately this method can only be applied to certain plants, mainly citrus, that possess a great many oil–producing glands. With the cold method the components present in the oils undergo only the slightest alteration, thus making it possible to produce essences of great purity, which can even be used internally. The two main methods of cold extraction are:

Expression

The former is carried out by putting the skins of the fruit into special containers where they are pressed, thus causing their glands to rupture and allowing the essence to be collected together with water and other substances. Essences extracted in this way are, inevitably, cloudy, although their fragrance and substance remain unaltered and they clarify when subsequently decanted. This method is mainly used now for homemade essences. Industry has adopted the

Ecuelle process

This involves the use of machines in which the fruit is revolved in metal cups or drums lined with spikes, which delicately rupture the oil–bearing glands to release their essences. As this is a fast process and the fruit are not identical in size or shape, there is considerable wastage of essence; this is, however, compensated for by the speed of the operation.

Cold enfleurage

This method alters neither the perfume nor the characteristics of the oils. This procedure is based on the special is based on the special quality possessed by some substances to condense essential oils on their surface area. These substances are purified waxes, which are spread over flat glass surfaces; the plants are placed on top and enclosed in special containers. After a day or two, the plants are removed and replaced by fresh ones; the process is then repeated over several months or until the wax has reached saturation point. The wax is then removed from the glass and the essence recovered by following the same procedure as for volatile solvents.

The problems involved in obtaining the products of essences producing plants are such that the methods described are only adopted for particular purposes.

Distillation

Normally, even though the process may change the composition of the essences due to the heat employed, *distillation* is used. This can be divided into three categories: simple distillation over direct heat, steam distillation and vacuum distillation. In distillation, heat both ruptures the oleiferous glands and, unfortunately, slightly modifies the essence. We shall only deal with the type of distillation in which water is the transporting vehicle. The distilled liquid will be a mixture of condensed water and essential oil, which will separate naturally because of their different specific gravities. The plants to be distilled must be used while still fresh and should have been gathered when most fragrant. In order to avoid fermentation, they should never be piled on top of one another.

The apparatus used for distilling is known as an alembic, from the Arab word *al–anbiq,* a vase. This is divided into three parts: boiler, distilling column and condenser. Vaporization of the water and volatization (rapid evaporation) of the essential oils are achieved in the distilling flask. The vapours then rise up the column and come down through the condenser, whence, having recondensed rapidly, the liquid falls into a receiver.

The boiler is usually made of copper or stainless steel, but may be of glass if laboratory apparatus is being used. It is generally cylindrical in shape and its base, to which the heat is applied, is never in direct contact with the plants, as these are kept slightly raised on wire mesh racks. Part of the space between the base and the first rack contains water, which produces the necessary steam. The column, which is firmly set in the neck of the boiler, leads to the condenser and allows for the expansion of the steam and for its initial cooling. If the boiler is metal, the column is clamped to it to form an airtight join, but if it is glass, either the foot of the column is shaped to fit the neck of the heater flask, or it is passed through a close–fitting stopper or cork. The condenser consists of a spiral tube, which is completely immersed in a vessel containing cold running water.

When the steam from the column comes into contact with the cold walls of the condenser, it condenses and, by force of gravity, runs down into a receiver, known as a 'Florentine flask', where the essence automatically separates from the water. If this type of flask is not used, separation has to be effected by means of a separatory funnel. Under normal conditions, boiling point is reached when the tension of the water equals the atmospheric pressure and to achieve this, the heat source is placed directly under the boiler; in this case distillation is brought about by direct heat.

In the laboratory the boiler is replaced by a glass distillation flask, and the heat is also applied from below to avoid breakages an asbestos, wire mesh or gauze mat is interposed so that the heat is not applied directly to the glass. In order to obtain uniform heating, the flask may be placed in a bed of sand or in water–bath. In this way the heat will be diffused evenly over the lower surface of the flask.

The two main types of condenser used in a laboratory for liquids with a low boiling point are the Liebig and the serpentine. If the steam, rather than being produced in the same container as the herbs, as described above, is produced in a separate boiler, this prevents the essence–containing plants form being 'cooked', which might adversely affect the result.

The method, known as *steam distillation,* makes it possible to distil those liquids, which have higher boiling point than water at temperatures lower than the boiling point of water. This method also makes it possible to obtain essences that are not excessively altered and is, therefore, preferable to the previously described system because of the greater purity of the resulting product.

Distillation can also be carried out at a pressure lower than that of the atmosphere. This is done by vacuum pumps and is known as 'distillation under reduced pressure' or 'vacuum distillation'. By decreasing the atmospheric pressure, the boiling point is also lowered, so enabling distillation to take place at a lower temperature to obtain a product that is even less modified than that produced by steam distillation.

Fractional distillation: Once the essences have been obtained, they are not always used in their complete state but are often broken down into their various components. This is done by fractional distillation, based on the already discussed principle of boiling, which occurs as a result of the equality between the atmospheric pressure and the sum of the vapour tensions of the components. The distillation temperature will initially be lower than that of the most volatile component and will then gradually rise. By carefully controlling the temperatures, the fractions of the essences can thus be collected. As the various components separate, they are retained individually by changing the receiving vessel when the appropriate temperatures are reached. To carry out such work in a laboratory, a special container in used, which is known as a Pauly apparatus or, more commonly a 'spider'. However, on an industrial scale such a method would be totally unsuitable because it is lengthy, laborious and, what is worse, discontinuous. For practical reasons, therefore, the *dephlegmator* or *fractionating column* is used. The most usual type is the Egrot dephlegmator, in which the essence vapours are cooled by a flow of water. This causes only the less volatile constituents to condense, thus effectively separating them from the more highly volatile ones.

Distilled water is the secondary product of distillation and is used a great deal in perfumery. It is, of course, merely water in which a very small amount of essence has remained and which gives it a fragrance and character of its own. Distilled waters do not keep well and are prone to alteration as they are subject of fungi and moulds. The only precaution possible is to store them away from the light in dark glass bottles. Their fragrance can be made more subtle by diluting a little of the essence itself in the water but this will deprive the water of its active volatile and other unknown principles that are typical of distillation. Distilled waters are widely used today in phytotherapeutic technology because they are readily available in large quantities. Although they contain only a low level of active principles, their medicinal effect is consistent with the concept of homoeopathic medicine.

PARTS OF MEDICINAL PLANT TO BE USED

Aerial Parts

These include all the parts of the plant growing above ground–stems, leaves, flowers, berries and seeds. The stems are normally cut 5–10 cm (2–4 in) above ground shortly after the plant has begun to flower, when it is putting most effort into growth. Perennials may be cut higher above ground to encourage further crops. Removes and dry large flowers crops. Remove and dry large flowers and leaves separately; smaller cones can be dried on the stem.

Large Flowers

In most cases, flowers are picked just after they have opened, usually during the spring or summer. Sometimes only specific parts of the flower are used, such as the petals of marigold (*Calendula officinalis*), while other flowers are used whole.

Fruit and Berries

Harvest fruit and berries in early autumn when rope but still firm. If allowed to become over–ripe, they may not dry properly. They can be picked individually or in bunches.

Roots, Rhizomes,Tubers and Bulbs

The underground parts of the plant are usually gathered in autumn after the aerial part have withered or because inactive and before the soil is waterlogged or frozen. Many roots may also be collected in early spring before the root loses its vitality to aerial growth. Dig deeply around the root, prising it carefully out of the ground. Some tap roots are very difficult to uproot completely. Remove the required amount and replant the remaining underground part.

Seeds

Collect ripe seed pods, capsules or flowering stems in late summer before the seed have been scattered.

Sap and Gel

Only harvest sap from your own garden. Collect sap in the spring as it rises, or as it falls in the autumn. Trees such as silver birch (*Betula pendula*) produce huge quantities of sap if tapped, although this reduces the tree's vitality. Bore a deep hole into the trunk of the tree–no more than a quarter of the diameter of the trunk–and place a collecting cup under the mouth of the hole. In spring, litres of sap may be produced and it is essential to stop the hole with resin or wood filler once about a little of fluid has been removed. Collect milky juices or latex from plants such as dandelion (*Taraxacum officinale*), by squeezing the stems over a bowl. Wear gloves as latex or sap can be corrosive. The gel from aloe vera (*Aloe vera*) is scarped out after slicing the leaf lengthwise and peeling back the edges.

Bark

Only harvest bark from your own shrubs or trees as it carries the risk of losing the whole plat through over–stripping or "ringing" (removing a whole band of bark). It is far better to collect bark from outlying branches, which can then be pruned back. If stripping bark from a plant, gather it in autumn when the sap is falling. Remove insects, lichen and moss from the bark, cut it into small pieces and place on a tray to dry.

Other Method of Processing

Apart from simply air–drying herbs, there are a number of other ways to preserve their medicinal benefits.

Dehumidifying

An effective but expensive way to dry herbs is to use a dehumidifer, which literally sucks water out of the plant. The dehumidifer should be placed in a more or less sealed small room in which the herbs are hung in loose bunches or placed on mesh trays. Herbs will dry quickly with this method and, as no heat is used, there is little deterioration or decay.

Freeze–Drying

Freeze–drying retains colour and flavour but is more suited to culinary than to medicinal herbs. Whole sprigs of herbs such as parsley (*Petroselinum crispum*) or sage (*Salvia officinalis*), can be frozen in plastic freezer bags. There is no need to defrost before use as the leaves crumble easily when still frozen. Chickweed (*Stellaria media*) can also be frozen and used topically for itchy and weeping skin conditions. Many plant may be juiced, frozen as ice cubes and thawed as required.

Storing Herbs

Storage method is very important for maintaining the quality of drys medicinal plants Leaves, flowers, roots and other parts should be stored in sterilized, dark glass containers with airtight lids. They may also be stored in new brown paper bags, which must be kept dry and away from light. Metal and plastic containers are inadvisable as they may contaminate the herb. If stored in a cool dark place, herbs can be kept for about 12 months after harvesting. Herbs frozen in plastic freezer bags can be used for up to 6 months. Make sure the container you use is labeled with the herb. Source, strength of preparation if appropriate, and date of harvesting. Watch out for insect infestation. If this occurs, put all affected material in a sealed plastic bag and discard. Sterilize the containers and check all other herbs for contamination.

PRESERVATION

Medicinal plants can be preserved in a number of ways, the most common and simple, being air or oven drying. A warm, dry place, for example an airing cupboard, is ideal. Use plain paper for drying herbs, never printed newspaper. Dried herbs can be stored for man months in a dark glass jar or a brown paper bag.

STANDARDIZATION OF MEDICINAL PLANTS

When a medicine is administered to a patient, the doctor who prescribes the medicine needs to be assured that the medicine contains the correct amount of the right substances as only then would the medicine induce its therapeutic effect. This is assured both to the doctors and the patient by the pharmaceutical company producing the medicine. In the laboratories of the pharmaceutical house, the medicine–or batches of the same–have been tested for quality and quantity and the drug is released for use only if the quality control laboratories of the pharmaceutical house approve the batch in question. Overseeing the situation nationally are national drug control laboratories run by government scientists who also monitor the equality of the drug being released by carrying out random checks to ensure that the results conform to the standards laid down by both the pharmaceutical house and the national drug regulatory authority at a time when the pharmaceutical house requests for the release of a particular drug in the market. This is known as standardization–a system to ensure that every packet of medicine that is being sold has the correct substance in the correct amount and will induce its therapeutic effect.

This system has worked well in developed countries and reasonably well in countries in the third world, particularly if the country has a strong drug regulatory agency with its own laboratories. However, the system has been developed for synthetic medicines and its has not been difficult to "fingerprint" the synthetic medicines and lay down standards. It is much more difficult to ensure that this system works in regard to herbal medicine.

It is very important that a system of standardization is established for every plant medicine in the market because the scope for variation in different batches of medicine is enormous. Plant material, as has already been mentioned earlier, may vary in its alkaloid content and therefore in its therapeutic effect according to different places of collection, with different times in a year for collection, with collection at the same time and place but in different years, and with different environmental factors surrounding the cultivation of a particular medicinal plant. Adding to this variability is the fact that in herbal medicine several plants may be used together in the same preparation. This means that there should be a quality control test for the entire preparation to ensure quality of the preparation.

As long as herbal medicines were grown locally, perhaps even in a kitchen garden and used fresh, for example, as a tea, whenever needed, it may not have been necessary to carry out extensive procedures of standardization. The Chinese scientists could not always fully comprehend the scope of standardization when he raised this topic since they were largely using freshly–prepared herbal medicines. However, the position changed and by the time of this next visit in 1985, most scientists involved with the development of herbal medicine were very concerned about standardization. Herbal medicines were now being prepared in factories and pharmaceutical houses and packed for use all over the country and also for export. Quality control had therefore to be carried out with their products and this could only be carried out if standards had been laid down to ensure quality. These standards had to be developed for different plants and for the final products and the whole issue of standardization of herbal remedies and medicinal plants came to the fore.

Before considering this issue in more detail, two things should be kept in mind. If plants are used fresh, after brewing as a tea or as a juice, it is probably not necessary to carry out tests for quality control. However, the moment plant substances are prepared for storage and subsequent use, it is essential to carry out tests to check that the standards are being maintained.

The second point to remember is that when plants are used fresh–and perhaps cultivated in the kitchen garden or village garden–these lead to cheap remedies. However, if tests for standardization of plant preparations has to be carried out and if standards are maintained, this requires the use of some sophisticated equipment and the time of suitably–trained technicians and supervisors. This inevitably means that this cost will be added on to the price of the herbal medicine which does not remain a cheap medicine any more. That is why it has often been stated that herbal medicines are, in fact, not cheap. This depends on the way herbal medicine is used. With elaborate quality control tests needed for four to five ingredients and the product, a herbal medicine may indeed be more expensive than a synthetic drug for the same purpose.

It is generally felt that standards can only be established for an isolated compound. Interest in developing extracts for use–both at the primary health care level and more widely–is therefore tempered by a feeling that these extracts cannot be standardized and therefore the extracts are not a marketable commodity. Development of therapeutic substances concentrates on isolated compounds and those plants in which an isolated compound cannot be obtained are not followed up. It has been stated earlier that biological activity present in some extract will be present when the plant is in an extract form only.

The full pharmacological effect will be decreased or even disappear if further extraction and fractionation is carried out. If specialists in the modern system of medicine want to use some of the medicinal plants in use today e.g. an extract of *Momordica charantia* for diabetes mellitus, they will need to consider working with extracts. It should be clearly stated that extracts can be standardized and the lack of standardization methodology today should not be a reason for not working with extracts. There may be other reasons for not working with extracts but the lack of standardization is not one of them. If the method of production of the extract is properly standardized and if there is an appropriate chemical assay method developed, there is no reason why standards cannot be developed for an extract or a fraction. Further, this will be augmented by a bioassay method, which would certainly be available. Once this reservation in thinking is overcome, a wide range of medicinal plants becomes available for investigation, for isolating maximum activity in an extract and for using the extract.

Another apparent consistent in standardization appears to be a preoccupation of chemists and pharmacologists with a medicinal plant having only one active principle which needs to be standardized. Again, if modern medicine is to take advantage of medicinal plants used in the traditional systems of medicine, then one has to accept that, in many instances, the pharmacological and therapeutic activity will not be residing in one active substance but may, in fact, be present in a combination of a few active substances. As far as standardization is concerned, this again need not be an insurmountable barrier because all the active substances could be identified and standards set for each of these.

Once scientists in the field of medicinal plants research accept these two "facts of life"–that standards have to be set for extract and that standards may have to be set for several active substances in a plant–and once they work towards these goals, there will certainly be advances in the field. Such advances have been lacking in the last two decades. Participants at two recent international meetings organized by Who have clearly pointed out the problems relating to standardization of herbal medicines and the tremendous need for urgent immediate work in this field. This first was an Interregional Meeting on Standardization and Use of Medicinal Plants, held in Tianjin, China, in November 1980, while the second was a Conference on Research in Traditional Medicine, held in Tokyo in March 1986. This meeting identified three areas of priority for research, and research on standardization was one of these. Standardization of a plant produce entails standardization of the raw material, standardization of the method of production and quality control of the final product.

Identification of the actual plant is not easy. Sometimes two plants are known by the same local name. When the plant is being collected, it is very possible that another plant is being collected at the same time and this will be mixed up with the plant which actually has the activity. One example of this is manifest when one collects the plant, *Boerhaavia diffusa*, which is used widely as a "quality of life enhancer" in the traditional systems of medicine. However, both *Boerhaavia diffusa* and the plant, *Trianthema portulacastrum*, are known as "Punarva", and so both plants may be collected at the same time.

A second area of concern is that plant collectors may substitute cheaper plant material that looks the same, for the actual plant material which has the therapeutic effect. In this case, it is not a case of inadvertent mistaking a non–medicinal plant for a medicinal plant, as described in the last paragraph, but one of adulteration and cheating. One example which is very well known concerns the bark of *Caesalpina sappen*. When this substance is collected, bark from other plants such as *Pterocarpus, Gluta Travancorea* and *Toona cilita* are substituted for the bark of *Caesalpina sappen*. Other examples with commonly–used medicinal plant sin India are substitution of the bark of *Saraca indica* by the bark of Trema orientalis and substituon of the plant, *Halarrhena antidysentarica*, by the plant *Wrightia tinctoria*. It is very important, therefore, when laying down standards for a herbal product–either for experimental research, clinical evaluation or widespread commercial use–to lay down clear–cut standard nomenclatures and clear–cut criteria to actually "finger print" that the substance being used in actually the substance which should be used. Once it has become clear that the substance being used is the substance being used is the substance meant to be sued, the first hurdle in standardization of the preparation is overcome. Every crude ingredient going into the herbal preparation must be clearly identified.

The next step is to standardize the method of production. This could be the method, as it usually is today, of isolating the compound which is to be used or the method for preparing the extract which is to be used. The steps leading up to this should be clearly described and the end points defined.

Finally, procedures have to be developed for laying down standards for laying down standards for the final product–if it is a single substance or for the final formulation–if it is a mixture of substance. These standards would attest to the quality of the final product and would comprise both physiochemical methods and biological tests of efficiency. If mixtures or extracts are to be used as the final product, then methods for standardization of the mixtures or extracts should be developed. These standards should be strictly adhered to.

It has been stated very often that the lack of standardization of herbal remedies and plant medicines is holding back the use of medicinal plants in the modern system of medicine. It has also been said that practitioners of the modern system of medicine cannot have confidence in the use of herbal the medicines and do not want to use such medicines because they are not certain that the substance being used is what it is supposed to contain. This sentiment is not confined to practitioners of the modern systems of medicine. At the III International Congress of Traditional Asian Medicine, held in Bombay from 4 to 9 January 1990, similar views were expressed by a large number of participants who die not belong to the allopathic medical profession. Botanists brought out of the difficulty in the identification of Artemesias as the herbs and shrubs belong to at least ten species of Artemesia. A group of Ayurvedic research workers stressed the importance of developing good methods for standardizing crude extracts, decoctions and compound formulations which consists of different ingredients. It was clearly stated that the technology currently available is not able to develop suitable quality control criteria for mixtures and compound preparations. Research, therefore, should be carried out to develop the methodology needed for the standardization of such preparations as otherwise these could never be used either for primary health care or more widely.

Another investigator suggested that extensive work be put into the methodology of standardization keeping in view the vary intricate and complicated system being dealt with. He pointed out the biological activity of a plant depended not only on the use of the proper plant and its contents but also on the presence of the required quality and nature of secondary metabolities in the raw drug.

The availability of these secondary metabolities depended on environmental and other factors such as time and season for collection, stage of plant growth, storage, drying procedure and geographical variation. Unless clear-cut standards are laid down for the evaluation of the final product, these factors could certainly modify and affect the efficiency of the product and lead to failures in therapy. Still another investigator stressed the need to develop methods for rapidly determining whether the plants being collected were authentic and whether the quality of the material used was up to the standard.

There appears, therefore, to be a general consensus that the lack of standardization constitutes a major constraint to the development and use of medicinal plants; that this need is felt by practitioners of both the modern and the traditional systems of medicine and that the area which needs attention is that for developing a methodology. It is very interesting to note that researchers and practitioners of the traditional systems of medicine do not have any reservation about the use of modern technology for developing methods for standardization. In fact, these workers have often stressed not only that all modern method should be used and that these methods are not always adequate and that more sophisticated and more advanced test should be devised.

ACTIVE CONSTITUENTS MEDICINAL PLANTS

Active ingradient are the main effective compounds of medicinal plants.Quantification of Active ingradients is the first step of stanndardiztion.Verious chemical test are available for quanitfication of active ingradients. Some of the main groups of active ingradients are described here.

Mucilage

Found in many plants, mucilage is made up of polysaccharides (large sugar molecules) that soak up water, producing a sticky jelly–like mass. Mucilage lines the mucous membranes of the digestive tract, protecting against irritation, acidity and inflammation. This soothing and protective action appears to extend to other areas, including the mucous membranes of the throat, lungs, kidneys and urinary tubules. Slippery elm (*Ulmus rubra*), is a typical mucilaginous herb.

Phenols

This group of compounds includes salicylic acid–the natural forerunner of aspirin. Salicylic acid is found in many plants, for example wintergreen (*Gaultheria procumbens*), and white willow (*Salix alba*). Another phenol is thymol–a constituent of thyme (*Thymus vulgaris*). Phenols are antiseptic and reduce inflammation when taken internally yet they have an irritant effect when applied to the skin.

Tannins

Tannins are produced to a greater or lesser degree by all plants. The harsh, astringent taste to tannin–laden bark and leaves makes them unpalatable to insects and grazing animals. Tannins contract the tissues of the body–hence their use to "tan" leather. They draw the tissues closer together and improve their resistance to infection. Oak bark (*Quercus robur*), and black catechu (*Acacia catechu*) are both high in tannins.

Coumarins

Coumarins of different kinds are found in many plant species and have widely divergent actions. The coumarins in melilot (*Melilotus officinalis*), thin the blood, while bergapten, found in celery (*Apium graveolens*), is used as a sunscreen, and khellin, found in visnaga (*Ammi visnaga*), is a powerful smooth muscle relaxant.

Anthraquinones

Anthraquinones are the main active constituents in herbs such as senna (*Cassia senna*), and Chinese rhubarb (*Rheum palmatum*), both of which are taken to relieve constipation. Anthraquinones have an irritant laxative effect on the large intestine, causing contractions of the intestinal walls and stimulating a bowel movement approximately 10 hours after being taken. They also make the stool more liquid, easing bowel movements.

Flavonoids

Found in many plants, flavonoids have a wide range of actions. They are anti–inflammatory and are especially useful in maintaining healthy circulation. Rutin, a flavonoid found in plants including buckwheat (*Fagopyrum esculentum*), and lemon (*Citrus limon*), strengthens capillary walls.

Anthocyanins

These pigments, which give flowers and fruits a blue, purple or red hue, help to keep the blood vessels healthy. Blackberry (*Rubus fruticosus*), and grapes (*Vitis vinifera*) contain appreciable quantities anthocyanins.

Glucosilinates

Found exclusively in species of the mustard family, glucosilinates have an irritant effect on the skin, causing inflammation and blistering. Applied as poultices of painful or aching joints, they increase blood flow to the affected area, helping to remove the build–up of waste products (a contributory factor in joint problems). Glucosilinates also help to reduce thyroid function. Both radish (*Raphanus sativus*), and mustard (*Sinapis alba*) contain significant quantities of glucosilinates.

Volatile Oils

Volatile oils–which are extracted from plants to produce essential oils–are some of the most important plant constituents of all. Tea tree (*Melaleuca alternifolia*), for example, is known to contain over 60 different volatile compounds within its volatile oil, many of them being strongly antiseptic. Some volatile oils contain sesquiterpenes, such as azulence, found in German chamomile (*Chamomilla recutita*). These constituents have an anti–inflammatory effect.

Saponins

There are two types of saponins–triterpenoid and steroidal saponins. The latter get their name from their similarity to the human body's own naturally occurring steroid hormones. Many plants containing steroidal saponins have a marked hormonal activity, liquorice (*Glycyrrhiza glabra*), being one of the best known. Triterpenoid saponins, for example those in cowslip root (*Primula veris*), are often strong expectorants, and may also aid in the absorption of nutrients.

Cardiac Glycosides

Found in various medicinal plants, most famously in common foxglove (*Digitalis purpurea*), yellow foxglove (*D. lutea*), and woolly foxglove (*D. lanata*), cardiac glycosides such as digitoxin, digoxin, and gitoxin have a strong, direct action on the heart, helping to support its strength and rate of contraction when it is failing. Cardiac glycosides are also significantly diuretic. They help to transfer fluids from the tissues and circulatory system to the urinary tract, thereby lowering blood pressure.

Cyanogenic Glycosides

Though these glycosides are based on cyanide, a very potent poison, they have a helpful sedative and relaxant effect on the heart and muscles in small doses. Wild cherry bark (*Prunus serotina*), and elder (*Sambucus nigra*), both contain cyanogenic glycosides, which contribute to both plants' ability to suppress and soothe irritant dry coughs.

Vitamins

Some plants contain significant levels of vitamins. Watercress (*Nasturtium officinale*), for example, contains an appreciable quantity of vitamin E, and the hips of dog rose (*Rosa canina*), have particularly high levels of vitamin C. Most other medicinal plants contain at least some vitamins. While the content may be small it contributes to overall daily intake. For other plants that are rich in vitamins.

Bitters

Bitters are a varied group of constituents linked only by their pronounced bitter taste. The bitterness itself stimulates secretions by the salivary glands and digestive organs. Such secretions can dramatically improve the appetite and strengthen the overall function of the digestive system. With the improved digestion system. With the improved digestion and absorption of nutrients that follow, the bodyis nourished and strengthened. Many herbs have bitter constituents, notably wormwood (*Artemisia absinthium*), and chiretta (*Swertia chirata*).

Alkaloids

A very mixed group, alkaloid mostly contains a nitrogen–bearing molecule ($-NH_2$) that makes them particularly pharmacologically active. Some are well–known drugs and have a recognized medical use. Vincristine, for example, derived from Medagascar periwinkle (*Vinca rosea*), is used to treat some types of cancer. Other alkaloids, such as atropine, found in deadly nightshade (*Atropa belladonna*), have a direct effect on the body, reducing spasms, relieving pain and drying up bodily secretions.

Minerals

Some herbs are particularly rich in minerals. Horsetail (*Equisetum arvense*), for example, has high levels of silica. Dandelion (*Taraxacum officinale*), has large quantities of potassium, and unlike other diuretics which flush this mineral out of the body, it helps to maintain high levels of potassium. These plants act as mineral supplements in their own right, while other herbs with a small concentration contribute to overall intake. For other plants with a high mineral content.

Tests for Standardization

Generally, the tests for standardization of plant medicines in use today are macroscopic, microscopic, physiochemical and biological. It is not the place to deal critically and exhaustively with these test nor is the author competent to do so. The list of tests generally used is given below.

- Macroscopic examination
- Microscopic examination, e.g.

Anatomical structure

Detailed study of fragments

- Physiological testing, e.g.

  Boling point

  Freezing point

  Absorption coefficient

  Loss on drying

  Ash value

  Refractory index

  Optical ratio

  Water/alcohol soluble solid

  Spectroscopic analysis

  Thin layer chromatography–R.F. value

  Gas liquid chromatography

- Biological testing where appropriate, e.g.

Bioassay

If a herbal remedy or a plant medicine is sought to be prepared for clinical trial or for wide use, it is essential that it passes the tests appropriate for the particular plant described above. Safety and efficiency need to be evaluated and documented. Only then will practitioners have confidence in the herbal medicine they use. Even these test methods are not adequate. More tests have to be developed to cope with enormous variability that may be, this has to be undertaken if we are interested in utilizing the heritage of medicinal plants available for use. If we are not prepared to expend the time, resources and superior calibre manpower needed, then we will never be able to develop more medicines from plants. The great effort and crusade for saving the rain forests–one reason for which is that these forests contain plants which would be the source of medicines in the future–would have been in vain and would remain a hallow sentiment. The best brains and sizable resources need to be put, not only in the areas of standardization but also in allied areas such as pharmacokinetic studies with plants, clinical evaluation methodology, development of toxicology models and development of clinical pharmacology in the third world where these plant are being used. Only then could we hope to use properly the herbal remedies we have or discover new medicines from plants in the coming century.

Preparation of Herbal Remedies

Identification

Before using medicinal plants that have been collected from the wild, it is essential that they are correctly identified. If inn doubt, do not use the herb. The wrong identification of herbs has led to many cases of poisoning. Foxglove leaves (*Digitalis purpurea*), for example, are often mistaken for comfrey (*Symphytum officinale*).

Utensils

Use glass, enamel or stainless steel pots and pans, wooden or steel knives and spatulas and plastic or nylon siees. A wine press is useful for making tinctures. Do not use aluminium utensils, as this potentially toxic element is easily absorbed by herbs.

Sterilization

All utensils used to make herbal remedies should be sterilized for at least 30 minutes in a well-diluted sterilizing solution, such as the type used for a baby's bottle. After soaking rinse thoroughly with boiled water and dry in a hot ovenor wash in a dishwasher. Proper sterilization maintain hygiene and prevents remedies, especially creams and syrups, from turning mouldy.

Weights and Measures

For most purposes, ordinary kitchen scales are suitable, although electronic scales are more accurate. Metric measurements of grams and litres are generally much easier to use than imperial measures when making remedies. If it is difficult to weight a small quantity, such as 10 g, on your scales, measure double the weight, i.e. 20 g, then halve the quantity. Liquids can be measured in a kitchen measuring jug, although conical or straight-sided glass measures are more accurate. Very small volumes of liquid can be measure in drops (*Measuring Remedies*, right).

Storage

Different preparation may be kept for varying periods of time before they begin to lose their medicinal properties. Infusions should be made fresh each day and decoctions must be consumed within 48 hours. Store both in a refrigerator or cool place. Tinctures and other liquid preparations, such as syrups and essential oils, need to be stored in dark glass bottles in a cool environment away from sunlight, but can be kept for a number of months or years. Ointments, creams and capsules are best kept in dark glass jars, although plastic containers are also acceptable..

Infusions

The medicinal value of many herbs lies chiefly in their volatile oils, which will disperse into the air if a lid is not used. This is especially important in the case of German chamomile (*Chamomilla rectita*). Use a teapot, or place lid or saucer over a cup if making a small quantity. Use water that has just boiled.

Popular herbal teas, such as German chamomile, are often taken as much for their refreshing taste as for their medicinal value and can be safely consumed in quantities of up to 5 or 6 cups a day. Some herbs, however, such as yarrow (*Achillea millefolium*), are significantly stronger and must be taken in less frequent doses. Other herbs, such as feverfew (*Tanacetum parthenium*), are so strong that they are not suitable for use in infusions. Always check the recommended dosage and quantity of herb to use, as infusions have medicinal actions and can produce unwanted effects at the wrong dosage.

Decoctions

Decoctions are generally made using roots, bark and barriers, but something, leaves and flowers may be included. Add these more delicate parts of a plant once the heat is turned off and the decoction has finished simmering and is beginning to cool. Then strain and use as required.

Chinese Decoctions

In traditional Chinese medicine, decoctions are the main way in which herbal medicines are the main way in which herbs medicines are prepared. Large quantities of herb are often used to produce a highly concentrated liquid, or the decoction is further reduced so that there is only 200 ml of liquid remaining. This increases the preparation's concentration. This process is useful for astringent barks such as babul (*Acacia arabica*), and common oak (*Quercus robur*), which may be used externally to tighten gums or wash weeping skin rashes. (Do not take internally.)

Infused oils

Got infused oils: Although hot infused oils can last up to a year, they are most potent when used fresh. If only using infused oils very occasionally, make a smaller quantity than the standard amount with the same proportion of herb to oil. The wine press may be replaced with a jug–when cool enough to touch, squeeze the oil through the jelly bag as illustrated in *Cold Infused Oils* below.

Many herbs make effective hot infused oils, especially spicy herbs such as ginger (*Zingiber officinale*), cayenne (*Capsicum frutescens*), and pepper (*Piper nigrum*). These oils can be rubbed into the skin to relieve rheumatic and arthritic pain, improve local blood flow and relax muscles. Other hot infused oil from leafy herbs, such as comfrey (*Symphytum officinale*), speed wound healing. Oil infused with mullein (*Verbascum thapsus*), is used for earache and ear infections, and chickweed (*Stellaria media*), ointment may be produced from a hot infused oil.

Cold infused oils: Making a cold infused oil is a slow process and involves leaving a jar packed with herbs and oil to stand for several weeks. Sunlight encourages the plant to release its active constituents into the oil. It is the most suitable method of oil infusion for fresh plant material, especially the more delicate parts such as flowers. St John's wort (*Hypercum perforatum*), marigold (*Calendula officinalis*), and melilot (*Melilotus officinalis*), are three of the most commonly produced cold infused oils. St John's wort oil is anti–inflammatory and analgesic and may be applied topically or taken internally (after consulting a herbalist) for peptic ulceration.

Olive oil is particularly suitable for cold infusion, as it rarely turns rancid. The intensity of sunlight and length of time a herb is infused for affects the concentration of its medicinal constituents. For greater strength, add the extracted oil to a fresh supply of herbs and infuse again.

Ointments: Ointments can be made with dozens of bases and they vary in consistency, depending on the constituents and proportions used. The simplest way to make a soft, all–purpose ointment is to use petroleum jelly or soft paraffin wax (other methods are explained below). Petroleum jelly is impermeable to water and provides a protective barrier for the skin. Single herbs or mixtures of herbs may be used as required, provided they are finely cut and essential oil can be stirred into the ointment just before straining.

Consistencies: A solid and relatively grease–free ointment will spread easily and is useful for preparations such as lip balms. This may be made by using alternatives to mineral oils. Melt 140 g of coconut oil with 120 g of beeswax and 100 g of powered herb. Simmer gently for 90 minutes in a glass bowl set in a pan of boiling water, or a double boiler, then strain and pour into jars.

A less solid ointment, for conditions such as skin rashes, may be made by combining olive oil and beeswax. Melt 60 g of beeswax with 500 ml of olive oil and 120 g of dried or 300 g of fresh herb in a glass bowl. Cover and place in a warm oven for 3 hours, then remove strain and pour into jars. This ointment can also be made by combining 500 ml of hot infused oil with 60 g of melted beeswax.

Creams: Small quantities of additional ingredients such as tinctures, powders and essential oils can be added to a cream before or after it is put in jars. Adding an essential oil, such as 1 ml of tea tree

(*Melaleuca alternifolia*) to 100 ml of cream, counters mould growth and lengthens shelf life, as does 5 ml of borax. Other recipes for making cream use infusions, tinctures or infused oils.

Compresses and lotions: After an accident or sports injury, bruising and swelling can often be reduced or prevented if a hot compress is swiftly applied, provided the skin is unbroken. Cold compresses are particularly useful in soothing inflammation, cooling fever and easing headaches. Both hot and cold compresses should be frequently soaked and re–applied for maximum benefit.

Other preparations

Stem Inhalations

Steam inhalations are an effective way to clear catarrh, and relieve sinusitis, hay fever and bronchial asthma. The combination of steam and antiseptic ingredients clears the airways throughout the respiratory system.

Baths and skin washes

Herbal baths and skin washes can relieve many conditions, including aching limbs and stuffy sinuses. They are made from diluted essential oils or infusions. Eyebaths soothe sore, inflamed or irritated eyes.

To make a herbal bath Add 500 ml of strained infusion or 5–10 drops of essential oil to a running bath.

To make a skin wash Make an infusion, strain it and bathe the affected area.

To make an eyebath Make a small quantity of an infusion or use a herbal teabag. Strain the liquid carefully into a sterilized eyebath. Alternatively, add 2–3 drops of a tincture to an eyebath filled with water that has just boiled. Allow to cool and place the eyebath firmly over the eye. Tip the head back and eye by continuously blinking. Repeat up to 3 times a day.

General caution Eyebaths should be very weak, so as not to sting the eyes. Always use boiled, cooled water in a sterilized container. Do not bathe eyes over a period of more than 2–3 weeks at a time. If bathing eyes frequently, add a tiny pinch of salt to each eyebath to counter leaching of salts and minerals from the eye.

Juices

The juices extracted from many herbs can be taken internally or applied externally. **To make** Pulp the plant preferably using a mechanical juicer. Otherwise use a food processor. Squeeze the pulp through a jelly bag to collect the juice. Some herbs need to be cooked in order to extract their juice.

STANDARDIZATION OF MEDICINAL PLANTS

When a medicine is administered to a patient, the doctor who prescribes the medicine needs to be assured that the medicine contains the correct amount of the right substances as only then would the medicine induce its therapeutic effect. This is assured both to the doctors and the patient by the pharmaceutical company producing the medicine. In the laboratories of the pharmaceutical house, the medicine–or batches of the same–have been tested for quality and quantity and the drug is released for use only if the quality control laboratories of the pharmaceutical house approve the batch in question. Overseeing the situation nationally are national drug control laboratories run by government scientists who also monitor the equality of the drug being released by carrying out random checks to ensure that the results conform to the standards laid down by both the pharmaceutical house and the national drug regulatory authority at a time when the pharmaceutical house requests for the release of a particular drug in the market. This is known as standardization–a system to ensure that every packet of medicine that is being sold has the correct substance in the correct amount and will induce its therapeutic effect.

This system has worked well in developed countries and reasonably well in countries in the third world, particularly if the country has a strong drug regulatory agency with its own laboratories. However, the system has been developed for synthetic medicines and its has not been difficult to "fingerprint" the synthetic medicines and lay down standards. It is much more difficult to ensure that this system works in regard to herbal medicine.

The system of standardization should be established for every plant medicine in the market because the scope for variation in different batches of medicine is enormous. Plant material, as has already been mentioned earlier, may vary in its alkaloid content and therefore in its therapeutic effect according to different places of collection, with different times in a year for collection, with collection at the same time and place but in different years, and with different environmental factors surrounding the cultivation of a particular medicinal plant. Adding to this variability is the fact that in herbal medicine several plants may be used together in the same preparation. This means that there should be a quality control test for the entire preparation to ensure quality of the preparation.

Following factors should be given due consideration while using plants:

1. If plants are used fresh, after brewing as a tea or as a juice, it is probably not necessary to carry out tests for quality control. When plant substances are prepared for storage and subsequent use, it is essential to carry out tests to check that the standards are being maintained.

2. When plants are used fresh–and perhaps cultivated in the kitchen garden or village garden–these lead to cheap remedies.

It is necessary that tests for standardization of plant preparations should be carried out and if standards are maintained, this requires the use of some sophisticated equipment and the time of suitably–trained technicians and supervisors. This inevitably means that this cost will be added on to the price of the herbal medicine, which does not remain a cheap medicine any more.

Herbal medicines are not cheap, it is more expensive than a synthetic drug for the same purpose. It also depends on the way herbal medicine is used. Quality control tests should be conducted for four to five ingredients and the products.

Standards can only be established for an isolated compound. Interest in developing extracts for use–both at the primary health care level and more widely–is therefore tempered by a feeling that these extracts cannot be standardized and therefore the extracts are not a marketable commodity. Development of therapeutic substances concentrates on isolated compounds and those plants in which an isolated compound cannot be obtained are not followed up. It has been stated earlier that biological activity present in some extract will be present when the plant is in an extract form only.

Standardization is the basic need of a chemists and pharmacologists to know the contents of active principle of medicinal plant. Pharmacological and therapeutic activity will not be residing in one active substance but may, in fact, be present in a combination of a few active substances. As far as standardization is concerned, this again need not be an insurmountable barrier because all the active substances could be identified and standards set for each of these.

Identification of the actual plant is not easy. Sometimes two plants are known by the same local name. When the plant is being collected, it is very possible that another plant is being collected at the same time and this will be mixed up with the plant which actually has the activity. One example of this is manifest when one collects the plant, *Boerhaavia diffusa*, which is used widely as a "quality of life enhancer" in the traditional systems of medicine. However, both *Boerhaavia diffusa* and the plant, *Trianthema portulacastrum*, are known as "Punarva", and so both plants may be collected at the same time.

It is observed that plant collectors may think for substitute for cheaper plant material. In this case, it is not a case of inadvertent mistaking a non-medicinal plant for a medicinal plant, as described in the last paragraph, but one of adulteration and cheating. One example which is very well known concerns the bark of *Caesalpina sappen*. When this substance is collected, bark from other plants such as *Pterocarpus, Gluta Travancorea* and *Toona cilita* are substituted for the bark of *Caesalpina sappen*. Other examples with commonly–used medicinal plant sin India are substitution of the bark of *Saraca indica* by the bark of Trema orientalis and substituon of the plant, *Halarrhena antidysentarica*, by the plant *Wrightia tinctoria*. It is very important, therefore, when laying down standards for a herbal product–either for experimental research, clinical evaluation or widespread commercial use–to lay down clear–cut standard nomenclatures and clear–cut criteria to actually "finger print" that the substance being used in actually the substance which should be used. Once it has become clear that the substance being used is the substance being used is the substance meant to be sued, the first hurdle in standardization of the preparation is overcome. Every crude ingredient going into the herbal preparation must be clearly identified.

Standardize for the method of production is also necessary for isolation of the compound, which is to be used or the method for preparing the extract which is to be used.

Standard procedures should be developed for getting the final product–if it is a single substance or for the final formulation–if it is a mixture of substance. These standards would attest to the quality of the final product and would comprise both physiochemical methods and biological tests of efficiency. If mixtures or extracts are to be used as the final product, then methods for standardization of the mixtures or extracts should be developed. These standards should be strictly adhered to.

For standardization of plant medicines macroscopic, microscopic, physiochemical and biological methods are used. It is not the place to deal critically and exhaustively with these test nor is the author competent to do so. Following test are to be conducted:

Macroscopic examination	
Microscopic examination	
Anatomical structure	Detailed study of fragments
Physiological testing	Boling point, Freezing point, Absorption coefficient, Loss on drying, Ash value, Refractory index, Optical ratio, Water/alcohol soluble solid, Spectroscopic analysis, Thin layer chromatography–R.F. value, Gas liquid chromatography
Biological testing	Digitalis bioassay

Decoction

Decoction is the method normally used for those medicinal herbs whose active principles are difficult to extract because they are contained in woody parts of the plant, or which require prolonged heating in order to pass into solution. The procedures dealt with here only involve water extraction, as more complex forms requiring various solvents are too technical for a book of this nature.

Extraction by decoction involves boiling the whole plant or a part of it in water for a given time and then allowing it to macerate for a further period before filtering. A slight variation of this method is to soak the plant beforehand in cold water for a specific time, depending on the drugs required, in order to soften the leathery part and thus make extraction easier at the decoction stage. This method is reserved for certain plants such as those with a high mucilaginous content.

Decoction is, understandably, quite a drastic method of extraction and one, which is capable of modifying some of the plant compounds. It is important to ensure that the main active principle to be extracted is not affected by other harmful compounds induced by the heat. The boiling process during, which water is added, nearly always destroys the volatile active principles, that is to say, those with a low boiling point. This means, therefore, that the resulting decoction will never possess all the original principles of the drug.

Filtering Operation

The filtering operation is equally important, as it serves to strain off not only the leathery residues of the plant but also the mucilage or deposits of amphorous substances that are carried in solution during the boiling. The liquid obtained is, therefore, always left to clear before the next stage when it is filtered through paper of finely woven linen.

Extraction

Extraction is much more suitable method for obtaining the active principles when the parts of the plant being used are soft and fragile, such as leaves bud or flowers. It is preferable, except in certain cases, to use herbs that have been slightly dried, as the reduction of water content will concentrate the principal constituents. Unlike decoction, this method allows retention of many of the volatile principles, which would otherwise be lost, but does not permit extraction of those requiring a continuously high temperature. An expert, with extensive knowledge of medicinal plants and their medical compounds, can decide, which of these two methods is more suitable for obtaining the active principles required.

Infusion

Infusion entails pouring boiling water over that part of the plant known to contain the required drug. The container should be made of pottery of glass to avoid the formation of tannate of iron, which due to the presence of tannin in almost all plants, would occur it metal were used. As soon a s the water ahs been poured over the plants, the container should be covered, thereby allowing the steam, rich in volatile compounds, to condense. After a given time, which varies for each plant used, the liquid is filtered before being used.

Maceration

The third simple method, known as maceration, is used for medicinal plants whose active principles are soluble in cold water for several hours during, which time all the principles that do not need heat to release them (i.e. that are not thermolabile) will be released into the solution. The yield of mucilage from certain plants, such as the mallow (*Malva*) and marsh mallow (*Althaea officinalis*), is in fact greater when extraction is carried out by means of cold maceration rather than by infusion.

The method of maceration described above is hardly ever used nowadays in the pharmaceutical industry. Instead, tinctures are prepared by diluting a certain amount of fluidextract of the requisite drug with alcohol of a predetermined strength. When, as is sometimes done, a sugar solution is added to spirit solutions, the resulting preparation is known as an *elixir* or *ratafia*. These preparations are, in fact, genuine liqueurs and have been almost abolished in pharmaceutical practice.

If the vehicle of maceration were to be a mixture of alcohol and ether, andethereal tincture' or, more scientifically, an ethereal spirit solution would be obtained. Many varieties of such preparations could once be found in all the pharmacopoeias, but are now little used. The best known is ethereal tincture of valerian.

Extraction

It is a straightforward method used for the extraction of juices. In this case the plants, which contain the required medicinal ingredients must be fresh and have high water content. The Juice, which can be extracted by various methods, contains the mineral salts and vitamins of the plant, together with all the other substances that can be obtained through pressure. Again, the juice will not contain all the active principles of the plant but, on the other hand, cold extraction does not modify the structure of those compounds, which as we have seen, can be altered by heat. In the home, juices can be produced by first parboiling the fresh plants very briefly and then applying pressure with an appropriate utensil such as a small press. Because of the additional heat used for parboiling, however, this method will modify some of the constituents.

Better still, of course, is the modern electric blender, which extracts almost the entire juice content of the plant.

All the methods described above have a time limit; hence they are considered short–term procedures. In fact, the decoction, the influsion, the maceration and the juice all contain biological compounds that immediately undergo processes of oxidization and fermentation that denaturalize the medicinal substance, often making the liquid taste repugnant and, therefore, unusable. To avoid this, it is possible to add preservatives but this, of course, would be quite contrary to the whole concept of non–adulteration, which is the aim of the methods described here. Additions of sugar and alcohol admittedly also enable juices to be kept for a slightly longer period and, if vacuum–bottled with sugars, their properties and the freshness of their components will remain unaltered; unfortunately, this kind of preservation is almost impossible in the average household because the apparatus required is often expensive.

The Problem

The problem of conserving medicinal principles, once extracted, is of the utmost importance. The pharmaceutical industry has, therefore, done much work in this field, producing further preservation techniques so that active principles can be used at any time and in any dosage. The difficulty of tracking down exotic or rare drugs, combined with the relatively short harvesting period of healing herbs, has necessitated the development and regulation of highly advanced methods of extraction and preservation.

Forms of Preparations

Such preparations are known as extracts. They are divided into semi–solid, dry and fluid types; another means of classifying them is by their vehicle of evaporation: water, water and alcohol, or ether. Strictly speaking, an extract is the concentration of all the substances and salts diluted in the juice obtained from it. This concentration is achieved by the use of two fundamental processes: the first is based on freezing and the other on evaporation. The latter, more generally used, consists of putting the juice into an evaporating dish from, which the water content is evaporated at a low heat. Obviously, depending on the length of the evaporation process, different concentrations of the juice will be obtained. Concentrations will thus range from those still possessing a high water content to concentrates in which water is no longer present. The extract obtained is termed soft extracts have a semi–solid honey–like consistency, while dry ones are often composed of solid masses that can be reduced to powder. A classic example of a dry extract is that of aloes, which has the appearance of black, solid lumps, almost vitrified, but which are friable and easily pulverized; an even better known instance is liquorice, which can be reduced to a powder or to liquorice sticks.

Water content of juice

The water content of juice is not, however, always the vehicle of evaporation used in obtaining an extract. Instead, to facilitate concentration through evaporation, a solution of water and alcohol is often used. Alternatively, ether may be used and then recovered through distillation. The addition of these substances to the water enables compounds to dissolve, which are hardly soluble at all in water alone, but which become very soluble in a combination of the two liquids.

The Solvants

Extracts in which ether is used are described as ethereal and those in which alcohol are used as hydroalcoholic. Certainly the most important type of extract is the fluidextract, which has only relatively recently been formulated and accepted in pharmaceutical practice. In comparison with the type of extract previously described it has one property, which makes it extremely useful: one gramme of fluidextract is equivalent to one gramme of the original plant material. In other words, all the active principles contained in a precise quantity of plant matter to be treated are present in the same quantity of fluidextract obtained. The fluid extract makes it possible to have any drug available at any given time (it does not deteriorate quickly and fluid extract obtained. The fluid extract makes it possible to have any drug available at any given time (it does not deteriorate quickly and is not modified, except very slowly, by external agents); it is of a purify and accuracy of tiration that would be impossible to achieve in drugs fresh from the plant.

Alcohol–soluble substances

When, for particular purposes, it is necessary to extract only the alcohol–soluble substances such as alkaloids, bitter principles, and organic acids and colouring substances, another specific method of preparation is used. This is generally known as an alcoholic tincture or, more correctly, spirit solution. Apart from the reason already given, these tinctures are produced because their high alcohol content makes them easy to preserve. A spirit solution can be prepared either by maceration, in which a measured amount of the medicinal plant is immersed in alcohol of a suitable strength for a predetermined length of time and subsequently filtered, or by digestion, passing it through a still. This apparatus is equipped with a cooling flask, which causes the alcohol that ahs been condensed in it to fall back into the receiver flask in which the drugs to be digested have been placed. Because tinctures are very sensitive to light they are always kept in bottles made of dark glass. The alcohol in which the plants have been macerated develops varying degrees of strength, depending on the drug being used and the ease with which it releases its essential constituents, but it is usually not less than 60% vol. Although these are alcoholic preparations they cannot.

The alcohol content is sufficient to obtain an extraction of the soluble compounds if the medicinal plants are allowed to macerate in the wine for the length of time appropriate to each type. Unfortunately, medicated wines are subject to acetic fermentation (that is, they go vinegary) and form sediment just like any other wine. It is, therefore, important to prepare only small quantities and to keep the wine completely airtight and away form the light.

Fixed Solvents

Essential oils are soluble in solvents that are described as fixed if they do not evaporate at a normal temperature, and as volatile if the reverse is the case. Fixed solvents consist of solid or liquid odouless fats such as lard, tallow or refined olive oil. These solvents enable essence to be extracted by means of a method known as *hot enfleurage*. The essence–producing plants are placed in copper containers and left to macerate in fat, which is brought up to a temperature of about 104° F. (40° C.), with more plants being added until the fat is saturated. The fat is then separated from the essence to give a good yield.

Volatile solvents

Extraction with volatile solvents, while presenting much greater difficulties in obtaining the essential oil, has the advantage of making it possible to extract essences from plants that have only very low percentage of the fragrant principle. The volatile solvents normally used are benzene and petroleum ether, which carry both the essence in solution and other products, making it necessary to carry our further, rather laborious tasks in order to obtain a pure products. The first phase of extraction by this method is the soaking of the flowers in an apparatus known as a *digester*. The solution obtained from this is distilled, during, which process the solvent is recovered. The essence' because of the traces of extraneous material contained in it. In order to purify the concrete essence, it is treated with pure alcohol, which takes up the essence, leaving many undissolved impurities. The alcohol is then brought to a low temperature, which enables the remaining impurities to become concentrate. As this stage, the alcohol can be called an extract. To complete the process, the extract is distilled to give the resulting essence a high degree of purity.

Uses of Extracts

These extracts can be used either by themselves or as the basic ingredient of various medicinal compounds, both of which are guaranteed as a homogenous product. Although the method of preparation varies according to the drug, it can be summarized as follows:

1,000 parts of the finely chopped dried plant are left to macerate for several hours in alcohol of the appropriate strength. This alcohol is then strained off and discarded. A similar amount of fresh alcohol is then poured over the same plant matter and a part of it strained off a day later. This alcohol, the weight of which is in direct relation to the type of herb used, is held in reserve. New alcohol is added until the dried plant material is exhausted of all the soluble extracts. The next stage is to distil this second liquid, recovering the alcohol and allowing the rest to evaporate until an extract is obtained, which, when mixed with the part held in reserve, will be of exactly the same weight as the original herb material. Some experts maintain that the solvent action of the alcohol can be improved by the addition of certain substances such as inorganic or organic acids, salts and ammonia. The various pharmacopoeias certainly use one or other these additives. The fluidextract will remain unaltered for a long time If kept in dark glass bottles, which are firmly stoppered.

The above explanation demonstrates the superiority of this method of extraction over the other methods described, and accounts for are almost unreserved use throughout the world.

Unlike fluidextracts, be preserved indefinitely. They react quickly to light and air, which cause flocculation and acetic fermentation.

Looking at the field of galenical preparations (those deriving from plant of natural origins) as a whole, there is one particular preparation reassessed by modern phytotherapy, both because of its successful results and its ease of preparation. It can even be made at home. This is medicinal wine. As long ago as the thirteenth century, Arnold of Villanova wrote his *Incipit* Tractatus de Vinis, the earliest published book on wines, which dealt particularly with 'methods of making preparations with wine basis'. Such wines are made by simply macerating plant drugs in wine, preferably white, with a high alcohol content, such as a fortified wine.

Examination of galenic products

These are examined are the *alcoholates* or *spirits*, produced by the distillation of spirit solutions. The difference between spirits and spirit solutions is that the former, through distillation, contain only the volatile principles of the drug and not the fixed principle, as do the latter. For the distillation, 70–80% vol. alcohols are generally used, after appropriate maceration. Only a certain part of the distillate is retained, so as not to change its characteristics with substances of low volatility, which remain in the flask, following the concentration of the watery part. Some of the best known spirit solutions still used today are aqua vitae of lemon balm and Hungary water, or spirit of rosemary, the former being used as a digestive antispasmodic and the latter as a perfume component. Spirits have excellent preservation qualities due to their high alcohol content.

Syrups Preparation

Instead of using alcohol as a preservative for garden herbs, sugar can be sued in a concentrated form. By adopting this alternative, sugary solutions can be made, which contain medicinal substances; they are known as *syrups*. Syrups also serve to disguise the unpleasant taste of many medicines.

Ordinary syrup is made by dissolving a certain quantity of sugar in water, at a low heat; the mixture needs to be stirred frequently and allowed to evaporate sufficiently to obtain the concentration necessary to achieve the characteristic density f syrup. The curative substances are then dissolved in it and it is these that determine the particular qualities of each type of syrup. If the resulting liquid is cloudy, it can be clarified. Syrups should be stored in hermetically sealed bottles and kept in a cool dry place, preferably away from the light. Despite such precautions, syrup is prone to alteration, especially when the additives are organic. In such cases, the syrup will have to be re–boiled in order to increase its density and, therefore, its preservation potential. Instead of sugar, honey can be substituted using the same procedure. Such preparations are called *mellitus* or honeyed syrups. For instance, 'melrosette' or 'honey of roses', which is still made for children, belongs to this category.

Electuaries of Conserves

Nowadays there is a growing demand for plants and vegetables that have not been contaminated with insecticides or fungicides, to be used in a natural form as natural form as possible. The interest in macrobiotics ash even brought back a number of preparations, which, due to their short shelf life, had become neglected. These confections are known as *electuaries* of *conserves* and are in the form of paste made by mixing the pulp of fruits, which have special nutritive of medicinal properties, with certain powders, honey of syrups. Some of these are sold commercially but, because of the high percentage of organic substances in them, preservatives have to be added. The macrobiotic diet makes use of several types of electuaries in this double role of supplementary food and medicine.

Use of Oil as solvent

When medicinal substances are dissolved in oil rather than the usual solvents, the preparations can be made either by dissolving one part of an oily fluid extract of a particular plant in a given quantity of refined olive oil or, alternatively, by boiling the plant itself in the oil and then filtering the as rheumatism, in which an oily preparation is required to facilitate localized massages.

Closely related to the medicated oils are the ointments, also known as *salves* or *unguents*, the base of which is usually a semi–solid, fatty or greasy substance such as lard or wool–fat (lanolin). They may be prepared simply by mixing powdered vegetal drugs into the fat, or the fat these ointments are all intended for external use.

At one time simple ointments such as these were very well known and widely used, but nowadays they have been largely replaced by commercial products containing chemical additives. The creams and liniments found on the market today tend to have quite different bases. Sometimes, however, we are reminded of remedies, which must have been familiar to our ancestors, when we see an old apothecary jar bearing a name such as unguent of polar or unguent of lily root. In Britain there is, increasingly, a tendency towards these simple creams containing no chemical additives.

Distillation Process

Distillation process is of fundamental importance for obtaining those ubiquitous ingredients of so many medicines and cosmetics known as essential oils or essences. These are not only used for their aromatic qualities, and s the main ingredients in perfumery, but also as the main medicinal ingredients in modern aromatherapy. The rest of this section, therefore, is devoted to a fairly detailed description of various processes necessary for the production of these oils.

Essences

Essences are complex substances, which are often fragrant and, although not oily, when placed on paper will produce a translucent effect. It is now possible to reproduce a great many essential oils chemically, and although this might suggest that distillation is an outdated method, that is not the case.

The essences derived from plants do not merely consist of open or more compounds, which it is possible to reproduce, but of a whole combination of substances, which are often undefined. It is not difficult to differentiate between the natural and the synthetic essences, because the natural perfume is altogether more delicate. There are also cases were chemistry has to make use of natural raw materials in order to reproduce some of the compounds synthetically produced.

The reasons why plants manufacture essential oils are still being investigated. A Few of the many theories formulated have some credibility, but what is certain, in any event, is that essences are beneficial to the economy of a plant, enabling it to manufacture other products. Some authorities maintain they are either waste materials, which have not yet been eliminated or that they are a means of protection against excessive sunshine. It is, in fact, true to say that nearly all–alpine plants are scented and the perfume that surrounds them serves as a filter through, which the solar rays must penetrate.

Essences are quite easily altered, and the least change in temperature or humidity is enough to allow the enzymes present to become activated. Another factor to be borne in mind when gathering herbs is the effect of light on the amount of essential oil contained in plants at different times of day. Experienced collectors, knowing just when the healing properties of each type of plant are at their peak, can decide exactly when to harvest it in order to derive the most benefit. Thus in some plants, the amount of essence will be reduced by light, whereas in others it will be concentrated. The composition of the soil may also affect the size of the yield.

Having made these points, it has to be said that the most satisfactory extraction is obtained when there is the least possible alteration to the characteristics of the essence itself. This type of extraction, which is described as *cold*, entails no change in the composition of the oil because no heat is involved. Unfortunately this method can only be applied to certain plants, mainly citrus, that possess a great many oil–producing glands. With the cold method the components present in the oils undergo only the slightest alteration, thus making it possible to produce essences of great purity, which can even be used internally. The two main methods of cold extraction are:

Expression

The former is carried out by putting the skins of the fruit into special containers where they are pressed, thus causing their glands to rupture and allowing the essence to be collected together with water and other substances. Essences extracted in this way are, inevitably, cloudy, although their fragrance and substance remain unaltered and they clarify when subsequently decanted. This method is mainly used now for homemade essences. Industry has adopted the

Ecuelle process

This involves the use of machines in which the fruit is revolved in metal cups or drums lined with spikes, which delicately rupture the oil–bearing glands to release their essences. As this is a fast process and the fruit are not identical in size or shape, there is considerable wastage of essence; this is, however, compensated for by the speed of the operation.

Cold enfleurage

This method alters neither the perfume nor the characteristics of the oils. This procedure is based on the special is based on the special quality possessed by some substances to condense essential oils on their surface area. These substances are purified waxes, which are spread over flat glass surfaces; the plants are placed on top and enclosed in special containers. After a day or two, the plants are removed and replaced by fresh ones; the process is then repeated over several months or until the wax has reached saturation point. The wax is then removed from the glass and the essence recovered by following the same procedure as for volatile solvents.

The problems involved in obtaining the products of essences producing plants are such that the methods described are only adopted for particular purposes.

Distillation

Normally, even though the process may change the composition of the essences due to the heat employed, *distillation* is used. This can be divided into three categories: simple distillation over direct heat, steam distillation and vacuum distillation. In distillation, heat both ruptures the oleiferous glands and, unfortunately, slightly modifies the essence. We shall only deal with the type of distillation in which water is the transporting vehicle. The distilled liquid will be a mixture of condensed water and essential oil, which will separate naturally because of their different specific gravities. The plants to be distilled must be used while still fresh and should have been gathered when most fragrant. In order to avoid fermentation, they should never be piled on top of one another.

The apparatus used for distilling is known as an alembic, from the Arab word *al–anbiq*, a vase. This is divided into three parts: boiler, distilling column and condenser. Vaporization of the water and volatization (rapid evaporation) of the essential oils are achieved in the distilling flask. The vapours then rise up the column and come down through the condenser, whence, having recondensed rapidly, the liquid falls into a receiver.

The boiler is usually made of copper or stainless steel, but may be of glass if laboratory apparatus is being used. It is generally cylindrical in shape and its base, to which the heat is applied, is never in direct contact with the plants, as these are kept slightly raised on wire mesh racks. Part of the space between the base and the first rack contains water, which produces the necessary steam. The column, which is firmly set in the neck of the boiler, leads to the condenser and allows for the expansion of the steam and for its initial cooling. If the boiler is metal, the column is clamped to it to form an airtight join, but if it is glass, either the foot of the column is shaped to fit the neck of the heater flask, or it is passed through a close–fitting stopper or cork. The condenser consists of a spiral tube, which is completely immersed in a vessel containing cold running water.

When the steam from the column comes into contact with the cold walls of the condenser, it condenses and, by force of gravity, runs down into a receiver, known as a 'Florentine flask', where the essence automatically separates from the water. If this type of flask is not used, separation has to be effected by means of a separatory funnel. Under normal conditions, boiling point is reached when the tension of the water equals the atmospheric pressure and to achieve this, the heat source is placed directly under the boiler; in this case distillation is brought about by direct heat.

In the laboratory the boiler is replaced by a glass distillation flask, and the heat is also applied from below to avoid breakages an asbestos, wire mesh or gauze mat is interposed so that the heat is not applied directly to the glass. In order to obtain uniform heating, the flask may be placed in a bed of sand or in water–bath. In this way the heat will be diffused evenly over the lower surface of the flask.

The two main types of condenser used in a laboratory for liquids with a low boiling point are the Liebig and the serpentine. If the steam, rather than being produced in the same container as the herbs, as described above, is produced in a separate boiler, this prevents the essence–containing plants form being 'cooked', which might adversely affect the result.

The method, known as *steam distillation*, makes it possible to distil those liquids, which have higher boiling point than water at temperatures lower than the boiling point of water. This method also makes it possible to obtain essences that are not excessively altered and is, therefore, preferable to the previously described system because of the greater purity of the resulting product.

Distillation can also be carried out at a pressure lower than that of the atmosphere. This is done by vacuum pumps and is known as 'distillation under reduced pressure' or 'vacuum distillation'. By decreasing the atmospheric pressure, the boiling point is also lowered, so enabling distillation to take place at a lower temperature to obtain a product that is even less modified than that produced by steam distillation.

Fractional distillation: Once the essences have been obtained, they are not always used in their complete state but are often broken down into their various components. This is done by fractional distillation, based on the already discussed principle of boiling, which occurs as a result of the equality between the atmospheric pressure and the sum of the vapour tensions of the components. The distillation temperature will initially be lower than that of the most volatile component and will then gradually rise. By carefully controlling the temperatures, the fractions of the essences can thus be collected. As the various components separate, they are retained individually by changing the receiving vessel when the appropriate temperatures are reached. To carry out such work in a laboratory, a special container in used, which is known as a Pauly apparatus or, more commonly a 'spider'. However, on an industrial scale such a method would be totally unsuitable because it is lengthy, laborious and, what is worse, discontinuous. For practical reasons, therefore, the *dephlegmator* or *fractionating column* is used. The most usual type is the Egrot dephlegmator, in which the essence vapours are cooled by a flow of water. This causes only the less volatile constituents to condense, thus effectively separating them from the more highly volatile ones.

Distilled water is the secondary product of distillation and is used a great deal in perfumery. It is, of course, merely water in which a very small amount of essence has remained and which gives it a fragrance and character of its own. Distilled waters do not keep well and are prone to alteration as they are subject of fungi and moulds. The only precaution possible is to store them away from the light in dark glass bottles. Their fragrance can be made more subtle by diluting a little of the essence itself in the water but this will deprive the water of its active volatile and other unknown principles that are typical of distillation. Distilled waters are widely used today in phytotherapeutic technology because they are readily available in large quantities. Although they contain only a low level of active principles, their medicinal effect is consistent with the concept of homoeopathic medicine.

9 CONSERVATION STRATEGIES OF MEDICINAL PLANTS

This universe is the creation of the supreme power meant for the benefit of all His creations. Individual species must, therefore, learn to enjoy its benefits by forming a part of the system in close relation with other species. Let not only one species encroach upon the other's rights.

(*Source*: **Ishopanishad**)

Native biodiversities a source of pride for each country, composing as it does a shining part of the national heritage.

Anon.

Our National Food Security depends on our ability to conserve all out biological wealth.

Dr. M.S. Swaminathan

WHY CONSERVATION

Harvesting Too Much, Growing And Protecting Too Little

Open access to medicinal plants in the wild is perhaps one of the main reasons for the current unsustainable levels of harvesting. Other factors contributing to unsustainability include lack of sufficient data on wild plant populations, marketing, and trading; inadequate regulations and legal protection (including intellectual property rights for local practitioners with local knowledge); and poor access to appropriate technology for sound harvesting and plantation development.

Government support for and supervision of medicinal plant development are often weak. In some countries, public sector agencies exercise monopoly control over the purchasing and processing of such plants and other forest products, fostering inefficiencies, thwarting commercial development, and preventing fair pricing for collectors. But even when they maintain such controls, exporting nations generally reap low returns, since royalty payments and permit requirements are usually not enforced. In Nepal, for instance, less than 25 per cent of the total medicinal plant trade is actually registered.

Nevertheless, attempts are now under way to cultivate some easily grown species and protect important natural habitats in order to reduce the pressure on these vital resources. Indeed, cultivation offers the best hope for conserving many medicinal plants found in the wild while maintaining harvested supplies at today's levels. Cultivation also permits better species identification, improved quality control, and increased prospects for genetic improvements.

According to Alexander McCalla, director of the Agriculture and Natural Resources Department of the World Bank, *What looks like a problem actually provides numerous opportunities for developing nations to advance rural well–being.* After all, medicinal plants are one of the few (legal) developing country natural products that sell at premium prices. Thus, the global clamor for more herbal ingredients creates possibilities for the local cultivation of medicinal crops as well as for the regulated and sustainable harvest of wild stands. Such endeavors could help raise rural employment in the developing countries, boost commerce around the world, and perhaps contribute to the health of millions.

If existing supplies of medicinal plants are to keep up with demand, they will need adequate protection through development of appropriate institutions, policies, and legislation. Local communities need support and encouragement to protect these resources. To complement cultivation of adaptable species, harvesting from the wild must be guided by accurate inventories and knowledge about the species concerned. Above all, overexploitation of rare and endangered species must be avoided.

WHAT IS CONSERVATION

Conservation, defined as management for the benefit of all life, is increasingly recognized throughout the world as one of the most important aspects of preserving biodiversity.

Biodicersity: The Natural Biological Capital of the Earth

Variation is the law of nature. It occurs everywhere and every moment. The variations take place at micro levels at short space and small time period, but these become apparent only over a large space and big a time gap. The variations may be linear or cyclic. The variety and variability of organisms and ecosystems is referred to as biological diversity or biodiversity. Similarly, the biological variations initiate at the micro level (bio–molecular level or genes) and become apparent at species and ecosystem level. The biological variations in nature over time and space form the basis of evolutionary processes. Thus, *biodiversity is the degree of variety in nature and not nature itself.* Similarly, the biological diversity is not the same as biological resource although mutually, they form part of each other. The conservation of biological diversity is distinct but related to biological resources. It is difficult to discretely distinguish the value of biodiversity as a distinct characteristic of biological resources (IUCN *et al.* 1990).

Biological diversity means the variability among living organisms from all sources including inter alia, terrestrial, marine and other aquatic ecosystems and the ecological complexes of which they are part. Biodiversity provides the basic biotic resource that sustains the human race. This includes diversity within species, between species and of ecosystems. Biodiversity is the most significant national asset and constitutes an enduring resource for supporting the continued existence of human societies. Biodiversity is not merely a natural resources, it is an embodiment of cultural diversity and the diverse knowledge traditions of different communities across the world. It includes diversity of forms, right from the molecular unit to the individual organism and then on to the population, community, ecosystems and biospheric levels.

The World Commission on Environment and Development (WCED) constituted by the General Assembly of the United Nations published its report in 1987 which provided a major boost and endorsement to the need for conserving the world's rich biodiversity, particularly that of the tropical areas. Despite conflicting views among nations, a broad consensus was reached after bitter negotiations, and 170 countries signed the Biodiversity Convention, which is now ratified by 104 countries (42 Articles were adopted). One of the prerequisite tasks as expressed by Article 7 of the Convention is the identification and monitoring the components of biological diversity. Article 12 calls for Research and Training and suggest programmes for identification, conservation and sustainable use of biological diversity.

In context of the Indian desert, conservation of biodiversity is essential not only to maintain the most fragile ecological processes and life support systems but also to ensure the sustainable utilization of the species as well as the ecosystem.

According to one estimate, at least one species is being lost every day and by 2000, one million species would have been lost. Extinction is a process that is continuous and irreversible. A number of plant species have already disappeared and others await a similar fate (WRI, IUCN, UNEP 1992).

Each forest or grassland has a particular form of each species and each form is specially adapted to a particular site where is grows. Differences between them can be identified and used for better management. Desert, is therefore, a tremendous storehouse of potential resources, not only for ecological or taxonomical research but also as a source of as yet unknown economic products from plants. Day in and day out, we read about a new antibiotic or a new drug from plant sources. The discovery of gugul gum *Commiphora wightii*, which reduced serum cholesterol, and diosgenin from *Balantities roxburghii* are two instances of such discoveries. We, therefore, need to keep inviolate samples of as many types of vegetation in as many situations as possible, and to keep from us who could evaluate the potentials of *Schwieinfurthia sphaerocarpa* or *Farsetia marcantha*? None of us can, for this scorph and this crucifer have almost disappeared from the Indian desert, and once extinct, no human effort can ever recreate these or nay other species, particularly because they are rare or even endemic to this desert.

An integrated conservational strategy needs to be followed for both saving the species and meeting the increasing demand of the medicinal plants.

TYPES OF CONSERVATION

In situ conservation

Since most of these threatened plants occur as components of biotic or bioedaphic communities in open sites, restoring climax vegetation in such habitats through judicious protection measures is required without further loss of time. Equally important would be to rehabilitate fast–depleting types in ecotonal zones since such sites provide wide ecological amplitude. Identification of such floristic niches within the biosphere reserve would assure their stability vis–à–vis preservation.

For *in situ* conservation, a biosphere reserve offers the best site of natural conservation of threatened flora. The concept of preserving biodiversity resulted in the Biosphere Reserve in 1974 as UNESCO MAB (Man and the Biosphere) Project no. 8 for the conservation of the natural areas and of the genetic material they contain. The driving force for the creation of such reserves was the realization that natural ecosystems throughout the world were being altered on a massive scale. Therefore, the setting aside of representative sites inclusive of major ecosystem types became absolutely necessary.

The Government of India conceived the idea of establishing 13 biosphere reserves; the DBR (Desert Biosphere Reserve) was one of them. A comprehensive document to that effect was prepared and submitted in 1988 by an expert committee of which the present writer happened to be a member. The proposed DBR has been envisaged to offer the best site for *in situ* conservation of the threatened flora of the desert. Unfortunately, to this date, this proposal has remained only on paper and has not seen the light of the day due to lack of political will on part of the state government.

Recalling that man and all animal are dependent for their survival on the plant kingdom; that plants (species, sub–species, varieties, etc.) form a genetic resource of immeasurable value to mankind; and that the economic potential of the plant kingdom is only partly realized, and also realizing that once a species becomes extinct, it cannot be recreated by man, it is important to ensure the conservation of as many species as possible for the economic, scientific, and cultural benefit of mankind. A proper survey of the entire flora will reveal which plants are threatened, which are rare, and which are endangered in this basis of literature and herbarium survey, as has been done in the past. This is necessary due to the fast–changing habitats and degradation of ecosystem, which ultimately result in desertification.

Therefore, detailed mapping and a floristic ecological survey need to be made within the biosphere reserve. In addition to the proposed biosphere reserve, small representative areas throughout the desert will have to be identified and recommended to be preserved against the destructive agencies through legislations. Such areas should be set aside as sanctum sanctorum for the total preservation of depleting germplasm.

In situ Production

Nature has immense potential for restoration of an ecosystem provided the conditions are favourable. The arid ecosystem has been sustained since time immemorial and it is only theover exploitation of natural resources which makes the system unsustainable. In general, man–made reforestation / replanting is difficult, as one would need to study the habitat and microenvironmental requirements of each and every species for their cultivation. Given these problems *in situ* conservation projects have been started, for example, a project near Jodhpur. The area has been protected by stone wall fencing, watershed soil and water conservation measures are in place and the participation of local people has been gained. The naturally regenerated plant population of *C. wightii* has increased by 813.3 percent in 7 years. *C. wightii* is an endangered medicinal plant in the region, however, despite much research into macro/micro propagation, experiments in cultivation have not been comparable with the *in situ* conservation project.

Ex situ Conservation or Domestication

However, the impracticability of advocating theories of plant reserves for the protection of the flora under climatic conditions of the arid region is quite obvious, especially because here the plants are represented by species scattered over hundreds of kilometers in the desert. An alternative to this is to start desert gardens, where conditions can be created that are more favourable for the conservation of those species, which are in critical state.

Though there are several botanical gardens in our country, the natural genetic wealth, including wild relatives of cultivated plants, and rare and threatened plants, is not given priority over ornamental plants and other exotic flora in these gardens. Therefore, for *ex situ* preservation, special purpose gardens should be established. The establishment of at least one desert garden, where all the desert plants could grow under semi–natural conditions and disseminate their seed and propagules for self–propagation, is of great practical value. Practical conservation can always be effective through restrictions in collection and preventing them from being damaged by accelerated human use. Therefore, a national desert botanic garden should be created, in which all plants growing in the desert can be cultivated, propagated, and kept under conditions similar to those in natural desert. Bulking up such plants in the garden and re–introducing them is essential to restore the critically low population.

AGRICULTURE PRODUCTION

Although it is better to increase the production of Medicinal Plants by conserving them *in situ* there are plants, which are required or demanded, in large quantity such as Senna and Psyllium. For meeting this demand, cultivation is necessary. Under the arid tropical conditions cultivation of medicinal plants has economic advantages for farmers, helps the conservation of natural resources and can ultimately contribute to the sustainability of this fragile ecosystem.

POSSIBILITIES AND POTENTIAL

India, specially arid region, has huge possibilities and potential for the cultivation of medicinal plants which should be exploited.

1. The Medicinal Plants of this region are drought hardy by nature, thus their production is less affected by drought compared to food grain crops. As the root, stem and leaf are the useful parts in most Medicinal Plants, rather than the fruits, the yields of these plants are less affected by drought.
2. The soils of the region are comparatively untouched by fertilizers, pesticides and irrigation (FPI). The use of FPI is highly risky due to climatic conditions, moreover the marginal farmers are unable to use costly inputs. On the other hand the farming systems of these regions are dominated by animals, and the excreta of animals can improve the properties of sandy soils. These, which are seen as limitations for food grain production, are opportunities for Medicinal Plants cultivation. Furthermore, in organic farming quality i.e. no residue of pesticides / fertilizers) is more important than the quantity.
3. A major part of the region is currently wasteland (12 million ha) due to various land forms e.g. deep and sand / sand dunes, gravely, rocky area, saline soils / water etc. where cultivation of food crops is not possible. Medicinal plants can, however, be grown in these areas, e.g. *Cassia angustifolia* (senna) in deep sand / and dunes; *Comiphora wightii* on rocky / gravely land; *Plantago ovata* and *Vinca rosea* in saline soils. Using wastelands for cultivation will not only increase the production of these plants but will also help halt desertification due to increased vegetative cover.
4. At present the farming community remains idle for 7–8 months, after the rainy season (Nov–June). Year round cultivation of Medicinal Plants would provide more work and additional income, thus providing support to the economies of drought prone regions.
5. Because of the climatic uncertainty agroforestry systems have developed in the Arid Tropics, Medicinal Plants can easily be accommodated in these systems.

CONSERVATION THROUGH GENE BANKS

In addition to *in situ* and *ex situ* conservation, long–term storage of seeds are gene banks can also be undertaken. The National Bureau of Plant Genetic Resources, New Delhi, has already developed cold storage modules. Therefore, seeds can be sent to the Bureau for maintaining this diversity.

The area of conserving rare and threatened plants through biotechnological approaches is vital to the conservational needs of the country. It is necessary to have a well–conceived production programme for the conservation of plants that usually do not produce viable seeds in large quantities and therefore are under constant threat of elimination. Clonal propagation is now gaining recognition as a quicker alternative in conservation. *In vitro* techniques are being increasingly applied to supplement conventional method of propagation.

SURVEY AND RESEARCH NEEDS

As already mentioned, apart from the needs of a survey, the whole question of biodiversity and its conservation in this region needs basic research. To carry out basic research, we must have natural or scientific areas, that are tracts of land in a natural state, set aside and permanently protected or managed to preserve natural plant or animal communities, free from any kind of interference that will destroy the community. Cultivated land as that of Ganganagar or grazed and overgrazed land as found throughout the desert; support different living things–the complex system has changed and with it the original value of the basic research is lost. Desert habitats need their own wilderness for comparative studies of used and unused lands. Of course it is too late now, particularly when man with his ever–sharp axe and hungry herds of camel, sheep, and goat has raped the desert for centuries, to salvage more than a lop–sided system of wilderness remnants, most of these far too small to retain their normality.

GOVERNMENTAL POLICY

A National Policy has to admit the needs of various user groups of medicinal plants and therefore one of the basic factors that should influence the design of the policy framework is the users' profile. In the case of medicinal plans it is important to note than there exist non–commercial users who constitute a much larger population that commercial users.

The policy framework has to include temporal consideration viz. long–term availability of medicinal plans, as well as the more immediate needs of the user groups. It needs to consider financial resources and were needed incentives for encouraging conservation actions.

The policy since it is formulated for the purpose of guiding implementation, has to review the need for strengthening and where necessary the building of new institutions in both the government and non–government sectors. It also needs to examine the need for national level co–ordination with appropriate representation of user groups.

Finally, there is legal matter specific to the subject of medicinal plants for e.g. regulation of collection of plants from the wild and the new issue of property rights over traditional knowledge and Indian biological resources. A national policy framework needs to take these legal matters into consideration.

GOALS OF NATIONAL POLICY

The goals of national medicinal plants conservation policy should include:

- To ensure long–term conservation *in situ*, of viable breeding populations of medicinal plants diversity in a range of natural habitats corresponding to their natural distribution.
- To encourage and support a range of *ex situ* conservation measures as a supplementary and complementary measure to the above.
- To encourage medicinal plant requirements of industry to be met sustainably through policy instruments that create a favourable economic environment for the large–scale cultivation of medicinal plants.
- To ensure access of medicinal plants to village communities for their primary health care needs and address issues relating to participation and empowerment of village communities in conserving and managing forest and non–forest resources.
- To regulate, improve and where necessary ban medicinal plants collection from the wild.
- To carry out appropriate legislation and/or modify existing ones to regulate internal and external trade in medicinal plants and to ensure adequate staff training of the agencies involved in regulation.
- To ensure community benefits arising from commercial utilization of indigenous medical knowledge of plant resources as provided for in the international "Convention on Bio–Diversity".
- To develop a cadre of taxonomists, para–taxonomists and forest scientists to support and sustain rapid, prioritized baseline surveys for medicinal plants conservation status and to monitor changes on a long–term basis.

- To identify, review and clearly mandate appropriate institutions, governmental and non-governmental to implement the national policy; and to strengthen/build adequate institutional structures and capacity in Government and Non–Government Organizations for research, training and conservation action which are essential to initiate and sustain effective policy implementation.
- To encourage and facilitate time–boud "projects" through governmental and non-governmental institutions, to further the goals of the policy.
- To create widespread public awareness on the importance and need for medicinal plants conservation.
- To encourage local processing and enterprise development for value addition at the local levels where plants are collected for the market.
- To continually monitor, evaluate and analyze the impact of this Medicinal Plants Conservation Policy and for this purpose to create and national–level co–ordination structure.

NATIONAL PROGRAMS THAT NEED TO BE IMPLANTED IN THE NEXT DECADE TO SAVE MEDICINAL PLANTS

In situ Conservation

It is only in Nature that plant diversity at the genetic, species and eco–system level can be conserved on a long–term basis. Unless plant populations are conserved in the wild, that is in natural habitats, in variable breeding populations, they run the risk of extinction. It is necessary to conserve in distinct, representative biogeographic zones intern and intraspecific genetic variation. This alone will ensure that species would have the necessary resilience to adapt to change in the future.

Medicinal plant populations have large and often disjunct areas of distribution, while there are also endemic species confined to a few pockets. Conservation of these disparate and widely separated populations is therefore possible only through setting up to a network of representative medicinal plants conservation reserves with a broadly common management framework. This network would ideally include areas within and outside the existing Protected Area network in the Country.

For long–term conservation and management of medicinal plants *in situ* network would need to be integrated into regular forestry and wildlife management in the country. But for this to happen appropriate changes in forest management priorities backed by intensive trainings at various levels including training of community leaders to involve them in the protection and management of the forest reserves is necessary.

Regulation on Wild Collection

An essential corollary to *in situ* conservation of medicinal plants is regulating the harvest of medicinal plants from the wild for commercial purpose. Particularly those species whose harvest inevitably involves destructive collection. The management of Medicinal Plants collection needs to be critically examined and redesigned, so that local communities can develop a stake in sustainably harvesting medicinal plants from the forest.

Ex situ Conservation

Ethno–medicinal plant gardens

A valuable *ex situ* conservation measure would be the creating of a network of regional and sub–regional ethno–medicinal plans gardens, which should contain accessions of all the medicinal plants known to the various ethnic communities in different regions of India. The chain of gardens will act as regional repositories of our cultural and ethno medicinal history and embody and living traditions of our society's knowledge of medicinal plants.

Gene Banks

While it is known that the largest proportion of local biodiversity in all our eco–system sis used for medicinal purposes, very little is known about their conservation status in the wild. What is likely is that a large number of medicinal plant species are under various degrees of threat. The 'Precautionary principle' would suggest that an immediate and countrywide exercise be taken up to deposit seeds of wild medicinal plants with a first priority to known Rare, Endangered, Threatened (RET), species and endemic species. A simultaneous effort should also be launched to evaluate the genetic variation of economic plants with a view to promoting their domestication and breeding.

Nursery Network

The most urgent task in order to ensure immediate availability of plants and planting materials to various user groups like farmers, the professional Indian System of Medicines (SM) community, plants breeders, industry and to conservation organizations, is to promote and nation–wide network of medicinal plant nurseries which will multiply all the regional–specific plants that are used in the current practice of traditional medicine. These nurseries should become the primary sources of supply of plants and seed material that can be subsequently multiplied by various users. The forest departments, agricultural extension agencies, village panchayats, Non–Governmental Organizations (NGOs) and private enterprises should be encouraged to establish these nurseries or grow medicinal plants in existing ones. In the initial years interest–free short–term loans or loans at different rates of interest can be offered by banking institutions to this nursery network.

In view of its importance and urgency, Government can promote national co–ordination of this program through a national nodal institution, which may be called NATIONAL MEDICINAL PLANTS DEVELOPMENT BOARD.

Cultivation

Figures projecting demand and trade in medicinal plants species globally indicate a steep upward trend in the near future. One estimate puts the figure of world trade in medicinal plants and related products at US$ 5 trillion by A.D. 2050 (World Bank Report, 1996). The demand so far has been met mainly from wild sources. This cannot go on much longer. Policy intervention is urgently needed to encourage and facilitate investments into commercial cultivation of medicinal plants.

Cultivation of medicinal plans, however, is inversely linked to prevalence of easy and cheap collection from the wild, leak of regulation in trade, cornering of the profits from wild collection by a vast network of traders and middlemen and absence of industry's interest in providing buy–back guarantees to growers. Cultivation of medicinal plants is also difficult due to lack of standardized agronomic practices for not species and unavailability of sources of quality planting materials.

Policy measures to promote cultivation of medicinal plants, therefore, need to facilitate industry's role by way of tax incentives, etc. for investments in cultivation and agricultural research and simultaneously regulate indiscriminate, destructive collection of medicinal plants from the wild, while improving their conservation status *in situ*. In the context of medicinal plants, there is a special case for encouraging organic systems and polyculture models instead of the conventional mono–culture models in agriculture and agroforestry.

There is also a special case for encouraging in an "organized" way, small, marginal farmers and tribals to grow medicinal plants in their household gardens, bunds, wastelands because this can encourage economic participation of the rural poor in the growth of the herbal industry.

Community Based Enterprises

Considering the low value of many medicinal plant species (in raw drug form), a strong case exists for promotion of community–level enterprise for value addition to medicinal plants through simple, on site techniques like drying, cleaning, crushing, powdering, grading, packaging, etc. This will also increase the stake of village communities in conservation.

Isolated micro enterprises on their own may find it difficult to manufacture standardized products and market them. Therefore, a care to promote a macro organization to network and provide financial, technical and marketing support to rural enterprises exists.

Research

In order to help conservation of medicinal plants, the thrust of research should focus on immediate field–related problems. Priority areas in medicinal plants research need to include inventorisation and distribution mapping; threat categorization based on IUCN guidelines; conservation biology, propagation of rare species for reintroduction into their natural habitats; agro–technology of economically and clinically important species along with effective and quick technology transfer.

Research on medicinal plants based on Indian System of Medicines (ISM) theories like *desh vichar*, traditional guidelines on suitable collection times and habitats and advice based upon indigenous texts like *Vrksh–ayurveda* and *krishi shastra* need to be promoted so that parameters for quality of plants can be evolved based on Indian System of Medicines (ISM) principles.

Training

In–service training programs for staff of various government and non governmental agencies ike forests, wildlife, botanic gardens, schools and colleges in taxonomy and conservation biology need to be developed and supported in a large way. Training of community–based parataxonomists is also relevant to encourage community involvement in conservation.

To encourage the use and sustainable economic benefit from medicinal plants so that local communities can develop a stake in their conservation, suitable training courses in sustainable harvest (specially for tribal collectors), value addition and marketing of medicinal plants, needs to be promoted.

One of the major user groups of medicinal plants is the community of practitioners of traditional medicine, both classical and folk. Unfortunately, this group is least involved with the conservation of medicinal plants. With adequate orientation and training, this large group could make a significant contribution to the conservation of medicinal plants and its sustainable use.

Databases

As the existence and accessibility of reliable information is crucial to organized development and growth of any sustained medicinal plants conservation effort, a project on the building up of a national medicinal plants conservation database is the need of the hour.

Herbarium

The role of herbarium in authenticating identity of plants is well known. There is, therefore, a need to establish a national herbarium and raw drug museum of the medicinal plants of India. A critical task in a medicinal plants herbarium is to have rigorously worked out correlations between vernacular names and botanical names based on both etymological analysis of vernacular nomenclature and field studies.

LEGISLATION FOR PROTECTION OF TRADITIONAL KNOWLEDGE AND RELATED NATURAL RESOURCES

Based on clause 27(ii) of TRIPs related to public interest, India should modify its 1970 Patents Act to exclude products, processes, extracts, derivatives and any modification of its plans and natural products (as known in the folk stream of medicine which is prevalent in its various ethnic communities and in its codified systems of medicine like Ayurveda, Unani, Siddha and Tibetan including their numerous manuscripts and literary works) from being granted patents in India, for uses similar to their traditional use.

In order to uphold traditional knowledge as a priceless national heritage, this knowledge of plant and plant products should continue to be in the public domain. The proposed biodiversity legislation (in the context of the Biodiversity Convention as per provisions 8j, 10(c), 15(v) must ensure that all our indigenous medicinal knowledge systems (both oral and codified) and their associated biological resources remain our sovereign property and that "informed consent" is taken from traditional communities.

Similar conditions of informed consent should be brought into the Plant Breeders Act for medicinal plant genetic materials. A national biodiversity fund needs to be created to receive contributions from industry and other sources in lieu of utilization of indigenous knowledge and native plants collected from non–cultivated sources.

MEETING IMMEDIATE NEEDS OF ALL USER GROUPS

National Agricultural and Rural Development Bank (NABARD) and representatives of industry in collaboration with Indian System of Medicines (ISM), Indian Council for Agricultural Research (ICAR) and Non–Governmental Organizations (NGOs) establish a fund to support a co–ordinated scheme for establishment of a national–wide network of medicinal plant nurseries to ensure supply of planting materials of medicinal plants and semi–processed materials to various categories of users like village communities, industry and farmers.

Council for Scientific and Industrial Research (CSIR), Industrial Development Bank of India (IDBI), Basic Chemicals, Pharmaceuticals and Cosmetics Export Promotion Council (CHEMEXCIL) and Finance Ministry work out schemes of financial (tax) incentives for industry and Research Institutes on investments for standardization of classical Indian System of Medicines (ISM) drugs to bring them upto international standards of marketability.

Transfer of technology and training should also be extended to community–based enterprises so as to increase stake of rural communities in conservation and sustainable use of medicinal plans.

Adequate standards currently do not exist for identification and quality control of raw drugs. Department of Indian System of Medicines (ISM) should take the initiative in collaboration with industry and Council for Scientific and Industrial Research (CSIR) to establish standards for priority plants that are currently used in formulations for domestic and export markets.

Reliable standards should also be set for plant formulations which are used for self–help, by rural and urban communities, with reference to identity of plants, part used, processing method, dosage, duration and limitations, so as to promote pubic health education based on medicinal plants and indigenous systems of medicine.

In general, the desert ecosystem poses difficult problems to man. Its extent is large, its nature is difficult, and its opportunities are limited or insignificant, particularly when we consider the effort and investment needed for its eco development. Originally, this area had but a scant population. More often than not, for reasons rooted in their history, the population does not command the advanced technological and managerial competence required for the utilization of so difficult an environment.

It is true that to preserve and regenerate the proposed desert biosphere reserve, we have to enlist the active participation of the local population, which has to be educated to preserve and develop the area sustainably.

10 ECONOMIC ASPECTS OF MEDICINAL PLANTS

The grower is always interested to look into the gain or loss in the business. He will grow only those medicinal plants, which can give him good economic return. Before selecting and planting the grower has to make an over all assessment of the total production cost, its sale potential, lossess and profit etc. We are presenting the economics of the few important medicinal plant for your assessment at a glance.

CAUTION

Though we are presenting the economic aspects of selective medicinal plants. However, the economics depends on the soil, climate, quality of seed, agronomic conditions, time of planting, use of organic manure, etc. Therefore, the authors are not responsible for the data presented in the following text. The amount (in Rs) presented in the text is the approximate expendature/return for cultivation, it may vary.

Abelmoschus moschatus

SN	Particulars	Expenditure (Rs.)	SN	Particulars	Income (Rs.)
	(A) Cost			**(B) Products obtained**	
1.	Preparation of Farmyard	1,100.00	1.	Roots (400 kg) (@ Rs. 200/kg)	80,000.00
2.	Planting material (Seeds 4 kg) (@ Rs. 250/Rhizome)	1,000.00			
3.	Sowing labour	1,500.00	2.	Other Important Part	11,000.00
4.	Fertilizers and Pesticides	850.00			
5.	Irrigation and hoeing–weeding etc.	350.00			
6.	Harvesting labour	2,000.00			
7.	Other expanses (Collection, Transportation, etc.)	500.00			
	Total Cost	**7,300.00**		**Total**	**91,000.00**

Net Profit: Total Production Obtained–Total Cost

Rs. 91,000.00–Rs. 7,300.00 = **Rs. 83,700.00**

Acorus calamus

SN	Particulars	Expenditure (Rs.)	SN	Particulars	Income (Rs.)
	(A) Cost			**(B) Products obtained**	
1.	Preparation of Farmyard	2,040.00	1.	Roots (4000 kg) (@ Rs. 25.00/kg)	1,00,000.00
2.	Planting material (1 lakh Rhizome) (@ Rs. 0.60/Rhizome)	60,000.00			
3.	Sowing labour	2,550.00	2.	Planting material	20,400.00
4.	Fertilizers and Pesticides	1,530.00			
5.	Irrigation and hoeing–weeding etc.	510.00			
6.	Harvesting labour	3,060.00			
7.	Other expanses (Collection, Transportation, etc.)	510.00			
	Total Cost	**70,200.00**		**Total**	**1,20,400.00**

Net Profit: Total Production Obtained–Total Cost
Rs. 1,20,400.00–Rs. 70,200.00 = **Rs. 50,200.00**

Aloe vera

SN	Particulars	Expenditure (Rs.)	SN	Particulars	Income (Rs.)
	(A) Cost			**(B) Products obtained**	
1.	Preparation of Farmyard	510.00	1.	Fresh leaves (50,000 kg) (@ Rs. 3.00/kg)	1,50,000.00
2.	Planting material (40–50 thousand plant) (@ Rs. 1.00/plant)	40,000.00			
3.	Sowing labour	1,224.00	2.	Planting material	25,500.00
4.	Fertilizers and Pesticides	510.00			
5.	Irrigation and hoeing–weeding etc.	816.00			
6.	Harvesting labour	1,530.00			
7.	Other expanses (Collection, Transportation, etc.)	510.00			
	Total Cost	**45,100.00**		**Total Production Obtained**	**1,75,500.00**

Net Profit: Total Production Obtained–Total Cost
Rs. 1,75,500.00–Rs. 45,100.00 = **Rs. 1,30,400.00**

Andrographis paniculata

SN	Particulars	Expenditure (Rs.)	SN	Particulars	Income (Rs.)
	(A) Cost			(B) Products obtained	
1.	Preparation of Farmyard	1,326.00	1.	Total yield (3,000 kg) (@ Rs. 52.00/kg)	1,56,000.00
2.	Planting material	6,120.00			
3.	Sowing labour	1,020.00	2.	Planting material	10,200.00
4.	Fertilizers and Pesticides	2,040.00			
5.	Irrigation and hoeing–weeding etc.	1,224.00			
6.	Harvesting labour	2,550.00			
7.	Other expanses (Collection, Transportation, etc.)	2,040.00			
	Total Cost	**16,320.00**		**Total**	**1,66,200.00**

Net Profit: Total Production Obtained–Total Cost
Rs. 1,66,200.00–Rs. 16,320.00 = **Rs. 1,49,880.00**

Asparagus racemosus

SN	Particulars	Expenditure (Rs.)	SN	Particulars	Income (Rs.)
	(A) Cost			**(B) Products obtained**	
1.	Preparation of Farmyard	4,000.00	1.	Dry Roots (9 ton) (@Rs. 22.00/kg)	1,98,000.00
2.	Planting Material (Seeds 12 kg) (@ Rs.500.00/kg)	6,000.00			
3.	Sowing labour	3,500.00	2.	Planting material (Seeds)	10,000.00
4.	Fertilizers and Pesticides	400.00			
5.	Irrigation and hoeing–weeding etc.	500.00			
6.	Harvesting labour	3,000.00			
7.	Other expanses (Collection, Transportation, etc.)	200.00			
	Total Cost	**17,600.00**		**Total**	**2,08,000.00**

Net Profit: Total Production Obtained–Total Cost
Rs. 2,08,00.00–Rs. 17,600.00 = **Rs. 1,90,400.00**

Atropa acuminata

SN	Particulars	1st year	2nd year	3rd year
	(A) Cost			
1.	Preparation of Farmyard	2,040.00	–	–
2.	Planting material (5 kg seeds) (@ Rs. 290/kg)	1,450.00	–	–
3.	Sowing labour	1,938.00	–	–
4.	Fertilizers and Pesticides	918.00	918.00	918.00
5.	Irrigation and hoeing–weeding etc.	1,224.00	1,224.00	1,224.00
6.	Harvesting labour	2,244.00	2,244.00	2,244.00
7.	Other expanses (Collection, Transportation, etc.)	1,020.00	1,020.00	1,020.00
	Total Cost	**10,834.00**	**5,406.00**	**5,406.00**
	(B) Production Obtained			
1.	Dry Leaves (@ Rs. 35.00/kg)	21,000.00 (6 quintal)	52,500.00 (15 quintal)	52,500.00 (15 quintal)
2.	Dry Roots (3 quintals) (@ Rs. 55.00/kg)			16,500.00
	Net Profit	**10,166.00**	**47,094.00**	**63,594.00**

Bombax ceiba

SN	Particulars	Expenditure (Rs.)	SN	Particulars	Income (Rs.)
	(A) Cost			**(B) Products obtained**	
1.	Preparation of Farmyard	2,000.00	1.	Dry Roots (30 quintals) (@ Rs. 30.00/kg)	90,000.00
2.	Planting Material (10 kg Seeds) (@ Rs.200.00/kg)	2,000.00			
3.	Sowing labour	1,500.00			
4.	Fertilizers and Pesticides	1,000.00			
5.	Irrigation and hoeing–weeding etc.	1,000.00			
6.	Harvesting labour	5,000.00			
7.	Harvesting & Storage (@ Rs. 100.00/kg)	1,000.00			
8.	Other expanses (Collection, Transportation, etc.)				
	Total Cost	**13,500.00**		**Total**	**90,000.00**

Net Profit: Total Production Obtained–Total Cost
Rs. 90,000.00–Rs. 13,500.00 = **Rs. 76,500.00**

Cassia angustifolia

SN	Particulars	Expenditure (Rs.)	SN	Particulars	Income (Rs.)
	(A) Cost			**(B) Products obtained**	
1.	Preparation of Farmyard	1,000.00	1.	Dried leaves (15 quintals) (@Rs. 20.00/kg)	30,000.00
2.	Planting Material (Seeds 10 kg) (@ Rs.100.00/kg)	1,000.00			
3.	Sowing labour	1,000.00	2.	Planting material (Seeds 3 quintals) (@ Rs. 100.00/kg)	30,000.00
4.	Fertilizers and Pesticides	300.00			
5.	Irrigation and hoeing–weeding etc.	500.00			
6.	Harvesting labour	1,000.00			
7.	Other expanses (Collection, Transportation, etc.)	500.00			
	Total Cost	**5,300.00**		**Total**	**60,000.00**

Net Profit: Total Production Obtained–Total Cost
Rs. 60,000.00–Rs. 5,300.00 = **Rs. 54,700.00**

Catharanthus roseus

SN	Particulars	Expenditure (Rs.)	SN	Particulars	Income (Rs.)
	(A) Cost			**(B) Products obtained**	
1.	Preparation of Farmyard	1,500.00	1.	Leaf (30 quintals) (@ Rs. 25.00/kg)	75,000.00
2.	Planting Material (Seeds 5 kg) (@ Rs.60.00/kg)	300.00			
3.	Sowing labour	1,500.00	2.	Stem (10 quintals) (@ Rs. 10.00/kg)	10,000.00
4.	Fertilizers and Pesticides	700.00			
5.	Irrigation and hoeing–weeding etc.	1,000.00	3.	Dried Roots (8 quintals) (@ Rs. 50.00/kg)	40,000.00
6.	Harvesting labour	1,500.00			
7.	Other expanses (Collection, Transportation, etc.)	500.00			
	Total Cost	**7,000.00**		**Total**	**1,25,000.00**

Net Profit: Total Production Obtained–Total Cost
Rs. 1,25,000.00–Rs. 7,000.00 = **Rs. 1,18,000.00**

Chlorophytum borivilianum

SN	Particulars	Expenditure (Rs.)	SN	Particulars	Income (Rs.)
	(A) Cost			**(B) Products obtained**	
1.	Preparation of Farmyard	4,500.00	1.	Dry Bulb (10 quintals) (@Rs. 1200.00/kg)	12,00,000.00
2.	Planting Material (Bulb 6 quintals) (@ Rs.450.00/kg)	2,70,000.00			
3.	Sowing labour	6,000.00	2.	Planting material (3 quintals bulb) (@ Rs. 450.00/kg)	1,35,000.00
4.	Fertilizers and Pesticides	5,000.00			
5.	Irrigation and hoeing–weeding etc.	5,000.00			
6.	Harvesting labour	15,000.00			
7.	Harvesting & Storage (@ Rs. 100.00/kg)	1,00,000.00			
8.	Other expanses (Collection, Transportation, etc.)	3,000.00			
	Total Cost	**4,08,500.00**		**Total**	**12,35,000.00**

Net Profit: Total Production Obtained–Total Cost

Rs. 12,35,000.00–Rs. 4,08,500.00 = **Rs. 9,26,500.00**

Coleus forskohlii

SN	Particulars	Expenditure (Rs.)	SN	Particulars	Income (Rs.)
	(A) Cost			(B) Products obtained	
1.	Preparation of Farmyard	1,224.00	1.	Dry Roots (2000 kg) (@ Rs. 42.00/kg)	84,000.00
2.	Planting material (50,000 cutting) (@ Rs. 0.50 per cutting)	25,000.00			
3.	Sowing labour	1,632.00			
4.	Fertilizers and Pesticides	918.00			
5.	Irrigation and hoeing–weeding etc.	510.00			
6.	Harvesting labour	1,326.00			
7.	Other expanses (Collection, Transportation, etc.)	510.00			
	Total Cost	**31,120.00**		**Total**	**84,000.00**

Net Profit: Total Production Obtained–Total Cost

Rs. 84,000.00–Rs. 31,120.00 = **Rs. 52,880.00**

Costus speciosus

SN	Particulars	Expenditure (Rs.)	SN	Particulars	Income (Rs.)
	(A) Cost			(B) Products obtained	
1.	Preparation of Farmyard	1,530.00	1.	Dry rhizome (8000 kg) (@ Rs. 15.00/kg)	1,36,000.00
2.	Planting material (20 kg seeds) (@ Rs. 152.00/kg)	3,040.00			
3.	Sowing labour	2,040.00	2.	Planting material (seeds 700 kg) (@ Rs. 17.00/kg)	11,900.00
4.	Fertilizers and Pesticides	1,020.00			
5.	Irrigation and hoeing–weeding etc.	816.00			
6.	Harvesting labour	2,244.00			
7.	Other expanses (Collection, Transportation, etc.)	510.00			
	Total Cost	**11,200.00**		**Total Production Obtained**	**1,47,900.00**

Net Profit: Total Production Obtained–Total Cost
1,47,900.00–11,200.00 = **Rs. 1,36,700.00**

Curculigo orchioides

SN	Particulars	Expenditure (Rs.)	SN	Particulars	Income (Rs.)
	(A) Cost			(B) Products obtained	
1.	Preparation of Farmyard	1,020.00	1.	Stem (1,000 kg) (@ Rs. 62.00/kg)	62,000.00
2.	Planting material	5,100.00			
3.	Sowing labour	2,550.00	2.	Planting material (seeds)	5,100.00
4.	Fertilizers and Pesticides	2,040.00			
5.	Irrigation and hoeing–weeding etc.	1,020.00			
6.	Harvesting labour	1,530.00			
7.	Other expanses (Collection, Transportation, etc.)	1,020.00			
	Total Cost	**14,280.00**		**Total Production Obtained**	**67,100.00**

Net Profit: Total Production Obtained–Total Cost
Rs. 67,100.00–Rs. 14,280.00 = **Rs. 52,820.00**

Cymbopogan nardus

SN	Particulars	1st year	2nd year	3rd year	4th year	5th year
	(A) Cost					
1.	Preparation of Farmyard	1,500.00	–	–	–	–
2.	Planting Material (50,000 sleeps) (@ Rs. 30.00/hundred sleeps)	15,000.00	–	–	–	–
3.	Sowing labour	6,000.00	–	–	–	–
4.	Fertilizers and Pesticides	5,000.00	5,000.00	5,000.00	5,000.00	5,000.00
5.	Irrigation and hoeing–weeding etc.	2,500.00	1,500.00	1,500.00	1,500.00	1,500.00
6.	Harvesting labour	6,000.00	6,000.00	6,000.00	6,000.00	6,000.00
7.	Processing & Oil production (@ Rs. 50.00/kg)	8,000.00	10,000.00	10,000.00	10,000.00	10,000.00
8.	Other expanses (Collection, Transportation, etc.)	1,500.00	1,500.00	1,500.00	1,500.00	1,500.00
	Total Cost	**45,500.00**	**24,00.00**	**24,00.00**	**24,00.00**	**24,00.00**
	(B) Obtained Oil	48,000.00	60,000.00	60,000.00	60,000.00	60,000.00
	(@ Rs. 300.00/kg)	(160 kg)	(200 kg)	(200 kg)	(200 kg)	(200 kg)
	Net Profit	**2,500.00**	**36,000.00**	**36,000.00**	**36,000.00**	**36,000.00**

Cymbopogon citrates

SN	Particulars	1st year	2nd year	3rd year	4th year	5th year
	(A) Cost					
1.	Preparation of Farmyard	2,040.00	–	–	–	–
2.	Planting material (30,000 sleeps) (@ Rs. 52.00/hundred)	15,600.00	–	–	–	–
3.	Sowing labour	5,100.00	–	–	–	–
4.	Fertilizers and Pesticides	3,570.00	3,570.00	3,570.00	3,570.00	3,570.00
5.	Irrigation and hoeing–weeding etc.	2,040.00	1,020.00	1,020.00	1,020.00	1,020.00
6.	Harvesting labour & Oil Extraction	10,200.00	10,710.00	10,710.00	10,710.00	10,710.00
7.	Other expanses (Collection, Transportation, etc.)	5,100.00	5,100.00	5,100.00	5,100.00	5,100.00
	Total Cost	**43,650.00**	**20,400.00**	**20,400.00**	**20,400.00**	**20,400.00**
	(B) Obtained Oil	81,000.00	1,21,500.00	1,21,500.00	1,21,500.00	1,21,500.00
	(@ Rs. 405.00/kg)	(200 kg)	(300 kg)	(300 kg)	(300 kg)	(300 kg)
	Net Profit	**37,350.00**	**1,01,100.00**	**1,01,100.00**	**1,01,100.00**	**1,01,100.00**

Cymbopogon martini

SN	Particulars	1st year	2nd year	3rd year	4th year
	(A) Cost				
1.	Preparation of Farmyard	2,000.00	–	–	–
2.	Planting Material (5 kg seeds) (@ Rs. 50.00/kg)	250.00	–	–	–
3.	Sowing labour	3,000.00	–	–	–
4.	Fertilizers and Pesticides	1,500.00	1,500.00	1,500.00	1,500.00
5.	Irrigation and hoeing–weeding etc.	2,000.00	2,000.00	2,000.00	2,000.00
6.	Harvesting labour	3,000.00	3,000.00	3,000.00	3,000.00
7.	Processing (Oil production) (@ Rs. 50.00/kg)	4,000.00	6,000.00	6,000.00	6,000.00
8.	Other expanses (Collection, Transportation, etc.)	1,000.00	1,000.00	1,000.00	1,000.00
	Total Cost	**16,750.00**	**13,500.00**	**13,500.00**	**13,500.00**
	(B) Product Obtained				
1.	Aromatic oil	40,000.00	60,000.00	60,000.00	60,000.00
	(@ Rs. 500.00/kg)	(80 kg)	(120 kg)	(120 kg)	(120 kg)
	Net Profit	**23,250.00**	**46,500.00**	**46,500.00**	**46,500.00**

Cyperus scariosus

SN	Particulars	Expenditure (Rs.)	SN	Particulars	Income (Rs.)
	(A) Cost			**(B) Products obtained**	
1.	Preparation of Farmyard	1,836.00	1.	Roots (1200 kg) (@ Rs. 35.00/kg)	42,000.00
2.	Planting material	1,020.00			
3.	Sowing labour	1,224.00	2.	Planting material	5,100.00
4.	Fertilizers and Pesticides	816.00			
5.	Irrigation and hoeing–weeding etc.	1,224.00			
6.	Harvesting labour	2,040.00			
7.	Other expanses (Collection, Transportation, etc.)	1,020.00			
	Total Cost	**9,180.00**		**Total Production Obtained**	**47,100.00**

Net Profit: Total Production Obtained–Total Cost

Rs. 47,100.00–Rs. 9,180.00 = **Rs. 37,920.00**

Digitalis lanata

SN	Particulars	Expenditure (Rs.)	SN	Particulars	Income (Rs.)
	(A) Cost			**(B) Products obtained**	
1.	Preparation of Farmyard	1,020.00	1.	Dry Leaves (3000 kg) (@ Rs. 20.00/kg)	60,000.00
2.	Planting material (2 kg seeds) (@ Rs. 510.00/kg)	1,020.00	2.	Planting material	5,100.00
3.	Sowing labour	1,224.00			
4.	Fertilizers and Pesticides	510.00			
5.	Irrigation and hoeing–weeding etc.	408.00			
6.	Harvesting labour	1,326.00			
7.	Other expanses (Collection, Transportation, etc.)	612.00			
	Total Cost	**6,120.00**		**Total Production Obtained**	**65,100.00**

Net Profit: Total Production Obtained–Total Cost
Rs. 65,100.00–Rs. 6,120.00 = **Rs. 58,980.00**

Emblica officinalis

SN	Particulars	Expenditure (Rs.)	SN	Particulars	Income (Rs.)
	(A) Cost			**(B) Products obtained**	
1.	Preparation of Farmyard	2550.00	1.	Fruit 5 ton (after four years) (@ Rs. 12.00/ kg)	60,000.00
2.	Material (@ Rs. 62.00/ cutting)	1224.00			
3.	Sowing labour	1224.00	2.	Fruit 20 ton (after eight years) (@ Rs. 12.00/kg)	2,40,000.00
4.	Fertilizers and Irrigation	1530.00			
5.	Hoeing and Weeding	612.00			
6.	Digging labour	2040.00			
7.	Other expanses (Collection, Transportation, etc.)	1020.00			
	Total Cost	**10,200.00**		**Total Production Obatined**	**3,00,000.00**

Net Profit: Total Production Obtained–Total Cost
Rs. 60,000.00–Rs. 10,200.00 = **Rs. 49,800.00** (After Four Years)
Rs. 2,40,000.00–10,200.00 = **Rs. 2,29,800.00** (After Eight Years)

Gloriosa superba

SN	Particulars	1st Year	2nd Year	3rd Year	4th Year	5th Year
	(A) Cost					
1.	Preparation of Farmyard	3,000.00	–	–	–	–
2.	Material (800 kg Bulb) (@ Rs. 102.00/ kg)	81,600.00	–	–	–	–
3.	Sowing labour	2,040.00	1,530.00	1,530.00	1,530.00	1,530.00
4.	Management (@ Rs. 1.00/plant)	17,340.00	–	17,340.00	–	17,340.00
5.	Fertilizers and Pesticides	2,550.00	2,550.00	2,550.00	2,550.00	2,550.00
6.	Irrigation and Hoeing–Weeding	816.00	816.00	816.00	816.00	816.00
7.	Sowing labour	510.00	510.00	510.00	510.00	510.00
8.	Other expenses (collection, transportation etc.)	510.00	510.00	510.00	510.00	510.00
	Total cost	**1,08,366.00**	**5,916.00**	**23,256.00**	**5,916.00**	**23,256.00**
	(B) Production obtained					
1.	Seeds (@ Rs. 510/kg)	76,500.00 (150 kg)	1,02,000.00 (200 kg)	1,27,500.00 (250 kg)	1,53,000.00 (300 kg)	2,04,000.00 (400 kg)
2.	Dry bulb) (2500 kg) (@ Rs. 52/kg)	–	–	–	–	1,30,000.00

Net Profit: Total Production Obtained–Total Cost (After Five Years)
Rs. 3,34,000.00–Rs. 23,256.00 = **Rs. 3,10,744.00**

Glycyrrhiza glabra

SN	Particulars	Expenditure (Rs.)	SN	Particulars	Income (Rs.)
	(A) Cost			**(B) Products obtained**	
1.	Preparation of Farmyard	2,100.00	1.	Roots (4000 kg) (@ Rs. 50.00/kg)	2,00,000.00
2.	Planting material (40 kg) (@ Rs. 50.00/kg)	2,000.00			
3.	Sowing labour	1,250.00			
4.	Fertilizers and Pesticides	900.00			
5.	Irrigation and hoeing–weeding etc.	1,550.00			
6.	Harvesting labour	3,200.00			
7.	Other expanses (Collection, Transportation, etc.)	350.00			
	Total Cost	**11,350.00**		**Total**	**2,00,000.00**

Net Profit: Total Production Obtained–Total Cost
Rs. 2,00,000.00–Rs. 11,350.00 = **Rs. 1,88,650.00**

Gymnema sylvestre

SN	Particulars	Expenditure (Rs.)	SN	Particulars	Income (Rs.)
	(A) Cost			**(B) Products obtained**	
1.	Preparation of Farmyard	1,428.00	1.	Pattiya (1500 kg) (@ Rs. 52.00/kg)	78,000.00
2.	Planting material (seeds 10 kg) (@ Rs. 72.00/kg)	720.00	2.	Planting material (seeds)	5,100.00
3.	Sowing labour	2,142.00			
4.	Fertilizers and Pesticides	612.00			
5.	Irrigation and hoeing–weeding etc.	816.00			
6.	Harvesting labour	1,530.00			
7.	Other expanses (Collection, Transportation, etc.)	408.00			
	Total Cost	**7,656.00**		**Total Production Obtained**	**83,100.00**

Net Profit: Total Production Obtained–Total Cost
Rs. 83,100.00–Rs. 7,656.00 = **Rs. 75,444.00**

Hyoscyamus niger

SN	Particulars	Expenditure (Rs.)	SN	Particulars	Income (Rs.)
	(A) Cost			(B) Products obtained	
1.	Preparation of Farmyard	1,020.00	1.	Yield (2,000 kg) (@ Rs. 22.00/kg)	44,000.00
2.	Planting material (2/kg seeds) (@ Rs. 204.00/kg)	408.00	2.	Planting material (seeds 40 kg) (@ Rs. 202.00/kg)	8,080.00
3.	Sowing labour	1,020.00			
4.	Fertilizers and Pesticides	408.00			
5.	Irrigation and hoeing–weeding etc.	1,020.00			
6.	Harvesting labour	1,020.00			
7.	Other expanses (Collection, Drying, etc.)	204.00			
	Total Cost	**5,100.00**		**Total Production Obtained**	**52,080.00**

Net Profit: Total Production Obtained–Total Cost
Rs. 52,080.00–Rs. 5,100.00 = **Rs. 46,980.00**

Jatropha curcas

SN	Particulars	1st years	2nd Year	3rd Year	4th Year	5th Year	6th Year
	(A) Cost						–
1.	Preparation of Farmyard	510.00	–	–	–	–	–
2.	Planting material (5 kg seeds) (@ Rs. 150.00/kg)	750.00	–	–	–	–	–
3.	Sowing labour	612.00	–	–	–	–	–
4.	Fertilizers and Pesticides	306.00	306.00	306.00	306.00	306.00	306.00
5.	Irrigation and hoeing–weeding etc.	255.00	255.00	255.00	255.00	255.00	255.00
6.	Harvesting labour	612.00	612.00	816.00	1,020.00	1,530.00	2,040.00
7.	Other expenses (Collection, Transporting etc.)	153.00	255.00	255.00	561.00	867.00	1,275.00
	Total Cost (Rs.)	**3,198.00**	**1,428.00**	**1,632.00**	**2,142.00**	**2,958.00**	**3,876.00**
	(B) Obtained Seeds	3,600.00	12,000.00	30,000.00	60,000.00	96,000.00	1,32.000.00
	Seeds (@ Rs. 12.00/kg)	300 kg	1000 kg	2500 kg	5000 kg	8000 kg	11000 kg
	Net Profit	**402.00**	**10,572.00**	**28,368.00**	**57,858.00**	**93,042.00**	**1,28,124.00**

Lawsonia inermis

SN	Particulars	Expenditure (Rs.)	SN	Particulars	Income (Rs.)
	(A) Cost			**(B) Products obtained**	
1.	Preparation of Farmyard	1,250.00	1.	Dry leaves (15 quintals) (@Rs. 25.00/kg)	37,500.00
2.	Planting Material (Seeds 50 kg) (@ Rs.35.00/kg)	1,750.00	2.	Planting material	5,000.00
3.	Sowing labour	1,000.00			
4.	Fertilizers and Pesticides	500.00			
5.	Irrigation and hoeing–weeding etc.	500.00			
6.	Harvesting labour	3,500.00			
7.	Other expanses (Collection, Transportation, etc.)	1,000.00			
	Total Cost	**9,500.00**		**Total Production Obtained**	**42,500.00**

Net Profit: Total Production Obtained–Total Cost

Rs. 42,500.00–Rs. 9,500.00 = **Rs. 33,000.00**

Matricaria chamomilla

SN	Particulars	Expenditure (Rs.)	SN	Particulars	Income (Rs.)
	(A) Cost			(B) Products obtained	
1.	Preparation of Farmyard	2,040.00	1.	Dry fruits (2000 kg) (@ Rs. 92.00/kg)	1,84,000.00
2.	Seed (500 gm) (@ Rs. 400.00/kg)	200.00			
3.	Sowing labour	3,264.00			
4.	Fertilizers and Pesticides	1,530.00			
5.	Irrigation and hoeing–weeding etc.	612.00			
6.	Harvesting labour	2,244.00			
7.	Other expanses (Collection, Transportation, etc.)	816.00			
	Total Cost	**10,706.00**		**Total Production Obtained**	**1,84,000.00**

Net Profit: Total Production Obtained–Total Cost
Rs. 1,84,000.00–Rs. 10,706.00 = **Rs. 1,73,294.00**

Mentha arvensis

SN	Particulars	1st years	2nd Year	3rd Year	4th Year	5th Year
	(A) Cost					
1.	Preparation of Farmyard	1,530.00	–	–	–	–
2.	Planting material (300 kg) (@ Rs. 52.00/kg)	15,600.00	–	–	–	–
3.	Sowing labour	5,100.00	–	–	–	–
4.	Fertilizers and Pesticides	4,080.00	4,080.00	4,080.00	4,080.00	4,080.00
5.	Irrigation and hoeing–weeding etc.	2,040.00	2,040.00	2,040.00	2,040.00	2,040.00
6.	Pruning	10,200.00	10,200.00	10,200.00	10,200.00	10,200.00
7.	Other expenses (Collection, Transporting etc.)	2,040.00	2,040.00	2,040.00	2,040.00	2,040.00
	Total Cost (Rs.)	**40,590.00**	**18,360.00**	**18,360.00**	**18,360.00**	**18,360.00**
	(B) Products obtained					
1.	Oil (200 kg) (@ Rs. 300.00/kg)	60,000.00	60,000.00	60,000.00	60,000.00	60,000.00
2.	Planting material	10,200.00	10,200.00	10,200.00	10,200.00	10,200.00
	Total Production Obtained	**70,200.00**	**70,200.00**	**70,200.00**	**70,200.00**	**70,200.00**
	Net Profit	**29,610.00**	**51,840.00**	**51,840.00**	**51,840.00**	**51,840.00**

Mucuna prurita

SN	Particulars	Expenditure (Rs.)	SN	Particulars	Income (Rs.)
	(A) Cost			**(B) Products obtained**	
1.	Preparation of Farmyard	1,530.00	1.	Seeds (3000 kg) (@ Rs. 22.00/kg)	66,000.00
2.	Planting material (seeds 50 kg) (@ Rs. 22.00/kg)	1,100.00	2.	Crop (500 kg) (@ Rs. 22.00/kg)	11,000.00
3.	Sowing labour	1,224.00	3.	Income from Propping Tree	10,200.00
4.	Fertilizers and Pesticides	1,020.00			
5.	Irrigation and hoeing–weeding etc.	816.00			
6.	Harvesting labour	1,836.00			
7.	Other expanses (Collection, Transportation, etc.)	714.00			
	Total Cost	**8,240.00**		**Total Production Obtained**	**87,200.00**

Net Profit: Total Production Obtained–Total Cost
Rs. 87,200.00–Rs. 8,240.00 = **Rs. 78,960.00**

Ocimum basilicum

SN	Particulars	Expenditure (Rs.)	SN	Particulars	Income (Rs.)
	(A) Cost			**(B) Products obtained**	
1.	Preparation of Farmyard	816.00	1.	Essential oil (150 kg) (@ Rs. 252.00/kg)	37,800.00
2.	Seed (800 gm) (@ Rs. 250.00/kg)	190.00	2.	Planting material	5,100.00
3.	Sowing labour	612.00			
4.	Fertilizers and Pesticides	357.00			
5.	Irrigation and hoeing–weeding etc.	408.00			
6.	Harvesting labour	816.00			
7.	Other expanses (Collection, Transportation, etc.)	408.00			
	Total Cost	**3,607.00**		**Total Production Obtained**	**42,900.00**

Net Profit: Total Production Obtained–Total Cost
Rs. 42,900.00–Rs. 3,607.00 = **Rs. 39,293.00**

Piper longum

SN	Particulars	Expenditure (Rs.)	SN	Particulars	Income (Rs.)
	(A) Cost			**(B) Products obtained**	
1.	Preparation of Farmyard	8,160.00	1.	Dry Piper (1500 kg) (@ Rs. 100.00/kg)	1,50,000.00
2.	Planting material (1 lakh cuttings) (@ Rs. 0.60/cutting)	60,000.00			
3.	Sowing labour	6,120.00			
4.	Fertilizers and Pesticides	3,060.00			
5.	Irrigation and hoeing–weeding etc.	2,550.00			
6.	Harvesting labour	5,100.00			
7.	Other expanses (Collection, Transportation, etc.)	1,530.00			
	Total Cost	**86,520.00**		**Total Production Obtained**	**1,50,000.00**

Net Profit: Total Production Obtained–Total Cost
Rs. 1,50,000.00–Rs. 86,520.00 = **Rs. 63,480.00**
Dry Roots (after 5 years) (5 quintal @ Rs. 150.00/kg)
63,480.00 + 75,000.00 = **Rs. 1,38,480.00**

Plantago ovata

SN	Particulars	Expenditure (Rs.)	SN	Particulars	Income (Rs.)
	(A) Cost			**(B) Products obtained**	
1.	Preparation of Farmyard	2040.00	1.	Seeds (1500 kg) (@ Rs. 42.00/kg)	63,000.00
2.	Material (seed 10 kg) (@ Rs. 42.00/kg)	420.00			
3.	Sowing labour	1224.00			
4.	Fertilizers and Pesticides	1020.00			
5.	Irrigation and Hoeing–Weeding	816.00			
6.	Digging labour	1224.00			
7.	Other expanses (Collection, Transportation, etc.)	612.00			
	Total Cost	**7356.00**		**Total Production Obtained**	**63,000.00**

Net Profit: Total Production Obtained–Total Cost
Rs. 63,000.00–Rs. 7,356.00 = **Rs. 55,644.00**

Polianthes tuberosa

SN	Particulars	1st years	2nd years	3rd years
	(A) Cost			
1.	Preparation of Farmyard	6,000.00	–	–
2.	Planting Material (Bulb 2.5 lakh) (@ Rs.1.00/bulb)	2,50,000.00	–	–
3.	Sowing labour	12,000.00	–	–
4.	Fertilizers and Pesticides	15,000.00	15,000.00	15,000.00
5.	Irrigation and hoeing–weeding etc.	13,000.00	13,000.00	13,000.00
6.	Harvesting labour	20,000.00	20,000.00	20,000.00
7.	Other expanses (Collection, Transportation, etc.)	2,000.00	2,000.00	2,000.00
	Total Cost	**3,18,000.00**	**50,000.00**	**50,000.00**
	(B) Production Obtained			
1.	Pushup (30 ton) (@ Rs. 20.00/kg)	6,00,000.00	6,00,000.00	6,00,000.00
2.	Planting material	20,000.00	20,000.00	20,000.00
	Total Product Obtained	**6,20,000.00**	**6,20,000.00**	**6,20,000.00**
	Net Profit	**3,02,000.00**	**5,70,000.00**	**5,70,000.00**

Rauvolfia serpentina

SN	Particulars	Expenditure (Rs.)	SN	Particulars	Income (Rs.)
	(A) Cost			**(B) Products obtained**	
1.	Preparation of Farmyard	1,500.00	1.	Dry Roots (25 quintals) (@Rs. 55.00/kg)	1,37,500.00
2.	Planting Material (Seeds 6 kg) (@ Rs.300.00/kg)	1,800.00	2.	Planting material (Seeds 50 kg) (@ Rs. 300.00/kg)	15,000.00
3.	Sowing labour	3,500.00			
4.	Fertilizers and Pesticides	1,100.00			
5.	Irrigation and hoeing–weeding etc.	1,000.00			
6.	Harvesting labour	2,500.00			
7.	Other expanses (Collection, Transportation, etc.)	500.00			
	Total Cost	**11,900.00**		**Total Production Obtained**	**1,52,500.00**

Net Profit: Total Production Obtained–Total Cost
Rs. 1,52,500.00–Rs. 11,900.00 = **Rs. 1,40,600.00**

Tephrosia purpurea

SN	Particulars	Expenditure (Rs.)	SN	Particulars	Income (Rs.)
	(A) Cost			**(B) Products obtained**	
1.	Preparation of Farmyard	1,100.00	1.	Herb (20 quintals) (@ Rs. 15.00/kg)	30,000.00
2.	Planting Material (Seeds 10 kg) (@ Rs.120.00/kg)	1,200.00	2.	Dried Roots (12 quintals) (@ Rs.35.00/kg)	42,000.00
3.	Sowing labour	1,000.00	3.	Planting material	5,000.00
4.	Fertilizers and Pesticides	500.00			
5.	Irrigation and hoeing–weeding etc.	300.00			
6.	Harvesting labour	1000.00			
7.	Other expanses (Collection, Transportation, etc.)	500.00			
	Total Cost	**5,600.00**		**Total Production Obtained**	**77,000.00**

Net Profit: Total Production Obtained–Total Cost
Rs. 77,000.00–Rs. 5,600.00 = **Rs. 71,400.00**

Tinospora cordifolia

SN	Particulars	Expenditure (Rs.)	SN	Particulars	Income (Rs.)
	(A) Cost			**(B) Products obtained**	
1.	Preparation of Farmyard	714.00	1.	Dry Stem (1,200 kg) (@ Rs. 22.00/kg)	26,400.00
2.	Planting material	1,020.00	2.	Planting material	5,100.00
3.	Sowing labour	510.00			
4.	Fertilizers and Pesticides	306.00			
5.	Irrigation and hoeing–weeding etc.	357.00			
6.	Harvesting labour	561.00			
7.	Other expanses (Drying & Collection etc.)	204.00			
	Total Cost	**3,672.00**		**Total Production Obtained**	**31,500.00**

Net Profit: Total Production Obtained–Total Cost
Rs. 31,500.00–Rs. 3,672.00 = **Rs. 27,828.00**

Valeriana jatamansi

SN	Particulars	Expenditure (Rs.)	SN	Particulars	Income (Rs.)
	(A) Cost			**(B) Products obtained**	
1.	Preparation of Farmyard	1,326.00	1.	Dry fruits (800 kg) (@ Rs. 80.00/kg)	64,000.00
2.	Seed (500 gm) (@ Rs. 2,000.00/kg)	1000.00	2.	Planting material (Seed 5 kg) (@ Rs. 2,040/kg)	10,200.00
3.	Sowing labour	1,224.00			
4.	Fertilizers and Pesticides	816.00			
5.	Irrigation and hoeing–weeding etc.	714.00			
6.	Harvesting labour	2,040.00			
7.	Other expanses (Collection, Transportation, etc.)	510.00			
	Total Cost	**7630.00**		**Total Production Obtained**	**74,200.00**

Net Profit: Total Production Obtained–Total Cost
Rs. 74,200.00–Rs. 7,630.00 = **Rs.66,570.00**

Vetiveria zizanioides

SN	Particulars	Expenditure (Rs.)	SN	Particulars	Income (Rs.)
	(A) Cost			**(B) Products obtained**	
1.	Preparation of Farmyard	1,224.00	1.	Essential oil (30 kg) (@ Rs. 2,040.00/kg)	61,200.00
2.	Planting material (5,000 cutting) (@ Rs. 52.00/hundred)	2,600.00	2.	Planting material (sleep)	10,200.00
3.	Sowing labour	1,938.00			
4.	Fertilizers and Pesticides	306.00			
5.	Irrigation and hoeing–weeding etc.	816.00			
6.	Harvesting labour	1,734.00			
7.	Other expanses (Drying, Storage, etc.)	510.00			
	Total Cost	**9,128.00**		**Total Production Obtained**	**71,400.00**

Net Profit: Total Production Obtained–Total Cost
Rs. 71,400.00–Rs. 9,128.00 = **Rs. 62,272.00**

Withania somnifera

SN	Particulars	Expenditure (Rs.)	SN	Particulars	Income (Rs.)
	(A) Cost			**(B) Products obtained**	
1.	Preparation of Farmyard	2040.00	1.	Dry roots (600 kg) (@ Rs. 62.00/ kg)	37200.00
2.	Material (seeds 10 kg) (@ Rs. 52.00/ kg)	520.00			
3.	Sowing labour	1020.00	2.	Seeds for sowing (seeds 50 kg) (@ Rs. 52.00/ kg)	2600.00
4.	Fertilizers and Pesticides	816.00			
5.	Irrigation, weeding etc.	612.00			
6.	Digging labour	2040.00			
7.	Other expanses (Collection, Transportation, etc.)	816.00			
	Total Cost	**7864.00**		**Total Production Obtained**	**39800.00**

Net Profit: Total Production Obtained–Total Cost
Rs. 39800.00–Rs. 7864.00 = **Rs. 31936.00**

Table 1: Ayurvedic, Unani, Homeopathic and Alkaloid Medicines in Export

Year	Ayurvedic & Unani Medicines		Homeopathic Medicines		Alkaloid	
	Quantity (Ton)	Rs. (Lakh)	Quantity (Ton)	Rs. (Lakh)	Quantity (Ton)	Rs. (Lakh)
1991–92	3360.56	3318.48	–	567.19	–	40.68
1992–93	4117.25	5022.43	–	164.56	–	68.17
1993–94	3112.34	5361.12	–	517.34	–	119.02
1994–95	4173.46	9338.94	–	180.02	–	115.01
1995–96	3716.29	9644.97	–	652.51	–	402.95
1996–97	12986.70	15503.58	56.32	128.53	154.80	179.39
1997–98	8939.52	6499.84	51.99	309.51	271.49	1989.65
1998–99	10898.79	7451.59	32.56	37.47	73.18	613.11
1999–2000	10399.20	5474.00	121.96	67.39	122.45	899.04

Table 2: Ayurvedic, Unani, Homeopathic & Alkaloids in Import

Year	Ayurvedic & Unani Medicines		Homeopathic Medicines		Alkaloid	
	Quantity (Ton)	Rs. (Lakh)	Quantity (Ton)	Rs. (Lakh)	Quantity (Ton)	Rs. (Lakh)
1991–92	1732.50	583.61	–	447.21	–	0.28
1992–93	914.95	442.83	–	427.53	–	–
1993–94	2201.95	268.14	–	581.67	–	1.65
1994–95	1814.29	236.94	–	524.91	–	11.96
1995–96	1287.37	1270.26	–	485.61	–	3.34
1996–97	3640.05	3395.02	126.21	496.96	–	–
1997–98	1637.19	507.04	102.13	572.49	6.41	97.94
1998–99	3761.57	1863.54	171.63	936.42	0.63	53.99
1999–2000	3934.49	3956.77	146.06	799.69	0.07	0.27

Table 3 (a): Analysis of useful part of Ayurvedic Medicines & Aromatic Plants is Export.

Useful part of Ayurvedic & Aromatic Plant	1991–92		1992–93		1993–94		1994–95		1995–96	
	Quantity (Ton)	Rs. (Lakh)	Quantity (Ton)	Rs. (Lakh)	Quantity (Ton)	Rs. (Lakh)	Quantity (Ton)	Rs. (Lakh)	Quantity (Ton)	Rs. (Lakh)
Abelmoschus moschatus	2.3	1.61	1.64	0.69	14.95	8.5	56.99	18.27	624.97	83.13
Alpinia sp.	72.5	11.77	75.61	15.56	98.5	22.01	22.44	6.25	83.47	22.28
Ammomum sp.	902.9	499.05	1236.23	879.11	1785.81	1247.92	1243.12	789.93	1582.96	1169.02
Aquilaria agallocha	320.46	73.99	186.41	43.09	121.13	16.78	219.53	12.43	18.35	8.64
Artemisia pallens	0.67	43.15	1.31	105.12	1.04	58.96	1.36	74.96	1.3	70.49
Atropa belladonna	–	–	2.00	0.53	–	–	–	–	3.16	0.99
Canana odorata	–	–	0.25	0.80	–	–	–	–	–	–
Cassia angustifolia	5121.22	1116.29	4476.56	1222.99	3658.28	819.76	400.48	850.99	6279.77	1391.61
Catharanthus roseus	270.77	91.47	128.2	49.14	150.11	67.73	151.7	43.89	191.92	64.97
Cinnamomum cassia	1.08	65.81	2.68	95.47	5.52	282.12	0.92	16.1	1.38	9.47
Cinnamomum tamala	0.09	0.02	9.08	1.36	0.95	0.17	–	–	12.68	3.6
Cinnamomum tamala	–	–	–	–	–	–	0.03	0.41	0.05	0.46
Cinnamomum zeylanicum	23.930	9.760	0.031	0.094	5.350	0.580	1.010	2.290	2.480	0.580
Cinnamonum cassia	2763.29	199.98	1570.26	156.12	2248.18	96.63	882.45	45.37	1612.93	108.27
Citrus aurantifolia	12.96	32.76	0.91	2.52	0.8	1.73	0.15	0.21	0.06	0.29
Citrus sinensis	0.2	0.09	0.9	0.77	0.11	0.14	0.01	0.2	0.15	1.76
Crocus sativus	11.9	180.95	5.14	112.1	7.03	169.77	4.08	134.61	7.69	126.84
Cuminum cyminum	1653.73	637.61	2620.48	1438.88	3224.9	1630.35	5617.96	2449.65	3871.23	1739.32

Useful part of Ayurvedic & Aromatic Plant	1991–92		1992–93		1993–94		1994–95		1995–96	
	Quantity (Ton)	Rs. (Lakh)	Quantity (Ton)	Rs. (Lakh)	Quantity (Ton)	Rs. (Lakh)	Quantity (Ton)	Rs. (Lakh)	Quantity (Ton)	Rs. (Lakh)
Curcuma zedoaria	46.95	4.63	48.72	7.93	46.69	5.03	33.1	4.63	30	3.74
Cymbopogan winterianus	0.98	1.48	6.9	17.98	–	–	29.51	73.34	92.09	323.73
Cymbopogon flexuosus	114.36	295.37	33.22	95.25	35.96	97.64	64.14	174.15	50.93	179.29
Cymbopogon martini	6.08	23.7	3.91	13.50	2.72	16.77	0.27	1.62	12.18	49.01
Elettaria cardamomum	543.98	1558.07	181.91	588.00	400.28	1459.31	265.77	769.51	407.57	851.61
Elettaria cardamomum	0.07	3.79	–	–	3.55	187.25	1.02	35.87	0.312	13.88
Eucalyptus globulus	–	–	0.95	3.69	2.76	15.20	15.34	22.58	3.79	11.53
Foeniculum vulgare	4.05	1.39	17.74	6.12	5.12	3.04	12.55	4.89	15.05	6.87
Garbled/ Ungarbled/ Dehydrated/ Crushed/ Piper nigrum	20460.47	7428.68	23540.60	7674.65	461056.10	18654.51	36851.42	23428.81	25888.56	19273.00
Garcinia indica	6.65	1.67	1.79	0.5	99.69	20.2	11.85	5.02	22.44	10.13
Glycyrrhiza glabra	–	–	0.31	0.82	1.26	0.66	–	–	0.96	0.70
Guizotia abyssinica	13161.25	2345.28	15504.8	2855.14	10857.76	1867.37	7804.12	1267.01	9323.13	2135.8
Hemidesmus indicus	0.24	0.07	12	4.67	11.76	4.57	20.61	13.31	1.1	0.3
Humulus lupulus	–	–	–	–	–	–	0.89	0.08	19.00	1.37
Jasminum grandiflorum	2.01	206.58	48.91	540.74	16.98	405.02	4.59	563.11	6.75	805.69

Useful part of Ayurvedic & Aromatic Plant	1991–92		1992–93		1993–94		1994–95		1995–96	
	Quantity (Ton)	Rs. (Lakh)	Quantity (Ton)	Rs. (Lakh)	Quantity (Ton)	Rs. (Lakh)	Quantity (Ton)	Rs. (Lakh)	Quantity (Ton)	Rs. (Lakh)
Juniperus communis	2.0	0.14	–	–	–	–	4.0	1.0	12.63	4.01
Lavandula angustifolia	–	–	–	–	–	–	–	–	5.01	14.96
Melaleuca leucadendron	–	–	–	–	–	–	–	–	–	–
Mentha piperta	991.28	1956.93	1231.86	2047.5	1131.75	1980.62	1301.05	3629.49	1188.36	4189.94
Mentha sp.	–	2461.22	–	1549.32	–	2059.72	–	2890.30	–	2075.78
Mentha spicata	22.03	84.89	66.25	167.1	111.15	636.01	37.37	139.47	67.83	292.56
Murriaya koenigii	3236.21	982.86	2599.07	898.34	3134.68	1101.28	3733.06	128.42	3823.87	1580.66
Myristica fragrans	0.3	0.59	2.07	1.99	11.41	5.23	5.02	5.69	5.88	6.82
Myristica fragrans	0.20	0.52	0.02	0.14	0.55	1.88	4.08	17.06	2.9	18.35
Other Aromatic oil	4.67	16.31	20.92	32.69	23.28	61.08	42.07	144.81	64.17	137.6
Other Medicines	6009.67	1026.45	8253.17	1449.89	5470.18	1018.67	4452.73	753.98	–	–
Panax ginseng	1325.73	386.67	2034.79	838.18	1911.32	774.55	2945.2	1314.94	3072.11	1627.55
Pandanus odoratissimus	–	–	–	–	4.25	18.82	2.66	11.89	1.83	9.03
Pandanus odoratissimus	35.44	8.64	11.22	3.71	10.48	4.01	21.21	11.36	19.20	8.15
Pimpinella anisum	32.50	10.47	138.45	14.23	285.75	20.77	112.24	18.85	104.59	20.11
Piper longum	4.180	1.140	15.720	1.470	88.660	41.360	45.660	30.830	38.530	17.020
Piper nigrum	20.11	130.04	22.53	160.04	16.23	110.5	38.16	305.47	34.73	358.88
Plantago psyllium	17544.40	6854.74	15347.99	7741.40	15475.44	7546.76	20889.43	11372.11	19120.27	15440.97
Pogostemom cablin	2.55	6.49	4.17	9.6	0.5	1.25	–	–	1.65	6.32
Polianthes tuberosa	0.24	50.06	0.32	37.53	0.26	82.42	0.44	116.38	0.27	63.21

Useful part of Ayurvedic & Aromatic Plant	1991–92		1992–93		1993–94		1994–95		1995–96	
	Quantity (Ton)	Rs. (Lakh)	Quantity (Ton)	Rs. (Lakh)	Quantity (Ton)	Rs. (Lakh)	Quantity (Ton)	Rs. (Lakh)	Quantity (Ton)	Rs. (Lakh)
Rauvolfia serpentina	0.33	3.23	0.11	0.17	3.93	3.2	NA	NA	0.19	0.17
Ricinus communis	–	3330.10	–	1514.95	–	3816.23	–	1125.22	–	19.64
Rosa indica	0.47	1.72	2.75	17.48	0.94	1.05	0.85	1.13	0.05	1.26
Rosa spp.	205.95	38.68	174.59	51.5	118.69	34.09	154.72	56.15	154	49.01
Santalum album	3112.52	4097.01	1085.08	3055.01	977.5	3038.41	456.04	2528.79	602.54	3671.39
Saussurea costus	–	–	2.00	0.75	2.50	0.55	–	–	8.00	1.52
Swertia chirayita	13.69	3.87	0.575	0.61	5.6	1.36	–	–	–	–
Syzygium aromaticum	0.035	0.090	0.000	0.000	0.01	0.02	35.78	11.07	0.29	0.56
Syzygium aromaticum	1.68	7.36	5.90	24.44	3.38	14.78	4.79	20.24	2.26	9.97
Tamarindus indica	3557.75	141.08	2726.72	129.31	2745.33	210.33	2736.89	174.37	2718.2	189.58
Thymus vulgaris	2.53	0.82	2.01	0.64	54.32	16.16	24.58	8.29	72.33	34.59
Vetiveria zizanioides	–	–	1.05	12.13	–	–	4.14	12.63	0.15	1.17
Vitis vinifera	1062.91	59.73	–	181.37	–	20.64	–	69.7	–	82.07
Zingiber officinale	5.13	47.23	3.7	36.86	3.87	43.71	5.82	80.89	5.26	142
Ziziphus mauritiana	8.67	3.22	61.5	13.53	86	2.69	21.16	8.12	29.45	13.44

Table 3 (b): Analysis of Ayurvedic and Aromatic plants are Import in India.

Useful part of Ayurvedic & Aromatic Plant	1996–1997		1997–1998		1998–1999		1999–2000	
	Quantity (Ton)	Rs. (Lakh)	Quantity (Ton)	Rs. (Lakh)	Quantity (Ton)	Rs. (Lakh)	Quantity (Ton)	Rs. (Lakh)
Abelmoschus moschatus	77.11	31.22	38.03	25.17	141.82	94.96	172.75	47.52
Alpinia sp.	64.3	12.8	29.00	6.59	75.42	29.62	201.53	74.94
Ammomum sp.	1574.62	1167.89	1652.20	1383.51	1460.10	1548.42	1155.03	1938.01
Aquilaria agallocha	19.71	41.44	68.05	32.55	25.56	30.93	25.63	35.43
Artemisia pallens	0.74	61.71	1.65	207.85	4.06	890.12	3.85	638.63
Atrops belladonna	99.35	21.31	5.83	1.29	44.27	18.52	22.74	8.19
Canana odorata	–	–	0.31	7.05	4.80	22.60	–	–
Cassia angustifolia	5948.61	1380.82	5011.84	1377.31	5180.58	2070.82	7466.33	2254.20
Catharanthus roseus	24.57	7.85	–	–	277.71	104.42	541.54	213.19
Cinnamomum cassia	0.74	3.99	1.62	49.67	0.81	27.45	1.44	22.30
Cinnamomum tamala	1.2	0.55	21.00	6.75	2.00	1.11	17.30	6.29
Cinnamomum tamala	0.08	0.60	0.09	1.02	1.43	24.83	0.02	0.23
Cinnamomum zeylanicum	9.930	8.180	111.53	62.24	3.31	2.69	–	–
Cinnamonum cassia	636.69	93.95	207.22	100.34	1060.25	781.89	710.85	430.68
Citrus aurantifolia	0.29	1.71	1.33	4.46	5.06	22.97	4.31	20.83
Citrus sinensis	0.58	1.98	0.12	0.31	2.09	6.66	–	–
Crocus sativus	2.13	70.44	6.57	250.03	9.77	355.25	8.14	274.22
Cuminum cyminum	6374.61	3437.80	356.54	244.67	7571.72	4279.35	5399.18	3238.64
Curcuma zedoaria	31.7	5.02	37.23	6.38	43.17	7.42	36.15	8.04
Cymbopogan winterianus	0.15	0.66	2.98	10.95	29.82	56.93	51.82	115.31
Cymbopogon flexuosus	50.37	233.49	87.04	515.04	46.27	244.08	40.31	232.03
Cymbopogon martini	8.62	50.95	7.96	49.22	14.02	98.05	11.05	89.04
Elettaria cardamomum	218.17	702.05	232.05	674.44	472.94	1389.34	624.43	2223.04
Elettaria cardamomum	0.43	22.07	0.35	24.26	0.056	1.63	4.94	131.50

Useful part of Ayurvedic & Aromatic Plant	1996–1997		1997–1998		1998–1999		1999–2000	
	Quantity (Ton)	Rs. (Lakh)	Quantity (Ton)	Rs. (Lakh)	Quantity (Ton)	Rs. (Lakh)	Quantity (Ton)	Rs. (Lakh)
Eucalyptus globules	0.70	4.90	0.79	5.03	39.39	142.73	108.44	377.48
Foeniculum vulgare	–	–	–	–	–	–	–	–
Garbled/ Ungarbled/ Dehydrated/ Crushed/Piper nigrum	46904.56	40865.36	34632.32	483035.27	32798.39	59055.42	33908.33	66816.66
Garcinia indica	38.42	25.55	12.18	6.24	7.11	3.05	8.85	4.52
Glycyrrhiza glabra	0.01	0.02	9.51	8.35	3.42	9.22	70.39	81.93
Guizotia abyssinica	11867.74	2930.42	14782.44	3033.94	–	–	–	–
Hemidesmus indicus	11.69	3.07	23.14	4.19	32.02	27.22	14.71	6.22
Humulus lupulus	0.02	0.04	–	–	–	–	20.00	3.41
Jasminum grandiflorum	6.67	587.59	5.78	657.67	7.24	707.10	10.57	1595.88
Juniperus communis	2.98	1.78	29.13	7.93	1.06	0.73	0.80	0.79
Lavandula angustifolia	0.02	1.36	0.22	1.96	–	–	14.48	58.61
Melaleuca leucadendron	–	–	0.16	0.53	14.40	48.02	–	–
Mentha piperta	2021.22	10878.32	2756.43	8543.58	2824.67	7053.66	2734.08	9673.25
Mentha sp.	633.45	7380.16	–	–	–	–	–	–
Mentha spicata	81.06	555.18	102.01	523.31	193.53	947.75	92.11	450.13
Murriaya koenigii	4218.24	1839.82	4729.93	2193.53	5252.81	3012.44	5699.08	3144.71
Myristica fragrans	5.25	4.61	31.40	5.69	2.81	6.09	130.58	83.99
Myristica fragrans	2.87	20.31	5.54	44.29	20.94	281.30	28.49	278.02
Panax ginseng	2768.38	2074.05	3787.40	2399.29	4470.56	2995.35	1379.46	1015.14
Pandanus odoratissimus	0.79	5.24	1.29	10.67	5.60	46.49	4.68	32.45
Pandanus odoratissimus	24.45	9.21	24.49	11.08	16.73	12.08	33.78	18.78
Pimpinella anisum	420.03	82.3	1559.17	287.40	347.34	108.34	432.58	92.33
Piper longum	348.780	204.930	611.00	354.80	272.66	395.47	319.23	660.22
Piper nigrum	36.16	419.93	53.91	1378.17	92.04	2316.91	31.00	918.28

Useful part of Ayurvedic & Aromatic Plant	1996–1997		1997–1998		1998–1999		1999–2000	
	Quantity (Ton)	Rs. (Lakh)	Quantity (Ton)	Rs. (Lakh)	Quantity (Ton)	Rs. (Lakh)	Quantity (Ton)	Rs. (Lakh)
Plantago psyllium	17842.63	13697.52	20634.25	15884.62	147852.76	13742.48	15295.31	10815.18
Pogostemom cablin	1.99	5.85	0.16	1.04	0.24	7.32	0.52	10.29
Polianthes tuberosa	0.24	85.24	0.55	40.86	0.39	164.88	–	–
Rauvolfia serpentina	–	–	NA	NA	0.19	0.17	9.03	5.70
Ricinus communis	11.89	12.38	124.79	51.92	270.29	97.26	136.50	78.49
Rosa indica	0.46	6.5	0.25	7.79	9.21	86.36	32.07	147.85
Rosa spp.	98.29	60.79	140.27	54.18	186.73	98.58	171.69	67.96
Santalum album	999.59	4114.17	322.52	2846.56	768.28	2970.24	260.97	1759.62
Saussurea costus	–	–	NA	NA	NA	NA	–	–
Swertia chirayita	45.03	33.1	16.24	4.65	1.62	0.50	50.29	37.74
Syzygium aromaticum	83.09	24.04	–	–	1.25	5.56	310.73	384.77
Syzygium aromaticum	0.79	3.77	1.50	11.69	0.82	7.01	2.22	6.83
Tamarindus indica	2415.76	222.16	1174.36	138.95	1179.03	166.71	2763.08	423.98
Thymus vulgaris	64.31	20.12	43.84	12.05	78.55	18.35	34.35	13.17
Vetiveria zizanioides	–	–	0.05	0.62	0.1	0.92	–	–
Vitis vinifera	104.85	59.21	61.04	34.75	84.708	61.16	66.91	49.63
Zingiber officinale	4.11	109.56	10.38	346.35	15.69	185.65	14.35	399.98
Ziziphus mauritiana	38.00	30.01	–	–	81.90	58.65	35.90	15.25
Other Ayurvedic	–	–	3062.69	1430.32	4736.34	2333.74	2734.60	1136.40
Other Aromatic oil	73.58	189.26	124.85	737.83	39.09	120.64	24.24	60.99

Table 4 (a): Analysis of useful part of Ayurvedic & Aromatic plants is export by India.

Useful part of Ayurvedic & Aromatic Plant	1991–1992		1992–1993		1993–1994		1994–1995		1995–1996	
	Quantity (Ton)	Rs. (Lakh)	Quantity (Ton)	Rs. (Lakh)	Quantity (Ton)	Rs. (Lakh)	Quantity (Ton)	Rs. (Lakh)	Quantity (Ton)	Rs. (Lakh)
Abelmoschus moschatus	0.34	1.23	–	–	14.19	2.33	–	–	–	–
Alpinia sp.	5.00	0.64	44.18	3.48	–	–	70.82	6.78	55.3	6.34
Ammomum sp.	1650.15	548.08	1831.29	654.43	2909.95	1034.15	2150.93	778.14	2658.87	1073.49
Aquilaria agallocha	33.04	8.45	26.33	58.47	7.45	7.61	9.48	8.12	12.09	11.89
Artemisia pallens	–	–	–	–	0.01	0.02	–	–	–	–
Canana odorata	4.21	23.02	6.45	58.31	1.83	17.66	4.51	7.10	3.95	14.52
Carum carvl	0.42	2.39	0.20	3.04	0.52	0.58	0.45	11.45	0.93	9.18
Cassia angustifolia	–	–	15.39	4.96	–	–	–	–	–	–
Catharanthus roseus	2.79	0.23	–	–	–	–	–	–	–	–
Cinnamomum cassia	–	–	0.32	0.74	0.02	0.20	1.18	4.18	1.12	7.42
Cinnamomum tamala	0.60	0.05	21.35	6.43	24.23	7.27	4.87	0.18	0.89	0.06
Cinnamomum tamala	–	–	6.00	11.59	3.10	6.01	3.27	11.59	2.43	12.14
Cinnamomum zeylanicum	62.38	21.25	194.55	61.50	98.60	38.02	11.55	2.55	–	–
Cinnamomum zeylenicum	–	–	0.07	0.17	0.79	1.38	–	–	0.01	0.32
Cinnamonum cassia	1241.75	416.20	1426.26	656.46	5891.7	265.33	649.97	261.68	1346.76	554.75
Citrus aurantifolia	40.33	88.37	41.57	137.64	33.96	64.03	23.37	64.49	31.58	81.27
Citrus sinensis	339.41	144.32	162.93	71.92	163.51	79.92	336.37	152.19	204.09	317.65
Crocus sativus	–	–	–	–	0.70	64.96	–	–	–	–
Cuminum cyminum	567.56	148.15	299.91	73.60	329.12	88.94	618.74	99.84	589.44	116.21
Curcuma zedoaria	–	–	–	–	–	–	–	–	–	–
Cymbopogan winterianus	15.12	10.24	45.51	52.27	45.63	41.59	1.21	1.61	2.37	9.09

Useful part of Ayurvedic & Aromatic Plant	1991–1992		1992–1993		1993–1994		1994–1995		1995–1996	
	Quantity (Ton)	Rs. (Lakh)	Quantity (Ton)	Rs. (Lakh)	Quantity (Ton)	Rs. (Lakh)	Quantity (Ton)	Rs. (Lakh)	Quantity (Ton)	Rs. (Lakh)
Cymbopogon flexuosus	1.49	2.96	0.15	0.59	0.23	0.81	0.03	0.29	–	–
Cymbopogon martini	2.16	7.17	–	–	1.50	6.62	0.40	2.31	–	–
Eucalyptus globules	0.52	2.21	12.31	16.72	47.81	56.30	225.78	189.28	24.81	240.08
Garbled/ Ungarbled/ Dehydrated/ Crushed/ Piper nigrum	1796.90	628.59	1166.06	351.76	436.36	116.22	1999.23	1112.17	1629.65	1235.00
Glycyrrhiza glabra	650.46	63.88	488.02	35.78	650.85	48.48	1285.92	97.50	581.15	49.03
Hemidesmus indicus	–	–	1.83	0.55	2.99	0.56	–	–	3.50	1.08
Humulus lupulus	14.42	36.89	57.25	41.24	56.47	208.07	118.49	263.85	45.68	114.50
Jasminum grandiflorum	5.61	16.98	1.68	3.15	3.32	9.19	7.25	25.88	3.56	19.58
Juniperus communis	0.16	0.42	–	–	–	–	–	–	12.42	0.87
Lavandula angustifolia	39.44	92.82	30.02	79.58	54.11	183.95	43.99	153.24	92.12	184.32
Melaleuca leucadendron	2.15	4.25	0.04	0.16	0.23	0.86	0.86	2.29	–	–
Mentha piperta	11.84	76.67	49.92	468.51	78.03	684.93	21.52	165.74	26.30	210.50
Mentha spicata	22.03	84.89	66.25	167.10	111.15	636.01	37.37	139.47	67.83	292.56
Murriaya koenigii	–	–	–	–	–	–	–	–	–	–
Myristica fragrans	92.15	32.21	154.99	48.12	396.53	120.79	196.57	82.28	1938.52	699.78
Myristica fragrans	4.34	9.83	3.91	8.58	6.44	15.41	20.60	17.01	4.63	19.41
Panax ginseng	66.07	23.36	29.46	26.72	15.55	2.73	61.82	13.28	324.30	24.10
Pandanus odoratissimus	–	–	–	–	4.02	18.6	5.77	19.20	4.65	17.94
Pimpinella anisum	133.71	28.05	463.91	106.46	270.94	77.78	562.17	173.85	467.50	154.37
Piper longum	369.02	27.83	519.50	44.97	436.98	52.97	42.73	5.93	558.30	76.92
Piper nigrum	–	–	–	–	0.30	4.98	3.42	20.85	–	–

Useful part of Ayurvedic & Aromatic Plant	1991–1992		1992–1993		1993–1994		1994–1995		1995–1996	
	Quantity (Ton)	Rs. (Lakh)	Quantity (Ton)	Rs. (Lakh)	Quantity (Ton)	Rs. (Lakh)	Quantity (Ton)	Rs. (Lakh)	Quantity (Ton)	Rs. (Lakh)
Plantago psyllium	–	–	–	–	–	0.55	0.82	–	–	–
Pogostemom cablin	80.86	220.13	70.50	162.75	57.12	177.25	83.07	205.17	73.78	234.26
Polianthes tuberosa	0.24	50.06	0.32	38.53	0.26	82.42	0.44	116.38	0.27	63.21
Rauvolfia serpentina	–	–	–	–	–	–	–	–	–	–
Reen seeds (Ellettaria cardamomum)	543.98	1558.07	181.91	588.00	400.28	1459.31	265.77	769.51	407.57	851.61
Resinoids	37.44	102.23	35.86	141.83	47.02	176.23	50.90	206.29	41.36	158.26
Rosa indica	4.62	18.04	2.68	21.51	3.68	24.04	5.92	27.84	6.62	18.07
Rosa spp.	–	–	–	–	0.03	1.09	–	–	–	–
Santalum album	2.77	5.69	0.03	0.16	0.16	0.86	0.003	0.02	–	–
Saussurea costus	–	–	–	–	–	–	14.07	2.81	243.00	14.69
Swertia chirayita	24.23	2.51	93.04	12.23	172.15	25.85	152.18	22.68	58.22	14.61
Syzygium aromaticum	1594.25	569.51	2924.45	950.08	4418.87	968.84	2507.43	661.21	3345.01	962.85
Syzygium aromaticum	184.96	121.97	143.40	129.70	195.39	148.71	101.11	81.71	184.18	234.81
Thymus vulgaris	–	–	–	–	–	–	–	–	–	–
Vetiveria zizanioides	9.71	41.01	–	–	1.50	18.47	1.25	12.36	0.10	1.92
Zingiber officinale	5.00	2.71	–	–	–	–	1.88	16.23	3.08	9.50
Ziziphus mauritiana	5.47	0.27	2.0	0.13	66.08	6.29	41.57	3.58	25.18	1.71
Other Ayurvedic	1063.55	142.46	1301.85	179.02	1175.88	171.25	907.63	170.19	–	–
Other Aromatic oil	26.67	78.12	697.86	185.27	76.59	161.12	28.60	107.95	70.98	259.64

Table 3 (b): Analysis of Ayurvedic and Aromatic plants are Import in India.

Useful part of Ayurvedic & Aromatic Plant	1996–1997		1997–1998		1998–1999		1999–2000	
	Quantity (Ton)	Rs. (Lakh)	Quantity (Ton)	Rs. (Lakh)	Quantity (Ton)	Rs. (Lakh)	Quantity (Ton)	Rs. (Lakh)
Glycyrrhiza glabra	1622.96	167.12	594.68	70.73	1077.74	157.34	1106.63	178.45
Alpinia sp.	92.81	14.31	55.18	10.19	48.49	9.76	65.00	24.29
Curcuma zedoaria	–	–	–	–	–	–	9.00	1.64
Rauvolfia serpentina	–	–	27.96	5.14	–	–	25.80	4.86
Saussurea costus	245.00	18.94	194.15	26.60	147.10	31.78	266.31	43.16
Panax ginseng	62.85	32.19	24.47	10.07	46.79	36.11	15.27	13.07
Plantago psyllium	–	–	3.28	5.72	1.73	2.31	–	–
Swertia chirayita	52.10	12.29	271.63	22.82	47.49	11.75	53.87	15.41
Cassia angustifolia	–	–	–	–	29.39	46.03	–	–
Catharanthus roseus	4.50	0.24	–	–	0.38	8.40	–	–
Hemidesmus indicus	1.03	0.28	8.53	1.80	2.90	0.63	–	–
Ziziphus mauritiana	8.2	0.68	187.44	34.36	97.60	24.97	–	–
Humulus lupulus	61.64	277.41	137.97	192.54	159.18	348.28	106.72	211.15
Piper longum	409.74	79.01	355.13	308.16	1166.46	1442.27	832.80	1092.62
Garbled/ Ungarbled/ Dehydrated/ Crushed/ Piper nigrum	1882.61	1761.66	1853.98	2590.22	2619.59	4617.03	2304.34	3928.00
Cinnamomum zeylanicum	25.69	9.14	–	–	21.50	1.69	48.22	22.37
Syzygium aromaticum	5207.37	1687.39	6725.18	2643.16	19466.49	7228.25	1620.75	1225.31
Myristica fragrans	1009.35	460.10	644.25	389.43	1274.89	2257.94	672.70	1223.68
Amomum sp.	1921.40	872.26	3142.64	1452.06	3491.46	1537.20	3094.37	1477.79
Reen seeds (Elettaria cardamomum)	218.17	702.05	232.05	674.44	472.94	1389.34	624.43	2223.04
Pimpinella anisum	985.08	419.79	436.36	264.10	1518.06	962.31	383.68	244.17
Cuminum cyminum	1667.56	434.59	1349.15	417.58	1159.31	491.52	1647.72	761.18
Juniperus communis	3.48	0.82	175.07	15.02	180.07	17.74	301.39	24.85

Useful part of Ayurvedic & Aromatic Plant	1996–1997		1997–1998		1998–1999		1999–2000	
	Quantity (Ton)	Rs. (Lakh)	Quantity (Ton)	Rs. (Lakh)	Quantity (Ton)	Rs. (Lakh)	Quantity (Ton)	Rs. (Lakh)
Crocus sativus	–	–	–	–	–	–	33.03	8.30
Murriaya koenigii	0.08	0.36	0.53	1.17	2.53	4.09	15.99	15.61
Cinnamomum tamala	–	–	–	–	0.70	0.11	28.97	2.72
Cinnamonum cassia	2243.46	1017.10	3047.95	1625.50	6951.22	3459.34	12700.31	5921.39
Thymus vulgaris	–	–	–	–	–	–	3.42	0.59
Aquilaria agallocha	24.28	25.11	39.45	50.74	36.78	68.50	255.72	206.29
Abelmoschus moschatus	–	–	0.94	0.69	–	–	–	–
Santalum album	6.58	7.10	1.89	4.37	17.78	23.38	18.64	24.44
Citrus sinensis	408.73	349.12	625.77	279.38	636.63	298.89	777.11	288.22
Citrus aurantifolia	30.18	91.15	27.85	106.48	46.03	202.26	52.13	169.01
Lavandula angustifolia	35.34	155.18	56.77	204.46	43.33	306.94	67.08	447.76
Mentha piperta	40.31	312.64	30.26	309.71	27.11	263.01	27.18	382.94
Jasminum grandiflorum	27.18	83.34	5.69	23.58	2.62	27.41	0.50	6.31
Eucalyptus globulus	83.79	72.79	205.43	323.88	91.19	146.74	296.79	393.27
Zingiber officinale	0.45	5.08	0.68	9.30	0.79	11.86	0.05	1.43
Vetiveria zizanioides	6.41	112.09	1.37	29.65	1.32	14.36	4.46	46.42
Mentha spicata	81.06	555.18	102.01	523.31	193.53	947.75	92.11	450.13
Cymbopogan winterianus	7.63	14.91	34.85	55.31	72.70	117.76	121.53	215.00
Pogostemom cablin	156.63	422.85	155.28	677.81	104.88	1242.45	165.88	977.62
Melaleuca leucadendron	–	–	–	–	0.008	0.28	0.81	11.69
Canana odorata	3.78	8.23	11.64	35.00	2.00	16.57	6.05	23.03
Carum carvl	0.01	0.17	0.13	0.95	0.14	0.38	–	–
Cinnamomum zeylenicum	0.57	2.82	0.03	0.15	0.39	2.25	–	–
Cinnamomum tamala	1.50	5.39	1.36	4.74	2.72	16.94	3.20	16.04
Cinnamomum cassia	0.10	1.89	3.01	24.61	6.19	62.55	3.63	14.00

Useful part of Ayurvedic & Aromatic Plant	1996–1997		1997–1998		1998–1999		1999–2000	
	Quantity (Ton)	Rs. (Lakh)	Quantity (Ton)	Rs. (Lakh)	Quantity (Ton)	Rs. (Lakh)	Quantity (Ton)	Rs. (Lakh)
Syzygium aromaticum	214.23	309.55	169.52	242.83	112.93	174.51	227.96	394.65
Pandanus odoratissimus	1.00	11.87	3.85	24.42	8.18	22.54	16.15	64.38
Myristica fragrans	5.51	27.19	3.96	11.33	7.29	33.02	14.81	154.06
Polianthes tuberosa	0.24	85.24	0.18	1.64	0.10	0.42	–	–
Cymbopogon flexuosus	1.23	3.91	0.14	0.74	8.07	13.90	0.35	5.16
Cymbopogon martini	–	–	–	–	0.40	6.55	–	–
Rosa indica	12.09	29.25	13.57	81.24	12.45	88.81	28.66	148.99
Rosa spp.	0.01	0.66	0.12	3.03	0.006	0.04	–	–
Piper nigrum	–	–	4.08	146.76	6.13	31.18	6.67	175.01
Artemisia pallens	–	–	–	–	–	–	0.26	5.28
Resinoids	60.18	255.41	50.76	263.39	97.73	278.35	–	–
Other Ayurvedic	–	–	588.53	203.15	956.85	617.97	1017.12	659.23
Other Aromatic oil	37.43	244.33	114.50	390.97	88.08	342.67	41.88	125.57

SECTION : II

Medicinal Plants: A to Z

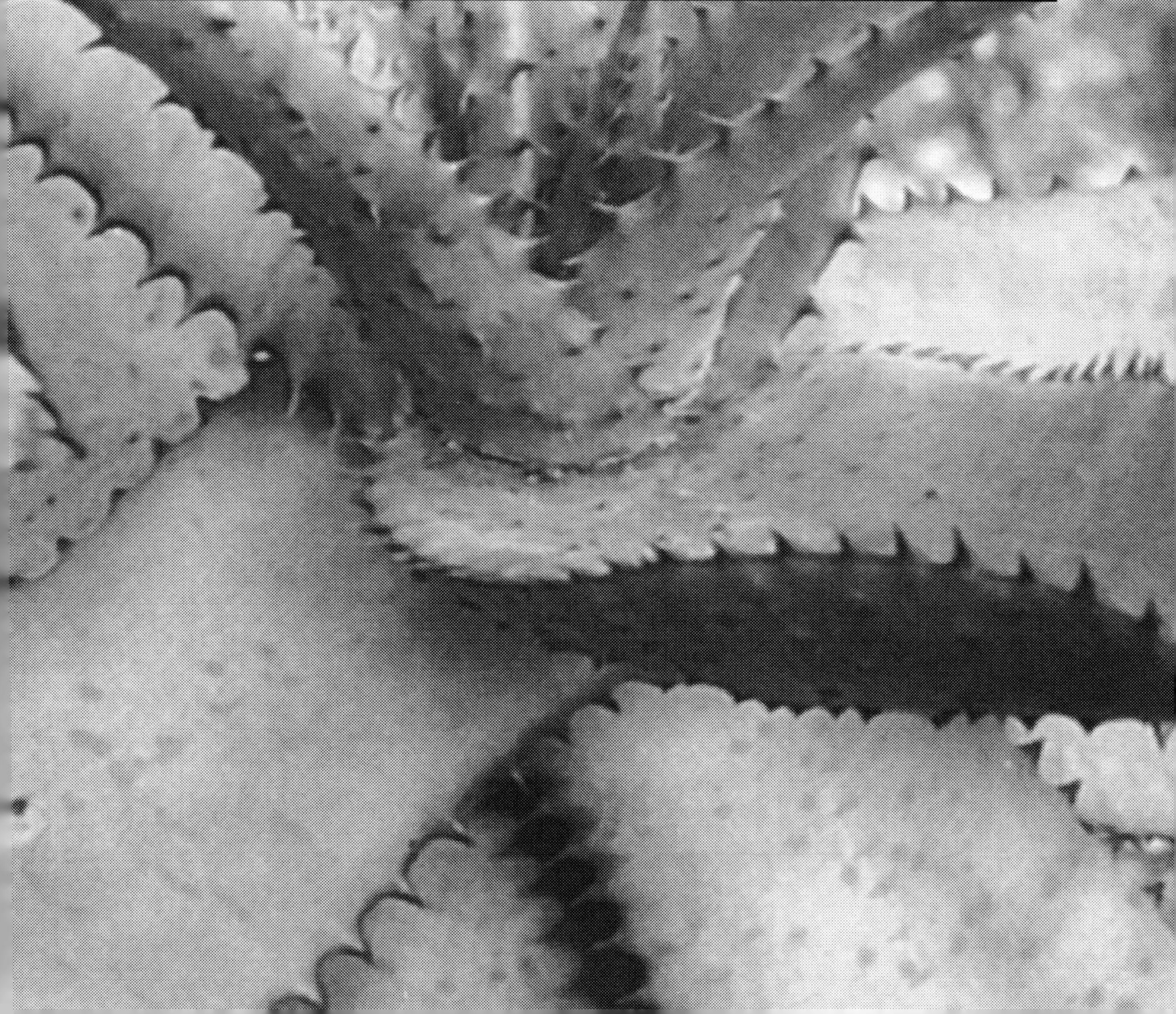

1. *Abelmoschus esculentus L. Moench* *(Malvaceae)*

Synonyms: *Hibiscus* esculentus Linn.

Vernacular Name: *San:* Bendakaya; *Eng:* Lady's finger, Okra; *Hin:* Bhindi-tori; *Kan:* Bendekayi and *Mal:* Venta.

Description: An annual erect herb, 0.9–2.1 m in height, covered with hair throughout; leaves simple, alternate, palmately 3-5 lobed, coarsely toothed, scabrous; flowers large, yellow with a purple center, staminal tube antheriferous throughout; fruits long, 6-8 ribbed, capsular; seeds many, rounded, striate.

Habitate: Throughout India, cultivated in areas upto 1200 m.

Propagation: By seeds.

Part Used: Fruits, seeds and root.

Chemical Constituents: The pods contain carotene, folic acid, thiamine, iboflavin, niacin, vitamin C, oxalic acid and the essential amino acids. The mucilage of the fruit on hydrolysis affords glucose, glucosamine and amino acids. The seeds afford protein lipids, gossypol, thiamine, riboflavin and α-tocopherol. Seed oil yields myristic, palmitic, palmitolcic, olcic, linolenic, tocopherols and acids.

Uses: Fruits: nutritious, demulcent, emollient, diuretic; a mucilaginous preparation used as a plasma replacement; decoction of immature capsules as aodyne, demulcent, diuretic, anticatarrhal and useful in dysentery, ardor urinae, dysuria and gonorrhoea; ***Seeds:*** stimulant, antispasmodic; infusion of roasted seeds sudorific.

2. *Abelmoschus moschatus* L. *(Malvaceae)*

Synonyms: *Hibiscus abelmoschus* Linn.

Vernacular Name: San: Latakasturika; *Eng:* Musk mallow; Hin: Latakasturi, Maskdana; Kan: Kadukasturi; Mal: Latakasturi, Kattukasturi, Kasturiventa; *Tam:* Vettrilaikkasturi, Kattukkasturi; *Tel:* Kasturibendavittu.

Description: An erect hirsute or hispid annual herb. 60-180 cm in height; leaves simple, of varying shapes, usually palmately 3-7 lobed, lobes narrow-acute or oblong-ovate, crenate, serrate or irregularly toothed, hairy on both surfaces; flowers large, yellow with purple center; fruits hairy, capsular; seeds many, subreniform, black or grayish brown, scented.

Habitate: Cultivated throughout India.

Propagation: By seeds.

Part Used: Seeds, leaves and root.

Chemical Constituents: Leaves, flowers and seeds of the plant contain β-sitosterol and its glucoside, campesterol, stigmasterol, cholesterol, ergosterol, higher fatty acids, Esters of acetic and amdrettolic acids, ambrettolide (musk-like odour), farnesol, farensylacetate, furfural, linoleic acid, plasmalogen, myricetin and its glucoside, cannabiscitrin, cyanidin–3-sambubioside and cyandin-3-glucoside.

Uses: ***Seeds:*** aphrodisiac, antispasmodic, carminative, demulcent, diuretic, stomachic and tonic; used as an inhalation in hoarseness and dryness of the throat; rubbed to a paste with milk known to cure scabies; infusion or decoction useful in nervous disorders and in hysteria; ***leaves*** and ***root***: efficacious in gonorrhoea and venereal diseases.

3. *Abies balsamea* (*Pinaceae*)

Vernacular Name: *Eng:* Balsam fir.

Description: Conical evergreen tree growing to 55m. Has aromatic needle-like leaves and purple fir cones.

Habitate: Native to North America.

Propagation: By Seeds.

Parts Used: Oleo-resin, leaves.

Chemical Constituents: Balsam fir leaves contain a liquid oleo-resin.

Uses: Balsam fir is antiseptic and stimulant, and has been used in North America and Europe for catarrh, chest infections such as bronchitis, and urinary tract conditions such as cystitis and frequent urination. Externally, balsam fir was rubbged on the chest or applied as a plaster for respiratory infections. It is little used in herbal medicine today.

4. *Abroma augusta* L. F. (*Sterculiaceae*)

Synonyms: *Ambroma augusta* Linn. F.

Vernacular Name: *San:* Pivari, Pisacakarpasa, Yosini; *Eng:* Devil's Cotton; *Hin:* Ulatkambal; Beng: Ulatkambal; *Kan:* Divvahatti, melpundigida; *Tam:* Sivapputtutti.

Description: A large, spreading, quick-growing hariy shrub or a small tree, roots found up to 1.5m depth; ***leaves:*** lower, cordate, 3-5 lobed; upper, ovate-lanceolate, non-lobed; flowers yellow, purple or dark red; capsules membranous, pentagonal, obpyramidal, winged, 4 cm long, seeds many, small, blackish, covered with silky hair.

Habitate: Found both wild and cultivated throughout hot and moist parts of India.

Propagation: By seeds.

Part Used: Root, root-bark, stem and leaves.

Chemical Constituents: Stem–bark contains β-sitosterol and friedelin. Seeds contain fixed oil composed of linoleic, oleic, hexadececenoic, palmatic and stearic acids. Root contains a fixed oil, resins, an alkaloid in minute quantity and water soluble bases.

Uses: The root and bark of Pivari are uterine tonic and emmenagogue. They contract the uterus and are used for treatment of congestive and nervous dysmenorrhoea, ammenorrhoea, sterlilty and other menstrual disorders. Powdered root act as an abortifacient and anti-fertility agent. Leaves useful in treating uterine disorders, diabetes, rheumatic paine of joints, and headache with sinusitis. Leaves and stem are demulcent and an infusion of fresh leaves and stems in cold water is very efficacious in gonorrhoea.

5. *Abrus precatorius* L. (*Fabaceae*)

Vernacular Name: *San:* Gunja; *Eng:* Jequirity, Indian liquorice; *Hin:* Ghugachi, Chirami, Ratti, Guncaci; *Kan:* Guruguni; *Mal:* Kunni; *Tam:* Kuntumani; *Tel:* Guruginja.

Description: A deciduous, wiry climber with tough branches; leaves abruptly pinnate with many pairs of leaflets, the rachis ending in a spine; the leaflets oblong, rounded at both ends, thinly membranous; flowers pink, clustered on tubercles arranged along the rachis of one-sided pedunculate raceme; fruits pods, turgid with a sharp deflexed beak; seeds usually scarlet with a black spot or sometimes pure white.

Habitate: Throughout India. On hedges and bushes in exposed areas.

Propagation: By seeds.

Part Used: Seeds, leaves and root.

Chemical Constituents: Roots and leaves contain glycyrrhizin. Precol, abrol, abrasine and precasine from roots. Gallic acid, abrine, hypaphorine, alanine, serine, valine, choline, trigonelline, precatorine, and methyl ester, 5B-cholanic acid, abrin A and abtrin B from seeds.

Uses: ***Seeds:*** purgative, emetic, tonic, antiphlogistic, aphrodisiac and used in nervous disorders; abortifacient; paste as local application in stiffness of sholder joints, sciarica and paralysis; ***leaves:*** decoction used for cough, cold colic pain; fresh juice mixed with a bland oil applied to painful swelling, in leucoderma (admixed with Plumbago zeylanica root) and in biliousness, itching and other skin diseases; ***root:*** tonic diuretic emetic, alexeteric; used in preparation for gonorrhoea, jaundice, haemoglobinuric bile. Leaves and root also used as substitute for liquorice in cattaral affections and cough.

6. *Abutilon hirtum* (Lam.) Sweet *(Malvaceae)*

Synonyms: *Abutilon graveolens.*

Vernacular Name: *Hin:* Barakanghi; Beng: Kanghani, jhanpi and *Kan:* Haktuti.

Description: Subshrub; branchlets viscid, indumentum stellate and tomentose; leaves broadly ovate-suborbicular, 4-8 x 3-6 cm, tomentose above, wooly bellow, base cordate, margin dentate-crenate, apex acute-acuminate; atipules falcate; flowers solitary, yeloe; calyx of 5 ovate sepals; petals5, inside base purplish, obovate; staminal column stellate-tomentose below, glabrous above; 20-25 celled; schizocarp globose, densely stellate; mericarps 20-25; seeds reniform, stallate-pubescent.

Habitate: Common in all districts in India, tropical regions of the Old World-tropical America and malesia.

Propagation: By seeds.

Part Used: Seeds, leaves, bark and root.

Chemical Constituents: Leaves contain mucilage, tannin, organic acid and traces of Asparagin and ash, containing alkaline sulphates, chlorides, magnesium phosphate and calcium carbonate. Roots also contain Asparagin.

Uses: ***Seeds:*** in piles; laxative, expectorant; in chronic cyatitis, gleet and gonorrhoea; ***leaves:*** demulcent, locally applied applied to boils and ulcers and as a fomentation to painful parts of the body; decoction used in toothache and tender gums; given internally for inflammation of bladder; infusion leaves or ***root:*** demulcent and diuretic; prescribed in fever, chest affection, and urethritis; ***bark:*** astringent and diuretic.

7. *Abutilon indicum* L. Sweet. *(Malvaceae)*

Synonyms: *Abutilon asiaticum* (L.) Sw.; *Sida guineensis* Schumach.

Vernacular Name: San: Atibala; Eng: Country mallow; Hin: Kanghi; Beng: Petari; *Tam:* Perum tutti; *Tel:* ; *Kan:* Tutti and *Mal:* Velluram.

Description: A perennial, softly tomentose, up to 3 m in height. Stems round, frequently tinged with purple. Leaves ovate to orbicular-cordate,1.9–2.5 cm long. Flowers solitary on jointed peduncles, orange-yellow or yellow; capsules hispid, hardly larger thin the calyx, awns erect. Seeds 3-5, reniform, tubercled or minutely stellate-hairy, black or dark brown. Flowers and fruits almost throughout the year.

Habitate: Found in the sub–Himalayan tract and hills up to 1,200 m and in hotter parts of India.

Propagation: By seeds.

Part Used: Seeds, leaves, bark and root.

Chemical Constituents: Leaves contain mucilage, tannin, organic acid and traces of Asparagin and ash, containing alkaline sulphates, chlorides, magnesium phosphate and calcium carbonate. Roots also contain Asparagin.

Uses: ***Seeds:*** in piles; laxative, expectorant; in chronic cyatitis, gleet and gonorrhoea; ***leaves:*** demulcent, locally applied applied to boils and ulcers and as a fomentation to painful parts of the body; decoction used in toothache and tender gums; given internally for inflammation of bladder; infusion leaves or ***root:*** demulcent and diuretic; prescribed in fever, chest affection, and urethritis; ***bark:*** astringent and diuretic.

8. *Abutilon theophrastii* Medic *(Malvaceae)*

Synonyms: *Abutilon avicennae* Gaertn.

Vernacular Name: San*:* Jaya; *Eng::* Indian mallow, China Jute and *Beng:* Jaya.

Description: An annual softy tomentose herb, attaining a height, up to 3.6 m. Leaves nearly entire, long-petioled, orbicular-cordate with a long point. Flowers solitary, axillary, yellow. Capsules with 15-20 carpels, larger than the calyx segment, oblong, hispid, each with two long horizontally spreading awns. Seeds pilose.

Habitate: Throughout India, up to an altitude of 1,500 m.

Propagation: By seeds.

Part Used: Seeds, leaves and root.

Chemical Constituents: Seed–oil has the following fatty acids: palmitic, atearic, oleic and linoleic, Mucilage from root contains pentoses, metthylpentoses, hexoses, pentosans, methylpentosans and uronic acids, rutin is present in the leaves.

Uses: ***Seeds:*** laxative demulcent and useful in coryza; decoction given in dysentery, fistula and eye sore; ***leaves:*** demulcent; juice antiphyretic; decoction applied in toothache; both leaves and seeds are valued in the treatment of gonorrhoea and urinary; ***root:*** decoction efficacious in cutaneous affections.

9. *Acacia catechu* L. F. Willd. *(Mimosaceae)*

Synonyms: *Acacia wallichiana.*

Vernacular Name: San: Khadirah; *Eng:* Cutch tree; Hin: Katha, Khair, Khaira; Kan: Kalu; Mal: Karinnali; *Tam:* Karunkali; *Tel:* Podalimanu.

Description: A maderate sized deciduous tree, 9-12 m in height with dark grayish or brown rough bark and hooked short spines, leaves bipinnately compound, leaflets 30-50 pairs, main rachis pubescent with a large conspicuous near the middle of the rachi; flowers pale yellow, sessile in peduncled spikes; fruits flat brown pods, shiny and with a triangular beak at the apex and narrowed at the base; seeds 3-10 per pod.

Habitate: Common in Indian forests, upto an elevation of 1,500m.

Propagation: By seeds.

Part Used: Bark and heartwood

Chemical Constituents: The chief constituents of the heartwood are catechin and catechutannic acid. The wood contains epicatechin, Afzelchin, catechin tetramer, dicatechin, gallochin, gossypetin, isorhamnetin, kaempferol.

Uses: ***Bark:*** astringent, useful in passive diarrhoea either alone or in combination with cinnamon or opium, decoction given internally in leprosy; heartwood: the concentrated aqueous exteact known as khayer gum or leprosy; cutch is astringent, cooling and digestive, beneficial in cough and diarrhoea, applied extermally to ulcers, boils and eruptions of the skin.

10. *Acacia farnesiana* L. Willd. *(Mimosaceae)*

Vernacular Name: *San:* Vitkhadira; *Eng:* Cassie flower; *Hin:* Gandh babul, Vilayati kikar; *Beng*: Guye babul; *Tam:* ladivel, Kadivel; *Tel:* Kasturi tuma.

Description: A thorny bush or small tree, attaining a height of 4.5 m. branches spread out from the main trunk. Bark with brown streaks. Leaves bipinnate with stipular spines. Flowers borne in axillary heads, fragrant, bright yellow. Pods dull brown, 5.0-7.5 cm long.

Habitate: In tropical part of India.

Propagation: By seeds.

Part Used: Leaves, bark and pod.

Chemical Constituents: It containt Eicosane, benzyl alcohol, farnesol, geranyl acetate, linalool, linalyl acetate, nerolided, pinitol, α-terpineol. The ripe pods contain gallic acid its derivatives, ellagic acid, tannin, aromadendrin, kaempterol, naringenin and their glucosides while apigenin and rutin glucosides have been found in the leaves. The oil of cassia flowers contains benzaldehyde; salicylic acid, methyl-salicylate, benzyl-alcohol analdehyde and essential oil.

Uses: Decoction of the bark together with ginger is an astringent wash for the teeth, and so it is useful in the bleeding of the gums etc. Tender leaves are bruised with a little water and swallowed in gonorrhoea. Pods of the round yellow heads constitute the cassia flowers, which when distilled yield a delicious perfume. Oil is employed as an adjunct to aphrodisiacs is spermatorrhoea.

11. *Acacia leucophloea* (Roxb.) Willd. *(Mimosaceae)*

Synonyms: *Acacia alba* Willd.

Vernacular Name: *San*: Arimedah; *Eng:* White babool, Distiller's acacia; *Hin*: Safed babul, Sarb ki kikar; *Kan*: Bilijali; *Mal*: Velvelam, Velvelakam; *Tam:* Velvelam, Pattaiccarayamaram; *Tel:* Tallatumma.

Description: A moderate sized tree upto 3 m in height with spreading branches, crooked stems, white spines and pale yellowish grey to nearly white bark with pale red inside; leaves bipinnate, 2.5-5 cm long, main rachis pubescent with a cup-shaped gland between each pair of pinnae, 5-15 pairs of pinnae of 12-30 pairs linear–oblong, obtuse; flowers in large terminal tomentose panicles, heads numerous, globose; fruits sessile, thin flat, slightly curved pods, covered with pale brown tomentum; seeds 10-20 per pod.

Habitate: Throughout India, in dry deciduous forests.

Propagation: By seeds.

Part Used: Bark.

Chemical Constituents: N.A.

Uses: The bark is astringent, bitter, thermogenic, styptic, alexeteric, anthelmintic, vulnerary, demulcent, constipating, expectorant and antipyretic, vulnerary, demulcent, constipating, bronchitis, cough, vomiting. Wounds, ulcers, diarrhoea, dysentery, internal and external haemorrhages, dental caries, oral ulcers, proctoptosis, stomatitis and intermittent fevers.

12. *Acacia nilotica* Delile *(Mimosaceae)*

Synonyms: *Acacia arabica* Willd.

Vernacular Name: *San:* Babbula; *Eng*: Indian gum Arabic tree; *Hin:* Babul; *Beng:* Babla; *Tam:* Karuvael; *Tel:* Nallatumma and *Mal:* Kruvelum.

Description: A medium sized tree with a short trunk, usually attaining a height of 15 m. bark almost black to dark brown, deeply cracked or longitudinally fissured; leaves bipinnate with spinescent stipules 2.5-5.0 cm long. Flowers crowded in long-peduncled globose heads, forming axillary clusters of 2-5 heads, fragrant, golden-yellow. Pods white, flat containing 8-12 seeds, 7.5-15.0 cm long.

Flowers during summer and fruits during winter.

Habitate: Throughout the drier regions of India.

Propagation: By seeds.

Part Used: Pods, leaves, bark and gum.

Chemical Constituents: ***Bark:*** yields several polyphenolic compounds, catechin, epicatechin, cpigallocatechin, quercetin, gallic acid, leucocyanidin gallate, sucrose and tannin, m–Digallic acid and chlorogenic acid; ***gum:*** contains galactose, L-rhamnose, L-arabinose and its derivatives along with four aldobiouronic acids. ***Seeds:*** contain amino acids, fatty acids and ascorbic acid along with tannin as the major constituent.

Uses: Pods: decoction beneficial in urinogenital diseases; ***leaves:*** infusion of tender leaves used as an astringent and remedy for diarrhoea and dysentery; ***bark:*** decoction used as a gargle in sore throat and toothache; dry powder applied exrernally in ulcers; ***gum:*** astringent and styptic.

13. *Acacia polyantha* Willd. *(Mimosaceae)*

Synonyms: *Acacia suma* (Roxb.) Buch.-Ham.

Vernacular Name: *San*: Kadarah, Somavalkah; *Eng:* White cutch tree, White catechu; *Hin:* Svetakhair; *Kan:* Kandaraha Mugali; *Mal*: Venkarinnali Somarayattoli; *Tam:* Kovil, Silaiyuncai; *Tel:* Tellatumma, Somavalkamu, Tellasundra.

Description: A medium sized tree with white bark exfoliating in papery flakes with horizontal patches of darker colour. Young shoots downy; leaves bipinnate, leaflets 30-50 pairs, linear-oblong, pubescent, nerves obscure, glands between many of the pairs of pinnae, stipular spines short, straight or slightly hooked; flowers sessile, white, in spikes; fruits pods, 7-12 cm long with a triangular beak at the apex; seeds many.

Habitate: Common in Indian forests.

Propagation: By seeds.

Part Used: Pods, leaves and bark.

Chemical Constituents: The seeds contain ascorbic acid, niacin and protein which on hydrolysis yields histidine, isoleucine, leucine, lysine, methionine, phenylalanine, tryptophan, tyrosine, and valine. It also contains catechu-tannic acid 35 per cent, catechuic acid or catechin; catechu red, tannin, gum and querecetin.

Uses: Pods: decoction beneficial in urino-genital diseases; ***leaves:*** infusion of tender leaves used as an astringent and remedy for diarrhoea and dysentery; ***bark:*** decoction used as a gargle in sore throat and toothache; dry powder applied externally in ulcers.

14. Acacia sinuata (Lour.) Merrill. *(Mimosaceae)*

Synonyms: *Acacia concinna* (Willd.) DC.

Vernacular Name: *San*: Saptala, Carmasahva; *Eng:* Soapnut-acacia; *Hin:* Satala, Kochi; *Kan:* Sege.

Mal: Chikaka; *Tam:* Cikaikkai, Cityakkai, Cikkai; *Tel:* Sikaya.

Description: A stout prickly climbing shrub with brown branches dotted with white; leaves bipinnate, main rachis bearing sharp hooked prickles and a large gland on the petiole, pinnae 8 pairs or more, leaflets subsessile, sensitive, unequal sided, glabrous; flowers small in globose heads polygamous; fruits short-stalked thin pods, flat, coriaceous, the sutures straight; seeds 6-10 per pod.

Habitate: Throughout India, in tropical forests.

Propagation: By seeds.

Part Used: Pods and bark.

Chemical Constituents: The ***bark:*** contains saponin, which on hydrolysis yields lupeol, α-spinasterol and acacic acid lactone. The sugars identified are glucose, arabinose and rhamnose. It also contains hexacosanol and α-spinasterone. The pods: yield saponins which have been reported to contain acacinin-C, -D and–E and a homologous series of oligosaccharides. The oligosaccharides have been identified as sucrose, raffinose, stachyose and verbascose.

Uses: The pods are bitter, astringent, cooling, diuretic, emetic, deobstruant, detergent, depurative and anthelmimitic. They are useful in vitiated condition of *pitta*, burning sensation, constipation renal and vesical cal culi strangury, haemorrhoids, erysipelas, leucoderma leprosy, prurigo, abscesses and eczema. The powdered pods are the best alternatives to soaps in all cases of skin diseases.

15. *Acacia tomentosa* Willd. *(Mimosaceae)*

Vernacular Name: *San:* Jalbarburaka and *Beng*: Salshai babla.

Description: A small tree, with branchlets and leaf-rachises densely covered with fine grey hairs, the latter with several glands. Bark grey-black, cracked into quandrangular pieces, 2 mm thick. Thorns spindle-shaped, blachish. Leaves crowded on arresting axillary branches, up to cm long; leaflets 8-16 pairs, sessile, oblong-linear, subcoriaceous, glabrescent. Flowers brone in axillary pedunculate heads, white. Pods thin, flat, ligulate, slightly falcate, short-stalked, 10-15 cm long and 1.0-1.5 cm wide. Seeds 6-10, flat, ovat, areolate, brownish-green.

Flowers in summer and fruits in rainy season.

Habitate: Found in Sunderbans and western part of Southern India.

Propagation: By seeds.

Part Used: Pods, leaves and bark.

Chemical Constituents: N.A.

Uses: Pods: decoction beneficial in urinogenital diseases; ***leaves:*** infusion of tender leaves used as an astringent and remedy for diarrhhoea and dysentery; ***bark:*** decoction used as a gargle in sore throat and toothache; dry powder applied extemally in ulcers; ***gum:*** astringent and styptic.

16. *Acalypha indica* L. *(Euphorbiaceae)*

Synonyms: *Acalypha spicata; Acalypha ciliata; Acalypha canescana.*

Vernacular Name: *San:* Haritamanjari; *Eng:* Indian acalypha; *Hin:* Khokli, Kuppi; *Beng*: Muktajhuri; *Kan:* Chalmari, kuppiidda, tuppakire; *Mal:* Kuppamani; *Tel:* Kuppichettu, moorkondachettu, mulakandachettu, pappantichettu.

Description: An erect, annual herb, 30-100cm in height, leaves ovate or rhombic-ovate, 2.5-7.5 cm long with slender petioles; spikes slender, erect, up to 7.6 cm, terminal or axillary with male flowers minute, clustered at the top, and female flowers with accrescent, broad, leafy bract; capsules often one-seeded, concealed in the bract; seeds pale-brown, ovoid, acute, smooth.

Habitate: Throughout the plains of India.

Propagation: By seeds.

Part Used: Whole plant.

Chemical Constituents: Plant contains kaempferol, sitosterol, triacetonamine. Leaves and twigs, acalyphine, acalypus, acalyphamide and other amides, quinone, sterols and cyanogenic glycoside.

Uses: Haritamanjari plant is bitter, acrid and possesses diuretic, cathartic, expectorant, emetic, anthelmintic, anodyne and hypnotic properties. But it causes gastro-intestinal irritation. It is used as a substtute for ipecac and senega. A decoction of the herb is used as a cure for tooth and ear ache and is safe and speedy laxative. It is useful in bronchitis, pneumonia and asthma. Root is cathatic. Leaves are laxative, used in scabies and in snake bite. Fresh leaf juice useful in rheumatoid arthritis and skin affections. Juice with salt applied on eczema. Paste of leaves applied on burns; with juice of lime, useful in early cases of ringworm. Powder of leaves for bed-sores and maggotinfested wounds.

17. *Acanthopanax trifoliatus* L. *(Araliaceae)*

Synonyms: *Acanthopanax aculeatum* seem.

Description: Rigid shrub, diffuse. Stems ascending, spiny. Leaves alternate, 3–5-palmifoliate; leaflets with margins toothed and spines on the nerves. Inflorescence in terminal panicle of some umbels; flowers small, greenish-white. Fruit globose, black when ripe. All parts of the plant are particularly fragrant.

Flowering period: September-November.

Habitate: Grows wild in mountainous regions & forests of eastern Asia, Malaysia.

Propagation: By seeds.

Part Used: Root bark and stem bark.

Chemical Constituents: The root bark and stem bark are contain triterpenoid saponins and oleanolic acid leaves contain potassium chloride, scyllitol, myoinositol, taraxerol, taraxeryl acetate, β-sitosterol, an unidentified steroid, triacontanol, dotriacontanol and a mixture of n-alkanes with hentriacontane as major component. The stems contain potassium nitrate, stigmasterol and sitosterol with their glucosides, a mixture of n-alkanes with nonacosane as major component, and n-pentadecanoic-palmitic-, margaric-, stearic-,and arachidic-acids.

Uses: The root bark and stem bark are prescribed in the treatment of rheumatism, lumbago, ostealgia and impotence. The drug is also considered as a central nervous system stimulant and tonic. It improves the memory.

18. *Acanthus mollis* *(Acanthaceae)*

Vernacular Name: *Eng:* Acanthus, Bear's breeches.

Description: Perennial growing to 1m. Has a black, branched taproot, white purple or blue flowers, and dark green basal leaves up to 1m in length.

Habitate: Native to Europe, acanthus is most commonly found as a garden plant. It prefers damp sites and low-lying ground.

Propagation: By Seeds.

Parts Used: Leaves and roots.

Chemical Constituents: Acanthus contains large quantities of mucilage and tannin.

Uses: Acanthus was well known in the ancient world. Callimacus, a Greek archtect of the 5th century BC, reputedly created the decorative pattern of foliage at the top of Corinthian columns after being inspired by the perfect symmetry of acanthus leaves. The Greek physician Dioscorides recommended the roots in the form of a plaster to treat burns and to wrap around dislocated joints. As an infusion, acanthus was thought to be diuretic. It was also used to relieve wind and spasms and to soothe damaged nerves.

19. *Achillea millefolium* L. *(Asteraceae)*

Vernacular Name: *Hin:* Gandana; *Guj*: Biramjasif; *Kan:* Roojamari.

Description: A small, perennial, tufted herb upto 50 cm tall, with a slender cropping rootstock throwing numerous roots and stolons with blunt succulent scale at each node. Leaves alternate, oblong-lanceolate, 3-pinnatisect, minutely divided into linear, dentate, mucronate more or less hairy segments. Flowers are numerous small, white in corymbose, ovoid flat topped heads at the ends of stems and branches. Fruits shining, with no pappus.

Habitate: Herb abounds in the Himalayas and Europe.

Propagation: By seeds.

Part Used: Whole plant.

Chemical Constituents: The herb contains an alkaloid, achilleine; aerial parts of the flowering herb, on distillation yield a yellowish green or dark blue essential oil, known as OIL OF MILFOIL; the herb contains; salicylic acid, β-sitosterol and its acetate, inositol, dulcitol, mannitol, betaine, choline, trigonelline, betonicine and stachydrine. The presence of folic acid, rutin and ascorbic acid in abundance has also been reported in the leaves.

Uses: It is diuretic, stimulant and haemostatic, a decoction of the leaves and flower heads is employed as a carminative, tonic and aromatic stimulant. Due to the presence of choline, it has hypotensive effect. The leaves and flower heads are also used as a tonic and vapour bath for fever. Its hot infusion is used as an emmenagogue in France. Medicated vapour bath containing yarrow, lavender flowers, wheat bran and milk is used in nasal catarrh and fever. It has a specific action on the pelvic organs and is used in amenorrhoea, menorrhagia and leucorrhoea. As a bitter tonic, it is given during convalescance from fevers and in atonic dyspepsia to promote appetite. Its chief use is in relaxation of the sphincter and with discharge of mucus or blood during defecation. The infusion is applied to relax throat and sore nipples with benefits. Local inhabitants chew the leaves to relieve tooth-ache as it produces a pungent, but tingling and cooling sensation bringing immediate relief.

20. *Achyranthes aspera* L. *(Amaranthaceae)*

Vernacular Name: *Eng*: Prickly Chaff Flower; *San:* Apamarga; *Hin:* Chirchira, chirchitta, Latjira; *Beng*: Apang, chirchiti; *Mal:* Kadaladi; Mar: Aghada, aghara; *Tam:* Chirukadaladi, naaurivi; *Tel:* Apamarganu, uttareeni and *Kan:* Utranigida, uttaraanne.

Description: Herbaceous plant about 1m to 2m. high. Stems erect, pubescent, swollen at the nodes. Leaves opposite, short-petioled, margins undulate. Flowers numerous, stiffly deflected against the pubescent rachis in elongate terminal spike, 20–30cm. long. Urticle oblong-cylindrical, enclosed in the hardened perianth, brown. Seeds oblong-ovoid.

Habitate: Throughout India wildly growing.

Propagation: By seeds.

Part Used: The whole plant, especially the roots and seeds.

Chemical Constituents: The roots contain triterpenoid saponins, betaine, achyranthine, hentriacontane, ecdysterone and two glycosides of oleanolic acid have been reported. The dried dehusked seeds contain amino acids.

Uses: The whole plant and especially the roots, characterized by their anti-inflammatory and uterine stimulant activity, are prescribed in the rheumatism, lumbago, osteodynia, dysuria, post-partum haematometra and dysmenorrhea. The seeds are nutritious when cooked with milk and are a potential source of food; the roots are astringent; their paste is applied to clear opacity of cornea, and to wounds as an haemostatic; it is reported to be useful in cancer. A decoction of the roots is used for stomach troubles, and an aqueous extract for stones in the bladder.

21. *Achyranthes bidentata* Blume *(Amaranthaceae)*

Vernacular Name: *Assam*: Apamarga, bankhat.

Description: Perennial herbaceous plant 60-80cm. high. Tuberous roots long, cylindrical. Stems angular, swollen at the nodes. Leaves opposite, elliptic to linear-lanceolate, short-petioled, with margins undulate. Inflorescence in terminal spike; flowers greenish-white, numerous, deflected against the rachis. Utricle oblong-cylindrical, one-seeded.

Habitate: It is cultivated in the plains.

Propagation: By seeds.

Part Used: Tuberous roots.

Chemical Constituents: The tuberous roots contain triterpeniod saponins, the genin of which is oleanolic acid; ecdysterone, inokosterone, β-sitosterol, stigmasterol.

Uses: The roots possess anti-inflammatory, hyprocholesterolaemic, hypotensive and uterotonic properties. The drug is indicated for rheumatism, lumbago, dysmenorrhoea, hypertension, hypercholesterolaemia, atherosclerosis, dysuria, haematuria, contusions, congestion and sore throat. It is also used as an oxytocic in dystocia, placenta retention and post-partum haematometra.

22. *Achyranthes japonica* (Miq.) Nakai *(Amaranthaceae)*

Vernacular Name: *Eng.*: Japanese chaff flower.

Description: Perennial herb, 50-100 cm tall, with thickened roots. Stems slightly pubescent, quadrangular, branched, nodes dilated. Leaves opposite, oblong or elliptic, slightly pubescent, 10-20 cm long, 4-10 cm wide, petiolate. Inflorescence spikes in axils and at terminals, elongate; bracts membranous, ovate-deltoid, with a green long-protruded midrib. Flowers horizontal, deflexed in ***fruit:*** bracteoles 3, subulate; perianth 5-parted; the segments linear-lanceolate, acuminate, 4-5 mm long, the inner ones slightly shorter; stamens 5, united at base; carpel 1; style 1, slender, erect, persistant in fruit. Fruit utricles oblong, about 2 mm long, 1 mm across, 1 seeded.

Habitate: Woody areas in lowlands and hills.

Propagation: By seeds.

Parts Used: Root.

Chemical Constituents: ***Seeds*:** insect moulting hormones like rubrosterone, ecdysterone, inokosterone. **Root:** triterpenoid, saponin.

Uses: Analgesic, antispamodic, uterine stimulating, diuretic, hypotensive, antiallergic, antioxidant (protocate chuic acid), anti-inflammatory, platelet aggregation inhibition. Traditionally used in Oedema, eheumatism, contraceptive, & abortifacient.

23. *Aconitum deinorrhizum* Stapf. *(Ranunculaceae)*

Vernacular Name: *Kash*: Dudhia bish; *Punj*: Sajed bikh and *Eng:* Indian aconite.

Description: A tall, glabrous, biennial herb with paired tuberous roots. The daughter tubers are conical rather elongate upto 15 cm long and 3.5 cm in diameter at the crown with few root fibres. The surface is dark brown and coarsely wrinkled. Mother tubers are similar, but have longer filiform root fibres; leaves are scattered, reniform or ovate reinform 5-10 cm long, acute or obtuse, 5 pedatipartite almost to the base. Cauline leaves, sharply toothed, lowest long petioled; flowers more than 2.5 cm long, bright blue to greenish blue with purple veins in terminal racemes which go upto 45 cm. long. Fruit is a capsule bearing numerous seeds.

Habitate: The plant is common in the sub-alpine and alpine zones of the Himalaya upto 2400 m–4500m.

Propagation: By seeds & tuber.

Part Used: Tuber roots.

Chemical Constituents: Alcaloid contain named as pseudoaconitine in larger proportions, its use in medicines required careful purification.

Uses: It is a poison and affects both the heart and central nervous system. In case of extreme toxicity, the heart stops and respiration is depressed. With large doses, death is almost instantaneous, resulting in paralysis of heart or the respiratory center. With moderate toxic doses, there is a tingling of the tongue, mouth, stomach, skin; followed by numbness, anaesthesia, nausea, vomiting, diarrhoea, excessive salivation, weak and irregular pulse, difficult respiration and muscular weakness may result. Externally, it is used with mustard oil as massage in neuralgia, paralysis and muscular rheumatism. Its application should be avoided in wounds or abrased skin as it may get absorbed and caused poisoning. Locally much used for removing body pains, but carefully. Root is smoked in toothache and body pains. Leaves are employed to improved the flavour of country liquor. Also used in leprosy, cholera, rheumatism, as tonic in diarrhoea and cough.

24. *Aconitum ferox* Wall. ex Ser. *(Renunculaceae)*

Vernacular Name: *San*: Vatsanava; *Hin:* Bish, Bacchanag; *Beng*: Katbish; *Tam:* Vashanabi; *Eng:* Indian aconite; *Tel:* Ativasanabhi; *Kan:* Vasanabhi and *Mal:* Vastsarabhi.

Description: A perennial herb. Roots tuberous, paired; daughter tuber ellipsoid to ovoid-oblong, 2.5-4.0 cm in length, with filiform root fibres. Leaves scattered, orbicular-cordate to reniform, palmately 5-lobed, resembling those of melon leaves; blade and petiole pubescent. Peduncle straight, bearing flowers on both sides. Flowers pale dirty blue, borne in a dense terminal raceme, 10-25 cm long, helmet-vaulted with a short sharp beak, resembling a pea flower. Follicles oblong; seeds long, obpyramidal to obovoid, winged along the raphe.

Habitate: The plant is common in the sub-alpine & alpine zone of Himalayas upto 3,600m.

Propagation: By seeds & vegetative methods.

Part Used: Undergound stem and root.

Chemical Constituents: It contain the alkaloids pseudaconitine, chasmaconitine, indaconitine and bikhaconitine recently two new alkaloids, veratroyl pseudaconitine and diacetyl pseudaconitine.

Uses: The root and undergound stems are highly toxic; but the toxicity may be reduced by suitable processing. In small doses they are beneficial in nasal catarrh, uvula hypertrophy, sore throat, gibbous, paralysis and chronic fever; in large doses it acts as narcotic poison and powerful sedative. Internally, the tincture of root is used in combination with other drugs for the treatment of fever and rheumatism. The root is considered to be cardiac stimulant, hypoglycemic, diaphoretic and antiphlogistic. Powdered roots in the form of liniment or paste is spread over the skin in case of arthritis and in scabies.

25. *Aconitum fortunei* Hemsl *(Renunculaceae)*

Description: Perennial herbaceous plant, 0.6-1m. high. Roots paired tuberous, conical with mother-tuber and daughter-tuber. Stem erect, cylindrical, glabrous. Leaves of two kings;

the lower cordate, crenated; the upper 3–palmatipartite, sharply denticulate. Inflorescence in terminal raceme; flower blue. Follicles: 5, sessile, oblong, divergent. Seeds winged.

Habitate: The plant is common in the sub-alpine & alpine zone of Himalayas upto 3,600m.

Propagation: By seeds & vegetative methods.

Part Used: Tuberous roots.

Chemical Constituents: N.A.

Uses: The tuberous roots are used in treating rheumatism, paresis, arthralgia, luxation, sprains and contusions. Their tincture is used as liniment. It must not be taken by mouth, because of its high toxicity.

26. *Aconitum heterophyllum* Wall.ex Royle *(Ranunculaceae)*

Vernacular Name: *Eng:* Atis roots, Indian Atis; *Hin*: Atis; *Kan:* Ativisa; *Mal:* Ativitayam; *San:* Ativisa *Tam*: Ativadayam; *Tel:* Ativasa.

Description: A perennial, erect, showy herb. Stem long, simple or branched from base, glabrous and puberulous above; leaves broad, ovate or orbicular or somewhat 5-lobed and toothed, upper 3-fid or entire. Flowers 2.5 cm long, helmet-shaped, bright, blue or greenish-blue with purple veins.

Habitate: Common in the alpine and sub-alpine belts of the Himalayan at altitudes between 1,800 and 4,500 m.

Propagation: By seeds & vegetative methods.

Part Used: Underground stem and root.

Chemical Constituents: Diterpenoid alkaloid atisine is the main constituent of the root. Others include atidine, histisine, hetisine, hetidine, heterophyllisine, heterophylline, heterlophylline, isoatisine, dihydroatisine, hetisinone and benzoyl heteratisine.

Uses: The roots are acrid, bitter, themogenic, expectorant, alexeteric, stomachic, digestive, antiperiodic and tonic. They are useful in dysentery, diarrhoea, stomach disorders, fever, malarial fever, vomiting, helminthiasis, haemorrhoids, haemorrhages, internal inflammatory conditions and general debility. They are highly recommended for diseases in children.

27. *Aconitum koreanum* R. Rkaymond *(Ranunculaceae)*

Vernacular Name: *Eng.*: Korean monk's hood.

Description: Erect, glabrous, perennial herb with thickened roots, to 1 m. tall. Leaves alternate, palmately 3-5 cleft, long-petioled, petioles of upper leaves shoter, almost sessile; leaflets deeply divided again to lanceolate, sharply acuminate. Flowers racemose at terminal, zygomorphic, pale yellow, sometimes purplish tint; pedicels short, densely pubescent; sepals 5, petal-like, the upper one clearly hooded, the others flat, the lower 2 narrower than the others; petals 2, small, hidden under the hood; stamens many; ovary 3-called, glabrous. Fruit of 3 follicles, sharp at tip.

Habitate: Grassy areas in mountain valleys or on slopes.

Propagation: By Roots.

Parts Used: Rhizome.

Chemical Constituents: Alkaloids: hypaconitines A, B, C, D, E, aconitine, mesaconitine, atisine, higenamine, coryneine, isoatisine, 19-epi-isoatisine.

Uses: Analgesic (aconitine alkaloids), cardiotonic (hygenamine, coryneine), uterine stimulant. Used in articular pain.

28. *Aconitum kusnezoffii* Reichb. *(Ranunculaceae)*

Vernacular Name: *Eng:* Kusnetzoff's monkshood.

Description: A perennial herb, 7-150 cm high. Stem erect smooth. Leaves alternate, petiolate; blade subcoriaceous, ovoid in outline, 6-14 cm long by 8-9 cm wide, tripalmatipartite, segments rhomic, pinnately parted again, the ultimate segments linear lanceolate or lanceolate; tip acute; both faces glabrous, sometimes puberulous. Inflorescence a terminal raceme or a dense pincle sepals 5, purplish-blue; upper sepal helmet-shaped, 1.5-2.5 cm high lateral sepal 1.4-1.7 cm long. Petals 2, glabrous, with long unguiculi, spur 1-4 mm long. Petals 2, glabros, with long unguiculi, spur 1.4 mm long. Stamens numerous. Carpels 4-5 glabrous. Fllicles 1-2 mm long. Seeds winged.

Habitate: In thickets, on slopes, in grassland and at forest edges of China. Korea, Mongolia.

Propagation: By seeds and vegetative method.

Part Used: The parent root tubers.

Chemical Constituents: N.A.

Uses: Rheumatic arthralgia, sciatica, hemiplegia, muscular spasm, contusions, local anesthetic.

29. *Aconitum napellus* L. *(Ranunaculaceae)*

Vernacular Name: *Eng:* Indian aconite, Monk's hood; *Hin*: Bachnag, Mithavis; *Kan:* Vatsanabhi; *Mal:* Vatsanabhi; *San:* Vatsanabhah; *Tam*: Vasanavi and *Tel:* Vatsanabhi.

Description: A perennial herb. Stem often decumbent in small states, glabrous or slightly pubescent. Leaves variable in size, palmatipartite, segments linear. Racemes simple or sparingly compound; bracts entire or 3-fid. Flowers borone on the upper portion of the peduncle and on both sides, bright, or dull greenish-blue; helmet thrice as long as high. Follicles 3-5, having many seeds inside.

Habitate: Alpine and sub-alpine belt of the Himalayas.

Propagation: By seeds and tuber.

Part Used: Roots.

Chemical Constituents: Aconitine is the principal constituent others are mesaconitine, neoline, songoramine, deoxyaconitine, hypaconitine and napelline (luciculine), 12-epidehydro-nepelline, 12-epiacetyldehydronapelline, 1,14-diacetylneoline. Roots contain vitamin C.

Uses: The roots are sweet, thermogenic, narcotic, anodyne, anti-inflammatory, diaphoretic, diuretic, expectorant, nervine tonic, stomachic, emmenagogue, anaphrodisiac, depurative, sedative and febrifuge. They are useful in vitiated conditions of *vata, pitta* and *kapha*, cephalagia, neuralgia, painful inflammations, strangury, cough, asthma, bronchitis, hypotension, dyspepsia, flatulence, colic, cardiac debility, dysmenorrhoea, amenorrhoea, spermatorrhoea, leprosy, skin diseases, sciatica, gout, paralysis, heptopathy, splenopathy, pharyngodynia, diabetes, nasal discharges, fever, inflammatory fevers and debility. Milk is prescribed as antidote for aconite poisoning.

30. *Acorus calamus* L. *(Araceae)*

Vernacular Name: *Eng:* Sweet flag, Calamus, Sweet root; *Hin*: Bach, Gorbacc; *Kan:* Baji; *Mal:* Vayampu; *San:* Vacha, Ugragandha; *Tam*: Vasampu; *Tel:* Vasa.

Description: A semi-aquatic rhizomatous perennial herb, rhizome creeping, much branched, as thick as the middle finger, cylindrical or slightly compressed, ligh brown or pinkish brown externally, white and spongy within; leaves bright green, distichous, ensiform, base equitant, thickened in the middle, margins wavy; flowers light brown densely packed in sessile cylindric spadix; fruits oblong turbinate berries with a pyramidal top; seeds fre, pendant from the apex of the cells.

Habitate: Throughout India in areas elevated upto 1,800 m. in marshes, also cultivated.

Propagation: By rhizome.

Part Used: Rhizomes.

Chemical Constituents: It yields a light brown to brownish yellow volatile oil known as CALAMUS OIL. The important constituents are asarone and its β-isomer. Other constituents are calamenol; calamene, calamenone, methyleugenol, eugenol and α-pinene and camphene, presence of small quantities of palmitic, heptylic and butyric acids, asaronaldehyde, calamol, calamone and azulene has also been reported. Sesquiterpenic ketones like acorone, calarene, calacone, calacorene, acorenone, acolamone, isoacolamone, epishyobunone, shyobunone, isoshyobunone and acoragermacrone, and alcohols like isocalamendiol and preisocalamendiol are also present.

Uses: The rhizome is acrid, bitter, thermogenic, aromatic, intellect promoting, emetic, laxative, carminative, stomachic, anthelmintic, emmenagogue, diuretic, alexeteric, expectorant, anodyne, antispasmodic, aphrodisiac, anticonvulsant, resuscitative, anti-inflammatory, sudorific, antipyretic, sialagogue, insecticidal, tranquillising, nervine tonic, sedative and tonic. It is useful in witiated conditions of *vata* and *kapha*, stomatopathy, hoarseness, colic flatulence, dyspepsia, helminthiasis, amenorrhoea, dysmenorrhoea, nephropathy, calculi, strangury, cough, bronchitis, odontalgia, pectoralgia, hepatodynia, otalgia, inflammations, gout, epilepsy, delirium, amentia, convulsions, depression and other mental disorders, tumours, dysentery, hyperdipsia, haemorrhoids, intermittent fevers, skin diseases, numbness and general debility.

31. *Acorus gramineus* Solander *(Araceae)*

Vernacular Name: *Eng*: Grass-leaved sweet rush.

Description: Perennial semi-aquatic herb. Rhizome aromatic, creeping and much-branched. Leaves long and amplexicaul, in fasciciles; principal nerves parallel. Inflorescence in spike on a compressed scape, surrounded by a long bract; flowers small, bisexual. Berry bright-red when ripe.

Habitate: Grows wild on the banks of mountain streams of China, Japan and Korea.

Propagation: By rhizome.

Part Used: Rhizomes.

Chemical Constituents: The rhizome contains an essential oil consisting of asaron and asaryl aldehyde; and a bitter glucoside, acorin.

Uses: The rhizome possesses pectoral, stomachic and sedative properties. It is utilized in the therapy of diarrhoea, gastralgia, cough, bronchial asthma, neurasthenia, fever, convulsions, rheumatism, osteodynia, and arrhythmia. External application is effective for dermatosis and haemorrhoids. It is also used as an insecticide for killing lice, bugs and fleas.

32. *Acronychia laurifolia* Blume *(Rutaceae)*

Synonyms: *Acronychia pedunculata* Linn., *Acronychia barberi* Gamble.

Vernacular Name: *Eng:* Claw flowered laurel; *Mal:* Mutta-nari; *Tam:* Mutta-nari and *Kan:* Bhutali, Soneman.

Description: Small tree, 1–3m. tall or more, much-branched. Leaves opposite, oblong or obovate, entire, coriaceous, glabrous; petiole long. Indlorescence in axillary or terminal corymb; flowers white, fragrant. Drupe globose, obscurely angular, pale-yellow when ripe, edible.

Habitate: Grows wild in the midlands and the mountainous regions.

Propagation: By seeds.

Part Used: Roots, twigs, stem bark and leaves.

Chemical Constituents: The stembark contains acrovestone, acronylin bauereno, potassium oxalate and traces of alkaloids. The rootbark yield 6-demethylacronylin and acrovestone.

Uses: The roots are utilized in the therapy of rheumatism, lumbago, paid in the limbs, post-partum blood stasis, furunculosis, impetigo and snake-bite. The torrefied roots or leaves are effective as a stomachic for dyspepsia in parturients. A poultice made of heated leaves and a wash with a decoction of the trunk bark are useful for furunculosis and impetigo.

33. *Actaea spicata* L. *(Ranunculaceae)*

Synonyms: *Actaea acuminata* Wall., *Actaea racemosa* Gilib.

Vernacular Name: *Eng:* Baneberry, Grapewort, *Kan:* Vishphala.

Description: A perennial herb, upto 60 cm. high, with a characteristic foetid smell, with stout obliquely ascending blackish rhizome, bearing underneath numerous fibrous roots. Leaves triternately compound, that is, the stalk of each leaf first divides into three small stalks, each of which again divides or redivides in threes, each leaf, thus, is composed of 18 or even 27 lobes or leaflets, having toothed margins. Inflorescence, with tiny, white flowers on a stalked raceme. Fruit egg shaped, berries, black, shining, many seeded; seeds arranged in two rows.

Habitate: Temperate regions in Asia and Europe.

Propagation: By seeds.

Parts Used: Roots and rhizomes.

Chemical Constituents: Transaconitic Acid. Absence of Protoanimonin.

Uses: Complaints specially rheumatism involving small joints with characteristic tearing, tingling pains. Wrist-rheumatism. Pulsation with tearing pain over the whole body, especially head, stomach, epigastrium, liver and renal region. Cardiovascular spasm/Angina pectoris. Early stages of Phthisis. Pains worse by touch or motion. Violent pain in upper jaw, running from teeth through molar bones to temple. Great oppression of breath. Shortness of breath on exposure to cold air. Dropsy. Hysteria.

34. *Adenanthera pavonina* L. *(Mimosaceae)*

Vernacular Name: *Eng:* Coralwood tree, Redwood tree; *Hin*: Baragunci; *Kan:* Manjatti; *Mal:* Mancati; *San:* kucandanah, Tamrakah; *Tam:* Yanai Kuntumani; *Tel:* Bandigurvina, Mansenikotta.

Description: A medium sized, unarmed deciduous tree about 20m in height with a clear bole of 6.0m having grayish brown bark with longitudinal fissures; leaves bipinnate, the pinnae 3-6 pairs, opposite, leaflets many, alternate, ovate-oblong, obtuse, glabrous, unequal sided, dark green above; flowers pale yellow, in short peduncled racemes; fruits falcately curved pointed pods, the valves spirally twisted after dehiscence; seeds shining brilliant scarlet, lenticular-globose.

Habitate: Throughout India, in deciduous forests, also cultivated.

Propagation: By seeds.

Part Used: Bark, leaves seeds, heartwood.

Chemical Constituents: The seeds contain non-protein amino acids, viz. γ-methylene glutamic acid, γ-methylene glutamine, and traces of γ-ethylidene glutamic acid. The kernels contain a pale yellow fat. The fatty acid composition of the fat is: palmitic, stearic, arachidic, lignoceri, octacosanoic, oleic, linoleic, eicosenoic, and uncharacterized, the kernels also contain stigasterol and its glucoside, dulcitol and a polysaccharide.the leaves contain octacosanol, dulcitol, glucosides of β-sitosterol and stigmasterol. Bark contains stigmasterol glucoside. The heartwood containsrobinetin, chalcone, butein, ampelopsin and dihydrorobinetin.

Uses: The bark and leaves are astringent, vulnerary and aphrodisiac, and are useful in colonorrhea, haematuria, ulcers, pharyngopathy, vitiated conditions of *vata* and gout. The seeds are bitter, astringent, sweet cooling, aphrodisiac, suppurative, antiemetic and febrifuge. They are useful in vitiated conditions of *vata* and *pitta*, gout, buring sensation, hyperdipsia, vomiting, fever and giddiness. The heart wod is astringent, aphrodisiac, haemostatic, and is useful in dysentery, harmorrhages and vitiated conditions of *vata*.

35. *Adenia hondala* (Gaertn.) W.J. de Wilde *(Passifloraceae)*

Synonyms: *Modecca palmate* Lam., *Adenia palmate* (Lam.) Engl.

Vernacular Name: *San*: Vidari, *Kan:* Kempu chendu hannina balli, *Mal:* Modecca, Muthukku, Palmothakku.

Description: Large climbing shrubs with prominent tubers. *Tubers* robust, in different shapes, usually larger, 10-50 cm long, 5-20 cm broad, greenish white inside. *Tendrils* arise in leaf axils and bear flowers. *Stems* swollen at nodes. *Leaves* alternate, palmately 3-5 lobed, broadly egg-shaped in outline, 10-18 x 8-20 cm, base heart-shaped, 3-5-nerved from the base, with 2 glands just at the base and another 2 glands seen above them; lobes elliptic to oblong-lanceolate, apex acute-acuminate, margin entire, shiny, hairless; leaf stalks up to 8 cm long. *Flowers* unisexual; male flowers many and female flowers solitary or few, arranged in axillary cymes, greenish yellow, 1 cm long, 1.5 cm across. *Capsules* globose or ellipsoid, 3-5 x 2-4 cm, orange-red when ripe, splitting into 3 valves, with leathery rind. *Seeds* numerous, egg-shaped or kidney-shaped, flat, covered with membranous white aril.

Habitate: Most deciduous to semi-evergreen forests in western Ghats of India and Sri Lanka.

Propagation: By tubers, seeds and stem cuttings.

Parts Used: Tubers.

Chemical Constituents: N.A.

Uses: This species has been used as medicine since the 17th century. Tubers are reportedly poisonous. It may be an adulterant or an unauthorised substitute. The roots are reportedly used as Ayurvedic plant drug *Vidari*. Tubers used for treating hernia.

36. *Adenophora stricta* Miq. *(Campanulaceae)*

Vernacular Name: *Eng:* Upright ladybell.

Description: A perennial herb 60-100 cm high. The whole plant is covered with white fine hairs. Root robust, long and conical stem simple, erect, branched in upper part. Basal leaves oval cauline leaves alternate, briefly petiolate or sessile; limp ovate or narrowly ovate, 3-7 cm long, dentate in margin. Flowers in summer auttumm, Raceme terminal narrowed. Sepals 5, petals 5, deeply campanulate, up to 2 cm long, blue. Capsule subspherical.

Habitate: On slopes, in crevices or in tussocks, China, Japan, Korea and Mongolia.

Propagation: By seeds.

Part Used: Roots.

Chemical Constituents: N.A.

Uses: Chronic bronchitis, cough, thick sputum.

37. *Adensoma indianum* (Lour.) Merr (*Scrophulariaceae*)

Synonyms: *Adensoma capitatum* Benth.

Description: Annual herb, 20–60cm. high. Stems erect. Young twigs at first pubescent, finally glabrous. Leaves opposite, short-petioles, lanceolate, pubescent; margins toothed. Inflorescence terminal in a sort of head; flowers wioled. Capsule with numerous seeds.

Habitate: Commonly found wild in mountainous regions.

Propagation: By seeds.

Part Used: Whole plant.

Chemical Constituents: The plants contain triterpenoid saponins, phenolic acids, coumarins and flavonoids. The volatile oil from the plant consists of L. fenchone 35%, limonene 22.6%, cineol 5.9%, piperitenon oxide and sesquiterpene oxide.

Uses: The whole plant, except the roots, constitutes an antibacterial, cholagogic, diuretic and stomachic remedy. It is useful for the treatment of jaundice in viral hepatitis, oliguria, biliuria, fever ophthalmalgia, vertigo nd dyspepsia in parturients.

38. *Adhatoda vasica* Nees (*Acanthaceae*)

Synonyms: *Adhatoda zeylanica* Medic., *Justicia adhatoda.*

Vernacular Name: *San*: Vasa, *Hin:* Adusa; *Kan*: Adusoge; *Mal*: Adalodakam; *Eng*: Malabarnut, Vasaka; *Tam*: Adhatodai; *Tel:* Addasaramu.

Description: It is a small evergreen, subherbacious bush. The *leaves* are 10 to 16 cms in length, minutely pubescent and broadly lanceolate. The *inflorescence* is dense, short pedunculate, bractate and spike terminal. The *corolla* is large and white with lower lip streaked purple. The *corolla* is a 4-seeded small capsule.

Habitate: The plant grows all over the plains of India and in the lower Himalayan ranges, upto 1000m above sea-level. It is also found in Sri Lanka, Burma and Malaysia.

Propagation: By stem cutting.

Parts Used: Leaves, roots, flowers and stem bark.

Chemical Constituents: The leaves of the plant contain an essential oil and Alkaloids vasicine, N-oxides of vasicine, vasicinone, deoxyvasicine, and maiontone. The roots are known to contain vasicinolone, vasicol, peganine and 2'-glucosyl-oxychalcone. The flowers contain β-sitosterol-D-glucoside, kaempferol, its glycosides and quercetin.

Uses: Bronchitis and bronchial asthma. Local bleeding and thrombocytopenia. Pyorrhea. The leaf extract has been used for treatment of bronchitis and asthma for many centuries. It relieves cough and breathlessness. It is also prescribed commonly in Ayurveda for bleeding due to idiopathic thrombocytopenic purpura, local bleeding due to peptic ulcer, piles, menorrhagia etc. large doses of fresh juice of leaves have been used in tuberculosis. Its local use gives relief in pyorrhea and in bleeding gums.

39. *Adiantum capillus-veneries* L. (*Polypodiaceae*)

Vernacular Name: *Eng:* The Maidenhair Fern; *Guj*: Hanspadi; *Hin*: Hansraj, Mubaraka, Pursha; *Kan*: Hansraj.

Description: Fern with delicate founds growing to 30 cm long.

Habitate: Native to Europe and north America, maidenhair fern Europe and North America, maidenhair fern grows in moist, shady sites.

Propagation: By seeds and cutting.

Parts Used: Aerial parts.

Chemical Constituents: Maidenhair fern contains flavonoids terpenoids, tannins and mucilage. It contains volatile oil, bitter principle (capillerin), tanning material mucin, gallic acid, sugars and heterosides of kaempferol, quercetol and luteolol.

Uses: Maidenhair fern is still used by Western herbalists to treat coughs, bronchitis, catarrh, sore throat and chronic nasal catarrh. The plant also has a longstanding reputation as a remedy for conditions of the hair and scalp.

40. *Adonis vernalis* L. *(Ranunculaceae)*

Synonyms: *Adonis helleborus* Crantz., *Adonis parviflora* Janka ex. Nym.

Vernacular Name: *Eng:* False hellebore, Yellow pheasant's eye, Spring Adonis rose.

Description: A deciduous perennial herb, upto 50 cm. high. Stem simple or branched, longitudinally grooved, soft, branched mostly from near the base, densely foliaceous above; leaves sessile, 4-6 pinnately-divided into several linear and acute lobes/leaflets; flowers terminal, bright yellow; sepals 5, weak brown to weak olive; hairy, ovate, obtuse; petals 10 to 20, dentate bright yellow to moderately greenish yellow, concave, oblong, obtuse, slightly longer than the sepals; stamens indefinite; carpels, apocarpous, forming an ovoid, obtuse, dense head of ovoid achenes each tipped with a small persistent style. Taste bitter and slightly acrid.

Habitate: On mountains in Central and South-Eastern Europe.

Propagation: By seeds.

Parts Used: Whole plant.

Chemical Constituents: Adonidin, Cimarin and adonin-Glycosides, Adonidoside, Adonivernoside, Choline, Adonitol, Vernadin, Vernadigin, Adonidinic acid and Strophanthidin.

Uses: For complaints, especially heart after rheumatism or influenza or bright's disease, where muscles of the heart are in stage of fatty degeneration. Regulates the pulse. Increases the power of heart contraction with increased urinary secretion. Most valuable in cardiac dropsy. Mitral and aortic regurgitation. Chronic aortitis. Fatty heart pericarditis. Rheumatic endocarditis. Marked venous engorgement. Cardiac asthma. Hydrothorax, ascites, anasarca. Headache from occiput around temples to eyes. Gnawing hunger with faint feeling in epigastrium. Oily pellicle on urine.

41. *Aegle marmelos* L. Corr. *(Rutaceae)*

Vernacular Name: *Eng:* Bael tree, Holy fruit tree; *Hin*: Bel, Sirphal; *Kan:* Belapatri; *Mal:* Kuvvalam, Kulakam; *San:* Vilvah, Sivadrumah, Sriphalah; *Tam:* Kuvilam, Vilvam; *Tel:* Bilvamu, Maredu.

Description: A medium sized armed deciduous tree upto 8.0 m high with straight, sharp, axillary thorns and yellowish brown shallowly furrowed corky bark; leaves trifoliate, aromatic, alternate, leaflets ovate of ovate-lanceolate, crenate, pellucid-punctate, the laterals subsessile and the terminal long-pertioled; flowers greenish white, e, sweet scented, in axillary panicles; fruits globose, woody berry with yellowish ring; seeds numerous oblong, compressed, embedded in orange brown sweet gummy pulp.

Habitate: Throughout India, in dry forests, also cultivated.

Propagation: By seeds and air-layering.

Part Used: Roots, leaves, fruits.

Chemical Constituents: Fruit contains marmalosin, young bark contains coumarin, and umbelliferone; old bark has umbelliferone and coumarin. Leaves are having essential oil, consisting of α and β-phellandrene. Matured bark contains fragrine, umbelliferone marmesin, sterols and triterpenoids. The leaves contain 0.6% essential oil mostly compound of d-limonene.

Uses: The roots are sweet, astringent, bitter and febrifuge. They are useful in diarrhoea, dysentery, dyspepsia, stomachalgia, cardiopalmus, vitiated conditions of *vata*, seminal weakness, uropathy, vomiting, intermittent fever, swellings and gastric irritability in infants. The leaves are astringent, laxative, febrifuge and expectorant, and are useful in ophthalmia, deafness, inflammations, catarrh, diabetes and asthmatic complaints. The unrips fruits are bitter, acrid, sour, astringent, digestive and stomachic, and are useful in diarrhoea, dysentery and stomachalgia. The ripe fruits are astringent, sweet, aromatic, cooling, febrifuge, laxative and tonic, and are good for the heart and brain and in dyspepsia.

42. *Aerva lanata* L. Juss. ex Schultes *(Amaranthaceae)*

Vernacular Name: *Hin*: Chaya, Gorakhganja; *Kan:* Bilihindisoppu; *Mal:* Cerula, Ceruvula, Cerupula; *San:* Bhadra, Astmabayda; *Tam*: Cerupulai, Sirupoolia; *Tel:* Pindicettu, Pindiconda.

Description: A much-branched herb, with the base hard as wood and the branches erect or creeping to the ground. Leaves alternate, wooly-tomentose, 1.3-2.5 cm long. Flower greenish-white, minute, borne in axillary panicles. Fruits greenish, roundish, compressed utricle; seeds kidney shaped with shining black.

Habitate: Throughout India, in waste lands.

Propagation: By seeds.

Part Used: Whole plant.

Chemical Constituents: α-Amyrin, campesterol, β-sitosterol and β-sitosteryl palmitate, chrysin and four flavonoid glycosides have been reported in the plant.

Uses: The plant is astringent, bitter, cooling emollient, vermifuge, suppurative, diuretic and lithontriptic. It is useful to treat boils, cephalalgia, cough, strangury, diabetes and lithiasis. Useful in catanh of bladder, tonic; flowers used for removal of kidney stone.

43. *Aesculus hippocastanum* *(Hippocastanaceae)*

Vernacular Name: *Eng:* Horese Chestnut.

Description: Stout deciduous tree growing to 25m, with a large domed crown. Has leaves with 5-7 narrowly oval leaflets, clusters of white and pink flowers, and spiny green fruit with up to 3 rounded, shiny brown seeds about 4 cm across.

Habitate: Native to mountain woods in the Balkans and western Asia, this tree is cultivated in temperate regions worldwide.

Propagation: By Seeds.

Parts Used: Seeds, leaves, bark.

Chemical Constituents: Horse chestnut contains triterpenoid saponins, coumarins and flavonoids. Aescin, the main active constituent, has anti-inflammatory properties. in Germany and other European countries, specialized aescin preparations are used because aescin is not easily absorbed from the gut.

Uses: Horse chestnut is astringent, anti-inflammatory and helps to tone the vein walls, which, when slack or distended, may become varicose, haemorrhoidal or otherwise proplematic. Horse chestnut also reduces fluid retention by increasing the permeability of the capillaries and allowing the reabsorption of excess fluid back into the circulatory system. The herb has been taken internally in small to moderate doses for leg ulcers, varicose veins, haemorrhoids and frostbite, and applied externally as a lotion, ointment or gel. An oil extracted from the seeds has been used as an external treatment for rheumatism. A decoction of the leaves has been given in cases of whooping cough.

44. *Aesculus indica.* Hook (*Hippocastanaceae)*

Vernacular Name: *Hin:* Bankhor, kandar, kanor, pangar; *Kash*: han, hane, hanudun; *Pun*: Bankhor, gu, gun, hazara, khanor.

Description: A large, deciduous tree, with a short, straight, cylindrical bole and spreading crown, 30 m in height bark grey when old, exfoliating upwards, in long and thin bands; leaves digitate: leaflets 5-9, oblanceolate or oblong; flowers white tinged with red and yellow in large thyrsoid panicles; capsules ovoid, rough outside, 5 cm long, leathery; seeds 2-3, dark brown, smooth, shining.

Habitate: Found in Himalayas upto 900 to 3,600m.

Propagation: By seeds.

Part Used: Seeds.

Chemical Constituents: The seeds contain a mixture of saponiins, one of which is described as aescine, which easily crystallizes. Also contains flavonoid glycosides, aesculine, albumin and fatty oils.

Uses: Aesculing is used medically and extracts from the seeds are used industrially. As medicine, it is especially used for the complaints of the veins, such as phlebitis, haemorrhoids, vari-cose veins; in ulcers; to prevent thrombosis; in some cases of migraine, effusions of blood; for limb complaints and forst bite. Fruits are given to horses in colic. Oil from the seeds is externally applied in rheumatism. The hydrosycoumarin glycoside aesculin from the bark of the branch absorbs ultra-violet rays and is an ingredient for suntan oil.

45. *Aethusa cynapium* L. (*Apiaceae)*

Synonyms: *Aethusa toxicaria* Salisb., *Aethusa cynica* Dulac., *Aethusa cicuta* Neck.

Vernacular Name: *Eng:* Fool's parsley.

Description: An annual poisonous herb upto 60 cm. high, nauseous smelling when rubbed, loathsome in taste, with roots spindle shaped, whitish. Stem erect with flat grooves or angular ribs, hollow and sometimes violet striped, often branching zigzag; leaves shining, dark green in colour, but light coloured on the under-surface and twice or thrice pinnatified. Inflorescence umbel, without involucre at the base but with three leaved pendulous bracts below each umblet which distinguishes this plant from the garden parsley. Flowers white, small on slender pedicels, the outer ones slightly radiant. Calyx absent. Petals obcordate, with a deep notch and a short incurved tongue, white. Disk board, flat; styles short reflexed; fruit small, about 3.3 mm. or little more in length, and about the same in width, nearly orbicular, smooth, pale greenish grey.

Habitate: Europe, New England to Pennsylvania.

Propagation: By seeds.

Parts Used: Whole plant.

Chemical Constituents: Cynapine, Cynapium, Essential oils; Polyine, Aethusin, Aethusanol A & B.

Uses: Colic. Cramps. Diarrhoea. Dysuria. Stomachache. Complaints especially of children during dentition in hot summer weather, children who cannot digest milk in any form, having great intolerance for milk with great weakness, cannot hold up the head. Milk is vomited out in large curds as soon as taken. Indigestion in teething children with violent sudden vomiting of frothy milky white substance followed by curdled milk and cheesy red face, eyes turned downwards, pupils fixed and dilated, with foam at mouth and jaws locked. Photophobia, swelling of Meibomian glands. Rolling of eyes on falling asleep. Herpetic eruption on tip of nose. Frequent ineffectual desire to sneeze. Undigested thin, greenish stool preceded by colic, tenesmus and exhaustion. Surface of body cold and covered with clammy sweat. Pimples in girls. Lymphatic glands swollen. Itching eruption around joints.

46. *Aframomum melegueta* Rosc. *(Zingiberaceae)*

Synonyms: *Amomum melegueta* Rosc.

Vernacular Name: *Eng:* Grains of paradise, Alligator Pepper, Meleguetta Pepper.

Description: Perennial growing to 2.5m with reed-like stems and narrow leaves. Single mauve flowers bear scarlet fruits growing to 10 cm across. Seeds are small, reddish-brown and oyster-shaped with a distinctly pungent, aromatic, taste.

Habitate: This plant grows in tropical West Africa and is gathered when ripe.

Propagation: By seeds.

Parts Used: Seeds.

Chemical Constituents: The seeds contain a volatile oil, a pungent principle called paradol and tannins.

Uses: Principally used as a condiment, the seeds also are a stimulant that strengthens and warms the stomach. Like other members of the ginger family, this plant is used to alleviate.indigestion, flatulence and bloating. Grains of paradise also help to ease abdominal discomfort due to colic or griping. The seeds can help to reduce or prevent vomiting and to bring relief from nausea. The plant's stimulant properties make it an invigorating herb, especially helpful for those with weak digestions.

47. *Agastache rugosa* (Fisch. Et Mey.) O. Kuntze *(Lameaceae)*

Vernacular Name: *Eng:* Wrinkle gaint hyssop.

Description: An annual or perennial fragrant herb, 30-120 cm high. Stem tetragonal. Leaves opposite, petiole 1-4 cm long. Blade ovate or elliptic-ovate, 2.8 cm long by 1-5 cm wide; tip acute or acuminate; base rounded or nearly cordate; margin obtusely dentate, usually with many oil-glands on upper surface, pubescent underneath. Inflorescence a dense, terminal spike, cylindrical, 7-10 cm long. Flowers purple, calyx campanulate, teeth 5, irregular. Corolla tubes as long as the calyx; limp bilabiate, the superior lip erect, bilobate, the inferior lip expanded, 3-lobed, the median lip broader and crenulate. Stamens 4, didymous, the superior pair declines; style bifed. Nutlets smooth. The taste of the leaves is sweet, the odour highly aromatic.

Habitate: On slopes or roadsides but mostly cultivated in gardens.

Propagation: By seeds.

Part Used: Leaves and stems.

Chemical Constituents: N.A.

Uses: Fever due to heat strokes; headache, distenstion of chest, poor appetite, Nausea. As an emetic, diarrhoea, Tinea on hands and feet.

48. *Agave americana* (*Agavaceae*)

Vernacular Name: *Eng:* Agave, Century plant; *Hin*: Banskeora, bara kanwar, kantala; *Kan*: Kalanaru; *San*: Kalakantala, Kantala; *Mal*: Panam-kattazha; *Tam*: Aanaikathaali; *Tel:* Kithanara, rakashima talu.

Description: Succulent perennial with large rosette of 30-60 fleshy, sharply toothed leaves that reach a height of 2m. Clusters of yellow flowers, growing to 7 cm across, bloom on a pole-like stem after 10 years or more.

Habitate: Agave is native to deserts of Central America. It is now grown as an ornamental plant in tropical and sub-tropical areas around the world.

Propagation: By vegetative methods.

Parts Used: Sap/Juice.

Chemical Constituents: Agave sap contains oestrogen-like isoflavonoids, alkloids, coumarins, vitamins pro-A, B^1, B^2, C, and also contains hecogenin, chlorogenin, rockogenin, figogenin and dehydrohecogenin.

Uses: Demulcent, laxative and antiseptic, agave sap is a soothing and restorative remedy for many digestive ailments. It is used to treat ulcers and inflammatory conditions affecting the stomach and intestines, protecting these parts from infection and irritation and encouraging healing. Agave has also been employed to treat a wide range of other conditions, including syphilis, tuberculosis, jaundice and liver disease.

49. *Ageratum conyzoides* L. (*Asteraceae*)

Vernacular Name: *Eng:* Goat weed, White weed, appa grass, conyzoid floss-flowers, bastard agrimony; *Beng*: Dochunty, uchunti; *Mal:* Appa, muryampacha; *Tam:* Pumpillu, sinnapoompillu; *Kan:* Uralgidda.

Description: Annual herb, 30-50cm. high. Stem erect hairy green or purple. Leaves opposite, broadly ovate, crenate, coarsely hairy on both sides, 3-nerved at the base. The inflorescence is a terminal corymb of many small heads; flowers violet or white. Achene minute, black 5-echinate.

Habitate: Common weed everywhere.

Propagation: By seeds.

Part Used: Whole plant.

Chemical Constituents: The plant yields 0.7-2% essential oil consisting of agratochromene, dimethoxy-ageratochromene, cadinene and caryophyllene; it also contains alkaloids and saponins.

Uses: The whole plant possesses anti-inflammatory and antiallergic properties. The juice from the fresh plant and the extract of the dried plant are used for the cure of allergic rhinitis and sinusitis, in aqueous solution for nasal instillation. The juice of the fresh plant is also useful in post-partum uterine haemorrhage. A hair-wash consisting of a decoction of the fresh plant makes the hair fragrant, soft and dandruff-free, prevents tetanus.

50. *Agrimonia eupatoria* L. (*Rosaceae*)

Synonyms*:* *Agrimonia pilosa.*

Vernacular Name: *Eng:* Agrimony, Stickle wort.

Description: Erect, downy and slightly aromatic perennial growing to 1m. Has paired leaves, green above and silvery-green beneath, and small 5-petalled yellow flowers growing on terminal spikes.

Habitate: Agrimony is a native European herb commonly found in marshes, wet meadows and on wasteground.

Propagation: By Seeds.

Parts Used: Aerial parts.

Chemical Constituents: Agrimony contains tannins, coumarins, flavonoids, including luterolin, a volatile oil and polysaccharides.

Uses: Agrimony has long been used by herbalists to heal wounds because it staunches bleeding and encourages clot formation. An astringent and mild bitter, it is a valuable remedy for cystitis and urinary incontinence, and has also been used for kidney stones, sore throats, hoarseness, rheumatism and arthritis.

51. *Agrimonia pilosa* Ledeb. *(Rosaceae)*

Vernacular Name: *Eng:*-Hairy agrimony.

Description: Hirsute perennial herb with erect stem, 30-100 cm tall. Leaves alternate, odd-pinnate, 5-7 foliolate; leaflets cuneate at base, pubescent beneath on veins only, gradually smaller in the lower ones, alternate with much smaller ones; the large leaflets obong, elliptic or obovate, coarsely dendate, hairy on both sides, 3-6 cm long, 1.5-3.5 cm wide. Inflorescence elkongated raceme at terminal. 10-20 cm long. Flowers small, pale yellow, short-pedicellate, small bracts leaflike; calyx persistent, calyx tube, deeply grooved, 5-toothed, with spines around edge, to 5 mm in diameter; petals 5, narrowly obovate, rounded at tip: stamens 5-10, carpels 2. Fruit a bristly burr, bristles incurved connivent apically.

Habitate: Roadsides, grassy areas in lowlands and mountains found in Korea, Japan, China, Siberia, Eastern Europe and North-East India.

Propagation: By seeds.

Parts Used: Herb.

Chemical Constituents: Agrimonolides, tannins, phenylpropanoids, coumarins, flavonoids, triterpenes.

Uses: Antitumour, bacteriostatic, immunostimulating, antidysentery action, antiyeast. Used in taenia, boils, eczema.

52. *Agropyron repens* Beauv. *(Poaceae)*

Synonyms: *Elymus repens.*

Vernacular Name: *Eng:* Couch grass, Dog graxss.

Description: Vigorous perennial growing to 80 cm. Has a long, creeping rhizome, slender leaves and erect spikes bearing green flowers aligned in two rows.

Habitate: Found in Europe, the couch grass is an invasive weed.

Propagation: By Seeds and Rhizome.

Parts Used: Rhizome, Seeds and Root.

Chemical Constituents: Couch grass, contains polysaccharides, a volatile oil, mucilage and mutrients. Agropyrene has antibiotic properties.

Uses: A gentle, effective diuretic and demulcent, couch grass is most commonly used for urinary tract infections such as cystitis and urethritis. It both protects the urinary tubules against infection and irritants, and increases the volume of urine, thereby diluting it. Couch grass seeds are used in a hot and moist pack that is applied to the abdomen for peptic ulcers, juice form the roots of couch grass has been advocated from treating jaundice and other liver complaints.

53. *Ailanthus altissima* Swingle. *(Simaroubaceae)*

Synonyms: *Ailanthus glandalosa* Desf.

Vernacular Name: *Eng:*-Tree-of-heaven, copal tree, varnish tree.

Description: Deciduous, polygamodioecious, rapidly growing tree, to 20 m or more. Leaves alternate, odd-pinnate, mostly 60-80 cm long; leaflets 13-25, 8-10 cm long, oblong to lanceolate or ovate, divided unequally by the midrib, entire except for 1-3 pairs of large gland-bearing or callus teeth at the base, glabrous beneath, ill-scented when bruised. Flowers small, 7-8 mm in diameter, greenish, in terminal panicles, 5-6 merous; petals woolly tomentose inside; stamens 10-12, but 5-6 in bisexual flowers; female flowers with deeply 2-5 parted ovary, style 1, stigmas 5-6, plumose. Fruit a 2-winged samara, 3.5-5 cm long, twisted, reddish-orange at maturity.

Habitate: Widespread urban weed, sometimes cultivated found in China, Korea and North-East India.

Propagation: By seeds.

Parts Used: Bark.

Chemical Constituents: Quercetin-3-glucoside, canthin-6-one and its derivatives, ailanthone, many other quassinoids, tannins, triterpene, saponins.

Uses: Antimalarial, amoebicidal. Used in granulating eruptions, naemorrhoids, mastitis.

54. Ajuga bracteosa Wall. ex Benth. *(Lameaceae)*

Vernacular Name: *San:* Nilkanthi and *Punj*: Khurbanti.

Description: A perennial, erect or ascending hairy herb, often prostrate, with oblanceolate or sub-spathulate, obtuse, sinuate toothed leaves; purplish violet tinged from lower surface. Flowers are purplish-violet, tinged from lower surface in distant, axillary whorls in a spike.

Habitate: Found as a weed in field borders, along roadsides, open slopes and even on rock crevice upto 1500 m.

Propagation: By seeds.

Part Used: Whole plant.

Chemical Constituents: Contains glycoside and tannin. Also yields ceryl alcohol β-sitosterol, Y-sitosterol, cerotic and palmitic acids alongwith a glucosidic constitutuent.

Uses: The aromatic leaves are regarded as stimulant, diuretic, tonic and apparient. It is said to be a bitter astringent given in the treatment of fervers and also used as febrifuge. As an aromatic tonic, it is useful in ague. Also used to kill lice, regarded as depurative and useful in cases of malarial fever as a substitute for cinchona. The herb is also used in gout, rheumatism, palsy and amenorrhoea. Ethyl alcohol extract has been found to have anticancer activity.

55. *Ajuga reptans* *(Lameaceae)*

Vernacular Name: *Eng:* Bugle.

Description: Low-growing, creeping perennial up to 30 cm in height. Has rooting runners, erect hairy stems, oblong to oval leaves and purplish-blue flowers.

Habitate: Native to Europe, North Africa and parts of Asia, bugle has become naturalized in North America. It prefers damp woods and grassy and mountainous areas, and is usually gathered when in flower in early summer.

Propagation: By Seeds.

Parts Used: Aerial part.

Chemical Constituents: Bugle contains iridoid glycosides, including harpagide, which is also found in devil's claw.

Uses: Bugle is bitter, astringent and aromatic, but opinion varies as to its value as a medicine. It has mild analgesic properties, and it is still used occasionally as a wound healer. It is also mildly laxative and traditionally has been thought to help cleanse the liver.

56. *Akebia quinata* Decne. *(Lardizabalaceae)*

Vernacular Name: *Eng:*-Five-leaf akebia, chocolate vine.

Description: Monoecious, woody, glabrous climber to 5 m tall. Leaves half-evergreen, alternate, palmately compound; leaflets 5, oblong, 3-5 cm long, 1-2 cm wide, entire, stalked, cuniate at the base, emarginated at the tip. Flowers purplish, in axillary racemes, fragrant, sepals 3; male flowers towards apex of the raceme, 12-16 mm across, the pedicels slender, sepals 7-8 mm long, stamens 6; female flowers below, much larger, 2-3 cm across, long-pedicellate, sepals broadly elliptic, 15-20 mm long. Fruit an ovoid-oblong, bluish or purple berry, 6-10 cm long, 2.5-3 cm in diameter, dehiscent along 1 side, seeds many, black.

Habitate: Thickets in hills and mountains found in Korea, Japan, and China.

Propagation: By seeds.

Parts Used: Stem, fruit.

Chemical Constituents: Many saponins of hederagenin and oleanolic acid glycosides. Flavonoids.

Uses: Diuretic, anti-inflammatory, lowers serum cholesterol level, antiulcer, antioxidant. Used in oedema, nephritis, dysuria, neuralgia.

57. *Alangium salviifolium* (Linn. f.) Wang. *(Alangiaceae)*

Synonyms: *Alangium lamarchii* Thw; *Grewia salvifolia* Linn.f.

Vernacular Name: *Eng:* Sage-leaved alangium; *Hin*: Angol, Dhera, Dhela; *Kan:* Ankolamara; *Mal:* Ankolam, Velittondi, Alinnil; *San:* Ankolah, Ankodah; *Tam*: Alangi and *Tel:* Ankolamu, Uduguceттu.

Description: A small deciduous tree or shrub, armed or not; leaves alternate, usually unequal at the base; flowers white or yellowish-white, fragrant, in axillary fascicles; fruits 1-2 seeded berries crowned by the calyx lobes, yellowish or red when ripe.

Habitate: In the forests of south India.

Propagation: By seeds.

Part Used: Roots & fruits.

Chemical Constituents: The rootbark contains the following alkaloids: alangine A and B, alangicine, desmethylpsychotrine, marckine, marckindine, lamarckinine, psychotrine, tubulosine, isotubulosine, cephaeline and emetine. The presence of protoemetinal and alangiosterol. The rootbark also contains fatty acid composition: myristic, palmitic, oleic, linoleic, and resin acid. The unsaponifiable matter contains stigmasterol and β-sitosterol. The fruit contains the alkaloids cephaeline, N-methylcephaeline, deoxytubulosine and alangiside. The seeds contain the alkaloids emetine, cephaeline, psychotrine, N-methylcephaeline and alangmide. Betulinic acid, betulinaldehyde, betulin, lupeol along with hydroxylactone-A of betulinic acid, and β-sitosterol have been isolated from the seed kernels.

Uses: The roots are acrid, astringent, emollient, anthelmintic, thermogenic, diuretic and purgative. Root bark is an antidote for several poisons. The roots are useful for external application in acute case of reumatism, leprosy and inflammation and for external and internal application in case of bites of rabid dogs. Fruits are sweet, cooling and purgative, and are useful in treating burning sensation and heamorrhages.

58. *Albizia julibrissin* Durazz *(Lamiaceae)*

Vernacular Name: *Eng:* Silk tree; pink siris.

Description: A large deciduous tree, 6-16 m high, bark dark grey, nearly smooth, young shoots and inflorescence clothed with yellowish-brown pubescence. Leaves bipinnate, stipules 7.5 mm long, linear, caduceus. Pinnae 4-16 pairs, 7.5-15 cm long; leaflets 10-30 pairs, 1.3-1.8 cm long by 0.4-0.6 cm wide, falcate-oblong, acute, oblique, dark-green on top, pale-green underneath, more or less aidpressed, hairy on both sides, midrib close to the upper edge, subsessile. Flowers reddish in peduncled heads, solitary or in fascicles of 2-3 arranged in a short terminal raceme, the lowest often axillary; peduncles 3.8-7.5 cm long; bracts 4-7.5 mm long linear, caduceus; peduncles 3.8-7.5 cm long; bracts 4-7.5 mm longl linear, caduceus; pedicles 1.25 mm long. Pod 9.5 cm by 1.5-2.5 cm thin, pubescent till mature, pale-brown or yellowish, with thickened sutures. Seeds 8-12.

Habitate: On waste ground and roadsides but mostly cultivated, China, Japan, Korea, Laos, North America, Soviet Union, Viet Nam.

Propagation: By seeds.

Part Used: Bark, flowers or floral buds.

Chemical Constituents: N.A.

Uses: Anxiety and insomnia, pulmonary abscess, expectoration, Trauma, flowers or floral buds; neurasthenia, insomnia, amnesia, feeling of construction in chest.

59. *Albizia lebbeck* Benth. *(Mimosaceae)*

Vernacular Name: *Eng:* Siris tree; *Hin*: Siris, Siris; *Kan:* Begemara; *Mal:* Nenmenivaka, Vaka; *San:* Sirisah, Bhandi; *Tam*: Vakai, Siridam; *Tel:* Dirisana.

Description: A medium to large sized unarmed deciduous tree about 20 m in height with an umbrella-shapedcrown and grey to dark brown rough irregularly cracked bark; leaves abruptly bipinnate, main rachis with a large gland above the base and one below the upper-most pair of pinnae, pinnae 2-4 pairs, leaflets 5-9 airs with glands between their bases, the lateral ones elliptic-oblong, the two terminal ovate-oblong, all unequal sided; flowers white, fragrant, in globose umbellate heads; fruits long, characteristic pods, bluntly pointed, tin, pale yellow, smooth, shiny, reticulately veined above the seed; seeds 4-12, pale brown, ellipsid, oblong, compressed.

Habitate: Throughout India, also cultivated.

Propagation: By seeds.

Part Used: Bark, flowers, seeds.

Chemical Constituents: The bark yields tannins of condensed type, viz. D-catechin, isomers of leucocyanidin and melacacidin and a new leucoantho-cyanidin, lebbecacidin. It also gives friedelin and β-sitosterol. Seeds gave crude protein, calcium, phosphorus, iron, niacin, and ascorbic acid, amino acid composition of the protein is: arginine, histidine, leucine & isoleucine lysine, methionine, phenylalanine, threonine, tyrosine, and valine. The flowers contain lupeol, α-and β-amyrin and a pigment similar to crocetin.

Uses: The bark is astringent, bitter, acrid, sweet, mildly thermogenic, expectorant, aphrodisiac, anti-inflammatory, anodyne, cephalic, ophthalmic, depurative, restorative and tonic. It is useful in vitiated conditions of *pitta* and *kapha*, cough and catarrh, asthma, enlarged cervical glands, ophthalmopathy, nyctalopia, strengthening gums, scrofula, skin eruptions, leprosy, leucoderma, sprains, wounds, ulcers, neuralgia, inflammations, erysipelas, diarrhoea and all types of poisning. It is also used as a dentifrice in odontopathy. The flowers are useful in chornic cough and bronchitis. The seeds are useful in inflammations. Scrofula, skin diseases, leprosy, leucoderma, chronic catarrh, seminal weakness, ophthalmopathy and poisoning.

60. *Albizia odoratissima* Benth. *(Mimosaceae)*

Vernacular Name: *Eng:* Black siris, Kala Siris; *Hin:* Kala siris; *Kan:* Bilvara; *Mal:* Pulivaka, Nellivaka, Karivaka, Kunnivaka; *San:* Bhusirisah; *Tam:* Karuvakai, Sittilavakai; *Tel:* cinduga, Sirisi, Telsu.

Description: A medium sized unarmed tree about 20 m in height with dark coloured young shoots and grey, rough, irregularly cracked bark with dark patches; leaved abruptly pinnate, alternate, main rachis with a gland on the upper side near its basal part and often with similar glands at the bases of the first two pairs of pinnae, leaflets unequal sided, rounded, or semicordate at base, obtuse or rounded at the apex, dark green, slightly pubescent above; flowers white, fragrant, sessile, numerous, in small globose 5-10 or more flowered heads, in corymbiform spreading panicles; fruits shortly stalked pods, brown, slightly reticulately veined; seeds flat yellow.

Habitate: Throughout India, upto an elevation of 1,500 m.

Propagation: By seeds.

Part Used: Bark.

Chemical Constituents: The bark yields tannins of condensed type, viz. D-catechin, isomers of leucocyanidin and melacacidin and a new leucoantho-cyanidin, lebbecacidin. It also gives friedelin and β-sitosterol. Seeds gave crude protein, calcium, phosphorus, iron, niacin, and ascorbic acid, amino acid composition of the protein is: arginine, histidine, leucine & isoleucine lysine, methionine, phenylalanine, threonine, tyrosine, and valine. The flowers contain lupeol, α-and β-amyrin and a pigment similar to crocetin.

Uses: The bark is astringent, acrid, cooling, depurative and expectorant, and is useful in ulcers, leprosy, skin diseases, erysipelas, cough, bronchitis, diabetes and burning sensation.

61. *Alchemilla vulgaris* *(Rosaceae)*

Vernacular Name: *Eng:* Lady's Mantle.

Description: Herbaceous perennial growing to 30cm. Has a basal rosette of lobed leaves and insignificant green flowers 3-5 mm across in loose clusters.

Habitate: Lady's mantle is native to Britain and continental Europe. It is gathered in summer.

Propagation: By Seeds.

Parts Used: Root.

Chemical Constituents: Lady's mantle contains tannins, a glycoside and salicylic acid.

Uses: Lady's mantle has always been prized as a wound healer. Its astringency ensures that blood flow is staunched and the first stage of healing soon gets under way. It has been used to facilitate childbirth, and is thought to act as a liver decongestant. It s astringent properties make it a useful herb for the treatment of diarrhoea and gastroenteritis.

62. *Aletris farinosa* *(Liliaceae)*

Vernacular Name: *Eng:* Star Grass, Ture unicorn root, Colic root.

Description: Perennial growing to 1m. Has a flowering stem, smooth lance-shaped leaves and white bell-shaped flowers that appear to be covered with forest.

Habitate: Native to eastern North America, star grass grows mainly in swamps and wet Sandy woodland, especially near the seashore. It is harvested commercially in Virginia, Tennessee and North Carolina.

Propagation: By Seeds.

Parts Used: Rhizome, leaves.

Chemical Constituents: Star grass contains steroidl saponins based on diosgenin, as well as a bitter principle, volatile oil an a resin.

Uses: Star grass is also a good digestive herb, proving beneficial in treating loss of appetite, indigestion, flatulence and bloating.

63. *Aleurites moluccana* L. Willd. *(Euphorbiaceae)*

Vernacular Name: *Eng:* candlenut tree.

Description: Tree to 25m high with soft wood. Leaves alternate petiolate, grey-green, ovate to palmately-lobed, up to 25cm. Long. Flowers unisexual, small 5-parted, white and borne in a dense terminal. Fruit a moderately-sized globose, green dry drupe upto 5cm long with rough mescarp and containing a single seed with a nut-like shell.

Habitate: Common in low land secondary and disturbed primary moist forests.

Propagation: By seeds and vegetative method.

Part Used: Seeds, leaves and bark.

Chemical Constituents: Moluccanin, moretenone, moretenol, alpha-amyrin, beta-sitosterol, alkaloids(fruits), lipids, proteins (seeds).

Uses: The seeds are applied externally to the male genitals as a contraceptive. The leaves are used to treat constipation and food poisoning. The bark is used to treat woonds. Leaves toxic, antitumour, cytotoxic, antiviral. Infertility in women is treated by daily dringking a decoction of the bark. The plant is used to treat pain in the bones and weakness after childbirth. A decoction of the leaves is used in treating coughs, diarrhoea, pains in the chest and hernia.

64. *Alisma orientalis* (Sam.) Juzep. *(Alismataceae)*

Vernacular Name: *Eng:* Oriental water-plantain.

Description: A perennial marsh herb 50-100 cm high. Corms up to 6 cm in diameter. Brownish, with many fibrous roots. Leaves all basal, ovoid-elliptic, 5-18 cm long by 2-10 cm wide, acuminate at apex, cuneate or slightly cordate at base, entire at margin, glabrous on both surfaces; longitudinal veins 5-7, petiole up to 54 cm long, sheath-like at base, June-August inflorescence in verticillate divisio, large, paniculate, bracteal. Flowers white, small. Sepals 3 petals 3, obovate, shorter than the sepals. Stamens 6. Carpels numerous, laterally compressed. Achenes abovate, compressed laterally.

Habitate: In fields, swamps and damp soil, China, India, Japan, Mongolia and Saviet Union.

Propagation: By seeds.

Part Used: Corms.

Chemical Constituents: N.A.

Uses: Nephritic oedema; pyelitis, dysuria, enteritis, diarrhoea.

65. *Alisma plantago-aquatica* L. *(Alismataceae)*

Synonyms: *Alisma plantago* L.

Vernacular Name: *Eng:* Common water plantain, mad-dog weed.

Description: Marsh herb, 40-50cm. high. Rhizome stout, globular. Leaves entire, long-petioled, forming a rosette; nerves curved. Inflorescence in terminal umbelliform cyme; scape long, flowers white, cylindrical. **Fruit:** an akene.

Habitate: Wild and cultivated species in rice-swamps and ponds.

Propagation: By seeds.

Part Used: Rhizomes.

Chemical Constituents: The rhizomes contain an essential oil consisting of alisol A, B, C and epialisol A: D-glucose, D-fructose, sucrose; β-sitosterol, lecithin, choline, resin, protein and starch.

Uses: The rhizome is diuretic and used in treating oedema, nepritis, dysuria, haematuria, pollakiuria, urodynia, urinary lithiasis, flatulence, vomiting and diarrhoea. It is likewise prescribed as an antidiabetic and as a galactagogue in hypogalactia.

66. *Allium ascalonicum* L. *(Liliaceae)*

Vernacular Name: *Hin:* Gandana and *Beng*: Gundhun.

Description: A hardy bulbous perennial native to Ascalon. It has been in cultivation from the remotest time in all the countries for the East. It is also cultivated in India. Bulbs about the size of a nut, white, leaves basal; flowers greenish white or purplish white in many-flowered, globose heads on a fistular scape.

Habitate: Naturalized throughout India.

Propagation: By bulbs.

Part Used: Bulbs.

Chemical Constituents: The major volatile constituents identified in the oil are methyl propyl trisulfide, dimethyl trisulfide, 1-methylthiopropyl ethyl disulfide, dipropyl trisulfide, propyl-trans-propenyl trisulfide, methyl-trans-propenyl disulfide, methyl propenyl trisulfide, propyl-cis-propenyl trirans-propenyl disulfide, methyl propenyl trisulfide, propyl-cis-propenyl trisulfide, propyl-trans-propenyl disulfide, dipropyl disulfide, methyl propyl trisulfide, propyl-trans-propenyl disulfide, dipropyl disulfide, methyl propyl disulfide, 2-n-hexyl-5-methyl-2, 3 dhhdrofuran-3-one, methyl-cis-propenyl disulfide, propyl-cis-propenyl disulfide, dimethyl disulfide, 3,4-propenyl disulfide, propyl-cis-propenyl disulfide, dimethyl disulfide, 3,4-dimethyl thiopeehen and 2-n-octyl-5-methyl-2-3-dhydrofuran-3-one.

Uses: The vlavour is similar to but milder than garlic and more delicate than onion. The bulbs are used for seasoning after deep-frying. There also pickled.

67. *Allium cepa* L. *(Liliaceae)*

Vernacular Name: *Eng:* Onion; *Hin*: Pyaj; *Kan:* Nirulli; *Mal:* Cuvannulli, Ceriya ulli; *San:* Palanduh, Raktakanda; *Tam*: Venkayam, Trulli; *Tel:* Ullipaya, Ulligadda, Erragadda.

Description: A biennial or perennial herb with aromatic fleshy underground bulb; leaves linear, hollow, cylindric and fleshy; flowers many white in globular umbels, spathe composed of 2-3 reflexed walls. The underground bulbs which are medicinally used very in size colour, shap, firmness, strength of flavour and keeping quality.

Habitate: Cultivated throughout India.

Propagation: By seeds.

Part Used: Bulbs.

Chemical Constituents: It contains essential amino acid compostion of arginine, histidine, lysine, tryptophan, phenylalanine, methionine, threonine, leucine, isoleucine. The bulbs on steam distillation yield an essential oil known as ONION OIL. The bulbs contain several phenolic acids, viz. protocatechuic acid, *p*-hydroxybenzoic acid, vanillic acid, caffeic acid, and o-and p-coumaric acids. Citric, mialic, abietic and oxalic acids are also present. It also conatins several oligosaccharides.

Uses: The bulbs are acrid, sweet, aromatic, thermogenic, antiperiodic, antibacterial, aphrodisiac, emmenagogue, emollient, expectorant, carminative, stomachic, diuretic, anodyne and tonic. They are useful in haemorrhoids, dysentery, flatulence, dyspepsia, colic, jaundice, splenopathy, hepatopathy, pneumonopathy, asthma, bronchitis, ophthalmia, vomiting, otalgia, pharyngodynia, malarial fever, lumbago, epilepsy, tumours, wounds paralysis, arthralgia, leucoderma and skin diseases.

68. *Allium fistulosum* L. *(Liliaceae)*

Vernacular Name: *Eng:* Japanese leek, Welsh onion, cibol, stone leek.

Description: Glabrous bulbous herb, 20-40cm. high, possessing a strong pungent aromatic odour. Leaves cylindrical, hollow, linear, oblong-acuminate at the apex. Inflorescence on the top of a long stalk in umbel forming a large globular head; flowers small, white. Capsule with numerous seeds, minute, trigonal, black.

Habitate: Extensively cultivated as a culinary herb throughout the country.

Propagation: By seeds and bulbs.

Part Used: Bulbs.

Chemical Constituents: The bulb contain essential oil. The constituents of the crude oil are allyl propyl disulfide, diallyl disulfide and sulfur compounds.

Uses: The whole plants, especially the bulbs, possess neurostimulant, stomachic and antibacterial properties. They are effective in the treatment of coryza, influenza, headache, fever, dyspepsia, intestinal infections, rheumatism, toothache, furunculosis and dysuria. A poultice of pounded fresh bulbs is effective in treating furunulosis, especially axillary and inguinal boils. Inhalation of the vapour from a boiling decoction is active on coryza, influenza and fever.

69. *Allium odorum* L. *(Liliaceae)*

Vernacular Name: *Eng:* Sweet leek, fragrant-flowered garlic, Chinese chives.

Description: Bulbous herb, 15-35cm. high, tufty. Leaves linear, flat, acuminate. Flowers white, in umbel on the top of a trigonal stalk, arising from the bulb. Capsule with black seeds. All parts of the herb are acrid-flavoured.

Habitate: Cultivated as a culinary and medicinal plant.

Propagation: By seeds and bulbs.

Part Used: Bulbs, leaves and seeds.

Chemical Constituents: The leaves and bulbs contain sulfur compounds, saponins and bitter substances. The seeds yield saponins and alkaloids.

Uses: The leaves and the bulbs possess antibacterial properties. They are useful for the treatment of haemoptysis, epistaxis, cough, sore throat, asthma, haematometra, dyspepsia, dysentery and oxyuriasis. They are also used in an anti-inflammatory poultice. The seeds are active on spermatorrhoea, haematuria, incontinence, lumbago, arthrodynia and metrorrhoea.

70. *Allium sativum* L. *(Liliaceae)*

Vernacular Name: *Eng:* Garlic; *Tel:* Velluli tella-gadda; *Beng*: Lashar, lashun, rasun; *Guj*: Lasan; *Hin:* Lahsan; *Kan:* Belluli; *San:* lashuna and *Tam:* Vallai-pundu.

Description: An annual glabrous, bulbous herb with pungent odour. Bulb short, consists of several smaller bulbs (called cloves) and is surrounded by a thin, white or pinkish sheath. Leaves flat and narrow, attenuate-acute at the apex; nerves parallel. Flowers white or pink with bulbils in globose head covered with a large bract.

Habitate: Cultivated all over the country.

Propagation: By cloves (Segments of bulbs).

Part Used: Bulbs.

Chemical Constituents: The essential oil obtained from the bulbs contains allicin, diallyl disulfide, allyl propyl disulfide and other sulfur compounds.

Uses: The bulb constitutes an antibacterial, anti-inflammatory amoebiasis, oxyuriasis and colitis. It cures cough, bronchitis and pertussis. The aqueous solution of bulb juice in a nasal instillation and a gruel made with the bulbs are active on coryza and influenza. It is also hypocholesterolaemic and thus useful in hypercholesterolaemia and atherosclerosis. A poultice of pounded bulb is used to treat boils, abscesses, phlegmons and centipede hites.

71. *Allium ursinum* *(Liliaceae)*

Vernacular Name: *Eng:* Ramsons.

Description: Bulbous perennial smelling strongly of garlic, growing to 28 cm. Has a triangular stem and broad elliptical leaves. Cluster of white, star-like flowers grow from a common stem.

Habitate: Ramsons are native to Europe and Asia. They crpet shady sites in damp woods any by streams.

Propagation: By bulbs.

Parts Used: Bulb.

Chemical Constituents: Ramsons contains volatile oil, aldehydes, vinyl sulphide and vitamin C.

Uses: Used mainly as a folk remedy and as a food, remsons are similar to garlic but weaker in action. They lower high blood pressure and help to prevent arteriosclerosis. As ramsons ease stomach pain and are tonic to the digestion, they have been used for diarrhoea, colic, wind, indigestion and loss of appetite. Ramsons are also thought to be beneficial for asthma, bronchitis and emphysema. The juice is used as an aid to weight loss, treating rheumatic and arthritic joints.

72. *Allophylus serratus* (Roxb.) Kurz *(Sapindaceae)*

Vernacular Name: *Hin*: Tippani; *Kan:* Togaratti; *Mal:* Mukkannapperuku, Mukkannanpelu, Mukkannanperera; *San:* Triputah; *Tam:* Amalai; *Tel:* Eravalu.

Description: A small tree or a large shrub with whitish bark; leaves 3-foliate, alternate, crowded at the ends of branchlets, pubescent, leaflets 5-12-5 cm long, ovate or elliptic, acute or acuminate, serrate-dentate, more or less hairy on both surfaces; flowers small, white in fascicles, on spicate axillary racemes, stamens 8, inserted on the receptacle inside the disc; fruits smooth, globose, red when ripe.

Habitate: Throughout south India and Assam hills.

Propagation: By seeds.

Part Used: Whole part.

Chemical Constituents: Leaves contains phenylacetamide and traces of alkaloids. The roots contain tannins and stem contains β-sitosterol.

Uses: The plant is astringent, bitter, sweet, anti-inflammatory, vulnerary, digestive, carminative and constipating. It is useful in bone fractures, dislocations, inflammations, ulcers, wounds, dyspepsia, anorexia and dislocations, inflammations, ulcers wounds, dyspepsia, anorexia and diarrhoea. The fruits are sweet, cooling and nourishing tonic.

73. *Alnus glutinosa* *(Betulaceae)*

Synonyms: *Alnus rotundifolia.*

Vernacular Name: *Eng:* Alder.

Description: Small tree with fissured bark, growing to 20m. Has notched oval leaves and male and female catkins.

Habitate: Alder is native to Europe, Asia and North Africa. It thrives in damp places an along riverbanks.

Propagation: By seeds.

Parts Used: Bark leaves.

Chemical Constituents: Alder contains lignans, tannin, emodin and glycosides.

Uses: The astringent alder is employed most often as a mouthwash and argle for tooth, gum and throat problems. The drying action of a decoction of the bark helps to contract the mucous membranes and reduce inflammation. A decoction may also be used to staunch internal or external bleeding, and to heal wounds. It is also used as a wash for scabies. In Spain, alder leaves are smoothed and placed on the soles of the feet to relieve aching. Leaves are used to help reduce breast engorgement in nursing mothers.

74. *Alocasia macrorrhiza* (L.) Schott *(Araceae)*

Synonyms: *Alocasia indica* Lour.

Vernacular Name: *Eng:* Big-rooted taro, giant alocasia, gaint taro, kopeh root; *Beng*: Mankachu; *Hin:* Mankanda; *Kan:* Maanaka, Marasani marasakage; *Mal:* Marambu, seema chembu, venal chembu; *San:* hastikarni manaka; *Tam:* Merukankilangu; *Tel:* Chara kanda, sara chema.

Description: Perennial herb, 0.5-1m. high. Rhizome cylindrical, long, stout, with many nodes. Leaves large, ovate–cordate with long stalks, surrounding the stem; margins wavy. Inflorescence in spadix, bearing male flowers above and female below. Berry ovoid, red when ripe.

Habitate: Grows wild in forest and mountains.

Propagation: By rhizome.

Part Used: Leaves and rhizomes.

Chemical Constituents: Oxalic acid, calcium oxalate, flavonoids, cyanogenic glycosides, alocasin, cholesterol, beta-sitosterol, stigmatosterol, camposterol, fucosterol, amino acids, citric acid, malic acid, ascorbic acid, succinic acid, glucose, fructose and sucrose, Arbabino-galactan proteins and betalectins.

Uses: The leaves and the rhizome are prescribed for the treatment of impetigo, furunculosis, phlegmon and snake-bite in the form of a liquid extract for administration by mouth, and their residue is used for poulticing. They are also used in treating colic and vomiting, their external use as a plaster is effective against furunculosis.

75. *Aloe barbadensis* Mill. *(Liliaceae)*

Synonyms: *Aloe vera* (Linn.) Burm., *Aloe perfoliata* L., *Aloe vulgaris* Lam., *Aloe chinensis* Baker., *Aloe indica,* Royle, *Aloe abyssinica* Lam.

Vernacular Name: *Eng:* Indian aloe, Curacao aloe, Barbados aloe, Jaffarabad aloe; *Hin*: Ghikuamr, Ghikumari; *Kan:* Kathaligida; *Mal:* Kattuvala, Kattarvala; *San:* Kumari, Ghartkumari; *Tam:* Kattalai, Sirukattalai; *Tel:* Kalabanda.

Description: A coarse perennial with short stem and shallow root system; leaves fleshy in rosettes, sessile, often crowded with horny prickles on the margins, convex below, 45-60 cm long tapering to a blunt point, surface pale green with irregular white blotches; flowers yellow or orange in racemes; fruits loculicidal capsule.

Habitate: Cultivated or seen wild in the drier part of India.

Propagation: By suckers.

Part Used: Fresh leave and leaf-juice.

Chemical Constituents: The leaves contain barbaloin, chrysophanol glycoside and the aglycone, aloe-emodin. The mucilage of the leaves contains glucose, galactose, mannose and galacturonic acid in addition to an unidentified aldopentose and a protein with 18 amino acids. The plant contains aloesone and aloesin.

Uses: The plant is bitter, sweet, cooling, anthelmintic, aperient, carminative, deobstruent, depurative, diuretic, stomachic, emmenagogue, ophthalmic and alexeteric. The juice is used in dyspepsia, amenorrhoea, burns, colic, hyperadenosis, hepatopathy, splenopathy, skin dieases, constipation, spanomenorrhea, vitiated conditions of *vata* and *pitta,* abdominal tumours, dropsy, carbuncles, sciatica, lumbago and flatulence.

The also is used for helminthiasis in children and is a purgative, anthelmintic and emmenagogue. It is used for local application in painful inflammations, chronic ulcers and catarrhal and purulent ophthalmia.

76. *Aloysia triphylla* (L. Herit.) Britton *(Verbenaceae)*

Synonyms: *Allium citriodora* Ort. ex. Pers; *Lippia citriodora* H. B. & K.

Vernacular Name: *Eng:* Lemon verbena.

Description: A graceful shrub or small tree, 3-6 m in height, indigenous to South America, and commonly grown in Indian gardens, especially in the hills, where it sometimes attains a considerable size. Leaves lanceolate, in whorls of three, densely covered beneath with glandular dots, lemon-scented; flowers small, pale purple, lilac or white, in whorled, axillary spikes or crowded in terminal panicles.

Habitate: Grown in Indian gardens.

Propagation: By seeds and vegetative method.

Part Used: Leaves.

Chemical Constituents: The oil contains citral, cineol, carvone, d-B-caryophyllene, isocaryophyllene and caryophyllene-2,6-B-oxide.

Uses: Verbea oil is used for seasoning food.

77. *Alphitonia zizphoides* (Sprenger) *(Rhamnaceae)*

Description: Tree upto 20m high. Leaves alternate, petiolate, blade ovate or lanceolate, often pale or red beneath. Flowers small, 5-parted, fragrant, white to cream coloured and borne on branching inflorescence with numerous flowers. Fruit purplish to black, globose and forming a small capsule-like drupe.

Habitate: Locally common in dry or dense lowland and foothill forests and thickets.

Propagation: By seeds.

Part Used: Bark and leaves.

Chemical Constituents: Zizphoisides A,C,D & E (triterpenoid saponins).

Uses: The sap of the bark is used to treat earache. The plant is also used to treat cancer. The inner bark is used in treating headaches and weakness after childbirth. In Samoa, the sap is used to treat swellings and feber. The leaves are used as an anhydrotic. A drink made from the bark is taken to treat constipation, cough and menstrual pain. Infertility is treated by drinking a decoction of the bark. Postpartum haemorrhage is treated with an infusion of the bark. The bark is used to make a lotion which is used to treat skin diseases like eczema.

78. *Alpinia galanga* L. Willd. *(Zingiberaceae)*

Synonyms: *Amomum galanga* (Linn.) Lour.

Vernacular Name: *Eng:* Greater galangal, Siamease ginger, Java galangal, Siamese galangal.; *Beng Hin* & *San:* Barakulanjar, kulanjan; *Kan:* Dumparasmi; *Mal:* Arattha, kolinji, peraratta; *Tam:* peraratthei; *Tel:* Peddadumparashtram.

Description: Perennial herbaceous plant, 1-2m. high. Rhizome cylindrical, stout, aromatic, covered with scales. Leaves alternate, lanceolate, lower part surrounding the stem, the upper face glabrous and shining. Inflorescence in terminal dense raceme 20-30cm. long; flowers white, lip veined with red. Fruit globose or ovoid.

Habitate: Grows wild in the mountains and is cultivated everywhere.

Propagation: By rhizome.

Part Used: Rhizomes.

Chemical Constituents: The rhizome yields an essential oil consisting of cineol, methyl cinnamate and flavones: galangin, alpinin, kaempferide and 3–dioxy 4-methoxy flavone.

Uses: The rhizome is an antibacterial agent and a digestive stimulant. It is indicated in the treatment of dyspepsia, flatulence, vomiting, gastralgia, colic, diarrhoea and malaria fever, it is also applied externally on carious teeth to cure toothache.

79. *Alpinia officinarum* Hance *(Zingiberaceae)*

Vernacular Name: *Eng:* Lesser galangal; small galangal.

Description: A perennial, leafy-stemmed herb 0.7-1.2 m high. Rhizome creeping, 12-18 mm in diameter, reddish-brown, glabrous, covered with fibrous scales which leave irregular rings. Leaves cartilaginous, glabrous, lanceolate, 29-40 cm long by 24 mm wide; sheath scariose. Inflorescence paniculate, enclosed in the superior sheaths before flowering. Bracts very small, caduceus. Calyx tubular, with 3 short teeth. Corolla longer than the calyx, lobes 15-20 mm long by 4-5 mm wide. Stamens awl-shaped, short labium white streaked with red, entire, 20 mm long, 15-18 mm wide. Ovary 3-called. Fruit a 3-valved capsule.

Habitate: On slopes in grassland, woods or thickets. Also cultivated in China and Viet Nam.

Propagation: By seeds and vegetative method.

Part Used: Rhizomes.

Chemical Constituents: N.A.

Uses: Epigastric pain; vomiting; indigestion, gastric and duodenal ulcer; chronic gastritis, acute gastroenteritis.

80. *Alpinia oxyphylla* Miq. *(Zingiberaceae)*

Vernacular Name: *Eng:* Sharp-leaved galangal.

Description: A perennial herb, 1-3 m high, Rootstock horizontal. Leafy stem elongated. Leaves lanceolate, 17-33 cm long by 3-6 cm wide. Raceme terminal. Calyx tubular, hairy, 3-toothed. Corolla tube about 1 cm long, 3-toothed, lip obovate, white with reddisn streaks. Anthesis March to May. The fruit, used as the drug, is capsule, oval; some capsules are ovate-oblong and a few nearly spherical, pointed at the extremities.

Habitate: In damp places in the tropics, China.

Propagation: By seeds and vegetative method.

Part Used: Fruit.

Chemical Constituents: N.A.

Uses: Stomachic, tonic in gastralgia, enuresis, spermatorrhoea.

81. *Alpinia purpurata* (Vieill.) K.schum. *(Zingiberaceae)*

Vernacular Name: *Eng:* Red ginger, Purple ginger.

Description: Erect herb upto 3 m tall with pseudostems and creeping fleshy rhizomes. Leaves distichous, long-petiolate, the basal leves sheathing to form a pseudobulb, blades green. Inflorescence terminal and arising from leafy pseudostem. Flowers (if present) whitish and substended by large pink to brigh red bracts.

Habitate: Cultivated as well as occurring in disturbed moist forest, old gardens, trail sides as well as along streams up to about 500m.

Propagation: By rhizome.

Part Used: Fruits and rhizome.

Chemical Constituents: Cyanidin, quercetin, amino acids.

Uses: The fruit is used to treat sores.

82. *Alstonia scholaris* L. R.Br. *(Apocynaceae)*

Vernacular Name: *San:* Saptaparna; *Eng:* Devil tree, Shaitan wood; *Hin*: Chattiyan, Saittan ka jat; *Kan:* Hale, Maddale; *Mal:* Elilampala, Yaksippala, Pala, Daivappala; *Tam*: Elilappalai, Palai; *Tel:* Phalagaruda, Edakularaticettu, Edakulaphala.

Description: A large evergreen tree upto 3.0 m in height, bark grayish brown, rough, lenticellate abounding in bitter, milky latex; leaves 4-7 in a whorl, coriaceous, elliptic-oblong, pale beneath; flowers small, greenish white, numerous in umbellate panicles, corolla tube shot, very strongly scented; fruits follicles, 30-60 cm long; seeds papillose with brownish hair at each end.

Habitate: Throughout India, in deciduous and evergreen forests.

Propagation: By seeds.

Part Used: Bark, leaves, milky exudate.

Chemical Constituents: The bark contains alkaloids: ditaine, echitenine, echitamine (ditamine) and echitamidine together with triterpenes: α-amyrin and lupeol.

Uses: The bark is bitter, astringent, acrid, thermogenic, digestive, laxative, anthelmintic, febrifuge, antipyretic, depurative, galactagogue, stomachic, cardiotonic and tonic. It is useful in fevers, malarial fevers, abdominal disorders, diarrhoea, dysentery, dyspepsia, leprosy, skin diseases, pruritus, tumours, chronic, and foul ulcers, asthma, bronchiltis, cardiopathy, helminthiasis, agalactia and debility. The tender leaves in the form of poultice are good for ulcers with foul discharges. The milky exudate is bitter and is good for ulcers, vitiated conditions of *vata* and otalgia.

83. *Alstonia venenata* R.Br. *(Apocynaceae)*

Vernacular Name: *San:* Visaghni, Anadana; *Mal:* Analivegam; *Kan:* Addasoppu and *Tam:* Sinnappalai.

Description: A large shrub or a small tree upto 6.0 m in height with grayish brown bark and bright yellow hard and woody root; leaves simple, in whorls of 3-6, memberanous, lanceolate, margins wavy, finely acuminate, main nerves numerous, close, parallel, united by intramarginal nerve; flowers white, in terminal, subumbellate cymes or in racemes; fruits fusiform, stalked and beaked follicles, tapering at both ends seeds many, flattened with a tuft of hair at each end.

Habitate: Throughout India in deciduous forests upto 1,800m elevation.

Propagation: By seeds.

Part Used: Roots, fruits.

Chemical Constituents: The plant is rich source of indole alkaloids. The stembark contains alkaloids belonging to yohimbinoid, aspido-fractinine and vincadifformine types. The contents of the various alkaloids in the stembark and in the root, respectively, are alstovenine, venenatine, 3-dehydroalstovenine, reserpine, venoxidine, and kopsinine.

Uses: The roots are bitter, astringent, thermogenic, depurative, antitoxic, febrifuge and anodyne. They are useful in skin diseases, erysipelas, leprosy, cobra bite and other venomous bites, epilepsy, fatigure, fever and otalgia. The fruits are useful in syphilis, insanity and epilepsy.

84. *Alternanthera sessilis* L. *(Amaranthaceae)*

Synonyms: *Alternanthera triandra* Lam., *Alternanthera denticulate* R. Br., *Alternanthera nodiflora* R. Br., *Alternanthera repens* Gmel.

Vernacular Name: *San:* Matsyaksi, Patturah; *Hin*: Gudrisag; *Kan:* Honugonesoppu; *Mal:* Minannani, Ponnannani, Ponnankannikkira; *Tam:* Ponnannkannikkirai; *Tel:* Ponnagantikura.

Description: A much branched prostrate herb, branches often purplish, frequently rooting at the lower nodes; leaves simple, opposite, somewhat fleshy, lanceolate, oblanceolate or linera-oblong, obtuse or subacute, sometimes obscurely denticulate, glabrous, shortly petiolate; flowers small, white, in axillary clusters; fruits compressed obcordate utricles, seeds suborbicular.

Habitate: Throughout India, in moist places upto 2,100 m.

Propagation: By seeds.

Part Used: Whole plant.

Chemical Constituents: β-Sitosterol, stigmasterol, campesterol, α-spinasterol, oleanolic acid rhamnoside, 24-methylene cycloartenol, cycloeucalenol, lupeol, 5-α-stigmasta-7-enol and its palmitate.

Uses: The plant is bitter, sweet, astringent, acrid, cooling constipating, depurative, digestive, cholagogue, galactagogue and febrifuge and is useful in vitiated conditions of *kapha* and *pitta*, buring sensation, diarrhoea, leprosy, skin disease, dyspepsia, haemorrhoids agalactia, splenomegaly and fever.

85. *Althaea officinalis* L. *(Malvaceae)*

Vernacular Name: *Eng:* Marshmallow; *Hin*: Gulkhairo; *Kan*: Seemetuti; *Tam:* Simaitutti; *Mar*: Gulkhair.

Description: Downy perennial growing to 2.2m. Has thick white roots, heart-shaped leaves and pink flowers.

Habitate: Native to Europe, marshmallow is naturalized in the Americas. It prefers marshy fields and tidal zones and is cultivated for medicinal use.

Propagation: By Seeds.

Parts Used: Root, leaves, flowers.

Chemical Constituents: Marshmallow root contains about 37% starch, 11% mucilage, 11% pectin, flavonoids, phenolic acids, sucrose and asparagines.

Uses: Useful whenever a soothing effect is needed, marshmallow protects and soothes the mucous membranes. The root counters excess stomach acid, peptic ulceration and gastritis. Marshmallow is also mildly laxative and beneficial for many intestinal problems. Including regional ileitis, colitis, diverticulitis and irritable bowel syndrome. Taken as a warm infusion, the leaves treat cystitis and frequent urination. Marshmallow's demulcent qualities bring relief to dry coughs, bronchial asthma, bronchial catarrh and pleurisy. The flowers crushed fresh or in a warm infusion, are applied to help soothe inflamed skin. The root is used in an ointment for boils and abscesses, and in a mouthwash for inflammation.

86. *Amaranthus hypochondriacus* *(Amaranthaceae)*

Vernacular Name: *Eng:* Amaranth.

Description: Sturdy, upright annual growing to about 1m. Has deeply veined, lance-shaped, purple-green leaves that grow to 15 cm and tufts of small, deep crimson flowers on long spikes.

Habitate: Native to India, amaranth grows wild in many countries.

Propagation: By Seeds.

Parts Used: Aerial parts.

Chemical Constituents: Amaranth contains tannins, including a red pigment used to dye foods and medicines.

Uses: Amaranth is an astringent herb that is used primarily to reduce blood loss and to treat diarrhoea. A decoction of amaranth is taken as a remedy in cases of heavy menstrual bleeding, excessive vaginal discharge, diarrhoea and dysentery. It is also used as a gargle to soothe inflammation of the pharynx and to hasten the healing of mouth ulcers.

87. *Amaranthus spinosus* L. *(Amaranthaceae)*

Vernacular Name: *San:* Tenduliyah; *Eng:* Prickly amaranth; *Hin*: Cauleyi, Kateli; *Kan:* Mulluhalavesoppu; *Mal:* Mullanicira, Cerucira; *Tam:* Mullukkirai; *Tel:* Mullutotakura.

Description: An erect, glabrous, spinous herb, varying in colour from green to red or purple, 30-60 cm in height with grooved branches and sharp divaricate spines in the leaf axils; leaves simple, alternate, ovate, lanceolate or oblong, entire, glabrous above, main nerves numerous, conspicuous below; flowers small, sessile, yellowish white or pale green, numerous, in dense axillary clusters and in terminal or interrupted spikes; fruits ovoid capsules, membranous, circumscissile about the middle.

Habitate: Throughout India, in waste lands.

Propagation: By seeds.

Part Used: Whole plant.

Chemical Constituents: Higher alkanes and their methyl derivatives, higher aliphatic alcohols, acids and esters, amino acids, β-sitosterol, stigmasterol, campesterol, cholesterol, α-spinasterol, α-spinasterol octacosanoate, glycosides of α-spinasterol and oleanolic acid have been reported in the plant.

Uses: The plant is sweet, cooling, alexeteric, laxative, diuretic, stomachic, antipyretic, febrifuge, sudorific, galactagogue, haematinic, appetizer and tonic it is useful in vitiated onditions of *pitta*, hyperdipsia, burning sensation, hallucination, leprosy, eczema, bronchitis, leucorrhoea, menorrhagia, haemorrhoids, abscesses, boils, burns, strangury, nausea, flatulence, colic anorexia, fever, intermittent fever, agalactia, anaemia and general debility. The roots are thermogenic and haemostatic. They are useful in vitiated conditions of *kapha*, menorrhagia, haemoptysis, haematemesis and leucorrhoea.

88. *Amaranthus tricolor* L. *(Amaranthaceae)*

Synonyms: *Amaranthus tristis* L., *Amaranthus gangeticus* L., *Amaranthus melancholicus* L., *Amaranthus polygamus* L.

Vernacular Name: *San:* Tanduliya; *Eng:* Chinese spinach; *Hin:* Lalsag; *Beng*: Lal-notya, dengue and *Tam:* Mulla-kirai.

Description: A diffuse or ascending herb, rooting at the nodes. Branches slender, not spiny. Leaves small, elliptic. Flowers unisexual, white, borne in clusters; male produced more than the female.

Habitate: Found in West Bengal, Bihar and Uttar Pradesh.

Propagation: By seeds.

Part Used: Whole plant.

Chemical Constituents: Leaf & seed is Analysis of the tender leaves gave: edible portion, moisture, protein, fat, fibre, carbohydrates, minerals, calcium, phosphorus, iron, thiamine, riboflavin, niacin, vitamin, energy and carotene. The amino acids reported to be rescent in the leaves are: arginine, cystine, histidine, leucine, isoleucine, lysine, methionine, phenylalanine, threonine, tryptophan, tyrosine, and valine. The leaves also showed the prescene of amarantin, isoamarantin and betanin. They are a good source of calcium and magnesium. They are a good source of calcium and manganese.

Uses: The plant is considered to be astringent, diuretic, appetizing, digestive and a wholesome diet. Decoction of the plant finds application in dynsentery and haemoptysis. Leaves are said to act as an antidote to poison. Root-paste, mixed with warm water, when given internally, induces vomiting and thereby purges out toxic matter from the bowel. Powdered root is effective in onychia; root-paste, in combination with honey and rice water, is useful in leucorrhoea.

89. Ammania baccifera L. *(Lythraceae)*

Synonyms: *Ammannia Vesicatoria, Ammania salicifolia.*

Vernacular Name: *San:* Kurandika; *Eng:* Blistering ammania; *Hin*: Dadamari, Kuranta; *Mal:* Nirummelneruppu, Kalluruvi; *Tam:* Kalluruvi, Nirummel neruppu; *Tel:* Agnivendrapaku.

Description: An erect glabrous reddish herb upto 60 cm in height, branches usually opposite; leaves lower opposite, upper sometimes alternate, oblong or narrow-elliptic, rounded or subcordate, usually obtuse or subacute; flowers reddish in dense axillary clusters, apetalous or with minute petals; fruits depressed globose capsules covered by calyx tube upto the middle.

Habitate: Throughout India, in marshy places.

Propagation: By seeds.

Part Used: Whole plant.

Chemical Constituents: Resin, glucose and vitamin-C.

Uses: The plant is bitter, acric, cooling appetizer, rubifacient, laxative, stomachic, diuretic, aphrodisiac and lithontriptic. It is useful in vitiated conditions of *kapha* and *pitta*, burning sensation, anorexia, dyspepsia, flatulence, colic, strangury, seminal weakness, renal and vesical calculi, rheumatism, intermittent fevers and herpetic eruptions.

90. *Ammi majus* *(Umbelliferae)*

Vernacular Name: *Eng:* Bishop's weed, Greater ammi,.

Description: Erect annual herb growing to 80 cm, with tangled leaflets and umbels of small white flowers.

Habitate: Bishop's weed is native to the Mediterranean region and as far east as Iran. It is cultivated for its seeds, which are harvested in late summer.

Propagation: By Seeds.

Parts Used: Seeds.

Chemical Constituents: The seeds contain furanocoumarins, flavonoids and tannins.

Uses: Used to treat asthma and angina. Bishop's weed reputedly helps treat patchy skin pigmentation in vitiligo. It has also been used for psoriasis.

91. *Ammi visnaga* *(Umbelliferae)*

Synonyms*: Daucus Visnaga.*

Vernacular Name: Eng; Visnaga, Khella.

Description: An erect annual growing to 1m, with leaves divided into wisps and clusters of small white flowers.

Habitate: Native to north Africa, visnaga grows wild in the Middle East and around the Mediterranean. It is naturalized in Australia and South America. Grown from seed, visnaga is widely cultivated.

Propagation: By Seeds.

Parts Used: Fruits and Seeds.

Chemical Constituents: Khellin (1%), Visnagin, Khellol glycoside, Volatile oil (0.2%), Flavonoids, Sterols.

Uses: Antispasmodic, Anti-asthmatic, Relaxant.

92. *Amomum aromaticum* Roxb. *(Zingiberaceae)*

Vernacular Name: *Eng:* Bengal cardamom, Nepal cardamom; *Hin:* Morang-elaichi; *Beng*: Morang-elaichi and *Assam*: Karpur.

Description: Tall perennial herb, 2-3m. high; root–stock horizontal with many nodes; leaves linear, sessile, lower part surrounding the stem; Inflorescence in radial spike; flowers red; fruit ovoid, 3–valved, crimson; seeds numerous, angular, with a pronounced fragrance.

Habitate: Wild or cultivated in wet places in the forest.

Propagation: By rhizome.

Part Used: Fruit.

Chemical Constituents: Essential oil form seeds 1-15%.

Uses: The seeds have antibacterial and somachic properties. They are used to alleviate dyspepsia, flatulence, colic, vomiting, diarrhoea and cough. They are also prescribed as a gargle or mouth-wash or for perlingual administration to treat toothache, gingivitis and parodontosis. They are also used for flavouring cakes.

93. *Amomum krervanh* Pierre ex gangnep *(Zingiberaceae)*

Vernacular Name: *Eng:* Round cardmom; cluster cardamon.

Description: Herbs with elongate leafy stems, 2-3 cm high and perennial spreading rootstocks. Leaves distichous, subsessile, lanceolate, 20-23 cm long by 7.5-10 cm wide, apex caudate, base narrowed, margin sub-undulate, glabrous. Flowers in dense spikes direct from the rootstock; early summerl bracts imbricate. The capsules are round, globular, smooth, ribbed, obscurely triangular, and of a brownish white colour. The seeds are packed together in a globular mass, easily broken into three portions, and have an aromatic flavour.

Habitate: In damp places in the tropics, Burma, Cambodia, China, Thailand, Viet Nam.

Propagation: By seeds and vegetative method.

Part Used: Fruit.

Chemical Constituents: N.A.

Uses: Abdominal distension, vomating due to stomach cold, indigestion.

94. *Amomum subulatum* Roxb. *(Zingiberaceae)*

Vernacular Name: *San:* Sthulaila, Bhadraila; *Eng:* Greater cardamom, Nepal cardamom; *Hin*: Badi llayaci, Bari llayaca; *Kan:* Doddayelakki; *Mal:* Perelam; *Tam:* Periya elam, Kattelam, Perelam; *Tel:* Pedda elakkaya, Adavielakkaya.

Description: A herb with leafy stem upto 90-100 cm in height, leaves oblong-lanceolate, bright green, glabrous on both surfaves; flowers white in globose shortly peduncled spikes, bracts reddish brown, lip ovate-cuneate, emarginated, yellowish white, filaments very short, anther crest small, truncate, entire, fruits reddish brown, densely echinate globose capsules; seeds many, held together by a viscid sugary pulp.

Habitate: In the Eastern Himalayas.

Propagation: By rhizome & seeds.

Part Used: Seeds.

Chemical Constituents: The seeds contain the glycosides, petunidin, 3.5-diglucoside, and leucocyanidin and a new aurone glycoside, subulin, chalcone, cardamonin and a flavanone, alpinetin is also reported.

Uses: The seeds are acrid, bitter, aromatic, thermogenic, deodorant, appetizer, carminative, digestive, stomachic, constipating, depurative, vulnerary, anodyne, cardiac and liver tonc, expectorant, diuretic, febrifuge, sudorific and hypnotic. They are userful in vitiated conditions of *kapha* and *vata*, halitosis, anorexia, dysentery, skin diseases, pruritus, wounds, ulcers, cephalalgia, odontalgia, neuralgia, cardiac debility, liver congestion, splenomegaly, cough, bronchiltis, strangury, fever proctoptosis, hyperdipsia and gonorrhoea.

95. *Amomum villosum* Lour. *(Zingiberaceae)*

Vernacular Name: *Eng:* Malabar cardamom, Tavoy cardamom.

Description: Perennial herb, 0.5-1.5m. high; root-stock horizontal, slender; leaves alternate, linear, amplexicaul, acute-attenuate at the apex; Inflorescence in radical raceme;

flowers white, lip yellowm spotted with purple. capsule 3-valved, with soft spines, brown red when ripe.

Habitate: Grows wild in shady places in the mountains.

Propagation:: By seeds & rhizome.

Part Used: Seeds.

Chemical Constituents: The essential oil from the seeds consists of D-camphor, D-bornoel, D-bornyl acetate, D-limonene, α-pinene, phellandrene, paramethoxyethyl cinnamate, nerolidol and linalool. The seeds also contain liquiritin and glucovanilli acid.

Uses: The seeds possess antibacterial and stomachic properties. They are utilized in dyspepsia, colic, flatulence, diarrhoea, vomiting and oedema. They are a constituent of composite recipes against threatened abortion. They are also active against toothache if the maceration or the powder are applied to carious patches on the teeth.

96. *Amorphophallus companulatus* Blume ex. Decne. *(Araceae)*

Synonyms: *Amorphophallus paeoniifolius* Dennst.

Vernacular Name: *San:* Suranah; *Eng:* Elephant foot yam; *Hin*: Suran, Jamikand; *Kan:* Suvarnagadda; *Mal:* Cena; *Tam*: Karunaikkilanku; *Tel:* kandagadda.

Description: A stout herbaceous plant with underground hemispherical depressed dark brown corm; leaves compound, large, solitary, petiole stout, mottled, 60-90 cm long, leaflets 5-12.5 cm long of variable width, obovate or oblong, acute, strongly and many-nerved; made and female inflorescences contiguous, neuters absent, appendage of spadix subglobose or amorphous, equaling or longer than the fertile region, spathe campanulate, pointed, strongly, closely veined, greenish pink externally, base within purple, margins recurved, undulate and crisped, male inflorescence subturbinate, female 7.5 cm or more long; fruits obovoid 2-3 seeded red berries.

Habitate: Throughout India, cultivated.

Propagation: By corm.

Part Used: Corms.

Chemical Constituents: The corms contain betulinic acid, β-sitosterol, stigmasterol, triacontane and β-sitosterol palmitate. Besides these, glucose, galactose, rhzmnose and exylose are also present. The corms are irritant due to the composition of the corms is as follows: arginine, histidine, leucine, isoleucine, lysine, methionine, phenylalanine, threonine, tryptophan, and valine.

Uses: The corms are acrid, astringent, thermogenic, irritant, anodyne, anti-inflammatory, antihaemorrhoidal, haemostatic, expectorant, carminative, digestive, appetizer, stomachic, anthelmintic, liver tonic, aphrodisiac, emmenagogue, rejuvenating and tonic. They are useful in vitiated conditions of *vata* and *kapha*, arthralgia, elephantiasis, tumours, inflammations, haemorrhoids, haemorrhages, vomiting, cough, bronchitis, asthma, anorexia, dyspepsia, flatulence, colic constipation, helminthiasis hepatopathy, splenopathy, amenorrhoea, dysmenorrhoea, seminal weakness, fatigue, anaemia and general debility. The roots are ophthalmic and emmenagogue, and are useful in ophthalmia, amenorrhoea and boils.

97. *Ampelocissus araneosa* Planch. *(Vitaceae)*

Synonyms: *Vitis araneosa* (Dalz. & Gibson) Lawson.

Vernacular Name: *San*:-Asvakathara, *Tam*:-Kattu thiratchai; *Hin*: Kauraj, Ghorvel,.

Description: A climbing shrub with flattened stems. Young parts densely covered with greyish brown woolly hairs. Leaves alternate, 3-foliolate, 10-20 cm long; leaf stalk 3-5 cm long; *leaflets* membranous, shortly stalked, margin doubly toothed with triangular teeth, hairless above, densely greyish brown tomentose below; terminal leaflets oblong or egg-shaped-lanceolate, 6-10 x 4-7 cm, base wedge-shaped, apex acuminate; the lateral leaflets egg-shaped-elliptic, 4-10 x 2-6, nearly heart-shaped, base unequal, apex acuminate. *Flowers* bisexual, minute, about 3 mm across, reddish orange, borne on tendrils as condensed cymes. *Tendrils* arise opposite to leaves, forked, densely woolly. *Cymes* up to 1.5 cm across borne on about 5 cm long peduncle. *Berries* globose, fleshy with rough surface, about 2 cm across. *Seeds* 2-4, with 2-furrows.

Habitate: Moist deciduous to evergreen forests found in Kerala, Karnataka, Tamilnadu.

Propagation: By seeds.

Parts Used: Roots.

Chemical Constituents: N.A.

Uses: Used in Ayurveda, Siddha and Unani system of medicne. The roots are used as a cooling agent and astringent.

98. *Ampelocissus indica* L. Planch. (*Vitaceae*)

Synonyms: *Ampelocissus arnottiana* Planch.

Vernacular Name: *Kan:* Sambara balli, Saavira sambara; *Hin*: Jangli Angoor,.

Description: A climbing shrub with young parts covered with brown-coloured wool. *Stems* hollow, cylindrical. *Leaves* alternate, simple, sometimes rarely shallowly 3-lobed, broadly egg-shaped or sub-orbicular, 10-25 x 8-20 cm, base deeply heart-shaped, apex acute or acuminate, margin coarsely toothed, hairless above when old, woolly-floccose, on the nerved beneath, 5-7 nerved from base; leaf stalks up to 10 cm long. *Flowers* bisexual, stalkless, minute, about 2 mm across, brownish red, occur in dense clusters or branched cymes; peduncles 6-20 cm long, woolly. *Berries* globose or ovoid-oblong, about 2 cm long, smooth, juicy, sweet, purple when ripe. *Seeds* 2-4, 3-angled, smooth, straw-coloured.

Habitate: Semi-evergreen to evergreen forests.

Propagation: By seeds.

Parts Used: Roots.

Chemical Constituents: N.A.

Uses: Juice of the roots is diuretic, aperient and a blood purifier. Used to cure eye troubles and ulcers.

99. *Ampelopsis japonica* (Thunb.) Makino (*Vitaceae*)

Vernacular Name: *Eng:* Japanese ampelopsis.

Description: A perennial climbing vine about 1 m long. Tuberous roots, clustered, robust, fleshy, long-fusiform or ovate, externally dark brown in colour, fracture white, stachy; stem ligneous at the base, much-branched; young branches glabrous, finely striate, slightly purplish. Tendrils opposite to the leaf. Leaves alternate, compound-palmate, 6-10 cm long by 7-12 cm wide; petiole shorter than the leaf blade, glabrous; leaflets 3-5, pinnatilobate; segments ovate or lanceolate, the middle segment being the longest one rachis broadly winged, both surfaces glabrous. Cymes small opposite to leaf. Summer. Flowers small, yellowish-green. Berry globose, blue or bluish-purple.

Habitate: On slopes or among grasses by roadsides, in China, Japan.

Propagation: By seeds.

Part Used: Tuberous roots.

Chemical Constituents: N.A.

Uses: Skin inflammationl pyogenic inflectional ulcerous disease of skin, burns. External use.

100. *Anacardium occidentale* L. *(Anacardiaceae)*

Vernacular Name: *San:* Vrkkabijah, Vrkkaphalah, Venamrah; *Eng:* Cashewnut tree; *Hin:* Kaju; *Kan:* Gerumara, Turakageru; *Mal:* Kasumavu, Parankimavu, Venamrah; *Tam:* Muntiri; *Tel:* Gidimavridi.

Description: A small tree with short, thick, crooked trunk. Leaves obovate or obovate-oblong, hard glabrous, obtuse-retuse or rounded at tip, cuneate at base, 10-20 cm long; flowers small, yellow, with pink stripes borne in 15-25 cm long, terminal panicles, with both staminate and hermaphrodite flowers; fruit, a kidney-shaped nut, 2.5cm long, borne and on 5.0-7.5 cm long, pyriform, fleshy receptacle, the cashew apple, having a thin bright yellow to scarlet skin and soft and juicy flesh. The nut is grayish green with a hard, smooth and shining oleaginous pericarp enclosing a curved white kernel covered with a thin reddish brown testa.

Habitate: Cultivated and wild especially on the sea coast.

Propagation: By seeds.

Part Used: Roots, bark leaves, fruits.

Chemical Constituents: The essential amino acides are as follows: arginine, histidine, lysine, phenylalanine, methionine, threonine, trytophan, leucine, isoleucine, and valine. Other amino acids present are alanine, aspartic acid, cystine, glutamic acid, glycine, serine, and tyrosine. The testa is a good source of condensedtpe of tannins. The polyphenols identified in the testa are catechin, epicatechin, ethylgallate, leucocyanidin, proanthocyanidin, leucodelphinidin and epiafazelchin.

Uses: The roots are considered purgative. The bark has alternative properties and is used along with the inflorescence for the treatment of snakebit. The bark and leaves are useful in odontalgia and ulitis. The gum from the bark is recommended in leprosy, ringworm, corns and obstinate ulcers. Fruits are acrid, sweet, thermogenic, aphrodisiac, trichogenous and anthelmintic, and are useful in vitiated conditions of *vata* and *kapha*, skin diseases, dysentery, haemorrhoids and anorexia. They are used for preventing hair loss and to increase the growth of hair. The kernels constitute a highly nutritious and concentrated food. A delicious drink is also derived from the spongy thalamus.

101. *Anacyclus pyrethrum* DC. *(Asteraceae)*

Synonyms: *Anacyclus officinarum* Hayne.

Vernacular Name: *San:* Agragrahi, Akarakarabhah; *Eng:* Pellitory; *Hin:* Akrakara; *Kan:* Akkalakara; *Mal:* Akkikkaruka, Akkravu; *Tam:* Akkirakkaram, Akkalkara; *Tel:* Akarakaramu.

Description: A perennial, procumbent plant with numerous stems and somewhat downy branches; leaves redical, stalked, smooth, pinnatisect into linear, subulate segments, cauline leaves sessile; branches one-headed, involucral scales lanceolate, acuminate, brown at the edge, receptacle convex; ray flowers white, purplish beneath.

Habitate: Indigenous to north Africa, introduced into south Europe.

Propagation: By seeds.

Part Used: Roots.

Chemical Constituents: The roots contain anacyclin, pellitorine, enetriyne alcohol, hydrocarolin, inulin, traces of volatile oil and seasamin. They also contain deca-, dodeca-, and tetradeca-trans-2, trans-4-dienamide, a new series of tyramine amides corresponding to the isobutylamides. The presence of polyacetyenic compounds is also reported in the plant.

Uses: Roots are acrid, astringent and are a valuable sialogogue and regarded as a tonic to the nervous system. It is anti-inflammatory, depurative and powerful irritant. A decoction of the root is useful as a gargle in dental caries, odontalgia, pharyngitis and tonsillitis. It is used to treatment of paralysis, hemiplegia, cephalalgia, chronic ophthalmia, epilepsy, cholera, rheumatism and typhus fever. Powdered root is given with honey for epilepsy.

102. *Anagallis arvensis* L. *(Primulaceae)*

Vernacular Name: *Eng:* Scarlet pimpernel; *Hin*: Jangamami, Jonkmari, Krishna-neel; *Guj*: Golophudi; .

Description: Creeping annual growing to 5cm with oval-to lance-shaped leaves and salmon-red flowers on long stems.

Habitate: Scarlet pimpernel is found in Europe and in temperate regions of Asia, North Africa, North America and Australia. It prefers wasteland and untended *San*dy ground, and is gathered in summer towards the end of its flowering period.

Propagation: By Stem cutting.

Parts Used: Aerial parts.

Chemical Constituents: The herb contains saponins, tannins and cucurbitacins. The latter are cytotoxic.

Uses: It has been used to treat epilepsy and mental problems for years but there is little evidence to support its efficacy.

103. Anamirta cocculus L. Wight & Arn. *(Menispermaceae)*

Synonyms: *Anamirta paniculata* Colebr.

Vernacular Name: *San:* Garalaphala, Kakamari; *Eng:* Levant berries, Fish berries, Crow killer; *Hin:* Kakamari; *Kan:* Kakamari, Kayamari; *Mal:* Polla, Kollakkaya, Pettumarunnu; *Tam:* Kakamari; *Tel:* Garalaphala, Kakinicampacettu.

Description: A large woody, climbing shrub with vertically furrowed ash-coloured bark and glabrous young parts; leaves large, simple, alternate, long-petioled, petioles thickened at the base and apex, broadly ovate, subcoriaceous, cordate or truncate at the base, acute or acuminate, 5-nerved with tufts of hairs in the axils of the nerves except the basal ones; flowers greenish in long panicles, drooping from the nodes of the old wood; fruits drupes, kidney shaped, turning red on ripening.

Habitate: Throughout India in forests.

Propagation: By seeds.

Part Used: Leaves, fruits & seeds.

Chemical Constituents: The seeds contain two alkaloids, menispermine and paramenispermine. Seeds yield fat with a pale yellow colour, an agreeable taste and the following constants: acid val, iod val, sap val, acetyl val, unsapon mater. The fatty acid compostion is as follows: palmitic, stearic, oleic, linoleic. The unsaponified matter contains sitosterol.

Uses: The fruits are bitter, astringent, thermogenic, expectorant, antifungal, anthelmintic and depurative. They are useful in vitiated conditions of *kapha* and *vata*, bronchitis, dermatophytosis, foul ulcers, inflammations, flatulence, chronic skin diseases and ringworm. The tender leaves are used by the tribals for the contraction of the uterus immediately after delivery.

104. Ananas comosus L. Merrill *(Bromeliaceae)*

Synonyms: *Ananas Sativus* Schultes f.

Vernacular Name: *San:* Anamnasam, Bahunetraphalam; *Eng:* Pineapple; *Hin:* Ananas; *Kan:* Anasahannu; *Mal:* Kaitaccakka, Kappaccakka, Ananas; *Tam:* Annasippalam; *Tel:* Annasapandu.

Description: A herbaceous perennial with a short stout stem; leaves numerous spirally and compactly arranged, linear-lanceolate, acuminate, margins spiny, toothed, shining on the upper surface, those subtending the inflorescence small, much reduced, reddish; heads terminal, ovoid, bracteoles reddish, numerous, triangular-ovate to oblong-ovate, imbricate; fruits composite, succulent, bearing a crown of leaves.

Habitate: Throughout India, cultivated.

Propagation: By suckers.

Part Used: Fruits, leaves.

Chemical Constituents: The fresh fruit is a good source of vitamins A and B, and is rich in vitamin C. it also contains some minerals, such as iron and phosphorus. It has low sugar and fat contents and is good for obsess people. Analysis of the fruit gave the following values: moisture, protein, fat, fibre, carbohydrates, and minerals, calciu, phosphorus, thiamine, riboflavin, niacin, vitamin and oxalic acid. Other than this is also contain sucrose, glucose, fructose, and citric and malic acids. The fruit also contain *p*-coumaric, caffeic, ferulic and sinapic acids and several amino acids.

Uses: The unripe fruits are sour, cooling, appetizer, digestive, anthelmintic, cathartic, cardiotonic, uterine tonic, emmenagogue and febrifuge. They are useful in vitiated conditions of *pitta*, anorexia, dyspepsia, helminthiasis, constipation, cardiac debility, haematemesis, sexually transmitted diseases, amenorrhoea, dysmenorrhoea and fever. The ripe fruits are sweet, cooling emollient, diuretic, carminative, digestive, cardiotonic, sudorific, styptic, lithontriptic, antiscorbutic, febrifuge and tonic. They are useful in vitiated conditions of *pitta*, strangury, dyspepsia, flatulence, colic, hyperacidity, cardiac debility, haematemesis, haemoptysis, jaundice, renal and vesical calculi, scabies, pruritus, fever and general debility. The leaves are anthelmintic, abortifacient and emmenagogue, and are useful in induction of abortion, helminthiasis, amenorrhoea, dysmenorrhoea and whooping cough.

105. *Andrographis paniculata* (Burm.f.) Nees *(Acanthaceae)*

Vernacular Name: *San:* Bhunimba, kirata; *Eng:* Creat, kariyat; *Hin:* Kalmegh, kirayat, mahatita; *Beng*: Kalmegh; *Kan:* Nelaberu; *Mal:* Kiriyattu, nelaveppu; *Tam:* Nilavembu; *Tel:* Neelaveemu.

Description: Erect annual herb, 0.4–1m. high. Stems quadrangular, much-branched. Leaves opposite, short-petioled, oblong-attenuate at both ends, glabrous, pale beneath. Inflorescence is axillary and terminal raceme or panicle; flowers white with pink spots. Capsule linear-oblong, acute at both ends, pubescent. Seeds numerous, oblong, glabrous.

Habitate: Species cultivated everywhere.

Propagation: By seeds & cutting.

Part Used: Whole plant.

Chemical Constituents: The plant contais bitter glucosides: andrographolide, neoandrographolide, panaculoside, flavonoids, andrographin, panicalin, apigeinin 7-4–dimethyl ether.

Uses: The whole plants, principally the leaves, possess antibacterial, anti-inflammatory and immunosuppressive properties. The leaves are used in treating dysentery, diarrhoea, enteritis, fever, coryza, cough, sore throat, tonsillitis, bronchitis, osteodynia, arthralgia, menstrual and post-partum haemtometra, scrofula, hypertension and snake-bite.

106. *Anemarrhena asphodeloides* *(Liliaceae)*

Vernacular Name: *Eng:* Common anemarrhena.

Description: A perennial herb, Rhixomes thick horizontal. Leaves basal, linear, 20-70 cm long by 3-6 mm wide, glabrous. Scape simple, erect 5-100 cm high, herminating in a long speciform cluster of small flowers in summer, fragrant, opening in the evening. Perianth white or light purple, in 6 divisions in 2 rows, lightly united at the base. Stamens 3, with a very short filament. Ovary 3-called. Style filiform. Fruit a hexagonal capsule, seeds 1-2, triangular, black.

Habitate: On exposed slopes and hills, in China.

Propagation: By seeds and vegetative method.

Part Used: Rhizomes.

Uses: Antipyretic in highly febrile diseases, feeling of thirst and irritation, cough due to heat in lungs, constipation.

107. *Anemone pulsatilla* *(Ranunculaceae)*

Synonyms*:* *Pulsatilla vulgaris.*

Vernacular Name: *Eng:* Pasque flower.

Description: Hairy perennial growing to 15cm. Has feathery leaves, and large, purple-blue bell-shaped flowers, with bright yellow anthers.

Habitate: Native to Europe, this herb thrives in dry grassland in central and northern parts of the continents, preferring chalky soil, the aerial parts are harvested when it flowers in spring.

Propagation: By Stem cutting.

Parts Used: Dried aerial parts.

Chemical Constituents: Pasque flower contains the lactone protoanemonin, triterpenoid saponins tannins and volatile oil.

Uses: Pasque flower is less commonly used now in herbal medicine than in the past, though it is still considered a valuable remedy for cramping pain, menstrual problems and emotional distress. It is considered a specific treatment for spasmodic pain of the reproductive system both male and female, and is given quite frequently for premenstrual tension and period pain, especially when these are accompanied by nervous exhaustion.

108. *Anethum graveolens* L. *(Apiaceae (Umbelliferae))*

Synonyms: *Peucedanum graveolens* Linn.

Vernacular Name: *San:* Satapuspa; *Eng:* Dill, Garden dill, Anet; *Hin:* Soya; *Kan:* Sabbasige; *Mal:* Satakuppa; *Tam:* Satakuppi; *Tel:* Satakuppivittulu.

Description: A glabrous aromatic annual herb, 30-90 cm in height with hollow finely grooved stem, striped dark green and white with blusih spots; leaves compound, 2-3 pinnate, blusih green, segments filiform, leafsheath surrounds the stem; flowers yellow, in flat compound umbels; fruits narrowly winged, vittae large and conspicuous.

Habitate: Throughout India, cultivated.

Propagation: By seeds.

Part Used: Fruits.

Chemical Constituents: The major constituents of the oil are carvone and *d*-llimonene, carvone, dihydrocar-vone, *d*-limonene, *d*-phellandrene α-terpinene, carveol, dihydrocarveol, iseugenol, and dill-apiol.

Uses: The fruits are acrid, bitter, thermogenic, deodorant, digestive, carminative, stomachic, anthelmintic, anodyne, anti-inflammatory, diuretic, emmenagogue, galactagogue, expectorant, cardiotonic, anaphrodisiac, febrifuge, sudorific, antispasmodic, antidysenteric, alexeteric and vulnerary. They are useful in halitosis, flatulence, colic, dyspepsia, intestinal worms, odontalgia, arthralgia, inflammation, strangury, amenorrhoea, dysmenorrhoea, agalactia, hiccough, cough, asthma, bronchitis, spermatorrhoea, fever ulcers, skin diseases, splenopathy, hepatopathy, uropathy, gleet, syphilis, haemorrhoids and cardiac debility.

109. *Anethum sowa* *(Apiaceae)*

Vernacular Name: *Eng:* Indian dill, sowa; *Hin:* Sotopha, sowa, soya; *Beng*: Shulupa, sooplpha; *Kan:* Sabbasige; *Mal:* Chatakuppa; *Tam:* Satakkuppi; *Tel:* Shatakupi-vitla.

Description: An annual aromatic herb; leaves decompound, aromatic; flowers pale yellow, in compound umbles; fruit sub-elliptical, the mericarps remaining joined togetherl vittae with irregular marginal walls.

Habitate: Cultivated throughout India, chiefly in Uttar Pradesh,Gujrat, Maharashtra, Assam and West Bengal.

Propagation: By seeds.

Part Used: Seeds, leaves.

Chemical Constituents: The major consttuents identified in the seed oil are carvone, dillapiole, limonene, and dihydrocarvone. The herb oil contains, less carvonethan the seed oil. It contains mainly d-a-phellandrene, eugenol, thymol, isoeugenol, linalyl acetate, and phellandral.

Uses: Sowa herb and oil are in great demand as a condiment for flavouring pickles, curries, soups and salads, and confectionery. They are also used for making tea.

110. *Angalis arvensis* L. *(Primulaceae)*

Synonyms: Anagalis caerulea Lam., Anagalis latifolia Linn.

Vernacular Name: *Eng:* Scarlet pimpernel.

Description: A trailing annual herb with stem 15-50 cm. high, branched from the base, more or less procumbent, quadrangular, glabrous, branched slightly winged. Leaves opposite, entire ovate, sessile, dotted on the lower surface. Flowers solitary, axillary on long peduncles, erect during flowering but curves backwards when seeds ripens, pentamerous. Petals scarlet, tubular below. Calyx 5. Stamens 5, opposite, petals, beset with a number of delicate violet hairs. Fruits a tiny capsule splitting into two halves, upper half lifts like a lid. Roots spindle shaped and contorted.

Habitate: Throughout Europe, particularly U.K. Also cultivated in India as protected plant.

Propagation: By seeds.

Parts Used: Whole plant.

Chemical Constituents: Glycosidic saponins and Cyclamin.

Uses: Diaphoretic, Diuretic, for Gallstones. Liver cirrhosis. Complaints especially of skin, characterized by great itching and tingling everywhere. Favours expulsion of splinters. An old remedy for hydrophobia and dropsy. Possesses power of destroying warts. Headache over supra-orbital ridges. Cramps in thumbs and fingers. Urethral irritation. Skin itches with dry bran like eruptions, especially of hands, fingers and palm. Vesicles in groups.

111. *Angelica archangelica* L. *(Apiaceae)*

Vernacular Name: *Eng:* Indian dill, sowa.

Description: An aromatic perennial herb leaves ovate, 2-3-pinnate; flowers white in compound umbels; schizocarps ellipsoid or subquadrate seeds compressed.

Habitate: Near water channels in Kashmir and Sikkim.

Propagation: By seeds.

Part Used: Roots, fruits.

Chemical Constituents: Root oil contains a-pinene, phellandrene and osthole and its musk-like odour is attributed to pentadecanolide. Fruit oil contains a-phellandrene, b-pinene, p-cymene, and dihydrocarvone.

Uses: Roots and fruits are used for flavouring wines, liqueur and confectionery. Root oil and fruit oil are used as flavouring, the former being richer in odour and flavour.

112. Angelica dahurica (Fisch. Ex Hoffm.) *(Apiaceae (Umbelliferae))*

Vernacular Name: *Eng:* Dahurian angelica.

Description: A large perennial herb, 2-2.5 m high. Stem hollow, pubescent, often purplish; Leaves basal, broad, tripinnatel leaflets oblong or oval-elliptical, tip acute, margin dentate; cauline leaf alternate, long-petiolate, petiole broadly dilated at the base. Inflorescence a large compound umbe, terminal, rays 22-38. White flowers in summer, bracts 1-2 dilated as a sheathl bracteoles small, often as long as or longer than the pedicels, each ray consisting of 10 pedicels or more. Petals 5, entire, incurvate at the tips. Fruit ovoid, compresed, edged with 4 membranous wings; mericarp, 5-ribbed, glabrate of spresely pubescent.

Habitate: In thickets, mostly cultivated in China, Japan Korea and Soviet Union.

Propagation: By seeds.

Part Used: Roots.

Uses: Common cold caused by the wind; headache, sinusitis, toothache, haemorhoids complicated by anal fistula, melaena; leucorrhea, skin inflammation and boils, burns.

113. *Angelica gigas* Nakai *(Umbelliferae)*

Vernacular Name: *Eng:*-Cham-dang-gui.

Description: Purpulish, glabrous, perennial herb, 1-2 m tall, with thickened rhizomes. Basal and lower leaves long-petiolated, odd 2-3 pinnate; leaflets deeply 3-lobed, sometimes 2-3 clefted again, segment long-elliptic or ovate, sharply double-serrate, terminal segment rhombic; upper leaves reduced to sharply double-serrate, terminal segment rhombic; upper leaves reduced to elliptic, dilated purplish brown hairs, rays 15-20, umbellets consisting of 20-40 flowers; bracts 1-2 enlarged like leaf sheath; bracteoles 5-7, linear-lanceolate. Flowers 8 mm long, 5 mm wide, with large wings.

Habitate: Along mountain streams, often cultivated in Korea found in Korea, Japan and Northern China.

Propagation: By seeds and stem cutting.

Parts Used: Root.

Chemical Constituents: Decursin, decursinol, nodakenin, angelinol, gigasol.

Uses: Increase duodenum motility. Anti-platelet aggregation (nodakenin).

114. *Angelica glauca* Edgeew. *(Apiaceae)*

Vernacular Name: *HP*: Chora, Choraka, Chamchora, Gandrayan, Chura; *Kas*: Chohore, chura; *Pun*: Chora, chura and *UP*: Chorak, gandhruayan.

Description: A, tall, robust, erect, aromatic, perennial herb 1 to 1.5 m tall with thick, stout, perennial rootstock. Roots are brownish, long fleshy branching, thick, annulate, fusiform, resinous and pungently aromatic. Leaves are pinnately divided, the basal ones are ternate pinnate. Leaflets oval to irregularly mucronate, serrate; upper surface dark green, lower glaucous. Flowers white or purple in long stalked compound umbels. Fruit; glabrous, flattened, oblong. the roots and rootstock become thick and increase with age.

Habitate: It is found in Western Himalaya upto 2700-3000 m.

Propagation: By seeds.

Part Used: Dried roots and rootstocks.

Chemical Constituents: The roots yield a pale to brownish yellow essential oil. The oil contains lactones, sesquiter-penes, *d*-α-pinene, d-α-phellandrene, selinene, d-α-cadinene, umbelliprenin and terpene alcohols. It has not yet been commercially exploited. The petroleum ether extract of the fruit contains a lactonic constituent.

Uses: The roots is pungent, aromatic, stomachic, tonic, stimulant, carminative, diphoretic, and diuretic. It increases appetite and combined with tonic, it is given in typhoid conditions, bronchitis, flatulence, colic and pain in the stomach. Roots are used as spice and conditment. Also used in obstinate constipation and biliousness. The aromatic root is a flavouring agent for food etc. Roots are also used in the preparation of gin and the liqueurs known as bitters.

115. *Angelica sinensis* (Oliv.) Deils *(Apiaceae)*

Description: Perennial herbaceous plant, 40–60cm. high. Stems striate, plae violet. Leaves alternate, amplexicaul, 3–4–pinnate; margins toothed. Inflorescence in dense terminal umbel; flowers small, white. Fruit compressed. All parts of the plant, especially the roots, have a special scent.

Habitate: Introduced species, cultivated in many places of India.

Propagation: By seeds.

Part Used: Root.

Chemical Constituents: The roots yield an essential oil consisting of ligustilid, butylidenephthalide, bergapten, safrol, p-cymene, scsquiterpene, dodecanol, tetradecanol and vitamin $B_{12.}$

Uses: The root has marked restorative, antinaemic and haemagogic properties. It is recommended for treating anaemia, general debitlity, headache, fatigue, lumbago, chest pains, colic, constipation, paresis, furunculosis, impetigo, contusions, menstrual disorders and dysmenorrhoea. In the case of menstrual disorders, the drug is taken a week before menstruation.

116. *Anisomeles malabarica* R.Br. ex Sims. *(Lameaceae)*

Vernacular Name: *San:* Vaikunthah, Mahadronah; *Eng:* Malabar catmint; *Hin:* Codhara; *Kan:* karitumbi; *Mal:* Karintumpa; *Tam:* Peyimarutti, Peyameratti; *Tel:* Mogabiraku.

Description: An erect shrub about 1.8 m in height with obtusely tetragonous and softly white-tomentose stems and branches; leaves simple, opposite, very thick aromatic, oblong-lanceolate, acute, pale above, white below, crenate-serrate, softly woolly; flowers purple, in dense whorls of more or less interrupted spikes; fruits nutlets, ellipsoid, compressed, the inner face slightly angular, the dorsal rounded, smooth, brown.

Habitate: Throughout south India.

Propagation: By seeds.

Part Used: Whole plant.

Chemical Constituents: The plant yields a light brown essential oil. It consists mainly of hydrocarbons, citral and geranic acid.

Uses: The plant is acrid, biiter, aromatic, intellect promoting, stomachic, anthelmintic, febrifuge and sudorific. It is useful in halitosis, epilepsy, hysteria, amentia, anorexia, dyspepsia, colic, flatulence, intestinal worms, fever arising from teething in children, intermittent fevers, vitiated conditions of *vata* and *kapha*, gout, swellings and diarrhoea.

117. *Annona muricata* L. *(Annonaceae)*

Vernacular Name: *Eng:* soursop, custard apple.

Description: Small tree to 7m tall. Leaves alternate, petiolate, the blades leathery and obolong-lanceolate. Flowers 3-merous, sepal and petals fleshy, and greenish in colour. Fruit a fleshy syncarp with a green exocarp covered with conspicuous long pseudo-spines, mescocarp a somewhat fibrous juicy sweet-sour flesh surrounding several large smooth black seeds. Flowers and fruit are usually available throughout the year.

Habitate: Cultivated at lower elevations.

Propagation: By seeds and vegetative method.

Part Used: Leaves and fruits.

Chemical Constituents: Annomonicin, annomontacin, annomruicins, annonacins and derivaties, annonacinone, anomuricine, anomurine anonaine, anoniine, atherospermine, atherosperminine, corepoxylone, corossolone, coclaurine, coreximine, epomuricenins, gigantetrocins, gigantetronenin, deacetyluvarcin, gomothalamicin, howiicins, montanacin, muricatacin, muricatetrocins, muricatocins, murihexocins, murisolin, rolliniastain, solamin, muricine, muricinine, reticuline, lipids, monotetrahydro-furan acetogenins, beta-sitosterol, stigmasterol, and tannins.

Uses: An infusion of the leaves is used in treating stomach ailments. Antimalarial, smooth muscle relaxant, uterine stimulant, anticrustacean, antiparasitic, cytotoxic, cardiac depressant, antiamoebic, antibacterial, antifungal, hypertensive, spasmogenic, vasodilator, insecticide, smooth muscle relaxant.

118. *Annona reticulata* L. *(Annonaceae)*

Vernacular Name: *San:* Ramphala, lavali, lavani, mruduphalam; *Eng:* Bullock's heart; *Hin:* Luvani, anta, nagnewa; *Beng:* Luvuni, nona; *Tam:* Ramasita; *Kan:* Raamaaphala; *Mal:* Manilanilam, parankich-chkka; *Tel:* Raamaaphalamu.

Description: A small deciduous or semi-deciduous tree. 6.1-7.6 m in height. Leaves acuminate, 12.7-20.3 cm long and 3.8-5.1 cm wide. Flowers cordate or subglobose, brownish or yellowish, with flat areoles, 7.6-12.7 cm diam. Flowers in the summer and fruits towards the end of rainy season. Ripe fruits are sweet and edible but inferior to those of A. squamosa.

Habitate: A native of West Indies, naturalized in eastern and south India.

Propagation: By seeds.

Part Used: Furits, seeds, leaves and bark.

Chemical Constituents: Anonaine, norushinsunine, tannic acid, oxoushinsunine and reticuline have been report.

Uses: Unripe and dried fruits are used in diarrhoea and blood dysentery; leaves considered insecticide, anthelmintic and externally useful as suppurant.

119. *Annona squamosa* L. *(Annonaceae)*

Vernacular Name: *San:* Sitaphalam; *Eng:* Custard apple, Sugar apple; *Hin:* Sitaphal; *Kan:* Sitaphala.

Mal: Sitappalam, Attaccakka; *Tam:* Sitappalam; *Tel:* Sitaapandu.

Description: A small tree about 6.0 m in height; leaves simple, alternate, bifarious, oblong-lanceolate or elliptic obtuse, glabrous above, lateral nerves 8-11 pairs ascending; flowers yellowish green, solitary, leaf-opposed or 2-4 on short extra exillary branchlets, sepals and petals three each; fruits yellowish green, globose with well marked areoles easily breaking into large pieces; seeds hard, brownish black, smooth.

Habitate: Throughout India, cultivated.

Propagation: By seeds.

Part Used: Roots, leaves fruits, seeds.

Chemical Constituents: Higenamine, anonaine, roemerine, norcorydiene, corydine, norisocorydine, isocorydine, glaucine, oxoushinsunine, norushinsunine, norlaureline, reticuline, amino acids, epicatechin, catechin, camphor, borneol, squamolone, five kaurane related diterpenes, α-and β-pinine, limonene, β-farnesene, β-sitoserol, rutin, hyperposide and squamocin, a new cytotoxic bis-tetrahydrofuran containing acetogenin.

Uses: The roots are powerful purgative, and are useful in mental depression and spinal disorders. The leaves are suppurative and insecticidal and are useful in destroying lice, proctoptosis in children and as a poultice to produce suppuration. The fruits are sweet, haematinic, cooling, sedative, stimulant, expectorant, maturant and tonic. They are useful in anaemia, burning sensation, vitiated conditions of *pitta,* vomiting, cough, malignant tumours, and for strengthening muscles. The seeds are abortifacient and insecticidal and are useful in destroying lice in the hair.

120. Anogeissus latifolia (Roxb.) Wall. ex Bedd. *(Combretaceae)*

Vernacular Name: *San:* Dahavah; *Eng:* Axle wood; *Hin:* Dhava, Dhaura, Bakali; *Kan:* Dinduge; *Mal:* Vellanava, Malukkanniram; *Tam*: Vellanagai, Vellanamai; *Tel:* Cerimanu, Sirikarra.

Description: A large deciduous tree upto 30 m in height with a clear bole of 15m and with greenish or grayish white smoth bark exfoliating in irregular thin scales; leaves elliptic or suborbicular, obtuse at the apex, rounded or sometimes cordate at base, glabrous when fully gorwn, midrib prominent, pink, main nerves 6-10 pairs arching, prominent on the lower side, leaves turning red before falling; flowers sessible in small dense heads; fruits small, many in a globular head, yellowishbrown, winged, beaked with the persistent calyx enclosing a single seed.

Habitate: Throughout India, in deciduous forests.

Propagation: By seeds.

Part Used: Roots, bark, leaves, fruits, gums.

Chemical Constituents: The gum is principally the calcium salt of a complex high molecular weight polysaccharide acid, ghattic acid conaining mainly L-arabinose, D-galactose, D-mannose, D-xylose and D-galacturonic acid. The dried young leaves and twigs contain hydrolysable or pyrogallol type of tannins. The acetone extract of the leaves on chromatographic analysis gave: a gallotannin, corilagin, gallic acid, chebulic acid, mtrigallic acid, shikimic acid, quinic acid and two unknown acids besides small amounts of ellagic acid. The bark contains tannins.

Uses: The roots are astringent, acrid, thermogenic and stomachic. They are useful in vitiated conditions of *kapha* and *vata*, and abdominal disorders. The bark is astringent, acrid, cooling vulnerary, anti-inflammatory, urinary astringent, haemostatic, constipating, depurative and reguvenating. It is useful in vitiated conditions of *kapha* and *vata*, wounds and ulcers, inflammations, diabetes, haemorrhages, haemoptysis, diarrhoea, dysentery, haemorrhoids, skin diseases, leprosy, hepatopathy, erysipelas, ophthalmia and general debility. The leaf juice is good for otopyorrhea. The fruits are acrid, astringent, sweet, cooling and constipating. They are useful in vitiated conditions of *kapha* and *pitta*, diarrhoea and dysentery.

121. *Anthemis cotula* *(Asteraceae)*

Vernacular Name: *Eng:* Mayweed, Stinking mayweed.

Description: Annual or perennial resembling German and Roman chamomile. Has slightly hairy stems and large solitary daisy-type flowers. As the name stinking mayweed suggests, this plant has an unplea*San*t smell and taste.

Habitate: This herb commonly grows wild in Europe, the Americas, Australia, New Zealand and Siberia. The flowers and leaves are gathered in summer.

Propagation: By Seeds.

Parts Used: Flowers, leaves.

Chemical Constituents: Mayweed contains sesquiterpene lactones.

Uses: Although it is similar in appearance to Roman and German chamomile, mayweed is far less effective as a medicine. It has been used as an antispasmodic and to induce menstruation, and was traditionally employed for supposedly hysterical conditions relating to the uterus. It is rarely used in contemporary herbal medicine.

122. *Anthocephalus chinensis* (Lam.) Rich. Ex. Walp *(Rubiaceae)*

Synonyms*:* *Neolamarckia cadamba* (Roxb.) Bosser, *Anthocephalus cadamba* (Roxb.) Miq.

Vernacular Name: *San*: Kadambah, Kutsitangah, *Eng*: Wild chinchona; *Hin*: Kadamb, *Kan*: Kaduavalatige, Arsenatige, *Mal*: Katampu, Attutekku, *Tam*: Vellaikkatampu, *Tel:* Rudrakskamba.

Description: A medium to large sized deciduous tree with clean cylindrical stem horizontal branches and rounded crown, bark dark grey with longitudinal fissures peeling off in thin scales; leaves elliptic-oblong or ovate, 30 cm long and 15 cm broad pubescent beneath; flowers yellow or orange in globose heads; fruits globose pseudocarps, yellow when ripe.

Habitate: Throughout the Western Ghats at low levels in wet places.

Propagation: By Seeds.

Parts Used: Bark, leaves, fruits.

Chemical Consistuents: Cadambine, cadamine, isocadamine, 3α-dihydrocadambine, 3α-isodihydro-cadambine, 3β-dihydrocadambine and 3β-isodihydro-cadambine. The leaves also yield hentriacontanol and β-sitosterol. The dried stembark gave the sapogenins cadambagenic acid and quinovic acid, β-sitosterol and four saponins, viz. saponins A, B, C and D. the saponins A and B on hydrolysis, gave cadambagenic acid, along with D-glucose and L-rhamnose in the case of A and L-fucose and L-rhamnose in B. the saponins C and D gave quinovic acid, with D-glucose, L-fucose and D-glucose as sugar moieties in C and L-rhamnose and L-fucose in D. the dried bark has been reported to contain steroids, alkaloids, fats and reducing sugars. The heartwood is reported to contain the alkaloids cadambine, 3α-dihydrocadambine, and isodihydrocadambine.

Uses: The bark is bitter, astringent, acrid cooling, anodyne, anti-inflammatory, digestive, carminative alexeteric, galactagogue, febrifuge, diuretic, expectorant, constipating, antiemetic, vulnerary and tonic. It is useful in vitiated conditions of *pitta*, inflammations, haemoptysis, gastropathy, fever, strangury, cough, diarrhoea, vomiting, burning sensation dipsia, ophthalmopathy, wounds, ulcers and debility. A decoction of the leaves is good for ulcers, wounds and metrorrhea. The fruits are useful in gastric irritability and fever.

123. *Anthriscus cerefolium* *(Apeaceae)*

Vernacular Name: *Eng:* Chervil.

Description: Annual herb growing to 60m. Has finely grooved stems, opposite leaves and many small white flowers arranged in compound umbels.

Habitate: Native to Europe, Asia Minor, Iran and the Caucasus, chervil grows freely on wasteground. It is cultivated throughout the world, including Australia and New Zealand.

Propagation: By Seeds.

Parts Used: Aerial parts.

Chemical Constituents: Chervil contains a volatile oil, coumarins and flavonoids.

Uses: Chervil is a good remedy for settling the digestion. It is also used to "purify the blood" and to help lower blood pressure, as well as being considered a diuretic. Juice from the fresh plant is applied to various skin conditions, including wounds, eczema and abscesses.

124. *Aphanamixis polystachya* (Wall.) Parker *(Meliaceae)*

Synonyms: *Amoora rohituka* (Roxb.) Wight & Arn.

Vernacular Name: *San:* Rohitakah; *Eng:* Rohituka tree; *Hin:* Harin-hara; *Kan:* Mullumuntala; *Mal:* Cemmaram; *Tam*: Malampuluvan, Semmaram; *Tel:* Sevamanu.

Description: A medium to large sized tree, 18-25 m height, bark grayish brown to dark brown, rough, exfoliating in circular flakes, wood reddish brown, leaves large, imparipinnate, leaflets opposite, 9-17 in number, elliptic-oblong or oblong-lanceolate, acuminate, glabrous on both surfaces; male flowers numerous in axillary panicles, female or bisexual flowers large than male in axillary or supra-axillary solitary spikes; fruits globular, smooth, yellow when ripe, opening by 3-valved; seeds with scarlet aril.

Habitate: Throughout India, in evergreen forests.

Propagation: By seeds.

Part Used: Bark, seeds.

Chemical Constituents: A limonoid, rohitukin has been isolated from the seeds. The fatty acid composition of the oil is as follows: palmitic, stearic, oleic, linoleic, and linolenic. Petroleum extract of the dried bark gave a new tetranortriterpenoid, aphanamixinin.

Uses: The bark is acrid, astringent, bitter, vulnerary, digestive, anthelmintic, depurative, urinary astringent, opththalimic and refrigerant. It is useful in splenomegaly, liver disorders, tumour, ulcer, dyspepsia, intestinal worms, skin diseases, leprosy, diabetes, ophthalmopathy, jaundice, haemorrhoids, burning sensation, rheumatoid arthritis and leucorrhoea. The seeds are acrid, refrigerant, laxative, anodyne and anthelmintic. They are useful in ulcers, ophthalmopathy, otopathy, myalgia, skin diseases intestinal worms, burning sensation and vitiated conditions of *vata*.

125. *Aphanes arvensis* *(Rosaceae)*

Vernacular Name: *Eng:* Parsley piert.

Description: Prostrate, hairy annual growing to 10cm. Has small wedge-shaped leaves and tiny green flowers in tufts.

Habitate: Parsley piert is native to Europe, North Africa and North America. It grows to an altitude of 500m, thriving in dry sites, including the top of walls.

Propagation: By Cutting.

Parts Used: Aerial parts.

Chemical Constituents: Parsley piert contains tannins.

Uses: Astringent, diuretic and demulcent, parsley piret is used to treat kidney and bladder problems, and is frequently used in the treatment of bladder stones, which cause irritation and obstruct urine flow. Best taken in an infusion, the herb is also a useful remedy for cystitis and recurrent urinary infections. It is combined with marshmallow in cases where a demulcent action is needed.

126. *Apium graveolens* L. *(Apiaceae)*

Synonyms: *Apium dulee* Mill., *Apium lobatum* Gilib.

Vernacular Name: *San*: Ajmoda, *Eng:* Celery, *Hin:* ajmod, *Kan:* Selerina.

Description: An annual or biennial herb. Stem upto 2-4 m. high, erect, branching. Radical leaves pinnate with deeply lobed segments, cauline 3-partite; segments once or twice trifid, coarsely toothed at the apex. Peduncle 6 mm. or less. Umbel rays 5-10, pedicels 6-16. Flowers white, very small; Fruit a cremocarp, each with 2 mericarps, 1-1.5 mm. long with narrow ridges, broad vittae.

Habitate: Cultivated in India, particularly Punjab & U.P. Europe and U.S.A.

Propagation: By seeds.

Parts Used: Fruits.

Chemical Constituents: Choline, Myristic acid, Myristicic acid, Myristoleic acid, Stearic acid; Apiin, Isoquercitrin, Apigenin; Apigravin, Apiumetin, Apiumoside, Bergapten, Celereoside, Rutaretin; α-eudesmol, β-eudesmol, santalol, 3-n-butyl phthalide, sedanenolide. ***Seeds:*** d-Limonene, Selinene, Oleoresin.

Uses: Used as Carminative, Stomachic, Anodyne, Nerve tonic, emmenogogue, Stomach trouble. For complaints of depression and sleeplessness. Obstinate retention of urine, throbbing headache, heartburn. Rheumatic pain in muscles of neck and sacrum. Dysmenorrhoea with short pains in both ovarian regions better by flexing legs, left ovarian pain better by lying on left side. Sharp sticking pain in left iliac region going over to right side. Intense constriction over sternum. Skin urticaria with shuddering. Itching blotches with burning.

127. *Apocynum cannabinum* L. *(Apocynaceae)*

Synonyms: *Apocynum hypercifolium* Ait., *Apocynum sibiricum* Jacq., *Apocynum pubescens* R.Br.

Vernacular Name: *Eng:* Hemp Dogbane.

Description: A perennial herb with stem erect, glabrous or downy, pubescent, upto 1.25 m. in height, having opposite or sub-opposite branches; root creeping, rarely branched, longitudinally wrinkled, grayish-brown externally; leaves pale green, short petioled on the main stem and nearly sessile on the branches, varying from nearly oval to blong and sometimes laneolate; flowers greenish white, bell shaped, in terminal and lateral Cymes; fruit a pair of follicles, 12.5 cm. long, slender and pendulous.

Habitate: Common in U.S.A. and Canada.

Propagation: By seeds.

Parts Used: Roots.

Chemical Constituents: Apocynamarin/Cymarin, Apocannoside. Cynocannoside, K-strophanthin, P-oxyaceto-phenone, Androsterol, Homoandrosterol, Harmalol.

Uses: Useful as cardiac stimulent, Expectorant, Diaphoretic, Emetic, Cathartic and Diuretic. It is one of the most efficient remedies in dropsies, ascites, anascara and hydrothorax and urinary suppression and stranguary. Arrhythmia. Mitral and tricuspid regurgitation. Relaxation of sphincters. Dropsy of serous membrances, after typhoid, scarlatina, cirrhosis. Acute hydrocephalus with open sutures, with stupor, sight of one eye lost. Long continued sneezing. Snuffles of children. Chronic nasal cararrh with tendency to stuffiness. Amenorrhoea in young girls with bloating or dropsical extension of abdomen. Metrorrhagia with continued or paroxysmal flow. Plant milk used for condylomata and warts.

128. *Aquilaria agallocha* Roxb. *(Thymeleaceae)*

Synonyms: *Aquilaria malaccensis.*

Vernacular Name: *San:* Aguruh, Krsnaguruh; *Eng:* Aloe wood, Eagle wood; *Hin:* Agar; *Kan:* Krisnagaru; *Mal:* Akil, Karakil; *Tam:* Agar Agalicandanam, Krsnaguru; *Tel:* Krsnagaru.

Description: A large evergreen tree about 21 m in height, leaves linear-lanceolate to ovate-oblong, 5-9cm long, silky glossy and faintly parallel nerved; flowers small, greenish on very slender pilose petioles in shortly peduncled umbles, on younder branchlets, perianth about 5 mm long, slightly hairy outside, stamens alternate the perianth, filaments red at the apex, ovary tawny-tomentose; fruits slightly compressed, hellowish tomentose capsules.

Habitate: In the forest of Bhutan, Assam and Myanmar.

Propagation: By seeds.

Part Used: Fragrant resinous wood and oil.

Chemical Constituents: The normal wood yields and essential oil which contains selinene, dihydroselinene, two unidentified sesquiterpene-hydrocarbons, agarol, a sesquiterpene alcohol, a hydroxy ketone, five isomeric decenes and rhombic as 5-isopropyl-7-methyl-5,5,5a, 6,7, 8-hexahydro-3H-naphtho. Agarwood, on distillation, yields an essential oil, known as AGAR OIL.

Uses: The wood is acrid, bitter, thermogenic, digestive, carminative, deodorant, sudorific, anodyne, anti-inflammatory, anti-leprotic, depurative, cardiotonic, rejuvenating and tonic. It is useful in vitiated conditions of *vata* and *kapha,* halitosis, dyspepsia, anorexia, cardiac debility, skin disease, leprosy, foul ulcers, hypothermia, inflammations, rheumatoid arthritis, cough, asthma, hiccough, albuminuria and general debility. An external application of agaru is very useful in vomiting in children, pectoralgia due to pneumonia and cephalalgia.

The oil is astringent, acrid, bitter, thermogenic, depurative, alexeteric and antileprotic. It is useful in vitiated conditions of *vata* and *kapha,* rhemunatoid arthritis, cough, asthma, bronchitis, leprosy, skin diseases and foul ulcers.

129. *Aquilaria sinensis* (Lour.) Gilg. *(Thymelaeaceae.)*

Vernacular Name: *Eng:* Chinese eaglewood.

Description: An evergreen large tree, upto 20 m high. Young shoots pilose. Leaves alternate, petiolate, elliptic or obovate-oblong, 5-9 cm long by 2.5-4.5 cm wide, apex briefly acuminate, base cuneate, entire, thin-chartaceous, slightly appressed-pilose on the nerves beneath or glabrous, with a silky gloss, faintly parallel nerved. Umbels, terminal or axillary, with 4-12 cm peduncle. Rather small greenish flowers in early summer, on very slender pilose pedicels 4.6 mm long or even longer. Capsules obovate suneate, slightly compressed, about 2.5 cm long, densely tawny or yellowish-tomentose, in a dried state shriveled and wrinkled.

Habitate: In China forests.

Propagation: By seeds.

Part Used: Wood.

Uses: Stomachic in gastralgia, colic, nervous vomiting.

130. *Arachis hypogaea* L. *(Fabaceae)*

Vernacular Name: *San:* Bhucanakah, Mandapi; *Eng:* Groundnut, Peanut, Monkeynut; *Hin:* Mung-phali; *Kan:* Nllakadali; *Mal:* Nilakkatala; *Tam:* Verkkatalai and *Tel:* Verusenagalu.

Description: A branched hairy annual herb with erect branches trailing on the ground; leaves compound, pulvinate, 8-12cm long, leaflets oblong to obovate, entire; flowers yellow, axillary, fascicled; fruits pods, ripening undergound, leathery, containing 1-3 seeds.

Habitate: Throughout India, cultivated.

Propagation: By seeds.

Part Used: Seeds, oil.

Chemical Constituents: The different constituents of follows: moisture, protein, lipids, crude fibre, N-free extr; reducing sugars, disaccharide sugars, starch and pentosans, Oil contains glycerides of palmitin and olein, hypogaeic, lignocerric, linolic and arachidic acids. The ground nut is also very rich in Vitamin-B_1, Nicotinic acid and riboflavin.

Uses: The seeds are sweet, oleaginous, aphrodisiac, galactagogue, constipating and tonic and are useful in agalactia, diarrhoea and general debitlity. The oil is sweet, purgative and emollient, and is used in nephropathy and dislocated joints.

131. *Aralia cordata* Thunb. *(Araliaceae)*

Vernacular Name: *Eng:*-Japanese spikenard.

Description: Spineless perennial herb, to 2 m tall, loosely short pilose throughout except the flowers. Leaves alternate, deltoid in outline, long-petiolate, 2-3 pinnate; leaflets of each pinna 5-7, ovate, acuminate at tip, 5-30 cm long, 3-20 cm wide, unequally serrate, sessile or short-petiolate. Inflorescence loosely branched raceme, arranged in large panicles terminal or axillary on upper part of stems. Flowers small, pale green, 3 mm across; petals 5, more or less imbricate; stamens 5; ovary 2-5 celled; styles 2-5, separate. Fruit a drupe, pyrenes 2-5.

Habitate: Thickets and woody areas, especially along streams. Sometimes cultivated found in Korea, Japan and China.

Propagation: By seeds and stem cutting.

Parts Used: Root.

Chemical Constituents: Essential oils. Various diterpene acids of pimarane and kaurane series. Methylesters of udosaponins A, B, C, D, E. Sesquiterpenes.

Uses: Anti-inflammatory activities(continentalic acid, kaurenoic acid). Analgesis. Antioedema. Antianaphylactic. Used in common cold, migraine.

132. *Aralia racemosa* L. *(Araliaceae)*

Vernacular Name: *Eng:* American spikenard.

Description: An aromatic perennial deciduous herb growing 1 to 2 m. in in height; stem ligneously, herbaceous, smooth, bifurcating, much branched and devoid of prickles; root large, thick, fleshy, aromatic, whitish internally; leaves very large oddpinnately compound, leaflets, cordate to ovate-cordate, doubly serrate, acuminate, usually glabrous beneath; flowers small greenish-yellow, monoeciously polygamous or perfect appearing in July; fruit globular, dark purplish to reddish brown, aromatic, drupes retaining the persistent calyx and divariacate styles.

Habitate: Rocky woods in North America.

Propagation: By Rhizomes and seeds.

Parts Used: Rhizomes and roots.

Chemical Constituents: Contains a volatile oil; a glycosidal seponin, called Araliin and Resin 3%.

Uses: Mainly asthmatic conditions with cough aggrevated on lying down. Prolapse of rectum with aching extending upwards. Dry cough coming on after first sleep, about midnight. Construction of chest, feels as if foreign body is lodged in throat, with frequent sneezing. Least current of air causes sneezing with copious watery, excruciating nasal discharge.

133. *Arbutus unedo* *(Ericaceae)*

Vernacular Name: *Eng:* Strawberry tree.

Description: Evergreen shrub growing to 6m. Has an upright stem with reddish bark, leathery serrated leaves, white or pink bell-shaped flowers and round warty red fruit resembling strawberries.

Habitate: Native to Mediterranean coasts, strawberry tree also grows in western Ireland, Australia and Africa. The leaves are gathered in late summer and the fruit in autumn.

Propagation: By Branch cutting.

Parts Used: Leaves fruit.

Chemical Constituents: Strawberry tree contains up to 2.7% arbutin, methylarbutin and other hydroquinones, a bitter principle, and tannins. Arbutin is powerfully antiseptic in the urinary system.

Uses: Strawberry tree is valued as an astringent and antiseptic herb. Its antiseptic action within the urinary tract makes it a useful remedy for treating cystitis and urethritis. Strawberry tree's astringent effect has been put to use in the treatment of diarrhoea and dysentery. Like many other astringent plants, it makes a gargle.

134. *Arctium lappa* L. *(Asteraceae)*

Vernacular Name: Jangli kuth, Burdock.

Description: An erect herb, branched, biennial to perennial; upto 1 m. or more tall. Leaves ovate, cordate, margins undulate, usually cottony beneath, stalked, 75-30 cm across. Flower heads globose, 1.8-3.7 cm across, in terminal clusters. Involucral bracts with rigid awl-like spreading barbed tips. Corolla and stamens purple-pink; style white, Achenes oblong, ribbed, angled.

Habitate: Occurs widely in Western Himalaya, 1800-3800m.

Propagation: By seeds.

Part Used: Root.

Chemical Constituents: The roots contain a hexasaccharide, arctose, a mucilaginous substance, tannis, volatile oil, stigmasterol and sitosterol. The presence of volatile and non-volatile fatty acids, various free amino acids including most of the essential one. And γ-guanidino-n-butyric acid, and a new sulphur-containing acetylenic acid called arctic acid has also been reported.

Uses: It has diuretic and arexigenic properties and it has been used for cutaneous eruptions, rheumatism, cystitis, gout and specifically for eczema and psoriasis. The plant extract has been found to cause sharp, long lasting reduction of blood sugar within increase in carbohydrate tolerance and less toxicity. 50% ethyl alcohol extract was found as cardiac, stimulant, diuretic and spasmolytic.

135. *Arctium majus* Bernh. *(Asteraceae)*

Synonyms: *Arctium lappa* Linn., *Lappa atrium* Hill., *Lappa major* Gaertn.

Vernacular Name: *Eng:* Great Burdock.

Description: A coarse, biennial seed with simple spindle-shaped externally brown roots; stem 1 m. high round furrowed, succulant and pubescent, erect, brunched and leafy. Leaves large, alternate, long-petioled, the upper ovate and the lower cordate, dentate, green above and whitish, cottony beneath. Flowers; purple in homogamous heads, with the imbricated scales of the involucre forming a hooked pouch.

Habitate: Europe and northern Asia; naturalized in United States and southern England.

Propagation: By seeds.

Parts Used: Root.

Chemical Constituents: Arctinone-a; Arctinone-b; Arctinol-a; Arctino-b; Arctinal; Arctic acid-b; Arctic acid-c; Methyl arctate-b; Arctionone-a-acetate; 1, 11-ridecadiene-3, 5, 7, 9-terayne; 1, 3, 11-tridecatrine-5, 7, 9-triyne; 1-tridecen-3, 5, 7, 9, 11-pentayne; Acids like cholrogenic acid, Acetic acid; Butyric acid, Gamma-guanidino-n-butyric acid, α-Guanidino-n-isovaleric acid, lauric acid, Myristic acid. Aldlhydes like valeraldehyde; Lactones e.g. Arctiopicrin, Lappatin, phytosterols. Inuline.

Uses: Very important in skin thereapeutics. Eruptions on head, face & neck. Pimples, Acne. Styes and ulcerations on the edge of eyelids. Profuse & frequent urination. Crops of boils & styes. Pain in hand, knees & ankles extending downwards to fingers & toes. Uterine displacement. An exceedingly sore bruised feeling in uterus with relaxed vagina. Traditionally it is used for cutaneous eruption, cystitis, gout, Anoraxia nervosa, eczema & psoriasis.

136. *Arctostaphylos uva-ursi* *(Ericaceae)*

Vernacular Name: *Eng:* Uva-ursi, Bearberry.

Description: Low-lying evergreen shrub growing to 50cm. Has long trailing stem, dark green leaves that are glossy on the upper side, bell-shaped pink flowers and small glossy red berries.

Habitate: Uva-uris is native to Europe, and naturalized throughout the northern hemisphere up to arctic. It grows in damp conditions in undergrowth, heathland and grassland.

Propagation: By Brach cutting.

Parts Used: Leaves berries.

Chemical Constituents: The leaves of uva-uris contain hydroquinones, phenolic glycosides and flavonoids. Arbutin and other hydroquinones have an antiseptic effect in the urinary tract.

Uses: Uva-uris is one of the best natural urinary antiseptics. It has been used extensively in herbal medicine to disinfect and astringe the urinary tract in cases of acute and chronic cystitis and urethritis. However, it is not a suitable remedy if there is a simultaneous infection of the kidneys.

137. *Areca catechu* L. *(Palmaceae)*

Vernacular Name: *San:* Gubak, poogiphalam, tantusara; *Eng:* Betal-nut palm, areca-nut palm, betel palm, areca palm, penang palm, catechu palm; *Hin:* Supari; *Beng*: Gau, supari; *Kan:* Adike, betta, chikaniyadike, puga; *Mal:* Adakkamaram, kavungu, kazhangu; *Tam:* Kamugu, paakkumaram, pugam; *Tel:* Gautupoka, kolapoka, oppuvakkulu, vakka.

Description: Slender palm about 10m tell. Stem erect, surmounted by a crown of pinnate leaves; petiole broadly expanded at the base. Inflorescence in spadix encased in a spathe; flowers yellowish-white in much-branched raceme, which bears both male and female flowers. Fruit ovoid; pericarp hard and fibrous; kernel (seed) brown.

Habitate: Under cultivation in south India and parts of North-East.

Propagation: By seeds.

Part Used: Pericarps and kernels.

Chemical Constituents: The kernels yield tannin, catechin (70% in the young fruit, 15–20% in the over-ripe fruit), lipids consisting of laurin, olein and myristin; glucides 50-60%; alkaloids: arecoline, arecaidine, arecaine, guvacine and guvacoline.

Uses: The pericarp is effective in the treatment of flatulence, oedema, dysuria and hyperaemesis of pregnancy. The kernel is used to treat diarrhoea and dysentery. It is also a taenifuge. It is also said to cure malaria. Arecoline induces papillary contraction and decreases ocular tension in glaucoma.

138. *Arenaria rubra* *(Carophyllaceae)*

Vernacular Name: *Eng: San*dwort, *San*d spurrey.

Description: Herbaceous, low-growing, sticky and hairy annual. Has small thin leaves and pale pink flowers growing to 6mm across.

Habitate: Found in the wild throughout Europe, Asia and Australia, *San*dwort thrives in *San*dy and gravelly places, especially close to the sea.

Propagation: By seeds.

Parts Used: Aerial parts.

Uses: *San*dwart is a diuretic herb that is thought to relax the muscle walls of the urinary tubules and bladder. *San*dwort is most commonly taken stones, acute and chronic cystitis, and other conditions of the bladder.

139. *Argemone mexicana* L. *(Papaveraceae)*

Vernacular Name: *San:* Svamaksiri, Brahmadanti; *Eng:* Mexican poppy, Yellow Mexican poppy, Prickly poppy; *Hin:* Satyanasi, Bhatbhamt, Pharamgi dhattura; *Kan:* Arasina, Ummatta, Datturigida; *Mal:* Ponnummattu, Kantankattiri; *Tam:* Kutiyotti, Ponnummattai; *Tel:* Brahmadandicettu.

Description: A strong, branched, prickly annual, 60-90cm in height with yellow latex; leaves simple, sessil, spiny, semi-amplexcaul, sinuate-pinnatified, variegated with white, spinous, veins white; flowers large, bright yellow, terminal on short leafy branches; fruits prickly capsules, oblong-ovoid, opening by 4-6 valves; seeds numerous.

Habitate: Throughout the hotter parts of India, in areas upto 1,500 m.

Propagation: By seeds.

Part Used: Whole plant.

Chemical Constituents: Allocryptopine, berberine, cheilanthifoline, chelerythrine, coptisine, cryptopine, dihydrosanguinarine, norchelerythrine, norsanguinarine, oxyhydrastinine, protopine, sanguinarine, β-scoiulerine methrohydroxide, α-and β-stylopine methohydroxide, 6-acetonyl-dihydrosanguinarine, α-tetrahydropalmatine methohydroxide, mexicanol and mexicanic acid have been reported. The flowers contain isorhamntin, isorhamnetin-3-glucoside and isorhamnetin-3, 7-diglucoside.

Uses: **The plant is bitter, acrid, cooling vulnerary, diuretic, depurative, anodyne, anthelmintic, antipyretic, ophthalmic, stomachic and sedative.**

The roots are useful in guinea-wrm infestation, skin diseases, leprosy, pruritus, blennorrhagia, inflammations, all types of poisoning, constipation, flatulence, colic, malarial fever and vesicular calculus. The leaves are useful in cough, wounds, ulcers and skin diseases. The seeds are useful in vitiated conditions of *kapha*, cough, asthma, pertussis, skin diseases, leprosy, ulcers, wounds odontalgia, dental caries, constipation, rheumatialgia, colic and flatulence. The latex is useful in dropsy, jaundice, skin diseases, leprosy, blisters, indolent ulcers, conjunctivitis, inflammations, burning sensation and malarial fever. The oil is useful in indolent ulcers, woulds, leprosy, skin diseases, constipation, flatulence, colic and rheumatalgia.

140. *Argyreia nervosa* (Burm.f.) Boj. *(Convolvulaceae)*

Synonyms: *Argyreia speciosa* Sweet.

Vernacular Name: *San:* Vrddhadarukah, Bastantri; *Eng:* Elephant creeper; *Hin:* Samandar-ka-pat, Samudrasos. Tameshar; *Kan:* Candrapada; *Mal:* Marikkunni, Marututari, Samudrappacca; *Tam:* Samuttirappaccai, Samuttirappalai; *Tel:* Candrapada.

Description: A very large climbing shrub with woody, white, tomentose stems; leaves simple, large, ovae, acute, base cordate, glabrous above, white tomentose beneath; flowers large, purple, silky-pubescent without in long-peduncled cymes, fruits dry, globose, apiculate.

Habitate: Throughout India, in areas upto 900 m elevation.

Propagation: By seeds.

Part Used: Roots & seeds.

Chemical Constituents: Tannin, and amber-coloured acid-resin soluble in ether, benzole and partly soluble in alkalies.

Uses: The roots are acrid, bitter, astringent, sweet, emollient, thermogenic, roborant, appetizer, disgetive, carminative, aperient, cardiotonic, anti-inflammatory, expectorant, diuretic, aphrodisiac, rejuvenating, intellect promoting, brain tonic, nervine tonic and tonic. They are useful in vitiated conditions of *kapha* and *vata*, emaciation, wounds, ulcers, anorexia, dyspepsia, flatulence, colic, constipation, cardiac debility, inflammations, cough, bronchitis, strangury, seminal weakness, nervous weakness, cerebral disorders, synovitis, heamorrhoids, obesity, hoarseness, syphilis, anaemia, diabetes, tuberculosis, arthritis, ascites, leucorrhoea and general debility.

141. *Arisaema amurense* Maxim. *(Araceae)*

Vernacular Name: *Eng:*-Jack-in-the-pulpit.

Description: Stemless, perennial herb, with well-developed tuber. Tuber depressed globose, 2-4 cm in diameter, bearing 2-3 small tubers; fibrous roots spreading from the top of tuber. Leaves pedate, segments 5, 10-20 cm long, middle one obovate, lateral ones oblong-lanceolate, petioles 15-30 cm long. Peduncle stout, shorter thanpetioles; spathe 10 cm long, tube pale green, margined with purple, blade erect, 5-6 cm long, greenish and sometimes purple-striped, or violet. Spadix with terminal appendage cylindrical, 4 cm long.

Habitate: Wet and shady areas in mountains found in Korea, Japan and China.

Propagation: By tubers.

Parts Used: Tuber.

Chemical Constituents: Saponins, diacylglycerylgalactosides.

Uses: Anticonvulsant. Platelet aggregation inhibition. Used in headache, expectorant, sputum, remedy.

142. *Aristolochia bracteolata* Lam. *(Aristolochiaceae)*

Synonyms: *Aristolochia bracteat.*

Vernacular Name: *San:* Kitamari; *Eng:* Worm killer, Bracteated birthwort; *Hin:* Kiramar, Kitamar; *Kan:* Sanajalihallu; *Mal:* Attukottappala, Atutinnappala; *Tam:* Atutinnappalai; *Tel:* Gadidagadapaku.

Description: A perennial prostrate herb with weak, glabrous stems; leaves simple, alternate reniform or broadly ovate, cordate at the base with a wide sinus upto 7.5 cm in diameter, finely reticulately veined; flowers solitary with a large sessily orbicular bract at the base, perianth tube cylindric with dark purple lip having revolute margins; fruits oblong-ellipsoid 12-ribbed glabrous capsules; seeds deltoid with slightly cordate base.

Habitate: Throughout India.

Propagation: By seeds.

Part Used: Roots, leaves.

Chemical Constituents: The leaves and fruits contain ceryl alcohol, β-sitosterol and aristolochic acid. The fatty-acid composition of the seeds is myristic, palmitic, stearic, lignoceric and oleic. Aristolochic acid, aristored, a nitrogen containing compound, and magnoflorine have also been reported from the seeds.

Uses: The roots and leaves are bitter, acrid, thermogenic, anthelmintic, cathartic, anti-inflammatory, emmenagogue, vulnerary, appetizer, sudorific and antiperiodic, and are useful in vitiated conditions of *kapha* and *vata*, intestinal worms, constipation, inflammations, amenorrhoea, dysmenorrhoea, foul ulcer, boils, syphilis, gonorrhoea, dyspepsia, colic, skin diseases, eczema, arthralgia and intermittent fevers.

143. *Aristolochia clematitis* *(Aristolochiaceae)*

Vernacular Name: *Eng:* Birthwort.

Description: Unpleasant-smelling perennial with heart-shaped leaves and tubular yellow flowers with flattened lips.

Habitate: Native to central and southern Europe, birthwort is also found in south-western Asia.

Propagation: By Seeds.

Parts Used: Roots.

Chemical Constituents: Birthwort contains aristolochic acids, a volatile oil and tannins. While stimulating white blood cell activity, aristolochic acid is also carcinogenic and damaging to the kidneys.

Uses: Little used today, birthwort was formerly used to treat wounds, sores and snake bite. It has been taken after childbirth to prevent infection and is also a potent menstruation-inducing herb and a abortifacient. A decoction was taken to encourage healing of ulcers. Birthwort has also been used for asthma and bronchitis.

144. *Aristolochia contorta* Bunge *(Aristolochiaceae)*

Vernacular Name: *Eng:*-Birthwort.

Description: Climbing perennial shrub, with stout elongated rhizomes. Stem slender, glabrous. Leaves alternate, cordate or broadly ovate-cordate, 4-10 cm long, 3.5-8 cm wide, acute or obtuse at tip, cordate at base, entire, petioles 1-7 cm long. Peduncles axillary, 1-4 cm long, with prominent bracts at base. Flowers few in axils, fascicled, the pedicels 1-4 cm long; the calyx tubular, inflated and globose at base, loosely pilose inside; the limb dilated, obliquenly truncate, narrowly deltoid, long-acuminate to a filiform point; stamens 6, ovary inferior. Fruit a capsule, globose, 3 cm in diameter, 6 valved.

Habitate: Edges of mountain woods found in Japan, Korea and China.

Propagation: By seeds.

Parts Used: Fruit, root.

Chemical Constituents: Aristolactam derivatives and their N-Glycosides: 8-desmethoxyaristolactam, 6-hydroxy-8-desmethoxy-aristolactam N-b-d-glucopyranoside. Oxoaporphines: dioxodehydroasisnilobine, lysicamine.

Uses: Antimicrobial, hallucinogen, immunostimulating, antitumour, antitumour, carcinogen (aristolochic acid and derivatives). Hypotensive (magnoflorine). Used in cough and sputum.

145. *Aristolochia debilis sieb.* Et. Zucc. *(Aristolochiaceae)*

Vernacular Name: *Eng:* Slender Dutchman's pipe.

Description: A perennial creping herb, up to 2 m long. Root cylindrical, often curved, yellowish-brown and aromatic. Stem slender, glabrous. Fresh stem and leaves possess a special odour. Leaves alternate, long-petiolate. Blade narrowly triangular-ovate, 3-8 cm long by 2-4.5 cm wide, base cordate and auriculate on both side Peduncles solitary, without bracts. Flowers irregular; summerl perianth simple, tube globular, inflated at the base, narrow, cylindrical at the top; limb oblique, descending, oval-lanceolate, acuminate, nearly as long as the tube. Fruit a rounded capsule, 6Ovalved; autumn; seeds berry numerous, compressed, winged.

Habitate: On slopes, at forest edges, in thickets or on gravely land in China and Japan.

Propagation: By seeds.

Part Used: Fruit, roots, herb.

Uses: Fruit, cough and dyspnaea, dyspnaea due to retention of sputum. Roots, stomach-ache, dizzines due to, hypertension, rheumatic arthritis, bruises and bone injuries, sore throat, toothache; eczemal poisonous snake bites, herb, cough due to inflammatioin in lung, dyspneae due to retention of sputum.

146. *Aristolochia roxburghiana* Klotsch *(Aristolochiaceae)*

Synonyms: *Aristolochia tagala.*

Vernacular Name: *Tel:* Nallayiswari and *Assam:* Belikol, Panipipuli.

Description: Slender climbing vine. Stems woody at the base, grooved, glabrous. Leaves alternate, long-petioled; base cordate, acuminate at the apex. Inflorescence in axillary raceme; bract small; flowers numerous, purplish-brown; perianth curved, mouth oblique. Capsule ovoid splitting into 6 valves. Seeds numerous, deltoid, flat and winged.

Habitate: Grows wild in mountainous regions.

Propagation: By seeds.

Part Used: Root.

Chemical Constituents: The leaves and fruits contain ceryl alcohol, β-sitosterol and aristolochic acid. The fatty-acid composition of the seeds is myristic, palmitic, stearic, lignoceric and oleic. Aristolochic acid, aristored, a nitrogen containing compound, and magnoflorine have also been reported from the seeds.

Uses: The roots are stomachic and are used in the treatment of colic, gastritis, entireties, diarrhoea, dysentery, food poisoning, furunculosis, rheumatism, oedema and dysmenorrhoea. A combination with some other plants is said to cure malaria. It is also used as tonic, carminative & immenagogue.

147. *Armeniaca valgaris* Lam. *(Rosaceae)*

Vernacular Name: *Eng:* Apricot.

Description: Small tree, 3-5m. high. Leaves alternate, obscurely cordate at the base, apex pointed; margins toothed. Flowers white, appearing before the leaves. Drupe round-ovate, velvety pubescent when young, nearly glabrous at maturity, with a yellow skin; stone hard, irregularly furrowed.

Habitate: Cultivated as a fruit-tree.

Propagation: By seeds.

Part Used: Fruit.

Chemical Constituents: The fruit contains organic acids: citric, tartaric, pangamic carotenoids: lycopene, α-carotene; flavonoids: quercetin, isoquercetin; vitamins A and C. The fruit kernels yield fixed oil enzyme, amygdalin and emulsin.

Uses: The salted fruit is used as an antiseptic and anti-inflammatory in respiratory and digestive diseases. It is used in the treatment of cough, dyspnoea, asthma, laryngitis, sore throat, ascariasis, dysentery and persistent diarrhoea. The liquid distilled from the seed kernels is toxic and active against cough, dyspnoea and gastralgia. The oil from the seed kernels is used as a laxative, in the form of an emulsion with water.

148. *Armoracia rusticana* *(Cruciferae)*

Synonyms: *Colchlearia armoracia.*

Vernacular Name: *Eng:* Horseradish.

Description: Perennial growing to 50 cm. Has a deep root, large leaves and cluster of 4-petalled white flowers.

Habitate: Native to Europe and western Asia, this herb is widely cultivated for its root.

Propagation: By Seed and cutting.

Parts Used: Root and leaves.

Chemical Constituents: Horseradish root contains glucosilinates, asparagines, resin and vitamin C. On being crushed, sinigrin produces allyl isothiocyanate, an antibiotic substance.

Uses: Now undervalued as a medicinal herb, horseradish has many healing properties. it strongly stimulates the digestion, increasing gastric secretions and appetite. It is a good diuretic and promotes perspiration, making it useful in fevers, colds and flu. It is also expectorant and mildly antibiotic, and can be of use in both respiratory and urinary tract infections. A *San*dwich of freshly grated root is a home remedy for hay fever. Externally, a poultice of the root can soothe chilblains.

149. Arnebia benthami (Wall. Ex G. Don.) Johnston *(Boraginaceae)*

Synonyms: *Macrotomia benthamii* DC.

Vernacular Name: Ratanjot, Laljari, Masreen.

Description: An erect, robust, herbaceous perennial, 30-90 cm tall with stout, woody, deep-red roots. Leaves narrow, lanceolate, hairy. Radical leaves are large, 28 cm x 1.3 cm; cauline leaves, 7.5 cm x 1.3 cm. Flowers pink purple in dense terminal spikes, bending downwards like a tail.

Habitate: Sub-alpine to alpine Himalayas upto 3,500 to 4,500 m.

Propagation: By seeds.

Part Used: Roots.

Uses: The plant is considered expectorant and used for cardiac disorders. Aqueous extracts, syrup, (Sharbat) and jam prepared from the flowering shoots are considered useful in diseases of the tongue, throat and is also useful in fever. Used as a colouring matter in hair oils, cookeries and for dyeing of silk. Root is frequently used as an antiseptic and antibiotic in healing of the wounds when applied as a poultice and also for subsiding water is applied to fireburns and is a quick healer.

150. Arnebia euchroma (Royle) Johnston Contr. *(Boraginaceae)*

Synonyms: *Macrotomia perennis* Boiss.

Vernacular Name: Ratanjot, Khanmet, Dimo.

Description: An erect caespitose, perennial, hairy herb, with thick purple roots. Stems many, arising from the axil of the leaves, which formed a sterile basal cluster the preceding year; fistular, striate, covered with white trichomes. Basal leaves lanceolae, acute; lower and middle cauline leaves sessile, lanceolate; upper ones usually shorter and broader. Flowers pink or purplish-White, in terminal, subglobular inflorescence. Bracts leaf-like, not exceeding the calys. Nutlets irrularly and coarsely tuberculate.

Habitate: Afghanistan to Central Nepal, Western and Central Asia between 3300-4500 m in drier areas.

Propagation: By seeds.

Part Used: Roots.

Uses: Roots are used in toothache, ear-ache, eye diseases, as healer of cuts and wounds and also the fire burns. It has been reported to be an antipyretic, anti-microbial and anti-inflammatory. The purple roots are used as hair tonic by the local people and often dug out for sale.

151. *Arnica montana* *(Asteraceae)*

Vernacular Name: *Eng:* Arnica.

Description: Aromatic perennial growing to 30cm. Has downy egg-shaped leaves and bright yellow daisy-like flowers.

Habitate: Arnica grows in mountain woods and pastures in central Europe, the Pyrenees, Siberia and north-western US and Canada. Its flowers are harvested when in full bloom; the rhizomes after the plant has died back in autumn.

Propagation: By Seeds and cutting.

Parts Used: Flowers and rhizomes.

Chemical Constituents: Arnica contains sesquiterpene lactones, flavonoids, and a volatile oil that includes thymol, mucilage and polysaccharides.

Uses: Best known as an effective ointment and compress for bruises, sprains and muscle pain, arnica improves the local blood supply and accelerates healing. It is anti-inflammatory and increases the rate of reabsorption of internal bleeding.

152. *Artemisia annua* L. *(Asteraceae)*

Vernacular Name: *Eng:* Sweet wormwood.

Description: An annual herb 30-90 cm high, very fragrant, stem furrowed, passing into an ample spreading brancheing compoung panicle. Basal leaves long-petiolate, in outline triangular-ovate bipinnatisect; primary segments petiolate, secondary ones oblong with acute, dentate pinnatipartite laciniate. Primary rachis without teeth. Floral leaves sessile, with linear setaceous teeth. Inflorescence a terminal, compound panicle; September-November. Flower heads hetrogamous, fruit an obvoid achene, smooth, 0.5 mm long.

Habitate: On waste land, roadsides, slopes, in grassland and by river banks in China, India, Japan, Korea, Soviet Union and Viet Nam.

Propagation: By seeds and vegetative method.

Part Used: Whole plant.

Uses: Fever due to summer heat; low fever without sweat, intermittent fever due to tuberculosis, malaria.

153. *Artemisia abrotanum* *(Asteraceae)*

Vernacular Name: *Eng:* Southernwood.

Description: Strongly aromatic, shrubby perennial, growing to 1m. Has woody stems, feathery silver-green leaves *S*and yellow flowers.

Habitate: Native to southern Europe, this he4rb is rare in the wild but is cultivated for the perfume industry and, to a lesser extent, for herbal medicine. The aerial parts are harvested in late summer.

Propagation: By Seeds and vegetative method.

Parts Used: Aerial parts.

Chemical Constituents: Southernwood contains a volatile oil, abrotanin and tannins.

Uses: Southernwood is a bitter tonic. It strengthens and supports digestive function by increasing secretions in the stomach and intestines. An infusion of southernwood has been given to children as a treatment for worms, but his is not recommended without professional supervision. Like other *Artemisias,* southernwood stimulates menstruation and is commonly taken to encourage the onset of irregular or absent periods.

154. *Artemisia absinthium* L. *(Astraceae)*

Synonyms: *Absinthium officinale* Lam.

Vernacular Name: *San:* Damara, Indhana, Aphasantin; *Eng:* Wormwood, Abisinthe, Madarwood, Ajenjo; *Hin:* Vilayathi ajsanthin; *Tel:* maachipati, tartiha; *Beng*: Mastaru; *Kan*: Urittige, uruvalu and *Mal:* Nilampala.

Description: An aromatic and bitter shrubby plant. Stems erect, angular, hoary and ribbed; leaves ovate to obovate, unequally 2-3 pinnatifidly cut into spreading linear or lanceolate-obtuse segments, hoary on both surfaces; flower heads heterogamous, numerous but hardly crowded, flowers yellow, ray florets dilated below; outer involucral bracts oblong, hoary, narrowly scarious; inner orbicular, broadly scarious; receptacular hair long, straight; achences elliptic-oblong.

Habitate: Native of Europe, found in Kashmir upto 1,500 to 2,000 m.

Propagation: By seeds and vegetative methods.

Part Used: Whole plant.

Chemical Constituents: Essential oil known as absinth or Wormwood oil. Artemisetin. Absinthin, artabasin, myrcene, a-pinene, thujyl alcohol and thujyi acetate.

Uses: Damara is tonic, stomachic, febrifuge and anthelmintic. It is useful for inflammation of liver and menstrual disorders. Tincture of the plant is used as tonic, digestive, febrifuge, anthelmintic and for brain concussions. It is a remedy for enfaabled digestions and debility. Flowers are vermifuge, tonic in intermittent fever. Drug "Afsanteen" used in chronic fever, swellings and inflammation of liver. It is also used as tonic and stimulant.

155. *Artemisia brevifolia* Wall. *(Asteraceae)*

Synonyms: *Artemisia maritime* Linn.

Vernacular Name: *San:* Gadadhari, gandha; *Hin:* Kirmala and *Kash*: Moorni.

Description: A strongly aromatic, much branched shrubby perennial with highly dissected, grayish to white leaves. Flower heads yellow to yellowish-red arranged in clusters of axillary spikes.

Habitate: Common in dry temperate and cold desert areas.

Propagation: By seeds and vegetative methods.

Part Used: Whole plant.

Chemical Constituents: It contain santonin, β-santonin, pseudosantonin and a bitter principal artemisin. The yellowish essential oil containt α-and β-pinens, comphene, cineol, thujone, dicyclic aldehyde camphor, bornyl acetate, citral, α-terpineol and βOcaryophyllene.

Uses: The drug is now rarely used as an aromatic, bitter for the loss of appetite, week digestion and stomach complaints. As a carminative, it is one of the strongly aromatic spice herbs used particularly with meat dishes, especially fatty roast goose, where taste and digestibility is improved. Also used in asthma and diseases of brain,. Santonin is very effective in action on round worms, less effective in thread worms and has no action on tape worms.

156. *Artemisia cina* *(Asteraceae)*

Vernacular Name: *Eng:* Levant Wormwood.

Description: Shrub by perennial with long thin leaves and tiny round tufts of flowers.

Habitate: This herb is native to the region stretching from the eastern Mediterranean to Siberia. The unopened flower heads are gathered from wild and cultivated plants.

Propagation: By Seeds and cutting.

Parts Used: Flower heads.

Chemical Constituents: Levant wormwood contains Santonin, artemisin and a volatile oil. Santonin is directly toxic to roundworms and, to a lesser extent, threadworms.

Uses: Used almost exclusively to expel worms, levant wormwood is strongly bitter and aromatic and has a tonic and stimulant effect on the digestion. The dried flowerheads are occasionally mixed with honey to disguise their bitterness.

157. *Artemisia dracunculus* L. *(Asteraceae)*

Vernacular Name: Dragon mugwort, estragon, tarragon.

Description: A perennial herb; stems grooved, leaves linear oblong; flower-heads almost round in branched racemes.

Habitate: Alpine regions of Kashmir and western Himalayas.

Propagation: By seeds.

Part Used: Aerial parts.

Chemical Constituents: The principal volatile component of tarragon oil is methyl chavicol. Other major compounds are sabinene, methyl eugenol, elemecin, Y-terpinene and ocimene.

Uses: Tarragon oil with its sweet, spicy-aromatic, anise-like odour is used for flavouring vinegar, sauces, pickles, salad dressings, canned soups, and liqueurs.

158. *Artemisia gmelini* Weber ex Stechm. *(Asteraceae)*

Vernacular Name: *Eng:*-Russian wormwood.

Description: Perennial herb from woody rhizomes to 50-100 cm tall. Stems tufted, slightly woody at base, branched. Leaves cauline; median leaves bi-pinnate, ovate, acute, base truncate, upper surface short pubescent, lower surface glandular dotted, petioles 2-3 cm long, segments 6-10 pairs, oblong, obtuse, the ultimate segment pinnately lobed, 1.5-4.5 mm wide; upper leaves gradually smaller. Heads 3-3.5 mm across, in panicles; involucre globose, 3-3.5 mm high; phyllaries in 3 series, nearly glabrous. Ray flowers female, corolla narrowly tubular, 1.3 mm long, density glandular dotted; disc flowers bisexual, corolla 1.8 mm long, tube 0.8 mm long. Achenes 1.5 mm long.

Habitate: Rocky slopes from coast to mountains found in Japan, Korea, China and Southern Russia to Siberia.

Propagation: By seeds and stem cutting.

Parts Used: Leaf, stem.

Chemical Constituents: Flavonoids, phenylpropanoids, scopoletin. Monoterpenes, sesquiterpenes.

Uses: Used in hepatitis, hyperlipaemia, infected cholecystitis.

159. *Artemisia nilagirica* (Clarke) Pamp. *(Asteraceae)*

Synonyms: *Artemisia vulgaris* auct. Non. Linn.

Vernacular Name: *San:* Damanakah, Damanah; *Eng:* Indian wormwood, Fleabane; *Hin:* Nagdona, Davana, Dauna; *Kan:* Urigattiga, Urruvalu; *Mal:* Makkippuvu, Masipatri; *Tam:* Masipattiri, Makkippu; *Tel:* Masipatri.

Description: A tall aromatic perennial shrub, often gregarious, pubescent or villous throughout; lower leaves ovate in outline deeply pinnatisect with small stipule-like lobes at the base, pubescent above, white-tomentose beneath, uppermost smaller, 3-fid or entire, lanceolate; flowers in subglobose heads, in spicate or suberect or horizontal panicled racemes, outer flowers female, very slender, inner disk flowers fertile, bisexual, bracts ovate or oblong, margins scarious, fruits fertile, bisexual, bracts ovate or oblong, margins scarious, fruits oblong-ellipsoid minute achenes.

Habitate: Throughout India, upto 2,400m elevation.

Propagation: By seeds.

Part Used: Leaves, flowering tops.

Chemical Constituents: The plant p-cymene, l-linalool, β-thujone, azulene, β-thujyl alcohol and an unidentified hydrocarbon. The plant contains a crystalline pentacyclic alcohol, fernenol, stigmasterol, β-sitosterol, and α-amyrin and its acetate.

Uses: Leaves and flowering tops are bitter, astringent, acrid, thermogenic, aromatic anodyne, anti-inflammatory, depurative, diuretic, emmenagogue, aphrodisiac, appetizer, digestive, stomachie, anthelmintic, febrifuge, deobstruent, alexeteric and haematinic. They are useful in vitiated conditions of *vata* and *kapha*, cough, asthma, bronchitis, cephalalgia, nervous and spasmodic affections, inflammations, leprosy, skin diseases, pruritus, strangury, amenorrhoea, dysmenorrhoea, anorexia, dyspepsia, flatulence, colic, intestinal worms, fever, hysteria, measles and anaemai.

160. *Artemisia vulgaris* L. *(Asteraceae)*

Vernacular Name: *San:* Nagadamani; *Eng:* Wormwood, mugwort, fleabane, felon herb, motherwort, sailor's tobacco; *Hin:* Nagdona; *Beng*: Nagdona; *Tel:* Davanamu and *Tam:* Machipatri.

Description: Aromatic, perennial herb, 04-1m. high. Young twigs pubescent. Leaves alternate, pinnately lobed, dark-green above, white-grey and pubescent beneath. Inflorescence in droping small head of terminal, compound raceme: flowers greenish-yellow. Achene minute, oblong-ellipsoid.

Habitate: Grows wild in mountainous regions and under cultivation.

Propagation: By seeds and vegetative methods.

Part Used: Whole plant.

Chemical Constituents: The essential oil from the plant consists of cineol, α-thujone, dihydro matricaria ester, tetradecatrilin, tricosanol, arachyl alcohol. In addition to the essential oil, it also contains adenine and choline.

Uses: The entire plant, except the roots, is used as a heamagogic, natispasmodic and haemostatic. It is used to treat menstrual disorders, leucorrhoea, threatened abortion, haemorrhagic dysentery, harmoptysis, epistaxis, metrorrhagia, vomiting, colic, neuralgia, rheumatism and impetigo. The young leaves are used as a cautery to relieve neuralgia. In treating menstrual disorders, the plant is administered a week before menstruation.

161. *Artocarpus altilis* (Parkinson) Fosb. *(Moraceae)*

Synonyms: *Artocarpus communis* Forst; *Artocarpus incisa* Linn. F.

Vernacular Name: *Eng:* Breadfruit; *Tel:* Seemapanasa and *Tam:* Seema pila.

Description: Tree 10 to 35 m tall with sticky, white latex and large spirally or alternately arranged lobed leaves. Flower monoecious. Mature fruits (syncarps) relatively large, yellow-green to yellow-brown, fleshy, with numerous moderate-sized seeds, exuding latex where damaged. Ripe fruit are often available throughout the year.

Habitate: Widely cultivated and occasionally naturalized from sea level to lower mountain.

Propagation: By seeds.

Part Used: Bark, leaves and root.

Chemical Constituents: Pectins, starch, artocarpin, hydrocynic acid, beta amyrin acetate, alpha amyrin; oleic, linoleic and linolenic acids (seed oil) cycloratenol, cycloartenone, cycloartenyl acetate, folic acid, cycloaltilisin, cyclomorusin, lectin, flavonoids.

Uses: Liquid squeened from the bark or leaves in given to remedy chest pain and vomiting resulting from heart trouble. Pressed liquid from the stem bark is employed in the treatment of pain in the bones and maternal postpartum infections. Pressed fluid of the root is used in the treatment of respirotory ailments which include difficult, painful breathing.

162. *Artocarpus communis* Forst. *(Moraceae)*

Synonyms: *Artocarpus incisus* (Thunb.) Linn.f.

Vernacular Name: *San:* Ksudrapanasah; *Eng:* Bread fruits; *Hin:* Kathal, Bilatti Kathal; *Mal:* Katappilavu, Simaplavu, Kataccakka; *Tam:* Simaippala; *Tel:* Simapavara.

Description: A tall, fast growing evergreen tree, 12-18m in height with thick yellowish grey bark; leaves large, simple incised, dark green; flowers in catkins; fruits prickly, globose, brownish or yellowish, composite, usually seedless, but sometime seed present.

Habitate: Cultivated throughout India.

Propagation: Root cutting, air layering.

Part Used: Fruits, latex.

Chemical Constituents: The fruit latex contains an ester of cerotic acid, probably the ceryl ester, α-amyrin and β-amyrin acetate. Dry edible matter of the fruit contains: iodine, 0.58 and fluorine, 4.2 pp. The unsaponifiable portion of the fruit fat is report to be a valuable source of eyclopropane containing sterols.

Uses: The fruits are bitter, sweet, acrid, cooling diuretic, stomachic, cardiotonic, appetizer and galactagogue. They are useful in vitiated conditions of *pitta*, anoresia, flatulence, colic, cardiac debility and agalactia. The fruit is a testy and nutritious vegetable. The latex is useful in external application for hyperadenosis and abscesses.

163. *Artocarpus heterophyllus* Lam. *(Moraceae)*

Synonyms: *Artocarpus integrifolia* auct. Non Lin.

Vernacular Name: *San:* Panasah; *Eng:* Jackfruit tree; *Hin:* Kathal, Cakki; *Kan:* Halasu; *Mal:* Plavu, Pilavu; *Tam:* Palamaram; *Tel:* Panasa.

Description: A large monoecious evergreen tree, 18-25 m in height, bark black mottled with green, rough with warty excrescences, leaves simple, alternate, coriaceous, entire, dark, shiny, green above, penninerved, lateral nerves 7-8 pairs, stipules sheathing, leaving a scar on falling; male flowers crowded on cylindrical receptacles; female flowers crowded on blogose receptacles-both cauliflorous; fruits multiple, large, flesgy, globose or oblong, covered with tubercles; seeds oval with a membranous testa, cotyledons unequal, tubercles; seeds oval, with a memberanous testa, cotyledons unequal.

Habitate: Throughout India.

Propagation: By seeds.

Part Used: Roots, leaves, fruits, seeds, wood, latex.

Chemical Constituents: Fruit constitutes a rich source of carbohydrates and essential amino acids. It also contains β-carotene. A dipeptide, aurantiamide acetate, has been isolated from the seeds. Latex from the fruits contains cycloartenone, cycloartenol, β-sitosterol, butyrospermol, leucine, isoleucine, tyrosine and valine. The heartwood contains morin, dihydromorin, cyanomaclurin, artocarpin, isoartocarpin, cycloartocarpin, artocarpesin, cycloartocarpesin, oxydihydroar-tocarpesin, artocarpetin, norartocarpetin, cycloartinone, artocarpanone, sucrose and ellagic acid. Bark contains betulinic acid, cycloheterophyllin, isocycloheterophyllin, cycloartenyl acetate, cycloartenol and cycloartenone. The leaves yield cycloartenone, cycloartenol, β-sitosterol and tannins. The roots contain β-sitosterol, ursolic acid, cycloartenone, and artoflavanone.

Uses: The roots are credited with antidiarrhoeal property. The leaves are useful in fever, boils, wounds, skin diseases and vitiated conditions of *pitta* and *vata*. The unripe fruits are acrid, astringent, carminative and tonic. They are useful in vitiated conditions of *kapha*, dyspepsia and debility. The ripe fruits are sweet cooling, oleaginous, laxative, aphrodiasiae and tonic, and are useful in vitiated conditions of *vata* and *pitta*, and ulcers. The seeds are sweet, diuretic, aphrodisiac and constipating. The wood is a nervine sedative, and is useful in vonvulsions. The latex is useful in dysopia, ophthalmitis and pharyngitis.

164. *Artocarpus hirsutus* Lam. *(Moraceae)*

Vernacular Name: *San:* Lakucah; *Eng:* Wild jack; *Kan:* Hebbalasu; *Mal:* Ayani, Ayaniplavu, Annali, Annili; *Tam:* Kattuppala; *Tel:* Pejuta.

Description: A tall, evergreen tree with a straight bole and dense foliage; bark grey, smooth, sapwood white, heartwood yellowish brown; leaves ovate, stipules yellow, hariy; fruits spinous, oblong or cylindrical, 7-7.5 cm long, yellow when ripe.

Habitate: Evergreen forests of the West Coast.

Propagation: By seeds.

Part Used: Bark, leaves, fruits.

Chemical Constituents: Fruit constitutes a rich source of carbohydrates and essential amino acids. It also contains β-carotene. A dipeptide, aurantiamide acetate, has been isolated from the seeds. Latex from the fruits contains cycloartenone, cycloartenol, β-sitosterol, butyrospermol, leucine, isoleucine, tyrosine and valine. The heartwood contains morin, dihydromorin, cyanomaclurin, artocarpin, isoartocarpin, cycloartocarpin, artocarpesin, cycloartocarpesin, oxydihydroar-tocarpesin, artocarpetin, norartocarpetin, cycloartinone, artocarpanone, sucrose and ellagic acid. Bark contains betulinic acid, cycloheterophyllin, isocycloheterophyllin, cycloartenyl acetate, cycloartenol and cycloartenone. The leaves yield cycloartenone, cycloartenol, β-sitosterol and tannins. The roots contain β-sitosterol, ursolic acid, cycloartenone, and artoflavanone.

Uses: Unripe fruits are sour, astringent, sweet, thermogenic, indigestible, anaphrodisiac and constipating, and cause flatulence, colic, tridosa and rakta vitiations. The ripe fruits are sweet, sour, appetizer, cooling aphrodisiac and indigestible. They are useful in vitiated conditions of *vata* and *pitta* and anorexia. An infusion of the bark is applied to cure small pimples and cracks on the skin, and the powdered bark is used to heal sores. Dry leaves are useful in treating buboes and hydrocele.

165. *Artocarpus lakoocha* Roxb. *(Moraceae)*

Vernacular Name: *Eng:* Monkey jack; *San:* Lakucha; *Hin:* Barhal; *Beng*: Dahua, dephal, dheu; *Tam:* Irapala; *Kan:* Esuluhuli vatehuli; *Mal:* Kattupilavu; *Tel:* Kammaregu.

Description: A large deciduous tree, up to 20 m in height. Bark dark-brown, exfoliating in small round woody peels, reddish inside, softy fibrous with faint streaks of white lates. Leaves elliptic, oblong or ovate, broadly cuneate, pinnatified, serrate, thick like a skin, rough, having venis in 8-12 pairs. Inflorescence axillary, solitary. Male heads ellipsoid; perianth of 2-3 free segments; bracts stoutly stalked. Female heads with styles exerted to 1.0-1.5 cm via low papilla everging between peltate bracts. Fruit a syncarp, sub-globose, shallowly lobed, 6-12 cm long, yellow and drying to brown; surface pubescent, irregularly papillate, with numerous persistent bracts.

Habitate: Occurs in evergreen, semi-evergreen and moist deciduous forests.

Propagation: By seeds and root suckers.

Part Used: Seeds and bark.

Chemical Constituents: Wood contain galangin, artocarpin, cycloartocarpin, norcycloartocarpin, norartocarpin and resoucinol. Bark yields β-sitosterol, cycloartenol, cycloartenone, α-amyrin and lupeol acetate. The heartwood contains artocarpin, norartocarpin, norcycloartocarpin, cycloartocarpin, resorcinol and oxyresveratol.

Uses: Externally powdered bark is applied to sores to draw out purulent matter; a paste of the bark found beneficial by local application in boils and small pimples. Seeds are purgative.

166. *Arum maculatum* L. *(Araceae)*

Synonyms: *Arum vulgare* Linn., *Arum vernale* Salisb.

Vernacular Name: *Eng:* Cuckoo pint.

Description: A perennial herb about 30 cm high; leaves usually red brown or blackspotted, hastate or sagitate, the front leaves triangular-ovate, about as high as the spathe; spathe somewhat contracted above the base, the margins of the limb becoming inrolled, spotted purple; spadix shorter than the spathe and purple. Tubers brown outside, white inside. Fruits few seeded, more or less round, red berries, sweetish in taste. Seeds oval or isodiametric.

Habitate: Middle & southern Europe including Germany.

Propagation: By seeds.

Parts Used: Root.

Chemical Constituents: Glucosidic saponins associated with starch, Aronine, nicotine and isobutylamine.

Uses: Diaphoretic. Expectorant. Sudorific. Excellent for paralysis. A good remedy for pharyngitis with sores. Inflammation and ulceration of mucous membranes. Violent nasal irritation wit polypus. Raw feeling at the roof and palate inside the mouth with burning and corners of the mouth sore and cracked. Ascarides.

167. *Asarum canadense* L. *(Aristolochiaceae)*

Synonyms: *Asrum carolinianum* Walt., *Asarum latifolium* Salisb.

Vernacular Name: *Eng:* Wild snake root, Canada snake root

Description: A soft, pubescent, perennial herb with creeping, fleshy, aromatic, ginger scented, somewhat jointed rhizome. Stem short hairy, forked into two, each bearing a reniform mucronate, ginger scented leaf, each provided with a conical or pointed apex. Leaves 7-10cm. long and 7-12.5 cm. broad with upper epidermal cells papillose; long, round petioles. A solitary brown or maroon, flower appears from the fork of stem on a pendulous peduncle. Calyx brownish-purple; corolla absent; style 6-lobed, fruit a capsule.

Habitate: North and Central United States.

Propagation: By Rhizomes.

Parts Used: Root and Rhizome.

Chemical Constituents: Asarol, Methyl eugenol, Asarin, Starch.

Uses: Abdominal pain. Cough. Toothache. Paralysis of mouth. Cold. In females cold followed by amenorrhoea and gastroenteritis.

168. *Asarum europaeum* L. *(Aristolochiaceae)*

Synonyms: *Asarum lucidum* Salisb., *Asarum officinale* Moench.

Vernacular Name: *Eng:* Asarabaca.

Description: A perennial pubescent herb consisting of a very short fleshy stem. Leaves kidney-shaped, evergreen, mostly notched or ridged at the apex, dark green, petiole 7.5 to 12.5 cm. flowers greenish-purple, solitary, with incurved 3-lobes; stamens 12, with tips of the filaments projecting beyond the anthers; styles 6, grooved or 2 parted, recurved; ovary inferior. Fruit a fleshy globular capsule, 6-celled.

Habitate: Central and South Europe, Temperate Asia and Asia minor.

Propagation: By stem cutting.

Parts Used: Whole plant.

Chemical Constituents: Asarine and asarone. Boryl acetate. Methyl eugenol.

Uses: Stimulant, diaphoretic. Emmenagogue. Emetic. Cathartic. A great remedy for nervous excitability, melancholy, over sensitiveness of nerves to the extent that scratching on linen or even crackling of paper is unbearable. A good remedy for alcoholic drunkards with unquenchable longing for alcohol. Horrible sensation of pressing, digging in morning after debauch. Sensation of pressing eyes inwards and outwards when reading. Yawning. Nervous deafness. All symptoms worse in cold dry weather, better in damp, wet, weather.

169. *Asarum maximum* Hemsl. *(Aristolochiaceae)*

Description: Perennial herb, 20–30cm. high; leaves long-cordate, glabrous, acute at the apex; petiole long, arising from the rhizome. Flowers tubular, brownish-grey, solitary in the axil of the leaves. Fruit enveloped in an accrescent perianth, bearing numerous seeds of dark-brown colour.

Habitate: Wild species in moist places.

Propagation: By vegetative methods.

Part Used: Whole plant.

Chemical Constituents: The flowers contain anthocyanoside.

Uses: Against dyspepsia and colic.

170. *Asarum sieboldii* Miq. *(Aristolochiaceae)*

Vernacular Name: *Eng:*-Wild ginger.

Description: Perennial, rhizomatous stemless herb. Rhizomes with short internodes. Leaves in pairs, cordate or reniform-cardate, to 8 cm wide, abruptly acute, petioles to 10 cm long. Flowers solitary on short pedicels, purplish, borne singly near surface of ground; perianth corolla-like , campanulate, the perianth tube depressed globose, the lobes 3-parted, deltoid-ovate, recurved on margin; corolla vestigial or none; stamens 12; styles 6. Fruit a fleshy, globose capsule.

Habitate: Shaded areas in mountain woods found in Korea and Japan.

Propagation: By roots and rhizomes.

Parts Used: Root.

Chemical Constituents: Essential oil: methyleugenol, eucarvone, 1-asarinin, limonene, sesamine, 1-pinene, safrole, sishinone, kakuol, borneol. Flavonoids. Phenylpropanoids.

Uses: Antipyretic, analgesic, tranquilizing, antibacterial, antitussive.

171. *Asclepia tuberosa* L. *(Asclepiadaceae)*

Synonyms: Asclepia decumbens Linn.

Vernacular Name: *Eng:* Pleurisy root.

Description: A perennial herb with erect, hirsute stem, frequently branched at the top. Leaves alternate, sessile or short petiolate, lanceolate or oblong-lanceolate with acute or obtuse apex and rounded or cordate base. Flowers yellow, orange or reddish orange, in terminal cymes of many flowered umbels, the peducles of which are shorter than the leaves. Calyx small and 5-parted; corolla deeply 5-parted, the segments greenish orange; corona of 5-erect, oblong, orange hoods, each bearing a filiform horn; stamens with filaments united to form a tube and winged anthers; stigma flat, 5-lobed. Fruit, fine-hairy, acuminate follicles, 2 in numbers, each containing numerous seeds.

Habitate: United States.

Propagation: By Rhizomes and seeds.

Parts Used: Root.

Chemical Constituents: Glycosides viz Afroside, Asclepiadin, Asclepin, Calactin, calotropin, Syriogenin, Syrioside, Uscharidin, Uscharin, Uzarigenin, Rutin, Isorhamnetin, choline & B-sitosterol.

Uses: Expectorant. Diaphoratic. Useful in bronchitis, pleurisy, catarrhal states from cold, irritation of laynx with huskiness and pleuritic pain. A general respiratory complaint's remedy acting specially on sudoriparous glands. Catarrhal frontal headache. Catarrhal dysentry with rheumatic pains all over. Stools smell like rotten eggs. Great abdominal flatulence.

172. *Asparagus adscendens* Roxb. *(Liliaceae)*

Vernacular Name: *Hin:* Satavar, safed-musli; *Mar*: Satavar, safed-musli and *Guj:* Ujli-musli, dholi-musali.

Description: A struggling or scandent, much branched spinous shrub with woody terete stems. Cladodes 0.6-1.2 cm long, linear; spines, stout, straight, densely crowded; flowers small, white mildly fragrant; 3-4 mm across, in solitary or fascicled, simple or branched, copious racemes; fruits 0.8 cm in diameter, golbose, often obscurely 3 lobed berry, with only one seed.

Habitate: Distributed throughout tropical and sub-tropical parts of India ascending upto 1300 m in the Himalayas.

Propagation: By seeds and tuber.

Part Used: Tuberous roots.

Chemical Constituents: Protein, saponins, total carbohydrates, crude fibre, inorganic matter and ash. The carbohydrates contain: free sugars, mucilage, hemicellulose, and insol polysaccharides. The tubers contain a mucilage which is composed of glucose and galacturonic acid. Polyfructosans and a disaccharideare are also reported.

Uses: Roots is used as appetizing, diuretic, aphrodisiac, laxative, astringent useful in dysentery, diarrhoea throat complaints and leprosy. Used as demulcent in veterinary medicines. Root bask is taken with milk for vitality and strength. It is an ingredient of GERIFORTE used against fatigue and senile pruritus.

173. *Asparagus cochinchinensis* (Lour.) Merr. *(Liliaceae)*

Description: Perennial scandent shrub with tuberous roots. Stems glabrous, spinous. Branchlets reduced to leaves (cadophylls), falciform, angular. Flowers white, small, arising in the leaf-axils. Berry globose, pale-green at first, finally white. Seeds black.

Habitate: Grows wild among shrubs on the sea-coast; also cultivated as an ornamental plant.

Propagation: By seeds and tuber.

Part Used: Roots.

Chemical Constituents: The roots contain asparagines, mucilage, starch and sugars.

Uses: The roots possesses pectoral, antitussive, diuretic and reconstituent properties. It is indicated in the treatment of persistent cough, haemoptysis, dry throat, fever, dysuria and constipation. It is also effective in neurasthenia.

174. *Asparagus officinalis* *(Liliaceae)*

Vernacular Name: *Eng:* Asparagus.

Description: Slender-stemmed perennial growing to 2m. Has long fronds of delicate needle-like leaves and bell-shaped yellow-green flowers that produce small bright red berries.

Habitate: Native to temperate regions in Europe, North Africa and Asia, asparagus is cultivated worldwide as a vegetable. The shoots grow into tender stems in spring. The root is gathered after the shoots have been cut.

Propagation: By Seeds and Roots.

Parts Used: Root, clump.

Chemical Constituents: Asparagus contains sterolidal glycosides, bitter glycosides, asparagines and flavonoids. Asparagines is a strong diuretic.

Uses: To judge from ancient Egyptian tomb drawings, asparagus was cultivated as long ago as 4000 BC. It has long been known to be diuretic. A decoction of asparagus root to improve urine flow and to treat kidney problems, jaundice and sciatica. Also recommended holding the chewed root against aching teeth.

175. *Asparagus racemosus* Willd. *(Liliaceae)*

Vernacular Name: *San:* Satavari, Abhiru; *Eng:* Wild asparagus; *Hin:* Satavar, Satamuli; *Kan:* Callagadda; *Mal:* Satavari, Satavali; *Tam:* Kilavari, Satavali; *Tel:* Satavari, Callagadda.

Description: An armed, climbing undershrub with woody terete stems and recurved or rarely straight spines, young stems very delicate, brittle and smooth; leaves reduced to minute chaffy scales and spines; cladodes triquitrous, curved in tufts or 2-6; flowers white, fragrant, in simple or branched racemes on the naked nodes of the main shoots or in the axils of the thorns; fruits globular or obscurely 3-lobed, pulpy berries, purplish black when ripe, seeds with hard and brittle testa. The tuberous succulent roots are 30 cm to a metre or more in length, fascicled at the stem base, smooth, tapering at both ends.

Habitate: Throughout India, in areas upto 1,400m elevations, also cultivated.

Propagation: By seeds and tuber.

Part Used: Tuberous roots.

Chemical Constituents: The plant contains four saponins, viz. shatavarin I to IV. Shatavarin IV is a glycoside of sarsasapogenin having two molecules of rhamnose and one molecule of glucose. It also contains mucilage and starch.

Uses: The roots are bitter, sweet, emollient, cooling, nervine tonic, constipating, galactagogue, ophthalimic, anodyne, aphrodisiac, diuretic, rejuvenating, carminative, appetizer, stomachic, antispasmodic and tonic. They are useful in nervous disorders, dyspepsia, diarrhoea, dysentery, tumours, inflammations, vitiated conditions of *vata* and *pitta*, burning sensations, hyperdipsia, ophthalmopathy, nephropathy, hepatopathy, strangury, scalding of urine, throat infections, tuberculosis, cough, bronchitis, gleet, gonorrhoea, leucorrhoea, leprosy, epilepsy, fatigue, hyperacidity, colic, haemorrhoids, cardiac debility, hypertension, abortion, agalactia and general debility.

176. *Asperula odorata* *(Rubiaceae)*

Synonyms: *Gallium odoratum.*

Vernacular Name: *Eng:* Sweet woodruff.

Description: Perennial growing to 45 cm. Has a square stem, whorls of narrow elliptical leaves, and small white flowers.

Habitate: Sweet woodruff is native to Europe, and is also found in Asia and North Africa. It grows in woodlands and shaded places.

Propagation: By seeds and cutting.

Parts Used: Aerial parts.

Chemical Constituents: Sweet woodruff contains iridoids, coumarins, tannins, anthraquinones and flavonoids. The flavonoids act on the circulation and are diuretic.

Uses: Sweet woodruff is considered tonic, with significant diuretic and anti-inflammatory effects. Its coumarin and flavonoid constituents make it helpful in treating varicose veins and phlebitis. It has been used as an antispasmodic, and it is given to children and adults for insomnia.

177. *Aspidosperma quebracho-blanco* *(Apocynaceae)*

Vernacular Name: *Eng:* Quebracho.

Description: Tree growing to 30m. Has thick corky bark, leathery leaves and tubular white flowers.

Habitate: Quebracho is found in the southern half of south America.

Propagation: By Seed and cutting.

Parts Used: Bark.

Chemical Constituents: Quebracho contains indole alkaloids and tannins.

Uses: With its antispasmodic effect on the bronchial tubes, quebracho is used therapeutically to treat asthma and emphysema. It is also a tonic and reduces fever. This is astringent and has been used externally on wounds and burns.

178. *Aster tataricus* L.F. *(Asteraceae)*

Vernacular Name: *Eng:*-Tartarian aster.

Description: Rhizomatous perennial herb, to 1.5 m tall, loosely situlose. Basal leaves spatulate-oblong, to 60 cm long including the long winged petiole, 6-10 cm wide, withering early; stem leaves long-petiolate, lanceolate, elliptic, or ovate-lanceolate, to 30 cm long including petiole; uppermost leaves nearly sessile, linear, gradually smaller. Heads 2.5-3.3 cm across, in large corymbs; pedicels 1.5-5 cm long, dense short-pilose; involucre hemispherical, 7 mm long, 13-15 mm across; phyllaries imbricate in three rows. Lanceolate, acuminate, short pilose, and margin hyaline. Ray flowers blue-purple, 16-17 mm long, 3-3.5 mm wide; disc flowers bisexual, yellow. Achenes 3 mm long, hairy, pappus 6 mm.

Habitate: Marshy areas in mountains found in Korea and Japan.

Propagation: By seeds.

Parts Used: Root.

Chemical Constituents: Triterpenes, shinone, friedelin, epifriedelinol. Monoterpenes.

Uses: Antitussive, antimicrobial, anticancer (epifriedelanol). Used in antitussine, asthma.

179. *Astragalus membranaceus* Bunge *(Leguminosae)*

Vernacular Name: *Eng:*-Milk vetch.

Description: Short-pubescent perennial herb, to 1 m tall. Stems tufted, woody at the base, sparsely branched. Leaves alternate, odd-pinnate petiolate, stipules broadly lanceolate to linear, 5-10 mm long; leaflets 6-11 pairs, ovate-ellipitic, 15-20 mm long, 5-8 mm wide, entire, obtuse, glabrous above, pubescent beneath. Inflorescence racemes in axils, pedicels 3 mm long. Flowers pea-like, yellowish white, 15-18 mm long; calyx tubulose, 5 mm long, 4 mm across, 5-toothed, the teeth 1 mm long; stamens 10, 9 united and 1 separate. Fruit a 1-2 celled legume, pendulous, inflated, 2-3 cm long, with scattered, minuted hairs.

Habitate: Mountain thickets, often cultivated in Korea.

Propagation: By seeds.

Parts Used: Root.

Chemical Constituents: Isoflavonoids: astraisoflavan, astrapterocarpan. Saponins: astragaloside I-IV.–Amino butyric acid. Lipids.

Uses: Antihypertensive, diuretic, macrophage stimulation, immunostimulation, antiulcer, uterine stimulant, interferon induction. Platelet aggregation. Used as tonic, energy-giving and haematic, night sweats.

180. *Astragalus mongholicus* Bunge *(Caecelpiniaceae)*

Vernacular Name: *Eng:* Mongolian milky-vetch.

Description: A perennial herb, 60-150 cm high. Leaves pinnate, leaflets 25-37, broadly elliptic, Raceme axillary, pod ovate-oblong, glabrous, reticulate.

Habitate: On slopes, grassland and roadsides in China and Mongolia.

Propagation: By seeds.

Part Used: Roots.

Uses: Perspiration caused by weakness or from no apparent cause, chronic diarrhoes; rectocele.

181. *Atrachylodes japonica* Koidz. ex Kitam. *(Asteraceae)*

Vernacular Name: *Eng:*-Japanese atractylodes.

Description: Perennial herb, 30-100 cm tall, with knotty rhizomes. Leaves radical and cauline; pinnately 3-5 segmented, 8-11 cm long, 1.5-2 mm wide, short-spinulose on margin, long-petioles 3-8 cm; segments elliptic or obovate-oblong; terminal ones larger, glabrous and lustrous above, prominent veins beneath; the upper leaves small and simple, subsessile. Heads terminal, 15-20 mm across, bracteal leaves 2-seriate, as long as head, bipinnate, segments bristle-like; involucre companulate, 17 mm high, 10-14 mm across; phyllaries in 7-8 rows, obtuse or rounded at tip. Female flowers narrowly tubular, corolla white, 10-12 mm long. Achenes cylindric, with denes haris; pappus brownish, 8-9 mm long.

Habitate: Woods in hills and mountains found in Korea, Japan and China.

Propagation: By rhizome.

Parts Used: Rhizome.

Chemical Constituents: Essential oil: hinesol, beta-eudesmol, elemol, atractylodin, acetoxy-atractylon, 3-hydroxyatractylon, carotenoid, sesquiterpenes. Polyacetylene: 1,4-diacetoxytetradeca-6,12-diene-8,10-diyne.

Uses: Stomachic, diuretic, diaphoretic, tranquilizing, hypoglycaemic, tonic activity, liver-protective activity against CC14-Induced hepatoxicity, glutamate-pyruvate transaminase inhibition, platelet aggregation inhibition, ATP-ase inhibition, tumour promotion inhibition. Used in gastrointestinal disorder, oedema, mastitis.

182. *Atractylodes lancea* Thunb. DC. *(Asteraceae)*

Vernacular Name: *Eng:* Swordlike atractylodes.

Description: A perennial herb, 30-70 cm high. Stem erect, simple. Cauline leaves alternate, petiolate or sessile, elliptic lanceolate, 4 cm long by 1-1.5 cm wide, entire or 3-7 pinnatilobate, margin serrate and spinulescent. Inflorescence a terminal head; involucre with scariose bracts, firm, imbricate, acuminate, ciliate. Flowers in autumn. Corolla of fertile flowers tubular, white, slightly tinged with purple.

Habitate: On slopes and in dry areas in China.

Propagation: By seeds.

Part Used: Rhizomes.

Uses: Water retention, vomating, diaarrhoea, oedema in lower extremities, loss of appetite, night blindness due to vitamin-A deficiency.

183. *Atractylodes macrocephala* Koidz. *(Asteraceae)*

Description: Perennial herbaceous plant, 40–60cm. high. Stems cylindrical, much-branched in the upper part. Leaves alternate, toothed, the lower 3-lobed with long petiole, the upper entire, short-petioled. Inlorescence in terminal head; flowers small, lilac, all tubulous. Acheme globose, with a coma of hairs.

Habitate: An introduced species, at an altitude of 1000-1500m.

Propagation: By seeds.

Part Used: Rhizomes.

Chemical Constituents: N.A.

Uses: The rhizome is used in treating various digestive disceases for its peptic, antiulcer, anti-inflammatory and cholagogic activity. It is used in the treatment of gastritis, peptic ulcer, hepatic hypofunction, dyspepsia, vomiting, lientery, chronic enteritis, colic in pregnant women and diaphoretic fever. It is also prescribed as a diuretic, antitussive and hypoglycaemic remedy, useful for the treatment of oedema and diabetes mellitus.

184. *Atropa belladonna* C.B. Clarke. *(Solanaceae)*

Synonyms: Atropa acuminata *Royle.*

Vernacular Name: *Eng*: Belladonna; Hin*:* Angurshefa, lukmuna sagangur; *Beng*: Yebruj; *Kan:* Nati belladonna.

Description: A tall, straight plant about 1 m high. Leaves are stalked, elliptic, lanceolate, acuminate 7-16 cm long and 5-10 cm broad. The aerial parts die every year in autumn and the new ones appear in the following year. The plant has a large tap root with many lateral rootlets. Flowers are yellowish coloured, solitary, shortly stalked. The fruit on ripening is a purple black berry of the size of a cherry.

Habitate: It grows in forest shade between 2500-3000 m.

Propagation: By seeds.

Part Used: Leaves and roots.

Chemical Constituents: The roots contain starch, tannin, asparagines, choline, succinic acid, scopoletin, a phytosterol and enzymes putrescine N-methyltransferase and N-methylputrescine oxidase, and ash with traces of copper. They are essentially free from flavonoids. The belladonna leaves contain choline, asparagines, succinic acid, a number of flavonoids, tannins, the glycoside methylaesculine yielding an aglycone β-methylaesculetin, β-sitosterol, nonacosane, ascorbic and dehydroascorbic acids, a number of enzymes including an oxides and two phosphatases, ash and nitrates. Leaves contain flavone glycosides A and B.

Uses: Indian belladonna is used in India for the manufacture of tinctures, plasters etc. and is used in the similar manner as the European A. belladonna in the treatment of intestinal and biliary colic and are often prescribed with vegetable laxatives to prevent gripping. Also used in asthma, whooping-cough, bladder and ureteral spasms. It is considered as sedative and narcotic. Ethyl alcohol extract (50%) of leaves is antiprotozoal, antiviral and hypoglycaemic.

185. *Avena sativa* *(Poaceae)*

Vernacular Name: *Eng:* Oats; *Hin*: Jei;.

Description: Annual grass growing to 1m. Has straight hollow stems, blade-like leaves and small spikes holding seeds.

Habitate: Native to northern Europe, oats are now grown worldwide in temperate regions as a cereal crop.

Propagation: By Seeds.

Parts Used: Seeds, straw.

Chemical Constituents: Oats contains saponins, alkaloids, sterols, flavonoids, silicic acid, starch, proteins, vitamins and minerals.

Uses: Pats are best known as a nutritious cereal, but they benefit the health in many other ways. Oat bran lowers cholesterol, and an oat-based diet many improve stamina. Oats, and oat straw in particulars, are tonic when taken medicinally. Oat straw is treat general debility and a wide variety of nervous conditions.

186. *Averrhoa carambola* L. *(Oxalidaceae)*

Vernacular Name: *San:* Karmarangah, Karukah; *Eng:* Carambola apple, Coromandel gooseberry; *Hin:* Kamarakh, Kamaramga; *Kan:* Derehuli; *Mal:* Caturappuli, Irumpanpuli; *Tam:* Tamarattai; *Tel:* Karamonga, tamaratama.

Description: A small, handsome evergreen tree about 9.0 m in height with close drooping branches; leaves compound, alternate, leaflets 5-11, glabrous, glaucous beneath, base oblique, acute; flowers variegated with white and purple in short racemes, chiefly axillary or sometimes springing from the stem; fruits ovoid, 5-angled, indehiscent.

Habitate: Throughout India, cultivated.

Propagation: By seeds and air layering.

Part Used: Leaves, fruits.

Chemical Constituents: They also contain oxalic acid and potassium oxalate. The presence of fluorine is also reported. A wide variation in vitamin content is recorded from different places in India. Sugar consists mainly of glucose with moderate quantities of fructose and traces of sucrose.

Uses: The leaves are antipruritic, antipyretic and anthelmintic. They are useful in scabies, various types of poisoning, pruritus, intermittent fevers and intestinal worms. The fruits are sweet, sour, thermogenic, constipating, febrifuge, antipyretic, antiscorbutic and tonic. They are useful in diarrhoea, vomiting, hyperdipsia, haemorrhoids, intermittent fever, hypatodynia, scabies, various kinds of poisoning and general debility.

187. *Azadirachta indica* A. Juss. *(Meliaceae)*

Vernacular Name: *San:* Nimbah, Prabhadrah; *Eng:* Neem tree, Margosa tree, India lilac; *Hin:* Nim, Nimb; *Kan:* Turakabevu, Huccabevu, Cikkabevu; *Mal:* Veppu, Aryaveppu, Aruveppu, Kaippanveppu; *Tam:* Vempu, Veppu; *Tel:* Kondavepa, Turakavepa.

Description: A medium to large sized tree, 15-20m in height with a clear bole of 7.0 m having grayish to dark grey tubercled bark; leaved compund, imparipinnate, leaflets, subopposite, serrate, very oblique at base; flowers cream or yellowish white in axillary panicles, staminal tubes conspicuous, cylindric, widening above, 9-10 lobed at the apex; fruits one-seeded drupes with woody endocarp greenish yellow when ripe, seeds ellipsoid, cotyledons thick, fleshy and oily.

Habitate: Throughout India, in deciduous forests, also under cultivated.

Propagation: By seeds.

Part Used: Bark, leaves, flowers, seeds, oil.

Chemical Constituents: The stembark contain: tannin, non-tannin and red dye. The bark exudes a clear, bright, amber-coloured gum, known as the EAST-INDIA GUM. The leaves contain nimbin, nimbinene, 6-desacetylnimbinene, nimbandiol, nimbolide and quercetin. The presence of β-sitosterol, n-hexacosanol and nonacosane is also reported. Analysis of the mature leaves gave moisture, protein, fat, fibres, carbohydrates, and minerals, calcium phosporus, iron, thiamine, niacin, vitamin carotene and cal val. The amino acids present are: glutamic acid, tyrosine, aspartic acid alanine, proline, and glutamine. The fruits contain gedunin, 7-deacetoxy-7α-hydroxy gedunin, azadiradione, azadirone, 17β-hydroxy-azadiradione, 17-epiazadiradione and nimbiol.

Uses: The bark is biiter, astringent, acrid, refrigerant, depurative, antiperiodic, vulnerary, demulcent, insecticidal, liver tonic, expectorant, urinary astrangent, anthelmintic, pectoral and tonic. It is useful in vitiated conditions of *pitta*, hyperdipsia, leprosy, skin diseases, eczema, leucoderma, preritus, intermittent and malarial fever, wounds, ulcers, burning sensation, tumour, tubercular glands, anoresia, vomiting dyspepsia, intestinal worms, hepatopathy, cough, bronchitis, urorrhea, diabetes, inflammation, amenorrhoea, lumbago, haemorrhoids, otalgia, syphilis and fatigue.

They leaves are bitter, astringent, acrid, depurative, antiseptic, ophthalmic, anthelmintic, alexeteric, appetiser, insecticidal, demulcent and refrigerant. They are useful in vitiated conditions of *pitta*, burning sensation, leprosy, skin diseases, leucoderma, pruritus, ophthalmopathy, intestinal worms, dyspepsia, ulcers, tuberculosis, boils, eczema and malarial and intermittent fevers.

188. Bacopa monnieri (L.) Pennell *(Scrophulariaceae)*

Synonyms: *Monniera cuneifolia* Michx.; *Herpestis monniera* (Linn.) H.B. and K.

Vernacular Name: *San:* Brahmi, Sarasvati; *Eng:* Thyme leaved gratiola; *Hin:* Barami, Jalnim; *Kan:* Nirbrahmi; *Mal:* Brahmi, Nirbrahmi; *Tam:* Nirpirami Piramiyapundu; *Tel:* Sambranicettu.

Description: A prostrate or creeping, juicy, succulent, glabrous annual herb rooting at the nodes with numerous ascending branches; herb simple, opposite, decussate, sessile, obovate-oblong or spatulate, entire, fleshy, obscurely veined, punctate; flowers pale blue or whitish, axillary, solitary, on long slender pedicles; fruits ovoid, acute, 2-celled, 2-valved capsules, tipped with style base; seeds minute, numerous.

Habitate: Throughout India, in wet places upto 1,200m elevation.

Propagation: By vegetative method.

Part Used: Whole plant.

Chemical Constituents: Alkaloid brahmine; its therapeutic action resembles strychnine, but is less toxic. Three bases isolated, B1 oxalate, B2 oxalate, B3 chloroplatinate and a sterol. Contains alkaloid herpestine. Plant saponins, bacoside A & B; monniern, hersaponin, betulic acid, d-mannitol, stigmasterol, β-sitosterol and stigmastanol. Hersaponin possesses cardiotonic, sedative and spasmodic properties.

Uses: The plant is astringent, bitter, sweet, cooling, laxative, intellect promoting, anodyne, carminative, digestive, anti-inflammatory, anticonvulsant, depurative, cardiotonic, bronchodilator, diuretic, emmenagogue, sudorific, febrifuge and tonic. It is useful in vitiated conditions of *kapha* and *vata*, biliousness, reuralgia, inflammations, epilepsy, insanity, amentia, tumours, ulcer, spenomegaly, ascites, dyspepsia, flatulence, constipation, asthma, bronchitis, skin diseases, leprosy, leucoderma, erysipelas, syphilis, hoarseness, strangury, elephantiasis, dysmenorrhoea, sterility, fever and general debility.

189. *Baeckea frutescens* L. *(Myrtaceae)*

Description: Small tufty shrub, about 1m. high. Stems slender, rigid, much-branched; bark brown. Leaves opposite, very narrow, caducous; main nerve conspicuous. Flowers white, solitary in the axil of the leaves. Capsule small; seeds angular. All parts of the plant are strongly scented.

Habitate: Grows wild on arid soils in the mountains and the midlands.

Propagation: By seeds.

Part Used: Whole plant.

Chemical Constituents: The whole plant yields 0.76% essential oil, consisting of cineol, pinene, linalol and limonene.

Uses: The whole plant, except the roots, possesses antibacterial, antiferile and haemostatic properties. It is indicated in the therapy of coryza, influenza, headache, measles, colic and jaundice, in the form of a fumigation of the dired plant or the inhalation of vapour from a boiling decoction of the fresh plant. It is also prescribed against apistaxis, impetigo, dyspepsia, haemorrahagic dysentery and menstrual disorders. It is applied externally as an antiseptic in treating furunculosis and impetigo. The essential oil tincture in cases of rheumatism.

190. *Balanites roxburghii.* Planch. *(Balanitaceae)*

Synonyms: *Balanites aegyptiaca* (Linn.) Delile.

Vernacular Name: *San*: Angavriksha, Beng: Hingol, hingon, *Hin:* Hingan, hingoli, *Kan:* Ingalore, *Mal:* Nanjunta, *Tam:* Nanjundan, Tal: Gara.

Description: A spiny, evergreen tree, up to 9 m in height, distributed in the drier parts of peninsular India, Western Rajasthan and from South-East Punjab to West Bengal and Sikkim. Bark grey, 6mm thick; leaves 2-foliolate, leaflets elliptic or obovate; flowers small, greenish white, fragrant, in axillary, few-or many-flowered fascicles; drupes ovoid, woody, 2.5-6.0 cm long, 5-grooved, enclosing an oily seed.

Habitate: Drier part of India, mainly in Rajasthan. M.P. and Gujarat.

Propagation: By seeds and root-suckers.

Part Used: Fruit pulp, leaves and seeds.

Chemical Constituents: It content steroidal saponin, balanitisn, tigmasterol, amino acid, diosgenin etc.

Uses: Unripe fruits cathartic; ripe ones used for whooping cough and skin troubles. Bark anthelmintic. Seeds expectorant, used in whooping cough and for colic; seed extract hypotensive. Seeds yield a fatty oil used for burns and freckles, and for soap making.

191. Baliospermum montanum (Willd.) Muell-Arg. *(Euphorbiaceae)*

Synonyms: *Balisopemum axillare* Bl.

Vernacular Name: *San:* Danti; *Hin:* Danti; *Kan:* Kaduharalu; *Mal:* Nagandanti, Danti; *Tam:* Nakatanti; *Tel:* Adaviamudamu, Kondaamudamu.

Description: A stout undershrub 0.9–1.8 m in height with herbaceous branches from the roots; leaves simple, sinuate-toothed, upper ones small, lower ones large, sometimes palmately 3-5 lobed; flowers numerous, in axillary racemes with male flowers above and a few females below; fruits capsules, 8-13mm long, obovoid, seeds ellipsoid, smooth, mottled.

Habitate: Throughout India.

Propagation: By seeds and vegetative method.

Part Used: Roots, leaves seeds.

Chemical Constituents: Roots yield 5 new phorbol esters belonging to diterpene hydrocarbo, tigliane skeleton viz. montain, balliospermin etc. Leaves contain β-stiosterol, B-D-glucoside and hexacosanol.

Uses: The roots are acrid, thermogenic, purgative, anti-inflammatory, anodyne, digestive, anthelmintic, diuretic, diaphoretic, rubefacient, febrifuge and tonic. They are useful in anasarca, dropsy, flatulence, constipation, jandice, haemorrhoids, leprosy, skin diseases, strangury, vesical cacculi, wounds, splenomegaly, anaemia, leucoderma, fever and vitiated conditions of *vata*. The leaves are good for asthma and bronchitis. The seeds are drastic purgative, rubefacient, hydragogue and stimulant, and are useful in vitiated conditions of *vata*, inflammations and flatulence.

192. *Ballota nigra* *(Lameaceae)*

Vernacular Name: *Eng:* Black Horehound.

Description: Straggling, strong-smelling perennial growing to 1m. Has Oval, toothed leaves and pink-purple flowers in whorls at the base of the upper leaves.

Habitate: This herb is found throughout much of Europe, in North America and in Asia. It thrives on wasteground, in pavement cracks and by roadsides, mostly near human habitation. It is harvested when in flower in summer.

Propagation: By Seeds and cutting.

Parts Used: Aerial parts.

Chemical Constituents: Black horehound contains diterpenoids, including marrubiin.

Uses: The herb is currently used by Anglo-American herbalists as an anti-emetic-preventing or reducing nausea or vomiting. It is perhaps most useful when nausea arises for disorders of the inner ear as opposed to those of the digestive system.

193. *Balsamodendron myrrha* *(Burseraceae)*

Vernacular Name: *San*: Vola, Rasagandha, *Hin:* Bol, Bal.

Description: A small tree or low bush about 3 m in height with a large trunk, many knotty irregular branches, terminating at right angles in sharp spines. *Leaves* trifoliate, *fruit* long and pyriform. *Gum resin* is obtained from phloem which contains ducts and cavities.

Habitate: Indigenous to North Eastern Africa. Collected in Southern Arabia, Abyssinia, Persia, Siam and sold in Indian market.

Propagation: By seeds and Stem cutting.

Parts Used: Gum from the bark of the tree.

Chemical Constituents: Myrrh contains volatile oil 2 to 10%, resin 25 to 40% and gum 57 to 61% and 3 to 4% impurities. Volatile oil is called as myrrhol and contains cuminic aldehyde, eugenol, m-cresol, pinene, limonene, dipentene and two sesquiterpenes.

Uses: Mouth, tooth infections. Dyspepsia. Local ulcers and wounds. Menorrhagia and dysmenorrhoea. Myrrh has stimulant and antiseptic properties and is mainly used in medicinal tooth powder and mouthwash. Useful in dyspepsia, it is also given in menstrual disorders and as a stimulating healing in ulcerated conditions and as a gargle for spongy gums and in ulcerated sore throat. It is used to prevent hair loss. Tincture of myrrh is useful in menstrual disorders and chlorosis in young girls.

194. *Bambusa arundinacea* (Retz.) Willd. (*Bambusaceae*)

Vernacular Name: *San*: Vamsah, Venuh, *Eng:* Thorny bamboo, *Hin:* Bans, Kantabans, *Kan:* Bedru, *Mal:* Mula, Illi, *Tam:* Mulmunkil, *Tel:* Vedurubiyyam, Veduruppu.

Description: A tall thorny bamboo upto 30 m in height with many stems, tufted on stout root stock, nodes prominent, the lowest rooting, internodes upto 45 cm long, stem sheath coriaceous, orange-yellow, streaked, glabrous or puberulous beneath, base rounded, ciliate, tip stiff, midrib narrow, leaf sheaths with a short bristly auricle, ligule short; spikelets glabrous, yellow or yellowish green, in very long panicles, often occupying the whole stem, floral glumes, 3-7 in number, the uppermost 1-3 male or neuter, lodicules 3, hyaline, 1-3 nerved, ciliate; fruits oblong grains, beaked by the style base, grooved on one side.

Habitate: Throughout India, in areas upto 2,100 m elevation.

Propagation: By seeds and rhizomes.

Parts Used: Roots, leaves sprouts, grains and bamboo manna.

Chemical Constituents: Analysis of tender shoots gave protein, carbohydrates, calcium, phosphorus, iron, magnesium, sodium, copper, chlorine, thiamine, vitamin-C, etc.

Uses: The roots are sweet, astringent, cooling, laxative, depurative, diuretic and tonic. They are useful in vitiated conditions of *kapha* and *pitta,* leprosy, skin diseases, burning sensation, discolourations, strangury, ringworm, ulorrhea, arthralgia and general debility. The leaves are sweet, astringent, cooling, emmenagogue, ophthalmic, vulnerary, constipating and febrifuge. They are useful in vitiated conditions of *pitta,* ophthalmopathy, lumbago, haemorrhoids, diarrhoea, gonorrhoea, amenorrhoea, dysmenorrhoea, wounds, skin diseases and fever. The sprouts are acrid, bitter, alxative, thermogenic, anti-inflammatory, digestive, carminative, anthelmintic and diuretic. They are useful in inflammations, ulcers and wounds, dyspepsia, nausea, intestinal worms, flatulence and strangury. The grains are acrid, sweet, thermogenic, anthelmintic, aphrodisiac, alexeteric and tonic. They are useful in vitiated conditions of *kapha,* urorrhea, intestinal worms and general debility.

The 'bamboo manna' or Banslochan is the siliceous secretion found in the internodes of the stems of various species of bamboo. It occurs in fragments or masses, and is translucent or transparent and of bluish white colour. It is astringent, acrid, sweet, cooling, expectorant, constipating, cardiotonic, haemostatic, aphrodisiac, diuretic, febrifuge and tonic. It is useful in vitiated conditions of *pitta* and *kapha,* vomiting, diarrhoea, hyperdipsia, burning sensation, leprosy, jaundice, cardiac diseases, haemoptysis, haematemesis, haemorrhages, bronchitis, cough, asthma, tuberculosis, strangury, stomatitis, syphilis, fever, ophthalmia and general debility.

195. *Banisteriopsis caapi* *(Malpighiaceae)*

Vernacular Name: *Eng:* Ayahuasca.

Description: Woody vine growing to 30m. Has smooth bark, oval leaves and bunches of small red or yellow flowers.

Habitate: Ayahuasca is native to jungles of the Amazon basin. It is cultivated by indigenous peoples, but the wild herb is preferred for medicinal use.

Propagation: By Seed and vegetative methods.

Parts Used: Bark.

Chemical Constituents: Ayahuasca contains betacarboline alkaloids which stimulate hallucinations.

Uses: Used as a remedy to cure a range of iagnosed conditions. In the shamanistic societies of the Amazon, ayahuasca allows the lealer to communicate with the spirit world where illness arises, interceding on behalf of the ill person and the community to restore health the individualized approach of western medicine. Beyond its ability to affect mood, the bark is emetic and purgative. At low doses it is used as a mild detoxifier.

196. *Baphicacanthus cusia* (Nees) Bremek. *(Acanthaceae)*

Synonyms: *Strobilanthes flaccidifolius* (Nees) Imlay.

Vernacular Name: *Eng:* Assam indigo.

Description: A subshrub, up to 1 m high. Rootstock terete. Stem erect. Both rootstock and stem with dilated nodes. Leaves opposite often unequal, elliptical, 5-16 cm long by 2.5-6 cm wide, tip acuminate, base attenuate, margin serrulate. Spikes forming somewhat dense panicles; flowers opposite, many remote; bracts leaf-like, 1-2 cm long, deciduous. Capsule stick-like, glabrous. Seeds much compressed, brownish.

Habitate: In low hills; often cultivated in India, China, Burma, Indonesia.

Propagation: By seeds and vegetative method.

Part Used: Roots and leaves.

Uses: Fever and headache due to influenza, febrile diseases with eruptions, sore throat, pharyngitis, tonsillitis, conjunctivitis, pyogenic infection.

197. *Baptisia tinctoria* *(Leguminosae)*

Vernacular Name: *Eng:* Wild Indigo.

Description: Herbaceous perennial growing to 1m. Has a smooth stem, clover-like leaves and purplish-blue flowers in small terminal clusters.

Habitate: Native to eastern parts of North America, wild indigo grows from North Carolina to southern Canada in dry, hilly woods.

Propagation: By seeds.

Parts Used: Root and leaves.

Chemical Constituents: Wild indigo contains isoflavones, flavonoids, alkaloids, coumarins and polysaccharides. The isoflavones are oestrogenic.

Uses: Wild indigo is a strong antiseptic and immune-stimulant. It is considered particularly effective for upper respirarty infections such as tonisillitis and pharyngitis, and is also valuable in treating infections of the chest, gastro-intestinal tract and skin.

198. *Barosma betulina* *(Rutaceae)*

Vernacular Name: *Eng:* Buchu.

Description: A bushy shrub growing to 2m with stemless, slightly leathery leaves dotted with oil glands.

Habitate: Buchu is native to South Africa, where is it widely cultivated on hillsides. It is also grown in parts of South America. The herb is grown from cuttings in late summer and requires well-drained soil and plenty of sun.

Propagation: By Stem cutting and Seeds.

Parts Used: Leaves.

Chemical Constituents: Volatile oil (1.5-2.5%), including pulegone, menthone, diosphenol, Sulphur Compounds, Flavonoids (diosmin, rutin), Mucilage.

Uses: Urinary antiseptic, Diuretic, Stimulant, Uterine stimulant.

199. *Barringtonia acutangula* (L.) Gaertn. *(Barringtoniaceae)*

Synonyms: .

Vernacular Name: *San:* Samudraphalah, *Eng:* Indian oak, *Hin:* Samudraphal, Hijjal, *Kan:* Holekavau, *Mal:* Nirpelu, Attupelu, Samudraphalam, *Tam:* Samuttirappalam, *Tel:* Kanapa, Kanigi.

Description: A medium sized glabrous tree 10-15 m in height with pale grey slender young branches and rough dark brown bark; leaves simple, alternate, obovate-oblong or elliptic-cuneate, the margins minutely denticulate or crenulate, main nerves 10-13 pairs; flowers fragran, dark scarlet, in pendulous many flowered racemes; fruits bluntly quadrangular, narrowed towards the ends, crowned by a small persistent calyx.

Habitate: Throughout India, in deciduous and evergreen forests, mostly along the banks of rivers, streams and tanks.

Propagation: By seeds.

Parts Used: Roots, leaves, fruits.

Chemical Constituents: Barringtogenin & berringtogentin in seeds and sapogenin in bark & leaves.

Uses: The roots are bitter, cooling, aperient, antipyretic, stimulant and emetic. They are useful in catarrh, intermittent fevers, splenomegaly and constipation. It is similar to 'cinchona' in action when administered in malarial fever. The leaves are bitter, constipating and tonic, and are useful in diarrhoea and dysentery. The fruits are acrid, bitter, cooling, anthelmintic, galactagogue, alexeteric, vulnerary, depurative, emetic, purgative, expectorant, diuretic, emmenagogue and antipyretic. They are useful in vitiated conditions of *pitta*, colic, intestinal worms, agalactia, wounds, ulcers, skin diseases, leprosy, splenomegaly, cough, bronchitis, strangury, dysmenorrhoea, intermittent fevers, ophthalmitis, cephalalgia, lumbago, syphilis, nasal catarrh and hallucinations.

200. *Barringtonia asiatica* (L.) Kurz. *(Barringtoniaceae)*

Synonyms: *Barringtonia speciosa.*

Description: Tree to 25 m. tall with glossy alternate, petiolate, entire leaves, obovate, 12-40 cm long, 10-20 cm broad. Flowers large and showy, white, Fruit a large fibrous drupe, shiny green, quardrangula, containing a large single seed. This tree usually forms large spreading branches as well as a large, spreading buttress root system.

Habitate: Common along the sea shore, edges of mangroves, lowland river margins and coastal forests.

Propagation: By seeds.

Part Used: Seeds, leaves and bark.

Chemical Constituents: Gallic acid, saponins (including barrinin A), hydrocyanic acid, monosaccharides, triterpenoids (bartogenic acid, 19-epibartogenic acid, and anhydrobartogenic acid).

Uses: The seed is greated, mixed with coconut cream and rubbed on to burns. A decoction of the leaves is used to treat hernia. A decoction of the bark is used to treat constipation and epilepsy. The fruit or bark is used to treat yaws, seed to treat ringworm and the bark is used in treating tuberculosis.

201. *Basella alba* (L.) Stewart *(Basellaceae)*

Synonyms: *Basella rubra* Linn.

Vernacular Name: *San*: Upodika, *Eng:* Indian spinach, *Hin:* Poi, Lalbaclu, *Kan:* Bansali, *Mal:* Vasalaccira, Basalaccira, *Tam:* Vasalakkirai, Sivappu Vasalakkirai, *Tel:* Baccali.

Description: The perennial succulent glabrous twining herb with white or red branches; leaves simple, alternate, broadly ovate, acute or acuminate, cordate at base, thick lamina narrowed into petiole; flowers white or red in spikes, bracteoles longer than perianth; fruits red, white or black, globose, utricle enclosed in the perianth.

Habitate: Throughout India, cultivated.

Propagation: By seeds and stem cuttings.

Parts Used: Stems, leaves.

Chemical Constituents: Iodine, fluorine, carotenoids, organic acids, vitamin-K.

Uses: The stems and leaves are sweet, cooling, emollient, aphrodisiac, laxative, haemostatic, appetizer, sedative, diuretic, demulcent, maturate and tonic. They are useful in vitiated conditions of *pitta,* burning sensation, constipation, flatulence, anorexia, haemorrhages, haemoptysis, sleeplessness, pruritus, leprosy, urticaria, ulcers, dysentery, gonorrhoea, balanitis, strangury, fatigue and general debility. They are especially useful as a laxative in children and pregnant women.

202. *Bauhinia variegata* L. *(Caesalpiniaceae)*

Synonyms: .

Vernacular Name: *San*: Kancnarah, Kovidarah, *Eng:* Buddhist Bauhinia, Orchid tree, *Hin:* Kachnar, Kancanar, *Kan:* Kempumandara , *Mal:* Mandaram, Cuvannamandaram, Malayakatti, Konnu, Konnumandaram, *Tam:* Sigappu mandaraii, *Tel:* Devakancanamu.

Description: A moderate sized deciduous tree with vertically cracked grey bark, wood moderately hard, greyish brown with irregular darker patches; leaves o f2 leaflets, connate for about two-thirds up, leaflets ovate, rounded at apex, 10-15cm long, pubescent beneath when young, coriaceous; flowers white or pink, the upper most petal darker and variegated, usually appearing before the leaves in short axillary or terminal racemes, stamens 5, staminodes absent, fruits flat dehiscent pods, seeds 10-15.

Habitate: Throughout India, in areas upto 1,800m elevation.

Propagation: By seeds.

Parts Used: Roots, bark.

Chemical Constituents: β-sitosterol, lupeol, kaempferol-3-glucoside and 5,7-dehydroxy, and 5,7-dimethoxyflavanone-4-O-a-L-rhamnopyranosyl-β-D-glucopyranosides.

Uses: The roots and bark are astringent, acrid, cooling, constipating, depurative, anthelmintic, vulnerary, anti-inflammatory and styptic. They are useful in vitiated conditions of *pitta* and *kapha,* diarrhoea, dysentery, skin diseases, leprosy, intestinal worms, tumours, wounds, ulcers, inflammations, scrofula, proctoptosis, haemorrhoids, haemoptysis, cough, menorrhagia and diabetes.

203. *Belamcanda chinensis* (L.) DC. *(Iridaceae)*

Vernacular Name: *Eng*: Leopard lily, leopard flower, blackberry lily and *Assam*: Surjakanti.

Description: Perennial herbaceous plant, 0.5–1m. high. Rhizome horizontal, creeping, much-branched. Leaves linear, amplexicaul and districhous, forming a fan; nerves closely parallel. Flowers orange, spotted with purple. Fruit avoid, bearing numerous seeds, shiny black.

Habitate: Cultivated as an ornamental plant.

Propagation: By seeds and cutting.

Part Used: Rhizome.

Chemical Constituents: The rhizomes contain flucosides: bleamcandin, tectoridin, shekanin and iridin.

Uses: The rhizome is well known for its antivacterial, antiinflammatory, antifebrile and expectorant properties. It is prescrived in the treatment of cough, sore throat, tonsillitis, laryngitis and pertusis. It is also effective for fever, dysmenorrhoea, dyschezia, dysuria, mastitis, galactophoritis, otalgia and snake-bite.

204. *Benincasa hispida* (Thunb.) Cogn. (*Cucurbitaceae)*

Synonyms: *Benincasa cerifera* Savi.

Vernacular Name: *San*: Kusmandah, *Eng:* Ash gourd, White gourd, *Hin:* Petha, Raksa, *Kan:* Budikumbala, *Mal:* Kum palam, *Tam:* Pusanikka, *Tel:* Budidagummadi.

Description: A large trailing gourd climbing by means of tendrils; leaves large, hispid beneath; flowers yellow, unisexual, male peduncle 7.5-10 cm long, female peduncle shorter; fruits broadly cylindric, 30-45 cm long, hairy throughout, ultimately covered with a waxy bloom.

Habitate: Cultivated throughout India in plains and hills.

Propagation: By seeds.

Parts Used: Fruits, seeds.

Chemical Constituents: Glucose, rhamnose, mannitol, n-triacontanol, lupeol and β-sitosterol are found in ash gourd. Seeds ad pure protein and arginine, histidine, lysine, tryptophan, phenylalanine, cystine.

Uses: The fruits are sweet, cooling, styptic, laxative, diuretic, tonic, aphrodisiac and antiperiodic. They are useful in asthma, cough, diabetes, haemoptysis, haemorrhages from internal organs, epilepsy, fever and vitiated conditions of *pitta.* The seeds are sweet, cooling and anthelmintic, and are useful in dry cough, fever, urethrorrhea, syphilis, hyperdipsia and vitiated conditions of *pitta.*

205. *Berberis aquifolium* Pursh. *(Berberidaceae)*

Synonyms: *Mahonia aquifolium* Nutt., *Berberis repens* Lindl.

Vernacular Name: *Eng:* Rocky mountain oregan grape.

Description: A shrub from 0.9-1.8 m in height with smooth stems and yellow wood. Leaves imparipinnate, each with 5-9 sessile leaflets, oblong or ovate, dark green and lustrous above, spinulose dentate but with no spine at base, 3.5-8.0 cm. long; racemes erect, fascicled. Berries blue and small. Flowers golden yellow in dense erect racemes often reddish tinged. Fruit berries, bluish pruinose with 2-5 shiny red brown seeds & dark red juice.

Habitate: Western United States, especially pacific coasts, Washington, California, United Kingdom.

Propagation: By seeds.

Parts Used: Root.

Chemical Constituents: Berberine, Oxycanthine, Berbadine, Candaine, Hydrastine, Isocorydine, Mahonine. Resin.

Uses: A great remedy for skin-care. Stimulates all glands and improves nutrition. Complaints like pimply, dry, rough, scaly skin, eruptions on scalp extending to face and neck, psoriasis, acne, eczema, pruritus, glandular induration. Chronic catarrhal affections, secondary syphilis. Hepatic torpor. Bilious headache. Clears face complexion. Stitching, crampy-pains in urination with thick mucous & red sediments.

206. *Berberis vulgaris* L. *(Berberidaceae)*

Synonyms: *Berberis canadensis* Mill., *Berberis cretica* Linn.

Vernacular Name: *Eng:* Pipperidge bush. *Eng* common berberry.

Description: A deciduous shrub having roots of pale yellow colour. The plant is 1-2.5 m. high and even higher under cultivation, with thorny alternate, angular branches. Leaves in tufts, somewhat shining, leathery petioled, elliptical, lanceolate, obovate with margins spinous, pointed serrated and fringed, and with three cleft spreading, sharp thorns at the base of each leaf bud. Flowers in drooping, many-flowered racemes, golden yellow with red dot of glands, Sepals 6, oblong in loose bunches with 2-3 finely wrinkled seeds. Fruit epidermis almost without stomata.

Habitate: India. North of Asia and Europe, especially U.K.

Propagation: By seeds.

Parts Used: Bark of root.

Chemical Constituents: Berberine, Oxyacanthine, Berbamine, berberubine, Chelidonic acid, Bervulcine, Columbamine, Jatrorrhizine. Resin.

Uses: For complaints predominantly of renal and gall stones. Renal calculi especially of left kidney with severe renal colic. Burning and soreness in kidneys with bubbling sensation. Stitching, cutting pain in the left back, radiating sidewards and then from left kidney following the course of ureter to the bladder and urethera. Urine greenish, blood red with thick, slimy mucus, transparent jelly like sediments. Fistula and. Neuralgia of spermatic cord and testicles. Smarting, burning, stitching in testicles, in prepuce and scrotum. Rheumatic paralytic pains in shoulders, fingers, legs and heels. Heels pain as if ulcerated. Stitching pain between metatarsal bones as from a nail when standing.

207. *Berberis wallich's* DC. *(Berberidaceae)*

Vernacular Name: *Eng*: Wallich's barbery, Wallich's berberis.

Description: Errect evergreen shrub, much branched, 2-3 m. high; bark greyish; wood yellow. Stems rigid, downy when young. Leaves in tufts of 2-5, narrow, subsessile, having branched spines at the base; margins sharply toothed. Flowers in short-stalked raceme, yellow, axillary. Berry ovoid, red at first, turning black on ripening.

Habitate: Grows wild in the hills upto 1500 m.

Propagation: By seeds.

Part Used: Root.

Chemical Constituents: The roots contain alkaloids: berberine, oxyacanthine and umbellantine.

Uses: The roots possess antibacterial properties and are useful for treating diarrhoea, dysentery, ophthalmia and dyspepsia. The alocholic maceration is employed as a gragle for toothache and is orally administered for headache, vertigo and photopsia.

208. *Bergenia ligulata* Wall. *(Saxifragaceae)*

Vernacular Name: *San*: Pashanabheda, *Hin:* Pashanabheda.

Description: It is a perennial climbing plant that grows well in moist The *stems* are short and thick and the *leaves* ovate and bright red seasonally. The *flowers* are white, pink or purple.

Habitate: And shady hilly areas, especially in the foothills of the Himalayas and the Khasi hills of Assam.

Propagation: By seeds.

Parts Used: Rhizomes.

Chemical Constituents: From the rhizomes of *B. ligulata* only bergenin and β-sitosterol have been isolated. The rhizomes of *B. ciliata* yield gallolylated leucoanthocyanidin-4-glucoside as well. The roots of *B. stacheyi* contain a new catechin derivative catechine-3-gallate.

Uses: Urinary calculi. Chronic ulcers and wounds. Diarrhoea. In Ayurvedic practice, *Pashanabheda*, as its name suggests, is used as a litholytic agent for urinary calculi. It is widely used in the treatment of dysuria and renal failure, cystitis and crystalluria. Its anti-inflammatory property finds a use in the treatment of abscesses and cutaneous infections. It is also used in the treatment of dysentery and diarrhoea.

209. *Beta vulgaris* L. *(Chenopodiaceae)*

Synonyms: .

Vernacular Name: *San*: Palakya, *Eng:* Beetroot, Garden beet, *Hin:* Chukkander, *Kan:* Biturutu, *Mal:* Bittruttu, cencira, Neycira, *Tam:* Cencirai, *Tel:* Bitrutu.

Description: An annual or biennial tuberous herb with condensed stem; leaves simple in rosettes, ovate, cauline; flowers 2-3 in a cluster or sometimes solitary on a long slender spike, appearing usually in the second year. The tuberous napiform taproot when fully grown is fleshy and purplish red in colour.

Habitate: Cultivated in many parts of India.

Propagation: By seeds.

Parts Used: Taproot, leaves, seeds.

Chemical Constituents: Fluorine, iodine, folic acid, biotin, asparagine, betalains, betanins.

Uses: The swollen roots are sweet, expectorant and tonic, and are useful in psychopathy, cough, inflammations and general debility. The leaves are sweet, acrid, cooling, diuretic, anti-inflammatory, purgative, anodyne and tonic. They are useful in cuts and burns, strangury, inflammations, paralysis, otalgia, cephalalgia, liver and spleen disorders, constipation, vitiated conditions of *pitta* and general debility. The seeds are bitter, expectorant, diuretic, aphrodisiac, carminative and emmenagogue, and are useful in cough, asthma, strangury, inflammation, flatulence, anorexia, amenorrhoea and dysmenorrhoea.

210. *Betula pendula* *(Betulaceae)*

Synonyms: *Betula verrucosa.*

Vernacular Name: *Eng:* Silver Birch.

Description: Handsome slender deciduous tree growing to a height of 30m. Has pale grey papery bark, toothed leaves, and catkins in spring.

Habitate: Silver birch is common in Europe, in temperate regions of Asia and North America. It flourishes in woods and thickets, and is also planted as a garden ornamental.

Propagation: By Seeds.

Parts Used: Leaves, bark, sap.

Chemical Constituents: Silver birch contains saponins, flavonoids, tannins, and a volatile oil that includes methyl salicylate.

Uses: An infusion made with silver birch leaves hastens the removal of waste products in the urine, and is beneficial for kidney stems and bladder stones, rheumatic conditions and gout. The leaves are also used, in combination with diuretic herbs, to reduce fluid retention and swelling. Silver birch sap is a mild diuretic. The oil distilled from the leaves is antiseptic and is commonly used in preparations the treat eczema and psoriasis.

211. *Betula platyphylla* *(Betulaceae)*

Vernacular Name: *Eng:*-Japanese white birch.

Description: Deciduous, monoecious tree to 20 m tall, with white bark. Branchlets dark purple-brown, grandular. Leaves alternate, ovate to triangular-ovate, 5-7 cm long, 4-6 cm wide, acuminate, mostly broadly cuneate at base, unequally serrate, glabrous or sparsely short-pilose beneath, with brownish axillary hairs, petioles 1.5-2 cm long. Flowers unisexual, borne in catkins, male catkins forming in autumn remaining naked during the winter, and opening in spring, female catkins becoming conelike, with 3-lobed scales. Nuts narrowly obovate to ovate, 1.2-2.2 mm long, puberulous, wings 1.5-2 times wider than the nuts.

Habitate: High mountain elevations found in Korea, Japan and China.

Propagation: By seeds.

Parts Used: Bark.

Chemical Constituents: Triterpenoids; lupeol, betulin, beetulafolianediol, betulafolienetriol, oleanolic acid, platyphyllin, platypyllonol, betuloside, betuligenol, paeonol, betulafolienetetraol, betulafolienepentaol. Flavonoids; myricetin, myricitrin, hemiphloin, hyperoside.

Uses: Antifungal activity. Tonic, haematic, internal disease, inflammation.

212. *Betula utilis* D. Don *(Betulaceae)*

Synonyms: *Betula bhojpathra* Wall.

Vernacular Name: *San*: Bhurjah, Bahulavalkalah, *Eng:* Himalayan Silver Birch, Indian Paper Birch, *Hin:* Bhojpatra, *Kan:* Burjjamara, *Mal:* Bhurjamaram, Bhujapatram, *Tam:* Bhurjjamaram, *Tel:* Burjapatramu

Description: A medium sized deciduous tree upto 20 m in height with white bark having horizontal lenticels and pink inner layers, peeling off in large papery layers; young shoots, petioles and leaves silky; leaves simple, ovate, acute, sharply irregularly serrate, base cuneate or rounded, sticky when young with yellow resinous scales; flowers in catkins, male catkins at the tip of the long shoots, female spikes solitary on the top of the dwarf shoots; fruits narrower than the bracts, the wings narrower than the nut.

Habitate: Himalayas, in areas upto 4,200 m elevation.

Propagation: By seeds.

Parts Used: Bark.

Chemical Constituents: Betulin, lupeol, oleanolic acid, betulic acid, lupenone, karachic acid.

Uses: The bark is astringent, acrid, thermogenic, alexeteric, deodorant, antibacterial, anticonvulsant, constipating, haemostatic, expectorant, carminative and tonic. It is useful in vitiated conditions of tridosa, convulsions, hysteria, epilepsy, bacteriall infections, wounds, diarrhoea, dysentery, haemorrhages, haemoptysis, haematemesis, cough, bronchitis, dyspepsia, otalgia, ottorrhea, jaundice, bilious fever, leprosy, skin diseases and general debility.

213. *Bidens tripartita* *(Asteraceae)*

Vernacular Name: *Eng:* Bur Marigold.

Description: Annual growing to a height of 60cm. Has toothed lance-shaped leaves, yellow button-like flowerheads and burr-like fruit.

Habitate: Bur marigold grows throughout Europe and in other temperate regions, including Australia and New Zealand. It is found in damp places and near fresh water.

Propagation: By Seeds.

Parts Used: Aerial parts.

Chemical Constituents: Bur marigold contains flavonoids, xanthophylls, volatitle oil, acetlenes, sterols and tannins.

Uses: Bur marigold is little used medicinally today, but it was once esteemed as a medicine. Astringent and diuretic, it may be employed to treat bladder and kidney problems. It also has a longstanding reputation for quickly. Bur marigold's astringency is beneficial in counteracting peptic ulceration, diarrhoea and ulcerative colitis.

214. *Bignonia catalpa* *(Bignoniaceae)*

Synonyms*:* *Catalpa bignonioides.*

Vernacular Name: *Eng:* Indian Bean tree.

Description: Deciduous tree growing to 20m. Has large oval leaves in whorls of 3, white flowers in conical clusters, and long thin fruits.

Habitate: Native to the south-eastern US, this tree is often planted in gardens in southern and western Europe.

Propagation: By Seeds.

Parts Used: Bark, fruit.

Chemical Constituents: The bark contains catalpine and oxylenzoic and protocatechetic acids.

Uses: The mildly sedative and narcotic bark is used to treat asthma, whooping cough and other spasmodic coughs in children. The distilled water of the fruits, in combination with herbs commonly used to treat eye problems, such as eyebright and rue makes an effective eyewash for conjunctivitis and other eye infections.

215. *Biophytum sensitivum* (L.) DC. (*Oxalidaceae*)

Synonyms: *Oxalis sensitiva* Linn.

Vernacular Name: *San*: Viparitalajjalu, Jhullapuspah, *Hin:* Lajjalu, Laksana, *Kan:* Horamuni, *Mal:* Mukkutti, *Tam:* Tintanall, *Tel:* Pulicenta.

Description: A slender erect annual with a rosette of leaves on top of the stem; leaves abruptly pinnate, sensitive, leaflets opposite, 6-12 pairs, the terminal pair being the largest, oblong, apiculate at the apex, glabrous, pale beneath; flowers yellow, dimorphic, peduncles many, slender upto 10 cm long, fruits ellipsoid capsules; seeds prominently ridged, transversely striate.

Habitate: Throughout the hotter parts of India as weeds in moist shady places. Tropical Asia, Africa and America.

Propagation: By seeds.

Parts Used: Whole plant.

Chemical Constituents: Insulin.

Uses: The plant is bitter, thermogenic, diuretic, lithonthriptic, suppurative, expectorant, stimulant and tonic. It is useful in strangury, urinary calculi, hyperdipsia in bilious fever, wounds, abscesses, gonorrhoea, asthma, phthisis, stomachalgia and snake bite.

216. *Biota orientals* (L.) Endl. (*Cupressaceae*)

Synonyms: *Thuja Orientalis* Linn.

Vernacular Name: *Eng*: Common Chinese arbor-vitae, oriental arbor-vitae and *Hin:* Morepankhi, mayurpankh.

Description: Small evergreen plant, much branched, with reddish-brown bark, Branches errect, wide-spreading, parallel to the stem. Leaves opposite, flat, scale-like and dark-green. Flowers monoecious, male catkin at the tip of branches, female cone at the base. Fruit ovoid.

Habitate: Cultivated as an ornamental plant.

Propagation: By seeds.

Part Used: Leaves and kernel.

Chemical Constituents: The leaves and fruits contain an essential oil. Consisting of L-borneol. Bornyl acetate, a-thujone, camphor and sesquiterpene alcohol. The leaves yield rhodoxanthin, amentoglavone, quercentin, myrcetin, carotene, xanthophyll and ascorbic acid.

Uses: The leaves and the fruid kernels are well known for their haemostatic properties. The leaves are utilized for the relief of haematemesis, dysentery, bloody stools, haematuria, haemoptysis, post-partum uterine haemorrhage, metrorrhagia, epistaxis, fever and cough. The fruit kernels are also effective against insomnia, palpitation, hyperhidrosis and constipation.

217. *Bischofia javanica* Blume (*Euphorbiaceae*)

Vernacular Name: *Hin:* Paniala; Beng: Kainjal; *Tel:* Nalupumushti; *Tam:* Thondi; *Kan:* Gobranerale and *Mal:* Nira, thirippu.

Description: Spreading tree upto 30 m tall with abundant clear latex when bruised. Leaves alternate, trifoliate, leaflets ovate-eliptic with toothed margins. Flowers minute, unisexual, cream to yellowish, borne in many-flowered axillary panicles. Fruit a small brown globose berry with thin flesh surrounding 3-6 seeds. Flowers apparently during the summer, but fruits can be found throughout the year.

Habitate: Moderately common from sea-level to mid-montane in primary or secondary forests, forest edges, grassy slopes and thickets.

Propagation: By seeds and vegetative method.

Part Used: Leaves, stem and bark.

Chemical Constituents: Tannins, beta-amyrin, betulinic acid, chrysoeriol, ellagic acid fisetin, friedelan-3-alpha-ol and acetate, epifriedelinol, friedelin, luteelin and glucoside, quercetin, quercitin, querctrin, sitostenone, beta-sitosterol, stigmasterol, ursolic acid.

Uses: Liquid from the stem of the plant is used to treat children who have not waled by two years of age. The bark is used to treat stomach ulcers, mouth ulcers and athelete's foot. The leaves are used in treating stomachache. Use an infusion of the bark to treat young children with mouth infections. The liquid from the leaves to treat pterygium as well as other eye infections. Apply the juice from the bark to burns. In the Solomon The plant is used to treat tuberculosis.

218. *Bistorta manshuriensis* Kom. *(Polygonaceae)*

Vernacular Name: *Eng:*-Asian bistort.

Description: Erect perennial herb with short thick rather large rhizome. Basal leaves long-petiolate, broadly ovate, acuminate, 5-10 cm long, 3-7 cm wide, cordate at base, whitish beneath; lower stem leaves similar as basal leaves, upper ones almost sessile, lanceolate. Spike solitary, terminal on peduncle 30-80 cm long, densely flowered, cylindrical, stamens 8, styles 3. Fruit achene, 3 mm long, enclosed in persistent perianth.

Habitate: Sunny areas in mountain valleys and lowlands in Korea and China.

Propagation: By rhizomes and seeds.

Parts Used: Rhizome.

Chemical Constituents: Tannins. Flavonoids.

Uses: Diarrhoea.

219. *Bixa orellana* L. *(Bixaceae)*

Synonyms: .

Vernacular Name: *San*: Sinduri, *Eng:* Annatto, Arnato, *Hin:* Sinduriya, Latkan, *Kan:* Kappumankala, Rangamali, *Mal:* Kappamannal, Kurannumannal, *Tam:* Sappira virai, Uragumanja, *Tel:* Jaffracettu.

Description: A small handsome evergreen tree; leaves large, cordate acuminate, glabrous on both surfaces; flowers white or pink in terminal panicles; fruits reddish brown or green capsules, clothed with soft bristles; seeds trigonous covered with a red pulp.

Habitate: Widely cultivated throughout India.

Propagation: By seeds.

Parts Used: Roots, bark, seeds.

Chemical Constituents: Bixin.

Uses: The roots, bark and seeds are antiperiodic, antipyretic and astringent. They are useful in intermittent fevers and gonorrhoea. The pulp surrounding the seed is a mosquito repellent, and is useful to treat dysentery. A non-toxic dye, 'Annatto dye', obtained from the pulp is used for colouring edible materials.

220. *Blumea balsamifera* (L.) DC. *(Asteraceae)*

Synonyms: *Blume densiflora* Hook. f.,.

Vernacular Name: *Eng*: Ngaii camphor; *Hin:* Kakaronda, Kalahad.

Description: Subshrub 1–2m. high. Stems striate-furrowed, much-branched at the top. Leaves alternate, bearing some linear segments at the base; margins toothed. Inflorescence in terminal corymb of many heads; flowers yellow. Achene hairy. All parts of the plant are clothed with a velvety tomentum and smell of camphor.

Habitate: Grows wild in the mountains and the midlands.

Propagation: By seeds.

Part Used: Leaves.

Chemical Constituents: The essential oil from the leaves contains L-borneol, d-camphor and cineol.

Uses: The leaves have antibacterial, antefebrile and anodyne properties. They are prescribed in the treatment of coryza, fever, influenza, cough and dyspepsia. Pounded leaves are used to treat haemorrhoids and an alcoholic maceration serves as a liniment for rheumatism. Borneol is administered chest pains, cough, sore throat, and toothache. External application is effective against impetigo.

221. *Blumea lacera* (Burm.f.) DC. *(Asteraceae)*

Vernacular Name: *San*: Kukundarah, Kukkuradry, *Hin:* Kukaraundha, Jangali muli, *Kan:* Kukkaradru, *Mal:* Kukkuravrksam, Rakkila, *Tam:* Kattumullanki, *Tel:* Kukundaramu.

Description: A herbaceous erect annual with a strong odour of turpentine upto 0.9 m in height, glandular, pubescent throughout; leaves simple, alternate, the lower petioled, often incised or lyrate, the upper sub-sessile, elliptic-oblong or obovate, 2.5-5 cm long; flowers yellow, numerous in heads, both terminal and axillary, corolla lobes glabrous; fruits subtetragonous achenes, not ribbed, crowned with white pappus hairs.

Habitate: Throughout India, in areas upto 600 m elevation.

Propagation: By seeds.

Parts Used: Whole plant.

Chemical Constituents: The leaves contain 5-hydroxy-3, 6, 7, 3'4-pentame-thoxyflavone, 5, 3'4'-trihydroxy-3, 6, 7-trimethoxyflavone, a thiophene derivative, a diester of coniferyl alcohol, an acetylenic compound, hentriacontane, hentriancontanol, α-amyrin and its acetate, lupeol and its acetate.

Uses: The plant is bitter, astringent, acrid, thermogenic, errhine, anti-inflammatory, styptic, ophthalmic, digestive, anthelmintic, liver tonic, expectorant, febrifuge, antipyrtic, diuretic, deobstruant and stimulant. It is useful in vitiated conditions of *pitta* and *kapha*, catarrh, cephalalgia, inflammation, ophthalmia, bruises, wounds, abdominal disorders intestinal worms, liver disorders, haemorrhoids, haemorrhages, haematemesis, cough, bronchitis, leucorrhoea, fever, intermittent fevers, burning sensation, hyperdipsia, halitosis and cholera.

222. *Boehmeria nivea* (L.) Gaud. *(Urticaceae)*

Vernacular Name: *Eng:* Ramie grass, Chaina grass, false nettle, Chinese silk-plant, Chinese nettle; *Beng*: Kankura; *Assam*: Rhea.

Description: Tall plant, 1m. or over in height, woody at the base. Young twigs and petioles violet-purple, pubescent. Leaves alternate, denticulate, covered with silver-white hairs beneath. Inflorescence in axillary panicle; flowers unisexual, monoecious. Achene with accrescent calyx.

Habitate: Cultivated in India, China and Taiwan.

Propagation: By seeds.

Part Used: Roots.

Chemical Constituents: The roots contain the flavonoid rutin. The whole plant yields cyanhydric acid and the seeds provide a fatty oil.

Uses: The root possesses antibacterial and diuretic properties. It is prescribed in the therapy of threatened abortion, colic of pregnancy, metroptosis, metritis, haemorrhoids, leucorrhoea & pollakiuria. The cure for pregnancy. The fresh root is pounded and applied externally as a poultice. The decoction is used as a wash.

223. *Boerhavia diffusa* L. (*Nyctaginaceae)*

Synonyms: *Boerhavia repens* Linn.

Vernacular Name: *San*: Punarnava, Sophaghni, *Eng:* Hogweed, Pigweed, *Hin: San*t, Bishkhapra, Gadahpurna, *Kan: San*adika, *Mal:* Tavilama, Talutama, *Tam:* Mukkurattai, Mukkarattai-kirai, *Tel:* Attamamidi.

Description: A perennial diffuse herb with stout root stock and many procumbent branches; leaves simple, opposite, short-petioled in unequal pairs, ovate-oblong, acute or obtuse, rounded or subcordate at base, glabrous above, and whitish beneath; flowers pale rose coloured, small, short-stalked, in irregular clusters of terminal panicles at the ends of branches; fruits highly viscid, easily detachable, one-seeded, indehiscent with a thin pericarp.

Habitate: Throughout India, as a weed in waste lands and road sides.

Propagation: By seeds.

Parts Used: Whole plant.

Chemical Constituents: The contain alkaloids, triacontanol hentriacontane, β-sitosterol, ursolic acid, 5,7-dihydroxy–3, 4-dimethoxy-6, 8-dimethyl flavone, glucose, fructose, sucrose and hypoxanthine-9-L-arabinoside, moulding hormone, β-ecdysone.

Uses: The plant is bitter, astringent, cooling, anthelmintic, diuretic, aphrodisiac, cardiac stimulant, diaphoretic, emetic, expectorant, anti-inflammatory, febrifuge, laxative and tonic. It is useful in all types of inflammations, strangury, leucorrhoea, ophthalmia, lumbago, myalgia, scabies, cardiac disorders, jaundice, anaemia, dyspepsia, constipation, cough, bronchitis and general debility.

224. *Bombax ceiba* L. (*Bombacaceae)*

Synonyms: *Salmalia malabarica* (DC.) SchottEndl., *Bombax malabaricum* DC.

Vernacular Name: *San*: Salmali, Moca, *Eng:* Red silk cotton tree, *Hin:* Semal, Semul, *Kan:* Burugadamara, *Mal:* Ilavu, Elavu, Pulamaram, Mullilavu, *Tam:* Ilavu, Mullilavu, *Tel:* Mulluburugacettu, Kondaburuga.

Description: A tall deciduous tree with a straight buttressed trunk having a clear bole of 24-30 m and spreading branches, bark grey or brown covered with hard, sharp, conical prickles; leaves large, spreading, glabrous, digitate, leaflets lanceolate, 3-7, entire; flowers red, numerous, appearing when the tree is bare of leaves, stamens many arranged in five bundles of 9-12 each and an inner bundle of 15; fruits capsules; dehiscing by 5 leathery or woody valves; seeds smooth, black or grey embedded in long white wool. A gummy exudate obtained from the bark is dried and sold as 'semul-gum' or 'mocharas'. The dried gum is light brown in colour resembling the galls, and gradually becomes opaque and dark brown.

Habitate: Throughout India, in forests upto an elevation of about 1,500m, also raised in plantations.

Propagation: By seeds.

Parts Used: Roots, gum, bark, leaves, flowers, young fruits, seeds.

Chemical Constituents: The bark on analysis gave: total water extr, 9.92; tannins, 3.01; and non-tannins, 6,91%. It also contains lupeol, β-sitosterol and its D-glucoside.

Uses: The roots are sweet, cooling, stimulant, tonic and demulcent, and are used in dysentery. The gum is astringent, cooling, stimulant, aphrodisiac, tonic, styptic and demulcent. It is useful in dysentery, haemoptysis of pulmonary tuberculosis, influenza, menorrhagia, burning sensation, strangury, haemorrhoids, blood impurities and vitiated conditions of *pitta*. The bark is mucilaginous, demulcent and emetic, and is used for fomenting and healing wounds. A paste of it is good for skin eruptions. Leaves are good for strangury and skin eruptions. Flowers are astringent and are good for skin troubles, splenomegaly and haemorrhoids. Young fruits are useful in calculus affections, chronic inflammations and ulceration of the bladder and kidney. Seeds are useful in treating gonorrhoea, chronic cystitis and vitiated conditions of *kapha*. A paste made out of the prickles is good for restoring skin colour especially on the face.

225. *Borago officinalis* *(Boraginaceae)*

Vernacular Name: *Eng:* Borage.

Description: Hairy annual growing to 60cm. Has a pulpy stem, large basal leaves, and attractive blue flowers.

Habitate: Borage is a common Mediterranean weed thought to originate from southern Spain and Morocco. Often grown as a garden herb.

Propagation: By Seeds.

Parts Used: Flowers, seeds, oil.

Chemical Constituents: N.A.

Uses: With its high mucilage content, borage is a demulcent herb and soothes respiratory problems. Its emollient qualities make it helpful for sore and inflamed skin–prepared either as freshly squeezed juice, in a poultice or as an infusion. The flowers encourage sweating and the leaves are diuretic. The seed oil is particularly rich in polyunsaturated fats, and is superior in this respect to evening primrose oil. Borage seed oil is used to treat premenstrual complaints, rheumatic problems, eczema and other chronic skin conditions.

226. *Borassus flabellifer* L. *(Arecaceae)*

Synonyms: *Borassus flabelliformis* Roxb.

Vernacular Name: *San*: Talah, Taladrumah, *Eng:* Palmyra palm, Brab tree, *Hin:* Tar, Tal, Tad, *Kan:* Talimara, *Mal:* Karimpana, *Tam:* Karumpanai, Nonkuppanai, *Tel:* Taducettu.

Description: A tall palm attaining a height of about 30 m, with a black stem with a crown of leaves at the top; leaves 0.9-1.5 m in diameter, palmately fan shaped, rigidly coriaceous, cleft into many lobes, petiole edges with ahrd horny spinescent serratures; flowers unisexual, male spadix branched, female spadix simple; fruits large, subglobose drupes, on the greatly enlarged perianth.

Habitate: Hotter parts of India, wild as well as cultivated.

Propagation: By seeds.

Parts Used: Roots, leaves, inflorescences, fruits.

Chemical Constituents: It contains all the nutritionally important minerals; iron, moisture, protein, sucrose, glucose, ash, thiamine, riboflavin, nicotinic acid and vitamin-C.

Uses: The roots are cooling, restorative, diuretic, stimulant and antiphlogistic. They are useful in hyperdipsia, burning sensation, strangury and inflammation. The juice of the leaf stalks and young roots is good for gastric catarrh and hiccough. The ash obtained by burning the inflorescene is a good antacid and antiperiodic, and is useful in hyperacidity, heart burn, bilious fever, splenomegaly, haepatomegaly and skin diseases. The fruits are sweet, cooling, laxative, sedative, anthelmintic, depurative, styptic, stomachic, aphrodisiac and tonic. They are useful in hyperdipsia, burning sensation, dyspepsia, flatulence, colic, constipation, intestinal worms, leprosy, skin diseases, haemorrhages, haemoptysis.

227. *Boswellia serrata* Roxb. ex Colebr. (*Burseraceae*)

Synonyms: *Boswellia glabra* Roxb.

Vernacular Name: *San*: Sallaki, Kunduruskah, *Eng:* Indian Olibanum tree, *Hin:* Salai, Kundur, Luban, *Kan:* Guggula, Madi, *Mal:* Kunturukkam, Samprani, *Tam:* Parankisampirani, *Tel:* Sambrani.

Description: A medium sized deciduous tree with ash coloured papery bark peeling off in thin flakes, young shoots pubescent; leaves alternate, imparipinnate, crowded at the ends of branches, leaflets opposite, pubescent, crenate-serrate; flowers small, white in axillary racemes; fruits trigonus drupes, three-valved; seeds compressed, pendulous.

Habitate: Throughout central and northern India on dry hills, the tree is common at the foot of the western Himalayas, in Rasjathan, Gujarat, Maharashtra, Madhya Pradesh, Bihar, Orissa, Andhra Pradesh and further south in the peninsula.

Propagation: By seeds and vegetative method.

Parts Used: Bark, gum-resin.

Chemical Constituents: The flowers and seeds are eaten. The seeds contain: moisture, crude protein, pentosans and water sol mucilage. In folk medicines the dried, powdered flowers are used in colds and fevers. The bark is reported to contain: tannins, pentosans, lignin, holocellulose, is β-sitosterol.

Uses: The bark is sweet, acrid, cooling and tonic. It is good for vitiated conditions of *pitta,* asthma, dysentery, ulcers, haemorrhoids and skin disease.s the gum-resin is sweet, bitter, astringent, antipyretic, antidysenteric, expectorant, diaphoretic, diuretic, stomachic and emmenagogue. It is useful in fevers, diaphoresis, convulsions, dysentery, urethrorrhea, orchiopathy, bronchitis, asthma, cough, stomatitis, syphilitic diseases, chronic laryngitis, jaundice and arthritis.

228. *Brassica juncea* Czern. & Coss. (*Brassicaceae*)

Vernacular Name: *Eng:* Indian mustard; *Hin:* Rayi; *Kan:* Sasive; *Mal:* Katuku, Cerukatuku; *San:* Sarsapah, Rajika; *Tam:* Katugu; *Tel:* Avalu.

Description: A glabrous annual with a few bristles at the base upto 1.5 m in height; basal leaves long, broadly ovate, coarsely dentate, persistent middle leaves oblong, 8-dentate, upper leaves broadly linear, entire; flowers yellow in racemes; fruits siliqua, breaking away from below upwards; seeds attached to the replum.

Habitate: Cultivated throughout India.

Propagation: By seeds.

Part Used: Seeds, oil.

Chemical Constituents: Seeds contain sinigrin, gluconapin, sinapine base and a volatile isothycoynate. Essential oil.

Uses: The seeds are acrid, bitter, thermogenic, anodyne, anti-inflammatory, carminative, digestive, anthelmintic, aperient, sudorific and tonic. They are useful in vitiated conditions of *vata* and *kapha*, dengue fever, abdominal colic, anorexia, dyspepsia, intestinal worms, flatulence, inflammations, morbid state of the cerebrospinal system, skin diseases, splenomegaly and persistent vomiting. Mustad is used in large doses as an emetic in cases of poisoning and it will cause hyperdipsia, burning sensation, and other disorders due to the vitiation of *pitta*.

229. *Brassica oleracea* L. *(Brassicaceae)*

Synonyms: .

Vernacular Name: *San*: Kembukah, Kemukh, *Eng:* Wild Cabbage, *Hin:* Bantgopi, *Kan:* Kobi-gaddi, *Mal:* Mottakkusu, Kyabej, *Tam:* Muttaikkos, *Tel:* Kosugadda.

Description: A suffruticose biennial 0.5 m in height, stems quite glabrous, branching in the upper part; leaves basal and lower cauline, large, stalked, nerves stout, white, especially prominent below, margins crenulate and undulate, the middle caulnie leaves amplexicaul, oblong-obovate, obtuse, the upper leaves oblong-linear, almost entire, all leaves fleshy, glabrous; flowers large, pale yellow, 20-40 in racemes; fruits irregularly spreading or ascending linear pods, tetragonous, often serpentine-flexuose with a beak, mostly one-seeded, seeds globose, obscurely brown, pendulous.

Habitate: Cultivated on hill-tops of India.

Propagation: By seeds.

Parts Used: Leaves.

Chemical Constituents: The essential amino acid composition of turnips and turnip greens. The leaf protein concentrates are rich in lysine and tryptophan and are a good supplement to food deficient in these amino acids. Dehydrated turnip root meal.

Uses: Leaves are sweet, cooling, stomachic, antiscorbutic, emollient, constipating, diuretic, anthelmintic and cardiotonic. They are useful in abdominal disorders, pruritus, skin diseases, diarrhoea, strangury, intestinal worms, cough, bronchial asthma, fever, warts, urorrhea, haemorrhoids, gout and vitiated conditions of *pitta* and *vata*.

230. *Brucea javanica* (L.) Merr. *(Simarubaceae)*

Vernacular Name: Eng.: Kosam.

Description: Evergreen shrub, about 2m. high. Young parts softly pubescent. Leaves unequally pinnate, alternate; leaflets coarsely crenate-toothed, villous on both sides, especially beneath. Inflorescence in tomentose axillary raceme; flowers small, unisexual, dioecious. Drupe ovoid, black when ripe; seeds compressed, rugose, blackish-brown.

Habitate: Grows wild, common on the sea-coast.

Propagation: By seeds.

Part Used: Seeds.

Chemical Constituents: The fruit yields fatty oil, a glucoside (kosamin) and saponins (brucein A,B,C,G and brusatol).

Uses: The seeds are used as a parasiticide. They are effective for amoebiasis, They are active in malaria. The oil is extracted from the seeds to avoid its vomitive effect. Rectal injection of an aqueous maceration is less toxic. A poultice of pounded seeds relieves haemorrhoids.

231. *Bruguiera gymnorhiza* (L.) Lam. *(Rhizophoraceae)*

Synonyms: *Bruguiera conjugata* Merrill; *Bruguiera eriopetala* Hensl.

Vernacular Name: *Beng*: Kankra; *Tel:* Thuddaponna; *Tam:* Singapukokandam.

Description: Mangrove tree 20m tall with a buttressed trunk and pneumatophores ("kness"). Leaves opposite, petiolate, ovate and glossy with leathery texture. Flowers borne singly, moderate-sized, with conspicuous basal cupule (calyx) that form a persistent crown-like structure surrounding the petals and ovary. Fruit an elongate brown, cigar-like drupe which germinates while still on the tree. Flowers and fruit available throughout the year.

Habitate: Common along the inland margin of mangrove swamps and occasionally along beaches.

Propagation: By fruit.

Part Used: Bark and root.

Chemical Constituents: Bark contains D-glucose, rhamnose, arabinose, tannins, a mixture of bruguierol and isobruguierol. Hydrolysis of the sterol esters of the leaves gives beta-sitosterol, cholesterol, campesterol, stimasterol, and 28-isofucosterol. Also present in the plant are alpha-amyrin, beta-amyrin, lupeol, oleanolic acid, ursolic acid, taraxerol, gymnorhizol. Ellagic acid and derivatives.

Uses: Syphilis is treated with the bark of the plant. The bark, with the bark of some other species is used to treat cancer. The root is used to restore lost appetite and is used to treat diabetes.

232. *Bryonia dioica* *(Cucurbitaceae)*

Synonyms: *Bryonia cretica.*

Vernacular Name: *Eng:* White Bryony.

Description: Perennial climbing vine with fleshy taproot. Has straggling stem with tendrils, greenish flowers and red berries.

Habitate: White bryony is native to southern England and part of Europe.

Propagation: By Seeds.

Parts Used: Root.

Chemical Constituents: White bryony contains cucurbitacins, glycosides, volatile oil and tannins. The cucurbitacins kill cells and so act on tumours.

Uses: A powerful cathartic and purgative, bryony is used with great caution in herbal medicine today. It is principally prescribed for painful rheumatic conditions. It may be taken internally, or applied as a counter-irritant, causing swelling and increased blood flow to the area. White bryony is also given for other inflammatory conditions such as duodenal ulcers, asthma, bronchitis and pleurisy, and may be used to reduce high blood pressure.

233. *Buchanania lanzan* Spreng. *(Anacardiaceae)*

Synonyms: *Buchanania latifolia* Roxb.

Vernacular Name: *San*: Priyalah, *Eng:* Cheronjee, Almondette tree, *Hin:* Piyar, Ciraumci, Achar, Chironji, *Kan:* Nurkala, *Mal:* Mural, Munnapelu, Priyalam, *Tam:* Murala, *Tel:* Sara.

Description: A medium sized tree about 18 m in height with dark grey or nearly black rough fissured bark and young branches clothed with silky hairs; leaves simple, broadly oblong, obtuse, base rounded, thickly coriaceous, main nerves 10-20 pairs, straight and parallel; flowers small, greenish white, in terminal and axillary panicles which are shorter than the leaves; carpels 5, only one perfect, other four reduced to cylindrical filaments, fruits black, lenticular drupes.

Habitate: Throughout India, in deciduous forests in areas upto 900 m elevation.

Propagation: By seeds.

Parts Used: Roots, leaves, fruits.

Chemical Constituents: The kernels contain: moisture, protein, minerals, calcium, phosphorus, iron, oxalic acid, magnesium, sodium, potassium, copper, sulphur, chlorine, thiamine, riboflavin, niacin, vitamin C.

Uses: The roots are acrid, astringent, cooling, depurative and constipating, and are useful in vitiated conditions of *pitta* and *kapha*, leprosy, skin diseases and diarrhoea. The leaves are cooling, digestive, expectorant, purgative, depurative and aphrodisiac, and are useful in hyperdipsia, burning sensation, cough, bronchitis, dyspepsia, flatulence, constipation, leprosy, skin diseases and seminal weakness. The fruits are sweet, sour, cooling, emollient, depurative, anti-inflammatory, nervine tonic, cardiotonic, stomachic, laxative, diuretic, expectorant, aphrodisiac, rejuvenating, febrifuge and tonic. They are useful in vitiated conditions of *pitta* and *vata*, leprosy, skin diseases, gleet, inflammations, nervous debility, hyperdipsia, burning sensation, cardiac debility, abdominal disorders, constipation, strangury, urinary calculus, cough, asthma, seminal weakness, fever, emaciation, ulcers and general debility.

234. *Bupleurum Chinese* DC. *(Apiaceae)*

Vernacular Name: *Eng:* Chinese throughwas.

Description: A perennial herb. Stem erect, slender, flexuous, 45-48 cm high, sometimes branching, sometimes not. The whole plant is glabrous and somewhat yellowish. Leaves alternate, sessile, broad-linear or broad-lanceolate, 3-9 cm long by 0.6-1.3 cm wide apex acuminate, entire, with a marginal vein; base attenuate. Umbels compound, axillary and terminal. Carpel with 5 projecting ribs.

Habitate: On slopes, or waste ground and on roadsides in China and Northern Asia.

Propagation: By seeds.

Part Used: Roots.

Chemical Constituents: N.A.

Uses: Common cold, fever, cholecystitis, irregular menstruation.

235. *Bupleurum falcatum* L. *(Apiaceae)*

Vernacular Name: *Eng:*-Hare's-ear.

Description: Glabrous perennial herb, 40-70 cm tall. Stems erect, slender, branched above. Radical leaves simple, linear to oblong-spatulate, to 20 cm long, the base narrowed to petiole-like; stem leaves rather thick and firm, broadly linear to lanceolate, narrowed at base, entire, 4-10 cm long, 5-15 mm wide, acuminate, with prominent parallel nerves. Flowers yellow, in compound umbels; umbels numerous, 2-7 rays, involucre 0-15 mm long, with linear-lanceolate bracts shorter than rays; umbellets 5-10 flowered, involucels with broadly liner to oblong bractlets, bractlets 2.5-4 mm long. Fruit 5 mm long, compressed.

Habitate: Grassy areas on hills and mountain slopes in Korea, Japan, China, Siberia to Europe.

Propagation: By seeds.

Parts Used: Root.

Chemical Constituents: Saiko-saponins, saikogenins A, C, D, E, G, P, saikodiynes A, B, C.

Uses: Antipyretic, sedative, analgesic, hepatotoniC, anti-inflammatory, anaesthetic, cAMP phosphodiesterase inhibition, antiallergenic. Used in fever, hepatitis, apoplexy.

236. *Butea monosperma* (Lam.) Taub. (*Fabaceae*)

Synonyms: *Butea frondosa* Koenig ex Roxb.

Vernacular Name: *Eng:* Flame of the forest, Bastard teak, *Hin:* Dhak, Palas, *Kan:* Muttagamara, *Mal:* Plasu, Camata, *San*: Palasah, *Tam:* Camata, *Tel:* Moduga.

Description: A medium sized deciduous tree, very conspicuous when in flower, 12-15 m in height with gum-containing grey bark exfoliating in irregular pieces, and somewhat crooked trunk; leaves 3-foliate, leaflets coriaceous, obtuse, glabrous above when old, finely silky and conspicuously reticulately veined beneath; flowers bright orange red, large, in rigid racemes; fruits pods, thickened at the sutures,.

Habitate: Throughout India, in deciduous forests in areas upto 1,200 m elevation, also in open areas.

Propagation: By seeds and vegetative method.

Parts Used: Bark, leaves, flowers, seeds, gum.

Chemical Constituents: The composition of the leaves varies with the place of origin. Analysis of the leaves from jammu: crude protein crude fibre, ether extr, N-free extr, minerals, calcium, and phosphorus.

Uses: The bark is acrid, bitter, astringent, thermogenic, emollient, aphrodisiac, appestiser, digestive, constipating, anthelmintic and tonic. It is useful in vitiated conditions of *pitta* and *kapha*, anorexia, dyspepsia, diarrhoea, dysentery, harmorrhoids, intestinal worms, bone fractures, rectal diseases, dysmenorrhoea, genorrhoea, hepatopathy, ulcers, tumours, hydrocele and diabetes. The leaves are astringent, anti-inflammator, anodyne and aphrodisiac, and are useful in pimples, boils, flatulence, colic, worm infestations, inflammations, arthralgia and haemorrhoids. The flowers are astringent, sweet, cooling, constipating, aphrodisiac, haemostatic, diuretic, febrifuge, depurative and tonic. They are useful in vitiated conditions of *pitta* and *kapha*, diarrhoea, haemorrhoids, menorrhagia, strangury, fever, leprosy, skin diseases, swellings, hyperdipsia, haemoptysis, arthritis, burning sensation, bone fractures, and are very efficacious in birth control. The seeds are purgative, ophthalmic, anthelmintic, rubefacient, depurative and tonic. They are useful in herpes, skin diseases, ringworm, ophthalmopathy, epilepsy, round worm, arthritis, flatulence, constipation and diabetes. The gum known as Bengalkino or Buteakino is astringent, constipating, haemostatic, aphrodisiac, depurative and tonic, and is useful in diarrhoea, haemorrhoids, haemoptysis, haematemesis, diabetes, leprosy, skin diseases, ulcer, pharyngodynia, general debility, hyperacidity, dyspepsia and fever. The ash of the tender branches is useful in abdominal disorders such as flatulence, colic, etc.

237. *Caesalpinia bonduc* (L.) Roxb. (*Caesalpiniaceae*)

Synonyms: *Caesalpinia crista* Linn.

Vernacular Name: *San*: Latakaranjah, Kuberaksi, Kantakikaranjah, *Eng:* Fever nut, Bonduc nut, Physic nut, *Hin:* Kantkarej, Kantikaranja, *Kan:* Gajikekayi, *Mal:* Kalanci, *Tam:* Kaliccikkai, *Tel:* Gaccakaya.

Description: A large straggling, very thorny shrub, branches armed with hooks and straight hard yellow prickles; leaves bipinnate, large, stipules foliaceous, pinnae 7 pairs, leaflets 3-8 pairs with 1-2 small recurved prickles between them on the underside; flowers yellow, in dense long peduncled supra-axillary racemes at the top; fruits inflated pods, covered with wiry prickles, seeds 1-2 per pod, oblong or globular, hard, grey with a smooth shiny surface.

Habitate: Throughout India, in the plains on waste lands and coastal areas.

Propagation: By seeds.

Parts Used: Root bark, leaves, seeds.

Chemical Constituents: The defated kernels contain α-, β-, γ-, δ-and ε-caesalpins, caesalpin F and a homoisoflavone, bonducellin.

Uses: The root bark is emmenagogue, febrifuge, expectorant, anthelmintic and stomachic. It is useful in amenorrhoea, dysmenorrhoea, fevers, cough, asthma, intestinal worms, colic, flatulence and dyspepsia. The leaves are anthelmintic, emmenagogue and febrifuge, and are useful in elephantiasis, intestinal worms, splenomegaly, hepatomegaly, amenorrhoea, dysmenorrhoea, fevers and pharyngodynia. The seeds are bitter, astringent, acrid, thermogenic, anodyne, anti-inflammatory, anthelmintic, digestive, stomachic, liver tonic, depurative, expectorant, contraceptive, antipyretic, aphrodisiac and tonic. They are useful in vitiated conditions of tridosa, arthralgia, inflammations, hydrocele, cough, asthma, leucoderma, leprosy, skin diseases, dyspepsia, dysentery, colic, haemorrhoids, intestinal worms, hepatopathy, splenopathy, diabetes and intermittent fevers.

238. *Caesalpinia sappan* L. *(Caesalpiniaceae)*

Vernacular Name: *San:* Pattaranjaka; *Eng*: Sappan wood, brazil-wood, bukkum wood; *Hin:* Bakam, patang; *Beng*: Bakam, patang; *Tam:* Patungam; *Tel:* Bakamu; *Kan:* Pattanga and *Mal:* Sappannam.

Description: Small tree, 5-7m. in height, with hard wood, brownish-red. Stems prickly. Young shoots tomentose, branches glabrousl covered with short spines. Leaves alternate, pinnatel leaflets trapeziform, glabrous above, tomentose beneath. Inflorescence in terminal raceme; flowers yellow peduncle clothed with a ferruginous tomentum. Pod compressed, with hard shell and sharp horn. Seeds yellowish-brown.

Habitate: Grows wild, in mountains and is cultivated in many places as a hedge plant.

Propagation: By seeds.

Part Used: Trunk wood.

Chemical Constituents: The woody part contains brasilin and brasilein and an essential oil consisting of D-a-phellandrene, ocimene, tannin gallic acid and saponin.

Uses: The trunk wood possesses antibacterial, demulcent and haemostatic properties. It is indicated for the treatment of bacillary dysentery, diarrhoea, intestinal and uterine haemorrhages, post-partum haematometra, contusions, wounds, dysmenorrhoea, colic furnuculosis, impetigo, leucorrhoea and anaemia.

239. *Cajanus cajan* (L.) Millsp. *(Fabaceae)*

Synonyms: *Cajanus indicus* Spreng.

Vernacular Name: *San*: Adhaki, Tuvari, *Eng:* Red gram, Pigeon pea, Congo pea, *Hin:* Tuvar, Arhar, *Kan:* Togari, *Mal:* Tuvara, Tuvarapparippu, *Tam:* Tuvarai, *Tel:* Kandipappu.

Description: An erect shrub, 1.5-3 m in height with many branches provided with silky hair; leaves compound, pulvinate, leaflets oblong-lanceolate, entire, densely silky beneath; flowers yellow in terminal panicles or corymbose racemes; fruits pods, tipped with the persistent lower half of the style, seeds vary in colour from yellow and red to brown or black.

Habitate: Throughout India, cultivated.

Propagation: By seeds.

Parts Used: Leaves, seeds.

Chemical Constituents: The amino acid composition of the total protein of raw red gram dhal is arginine, alanine, asparagines, cystine glutamic acid, glycine, histidine, leucine, isoleucine, lysine, methionine, phenylalanine, proline, serine, threonine, tyrosine, tryptophan, and valine. The globulines are major storage peoteins in the seed and consist of three fractions, α, β and γ. The seeds also contain two α-galactosidase, three β-galactosidase isoenzymes, β-L-arabinosidase and nicotinamide deamidase.

Uses: The leaves are astringent, sweet, diuretic, laxative, cooling, anti-inflamamtory and anodyne, and are useful in oral ulcers, odontalgia, gingivitis, strnagury and inflammations. The seeds are astringent, acrid, sweet, cooling, anthelmintic, resolvent, pectoral, constipating, alexeteric, febrifuge and expectorant. They are useful in vitiated conditions of *pitta*, intestinal worms, oral ulcers, tumours, bronchitis, cough, vomiting, haemorrhoids, fever and cardiac diseases. The leaves and seeds when applied as a poultice over the breast may induce lactation.

240. *Caladium seguinum* Vent. *(Araceae)*

Synonyms: *Dieffenbachia seguine* (L.) Schott., *Dieffenbachia maculata* Sweet.

Vernacular Name: *Eng:* Poison American Arum.

Description: A low soft stemmed shrubby perennial, with stem, thick, inclined or creeping at the base, finally erect with leaf top. Leaves dark green, with white stripes and spots, white midrib, mottled leafstalk, obling or ovate-oblong, large, about 30 cm. or so, rounded or slightly cordate at the base, narrowed towards apex, short cuspidate; primary veins 9-15; lower spreading. Virtually stemless. Flowers white. Spathe axillary, 12.5-15 cm. long, oblong, stalked convolute with the apex of spadix just protruding. Spadix cylindrical; male wholly at apex; female with abortive stamens intermixed at base naked in middle.

Habitate: West Indies and South America.

Propagation: By seeds.

Parts Used: Whole plant.

Chemical Constituents: Calcium oxalate, L-asparagine. Proteolytic enzyme: Dumbcain.

Uses: For prurigo, dumbness, Rheumatism. Juice used as a contraceptive, Aphrodisiac, in Angina, dysmenorrhoea. Complaints mainly of genital organs and pruritus of this region. Impotence with mental depression, relaxed penis with pruritus, sexual desire and excitement. No erections, even after caress; no orgasm even during embrace. Erections when half-asleep but ceases when fully awake. Pruritus vulva and vagina during pregnancy inducing onanism. Sweet attracting flies. Burning sensation and erysipelatous inflammation of skin. A good remedy to destroy craving for tobacco. Eructation and flatulence.

241. *Calamintha ascendens* *(Lamiaceae)*

Synonyms: *Calamintha sylvatica, Calamintha officinalis.*

Vernacular Name: *Eng:* Calamint.

Description: Mint-scented perennial growing to 60cm. Has hairy oval leaves, and purple flowers in late summer.

Habitate: Calamint grows wild in Europe and Asia from the British Isles eastward to Iran, especially in the Mediterranean region. It flourishes along roads and in dry places.

Propagation: By vegetative method.

Parts Used: Aerial parts.

Chemical Constituents: Calamint contains a volatile oil consisting mainly of pulegone.

Uses: Calamint stimulates sweating and hence helps lowers fever. It also settles wind and indigestion. It is expectorant and is good cough and cold remedy. The range of applications makes it a good medicinal herb for mild respiratory infections. It should preferably be mixed with other herbs such as yarrow and thyme.

242. *Calamus rotang* L. (*Arecaceae*)

Synonyms: *Calamus roxburaghii*. Griff.

Vernacular Name: *San*: Vetrah, *Eng:* Common rattan, Rattan, *Hin:* Bet, Bemt, *Kan:* Betasu, *Mal:* Cural, *Tam:* Pirampu, *Tel:* Jatayurkuli.

Description: A scandent slender shrub with cylindrical uniformly thick yellowish white stems armed with short flat spines on leaf sheaths, leaf sheaths, glabrous, hollowed below, ochrea short, truncate, margined with small straight or recurved spines having laterally compressed bases, rachis near the base flat and smooth above, channeled at the sides to receive the leaflets, trigonous upwards armed below along the middle, leaflets very numerous, equidistant, 1-ribbed, the rib bearing scattered bristles; flowers unisexual, male spadix very long, flagelliferous, spaths elongate tubular, female flowers scattered along the slender branches of the spadix; fruits seated on the minute perianth, subglobose, mucronate, scales many, pale yellow in vertical series.

Habitate: Central and south India in dry tracts in areas upto 450 m elevation.

Propagation: By seeds and vegetative method.

Parts Used: Whole plant.

Chemical Constituents: Saponin, alkaloid, flavonoid.

Uses: The roots are astringent, acrid, bitter, cooling, expectorant, alexeteric, antidysenteric, hypotensive, depurative, anti-inflammatory, diuretic, febrifuge and tonic. They are useful in vitiated conditions of *pitta*, burning sensation, hyperdipsia, cough, bronchitis, dysentery, leprosy, skin diseases, erypsipelas, inflammations, strangury, vesical calculi, chronic fever and general debility. The leaves are acrid, bitter, cooling, astringent and laxative, and are useful in vitiated conditions of *kapha*, cough, skin diseases and pruritus. The sprouts are acrid, sweet and thermogenic, and are useful in vitiated conditions of *vata* and *kapha*.

243. *Calendula officinalis* (*Asteraceae*)

Vernacular Name: *Hin*: Zergul; *Eng:* Marigold, Pot Marigold.

Description: An aromatic, erect, annual herb, upto 60 cm in high; stem angular glandular, hairy; leaves long; lower spathulate, entire, upper lanceolate. With cordate-amplexicaul base; flowers heads terminal, heterogamous, light yellow to deep orange; ray florets fertile.

Habitate: Marigold, native to southern Europe, is cultivated in temperate regions around the world.

Propagation: By seeds.

Parts Used: Flowers.

Chemical Constituents: Triterpenes, Resins, Bitter glycosides, Volatile oil, Sterols, Flavonoids, Mucilage, Carotenes.

Uses: Anti-inflammatory, Relieves muscle spasms, Astringent, Prevents haemorrhaging, Heals wounds antiseptic, Detoxifying, Mildly oestrogenic.

244. *Callicarpa macrophylla* Vahl (*Verbenaceae*)

Vernacular Name: *San*: Priyangu, Phallini, *Hin:* Priyamgu, Daiya, *Kan:* Priyangu, *Mal:* Nalal, *Tam:* Nalal, *Tel:* Priyangu.

Description: An erect shrub, 1.2-2.4m in height with branches having tomentose tips; leaves simple, opposite, ovate or ovate-lanceolate, acumniate, base cuneate or rounded, white tomentose beneath, main lateral nerves 12-16 pairs; flowers rose-coloured, crowdedin axillary peduncled globose cymes; fruits white drupes.

Habitate: Bengal, Assam and sub-Himalayan tracts upto 1,800m elevation.

Propagation: By seeds and stem vegetative method.

Parts Used: Flowers, fruits.

Chemical Constituents: The leaves contain C_{22}-C_{24} fatty acids, ethyl ester of C_{23} fatty acid, 7, 3, 3′-trimethylquercetin, 7-O-glucuronides of luteolin and apigenin, and ursolic, 2α-hydroxyursolic, L-α-amino-β-propionic and crategolkic acids, and β-sitosterol and its β-D-glucoside.

Uses: The flowers and fruits are bitter, sweet, astringent, acrid, cooling, anodyne, deodorant, digestive, constipating, depurative, styptic, alexeteric and febrifuge. They are useful in vitiated condition of *pitta* and *vata*, rheumatoid arthritis, burning sensation, cephalalgia, diaphoresis, foul ulcers, dyspepsia, flatulence, colic, diarrhoea, dysentery, haemorrhages, haemoptysis, poisonous bites, skin diseases, diabetes, vomiting, fever and general weakness. The leaves are useful in gout and arthralgia.

245. *Calluna vulgaris* *(Ericaceae)*

Vernacular Name: *Eng:* Heather.

Description: Small, branched shrub growing to 60cm. Has tiny leaves and white or pink to pale-purple flowers growing on spikes.

Habitate: Heather grows in temperate regions of the northern hemisphere. It is found on heaths, moors, bogs and in open woods.

Propagation: By Seeds.

Parts Used: Flowering tips.

Chemical Constituents: Heather contains flvonoids, arbutin, tannin and an alkaloid, ericodin. This constituent has a strongly disinfectant effect within the bladder and urinary tubules.

Uses: Heather is a good urinary antiseptic and diuretic, disinfecting the urinary tract and mildly increasing urine production. Besides its role in treating cystitis and inflammatory bladder conditions, heather has been used to treat kidney and bladder stones. Cleansing and detoxifying, it is helpful for rheumatism, arthritis and gout. The macerated flowering tips produce a liniment to be rubbed on affected joints. A hot poultice of heather tips is a traditional remedy for chilblains and rheumatism.

246. *Calophyllum apetalum* Willd. *(Clusiaceae (Guttiferae))*

Synonyms: *Calophyllumcalaba* L., *Calophyllum decipiens* Wight, *Calophyllum wightiana* Wall. ex Planch. & Triana.

Vernacular Name: *Eng:* Poonspar of Travancore, *Hin:* Sarpuna, *Kan:* Irai, Kal punne, Kirihonne, *Mal:* Cheru punna, Manja punna, Attu punna, Mar: Bobbi, *San*: Jothish mathi, *Tam:* Siru pinnai.

Description: Large trees, 10-30 m tall, about 2.5 m girth. Trunk cylindrical. Wood dull reddish brown. Bark rough, about 2 cm thick, yellowish brown outside, with prominent deep vertical boat-shaped furrows, exuding sticky dull white resinous fluid when cut. Branchlets 4-angled, hairless, shiny. Blaze reddish pink. Leaves opposite, egg-shaped to oblong, 5-8 x 4-5 cm, base acute or rounded, apex rounded, margin entire, hairless, glossy, shortly stalked; lateral nerves numerous, close and parallel at right angles to the midrib. Flowers bisexual, arranged in axillary panicles, about 1.5 cm across, distinctly stalked;

petals absent, sepals modified into petal-like, white. Drupes ovoid to ellipsoid, about 1.5 cm long, smooth, red when ripe.

Habitate: Along the riverbanks (riparian) of moist deciduous to evergreen forests and backwaters along west coast low elevations.

Propagation: By seeds.

Parts Used: Seeds, flowers.

Chemical Constituents: Its contain friedelin, β-amyrin, betulinic acid, apetalic acid and β-sitosterol, jacareubin, l-methoxy-3, 5, 6-trihydroxyxanthone, 2-1, 3, 5, 6-tetrahydroxyxanthone and 1, 3, 5, 6-tetrahydroxyxanthone.

Uses: The seed oil is used to cure leprosy, rheumatism and septic poison. Resin used as vulnerary resolutive, antiphlogistic and anodyne. Flowers are used to relieve itching, eczema and scabby eruptions. Seeds are used to treat menstrual disorders and ear ulcers.

247. *Calophyllum inophyllum* L. *(Clusiaceae)*

Vernacular Name: *San:* Nagachampa,. Punnaga; *Hin:* Sultanachampa; *Beng*: Sultanachampa; *Tel:* Pouna; *Tam:* Punnai, pinnay; *Kan:* Vuma, hone; *Mal:* Punna.

Description: Tree to 25 m tall with robust trunk which exudes white latex when bruised. Leaves opposite, petiolate, thick and shiny with numerous parallel secondary veins. Flowers borne in axillary cymes, flowers moderate-sized, white, fragrant, with variable numbers of perianth parts and yellow anthers. Fruit a purplish-black globoid-to-ovoid drupe when mature with a single seed.

Habitate: Common in lowland coastal areas such as along beaches, in thickets and along rivers. Occasionally planted in other areas up to 500 m ineleavation.

Propagation: By seeds.

Part Used: Leaves, fruit-oil and bark.

Chemical Constituents: Seeds contain essential and vegetable oils amentoflavone, beta amyrin, apetalodie, pseudobrasilic acid, sixteen xanthones including buchanaxanthone, butyl citrate, calaustralin, calophylic acid, isocalophyllic acid, calo-pohylloide, calophynic acid, caloxanthones A-E, campesterol, canophyllal, canophylic acid, canophyllol, canophyllum, epicatechin, cinnamic acid, costatolide, erucic acid, erythro-diol-3-acetate, euxanthone, epifriendelanol, frieedelin, inophenic acid, inophyllic acid, inophyllolide, 12-dihydro-inophyllolide, trans-inophyllolide, inophyllums, jacarebuin and derivatives, leucocyanidin, macluraxanthone, myricetin and glucoside, ponnalide, pyranoamentoflavone, quercetin, beta-sitosterol, stigmasterol.

Uses: The leaves of the plant are soaked in water to make an eyewash for removing foreign objects from the eyes. The eyewash is also used to treat eye pains. The leaves are softened by heating and then applied to sores and cuts. Boiled leaves are used to make a solution used for bathing skin rashes. Oil from the fruit is rubbed onto joings to cure rheumatism. Wounds are treated with fum from the bark. An infusiton of the leaves is ingested for diarrhoea. Oil is used in massaging rheumatic aches.

248. *Calotropis procera* (L.) R. Br. *(Asclepiadaceae)*

Vernacular Name: *San*: Arkah, Aditya, mandare, *Eng:* Gigantic swallow wort, Madar milk-weed, *Hin:* Madar, AK, *Kan:* Ekkameli, *Mal:* Erukku, *Tam:* Erukku, *Tel:* Jilledu.

Description: A large hard much-branched milky shrub, very pale in colour, the branches, leaves and inflorescence covered with loose soft white wool; leaves opposite, subsessile, ovate, cordate at base; flowers beautiful lilac, rosy or purple tinted in umbellate lateral cymes; fruits fleshy follicles, green, seeds with abundant with coma.

Habitate: Throughout India, in dry waste places.

Propagation: By seeds.

Parts Used: All parts of the plant.

Chemical Constituents: Cardiac glycosides, calotropin, uscharin, calotoxin, calactin and uscharidin; gigantin.

Uses: The dried whole plant is good tonic, expectorant, depurative and anthelmintic. The dried root bark is a substitute for ipecacuanha. The root bark is febrifuge, anthelmintic, depurative, expectorant and laxative, and is useful in cutaneous diseases, intestinal worms, cough, ascites and anasarca. The powdered root promotes gastric secretions and is useful in asthma, bronchitis and dyspepsia. The leaves are useful in the treatment of paralysis, arthralgia, swellings and intermittent fevers. The flowers are bitter, digestive, astringent, stomachic, anthelmintic and tonic. They are useful in asthma, catarrh, anorexia, inflammations and tumours. In large doses it is purgative and emetic.

249. *Caltha palustris* L. *(Ranunculaceae)*

Synonyms: *Caltha glabra* Gilib., *Caltha himalensis* D. Don.

Vernacular Name: *Eng:* Marsh marigold.

Description: A perennial herb. Stem hollow, 20-60 cm. long, branched above, basal leaves long petioled, the upper one progressively short petioled and uppermost nearly or quite sessile. Leaves kidney-shaped with toothed or crenate margins and wide notch at the base. Petiole longitudinally ridged and grooved. Flowers bright yellow, on short or elongated peduncles. Sepals, 5, petaloid, golden yellow, elliptic to obovate. Stamens numerous with anthers linear-oblong or lace-oblong, about 2 mm. long. Follicles 4-12, 10-15 mm. long, abruptly or gradually narrowed into divergent style.

Habitate: India, in Himalayas at high altitudes; England, North America, Canada and temperate Asia, but adjacent brooks.

Propagation: By seeds.

Parts Used: Whole plant.

Chemical Constituents: Helleborin, Veratrin, Protoanemonin.

Uses: For complaints like pemphigus of skin with bullae surrounded by a ring and much itching. Itching eruptions on thighs. Dysuria. Diarrhoea, Anascara. Sexual debility depression, diabetes, bronchitis. Excellent for uterine cancer in tincture form in repeated long intervals.

250. *Calycopteris floribunda* Lam. *(Combretaceae)*

Vernacular Name: *San*: Susavi, Shveta-dhataki, *Hin:* Kokkarai, *Kan:* Marsadabaguli, *Mal:* Pullani, Varavalli, *Tam:* Minnarkoti, *Tel:* Bandimurududu.

Description: A scandent woody shrub with slender brown streaked diffuse branches occasionally twining around supports and storing water abundantly; leaves simple, opposite, elliptic or ovate, acute or acuminate, surfaces tomentose, main nerves 5-8 pairs; flowers yellowish green, apetalous, in fulvous pubescent terminal panicles, ovary 1-chambered with pendulous ovules; fruits 5-ribed, one seeded, crowed with strongly 3-nerved persistent calyx lobes.

Habitate: Throughout India in deciduous forests in areas upto 750 m elevation, as well as along water courses and in waste lands.

Propagation: By seeds.

Parts Used: Leaves, fruits.

Chemical Constituents: Helleborine, veratrine, jervine and magnoflorine, carotene, isorhamnetin, quercetin helleborine, veratrine, pentosan, wax, a fatty oil and calcium oxalate.

Uses: The leaves are bitter, astringent, laxative, anthelmintic, depurative, diaphoretic and febrifuge. They are useful in intestinal worms, colic, leprosy, malarial fever, dysentery, ulcers and vomiting. The fruits are useful in jaundice, ulcers, pruritus and skin diseases.

251. *Camellia sinensis* (L.) O. Kuntze *(Theaceae)*

Synonyms: *Camellia theifera* Griff.

Vernacular Name: *Eng:* Tea plant, *Hin:* Chai, *Kan:* Teyaku, *Mal:* Teyila, *San*: Syamaparni, Caha, *Tam:* Teyilai, *Tel:* Teyaku.

Description: An evergreen shrub or tree, 9-15 m in height (60-150 cm in height owing to purning in cultivation); leaves simple, alternate, elliptic-ovate or lanceolate with serrate margins, usually glabrous, leathery; flowers white, fragrant, solitary or 2-4 together; fruits depressed capsules, 3-cornered, 3-seeded.

Habitate: Throughout India, cultivated at high altitudes.

Propagation: By seeds.

Parts Used: Leaves.

Chemical Constituents: Its contain carotene, riboflavin and nicotinic, pantothenic and ascorbic acids, malic and oxalic acids, theophylline, theobromine, xanthine, hypoxanthine, adenine, gums, dextrins and inositol.

Uses: The leaves are astringent, bitter, thermogenic, appetizer, digestive, carminative, diuretic, diaphoretic, detergent, resolvent and nervine tonie. They are useful in hyperdipsia, hemicrania, cardiodynia, ophthalmia, haemorrhoids, inflammations, abdominal disorders, strangury, fever and fatigue.

252. *Canarium strictum* Roxb. *(Burseraceae)*

Vernacular Name: *San*: Mandadhupa, Raladhupa, Eng: The black dammar tree, *Hin:* Kala-damar, *Kan:* Hale maddu, Mada dhup, Kari dhoopa, *Mal:* Thelli, Pantham, Kunthirikkam, Mar: Dhup, Raldhup, *Tam:* Sambrani, Karunkungilium, *Tel:* Nalla rojanamu.

Description: A large resinous tree, reaching 40 m tall. *Trunk* straight, cylindrical, about 4 m girth. *Bark* about 1 cm thick, rough, greyish brown exfoliating into small irregular flakes; outer bark brittle and inner bark fibrous, inner surface slimy to touch, exudes gummy sap when cut, which turns black and hard later. *Blaze* fragrant, dull yellow. Young branchlets densely brown tomentose. Leaves alternate, simply odd-pinnate, large, reaching 1.2 m length; *leaflets* 9-11, egg-shaped-elliptic to egg-shaped-lanceolate, opposite or alternate, 7-30 x 5-15 cm, base unequal and rounded, apex acuminate, margin finely toothed with saw-like teeth, leathery, densely brown tomentose beneath, deep red when young with dense velvety tomentose hairs; lateral nerves 10-20 pairs, very prominent below. *Flowers* bisexual or polygamous, in shortly branched axillary panicles, about 1 cm long, yellow to dull white, shortly stalked and mildly fragrant. *Drupes* ellipsoid or oblongoid, 3-5 x 1.5-2 cm, tapering at both ends, dark blue when ripe. *Seeds* 1-3.

Habitate: Moist deciduous to evergreen forests.

Propagation: By seeds.

Parts Used: Resin.

Chemical Constituents: Its contain–junenol, canarone, epi-khusinol, α-amyrin, 11-keto-α-amyrin β-amyrin and its acetate, ψ-taraxasterol, epi-ψ-taraxastanonol, and epi-ψ-taraxastenediol.

Uses: Decoction or powder of the resin is given orally as a remedy for rheumatism, cough, fever, epilepsy, asthma, syphilis, blood impurities, various poisons, hernia, chronic skin diseases and haemorrage. Also the improve complexion.

253. *Canavalia gladiata* (Jacq.) DC. *(Fabaceae)*

Synonyms: *Canavalia ensiformis* sensu Baker, non DC.

Vernacular Name: *Eng:* Sword bean, Broad bean, Patagonian bean, *Hin:* Lalkudusumpal, Khadsampal, *Kan:* Tumbekonti, Sembi, Avare, *Mal:* Valvara, Valpayar, Valamara, *San*: Asisimbi, Mahasimbi, *Tam:* Segapputampattai, *Tel:* Tamma, Karocikadu.

Description: A stout perennial twiner with glabrous stems and branches; leaves compound, leaflets membranous, acute or shortly acuminate, apiculate, base rounded, nearly glabrous on both surfaces; flowers large, white or lilac, in lax few-flowered curved axillary racemes; fruits large sword shaped flattened pods, seeds reddish brown or white, strongly compressed.

Habitate: Throughout India, cultivated.

Propagation: By seeds.

Parts Used: Fruits and seeds.

Chemical Constituents: Its contain is Lupeoside, arginine, desaminocanavanine, canavanine, α, γ-diaminobutyric acid, α-amino-δ-hydroxyvaleric acid, *l*-homoserine, cysteine, choline, trigonelline, betonicine, caneine, kitogine, pentosan, phytosterol, enzymes, amylase arginase, argininosuccinate lyase, β-N-acetylglucosaminidase, catalase, α-and β-galactosidases, β-glucosidase, homocysteine, methyltransferase, traces of lipase, α-mannosidase, pectase, peroxidase, phosphorylase, protease and β-xylosidase, canavanine as a predominant amino acid presence of sucrose, raffinose, stachyose, verbascose and the gibberellins, GA_{21}, GA_{22}, and GA_{59}, D-α-amino-*n*-butyric acid, γ-guanidinooxypropyl-amine and 6, 8-di-C-glycosyl apigenin.

Uses: The fruits are sweet, astringent, cooling, appetizer, digestive and vulnerary. They are useful in burning sensation, hyperdipsia, anorexia, dyspepsia, wounds, ulcers and vitiated conditions of *kapha* and *pitta.*

254. *Canella winterana* *(Canellaceae)*

Synonyms*:* *Canella alba.*

Vernacular Name: *Eng:* Canella, Wild cinnamon.

Description: An aromatic tree, upto 15 m in height, leaves obovate, leathery. Sometimes dotted, flowers purple or violet, scented, terminal; berries black.

Habitate: Native to the Caribbean and Florida, canella is found in coastal swamps and scrubland.

Propagation: By Seeds.

Parts Used: Bark.

Chemical Constituents: Canella contains about 1% volatile oil, alpha-aldehydes, resin and mannitol.

Uses: Canella is cytotoxic, antifungal and repels insects. It is also strongly aromatic, stimulant and antiseptic. Canella is often used in the West Indies and Latin America as a substitute for cinnamon. The infusion is drunk for its plea*San*t flavour and tonic effect. Canella is also used for stomach problems, indigestion and puerperal fever, an infection that develops after childbirth.

255. *Cannabis sativa* L. *(Cannabinaceae)*

Synonyms: .

Vernacular Name: *San*: Bhanga, Vijaya, *Eng:* True hemp, Soft hemp, Indian hemp, *Hin:* Bhang, Ganja, Charas, *Kan:* Bhangi, *Mal:* Kancavu, Sivamuli, *Tam:* Ganca, Bhamgi, *Tel:* Ganjayi.

Description: A large aromatic resinous annual herb 1.2-4.8 m in height with erect angular stem, the female plant usually taller than the male; leaves palmately divided, lower 3-8 foliate with long petioles, upper 3-1 foliate passing into bracts; male flowers in short drooping panicles, females in short axillary crowded spikes; fruits achenes seeds black, flattened.

Habitate: Throughout India, wild (North west Himalayas).

Propagation: By seeds.

Parts Used: Dried leaves and flowering shoots.

Chemical Constituents: Its contain is tetrahydrocannabinol, cannabidiol, cannabinol, cannabichromene, cannabicitran, cannabicyclol, cannabigerol, cannabielsion, stereo isomers of cannabitriol, cannabinodiol, cannabicumaronone, cannabiglendol and cannabitetrol.

Uses: Leaves are bitter, astringent, tonic, aphrodisiac, antidiarrhoeic, intoxicating, stomachic, analgesic and abortifacient. They are used in convulsions, otalgia, abdominal disorders, diarrhoea, stomatalgia and haematorrhoea. Its excessive use causes dyspepsia, cough, impotence, melancholy, dropsy, hyperpraxia and insanity. The bark is tonic, and is useful in inflammations, haemorrhoids and hydrocele. Seeds are carminative, astringent, aphrodisiac, antiemetic and anti-inflammatory.

256. *Cannaga odorata* (Lam.) Hook. F & Thoms. *(Annonaceae)*

Vernacular Name: *Eng:* Ylang-ylang, kenanga.

Description: Tree up to 20m tall. Leaves alternate, entire and elliptical flowers very fragrant, often growing in culsters. Fruit oblong and indehiscent with 3-13 pale brown, seeds embedded in a yellow and oily pulp.

Habitate: Cultivated or naturalized in forests, slopes, or gullies from sea-level to mid-montane.

Propagation: By seeds and vegetative method.

Part Used: Leaves and bark.

Chemical Constituents: Essential oils, sesquiterpenoids, isoquinoline alkaloids, lignans, aromatic compounds (benzyl alchol, phenols, benzoic and salicylic acid esters), lipids and cyanogenic material.

Uses: Remedy for headaches, high blood pressure, coughs, dizziness, skin irritations. Anticonvulsant, cures earaches. Used in to treat gonorrhoea and back pain. Given to women to promote fertilify. Fluid from the pressed bark is used in treating toothaches and migraine headaches. use an infusion of the bark for treating stomach ailments such as pains, indigetion and colic. The leaves are used in treatment for diarrhoea in infants & used in treating boils.

257. *Canscora decussata* (Roxb.) Schult. *(Gentianaceae)*

Synonyms: .

Vernacular Name: *San*: *Sankhini*, *Sankhapuspi*, *Eng:* Canscora, *Hin:* Samkhaphuli, *Kan:* *Sankinisoppu*, *Mal:* Samkhapuspi, Kancankora, *Tel:* Kanapa, Kanigi,.

Description: An erect dichotomously branched annual upto 60 cm in height with 4-winged stems and decussate branches; leaves simple, ovate or lanceolate, acute, sessile, upto 5 cm long, prominently 3-nerved; flowers white, those in the forks, long pedicelled lax terminal dichasial cymes; fruits cylindric membranous septicidal capsules; seeds very small, brown, reticulate.

Habitate: Throughout India, in moist areas upto 1,500 m elevation. South East Asia, Australia and Africa.

Propagation: By seeds.

Parts Used: Whole plant.

Chemical Constituents: Contain loliolide, gluanone, canscoradione, friedelin, friedelan-3β-ol, β-amyrin, sitosterol, stigmasterol, campesterol, *n*-alkanes, and*n*-alkanols.

Uses: The plant is bitter, acrid, astringent, thermogenic, laxative, vulnerary, emollient, alexeteric, anthelmintic, appetizer, intellect promoting, aphrodisiac, depurative, rejuvenating and tonic. It is useful in vitiated conditions of *kapha*, inflammation, ascites, abdominal disorders, intestinal worms, insanity, epilepsy, nervous debility, forgetfulness, leucoderma, leprosy, skin diseases, tuberculosis, ulcers and general debility.

258. *Canthium parviflorum* Lam. *(Rubiaceae)*

Vernacular Name: *San*: Gangeruki, Chayatinisah, Naga-vala, *Eng:* Carray cheddie, Wild Jessamine, *Hin:* Kirma, Kadbar, *Kan:* Kakegida, *Mal:* Cerukara, Kantankara, Karamullu, Kara, *Tam:* Karaicceti, *Tel:* Balusu.

Description: A thorny subscandent shrub with spreading branches; leaves simple, small, opposite with interpetiolar stipules and axillary spines; flowers yellowish white, 4-merous, small, in axillary cymes, corolla tube short; fruits oblong-ellipsoid or compressed drupes, yellow when ripe.

Habitate: Throughout India, in scrub forests and dry plains.

Propagation: By seeds.

Parts Used: Roots, leaves.

Chemical Constituents: Mannitol and alkaloids.

Uses: The roots and leaves are astringent, sweet, thermogenic, diuretic, febrifuge, constipating, anthelmintic and tonic. They are useful in vitiated conditions of *kapha*, diarrhoea, strangury, fever, leucorrhoea, intestinal worms and general debility.

259. *Capits chinensis* *(Ranunculaceae)*

Vernacular Name: *Eng:* huang lian, Chinese goldthread.

Description: Perennial herb growing to 50cm. Has basal leaves and small whitish-green flowers.

Habitate: This herb is native to the mountains of China, and is most commonly cultivated in Szechwan province.

Propagation: By Seeds.

Parts Used: Root.

Chemical Constituents: Contains isoquiniline alkaloids, including berberine, coptisine and worenine. B erberine is antibacterial, amoebicidal and antidiarrhoeal.

Uses: A bitter-tasting herb, *huang lain* is given in the Chinese herbal tradition as a decoction to "clear heat" and "dry dampness", relieving fever, red and sore eyes, and sore throats. The herb is particularly helpful for diarrhoea and dysentery, and has been used to quell vomiting. Skin problems such as acne, boils, abscesses and burns are also treated with *huang lain.* Like the root of goldthread *huang lain* is taken as a gargle for mouth and tongue ulcers, and for swollen gums and toothache. Both herbs are also used as an eyewash to treat acute conjunctivitis.

260. *Capparis deciduas* (Forsk.) Edgew. (*Capparidaceae)*

Synonyms: *Capparis aphylla* Roth.

Vernacular Name: *San*: Karira, *Eng:* Caper, Berry, *Hin:* Karil, Kurel, Ker, *Kan:* Nispatige, *Mal:* Karimulli, Karimullu, *Tam:* Senkam, Sirakkali, *Tel:* Enugadanta.

Description: A densely branching straggling glabrous shrub with smooth terete reen branches; leaves simple, caduceus, found only on young shoots, linear-oblong, acute, spinous pointed, stipular thorns long, sharp, straight, orange yellow; flowers red, in many flowered corymbs on old branches or short lateral shoots, gynophore about 12 mm long; fruits globular, glabrous, beaked; seeds numerous embedded in the pulp.

Habitate: Throughout India, in dry areas.

Propagation: By seeds and vegetative method.

Parts Used: Roots, fruits.

Chemical Constituents: Its contain is capparin, capparilin, and capparinin, *l*-stachydrine, capparidisine, capparisine, capparisinine, *n*-pentacosane, *n*-triacontanol and β-sitosterol.

Uses: The roots are acrid, bitter, thermogenic, anodyne, sudorific, expectorant, digestive, carminative, anthelmintic, purgative, antibacterial, vulnerary, alexeteric, stimulant, emmenagogue, aphrodisiac and tonic. They are useful in boils, eruptions, swelling, chronic and foul ulcers, cough, hiccough, asthma, vomiting, haemorrhoids, intermittent fevers, arthritis, odontalgia, lumbago, dyspepsia, flatulence, constipation, intestinal worms, cardiac debility, gout, amenorrhoea, dysmenorrhoea and general debility. The fruits are bitter, sweet, astringent, acrid, thermogenic and constipating. They are useful in halitosis, cardiac disorders, urethrorrhea and vitiated conditions of *pitta.*

261. *Capparis spinosa* *(Capparidaceae)*

Vernacular Name: *Eng:* Caper.

Description: Shrub growing to 1m, with spiny trailing stems, fleshy oval leaves, green buds, large white flowers, and red berries in autumn.

Habitate: Native to the Mediterranean region, caper thrives in wasteland, often growing on stony terrain.

Propagation: By Seeds and vegetative method.

Parts Used: Root bark, bark, flowers buds.

Chemical Constituents: Caper contains capric acid.

Uses: The unopened flower buds are laxative and, if prepared correctly with vinegar, are thought to ease stomach pain. The bark is bitter and diuretic and can be taken immediately before meals to increase the appetite. The root bark is purifying and stops internal bleeding. It is used to treat skin conditions, capillary weakness and easy bruising and is also used in cosmetic preparations. A decoction of the plant is used to treat vaginal thrush.

262. *Capsella bursa pastoris* Moench. *(Cruciferae)*

Synonyms: *Capsella bursa* Rafin., *Capsella pastoris* Rubr.

Vernacular Name: *Eng:* Shephered's Purse.

Description: A glabrous or hairy herb 15-20 cm. tall with long and tapering root, with both radical and cauline leaves. Radical leaves oblong, acute or oblanceolate, tapering into petiole, emarginated, dentate or pinnatified-parted with narrow triangular pointed lobes, sometimes entire; while the stem leaves alternate, sessile, oblong-lanceolate, amplexicaul, hestate or sagitate at the base with acute parallel or diverging auricles. Flowers small, white in raceme; calyx 4 corolla 4, corolla tube as long as calyx, stamens 6 of which 4 longer than the rest two. Stem simple or branching with angular and ribbed surface. Fruit inversely triangular or triangular cordate with a notch at the apex, flattened from sides, 5-8 cm. by 4-5 cm.

Habitate: India, N-W temperate Himalayas.

Propagation: By seeds.

Parts Used: Whole plant.

Chemical Constituents: Acetylcholine, Choline, Proline, Histamine, Rutin, Hesperidin. Bursinic acid. Fumaric acid. Ascrobic acid and Vit-K. Camphor. Bursin. Diosmin. Thiocyanic acid.

Uses: It is used as an anti-haemorrhagic and anti-uric acid remedy. Used in complaints of haemorrhage from uterine fibroids with aching in back. Uterine haemorrhage with cramps, expulsion of clots. Menses too early, too profuse, 8-10-15 days early, tardy in starting, flowered by colic, vomiting & bleeding in large clots. Metrorrhagia with violent cramps and uterine colic with brick-dust sediments in urine. Urethritis very useful. Cystitis. Frequent epistaxis. Sharp pain over the right eye, while moving the eye upwards.

263. *Capsicum annuum* *(Solanaceae)*

Vernacular Name: *Eng:* Chilli, purple red or yellow chilli; *Hin:* Lamirch, gachmarich; *Beng*: lankamorich, lalmorich; *Tel:* Mirapa, kaya; *Tam:* Milagay; *Kan:* Mensina kai and *Mal:* Mulaku.

Description: A herbaceous, short-lived perennial, upto 1 m in height; leaves oblong, glabrous, flowers solitary, rarely in pairs, white to bluish white, berries green, maturing into yellow than red; seeds white or cream to yellow, thin, almost circular, having long placental connections.

Habitate: Cultivated throughout India.

Propagation: By seeds.

Part Used: Fruits.

Chemical Constituents: The fruits yield an oleoresin containing the characteristic odour and flavour of the spice. The major constituent of the oleoresin is capasaicin. The vacuum isolated bellpepper oil contains 2-methoxy-3-isobutylpyrazine, trans-b-ocimene, limonene, methyl salicylate, linalool, and hex-cis-3-enol as major constituents. Additional components detected in larger amounts in oil isolated at atmospheric pressure are non-1-en-4-one, non-trans-2-en-4-one, nona-trans, trans-2,5-dien-4-one, 2-entyl-furan, and benzaladehyde. 2-isobutyl1-3-methoxy pyraxine is an important flavour component of bell and Jalapeno peppers. Other important aroma components of bell-pepper are nona-trans, cis-2,6-dienal and deca-trans, trans-2,4-dienal.

Uses: The green chillies are used fresh for garnishing or flavouring savorry dishes. Bell pepper or capsicum is extensively used as food flavouring in processed foods, meat and vegetable soups, etc, Milder varieties or red chilli, as powder are used for garnishing an flavouring meat and fish dishes, salad-dressing, hot chilli sauces, tomato ketchup and as ingredients of ground spice powders. It is also used to enhance the pungency of black pepper, ginger and mustard. The oleoresin, a dark red viscous liquid, with the characteristic aroma of the spice, is used for blending flavours, particularly in the West. Three grades of oleoresin, classified on the basis of pungency, are available, of which oleoresin capsicum is used to impart pungency to manufactured food and some beverages and oleoresin red-pepper is chiefly used as a flavouring.

264. *Capsicum frutescens* L. *(Solanaceae)*

Synonyms: *Capsicum minimum.*

Vernacular Name: *Eng:* Chili pepper, red pepper, paprika.

Description: Perennial erect herb or small subshrub to 2 m high. Leaves alternate, petiolate, simple, ovate and pointed with entire margins. Flowers borne usually singly in leaf and branch axils, white to violet, five-parted. Fruit a dry to fleshy red elongated berry with numerous lattened seeds which are hot tasting.

Habitate: Commonly cultivated, as well as naturalized in weedy habitates from sea-level to lower montane.

Propagation: By seeds.

Part Used: Fruits and leaves.

Chemical Constituents: Ascorbic acid, caffeic acid, caproic acid, capsaicin, dihydrocapsaicin, cinnamic acid, para-coumaric acid, ferulic acid, mevalonic acid, pyrazine derivative, capsidiol, kaempferol derivative, quercetin derivative, lipids. Vitamins A 7 B, capsicin, volatile and fatty oils, pentosans, pectins. Acetic, butyric and isobytyric acids.

Uses: Is used as a remedy for diseases of the skin, tuberculosis, mild conjuctivitis and jauncie. Also used to treat boils, abscesses and wounds. Used to treat inflammations and coughs. Coconut oil mixed with the crushed leaves is applied to boils. The fruit contains a strong stimulant which causes a sensation of warmth when applied to the skin. The stronger doses, it causes a burning sensation without blistering. When taken internally it causes a sensation of warmth without any narcotic effect.

265. *Caragana sinica* (Buc'hoz) Rehder *(Fabaceae)*

Vernacular Name: *Eng:* Chinese pea shrub.

Description: Hardy shrub, to 2 m tall. Leaves alternate, even-pinnate; rachis turned into bristle at tip; leaflets in 2 pairs, remote from one another, obovate or elliptic, 1-3 cm long, slightly retuse or rounded at tip, dark green, glossy, small, entire; stipules 4-8 mm long spines. Flowers reddish-yellow, solitary at axils, 2.5-3 cm long, papilionaceous, long-claewed; pedicels 1 cm long, ring-like node in the middle; stamens 10, 9 united and 1 separate. Fruit linear, straight, glabrous, cylindrical legume.

Habitate: Open stops on mountains in Korea and North China.

Propagation: By seeds.

Parts Used: Root.

Chemical Constituents: Stilbenes. Saponions; caraganosides.

Uses: Anti-inflammatory, protein kinase C inhibition. Used in arthritis, neuralgia, diarrhoea, bone weakness.

266. *Cardiospermum halicacabum* L. *(Sapindaceae)*

Vernacular Name: *San*: Sakralata, Indravalli; *Eng:* Ballon vine, Heart pea, *Hin:* Kanphuti, Kapalphoti, *Kan:* Kanakayya, *Mal:* Ulinna, *Tam:* Mudukkottan, Modikkottan, *Tel:* Vekkudutiga.

Description: A pubescent or nearly glabrous annual or perennial with slender branches climbing by means of tendrillar hooks; leaves ternately bicompound, leaflets acuminate at the apex; flowers white, small; fruits membranous, depressed, pyriform capsule winged at the angles; seeds black with a large white heart-shaped aril.

Habitate: Throughout India, in the plains.

Propagation: By seeds.

Parts Used: Roots, leaves, seeds.

Chemical Constituents: Its contain alkaloid, l-triacontanol, and n-pentacosane, n-triacontane, n-triacontanol, n-non-acosane, pelargonidin-3-galactoside, glucocappasalin, β-sitosterol and phthalic acid.

Uses: The roots are diuretic, diaphoretic, emetic, mucilaginous, laxative and emmenagogue. They are useful in strangury, fever, arthritis, amenorrhoea, lumbago and neuropathy. The leaves are rubefacient and are good for arthritis, otalgia and ophthalmodynia. The seeds are tonic and diaphoretic, and are good for arthritis and fever. The plant has sedative action on the central nervous system.

267. *Carduus marianus* *(Asteraceae)*

Synonyms*:* *Silybum marianum.*

Vernacular Name: *Eng:* Milk Thistle, Mary Thistle.

Description: A spiny biennial, growing to 1.5 m, with white-veined leaves and purple flowerheads.

Habitate: Native to the Mediterranean, milk thistle grows throughout Europe but is rare in Britain. Now also cultivated in India.

Propagation: By Seeds.

Parts Used: Flowers and Seeds.

Chemical Constituents: Flavonlignans (1-4%) (Silymarin), Bitter principles, Polyacetylenes.

Uses: Protects the liver, Stimulates secretion of bile, Increases breast-milk production, AntidepresSant.

268. *Carica papaya* L. *(Caricaceae)*

Synonyms: .

Vernacular Name: *San*: Brahmairandah, Erandakarkati, *Eng:* Papaw tree, Papaya, *Hin:* Pappaya, Pappita, *Kan:* Pappaya, Peragi, Piranji, *Mal:* Pappaya, Karmmusu, Pappali, Karmmatti, *Tam:* Pappali, *Tel:* Bappayi, Bobbasi.

Description: A small, soft-wooded, fast growing, short lived laticiferous tree upto 8.0m in height with a straight cylindric stem bearing characteristic leaf-scars throughout and with a tuft of leaves at the top; leaves deeply lobed, palm-like with characteristically long, hollow petiole; flowers unisexual, white or yellowish white, rarely bisexual, males in long drooping panicles; females in short clusters; fruits one-chambered, succulent, indehiscent, spherical or cylindrical; seeds many, yellowish brown, ash coloured or black.

Habitate: Throughout India, cultivated.

Propagation: By seeds.

Parts Used: Fruits, latex.

Chemical Constituents: Cryptoxanthin, 48.16; β-carotene, 29.56; cryptoflavin, 12.85; and violaxanthin, 3.42%, phytoene, phytofluene, cis-β-carotene, ζ-carotene, γ-carotene, 5, 6-monoepoxy-β-carotene, mutatochorme, aurochrome, cis-violaxanthin, antheraxanthin, chrysanthemaxanthin, and neoxanthin.

Uses: The fruits are bitter, acrid, thermogenic, anodyne, aphrodisiac, stomachic, appetizer, digestive, carminative, anthelmintic, styptic, anti-inflammatory, antifungal, demulcent and diuretic. They are useful in vitiated conditions of *vata*, cough, bronchitis, stomachalgia, dyspepsia, anorexia, intestinal worms, haemoptysis, haemorrhoids, inflammations, splenomegaly, ringworm, skin diseases, psoriasis, urinary calculus and injures of the urinary tract. The latex is anthelmintic, anodyne, laxative, digestive, emmenagogue, galactagogue, depurative, sudorific, febrifuge and tonic. It is useful in round worm infestation, stomachalgia, dyspepsia, constipation, amenorrhoea, dysmenorrhoea, agalactia, skin diseases, leprosy, haemorrhoids, fever, strangury and general debility.

269. *Carissa carandas* L. *(Apocynaceae)*

Synonyms: .

Vernacular Name: *San*: Karamardah, Avighnah, *Eng:* Karaunda, Jasmine flowered carrisa, *Hin:* Karaunda, *Kan:* Karikayi, *Mal:* Klavu, Perumklavu, Karanta, *Tam:* Kalakkai, Perumkla, *Tel:* Peddakalavi, Vaka.

Description: A large dichotomously branched evergreen shrub with short stem and strong thorns in pairs, bark light grey, scaly; leaves simple, opposite, elliptic or obovate, shortly mucronate, glabrous, shining and coriaceous; flowers white, in pubescent terminal corymbose cymes; fruit ellipsoid or globose berry, purplish black when ripe enclosing two or more seeds.

Habitate: Throughout India, in dry forests, also cultivated.

Propagation: By seeds.

Parts Used: Roots, fruits.

Chemical Constituents: Contain carissone, carindone, carinol and four crystalline substances, viz. A; B; a cardioactive and β-sitosterol.

Uses: The roots are anthelmintic, stomachic and antiscorbutic, and are useful in stomach disorders, intestinal worms, scabies and pruritus. The unripe fruit is sour, astringent, bitter thermogenic, constipating, anaphrodisiac, appetizer and antipyretic, and is useful in vitiated conditions of *pitta* and *kapha*, hyperdipsia, diarrhoea, anorexia, and intermittent fevers. The ripe fruit is sweet cooling, appetiser and antiscorbutic, and is useful in anorexia, vitiated conditions of *pitta* and *vata*, burning sensation, skin diseases scabies and pruritus.

270. *Cartemisia maritime* L. *(Asteraceae)*

Synonyms: *Artemisia anglica* Hort ex. D.C., *Artemisia acetica Jacquem* ex. Bess., *Artemisia cina* Berg.

Vernacular Name: *Eng:* Wormseed. Sea wormwood seed.

Description: A strongly aromatic evergreen perennial under shrub with clusters of spreading to erect, partly woody stem, upto 60 cm. high, grey or white downy. Lower leaves 2-pinnate with very narrow blunt segments, white wooly on both sides, withering at flowering. Upper leaves similar but smaller and short stalked. Flower heads about 2-3 mm. in diameter, ovoid, sessile, in long leafy branched inflorescence. Florets yellow, yellowish-orange, pale brown.

Habitate: Western temperate Himalayas of India and mainly coastal regions of Europe.

Propagation: By seeds.

Parts Used: Flowers heads.

Chemical Constituents: *San*tonin and Artemisin.

Uses: A very good anthelmintic. For complaints of children suffering from worms with great irritability, grinding teeth, screaming during sleep, Ascarides, constant digging and boring at the nose, picking the nose all the time, itching of nose, sickly white and bluish appearance around mouth, with dark rings under the eyes, one cheek red and other pale. Canine hunger due to worms. Turbid urine turning milky and semisolid after standing. Twitching, jerking and trembling of limbs.

271. *Carthamus tinctorius* L. *(Asteraceae)*

Vernacular Name: *Eng:* Safflower; American saffron; false saffron.

Description: An annual, erect, branching herb 0.6-1.0 m high, glabrous; stem whitish, striate. Leaves sessile, somewhat clasping, broad-laneolate or lanceolate-oblong, attenuated at both ends, strongly dentate, slightly spinous; ventation pinnate and netted. Inflorescene a broad corymb, heads 3-5 borne on leafy peduncles. Flowers orange-red, fruit a white achene, obovoid, 4-angled, truncate at the top with 4 bosses; no pappus.

Habitate: Commonly cultivated in the fields in Cambodia, China, India, Laos, Middle East, Viet Nam.

Propagation: By seeds.

Part Used: Flowers.

Chemical Constituents: N.A.

Uses: Dysmennorhoea; amennorhoea, coronary heart diseases; angina pectoris, injuries; pains due to blood stasis.

272. *Carum carvi* L. *(Apiaceae)*

Vernacular Name: *San:* Sushavi; *Eng:* Caraway; *Hin:* Shia-jira, zira; *Beng*: Jira; *Tam:* Shimai-shembu; *Tel:* Shimaisapu.

Description: Annual or biennial herb; leaves pinnately dissected; flowers in dense white umbels; schizocarps oblong-oval, yellowish brown, mericarps aromatic.

Habitate: Himachal Pradesh; cultivated in the hills and plains of North India, and hills of south India.

Propagation: By seeds.

Part Used: Fruits.

Chemical Constituents: The chief constituents of the oil are carvone and limonene to which the odour and flavour are attributed. Other important consituents in the oil are a-and b-pinenes and p-cymene.

Uses: Caraway seeds (fruits) are widely used for flavouring bread, biscuits, cakes, candies, cheese, pickles, curries, sausages, meat products, confectionery, cordials, and liqueurs. Caraway oil is used like seeds for flavouring food products.

273. *Carum copticum* Benth, & Hook. f. *(Apiaceae)*

Vernacular Name: *San*: Yavanika, *Hin:* Ajowan.

Description: *Carum copticum* grows as a herb whose roots are fusiform. Stems are 30 to 90 cms long. *Leaves* are 2-3 pinnate bracts several and linear. The *fruit* is ovoid in shape and grayish brown in colour.

Habitate: The plant is largely cultivated in Eastern India. It is particularly abundant in and around Indore and in Andhra Pradesh. It also grows in Iran, Afghanistan, Pakistan and Egypt.

Propagation: By seeds.

Parts Used: Fruits, leaves, seeds, oil and essence.

Chemical Constituents: Contstituents of the seeds are: an aromatic volatile essential oil, and a crystalline substance stearoptene. It also contains cumene and terpene–'thymene'. The stearoptene is known as ajown-ka-phul. A phenolic glucosde has been isolated and identified as 2-methyl-3-glucosyoxy-5-isopropylphenol. The fruit yields 2 to 4% of a colourless brownish essential oil in which thymol is present to the extent of 35 to 60%. Theymol crystallizes easily from the oil. The remainder of the oil consists of p-cymene, β-pinene, dipentene, β-terpinene and carvacrol. The mixture is commercially known as thymene. TLC patterns have been studied.

Uses: Flatulence and colic, diarrhoea, urticaria, helminthiasis. The seeds are useful in flatulence, indigestion, colic, dyspepsia and diarrhoea. Fried seeds are particularly used in the control of diarrhoea. Volatile oil too is used in flatulence, colic, atonic dyspepsia or diarrhoea, hysteria and indigestion. The oil is mainly carminative and anti flatulent. It is also applied to relieve rheumatic and neuralgic pain. It is also used to eradicate worms and in urticaria.

274. *Caryota urens* L. *(Arecaceae)*

Vernacular Name: *San*: Sritalah, Dirgha, meda, *Eng:* Fish-tail palm, Elephant's palm, *Hin:* Mari, Bankhajur, *Kan:* Kondapana, *Mal:* Cuntappana, Anappana, Irampana, *Tam:* Kuntalpanai, Kuntarpanai, *Tel:* Jilugujattu, Kondajilugu.

Description: A lofty handsome palm with a smooth, cylindrical, shiny, annulate trunk, bearing a crown of large leaves; leaves 5-6m long, drooping, bipinnate with leaflets shaped like the tail of a fish, monoecious; flowers on pendulous spadix, inflorescence 3-4m long resembling a huge docked horse tail, flowers in groups of three, female in the center and males on sides; fruits globose, reddish when ripe.

Habitate: Throughout India from sea level to 1,200m, in Sri Lanka and Malaysia.

Propagation: By seeds.

Parts Used: Tender bud leaves and nuts.

Chemical Constituents: Its contain l-epicatechin, l-gallocatechin and l-epicatechingallate.

Uses: The tender leaves are sweet and cooling, and are useful in vitiated conditions of *pitta*. The pulp of the fruit is good for hyperdipsia and fatigue. A paste made from the nut is good for hemicrania.

275. *Cassia absus* L. *(Caesalpiniaceae)*

Vernacular Name: *San*: Kulatthika, Caksusya, *Hin:* Chaksu, Bankultthi, *Kan:* Kuti; *Mal:* Karinkolla, *Tam:* Mulaippalvirai, Kattukkol, *Tel:* Campalavittulu.

Description: A viscid erect annual or biennial upto 45cm in height with spreading branches clothed with glandular hairs; leaves compound, rachis viscous hairy, leaflets two pairs, very oblique, elliptic-oblong or elliptic-obovate, the terminal pair the largest; flowers reddish yellow in terminal or leaf-opposed, erect, few flowered racemes, stamens five, all equal and perfect; fruits ligulate, dehiscent, compressed pods, clothed with bristly hairs, seeds 4-6, trapezoid-ovoid, black, shining.

Habitate: Throughout India, in dry wastelands and open areas in forests.

Propagation: By seeds.

Parts Used: Leaves, seeds.

Chemical Constituents: Aloe-emodin, chrysophanol, isochrysophanol, rhein, physicion-l-glucoside, and β-sitosterol.

Uses: The leaves are bitter, astringent, acrid, thermogenic, haematinic, constipating and expectorant. They are useful in vitiated conditions of *kapha*, tumours, anaemia, diarrhoea, nasitis, cough, asthma and hiccough. The seeds are bitter, astringent, acrid, cooling, ophthalmic, haemostatic, diuretic, revulsive, constipating, alexeteric and vulnerary. They are useful in vitiated conditions of *kappa* and *pitta*, ophthalmopathy such as conjunctivitis, dysopia, ophthalmia, cataract, etc., epistaxis, haematemesis, haemorrhages, strangury, obesity, diarrhoea, dysentery, nephrolithiasis, poisonous bites, wounds, ulcers and bruises.

276. *Cassia alata* L. *(Caesalpiniaceae)*

Vernacular Name: *Eng*: Ringworm shrub, winged senna, ringworm senna, candelabra bush, craw-craw plant.

Description: Small shrub, about 1.5m. high, with horizontal branches leaves paripinnate, alternate; leaflets 8-12 pairs, broadly rounded, oblique at the base. Twigs and petioles usually reddish-brown. Inflorescence in axillary and terminal erect spike; flowers yellow. Pod long, slightly compressed, with winged margin. Seeds numerous, black.

Habitate: Grows wild in wet places and is also cultivated for its ornamental foliage and showy flowers.

Propagation: By seeds.

Part Used: Leaves.

Chemical Constituents: The leaves contain anthraglucosides, chrysophanic acid and rhein.

Uses: The leaves and the stem have antiseptic and laxative properties. They are prescrived for constipation, oedema, hepatitis and icterus in a tea-like infusion. Dermatomycosis, tinea imbricata, ringworm, scabies and impetigo are treated externally by rubbing with pounded fresh leaves or by applying fresh leaf juice on the diseased parts.

277. *Cassia angustifolia* Vahl. *(Caesalpiniaceae)*

Vernacular Name: *San:* Swarnpatri, Bhumiari, bhupadma; *Hin:* Sanaya; *Beng*: Sanna-makki, son-pat; *Tam:* Nila virai; *Tel:* Nela-tangedu; *Kan:* Nelavarike and *Mal:* Nila vaka.

Description: A small shrub, 61-91 cm in height. Leaves paripinnate; leaflets in 7-8 pairs, glabrous, yellowish-green, 2.5-5.1 cm x 0.4-1.3 cm. Flowers yellow. Pods greenish-brown to dark-brown, 3.4-6.8 cm long and 1.9 cm broad. Seeds 5-7, obovate, smooth, dark-brown.

Habitate: Cultivated in South India, Rajasthan (Jodhpur) and Gujarat.

Propagation: By seeds.

Part Used: Leaves and pods.

Chemical Constituents: The pods contain sennosides A and B, sennidin-8.8-diglucoside, glycosides of rhein and chrysophanic acid, aloe-emodin, its dianthrone diglucoside and emodin glucoside. Occurrence of oxymethyl-anthraquinone has been reported from the fruits. Leaves contain flavanols, isorhamnetin, kaempferol, rhein, emodin and sennosides A, B, C and D.

Uses: Laxative and purgative, used in contipation, loss of appetite, hepatomegaly, spleenomegaly, indigestion, malaria, skin diseases, jaundice and anaemia.

278. *Cassia auriculata* L. *(Caesalpiniaceae)*

Synonyms: .

Vernacular Name: *San*: Avarttaki, Hemapushpam, *Eng:* Tanner's cassia, Tanner's Senna, *Hin:* Tarval, Anwal, *Kan:* Tangedu, Taravadagida, *Mal:* Aviram, Avara, *Tam:* Avarai, Avirai, *Tel:* Tangedu.

Description: A much branched shrub with reddish brown branches; leaves with subulate glands between all the 8-12 pairs of leaflets and a pair of large obliquely cordate stipules at their bases; flowers bright yellow in sub-terminal axillary corymbs; fruits pods, flat, thin, papery, pale brown, deeply depressed between the seeds, transversely veined; seeds 10-20 per pod, obovate, dark brown with hard shiny seed coat.

Habitate: Throughout central and south India, in most districts on dry stony hills and black cotton soil.

Propagation: By seeds.

Parts Used: Roots, bark, leaves, flowers, seeds.

Chemical Constituents: Emodin, chrysophanol, rubiadin.

Uses: The roots are astringent, cooling, alterative, depruative and alexeteric, and are useful in skin diseases, leprosy, tumours, asthma and urethrorrhoea. The bark is astringent and alternative, and a decoction of this is used as enemas and gargles. The leaves are depurative and anthelmintic, and are recommended for leprosy, skin diseases and ulcers. The flowers are used in diabetes, urethrorrhoea, nocturnal emissions and pharyngopathy. The seeds are astringent. Sour, cooling, constipating, depurative, aphrodisiac, anthelmintic, stomachic and alexeteric, and are useful in diabetes, chyluria, ophthalmia, dysentery, diarrhoea, swellings, abdominal disorders, leprosy, skin diseases, worm infestations and chronic purulent conjunctivitis.

279. *Cassia fistula* L. *(Caesalpiniaceae)*

Synonyms: *Cassia rhombifolia* Roxb.

Vernacular Name: *San*: Argvadhah, Krtamalah, *Eng:* Indian laburnum, Purging fistula, Golden-shower, *Hin:* Amaltas, Girimala, *Kan:* Kakke, Kakke mara, *Mal:* Konna, Kanikkonna, *Tam:* Konnai, *Tel:* Rela, Kondrakaya, Aragvadamu.

Description: A moderate sized handsome deciduous tree, 8-15m in height with greenish grey smooth bark when young, and rough when old, exfoliating in hard scales; leaves pinnately compound, leaflets 4-8 pairs, ovate, acute, bright green, glabrous above, paler and silvery-pubescent beneath when young, main nerves numerous; flowers bright yellow in lax pendulous racemes; fruits cylindric pods, 30-60cm long, shortly stipitate, nearly straight, smooth, shiny, brownish black; seeds broadly ovate, horinzontally immersed in dark coloured sweetish pulp.

Habitate: Throughout India in deciduous forests.

Propagation: By seeds.

Parts Used: All parts of plant.

Chemical Constituents: The contains sennosides A and B, rhein and its glucoside, barbaloin, aloin, formic acid, butyric acid, their ethyl esters and oxalic acid, sap, acetyl acid, iod, thiocyanogen and unsapon matter, tannins, phlobaphenes, reducing sugars and oxyanthraquinones.

Uses: The roots are astringent, cooling, prugative, febrifuge and tonic, and are useful in skin diseases, tuberculous glands, syphilis and burning sensation. The bark is laxative, anthelmintic, emetic, febrifuge, diuretic and depurative, and is useful in boils, pustules, leprosy, ringworm, colic, dyspepsia, constipation, fever, diabetes, strangury and cardiopathy. The leaves are laxative, antiperiodic and depurative, and are useful in vitiated conditions of *vata*, skin diseases, leprosy, ulcers and intermittent fevers. The flowers are bitter, acrid, cooling, emollient, expectorant and demulcent, and are useful in vitiated conditions of *pitta*, skin diseases, pruritus, burning sensation, dry cough and bronchitis. The fruits are sweet, cooling, emollient, purgative, anodyne, anti-inflammatory, depurative, antipyretic, abortifacient, diuretic and ophthalmic, and are useful in vitiated conditions of *pitta*, burning sensation, leprosy, skin diseases, pruritus, flatulence, colic, inflammations, rheumatism, gout, anorexia, hepatomegaly, jaundice, cardiac disorders, intermittent fever, strangury, opthalmopathy and general debility.

280. *Cassia occidentalis* L. *(Caesalpiniaceae)*

Synonyms: .

Vernacular Name: *San*: Kasamardah, *Eng:* Negro coffee, Stinking weed, Coffee-senna, *Hin:* Kasaumdi, Barikasaumdi, *Kan:* Doddaagace, *Mal:* Ponnaviram, Ponnariviram, *Tam:* Ponnavirai, Peravirai, Nattam takarai, *Tel:* Kasinda.

Description: A diffuse offensively odorous undershrub with furrowed subglabrous branches; leaflets 3-5 pairs; flower yellow, in short peduncled few flowered racemes; fruits cylindrical or compressed, transversely septate glabrous pods containing 20-30 seeds, seeds ovoid, compressed, hard, smooth and shiny dark olive-green or pale brown.

Habitate: Throughout India, growing abundantly on wastelands immediately after the rains.

Propagation: By seeds.

Parts Used: All parts of plant.

Chemical Constituents: Chrysophanol, emodin, glycosides, physcion, metteucinol-7-rhamnoside, jaceidin-7-rhamnoside, and 4, 4, 5, 5-tetrahydroxy-2, 2-dimethyl-1, 1-bianthraquinone, curde protein, ether extra, crude fibre, ash, calcium phosphorus, iron, niacin, and ascorbic acid, β-sitosterol, emodin, physcion.

Uses: The plant is bitter, sweet, thermogenic, purgative, expectorant, and febrifuge, and is useful in vitiated conditions of *vata* and *kapha*, cough, bronchitis, constipation, fever, epilepsy and convulsions. The roots are bitter, acrid, thermogenic, diuretic, anti inflammatory, digestive, stomachic, and tonic. They are useful in vitiated condition of *vata*, inflammation, diabetes, strangury, elephantiasis, ring worm, colic flatulence, dyspepsia, epilepsy, convulsions and scorption sting. The leaves are bitter, acrid, sweet, thermogenic, depurative, vulnerary, anodyne, expectorant, alexeteric and aphrodisiac, and are useful in vitiated conditions of *vata* and *kapha*, leprosy, erysipelas, pruritus, wounds and ulcers, cough, bronchitis, hiccough, asthma, pharyngodynia, fever and hydrophobia. The seeds are bitter, sweet, acrid, depurative, diuretic, expectorant, vulnerary, purgative, stomachic and febrifuge, and are useful in leprosy, erysipelas, ulcers, strangury, cough, bronchitis, hiccough, constipation, flatulence, dyspepsia and fever.

281. *Cassia tora* L. *(Caesalpiniaceae)*

Vernacular Name: *San:* Dadamari; *Eng*: Sickle senna, sickle pod, cofee weed, tavara; *Hin*: Chakunda, panevar; *Beng*: Chakunda, panevar; *Tel:* Tantemu; *Tam:* Tagarai.

Description: Annual shrubby weed, 30-90cm. In height. Leaves alternate, pinnate, with 3 pairs of obovate leaflets. Inflorescence in axillary raceme, shorter than the leaf; flowers yellow: 1-3. Pod slender, very long, curved Seeds numerous, dark-brown, shining.

Habitate: Grows wild on roadsides and field margins in the midlands and mountains.

Propagation: By seeds.

Part Used: Seeds.

Chemical Constituents: The whole plant contains anthraglucosides that on hydrolysis yield emodin and glucose, chrysophanol and rhein. The seeds yield a fatty oil consisting of oleic, linolic, palmitic and lignoceric acids and sitosterol.

Uses: The raw seeds are utilized as a laxative. The torrefied seeds are effective for insomnia, headache, constipation, oliguria, cough, ophthalmia, dacryoliths, amblyopia, ocular congestion and hypertension. The alcoholic or vinegar maceration of pounded fresh leaves is used externally to treat eczema and dermatomycosis.

282. *Cassytha filiformis* L. *(Lauraceae)*

Vernacular Name: *San:* Akashavalli; *Hin:* Amarbeli; *Beng*: Akasbel; *Tel:* Nulu, tega; *Tam:* Erumaikkottan; *Kan:* Akasa balli, beluballi and *Mal:* Akasavalli.

Description: Parastic twining vine with thin, leafless yellow to orangish stems. Flowers small, white, solitary, borne in axils of small bracts. Fruit a small shitish-yellow drupe surrounded by a cupule with a single hard seed within.

Habitate: Common on many trees in neglected plantings, light bush, weedy areas, and on coastal vegetation.

Propagation: By seeds.

Part Used: Whole plant.

Chemical Constituents: Cassyfiline (alkaloid) and its O-methyl derivative (cassythidine), cassythine, nantenine (alkaloid), ocoteine, gentisic acid, para-hydrooxybenzoic acid, exo-polygalacturonase, exo-pectin, methylgalacturonase 15, amino acids, laurotetanine, dulcitol, essential oil.

Uses: The plant is used to treat jellyfish stings. An infusion of the crushed stem is used to treat dysmenorrhoea and postpartum bleeding in women. Use an infusion of the crushed stem to treat a disease whose symptoms include convulsions or twitches. The plant is used in a remedy for haemorrhoids.

283. *Castanea sativa* *(Fagaceae)*

Vernacular Name: *Eng:* Sweet chestnut.

Description: Deciduous tree growing to a height of 30m. Has smooth silver-grey bark, lance-shaped dark green leaves, male and female catkins, and spiny yellow0-green seed cases containing 2-3 glossy brown nuts.

Habitate: Native to the Mediterranean, Asia Minor and the Caucasus, sweet chestnut grows freely across Europe, including Britain.

Propagation: By Seeds.

Parts Used: Leaves, bark.

Chemical Constituents: Sweet chestnut contains tannins, plastoquinones and mucilage.

Uses: An infusion of sweet chestnut leaves is taken to treat whooping cough, bronchitis and bronchial catarrh. The preparation tightens the mucous membranes and inhibits racking coughs. the leaves are used in the treatment of rheumatic conditions, to ease lower back pain and also to relieve stiff joints or muscles.

284. *Casuarina equisetifolia* L. *(Casuarinaceae)*

Vernacular Name: *Eng:* Ironwood, she-oak, beefwood tree; *Hin:* Jangli, saru; *Beng*: Jau; *Tel:* Sarugudu, chavuku; *Tam:* Savukku; *Kan:* Sarve, mara, chabaku; *Mal:* Chavukku.

Description: Tree to 25 high with drooping brancehs and needle like branchlets. Leaves highly reduced and scale-like giving the branchlets a pine-needle-like appearance. Flowers anemophilous (wind-pollinated), male flowers borne in spikes, each flower relatively inconspicuous, female flowers borne in globose heads. Fruit a globose woody aggregate (somewhat resembling a small pine cone) enclosing many small winged nuts.

Habitate: Common along the coast on beaches, rocky coasts, limestone outcroppings, dry hillsides and open forests in both wet and dry zones from sea-level t mid-montane.

Propagation: By seeds.

Part Used: Bark.

Chemical Constituents: Ellagic acid, beta-sitosterol, kaempferol and glycosides, quercetin, cupressuflvone, isoquerctrin, several common triterpenoids, trifolin, catechin and epicatechin, cholesterol, stigmasterol, campesterol, cholest-5-en-3-beta-ol derivatives, tannin, proantho-cyanidins, juglanin, citrulline and amino acids, afzelin, casuarine, gallicin, catechol derivatives, gentisic acid, hydroquinone, nictoflorine, rutin, trifolin.

Uses: The plant is used to treat nervous disorders, diarrhoea and gonorrhoea. Use it to treat coughs, ulcers, stomachaches and constipation. Dysuria and menorrhagia are treated with an infusion of the bark. Secondary amenorrhoea is treated with a decoction of the bark. An infusion of the bark, is used as an emetic to treat throat infections, coughs and stomachaches are also noted. An infusion of the bark is used as a remedy for coughs, asthma and diabetes. Use an infusion of the grated bark to treat mouth infections and urinary tract infections.

285. *Catha edulis* *(Celastraceae)*

Vernacular Name: *Eng:* Khat, Catha.

Description: A shrubs or small tree, upto 7 m in hight; stem straight, slender, bark white; leaves ovate-lanceolate to elliptic; flowers small, white in short ujmes; capsules woody, oblong, splitting into 3 values; seeds small, brown with oil-containing testa.

Habitate: Native to the Middle east and the Horn of Africa, khat prefers grassland and arid conditions.

Propagation: By Seeds.

Parts Used: Leaves, twigs.

Chemical Constituents: Khat contains alkaloids similar to those in *Ephedra* species-norpseudoephedrine and ephedrine, tannins and a volatile oil. Ephedrine-type alkaloids strongly stimulate the central nervous system, are anti-allergenic and suppress the appetite.

Uses: Mainly used as a social drug, khat is also chewed fresh or taken in an infusion to treat ailments such as malaria. In Africa, it is taken in old age, stimulating and improving mental function. Khat is used Germany to counter obesity.

286. *Catharanthus roseus* (L.) G. Don. *(Apocynaceae)*

Synonyms: *Lochnera rosea* (Linn.) Reichb; *Vinca rosea* Linn.

Vernacular Name: Eng.: Madagascar perwinkle, red perwinkle, pink periwinkle, rosy-flowered Indian perwinkle, cape perwinkle, old maid; *Hin:* Sadabahar; *Beng*: Nayantara; *Tel:* Billaganneru; *Tam:* Sudukadu mallikai; *Mal*: Ushamalari.

Description: Perennial herb, 30-80cm. High stems pinkish-red, much-branched, Leaves opposite, obovate, glabrous on both sides, dark shining above flowers pink or white in the axil of the leaves. Follicle cylindrical, narrow, slightly arched-recurved in pairs; seeds numerous, tiny, blackish-brown.

Habitate: Common wild plant in coastal areas and is also cultivated.

Propagation: By seeds.

Part Used: Leaves and root.

Chemical Constituents: The leaves contain alkaloids: serpentine, ajmaline, ajmaliine, catharanthine, catharanthinole, vindoline, vindolinine, vincaleucoblastine, leurosidine, vincristine.

Uses: The leaves are useful in treating oliguria, haematuria, diabetics mellitus and menstrual disorders. The roots and the leaves in the form of a decoction or extract are active on hypertension. The purified alkaloids extracted from the leaves are effective in treating leukaemia, and those from the roots are used to induce cerebrovascular dilatation and for hypertension.

287. *Catunaregam spinosa* (Thunb.) *(Rubiaceae)*

Synonyms: *Xeromphis spinosa* (Thunb.) Keay, *Randia dumetorum* (Retz.) Lam.

Vernacular Name: *San*: Madana, *Eng:* Emetic nut tree, Common emetic nut, *Hin:* Mainphal, Madan, *Kan:* Banegaru, Kare, Mangarike, Mangri, *Mal:* Malankara, Karacculli, *Tam:* Madkarai, Marukkalankay, *Tel:* Manga, Marrga, Manda.

Description: A large deciduous armed shrub upto 9.0m in height with strong straight spines, horizontal rigid branches and dark brown or grey rough scaly bark; leaves simple, usually fascicled on the suppressed branches, obovate, obtuse, wrinkled, shining or more or less pubescent above and on nerves beneath, main nerves 6-10 pairs; flowers at first white, later turning yellow, fragrant, solitary or 2-3 together at the ends of short leaf-bearing branchlets; fruits globose or broadly ovoid, smooth or obscurely longitudinally ribbed berries, yellow when ripe, crowned with the large calyx limb; seeds many, angular, embedded in the pulp.

Habitate: Throughout India in deciduous forests and exposed areas upto an elevation of 1,350 m.

Propagation: By seeds.

Parts Used: Bark, fruits.

Chemical Constituents: Saponins, dumetoronins A, B, C, D, E and F; olean 3-Orandioside A and ursoasaponin.

Uses: The bark is astringent, emetic, abortifacient, anodyne, constipating and antiseptic, and is useful in ostalgia during fever, diarrhoea, dysentery, bruises, cuts and vitiated conditions of *vata*. The fruits are bitter, astringent, acrid, sweet, thermogenic, emetic, anodyne, anti-inflammatory, carminative, anthelmintic, depurative, vulnerary, emmenagogue, expectorant, febrifuge, sudorific, abortifacient and antispasmodic, and are useful in vitiated conditions of *pitta* and *kapha*, pains and sprains, inflammations, gout, helminthiasis, leprosy, skin diseases, wounds, ulcers, tumours, amenorrhoea, dysmenorrhoea, cough, asthma, bronchitis, flatulence, colic, constipation and fever.

288. *Caulophyllum thalictroides* Michx. *(Berberidaceae)*

Synonyms: *Leontice thalictroides* Linn.

Vernacular Name: *Eng:* Blue cohosh, Pappoose root

Description: A perennial herb with thickened root-stocks, stem upto 1 m. in height with a large triternate almost sessile leaf near the summit and smaller usually biternate leaf near the base of the panicle; leaflets oval to obovate, 3-5 lobed, 2.5-10 cm. long. Flowers in terminal panicles, yellow-green, or greenish purple, 1.25 cm. across; sepals 6; petals 6, reduced to small gland like bodies, opposite the sepals, stamens 6; pistil forming head smaller than sepals, seeds 8 mm. thick, blueblack.

Habitate: U.S.A., Canada.

Propagation: By seeds.

Parts Used: Rhizome including roots.

Chemical Constituents: Caulosapoin, Cauloside; Anagyrine, Magnoflorine, Methylcytisine, Baptifoline; Starch; Citrullol, gum, resins, phytosterols.

Uses: Diuretic, Emmenagogue. Antispasmodic. For complaints of women especially for restoring tonicity of the uterus; extraordinary rigidity of the uterine-Os, which ca**Uses** spasmodic and severe pain during labour & makes the patient exhausted & fretful with pain radiating in all directions. Revives labour pains and further progress of labour. Leucorrhoea with MOTH-SPOTS on forehead. Habitual abortion. Needle like pain in cervix. Dysmenrrhoea with pains flying in all direction. Lochia, Chorea, hysteria or epilepsy at puberty. Dyspepsia with spasm. Stiftness of small bones.

289. *Cayratia carnosa* (Wall. ex Wight). *(Vitaceae)*

Synonyms: *Vitis carnosa* Linn., *Cayratia auriculata* (Roxb.).

Vernacular Name: *San*: Gandirah, *Eng:* Fox-grape, *Hin:* Amalbel, Ramchana, Gidardrak, *Kan:* Heggoli, *Mal:* Amarcakkoti, Corivalli, Kattuperanta, *Vatakkoti*, *Tam:* Kattuppirandai, *Tel:* Kurudinne, Kamputige.

Description: A somewhat fleshy climbing shrub, usually pubescent when young; tendrils short, slender and branched; leaves trifoliate, usually pubescent, leaflets dentate; flowers in branched; long peduncled cymes, flower buds globose; fruits fleshy berries; seeds pyriform or trnagular, rounded and rugose on the back.

Habitate: Throughout India on the hills, west coast and Western Ghats in India.

Propagation: By seeds.

Parts Used: Whole plant.

Chemical Constituents: Hydrocyanic acid, delphinidin, cyaniding.

Uses: The plant is sour, astringent and diuretic and is useful in vitiated conditions of *vata* and *kapha*, tumours, fever, neuralgia and splenopathy. It purifies the blood and is given for hepatopathy, cardiac disorders, ulcers, wounds, dropsy, haemorrhoids and strangury. A poultice prepared from the leaves from the leaves is used in the treatment of 'yolk sores' on the necks of bullocks.

290. *Cayratia pedata* (Laur.) Juss. ex Gagnep. *(Vitaceae)*

Synonyms: *Vitis pedta* Vahl ex. Wight & Arn.

Vernacular Name: *San*: Suvaha, Godhapadi, *Kan:* Kaama pattige balli, *Mal:* Velutta sori valli, Mar: Gorpadvel, *Tam:* Pannikkodi, Tiripatakam, Kattu pirandai, *Tel:* Gummadi tige.

Description: A large but week climbing shrub completely hairless. *Tendrils* leaf-opposed, branched, wiry, coiled. Leaves alternate, pedately 5-7 foliolate, hairless; leaf stalks 2-7 cm long; *terminal leaflets* elliptic to egg-shaped-lanceolate, 5-12 x 3-6 cm, base rounded or acute, apex acuminate, margin toothed with saw-like teeth, stalk 1-2 cm long; *lateral leaflets* 2.5-9 x 1.5-5 cm, base unequal, stalk up to 1 cm long. *Flowers* bisexual, hairless, greenish yellow or yellowish white, about 3 mm across, placed on about 10 cm long branched, axillary corymbs. *Berries* globose, about 1 cm across, creamy white. *Seeds* 1-2, flat, semicircular, smooth.

Habitate: Semi evergreen to evergreen forests.

Propagation: By seeds and vegetative method.

Parts Used: Leaves.

Chemical Constituents: Green waxyoil, sterol.

Uses: The whole plant of (excluding the roots) has low diuretic activity and has been a reputed remedy for cough, bronchitis, asthma, joint pain and to check uterine reflexes. The leaves are a stringent and refrigerant and are used as a remedy for ulcers and diarrhoea. A decoction of leaves is given to check uterine and other fluxes.

291. *Ceanothus americanus* L. *(Ranunculaceae)*

Synonyms: *Ceanothus officinalis* Refin., *Ceanothus trinerous* Moench., *Ceanothus herbaceous* Rafin.

Vernacular Name: *Eng:* New Jersey Tea.

Description: A low growing shrub, under 2 m. in height. Leaves alternate ovate, to ovate-oblong, 4-10 cm. long, acute or acuminate, glandular serrate or toothed, 3-veined from base, dull green above, pubescent beneath with lateral nerves commonly naked for 1-3 mm. at the base; petiole 6-12 mm. long. Flowers off white, in long-stalked cluster, 2.5-5 cm. long, forming large panicles at the end of branches. Flowers, fragrant, small, each with a calyx of five sepals and a regular corolla. Roots dark red. Fruit a triangular seed pod.

Habitate: Southern Canada, North America and Texas.

Propagation: By seeds.

Parts Used: Leaves.

Chemical Constituents: Ceanothic acid and Emolic acid.

Uses: As Hemostatic. Blood coagulent. Lung haemorrhages. For complaints specifically of spleen, left sided complaints. Anaemic patients where liver & spleen are at fault. Chronic bronchitis with profuse secretion. High blood pressure. Enormous enlargement of spleen, splenitis with pain radiating all up left side. Deep seated pain in left hypochondrium. Hypertrophy of spleen. Leucaemia. Constant urging to urinate., green, frothy, containing bile.

292. *Cebera Manghas* L. *(Apocynaceae)*

Vernacular Name: *Eng*: Odollam tree, pink-eyed cerbera, dog-bane.

Description: Medium-sized tree, nearly 10m. high. Bark thick and scabrous. Leaves alternate, usually crowded at the end of branches, shining glabrous on the upper side. Inflorescence in terminal cyme; flowers white with a reddish-pink centre, fragrant. Drupe oval, with two flattened seeds. All parts of the plant contain a milky latex.

Habitate: Grows wild in coastal areas.

Propagation: By seeds.

Part Used: Seeds.

Chemical Constituents: The seeds contain glucosides: cerberine, cerberoside, neriifolin and thevetin.

Uses: The seed oil in plasters applied to the skin is effective for scabies and prurigo, and applied to the hair kills head-lice. The glycosides extracted from the seeds are active on heart failure. The trunk bark or the leaves are occasionally used as a purgative, but strict precautions must be taken because of their high toxicity.

293. *Cedrus deodara* (Roxb. ex D. Don) G. Don *(Pinaceae)*

Vernacular Name: *San*: Devadaru, *Eng:* Deodar, Himalayan cedar, true cedar, *Hin:* Debdar, Deyodar, *Kan:* Devadaru, *Mal:* Devataram, *Tam:* Tevataram, Tevataru, *Tel:* Devadaru.

Description: A large handsome evergreen conifer tree reaching upto 85 m in height, with almost rough, black, furrowed bark and spreading branches; shoots dimorphic; leaves needle-like, triquetrous, sharp, pointed; male cones solitary, cylindric at the ends of branchlets, female cones solitary at the ends of branchlets, composed of imbricating thin woody placental scales; seeds pale brown, wings longer than the seeds.

Habitate: Himalayas, in areas of elevation from 1,050-3,600 m.

Propagation: By seeds.

Parts Used: Leaves, heartwood, oil.

Chemical Constituents: Its contain himachalol, allohimachalol, himadarol, centdarol, isocentdarol, dewarene, dewarol, dewardiol, dewarenol, taxifolin, cedeodarin,, dihydromyricetin, cedrin, cedrinoside dihydrodehydrodiconiferyl alcohol.

Uses: The leaves are bitter, acrid and thermogenic, and are useful in inflammations and tubercular glands. The heartwood is bitter, acrid, thermogenic, emollient, anodyne, anthelmintic, digestive, carminative, cardiotonic, galacto-purifier, anti-inflammatory, diuretic, expectorant, diaphoretic, antiseptic, laxative and febrifuge, and is useful in inflammations, dyspepsia, cephalalgia, haemorrhoids, insomnia, epilepsy, hiccough, bronchitis, tubercular glands, diabetes, urethrorrhea, renal and vesical calculi, elephantiasis, fever, cardiac disorders, leucoderma, skin diseases, proctoptosis and vitiated conditions of *vata* and *kapha*. The oil is antiseptic, diaphoretic, depurative and diuretic, and is useful in leprosy, syphilis, skin diseases, wounds and ulcers, fever and strangury.

294. *Cedrus* Libani *(Pinaceae)*

Vernacular Name: *Eng:* Cedar.

Description: Cedar of Lebanon is a majestic flat-topped tree growing to 40m. It has dark green needle-like leaves and oval cones.

Habitate: Cedar of Lebanon is native to mountain forests in Lebanon and south-west Turkey. Himalayan cedar is native to the Himalayan region, growing to 1,050 to 3,600m above sea level.

Propagation: By Seeds.

Parts Used: Leaves, wood, essential oil.

Chemical Constituents: The volatile oil contains cedrene, atlantol and atlantone.

Uses: Cedar of Lebanon is antiseptic and expectorant, acting to disinfect the respiratory tract. In Indian herbal medicine. Himalayan cedar leaves as used to treat tuberculosis. The heartwood is also given as a decoction for feverish chest ailments such as acute bronchitis, and for insomnia and diabetes. Cedarwood essential oil is generally distilled from the atlas or African cedar and the red cedar. The oil is strongly antiseptic, astringent, diuretic, expectorant and sedative. Diluted and massaged into the skin, it treats catarrh, chest infections and cystitis. It is also used to treat skin wounds and ulcers. In Ayurvedic medicine, cedarwood essential oil is prescribed for syphilis and leprosy.

295. *Ceiba pentandra* (Linn.) Gaertn. *(Bombacaceae)*

Synonyms: *Bombax pentandrum* Linn.

Vernacular Name: *San*: Kutasalmali, Svetasalmali, *Eng:* Sinhaporekapok, True kopok tree, *Hin:* Saphed simal, *Kan:* Burga, Biliburuga, *Mal:* Pannimaram, *Tam:* Pancu, *Tel:* Tella buruga, Buruga sauna.

Description: A medium sized to tall deciduous tree, trunk prickly when young and smooth when old, branches green, horizontal usually in whorls of three; leaves digitately compound, glabrous, petioles 10-15 cm long, leaflets lanceolate, entire; flowers white or yellowish appearing at the ends of the branches along with the leaves, petals twice the length of the calyx, wooly outside; fruits oblong or fusiform capsules; lined with long silky white hairs; seeds black, glabrous, enveloped in silky wool.

Habitate: Planted mainly in south India in areas upto 450 m elevation. Tropical America, Asia and Africa.

Propagation: By seeds.

Parts Used: Root, bark.

Chemical Constituents: Its contain cellulose, hemicellulose, pectin, lignin, and ash, sesquiterpene lactones, 2,7-dimethoxy-5-isopropyl-3-methyl-8-l-naphthalene carbolactone and 2-hydroxy-5-isopropyl-7-methoxy-3-methyl-8-l-naphthalene carbolactone.

Uses: The roots are diuretic, aphrodisiac, antipyretic and tonic, and are useful in gonorrhoea, dysuria, intermittent fevers and vitiated conditions of *pitta*. The bark is acrid, bitter, thermogenic, diuretic, febrifuge, emetic, purgative and tonic, and is useful in hepatopathy, splenopathy, abdominal complaints, tumours, constipation, strangury, flatulence, lochiorrhoea, colic and vitiated conditions of *vata* and *kapha*.

The leaves are used as an emollient and the decoction of the flowers as a laxative.

296. *Celastrus paniculatus* Willd. *(Celastraceae)*

Synonyms: .

Vernacular Name: *San*: Jyotismati, Pitataila, *Eng:* Climbing staff tree, Balck oil plant Intellect tree, *Hin:* Malkangani, Malkunki, *Kan:* Kariganne, *Mal:* Ceruppunna, Valulavam, Palulavam, *Tam:* Valuluvai, Siruvaluluvai, *Tel:* Danti cettu, Gundumida.

Description: A large climbing unarmed shrub with long slender elongating branches which are reddish brown and covered with elongate white lenticles; leaves simple, alternate, ovate or obovate, crenulate, coriaceous, glabrous, lateral nerves arching; flowers greenish white in terminal drooping panicles; fruits capsules, depressed-globose, 3-lobed, bright yellow when ripe, opening to expose the brown seeds covered with orange red aril.

Habitate: Throughout India, on hills upto and altitude of 1,200 m.

Propagation: By seeds.

Parts Used: Bark, leaves, seeds.

Chemical Constituents: Sesquiterpene alkaloids, celapagine, celapanigine and celapanine, hydrolysis gave polyalcohol A, polyalcohol C, polyalcohol D.

Uses: The bark is abortifacient, depurative and a brain tonic. The leaves are emmenagogue and the leaf sap is a good antidote for opium poisoning. The seeds are acrid, bitter, termogenic, emollient, stimulant, intellect promoting, digestive, laxative, emetic, expectorant, appetiser, aphrodisiac, cardiotonic, anti-inflammatory, diuretic, emmenagogue, diaphoretic, febrifuge and tonic, and are useful in vitiated conditions of *vata* and *kapha*, abdominal disorders, leprosy, pruritus, skin diseases, paralysis, cephalalgia, arthralgia, asthma, leucoderma, cardiac debility, inflammation, strnagury, nephropathy, amenorrhoea, dysmenorrhoea and fever and for stimulating the intellect and sharpening the memory. The seed oil is bitter, thermogenic and intellect promoting, and is useful in abdominal disorders, beri-beri and sores.

297. *Celosia argenta* L. *(Amaranthaceae)*

Vernacular Name: *Eng:* Feather cockscomb, quil grass.

Description: An annual erect tropical herb, 0.3-1.0 m high, glbrous, more or less branching, Leaves variable, linear or lanceolate, 8-10 cm long by 2-4 cm wide; tip acuminate, entire glabrous; base tapering sharply into a short petiole or leaves sessile. Flowers at firs pinkish, afterwards glistening white, crowded and imbricate, in close cylindrical blunt or acuminate terminal spikes. Capsules 3-4 mm long, ellipsoid, tapering at the apex into the style circumscisile. Seeds black, subreniform, shining, flat small taste bitter.

Habitate: On slopes and roadsides in dry, exposed areas in Africa and India.

Propagation: By seeds.

Part Used: Seeds.

Chemical Constituents: Vitamins, fats, carbohydrate, oxalicacid.

Uses: Acute conjunctivitis; keratitis, chronic uveitis, dizziness due to hypertension.

298. *Celosia cristata* L. *(Amaranthaceae)*

Vernacular Name: *Eng:* Cockscomb.

Description: A cultivated sport of C. argentea L. Leaves often broad, sometimes up to 23 cm long by 5 cm wide. Flowers from July to September. The spikes are flattened, truncate, often 15 cm wide. The purple spikes are officinal.

Habitate: Commonly cultivated as an ornamental plant in Burma, China, India, Japan, Malaysia, Mexico, Philippines.

Propagation: By seeds.

Part Used: Inflorescence.

Chemical Constituents: Lauric, myristic, palmitic, stearic, oleic, linoleic, lindenic and alkaloids.

Uses: Epistaxis; haemoptysis; haematemesis; haemorrhoidial, bleeding, haematuria; functional uterine bleeding, diarrhoea, leucorrhoea, urinary tract infection.

299. *Celtis australis* *(Ulmaceae)*

Vernacular Name: *Eng:* Southern nettle tree.

Description: Dome-shaped deciduous tree growing to 25m. Has lance-shaped leaves, green glowers and small round purple-black fruits.

Habitate: Native to Mediterranean region and south-western Asia, southern nettle tree is also planted as a border tree in Italy and France.

Propagation: By Seeds.

Parts Used: Leaves, fruit.

Chemical Constituents: Southern nettle contains tannins and mucilage.

Uses: Leaves and fruit both is taken to reduce heavy menstrual and intermenstrual uterine bleeding. The fruit and leaves may be used to astringe the mucous membranes in peptic ulcers, diarrhoea and dysentery.

300. *Centaurea cyanus* *(Asteraceae)*

Vernacular Name: *Eng:* Cornflower.

Description: Annual or biennial plant growing to 90 cm. Hs a multi-branched stem a basal rosette of leaves and sky-blue flowers in summer.

Habitate: Native to the near east, cornflower grows wild in al temperate regions, often in cornfields. The flowers are gathered just after they open.

Propagation: By Seeds.

Parts Used: Flowers, seeds, leave.

Chemical Constituents: Cornflower contains flavonoids, sesquiterpene lactones, acetylenes and coumarins. Cnicin is slightly antibiotic.

Uses: Cornflower is still used in French herbal medicine as a remedy for the eyes, but opinion differs as to its efficacy. The petals are also taken as a bitter tonic and stimulant, improving digestion and possibly supporting the liver as well as improving resistance to infection. The seeds have been used as a mild laxative for children.

301. *Centella asiatica* (L.) Urban *(Apiaceae)*

Vernacular Name: *San:* Mandukaparni; *Eng:* Indian pennywort, *Hin:* Brahmamanduki, Bemgsag, *Kan:* Urage, Vondelaga, *Mal:* Muttil, Kutannal, Kutakan, *San*: Mandukaparni, Manduki, *Tam:* Vallarai, *Tel:* Brahmi, Saraswataku.

Description: Small trailing herb. Stems slender, prostrate, rooting at the joinds. Leaves alternate or tufted at each node, orbicular, round or kidney-shaped, obviously crenate. Inflorescence in single umbel, bearing 1-5 small flowers, white or reddish, without stalks, Fruit very small, compressed.

Habitate: Grows wild in wet places.

Propagation: By seeds and vegetative method.

Part Used: Whole plant.

Chemical Constituents: Asiaticoside, madecassoside, brahmoside, bicycloelemene, centelloside, indocentelloside, oxyasiatiocoside, thankuniside, asiatic acid, betulinic acid, centellic acid, madecassic acid, centellose, kaempferol, hydrocotyline, phellandrene, vitamin C, linamarase, triterpenoid trisaccharides.

Uses: The whole plant possesses antibacterial, anti-inflammatory, antifebrile, diuretic and galactagogic activity. It is used in the therapy of feber, measles, haematemesis, epistaxis, diarrhoea, dysentery, constipation, leucorrhoea, jaundice, dysuria, furunculosis, dysmenorrhoea and varices. External application in the form of poultices is prescrived for contusions, closed fractures, sprains and furunculosis.

302. *Cephaelis ipecacuanha* (Bort.) A. rich. *(Rubiaceae)*

Synonyms: *Psychotria ipecacuanha* Stokes., *Callicocca ipecacuanha* Brot., *Urgoga ipecacuanha* Baill.

Vernacular Name: *Eng:* Ipecac

Description: A half shrubby perennial plant. Stem upto 1 m. long, partly underground, smooth grey at base, pubescent and green above. Leaves opposite, petiolate, obovate, acute, entire, blackish-green, somewhat rough above, pale downy and veined beneath, 7-10 cm. long, 2.5-5 cm. broad with large stipules. Flowers small, white, sessile, in dense head on axillary, but apparently terminal peduncles, surrounded by an involucre of four bracts. Fruits, blue berries, each with 2-seeds.

Habitate: Cultivated in India, Brazil, South America, Malaysia.

Propagation: By vegetative method.

Parts Used: Roots.

Chemical Constituents: Emetine, Cephaeline, Psychotrine, Saponins, Emetamine, O-methyl psychotrine, Ipecamine, Hydroipecamine.

Uses: For complaints specially accompanied with constant & continuous nausea. Nausea with saliva, vomiting of white, glairy mucus in large quantities without relief, sleepy afterwards. Flatulence with cutting colic about umbilicus. Grassy-green, slimy, foamy, frothy stool. Cutting pain across abdomen from left to right. Tearing pain in bones. Haemorrhages from all orifices of the body. The drug therefore puts good control over pneumogastric nerves to bring relief.

303. *Cephalonoplos segetum* (Bunge) Kitam. *(Asteraceae)*

Vernacular Name: *Eng:* Common cephalanoplos.

Description: A perennial herb, 25-50 cm high. Rhizome creeping, slender, white, fleshy. Stem erect, slightly purplish, with longitudinal furrows and white pubescent patches, upper part branching, leaves alternate, sessile, long-elliptic or elliptic-lanceolate, 7-10 cm long by 1.5-2.5 cm wide, apex obtuse, spinulate; base rounded-obtuse, margin entire and much spinulat, both faces covered with cottony hairs; lower leaves deciduous after flowering. Inflorescence a terminal head, erect. Flowers in summer, unisexual dioecious. Achene elliptic of long-ovate.

Habitate: In field margins, by roadsides, near villages and on waste land China, Korea, Mongolia.

Propagation: By seeds and vegetative method.

Part Used: Whole plant.

Chemical Constituents: N.A.

Uses: Epistaxis; haematuria and other haemorrhagic conditions, pyogenic infection.

304. *Ceratonia siliqua* *(Caesalpiniaceae)*

Vernacular Name: *Eng:* Carob.

Description: A small, evergreen, usually dioecious tree 10-17 m in hight; leaves paripinnate, leaflets 3-4 pairs, elliptic or broadly obovate, coriaceous, 3-5 cm long; inflorescence in axillary racemes, majority of flowers unisexual with male and female flowers on different trees, white, yellow-green or red; pods curved, compressed; seeds 3-6 or more, pale or red-brown.

Habitate: Native to south-eastern Europe, western Asia and North Africa, carob flourishes in poor soil in warm temperate climates.

Propagation: By Seeds.

Parts Used: Fruit, bark.

Chemical Constituents: The fruit contains up to 70% sugars, fats, starch, proteins, vitamins and tannins.

Uses: Carob pods are nutritious and, due to their high sugar content, sweet-tasting and mildly laxative. These appear to be contradictory effects, but carob is an example of how the body responds to herbal medicines in different ways, according to how the herb is prepared, and according to the specific medical problem.

305. *Ceratophyllum demersum* L. *(Ceratophyllaceae)*

Vernacular Name: *San*: Saivalah, Jalanili, Ambuluta, *Eng:* Hornwort, Coontail, *Hin:* Sevar, Sivara, *Kan:* Cande, Nonde, Honde, Naval, *Mal:* Karimpayal, *Tam:* Velampasi, *Tel:* Nasu.

Description: A fragile hydrophyte, 20-90cm long, forming a much branched tangle of slender branches and leaves which collapse in a tassel when taken out of the water; leaves upto 2.5 cm long, segments variable in thickness and amount of toothing; male flowers solitary, axillary in separate axils from the female but on the same plant; fruits ovoid or ellipsoid nutlets with persistent style.

Habitate: Throughout India, in still waters.

Propagation: By vegetative method.

Parts Used: Whole plant.

Chemical Constituents: Ferredoxin, plastocyanin.

Uses: The plant is astringent, bitter, sweet, oleaginous, fragrant, constipating, refrigerant, haemostatic and antipyretic, and is useful in vitiated conditions of *pitta*, diarrhoea, dysentery, burning sensation, hyperdipsia, epistaxis, haematemesis, haemoptysis, haemorroids, ulcers and intermittent fevers.

306. *Cetraria islandica* *(Parmeliaceae)*

Vernacular Name: *Eng:* Iceland moss.

Description: Yellow-green lichen growing in undulating, leathery tufts up to 8cm across.

Habitate: Iceland moss is native to northern and alpine areas of Europe. It flourishes in sub-arctic and mountainous regions on rocks and on the bark of trees.

Propagation: By Seeds and vegetative method.

Parts Used: Whole plant.

Chemical Constituents: Iceland moss contaons lichen acids and about 50% polysaccharides. Usnic acid and the other lichen acids are powerfully antibiotic.

Uses: Strongly demulcent, Iceland moss soothes the mucous membranes of the chest, counters catarrh, and calms dry and paroxysmal coughs, being particularly helpful as a treatment of elderly people. Iceland moss is also very bitter and, within the gut, has both a demulcent and bitter tonic effect–a combination almost unique in medicinal herbs. It is thus of value in all kinds of chronic digestive problems. For instance irritable bowel syndrome.

307. *Chaenomeles sinensis* (Thouin) koehne *(Rosaceae)*

Vernacular Name: *Eng:* Chinese quince.

Description: Thornless, deciduous tree, to 10 m tall. Branchlets pubescent, but becoming glabrous in the second year. Leaves alternate, entire, elliptic ovate or lanceolate, 7-10 cm long, gland-toothed, pubescent beneath and becoming glabrous later; stipules linear, with glandular hairs at margins. Flowers solitary, pink, 2.5-3 cm across, sepals 5, glandular-serrate, woolly above; calyx with whitish hairs inside, glabrous outside; petals 5, obovate, short pilose at base; stamens 20 or more, in 1 row; carpels fused along the inner side only, styles 5, Fruit fragrant subglobose pome, yellow, 8-15 cm long. May. Fruit ripening in September.

Habitate: Mostly planted for fruit in Korea and China.

Propagation: By seeds.

Parts Used: Fruit.

Chemical Constituents: Organic acids: malic acid, ascorbic acid, hydrocyanic acid. Flavonoids: quercetin, rutin. Isozedoarondiol, isofuranogermacrene.

Uses: Mutagenic, anti-HIV activity (Quercetin), aldose reductase inhibition. Antianaphylactic activity. Used in Asthama, common cold, harsh throat, tuberculosis, mastitis, liver protection.

308. *Chaenomeles speciosa* (sweet). Nakai *(Rosaceae)*

Synonyms: *Chaenomeles lagenaria* koidx.

Vernacular Name: *Eng:* Common floweringquince.

Description: A spiny deciduous shrub, 2,3 m high, glabrous. Spines up to 2 cm long. Leaves alternate, petiolate, simple, ovate, long-elliptic of elliptic-obolanceolate, often reddish, 3-9 cm long by 2-5 cm wide, apex acuminate, base cuneate, margin biserrate, pubescent underneath when young. Flowers 3-5 in clusters, fruit a fleshy pome, ovoid, ligneous, yellow or yellowish-green, smooth.

Habitate: Mostly cultivated in China, Iran, Japan.

Propagation: By seeds.

Part Used: Fruit.

Chemical Constituents: N.A.

Uses: Numbeness and tiredness of the lower part of the body, vomiting and diarrhoea; abdominal pain.

309. *Chamaelirium luteum* *(Liliaceae)*

Synonyms: *Helonias dioica.*

Vernacular Name: *Eng:* Helonias, False Unicorn Root, Blazing Star.

Description: A herbaceous perennial growing to 1m, with long green leaves and green-white flowers.

Habitate: Native to North America, helonias grows in low, moist, well-drained ground east of the Mississippi river. It is generally harvested from the wild and is rarely cultivated.

Propagation: By seeds.

Parts Used: Root.

Chemical Constituents: Steroidal saponins, Glycosides.

Uses: Uterine & ovarian tonic, Promotes menstrual flow, Diuretic.

310. *Chamaemelum nobile* *(Asteraceae)*

Synonyms: *Anthemis nobilis.*

Vernacular Name: *Eng:* Roman chamomile.

Description: Aromatic perennial growing to 50cm. Has feathery leaves and daisy-like flowerheads.

Habitate: Native to western Europe, Roman chamomile is now cultivated across Europe, and also in other temperate regions.

Propagation: By Seeds.

Parts Used: Flowers.

Chemical Constituents: Roman chamomile contains up to 1.75% volatle oil, sesquiterpene lactones, flavonoids, coumarins and phenolic acids.

Uses: A remedy for the digestive system, Roman chamomile is often used interchangeably with German chamomile. It is an excellent treatment for nausea, vomiting, indigestion and loss of appetite. It is also sedative, antispasmodic and mildly analgesic, and will relieve colic, griping and other cramping pains. By stimulating digestive secretions and relaxing the muscles of the gut, it helps normalize digestive function.

311. *Chamaenerion angustifolia* *(Onagraceae)*

Synonyms: *Epilobium angustifolium.*

Vernacular Name: *Eng:* Rose bay willow herb.

Description: Perennial growing to 2m. Has an erect stem, narrow leaves and long spikes of pink-purple flowers.

Habitate: This herb is found in Europe and western Asia, and grows in clearing, in hedgerows and on wasteground. It is picked when in flowers in late summer.

Propagation: By Seeds.

Parts Used: Aerial parts.

Chemical Constituents: Rose bay willow herb contains flavones and tannins.

Uses: Demulcent and astringent, rose bay willow herb treats diarrhoea, mucous colitis and irritable bowel syndrome. It has also been made into an ointment to soothe skin problems in children. Rose bay willow herb has been used Germany and Austria to treat prostate problems.

312. *Chamomilla recutita* *(Asteraceae)*

Synonyms: *Matricaria recutita.*

Vernacular Name: *Eng:* German Chamomile.

Description: A sweetly aromatic annual growing to 60cm, with finely cut leaves and white flowerheads.

Habitate: German chamomile grows wild and is cultivated in much of Europe and other temperate regions. The seeds are sown in spring or autumn and the flowerheads are picked in full bloom, in summer.

Propagation: By Seeds.

Parts Used: Flowers.

Chemical Constituents: Volatile oil, Flavonoids, bitter glycosides, Coumarins, Tannins.

Uses: Anti-inflammatory, Antispasmodic, Relaxant, Mild bitter, Anti-allergenic.

313. *Cheiranthus cheiri* *(Cruciferae)*

Vernacular Name: *Eng:* Wallflower.

Description: Evergreen perennial growing to 45 cm. Has lance-shaped leaves and yellow-orange flowers appearing in spring.

Habitate: Native to southern Europe, wallflower is now found throughout the continent. It grows on cliffs and old wall, and is a common garden plant.

Propagation: By seeds.

Parts Used: Leaves, flowers.

Chemical Constituents: The herb contains cheiranthin and other cardioactive glycosides.

Uses: Although wallflower was formerly used as a diuretic, there was no understanding of its powerful effect on the heart. In small doses it is cardio tonic, supporting a failing heart in a manner similar to foxglove. In more than small doses it is toxic, and is therefore rarely used in herbal medicine.

314. *Chelidonium jajus* var. *asiaticum* (Hara) Ohwi. *(Papaveraceae)*

Vernacular Name: *Eng:* Celandine.

Description: Biennial herb, with multicellular curled hairs early, becoming glabrate later. Stems, erect, branched, 30-80 cm tall, with orange-coloured sap secreted when stems cut. Leaves deeply 1-2 pinnatifid, 7-15 cm long, 5-10 cm wide, obtuse, glaucous beneath, obtusely toothed and incised. Inflorescence axillary umbels, pedunculate, few-flowered. Flowers yellow, pedicelled, to 2 cm acroos, sepals 2, 6-8 mm long, yellow-green, often hairy outside, falling early; petals 4, 10-12 mm long; stamens many; pistils 1. Fruit a cylindrical capsule, 3-4 cm long, 2 cm wide. May-August.

Habitate: Sunny open places in Asia & Europe.

Propagation: By seeds and vegetative method.

Parts Used: Herb.

Chemical Constituents: Alkaloids: sanguinarine, chelerythrine, chelidamine, chelidonine, berberine, coptisine, protopine, stylopine.

Uses: Cytotoxicity, analgesic, antioxidant. Used in anodyne, antitussive detoxicant, stomach cancer.

315. *Chelone glabra* L. *(Scrophulariaceae)*

Synonyms: *Chlelone alba* Moench., *Chelone capitata* Rafin., *Chelone maculata* Rafin.

Vernacular Name: *Eng:* Balmony.

Description: A perennial herb about 1m. high, erect, simple, branched above. Leaves elongated, lanceolate, acuminate, appressed, serrate, nearly sessile or very short petioled with slightly channeled petioles. Spikes 3 to 8 cm. long, subtended by scarcely reduced foliage leaves; bracts not ciliated. Flowers white or rose-tinged; corolla bilabiate, the lower lip bordered in the throat; anthers heart shaped with filaments wooly. Odour slight somewhat tea-like; taste bitter.

Habitate: Eastern United State and Canada.

Propagation: By seeds.

Parts Used: Whole plant.

Chemical Constituents: Chelonin.

Uses: As Tonic, Cathartic, to expel worms. For complaints specifically liver affections with pain or soreness of left lobe of the liver, extending downwards. Dumbague. Mialaise, following intermittents. Dyspepsia with hepatic torpor. Jaundice.

316. *Chenopodium album* L. *(Chenopodiaceae)*

Vernacular Name: *San*: Vastukah, Agaralohita, Chilika, *Eng:* Lamb's Quarters, Wild spinach, *Hin:* Cheel, Bathua Sag, *Kan:* Hancike, *Mal:* Vastuccira, *Tam:* Paruppukkirai, Cakkaravarttikkirai, *Tel:* Pappukura.

Description: A small odourless herb upto 3.5 m in height, erect or ascending, stems often striped; leaves simple, very variable, upto 15 cm long, oblong, deltoid or lanceolate, obtuse or acute, entire, toothed or irregularly lobulate; flowers in clusters in spikes; fruits membranous utricle; enclosed in the perianth, seeds smooth, shiny, compressed.

Habitate: Throughout India, in areas upto 4,200 m elevation, wild as well as cultivated.

Propagation: By seeds.

Parts Used: Seeds.

Chemical Constituents: Leucine, isoleucine, lysine, methionine, phenylalanine, threonine, valine and tryptophan, alkaloids, trigonelline and chenopodine. Ecdysteroids, hydroxyecdysone, and polypodine B.

Uses: The plant is sweet, acrid, oleaginous, digestive, carmiantive, laxative, anthelmintic, diuretic, aphrodisiac and tonic, and is useful in vitiated conditions of *pitta*, peptic ulcer, helminthiasis, dyspepsia, flatulence, strangury, seminal weakness, pharyngopathy, splenopathy, haemorrhoids, ophthalmopathy, cardiac disorders and general debility.

317. *Chenopodium ambrosioides* *(Chenopodiaceae)*

Vernacular Name: *Eng:* Wormseed; *Mal*: Kattayamodagum; *Hin*: Khatua; *San*: Kshetravastuka; *Kan*: Kaaduvoma; *Tam*: Kattasambadan.

Description: Annual or perennial herb, 0.5-am. high Stems and twigs striate, glandular-pubescent, green or purple. Leaves alternate, sinuate-dentate, glandular-pubescent beneath. Flowers minute, in simple or paniculate axillary leafe spike. Utricle globular, membranaous, pale-green. Seeds black, shining. All parts of the herb have a disagreeable strong smell.

Habitate: Wormseed is native to Central and South America and the Caribbean. It has been extensively cultivated in Maryland, US and in China.

Propagation: By Seeds.

Parts Used: Flowers.

Chemical Constituents: Wormseed contains a volatile oil and triterpenoid saponins. Ascaridol is a powerful worm-expellent.

Uses: Wormseed is principally known for its ability to expel worms, especially roundworms and hookworms. However, it also used in the Americas as a digestive remedy, being generally taken to settle colic and stomach pains. wormseed leaves have antispasmodic properties. a wormseed's muscle-relaxing action has led to its use in the treatment of spasmodic coughs and asthma. The plant also has external uses. Juice expressed from the whole herb is applied as a wash for haemorrhoids.

318. *Chimaphila umbellate* (L.) Barton. *(Ericaceae)*

Synonyms: *Chimaphila corymbosa* Pursh., *Chimaphila cymosa* J & C.

Vernacular Name: *Eng:* Spotted American winter-green.

Description: A small evergreen, perennial shrub creeping yellow rhizome. Aerial stems creeping, erect or semi-procumbent, slender, possessing scars of former leaves, woody at base, 10-30 cm. high. ***Leaves:*** oblanceolate or cuneate-lanceolate, sharply dentate in upper half, entire in lower half, tapering, 3-6 cm. long, short petioled, in whorls; upper surface dark-green shining and coriaceous, undersurface pale. Flowers 2-8, white or pinkish, 10-15 mm. wide, corymbose or sub-umbellate; depressed, anthers violet, filament swollen and ciliolate at part. Fruit a capsule, five-celled.

Habitate: Temperate Asia, North America, Canada, Mexico, Japan, Siberia and Europe.

Propagation: By seeds.

Parts Used: Whole plant.

Chemical Constituents: Ericolin, Arbutin, Chimaphilin, Urson, Tannin.

Uses: For complaints principally of kidneys, genitourinary tract, bladder stone, lymphatic and mesenteric glands, female mammae. Dysuria. Large breasts with painful tumors. Hepatic and renal dropsies. Scanty urine, loaded with ropy, muco-purulent sediments with burning and scalding. Have to strain before and after micturation. Prostatic enlargements.

Itching of eyelids with stabbing pain in left eye with lachrymation. Labium inflammation in females with painful vagina, painful tumor of mammae.

319. *Chionanthus virginica* L. *(Oleaceae)*

Synonyms: *Chionanthus angustifolia* Rafin., *Chionanthus heterophyla* Rafin.

Vernacular Name: *Eng:* Fringe tree, Chionanthe.

Description: A low deciduous, dioecious tree with opposite, petiolate, ovate to obovate-lanceolate leaves and drooping panicles of white flowers, each with 5 to 6 white linear elongated, about 2.5 cm. long, petals. Stamens 2, ovary superior, 2-celled. **Fruit:** ovoid, purple drupe, one seeded.

Habitate: Southern United States, Pennsylvania, New Jersey, Texas, Florida.

Propagation: By seeds.

Parts Used: Root bark.

Chemical Constituents: Phyllyrin glycosides: Chionanthin, Phyllyroside and Forsythin; Agluane phillygenins.

Uses: Catarrhal jaundice. Hepatitis. Acts as a prominent liver remedy for enlarged liver and jaundice. Complaints specifically of enlarged spleen, gallstones, diabetes mellitus and paroxysmal abdominal pain. Habitual severe headache, neurasthenic, periodic, menstrual and bilious, with pain in forehead chiefly over eyes. Aching and gripping pain in umbilical and liver region due to enlarged and sore liver. Tenderness of hepatic region.

320. *Chloranthus japonicus* Siebold *(Chloranthaceae)*

Vernacular Name: *Eng:* Chloranthus.

Description: Glabrous perennial herb from short, creeping rhizomes, to 20-30 cm tall. Stems erect, simple. Leaves small, membranaceous and scalelike toward the base; the uppermost consisting of 2 ordinary pairs simulating a whorl of 4 leaves, ovate or elliptic, 4-12 cm long, 2-6 cm wide, abruptly acute, sharply serrate; petioles 10-15 mm long. Spikes usually simple, solitary, 2-3 cm long, erect; peduncle 2-5 cm long. Flowers white, sessile; filaments white and conspicuous, shortly connate below and adnate to the ovary, linear, obtuse, spreading 4-5 mm long.

Habitate: Mountain woods in Korea. Japan and China.

Propagation: By seeds.

Parts Used: Rhizome.

Chemical Constituents: Sesquiterpenes. Coumarins.

Uses: None reported. Used in dermatopathia and enteric fever.

321. *Chondrodendron tomentosum* *(Menispermaceae)*

Vernacular Name: *Eng:* Pareira.

Description: Vine climbing to a great height in tropical rainforests. Reaches 30m. Has large leaves up to 30cm long, and trailing clusters of flowers.

Habitate: Pareira grows wild in rainforests in the upper Amazon region and in Panama.

Propagation: By Seeds and vegetative method.

Parts Used: Root, stem.

Chemical Constituents: Pareira contains alkaloids, including delta-tubocurarine and L-curarine. Tubocurarine is a potent muscle relaxant.

Uses: Pareira's notoriety as a poison hinges on the effect of its toxic derivative entering directly into the bloodstream. Provided there are no cuts or sores in the mouth, the plant is reasonably safe taken orally as a medicinal remedy. The bitter and slightly sweet-tasting roots and stems are mildly laxative, tonic and diuretic, *S*and also act to induce menstruation. The plant is chiefly used to relieve chronic inflammation of the urinary tubules. In Brazil, purpose an infusion of the root is taken internally while the bruised leaves are applied externally.

322. *Chondrus crispus* *(Gigartinaceae)*

Vernacular Name: *Eng:* Carragheen, Irish moss.

Description: Reddish-brown seaweed growing to 25 cm. Plant body is flat and forked, with a fan-shaped outline.

Habitate: Carragheen is found on the Atlantic coasts of Europe and North America. It grows just below the waterline, attached to rocks and stones.

Propagation: By Seeds and Vegetative method.

Parts Used: Whole plants.

Chemical Constituents: Carragheen contains large amounts of polysaccharides, proteins, amino acids, iodine and bromine. The polysaccharides become jelly-like and demulcent when the plant is immersed in water.

Uses: A useful demulcent and emollient, carragheen is mainly taken for coughs and bronchitis. Its expectorant effect encourages the coughing up of phlegm and it soothes dry and irritated mucous membranes. It is of value for acid indigestion, gastritis and urinary infections such as cystitis. For these conditions it is normally combined with other appropriate herbs. Mucilaginous in make s a valuable nutrient in convalescence. Applied externally, this emollient herb soothes inflamed skin. Carragheen also acts to thin the blood.

323. *Chonemorpha fragrans* (Moon) Alston *(Apocynaceae)*

Synonyms: *Chonemorpha macrophyllа* (Roxb.) G. Don.

Vernacular Name: *San*: Murva, Morata, *Eng:* Wood vine, *Hin:* Garbhedaro, *Kan:* Manjinaru, *Mal:* Perunkurumpa, *Tam:* Perumkurumpa, *Tel:* Chaga.

Description: A stout spreading laticiferous shrub with soft greyish to rusty-brown bark which yields fibre of good quality; leaves simple, opposite, large, orbicular, fulvous tomentose beneath, prominently veined; flowers large, whitish to cream-yellow, fragrant, in terminal or pseudo-axillary cymose panicles; fruits long, straight, woody, parallel, follicular mericarps; seeds many, flat, shortly beaked with long white silky coma.

Habitate: Throughout India, in moist forests in Andman Islands.

Propagation: By seeds.

Parts Used: Roots and stems.

Chemical Constituents: Japindine, N-formylchonemorphine, N-methyl-chonemorphine and funtumafrine-C. chonemorphine dihydrochloride.

Uses: The roots are sweet, bitter, astringent, laxative, thermogenic, depurative, carminative, anthelmintic, digestive, antiscorbutic, sudorific, anodyne, expectorant and febrifuge. They are useful in vitiated conditions of *vata* and *kapha*, skin diseases, leprosy, scabies, syphilis, dyspepsia, flatulence, colic constipation, helminthiasis, hyperdipsia, urethrorrhea, hyperacidity, cardiac debility, diabetes, jaundice, cough, bronchitis and intermittent fevers.

324. *Chrysanthemum indicum* L. *(Asteraceae)*

Vernacular Name: *San:* Sevanti; *Eng*: Indian chrysanthemum; *Hin:* Guldaudi; *Tam:* Akkarakkaram; *Tel:* Chamunti.

Description: Annual or perennial herb, 20-50 cm. High. Stems sulcate, glabrous. Leaves alternate, deeply lobed and irregularly toothed. Inflorescence is an axillary or terminal corymb of many heads; flowers yellow.

Habitate: Grown everywhere.

Propagation: By seeds.

Part Used: Flowers.

Chemical Constituents: The flowers yield the glycoside chrysanthemin that yields glucose and cyanidin on hydrolysis, together with stachydrine, an essential oil and vitamin A. the semidried seeds contain 15.8% oil.

Uses: The flowers possess antibacterial and antihypertensive properties. They are utilized in medication for photopsia, vertigo, fever, headache, ophthalmia, dacryolithiasis, xerophthalmia, amblyopia, hypertension. Furunculosis and phelgmon. Their long-term use is rejuvenating. They are also a constituent of composite prescriptions. Washing with the decoction and poultices of pounded flowers are effective in furunculosis and impetigo.

325. *Chrysanthemum morifolium* Ramat *(Asteraceae)*

Vernacular Name: *Eng:* Florists chrysanthemum.

Description: A perennial herb. 60-150 cm high. Stem erect, striate, hairy, leaves alternate, petiolate, ovate or oblong, 3.5-5 cm long by 3-4 cm wide, variously loved and divided. Inflorescence small head, 5 cm in diameter. Flowers yellwish-white. Fruit a one-seeded cypsela, crowned. Seeds fills the fruit.

Habitate: Widely distributed, occurring in almost all habitats.

Propagation: By seeds.

Part Used: Inflorescences.

Chemical Constituents: N.A.

Uses: Vertigo, opthalmia with swelling and pain, headache with fever.

326. *Cicer arietinum* L. *(Fabaceae)*

Synonyms: .

Vernacular Name: *San*: Canaka, *Eng:* Bengal gram, Chick pea, *Hin:* Chana, *Kan:* Kadale, *Mal:* Kadala, *Tam:* Kadalai, *Tel: San*agalu, Canakamula.

Description: An erect or spreading, much branched annual; leaves imparipinnately compound, leaflets small, oval, all parts covered over with glandular hairs, inflorescence stalk jointed about the middle; flowers pink, blue or white; fruits turgid, pubescent pods; seeds reddish brown, black or white, subglobose or obovate with a beak.

Habitate: Cultivated throughout India.

Propagation: By seeds.

Parts Used: Leaves, seeds.

Chemical Constituents: Saccharose, glucose, fructose, polysaccharides including starch, γ-galactan, levulose and *p*-galactoaraban, betaine, choline, adenine, inositol, phytin, saponin and citric and oxalic acids. The total carbohydrate content of seeds ranges from 52.4 to 70.9 per cent. Starch being the major constituent. The starch content in whole seed ranges from 37.2 to 50.8 per cent.

Uses: Leaves are purgative, abortifacient and trichogenous and are useful in anorexia, dyspepsia and bronchitis. The seeds are sweet when raw, indigestible, tonic, aphrodisiac, expectorant and cooling, and are useful in hyperdipsia, burningsensation, splenohepatomegaly, leprosy, pharyngopathy, vitiated conditions of *pitta*, bronchitis, inflammations and skin diseases.

327. *Cichorium intybus* L. *(Asteraceae)*

Vernacular Name: *San*: Kasani, *Eng:* Chicory, Endive, succory, *Hin:* Kasni, *Kan:* Kacani, *Mal:* Cikkari, *Tam:* Cikkari, Kasini, *Tel:* Cicori, Kasini vittulu.

Description: An erect glandular perennial milky herb upto 90 cm in height, with tough, rigid, spreading branches; leaves radical and lower pinnatifid lobes toothed, upper alternate, small, entire; flowers bright blue in ligulate heads, terminal, axillary and clustered; fruits smooth angled achenes, crowned with a ring of erect pappus scals.

Habitate: Cultivated throughout India, also grows wild in Punjab, northwest India and Hyderabad in areas upto 1,800 m elevation.

Propagation: By seeds.

Parts Used: Whole plant.

Chemical Constituents: The roots contain the sesquiterpene lactones, viz., lactucin, 8-deoxylactucin, lactucopicrin, crepidiaside B, sonchusides A and C, cichoriolide A and cichoriosides B and C. they also contain a cytokinin, ribosylzeatin, a nucleotide sugar, uridine-5′-diphosphoglucose, and chlorogenic, neochlorogenic isochlorogenic, caffeic and chicoric acids. The carbohydrates prescent in the roots include a series of glucofructosans between sucrose and insulin besides glucose and fructose. During storage the inluin present in the roots is converted into inulide and finally into fructose due to the presence of an enzyme. Presence of an enzyme, inulocoagulase, which coagulates inulin is also reported in the expressed root juice.

Uses: The plant is bitter, acrid, thermogenic, anti-inflammatory, appetiser, digestive, stomachic, liver tonic, cholagogue, cardiotonic, depurative, diuretic, emmenagogue, febrifuge, alexeteric, and tonic. It is useful in vitiated conditions of *kapha* and *pitta*, cephalalgia, hepatomegaly, inflammations, anorexia, dyspepsia, flatulence, colic, gout, burning sensation, allergic conditions of the skin, insomnia, jaundice, splenomegaly, hyperdipsia, skin diseases, leprosy, strangury, amenorrhoea, dysmenorrhoea, chronic and bilious fevers, ophthalmia, pharyngitis, vomiting, diarrhoea, arthralgia, lumbago, asthma and general debility.

328. *Cichorum endivia* L. *(Asteraceae)*

Vernacular Name: *San*: Ka*Sani*, *Hin:* Hinduba, Kashi.

Description: Erect, glabrous or hispid herb, with diariacte branches, occasionally spinescent. *Leaves* upper subsentire, lower pinnatifid. Head sessile on the branches or on thickened peduncles, homogamous, blue. *Flowers* all ligulate. *Bracts* involucral, inner 1-serrate, at length concave at the base with outer flowers in the concavity. Outer few shorter: receptacle flat, naked or sub-fimbrillate. *Achenes* glabrous, sub-5-angled, base contracted, tip truncate or the margin slightly producted: *pappus* pale short, 2-3 serrate.

Habitate: Grows in North west India, the Deccan plateau, Punjab, Kashmir and in Iran and many parts of Europe.

Propagation: By seeds.

Parts Used: Seeds, roots, flowers.

Chemical Constituents: The leaves and pods contain 6-hydroxymusizin glucoside, tinnevellin glucoside, kaempferol glucoside, kaempfero-3-D-glucuronide, kaempferol-3-β-

D-glucoside, kaempferol-3-D glucuronide luteolin, DC+7-dicaffeoultartaric acid, methyl caffeinate, ethyl caffeinate, ethyl 4-coumarate, methyl protocate chinate, methol and ethyl esters of hydroxy cinnamic and benzoic acids, malic acid, citric acid, fumaric acid, succinic acid, quininic acid, nitrites and nitrates. The oil extracted from endive contains camphor, campene, phellodrene, immonene, β-pinene, diterpene, cineole, terpinol and caryophyllene. The flowers contain the glycoside cichorin.

Uses: Cough with dyspnoea, hepatitis, as a mild diuretic, inflammatory swelling. The powder of dried root is used in the treatment of liver congestion, as a demulcent, and as an antidiarrhoeal.

329. *Cimicifuga foetida* L. *(Ranunculaceae)*

Vernacular Name: *Eng:* Skunk bugbane; stinking bugbane.

Description: A perennial, more or less pubescent, herb. Stems erect, leafy, branched. Leaves pinnately compoundl leaflets ovate or lanceolate, deeply and sharply toothed, terminal leaflet 3-lobed. Flowers nearly regular, barely 6 mm in diameter, white, crowned by short or long racemes. Follicles 12 mm long, flat, tipped with the persistent styles. Seeds 6-8.

Habitate: On slopes and in grassland in China, India, Japan.

Propagation: By seeds.

Part Used: Rhizomes.

Chemical Constituents: N.A.

Uses: Toothache; headache; sore throad, chronic diarrhoea and rectocele; prolapsed womb.

330. *Cimicifuga heracleifolia* Kom. *(Ranunculaceae)*

Vernacular Name: *Eng:*-Bugbane, rattletop.

Description: Upright, perennial herb with thickened, dark-purple root, to 1 m tall. Leaves large, ternately 1-2 clefted, long-petiolate; leaflets petiolulate, ovate, acuminate, slightly cordate at base, irregulary toothed, glabrous. Flowers small, white, many, in long compound racemes; sepals 4-5, petaloid, falling early; petals 3-4, small, clawed; stamens many; pistils 1-8, sessile, many-ovuled. Fruit of follicles. August-September.

Habitate: Mountain woods in China and Korea.

Propagation: By Seeds and Vegetative method.

Parts Used: Rhizome.

Chemical Constituents: Cycloartenol triterpenes.

Uses: Antioxidant. Interleukin-8 induction inhibition. Used in fever and headache. The plant is possess insect-repellent, insecticidal and piscicidal properties. The proofs are sudorific, antipenodic and emeto-purgative. It is also given in rheumatic affections, dropsy and bronchial diseases.

331. *Cimicifuga racemosa* Nutt. *(Ranunculaceae)*

Synonyms: *Actaea racemosa* Linn., *Cimicifuga serpentaria* Pursh.

Vernacular Name: *Eng:* Black Snake root, Black Cohosh.

Description: An erect herb, 1-2.5 m. in height. Leaves ternate, the three divisions again tripinnately compound. Leaflets ovate or oblong, incisely toothed, mostly 4-8 cm. long, cuneate to cordate at base. Flowers cream coloured, in 4rect, tall spike-like, curved racemes. Sepals 4 or 5, short lived. Petals none. Stamens many with elongated white filaments, few outer transformed in 2 horned staminodia. Stigma truncated. Fruits are follicles on long pedicels with intact recurved style.

Habitate: U.S.A. and Canada.

Propagation: By seeds.

Parts Used: Rhizome.

Chemical Constituents: N-methylcytisine, quinolizidine type alkaloid; Actein, 12-acetylactein, Cimigoside; Tannic and Gallic acids; Formic acid, Isoferulic acid, Oleic acid, Salicylic acid, Racemosin, formononetin, Climicifugin, Acteina. Cimigenol.

Uses: Acts as Sedative, Emmenagogue and antitussive. Used for complaints of cerebrospinal and muscular system, uterus and ovaries, ovarian irritation, uterine cramps. Muscular and crampy neuralgic pain characteristic of the drug occurring in every part of the body. Migraine. Amenorrhoea with pain in ovarian region, shooting upward and pain in ovarian region, shooting upward and with profuge flow, ovarian neuralgia, pain across pelvis, from hip to hip, great sensitiveness. Infra-mammary pains worse left side. Great mental depression with evil dreams. Visions of rats and mice. Neuralgic headache. Neuralgic, throbbing pain in eyes. All complaints worse morning, cold and during menses.

332. *Cinchona officinalis* L. *(Rubiaceae)*

Vernacular Name: *San*: Sinkona, Kunayanah, *Eng:* Quinine bark, Peruvian bark, *Hin:* Quinine, *Kan:* Sinkona, Barkino, *Mal:* Sinkona, Koyina, *Tam:* Cinkona, Konia, *Tel:* Cinkona, Jaddapatta.

Description: A slender tree, 6-9 m in height with brown bark marked with black and whitish lines; leaves simple, opposite, lanceolate or ovate-lanceolate, shining, petioles reddish, secondary nerves 8-10 pairs with hairy pits in their axils; flowers pink or purple coloured in short corymbiform terminal and axillary compound cymes; fruits ovoid-oblong capsules.

Habitate: Cultivated in India in Nilgiris at an elevation of 1,800-2,400 m.

Propagation: By seeds.

Parts Used: Quinine isolated from bark.

Chemical Constituents: Chinchonidine, cinchonine, javanine, quinamine, quinidine, quinine.

Uses: The quinine is bitter, astringent, acrid, thermogenic, febrifuge, oxytocic, anodyne, anti-bacterial, anthelmintic, digestive, constipating, depurative, antipyretic, cardiotonic, anti-inflammatory, expectorant, calefacient and tonic. It is useful in malarial and intermittent fevers, dystocia, brachial neuritis, lumbago, sciatica, intercostals neuralgia, bacterial infections, helminthiasis, dyspepsia, chronic dysentery, skin diseases, cardiac debility, arthralgia, hepato-splenomegaly, vitiated conditions of *kapha*, cough bronchitis, pharyngopathy, stomatopathy, otorrhoea, internal haemorrhoids, amenorrhoea and dysmenorrhoea.

333. *Cineraria maritima* *(Asteraceae)*

Synonyms: *Senecio cineraria.*

Vernacular Name: *Eng:* Silver ragwort.

Description: Evergreen shrub growing to 30cm Has oblong, toothed leaves covered in a silver-white felt, and yellow composite flowers about 1cm across.

Habitate: Native to the West Indies, silver ragwort has become naturalized throughout the Mediterranean and occasionally grows in more northerly parts of Europe. It prefer cliffs and rocks, and is widely cultivated as a garden plant. It is gathered when in flower in summer.

Propagation: By Root cutting.

Parts Used: Whole plant.

Chemical Constituents: Contains pyrrolizidine alkaloids and tannins. Pyrrolizidine alkaloids in isolation are highly toxic to the liver.

Uses: The juice of the whole plant is mainly used for conjunctivitis and other eye problems. Applied to the eyes, it has a mildly irritating effect that increases blood flow to the area, helping to strengthen resistance and clear away infection. It is also used for weak eyesight, and for the early stages of cataracts.

334. *Cinnamomum camphora* (L.) Presl *(Lauraceae)*

Vernacular Name: *Eng*: Camphor tree, Formosan wood; *Hin:* Kapur, karpur; *Tel:* Karppuram; *Tam:* Karpurammu.

Description: Evergreen treen about 15m. tall. Trunk bark thick and grooved. Leaves alternate, coriaceous, long-petiolate, shining on the upper side, 3-nerved at the base. Inflorescence in axillary panicle, shorter than the leaf; flowers small, greenish-yellow. Berry globose, black when ripe.

Habitate: Cultivated as a shade-tree in sub-tropical and tropical region.

Propagation: By seeds.

Part Used: Roots and wood.

Chemical Constituents: The stem wood and leaves contain an essential oil consisting of camphor, D-a-pinene, cineol, terpineol, caryophyllin, safrole, limonene, phellandrene, carvacrol, camphorene and azulene.

Uses: The camphor from the trunk wood possesses cardiac, analeptic, antivacterial, demulcent and anodyne properties. Injections of camphor oil and sodium camphosulfonate are prescrived in case of cardiovascular collapse. The peroral administration of camphor is effective for fever, colic, sore throat and impotence. It is applied externally as an antiseptic, demulcent and anodyne for impetigo, boils, neuralgia and rheumatism, in the form of a tincture, an aqueous solution or an ointment.

335. *Cinnamomum cassia* Blume *(Lauraceae)*

Vernacular Name: *Eng*: Camphor tree, Formosan wood.

Description: Evergreen treen about 15m. tall. Trunk bark thick and grooved. Leaves alternate, coriaceous, long-petiolate, shining on the upper side, 3-nerved at the base. Inflorescence in axillary or terminal cymose panicle; flowers white. Drupe ovoid, glabrous, purplish-brown when ripe.

Habitate: Occurs wild in mountainous regions; also cultivated.

Propagation: By seeds.

Part Used: Bark.

Chemical Constituents: The whole plant, especially the stem bark and twig bark, contain an essential oil. Cinnamic aldehyde, coumarin.

Uses: The bark possesses antibacterial circulatory, respiratory, uterotonic and stomachic properties. It is applied in the therapy of dyspepsia, colic, diarrhoea, cholera, dysentery, menstrual haematometra, croyza, influenza, cough, asthma, paresis and snake-bite. It is also recommended as a tonic. The essential oil from the bark is constituent of balasams.

336. *Cinnamomum macrocarpum* Hook.f. *(Lauraceae)*

Vernacular Name: *San*:-Tamalapatra, *Kan*:-Kadu dalchini, Lavanga patre, *Mal*: -Karuva, *Tam*:-Periya lavanga pattai, *Tel*:-Talisapatramu.

Description: A medium sized tree, up to 15 m tall and about 75 cm girth. *Bark* smooth, grey to light brown, about 5 mm thick, smelling like clove when cut. Branchlets thick, angular hairless. *Leaves* opposite and sub-opposite, thick-leathery, hairless, egg-shaped-elliptic to oblong-lanceolate, 7-25 x 2-12 cm, base wedge-shaped, apex rounded to shortly acuminate, glossy, fragrant; nerves 3-5, arising from the base of the leaf, prominent, reaching nearly to the apex; leaf stalks stout, 1-2 cm long. *Flowers* bisexual, dull yellow, distinctly stalked, arranged in axillary paniculate cymes. Panicles branched, 5-7 cm long, stout, hairless with flattened peduncle; each cyme about 3-flowered. *Berries* ellipsoid, about 2 x 2.5 cm, hairless, greenish pink ripening purplish brown, seated on a fleshy inverted cone-like disc, which is about 1.5 cm long.

Habitate: Moist deciduous to shoal forests.

Propagation: By seeds and vegetative method.

Parts Used: Bark, leaves, root-bark.

Chemical Constituents: Eugenol, camphor, cineol, linalool.

Uses: The bark is used for cough, diarrhoea and dysentery. Oil from the root bark and leaves is applied externally in rheumatic affections.

337. *Cinnamomum sulphuratum* Nees *(Lauraceae)*

Vernacular Name: Kan:-Pinga dalchinni, Matta dalchinni, Mal: -Kattu karuva, *Tam*:-Kattu lavangam.

Description: A small to medium sized tree, about 8 m tall and about 70 cm girth. *Bark* smooth, reddish brown outside, dull red inside, with a strong aromatic smell. Young branches slender, angular, with dense minute yellowish-brown addressed tomentose hairs. *Leaves* opposite and sub-opposite, 4-12 x 2-4.5 cm, oblong or elliptic-oblong, base rounded or acute, apex acute, slightly leathery, airless, glossy, tomentose, bluish grey beneath, with 3 basal nerves; young leaves with tomentose hairs below, gradually becoming hairless when old, distinctly stalked. *Flowers* bisexual, about 2-4 mm long, distinctly stalked, greenish yellow, in terminal and axillary 10-14 cm long panicles. *Berries* oblong-ellipsoid, 1 x 1.5 cm, smooth, hairless, seated on about1 cm across cup-shaped fleshy disc.

Habitate: Moist deciduous to shoal forests.

Propagation: By seeds and vegetative method.

Parts Used: Leaves, bark, roots bark.

Chemical Constituents: N.A.

Uses: Bark and leaves are used like that of its relative species, *C. zeylanicum*, which is used to cure cough, headache, spider poison and as a mouth refresher.

338. *Cinnamomum tamala* Nees & Eberm. *(Lauraceae)*

Vernacular Name: *Eng:* Indian cassia lignea, Cassia cinnamon, *Hin:* Tejpatt, *Kan:* Kadu lavanga patte, *Mal:* Paccila, *San*: Tamalapatram, *Tam:* Tamalapattirii, *Tel:* Talisa patri, Adavi-lavanga patri.

Description: A moderate sized evergreen tree 7.5 m in height with dark brown or blackish rough bark and pinkish or reddish brown blaze; leaves simple, opposite, sub-opposite or alternate, ovate-lanceolate or ovate-oblong, acuminate, coriaceous, glabrous, 3-nerved from base to apex; flowers pale yellowish in axillary and terminal, lax puberulous panicles; fruits ovoid, fleshy, black drupe, supported by enlarged perianth tube.

Habitate: Himalayas, in areas of 900-2,400 m elevation.

Propagation: By seeds.

Parts Used: Leaves.

Chemical Constituents: Cinnamic aldehyde, linalool, eugenol, eugenol acetate, β-caryophyllene, benzaldehyde, camphor, cadinene, α-terpineol, α-and β-pinene, *p*-cymene, limonene, geraniol, ocimene, γ-terpinene, β-phellandrene, benzyl cinnamate, benzyl acetate.

Uses: The leaves are bitter, sweet, aromatic, thermogenic, alexeteric, anthelmintic, diuretic, stimulant, carminative and tonic. They are useful in cardiac disorders, inflammations, helminthiasis dyspepsia, strangury, colic, hyperptyalism, ophthalmia, vitiated conditions of *vata*, diarrhoea, proctitis, proctalgia, hepatopathy and splenopathy.

339. *Cinnamomum verum* Presl (*Lauraceae*)

Synonyms: *Cinnamomum zeylanicum* Blume.

Vernacular Name: *San*: Tvak, Darusita, *Eng:* Cinnamon, cylon cinnamom, *Hin:* Dalcini, Darucini, *Kan:* Dalcini, *Mal:* Ilavangam, Elavangam, Karuva, Vayana, *Tam:* Ilavangam, Karuva, *Tel:* Dasini cekka, Dalcini.

Description: A moderate sized evergreen tree, 8-18 m in height and 50 cm in diameter with reddish brown soft bark, having numerous small warts; leaves ovate or elliptic-ovate, shiny above, 3-5 ribbed from a little above the base, the side ribs ending about three-fourths up, the base usually rounded; flowers small in axillary or sub-terminal cymes or panicles; fruits ovoid berry, dark purple in colour having persistent perianth.

Habitate: West coast tropical evergreen and semi-evergreen forests.

Propagation: By seeds.

Parts Used: Bark, oil.

Chemical Constituents: Eugenol, O-methyl eugenol, benzaldehyde, cinnamaldehyde, I-α-pinene, I-α-and I-β-phellandrene, p-cymene, caryophyllene, benzyl benzoate and linalool. Presence of safrole, acetyleugenol, cinnamyl acetate and cinnamyl alcohol.

Uses: The bark is acrid, bitter, sweet, aromatic, astringent, aphrodisiac, deodorant, stimulant, alexeteric, expectorant, febrifuge, diuretic, and carminative. It is useful in bronchitis, asthma, cephalalgia, odontalgia, cardiac diseases, diarrhoea, uropathy, nausea and vomiting, flatulence, fever, halitosis and restoring normal skin colour on the face.

Cinnamon oil is stomachic, carminative, emenagogue and styptic, and is useful in anorexia, inflammations, stomachalgia, vitiated conditions of *vata*, odontalgia, vomitingand tubercular ulcers.

340. *Cinnamomum wightii* Meisn. (*Lauraceae*)

Vernacular Name: Kan:-Kadu dalchini, Mal: -Kattu karuva, *San*:-Tejpatra, *Tam:*-Sempala, Vattadu, Kattu lavangam.

Description: Densely foliaceous shoal trees, up to 30 m tall and about 2 m girth. *Outer bark* smooth, grey, thin; *inner bark* about 1 cm thick, whitish yellow, strongly aromatic. *Crown* compact, nearly ball-shaped. Branchlets slightly 4-angled, hairless. *Leaves* opposite or alternate, broadly elliptic to egg-shaped, 7-12 x 3-7 cm, base rounded to truncate, apex acute, leathery, smooth and shiny, bluish grey below, hairless, with 3-5 strong basal nerves, distinctly stalked. *Flowers* bisexual, about 5 mm long, shortly stalked, yellowish, arranged in 6-10 cm long axillary brown tomentose panicles. *Berries* ellipsoid, about 1.5 x

1 cm, smooth, ripening brown, seated on a fleshy inverted cone-shaped about 1 cm long cup.

Habitate: Shola forests to evergreen forests.

Propagation: By seeds and vegetative method.

Parts Used: Bark, leaves, oil.

Chemical Constituents: N.A.

Uses: Bark, leaves and oil used to treat paralytic disorders, deficiency in digestive power, abdominal disorders, cough, dysuria and gynaecological disorders. Tender fruits, including stalk and calyx, are astringent, aromatic, stimulant and carminative.

341. *Cirsium japonicum* var. *ussuriense* Kitamura *(Asteraceae)*

Vernacular Name: *Eng:*-Japanese thistle.

Description: Perennial herb, to 50-100 cm tall. Basal leaves obovate-oblang, pubescent on herves beneath; stem leaves alternate, oblong, pinnately cut, clasping, margins spiny. Heads of 4 cm across, solitary or in clusters of 2-3 on the ends of branches; involucre companulate, ovoid; involucral bracts imbricate in several rows, spine-tipped, receptacle densely bristly. Flower all tubular, purplish or rose, anthers tailed. Achenes 4-angled, glabrous, pappus of plumose bristles united basally in a ring and falling as a unit.

Habitate: Open sunny places in Korea, Japan.

Propagation: By seeds.

Parts Used: Whole plant.

Chemical Constituents: Flavonoids.

Uses: Used in cough, headache, lassitude, pneumonia, swelling.

342. *Cissus quadrangularis* L. *(Vitaceae)*

Synonyms: *Vitis quadrangularis* (Linn.) Wall. ex Wight & Arm.

Vernacular Name: *Eng:* Edible-stemmed vine, Adamant creeper, Bone-setter, *Hin:* Hadjod, Hadjora, *Kan:* Mangarahalli, *Mal:* Cannalamparanta, Peranta, *San*: Asthisrnkhala, Vajravalli, *Tam:* Pirantai, Vajjiravalli, *Tel:* Nalleru, Nulleratiga.

Description: A tendril climber with stout fleshy jointed quadrangular stems, tendrils simple, long, slender and leaf-opposed, in addition to the normal roots, some aerial roots arising from the jointed nodes grow downwards and strike the soil; leaves simple, broadly reniform, entire or toothed, rounded, truncate or cuneate at the base; flowers small, greenish, in shortly peduncled cymes, petals 4, hooded at the apex; fruits ovoid or globose, red berries, seeds ellipsoid.

Habitate: Throughout the hotter parts of India.

Propagation: By vegetative method.

Parts Used: Whole plant.

Chemical Constituents: The stem contains two unsymmetric tetracyclic triterpenoids, onocer-7-ene-3α-, 21 β-diol and onocer-7-ene-3 β, 21 α-diol and two steroidal principles I and II. Prescene of β-sitosterol, δ-amyrin and δ-amyrone is also reported.

Uses: The plant is bitter, sweet, sour, thermogenic, alternate, laxative, anthelmintic, carminative, digestive, stomachic, depurative, haemostatic, aphrodisiac, anodyne, ophthalmic and union-promoting and is useful in vitiated condition of *vata*, helminthiasis, anorexia, dyspepsia, colic, flatulence, skin diseases, leprosy, haemorrhages, haemoptysis, ophthalmopathy, otorrhoea, chronic ulcers, tumours, haemorrhoids, epilepsy, convulsions, spanomenorrhea, fractures, swellings and vitiated conditions of *kapha*. The shoots are useful in colonopathy, scurvy, otorrhoea, asthma, burns and wounds. Powdered roots as well as the stem paste are very specific for bone fractures.

343. *Citrullus colocynthis (Linn.) Schrad* *(Cucurbitaceae)*

Vernacular Name: *San*: Visala, Mahendravaruni, *Eng:* Colocynth, Bitter apple, *Hin:* Badi indrayan, Makkal, Tumba, *Kan:* Tuntikaye, Meekkikayi, *Mal:* Kattuvellari (Valutu), Valiya pekkummatti, *Tam:* Paitummatti, Petummatti, *Tel:* Verripuccha, Etipucchala.

Description: An extensively trailing annual herb with bifid tendrils, angular branching stems and woolly tender shoots; leaves deeply divided, lobes narrow, thick, glabrous or somewhat hairy; flowers monoecious, yellow, both males and females solitary, corolla pale-yellow; fruit a globose or oblong fleshy indehiscent berry, 5-7.5 cm in diameter and variegated with green and white; seeds pale brown.

Habitate: Cultivated and wild, throughout India in warm areas.

Propagation: By seeds and vegetative method.

Parts Used: Roots, fruits.

Chemical Constituents: The juice of the fruit contains α-elaterin, citrulluin, citrulluene, and citrulluic acid. A dihydric alcohol, citrullol and p-hydroxybenzyl, methylether have been isolated from the dried pulp and the unripe fruit, respectively. The peel-free flesh of ripe fruits contains a yellow, bitter oil, citbittol.

Uses: The roots are purgative and are used for treating uteralgia, mammillitis, rheumatalgia, visceromegaly in children, ophthalmia, ascites, jaundice and uropathy. The fruits are bitter, acrid, cooling, carminative, purgative, antipyretic and anthelmintic, and are useful in tumours, ascites, leucoderma, ulcers, asthma, bronchitis, urethrorrhea, jaundice, dyspepsia, constipation, elephantiasis, tubercular glands of the neck and splenomegaly.

344. *Citrullus vulgaris* *(Cucurbitaceae)*

Vernacular Name: *Eng:* Watermelon.

Description: Annual vine with hairy, 3-5 lobed leaves, yellow flowers, and green fruit typically growing to 25 cm across.

Habitate: Native to tropical Africa, watermelon is grown throughout warm temperate to tropical region. The fruit is gathered when ripe.

Propagation: By seeds and vegetative method.

Parts Used: Fruits, Seeds.

Chemical Constituents: Watermelon contains citrullin and arginine, both of which are thought to increase urea production in the liver, so increasing the flow of urine.

Uses: Used characterized by excessive sweating, thirst, raised temperature, scanty urine, diarrhoea and irritability or anger. Watermelon fruit and juice soothe these symptoms, increasing urine flow and cleansing the kidneys. The fruit's refreshing properties extend to the digestive system, where it clears wind. Watermelon may also be used in the treatment of hepatitis. In hot, stifling weather it is helpful for those suffering from bronchitis or asthma. The cooling fruit pulp may be applied to hot and inflamed skin and to soothe sunburn. The seeds can be mashed and used to expel worms.

345. *Citrus aurantifolia* (christn) Swingle. *(Rutaceae)*

Vernacular Name: *Eng:* Acid or sour lime; *Hin:* Kaghzi nimbu; *Beng*: Kaghzinimbu, patinebu; *Tam:* Elumichai; *Tal*: Nimma; *Kan:* Limbe, nimbe; *Mal:* Erumichinarakam.

Habitate: Cultivated all over india.

Propagation: By seeds and vegetative method.

Part Used: Fruit peel, juice.

Chemical Constituents: The major constituents of the distilled oil are d-limonene, a-and b-pinenes y-terpinene, terpinolene, a-terpineol, b-bisabolene, 1,4-cineol, terpinen-4-ol, and myrcene.

Uses: The oil is fresh and sharp and is used to flavour soft drinks, especially cola and lemon-lime types, ice-cream, candy, baked goods, gelatins, puddings, chewing gum, condiments, etc. It is also used as amodifier in citrus formulations.

346. *Citrus aurantium* L. *(Rutaceae)*

Vernacular Name: *Eng:* Seville or sour orange; *Hin:* Khatta; *Tam:* Narangam, narattai; *Tel:* Mallikanarangi; *Kan:* Heralay and *Mal:* Karna.

Description: Small tree to 10m tall with large spines on younger branches. Leaves alternate with winged-petioles, the blade ovate, bluntly toothed, emitting astrong citrus odour due to the presence of copious oil glands. Flowers axillary, borne singly or a few, white and very fragrant. Fruit a yellow-orange hesperidium, several to numerous seed within. Flowers usually during warmer months and fruit available later in the year.

Habitate: Cultivated and possibly naturalized in some locations.

Propagation: By seeds and vegetative method.

Part Used: Leaves, bark and fruits.

Chemical Constituents: 4-methulacetophenone, carotenoids, essential oil containing more than 60 monoterpenses and 25 sesquiterpenes. Several coumarins, caffeinel isoquinoline alkaloids synerphrine, 5-methyl and N-methul tyramines. Forty flavonoids, sixteen triterpenoids, and common steriods such as desmosterol, ergosterol, beta-sitosterol and stigmasterol.

Uses: Headaches is treated with tea made from the leaves or the bark of the plant. Vermin of the head are treated with the leaves. The bark is used to treat sunstroke. The juice or the fruit is mixed with coconut oil or castor oil and given as a laxative. The new leaves are used to treat abdominal pain. The fruit is eaten if a fishbone gets caught in one's throat. The bark or leaves are boiled and taken to treat urinary tract infections.

347. *Citrus grandis* (L.) Osbeck *(Rutaceae)*

Synonyms: Citrus maxima.

Vernacular Name: *Eng*: Pomelo, shaddock, paradise apple, forbidden fruit, pompelmoose; *Hin*: Chakotra, mahanibu, sadaphal; *Beng* Chakotra, mahanibu, sadaphal; *Mal:* Pamparamasam; *Kan:* Chakotre, sakkota; *Tam:* Pambalimasu; *Tel:* Pampalamasam.

Description: A tree about 10m. high. Young shoots thorny. Leaves alternate dark-green, shining above, obscurely puberulent beneath; petiole broadly winged. Inflrescence in axillary cyme; flowers white, fragrant, fruit large, globose, pale-yellow; rind thick; vesicles numerous, distinct. Seeds angular.

Habitate: Widely cultivated every where as a domestic fruit.

Propagation: By seeds & vegetative propagation.

Part Used: Leaves, skin of fruit, flowers.

Chemical Constituents: The essential oil from the leaves consists of dipentene. Linalol, citral. Limonene, flavonoids, vitamins A,C,B_1, rhamnose, citric acid, pectin and fatty oil.

Uses: The fresh leaves in combination with leaves from some other aromatic plants are used in treating coryza, influenza and headache by inhalation of the vapour from the boiling decoction. The fruit rind is effective for dyspepsia, colic and cough. The seed envelopes contain pectin, which is a haemostatic. The seeds, stripped of their envelope and charred, are applied externally for impetigo. Massage with heated young leaves is effective for treating bruises.

348. *Citrus japoncia* Thunb. *(Rutaceae)*

Synonyms: *Fortunella japonica* Thunb.

Vernacular Name: *Eng*: Kumquat, cherry orange.

Description: Shrubby plant 1-3m. high, much-branched. Leaves alternate, short-petioled, oval or obovate, rounded at the apex, glabrous, with shining upper surface. Flowers white, axillary or terminal. Fruit globose, orange-red when ripe, with a leathery rind.

Habitate: Species cultivated in sub-tropical and tropical region.

Propagation: By seeds and vegetative methods.

Part Used: Fresh fruit.

Chemical Constituents: The leaves and fruit contain an essential oil. The juice of the fruit contains sugars and organic acids.

Uses: The fesh fruit has an antitussive and expectorant action.It is also effective in sore throat. It is very goods for infants.

349. *Citrus limon* (Linn.) Burm. f. *(Rutaceae)*

Vernacular Name: *San*: Jambirah, *Eng:* Lime, *Hin:* Jamiri nimbu, Bara Nimbu, *Kan:* Limbe, *Mal:* Cerunarakam, *Tam:* Elumiccai, *Tel:* Peddanimma, Nimma.

Description: A much branched thorny shrub with spreading branches; leaves unifoliately compound, rachis winged, leaflet elliptic-oblong, alternate, coriaceous, entire or crenulate; flowers white in short racemes; fruits large, globose berries with thick or thin rind, pulp pale, very acid, seeds many, horizontal, testa coriaceous.

Habitate: Throughout India, cultivated in plains and hills in areas upto 1,200 m elevation.

Propagation: By seeds and vegetative method.

Parts Used: Fruits.

Chemical Constituents: Citric acid, pectin, lemon oil, carotene.

Uses: The fruits are sour, thermogenic, digestive, carminative, stomachic, laxative, anthelmintic, antiscorbutic, stimulant, antiseptic and mosquito repellent, and are useful in viatiated condition of *kapha* and *vata*, dyspepsia, flatulence, colic, constipation, anorexia, helminthiasis, scabies, fatigue, halitosis, vomiting, trembling of the limbs, hemicrania, psychopathy pharyngopathy, cough, bronchitis and heartburn.

350. *Citrus limonia* Osbeck *(Rutaceae)*

Vernacular Name: *Eng*: Canton lemon, ninmeng, Japanese citron; *Hin:* Baranibu, jambira; *Beng*: Baranebu, goranebu; *Kan:* Bijapura, bijori; *Tam:* Periya yelumichai; *Tel:* Bijapuram.

Description: Evergreen shrub, armed with long, sharp, axillary thorns. Leaves alternate, coriaceous, glabrous, dark green above, obscurely crenate–serrate. Flowers white, solitary or in a few-flowered raceme. Fruit globose, rind smooth and thin, yellow when ripe.

Habitate: Cultivated everywhere as a spice and medicinal plant.

Propagation: By seeds and vegetative methods.

Part Used: Leaves & fruit.

Chemical Constituents: The leaves contain essential oil 0.3-0.5% strachydrine. The skin of the fruit yields an essential oil consisting of D-liminone, A-pinene, B-phellandrene, camphene, citral and pectin. The juice of the fruit contains citric acid 5-10%, calcium and potassium citrate 1-2% vitamins C,B_1, riboflvin.

Uses: The leaves, the roots and the fruit rinds possess antibacterial and demulcent properties. The boiling decoction of fresh leaves is indicated for inhalation against coryza and influenza. The leaves, the roots and the fruit rinds are used to treat cough, sore throat, dyspnoea, headache, ophthalmagia, mastitis, galactophoritis, anorexia, vomiting and snake-bite.

351. *Citrus medica* L. *(Rutaceae)*

Vernacular Name: *San*: Matulungah, *Eng:* Citron, *Hin:* Baranimbu, Bijaura, *Kan:* Madala, Mahaphala, *Mal:* Ganapatinarakam, *Tam:* Kadaranarattai, *Tel:* Madiaphalamu, Lungamu.

Description: An evergreen armed shrub with straggling thorny branches and smooth yellowish brown bark; leaves oblong or elliptic with acute or rounded apex, coriaceous, glabrous, pellucid-punctate, dull dark green above; flowers white tinged with pink, scented, in axillary cymes; fruits large berries oblong or globose, fleshy, rind thick, rough, irregular or warted, yellow when ripe; seeds few, smooth.

Habitate: Throughout India, on forests along streams, in areas upto 1,200 m elevation.

Propagation: By seeds and vegetative method.

Parts Used: Fruits, roots.

Chemical Constituents: Campesterol, stigmasterol, sitosterol, cholesterol.

Uses: The roots are laxative, anthelmintic and diuretic and are useful in constipation, colic, flatulence, stranguary, renal and vesical calculi, tumours, vomiting, helminthiasis and dental caries. The buds and flowers are astringent, stimulant, antiemetic and appetiser, and are useful in anorexia, vomiting, tumorus, abdominal disorders, asthma, cough and hiccough. The ripe fruits are sweet, emollient, sour, astringent, stimulant, refrigerant, anthelmintic, carminative, digestive, cardiac stimulant, haemostatic, emmenagogue and tonic, and are useful in pharyngodynia, cough, asthma, hiccough, hyperdipsia, otalgia, anorexia, vomiting, hepatopathy, flatulence, haemorrhoids, haemoptysis, amenorrhoea, dysmenorrhoea, dysentery, leprosy and skin diseases. The seeds are stimulant, anti-inflammatory, emmenagogue and tonic, and are useful in inflammations, skin diseases, amenorrhoea, dysmenorrhoea and haemorrhoids. The leaves are anodyne.

352. *Citrus paradisi* Macf. *(Rutaceae)*

Vernacular Name: *Eng:* Grapefruit; *Hindi*: Chakotra.

Description: A spreading tree; leaves large, petioles winged; flowes in clusters; fruit in clusters, ligh yellow, flesh yellow or pink, sweet with bitter after-taste; seeds white.

Habitate: Cultivated in India.

Propagation: By seeds and vegetative method.

Part Used: Fruit peel.

Chemical Constituents: Grapefruit oil contains limonene, myrcene, a-pinene, sabinene, p-cymene, caryophyllene, y-terpinene, terpinene-4-ol, octanal, linalool, and nootkatone as its major components.

Uses: Grapefruit oil has a sweet, plesant odour intermediate between orange and lemon. It is largely employed in flavours for soft-drinks, ice-cream, candy, baked goods, gelatins and puddings, chewing gum and toppings.

353. *Citrus reticulata* Blanco (*Rutaceae*)

Synonyms: *Citrus chrysocarpa* Lushington; *Citrus aurantium*; *Citrus nobilis* Watt.

Vernacular Name: *Eng*: Tangerine, Maltese o\orange, loose–skinned orange, Satsuma; *Hin:* Santara; *Beng*: Kamala.

Description: Medium–sized plant, 5-8m. high naked or with short spines. Leaves alternate with rounded or acute coriaceous apex, entire, glabrous; petiole obscurely winged. Flowers white in axillary raceme. Bery globose or subglobose, deep-orange when fuly ripe; pulp juicy, sweet.

Habitate: Cultivated every where.

Propagation: By seeds and vegetative methods.

Part Used: Green fruit, the rind of ripe fruit and seeds.

Chemical Constituents: The leaves and the skins of the fuit yield an essential oil consisting of D-limonene, D-Limonene, linalool, citral, nonylic and decylic aldehyde, methyl anthranilate.The juice of the fruit contains sugars, citric acid, vitamin C and carotene.

Uses: The dried rind of the fruit is effective in treating cough, chest pain, excessive exceptoration, dyspepsia, colic, diarrhoea, eructations and vomiting.It is also an antirheumatic and diuretic drug. External application of a poultice made of heated fresh leaves and a decoction of dried leaves taken by mouth are prescrived for the treatment of colic and mastitis.

354. *Citrus sinensis* (L.) Osbeck (*Rutaceae*)

Synonyms: *Citrus aurantium.*

Vernacular Name: *Eng:* Orange, sweet orange; *Hin:* Musambi, narangi, kamala nembu; *Beng*: Musambi, narangi, kamala nembu; *Kan:* Kittile, sathgudi; *Tam:* Sathagudi, chini; *Tel:* Battavin, arinja, buddasini, naranji, satghudi, sini.

Description: Small tree to 12 m tall with large spines or younger branches. Leaves alternate with narrowly winged-petioles the blade ovate, bluntly toothed, emitting a strong citrus odour due to the presence of copious oil glands. Flowers axillary, borne singly or in a small bunch, white and very fragrant. Fruit a green or orange hesperidium somewhat thin skin containing usually sweet pulp and several to numerous seeds within.

Habitate: Cultivated and possibly naturalized in some locations.

Propagation: By seeds and vegetative method.

Part Used: Leaves, bark and fruits.

Chemical Constituents: 14 monoterpenses, 15 sesquiterpenes, gibberellic acid, phytol, amyrin, limonin and its glucosides, nomilin derivatives, seventeen flavonoids, cartenoids, thirteen alkaloids, brassinolide, castesterone, sitosterol, hydroquinone, sinapic acid, anethole, frrulic acid, etrogol, vitamin C, coumaric acid, citrusins (proteid), caffeic acid, eleven coumarins, pectin, and stigmasterol.

Uses: An infusion of the leaves is used to treat relapse sickness which mainly affects women who return to strenuous work too soon after giving birth. An infusion of the bark is used to treat an illness similar to relapse sickness, as well as to treat postpartum sickness. The juice of the fruit together with coconut oil or castor oil is used as a purgative. They also ingest the crushed leaves of the plant to treat abdominal pains. A whole peeled orange is swallowed to remove a fishbone stuck in the throat. The leaves of the plant are used as remedies for internal ailments and fractures as well as other sicknesses.

355. *Citrus unshiu* Markovich (*Rutaceae*)

Vernacular Name: *Eng:*-Japanese sweet orange.

Description: Evergreen, small tree, to 5 tall, without spines. Leaves alternate, lanceolate, or broad lanceolate, obtuse at base, 5-7 cm long entire or serrulate, petioles narrowly winged or wingless, glandular-dotted. Flowers white, fragrant, bisexual; calyx 5-lobed; petals 5; stamens about 20, united in bundles; carpel; 1. Fruit an aromatic, leathery-skinned berry (a hesperidium).

Habitate: Cultivated in the southernmost part of Korea.

Propagation: By seeds and vegetative method.

Parts Used: Pericarp.

Chemical Constituents: Phenylpropanoids. Monoterpenes, sesquiterpenes, Flavonoids, synephrine, citroside A, B.

Uses: Stimulation of gastric secretion and movement, serotonin antagonism, tyrosinase inhibition, antibacterial, smooth muscle relaxant activity. Used in Dyspepsia, cough, phlegm, common cold, liver disease.

356. *Clematis hexapetala* Pall. (*Ranunculaceae*)

Vernacular Name: *Eng:* Six-petalled clematis.

Description: A perennial erect herb, up to 65 cm high. It has a group of long blackish roots, which run blacker when dry, 7-15 cm long, 1-3 mm in diameter. Leaves opposite, pinnate; leaflets bipartite or tripartite, leathery; segments lanceolate, entire; petioles 0.5-3.5 cm long. Flowers panicled, grouped in ramified cymes, axillary or terminal. May-June. Fruit a head of stalked achenes with long, usually feathery, styles.

Habitate: On slopes and by roadsides in China, Korea.

Propagation: By seeds.

Part Used: Roots.

Chemical Constituents: N.A.

Uses: Rheumatic arthritis, acute tonsillitis, throat inflammation, jaundice due to acute infectious hepatitis, toothache.

357. *Clematis mandschurica* Rupr. (*Ranunculaceae*)

Vernacular Name: *Eng:* Virgin's bower, leather flower, vase vine.

Description: Herbaceous climbing vine, to 2m tall. Leaves opposite, pinnately compound; leaflect 5-7, ovate, acuminate at apex, rounded at base, entire, glabrous. Flowers in axillary panicles, white, fragrant, opening flat; sepals petalotid, 4-5, 1-2 cm long, obovate-elliptic, glabrous; petals none; stamens many. Fruit an ovoid achene, with a long feathery style of 2 cm.

Habitate: Low elevations in mountains in Korea and China.

Propagation: By seeds and vegetative method.

Parts Used: Root.

Chemical Constituents: Clematosides A, A', B, C, hederagenin, anemonin.

Uses: Antibacterial, antifungal, hypotensive, analgesic, antidiuretic, platelet aggregation inhibition. Used in leucorrhoea, dysentery, neuralgia, menostasis, sputum remedy.

358. *Clematis vitalba* *(Ranunculaceae)*

Vernacular Name: *Eng:* Traveller's joy.

Description: Robust perennial climber growing to 30m in length. Has lance-shaped compound leaves, small white fragrant flowers and fluffy seedheads.

Habitate: This herb is found throughout Europe, and also in western Asia and North America.

Propagation: By seeds and vegetative method.

Parts Used: Leaves.

Chemical Constituents: Traveller's joy contains protoanemonin and saponins. Protoanemonin is caustic and irritant.

Uses: The leaves of traveller's joy irritate the skin, causing it to redden and blister, but they are also strongly analgesic. Applied to arthritic joints, they help relieve pain and encourage the removal of waste products. The plant is also diuretic, and in the past was taken internally to counter urinary problems. However, the mature plant is now known to be toxic and should not be ingested. The juice is reputed to relieve headaches and migraine if sniffed, but as this might destroy the mucous.

359. *Cleome viscosa* L. *(Capparideaceae)*

Synonyms: *Cleome ico Sandra* Linn.

Vernacular Name: *Eng:* Wild mustard, Dog mustard, Sticky cleome, *Hin:* Hulhul, Hurhur, *Kan:* Nayibelu, Kadu sasive, *Mal:* Atunarivela, Vela, Aryavela, Naivela, *San*: Pasugandha, *Tam:* Naivelai, Naikkaduku, *Tel:* Kukkavaminta, Nallavaminta.

Description: An annual, sticky herb with strong penetrating odour and clothed with glandular and simple hairs; leaves 3-5 foliate, gradually becoming shorter upwards; flowers yellow in lax raceme; fruits capsules, compressed, hairy throughout; seeds brownish black when ripe.

Habitate: A weed throughout the plains in India.

Propagation: By seeds and vegetative method.

Parts Used: Whole plant.

Chemical Constituents: The aerial parts contain a macrocyclic diterpene, -20-oxocembra-3, 7, 11, 15-tetra en-19-oic acid and a bicyclic diterpene, cleomeolide. The seeds contain coumarino-lignans, cleomiscosin, A, B, C and D.

Uses: The plant is acrid, thermogenic, anthelmintic and sudorific. The roots are stimulant, antiscorbutic and vermifuge. The leaf juice is digestive and is good for otalgia. The seeds are anthelmintic, carminative, constipating, febrifuge and cardiac stimulant and are useful in fever, diarrhoea, worm infestations, cardiac disordes and dyspepsia.

360. *Clerodendrum fragrans* (Vent.) Willd. *(Verbenaceae)*

Vernacular Name: *Eng:* Chinese glory tree.

Description: Small shrub, 0.5-1.5m high. Young twings quadrangular, pubescent, Leaves opposite, long-petioled, cordate or flat at the base, tomentose on both sides; margins toothed or wavy, Inflorescence in terminal head of dense, white flowers, berry globose, calyx persistent.

Habitate: Grows wild; common in many places.

Propagation: By seeds and vegetative methods.

Part Used: Roots.

Chemical Constituents: N.A.

Uses: The roots have antivacterial and anti-inflammatory activity. They are utilized in treating metritis, metrrohoea, menstrual disorders, furunculosis, impetigo, osteodynia, lumbago, hypertension and icterus. The decoction serves also as an external antiseptic for the washing of infected wounds, burns and impetigo.

361. *Clerodendrum serratum* (L.) Moon *(Verbenaceae)*

Vernacular Name: *San*: Bharngi, Kharasakah, *Hin:* Bharangi, Kan: Gantabarangi, *Mal:* Cerutekku, *Tam:* Sirutekku, *Tel:* Gantubarangi.

Description: A slightly woody shrub with bluntly quadrangular stems and branches; leaves usually three at a node, sometimes opposite, oblong or elliptic, coarsely and sharply serrate; flowers blue, many, in long cylindrical thyrsus with a pair of acute bracts at each branching and a flower in the fork; fruit a 4-lobed purple durpe, somewhat succulent with one pyrene in each lobe.

Habitate: Throughout India, in forests upto 1,500 m elevation.

Propagation: By seeds and vegetative method.

Parts Used: Roots, leaves.

Chemical Constituents: N.A.

Uses: The roots are bitter, acrid, thermogenic, anti-inflammatory, digestive, carminative, stomachic, anthelmintic, depurative, expectorant, sudorific, antispasmodic, stimulant and febrifuge, and are useful in vitiated condition of *kapha* and *vata*, inflammations, dyspepsia, anorexia, colic, flatulence, helminthiasis, cough, asthma, bronchitis, hiccough, tumours, tubercular glands, dropsy, consumption, chronic nasitis, skin diseases, leucoderma, leprosy and fevers. The leaves are useful as an external application for cephalalgia and ophthalmia. Seeds aperient, used in dropsy.

362. *Clerodendrum squamatum* Vahl *(Verbenaceae)*

Description: Small shrub about 1m.high. Stems and branches glabrous, quadrangular. Leaves opposite, long-petioled, round cordate, entire or slightly dentate. Inflorescence in terminal cymose panicle flowers tinged red, stamens and style very long, exserted. Berry globose.

Habitate: Widely grown everywhere.

Propagation: By seeds and vegetative methods.

Part Used: Leaves and roots.

Chemical Constituents: N.A.

Uses: The entire plant has antibacterial and anti-inflammatory properties. It is indicated in the treatent of leucorrhoea, metritis, menstrual disorders, jaundice, furnuculosis, impetigo, arthralgia, osteodynia, lumbago and hypertension. A poultice of pounded fresh leaves and washing with their juice help to heal wounds, burns, boils and impetigo.

363. *Clerodendrum trichotomum* *(Verbenaceae)*

Vernacular Name: *Eng:* Chou wu tong.

Description: Upright, deciduous shrub growing to 3m. Has large leaves, clusters of white flowers and blue berries.

Habitate: This herb grows in central and southern china.

Propagation: By seeds and vegetative method.

Parts Used: Leaves.

Chemical Constituents: *Chou wu tong* contains clerodendrin, acacetin and mesoinositol.

Uses: In Chinese herbal medicine, *chou wu tong* is prescribed for joint pain, numbness and paralysis, and occasionally for eczema. Traditionally regarded as a plant that "dispels wind-dampness", it is now also being used to help lower blood pressure. The plant is mildly lower blood pressure. The plant is mildly analgesic and, when used with the herb *siegesbeckia puescens,* is anti-inflammatory.

364. *Clerodendrum viscosum* Vent. *(Verbenaceae)*

Synonyms: *Clerodendrum infortunatum* auct. non Linn.

Vernacular Name: *Hin:* Titabhamt, Bhates, *Kan:* Basavana pada, Ibbane, *Mal:* Peruku, *San*: Bhandirah, *Tam:* Perukilai, *Tel:* Gurrapu katliyaku.

Description: A large gregarious tawny-villous shrub upto 9.0 m in height with bluntly quadrangular branchlets; the leaves large, 10-25 cm/9-20 cm, ovate, acuminate, entire or denticulate, base cordate, hairy on both sides; flowers white, tinged with pink in terminal panicles; fruits somewhat globose drupes, seated on the enlarged pink calyx containing 1-4 pyrenes.

Habitate: Throughout India, as undergrowth in forests upto 1,800 m and as weed along roadsides and wastelands.

Propagation: By seeds and vegetative method.

Parts Used: Leaves.

Chemical Constituents: The alcoholic extract of the roots yields sterol glycoside which is mixture of β-sitosterol and Δ^5-25-stigmastadien-3-β-ol. The aerial parts yield several sterols, viz. clerosterol and its 22E-dehy-dro derivative, 24β-ethylcholesta-5, 22E, 25-trien-3β-ol as major sterols in addition to campestrol, cholesterol, sitosterol, 24α-stigmasterol and 24β-stigmasterol.

Uses: The leaves are bitter, acrid, thermogenic, laxative, cholagogue, antiseptic, demulcent, anti-inflammatory, depurative, vermifuge, expectorant, antipyretic and tonic, and are useful in vitiated condition of *kapha,* helminthiasis, ascarides, abscesses, tumours, leprosy, skin diseases, indolent ulcers, cough, bronchitis, inflammations, intermittent fevers, malarial fever, general debility and proctoptosis.

365. *Clitoria ternatea* L. *(Fabaceae)*

Vernacular Name: *San*: Aparajita, Girikarnika, *Eng:* Clitoria, Butterfly-Pea, Conchflower, *Hin:* Aparajita, *Kan: San*ka puspo, Karnike, *Mal:* Samkhupuspam, Aral, Malayamukki, *Tam:* Kannikkoti, Girikanni, *Tel:* Gilagarnika, Tella-dintana.

Description: A good-looking perennial twining herb with terete stems and branches, leaves compound, imparipinnate, leaflets 5-7, sub-coriaceous, elliptic-oblong, obtuse; flowers blue or white, solitary, axillary or in fascicles, corolla papilionaceous; fruits nearly straight, flattened pods, sharply beaked; seeds 6-10, smooth, yellowish brown.

Habitate: Throughout India in hedges and thickers, also cultivated in gardens.

Propagation: By seeds.

Parts Used: Roots, leaves, seeds.

Chemical Constituents: The high calcium concentration in the plant showed that it can be exploited as a significant source of calcium brewed as herbal drink. The presence of stigmast-4-ene-3, 6, diene is reported from the plant. The roots contain taraxerol and teraxerone. The leaves contain 3-monoglucoside, 3-rutinoside, 3-neohesperidoside, 3-O-rhamnosyl-glucoside, 3-O-rhamnosyl-galactoside of kaempferol, besides kaempferol-3-O-rhamnosyl-O-rhamnosyl-glucoside. The also contain aparajitin and β-sitosterol. The blue flowers contain delphinidin-3,5-diglucoside, delphinidin-3β-glucoside and its 3-methyl derivative, malvidin -3βglucoside, kaempferol and cyanin chloride; the white flowers yield only kaempferol.other substances present in the seeds are: *p*-hydorxycinnamic acid, flavonol-3-glycoside, ethyl-α-D-galactopyranoside, adenosine, 3, 5, 7, 4'-tetrahydroxyflavone-3-rhamnoglucoside, a polypeptide, hexacosanol, β-sitosterol and an anthoxanthin glucoside. The seeds also contain oligosaccharides or flatulene.

Uses: The roots are bitter, refrigerant, ophthalmic, laxative, intellect promoting, alexeteric, diuretic, anthelmintic, depurative, aphrodisiac and tonic, and are useful in ophthalmopathy, tubercular glands, amentia, hemicrania, burning sensation, strangury, helminthiasis, leprosy, leucoderma, elephantiasis, inflammation, vitiated conditions of *pitta*, bronchitis, asthma, pulmonary tuberculosis, ascites, ulcers, visceromegaly and fevers. The leaves are useful in otalgia, hepatopathy and eruptions. The seeds are cathartic and are useful in visceralgia.

366. *Cnicus benedictus* *(Asteraceae)*

Synonyms: *Carbenia benedicta, Carduus benedictus.*

Vernacular Name: *Eng:* Holy thistle.

Description: Erect, red-stemmed annual growing to 65cm. Has spiny leathery leaves, a spiny stem, and yellow flowers in summer and autumn.

Habitate: This Mediterranean plant flourishes on dry stony ground and wasteland.

Propagation: By seeds and vegetative method.

Parts Used: Leaves, flowers.

Chemical Constituents: Holy thistle contains lignans, vsesquiterpene lactones, volatile oil, polyacetylenes, flovonoids, triterpenes, phytosterols and tannins. Cnicin is bitter, anti-inflammatory and antibiotic.

Uses: Holy thistle is a good bitter tonic, stimulating the secretions of the stomach, intestines and gallbladder. It is taken, generally as a tincture, for minor digestive complaints. It has also been a treatment for intermittent fevers. Holy thistle is mildly expectorant, and is antibiotic. It makes a healing balm for wounds and sores.

367. *Cnidium monnieri* *(Apiaceae)*

Vernacular Name: *Eng:* She chuang zi.

Description: Upright plant typical of the carrot family. Has ridged stem, compound leaves and clusters of flowers.

Habitate: *She chuang zi* is cultivated in China.

Propagation: By seeds and vegetative method.

Parts Used: Seeds.

Chemical Constituents: The volatile oil of *she chuang zi* contains pinene, camphene, bornyl isovalerate and isoborneol.

Uses: The seeds of *she chuang zi* appear to have an antifungal action. *She chuang zi* is most often prescribed externally as a lotion, powder or ointment for skin conditions such as eczema, ringworm and scabies. The seeds are considered particularly helpful for problems affecting the genital area, for example vaginitis and vaginal discharge. *She chuang zi* is also taken internally for impotence, and infertility in both men and women, often in combination with schi*San*dra.

368. *Cnidium officinale* Makino *(Apiaceae)*

Vernacular Name: *Eng:*-Cnidium.

Description: Erect perennial herb with thickened root, 30-60 cm tall. Leaves petiolate, long-sheathed at base, 2-pinnately compound; leaflets ovate or lanceolate, incised, sharply serrate. Umbels compound, rather large, with many rays; involucre and involucel bracts 5-6 respectively, linear. Flowers white; calyx-teeth obsolete; petals 5, obovate with an incurved apex; stylopodium elongated-conical. Fruit ovoid-globose; carpels subterete in cross-section; ribs thick, obtuse, unwinged.

Habitate: Mostly cultivated in China and Korea.

Propagation: By seeds and vegetative method.

Parts Used: Rhizome.

Chemical Constituents: Phthalides; cnidilide, neocnidilide, ligustilide, senkyunolide, butylphthalide, butylindenephthalide. Senkyunolides B-J. pregnenolone, vanillin, coniferyl ferulate, ferulic acid.

Uses: Vasodilating, sedative, intestinal blood flow increasing, analgesic, anti-inflammatory, antifebrile, antispasmodic, antibacterial, inotropic effect, antioxidant activity. Used in women's diseases anaemia, weakness & Pains.

369. *Coccinia grandis* (L.) Voigt *(Cucurbitaceae)*

Synonyms: *Cephalandra indica* (Wight & Arn.) Naud., *Coccina cordifolia* Cogn.

Vernacular Name: *San*: Bimbi, Bimbika, *Eng:* Ivy gourd, *Hin:* Bimb, Kanturi, *Kan:* Tondikayi, *Mal:* Kova, Koval, *Tam:* Kovai, *Tel:* Donda Kaya.

Description: A perennial, much branched handsome tendril climber, roots sometimes tuberous; leaves deltoid or subrotund, angled or lobed, bright green above and pale beneath, palmately 5-nerved from a cordate base with circular glands between the nerves; flowers white, large, unisexual; fruits ovoid or oblong or ellipsoid berries with white streaks, bright scarlet red when ripe; seeds ovoid, compressed, yellowish grey.

Habitate: Throughout India, cultivated as well as found growing wild.

Propagation: By seeds and vegetative method.

Parts Used: Roots, leaves, fruits.

Chemical Constituents: Petroleum ether extract of the mature fruits yields taraxerone, sitosterol, taraxerol and–24-ethylcholest-5-en-3β-ol. The triterpene alcohols from aerial parts are composed of acetates of cycloartanol, α-& β-amyrin, isomulti-florenol, cycloartanol, lupeol and 24-methylenecy-cloartanol. The drug also contain caffeic acid, quercitin, kaempferol and β-sitsoterol.

Uses: The roots are cooling and aphrodisiac and are useful in vomiting, burning sensation and uterine discharges. The leaves are bitter, sweet, astringent and cooling, and are useful in vitiated conditions of *kapha* and *pitta*. The fruits are cooling, sweet, astringent, depurative, antipyretic, galactagogue and expectorant, and are useful in burning sensation, leprosy, skin diseases, intermittent fever, agalactia, asthma, cough, bronchitis, consumption and jaundice. The fruits and leaves of the bitter variety are bitter, acrid, thermogenic, emetic, purgative, vulnerary, anti-inflammatory, anthelmintic, digestive, liver tonic, alexeteric, depurative, febrifuge, sudorific and expectorant, and are useful in vitiated conditions of *kapha* and *pitta*, wounds ulcers, inflammation, helminthiasis, dyspepsia, hepatopathy, jaundice, skin diseases, leprosy, fever, asthma, cough, diabeties, stomatitis and anaemia.

370. *Cocculus hirsutus* (L.) Diels *(Menispermaceae)*

Synonyms: *Cocculus villosus* Lam.

Vernacular Name: *San*: Patalagarudah, Chilihindah, *Eng:* Broom creeper, Ink berry, *Hin:* Patalagarudi, Jaljamni, *Kan:* Sogadiballi, Dusariballi, *Mal:* Patalagarudakkoti, *Tam:* Kattukkoti, *Tel:* Dusaratiga.

Description: A straggling scandent shrub with softly villous young parts; leaves simple; alternate, ovate-oblong, obtuse, spiculate, subcordate or truncate at the base, softly villous on both surfaces, petioles densely villous; male flowers small, in axillary cymose panicles; female flowers 2-3 together in axillary clusters, petals thick and fleshy, divided at the apex into two triangular lobes, claw hairy; fruits transversely rugose, purplish black drupes.

Habitate: Throughout India in dry localities.

Propagation: By seeds and vegetative method.

Parts Used: Roots, leaves.

Chemical Constituents: Cohirsine, haiderine, jamtine N-oxide, trilobine, isotrilobine, -syringaresinol and protoquercitol. The triterpenoid alcohols, hirsudiol and nonacosan-10-ol have been reported from the plant. Cohirsitinine, hirsutine, shaheenine, cohirsinine and jamtinine. The plant also cintaons coclaurine, magnoflorine, sitosterol, ginnol and monomethyl ether of inositol.

Uses: The roots are bitter, acrid, thermogenic, laxative, alternate, emollient, alexeteric, depurative, demulcent, digestive, carminative, diuretic, aphrodisiac, expectorant, anodyne, antipyretic and tonic, and are useful in vitiated conditions of *kapha* and *vata*, poisonous bites, leprosy, skin diseases, pruritus, dyspepsia, flatulence, colic, stranguary, cough, bronchitis, gout, cephalalgia, intermittent fevers, spermatorrhoea, urethrorrhea, burning sensation, tubercular glands, fractures, hypertension and general debility. The leaves are mucilaginous, cooling, demulcent, anodyne and expectorant, and are useful in eczema, gonorrhoea, prurigo, impetigo cough, ophthalmia, cephalalgia and neuralgia.

371. *Cochlearia officinalis* *(Cruciferae)*

Vernacular Name: *Eng:* Scurvy grass.

Description: Low-growing perennial with fleshy heart-shaped leaves, dense clusters of white 4-petalled flowers and rounded swollen seedpods.

Habitate: Native to Europe and temperate regions of Asia and North America, but now rare, scurvy grass thrives in the salty soil of coastal areas and salt marshes.

Propagation: By seeds and vegetative method.

Parts Used: Leaves.

Chemical Constituents: Scurvy grass contains glucosilinates, a volatile oil, a bitter principle, tannina, vitamiun C and minerals.

Uses: Besides having a high vitamin C content, scurvy grass has antiseptic and mild laxative actions. The young plant, which has a general detoxicant effect and contains a wide range of minerals, is taken as a spring tonic. Like watercress, it has diuretic properties and is useful for any condition in which poor nutrition is a factor. It can be used in the form of a juice as an antiseptic mouthwash for mouth ulcers and can also be applied externally to spots and pimples.

372. *Cochlospermum religiosum* (L.) Alston (*Cochlospermaceae*)

Synonyms: *Cochlospermum gossypium* DC.

Vernacular Name: *San*: Girisalmalika, Silakarpasika, *Eng:* Yellow-flowered cotton tree, *Hin:* Galgal, Kumbi, *Kan:* Arasina buruga, *Mal:* Appakkutukka, Cempanni, Parappanni, *Tam:* Kattupparutti, Malaipparutti, *Tel:* Konda Gogu, Kongu.

Description: A small deciduous tree, 2.4-5.4 m in height with smooth, ash coloured, fibrous, deeply furrowed bark containing a gum; leaves palmately 5-lobed, tomentose beneath; flowers large, golden yellow in terminal panicles appearing after the leaf fall; fruits large, pear shaped, 3-5 valved capsules; seeds numerous covered over the woolly hairs.

Habitate: Throughout India, in dry forests, especially on stony hills.

Propagation: By seeds.

Parts Used: Leaves, flowers, gum.

Chemical Constituents: N.A.

Uses: Dried leaves and flowers are used as stimulant, and the young leaves are used as a cooling wash for the hair. The gum-known as 'Katira gum' is sweet, thermogenic, anodyne and sedative, and is useful in cough, diarrhoea, dysentery, pharyngitis; gonorrhoea, syphilis and trachoma.

373. *Cocos nicifera* L. (*Arecaceae*)

Vernacular Name: *San:* Narikela; *Eng:* Coconut; *Hin:* Nariyal; *Beng*: Dab, narikel; *Tel:* Kobbarichettu, narikelamu, tenkaya; *Tam:* Tennaimaram, tenkai; *Kan:* Tengu; *Mal:* Thenna, thenga, narikelam.

Description: Monopodial tree with long, narrow, often curved trunk upto 30 ml tall. Foliage leaves all confined to apex of trunk, each leaf paripinnate and up to or exceeding 6 m in length. Flowers and fruit borne in drooping clusters arising from between the lower leaf petioles. Fruit large green brown, or reddish fibrous drupe up to or exceeding 30 cm in length.

Habitate: Common along the sea shore to moderate elevations in inland areas, most abundant near human settlements.

Propagation: By seeds and vegetative method.

Part Used: Fruit, stem, leaves and root.

Chemical Constituents: Saccharose, myonostol, scyllo-inositol, sorbitol, diphenylurea, alipahatic alcohols, ketones, leucoanthocyanins, 2-prppyleneglycol, glycerol, sucrose, glucose, stachyose, bongrek acid, xylan, glucosan, aliphatic fatty acids, polyphenols, ferricopnin, cocositol, mono and sesquiterpenes, alpha and betw-amyrin, campesterol, cycloartenol, beta-sitosterol, squalene, stigmasterol, alpha-tocopherol, and alkaloids: ligustrazine and 2,3,5-grimethylpyrazine.

Uses: Weakness after childbirth in treated with liquid extracted from the stem. Juice from the midrib at the lower base of the leaf isused in treating maternal postpartum illness. Coconut milk is used to treat fish poisoning. In new guinea sores and scabies are treated with parts of the plant. The root may be used as a toothbrush. The root is also employed in treating stomachache and blood in the urine. Oil from the kernel is rubbed onto stiff joints. The oil is also used to treat rheumatism and back pains or as an ointment to maintain smooth, soft skin. The oil mixed with turmeric, is used to treat sick new born infants and women who have just given birth. To place a baby from a breech to a normal position in the mother's womb, the abdomen is massaged with coconut oil. The oil is used as an emetic and as a purgative. The juice from a green coconut is given to women who have difficult pregnancies. Juice from the fruit is taken to treat kidney problems. The coconut is said to have vermicide properties. Haemorrhaging is stopped with the use of the dry, spongy kernel. Diarrhoea and dysentery are treated with parts of this plant.

374. *Codiaeum variegatum* (L.) Blume *(Euphorbiaceae)*

Vernacular Name: *Eng:* Croton.

Description: An ornamental shrub 2-6 m high. Leaves alternate, simple often multi-coloured with a myriad of various shapes and sizes depending upon the cultivar. Flwoers (if present) are small, unisexual and borne in racemes. Fruit a sub-globose, 3-lobed schizocarp. Flowers and fruit may not develop on some forms, whereas others may bear flowers and fruit throughout the year.

Habitate: Cultivated only, from sea-level to mid-montane.

Propagation: By vegetative method.

Part Used: Leaves and roots.

Chemical Constituents: Phenolic compounds, cis and trans-pcoumaric acids, tran-ferulic acid, ellagic acid, vanilla acid, protocatechuic acid, carbohydrates and alkanes.

Uses: The venereal disease gonorrhea is treated with a preparation of liquid pressed from the leaves. The root is applied to tooth cavities for temporary relief o pain. A fever may be relieved by bathing the patient in green solution of boiled leaves. Sores are treated with a direct application of sap, and a preparation of the root is used to treat wounds. The leaves are chewed and swallowed to promote miscarriage. Used mainly to treat swellings, toothache and diseases caused by spirits.

375. *Codonopsis javancia* (Blume) Hook f. *(Campanulaceae)*

Description: Slender perennial twining herb with tuberous roots and milky juice. Leaves opposite, cordate; margins entire or denticulate. Flowers campanulate, ivory-yellow, violet-veined inside, solitary at the leaf-axi. Berry globose, violet; seeds numerous.

Habitate: Grows wild on meadows and waste lands or at forest edges in mountainous areas.

Propagation: By seeds and vegetative method.

Part Used: Roots.

Chemical Constituents: The roots contain sugars, fatty sbustances, essential oil, the glucoside scutellarin and a small amoung of alkaloids.

Uses: The root is stomachic, expectorant and diuretic. It is recommended in treating general debility, anaemia, fatggue, cough jaundice, dyspepsia, diarrhoea, nephritis, albuminuria, oedema, haemorrhoids, metroptosis, metrorrhagia and lymphatic system diseases.

376. *Codonopsis pilosula* (Franch.) Nannf. *(Campanulaceae)*

Vernacular Name: *Eng:* Tanghesen; pilose-Asia-bell.

Description: A perennial herb, the stem herbaceous, twinge, 1-2 m long, young parts hairy, usually with milky juice. Leaves alternate or opposite. Long-petiolate, ovate or broadly ovate, 1-7 cm long by 0.8-5.5 cm wide; tip obtuse or acute; base rounded or slightly cordate; margin sub-entire or repand, green on top and pale green underneath, both surfaces pubescent. August-September. Flowers hermaphrodite, axillary or terminal, solidary, stalked, calyx deeply divided. Fruit an obconical capsule. Seeds numerous small.

Habitate: In thickets, on the edges of forests, or in mountain woods in China, Korea, Soviet Union.

Propagation: By seeds.

Part Used: Root.

Chemical Constituents: N.A.

Uses: Poor appetite, loose bowels, weakness lassitude, cough and shortness of breath, feeble voice, deficiency of blood accompanied by dizziness and palpitations; thirst due to deficiency of the body fluid, prolpase of the rectum, prolapse of the uterus.

377. *Coffea arabica* L. *(Rubiaceae)*

Vernacular Name: *Eng:* Coffee, Arabian coffee, *Hin:* Caphi, Pilu, *Kan:* Kafi, Bunna, *Mal:* Kappi, *San*: Rajapiluh, *Tam:* Kappi, *Tel:* Kaphi.

Description: A glabrous large shrub with spreading branches; leaves simple, opposite with interpetiolar stipules, oblong, acuminate, main lateral nerves 6-10 pairs jointed by interamarginal veins; flowers numerous, white, in axillary fascicles, corolla tube short; fruits obovoid, fleshy berries, purple when ripe; seeds concave or grooved ventrally.

Habitate: Cultivated in shade on hills.

Propagation: By seeds and vegetative method.

Parts Used: Seeds.

Chemical Constituents: 2-methyl-3-furanthiol, 2-furfuryl thiol, prenylmercaptan, 3-mercapto-3-methyl butanol, 3-mercaptan, 2-heptanol, acetoin, α-terpineol, 2-methyltetra-hydrofuran-3-one, -2-methyl butyric acid methyl ester, limonene, methional, 3-isopropyl–2-methoxypyrazine, 2-ethyl-3, 5-dimethyl pyrazine, 2, 3-diethyl-5-methyl pyrazine, 3-isobutyl-2-methoxyprazine, 3-hydroxy-4, 5-dimethyl-2-furanone, 4-ethyl guaincol, 5-ethyl-3-hydroxy–4-methyl-2-furanone, 4-vinyl guaiacol and β-damascenone. Important furan derivtes as flavour components in coffee are furfural, 5-methyl-furfural, acetylfuran and furan-carboxylic acid methyl etser. 2-Hydroxy-2-cyclopenten-l-ones are also detected in roasted coffee. Coffee berries contain the enzyme, β-galactosidase, which increases during fruit ripening. Japanese coffee beans contain tocopherols.

Uses: The seeds are bitter, stimulant, diuretic, antipyretic and aromatic, and are used as a medicinal beverage for the sick and convalescent. It stimulates the flow of digestive juices and intestinal peristalsis. The infusion of unripe seeds is good for migraine, fever and gout, whereas infusion of ripe roasted seeds is good for diarrhoea. Coffee is a palliative in spasmodic asthma, whooping cough, hysteria and cardiopalmus. A strong coffee is a remedy for poisoning by opium, alcohol and other narcotics.

378. *Coix lacryma-jobi* L. *(Poaceae)*

Synonyms: *Coix lacryma* Linn.

Vernacular Name: *Eng:* Job's tears, *Hin:* Gurlu, Samkru, *Kan:* Majutti, *Mal:* Kattugotampu, Kakkappalunku, *San*: Gavedhukah, *Tam:* Kattukuntumani, *Tel:* Adavi guruginja.

Description: An erect perennial grass upto 1.5 m high with basal rooting nodes; leaves linear-lanceolate, narrowed up from a broad cordate base, midrib stout, ligule narrow, membranous; racemes nodding or drooping from long peduncles carrying male and female spikelets; fruits subglobose or ellipsoid, bluish grey, smooth, polished, tear-shaped grains.

Habitate: Throughout India, except the hottest and driest localities, in areas upto an elevation of 2,100 m.

Propagation: By seeds and vegetative method.

Parts Used: Roots, seeds.

Chemical Constituents: The seeds contain trans-ferulyl stigmastanol and trans-ferulyl campestanol which form part of an ovulation-inducing or fertility drug. Seed extract can be used as immuno-enhancer and for prevention of cancer and infections. The roots contain adenosine and phenolic compounds, 4-ketopinoresinol, threo-and erythro-1-C-syringylglycerol, and 2,6-dimethoxy-p-hydroquienone 1-O-β-D-glucopyranoside.

Uses: The roots are used in menstrual disorders and strangury. The seeds are bitter, sweet, tonic, diuretic, cathartic and depurative, and are used as diet drinks for invalids and also for pnuemonosis and pectoral diseases.

379. *Cola acuminata* *(Sterculiaceae)*

Vernacular Name: *Eng:* Kola nut, Cola nut.

Description: Evergreen tree growing to 20m with dark green leaves and yellowish-white flowers. Large woody seed pods contain 5-10 white or red seeds.

Habitate: Native to West Africa, kola nut is cultivated widely in the tropics especially in Nigeria, Brazil and the West Indies.

Propagation: By seeds and vegetative method.

Parts Used: Seeds.

Chemical Constituents: Kola nut contains up to 2.5% caffeine, theobromine, tannins, phlobaphene and an anthocyanin.

Uses: Kola nut stimulates the central nervous system and the body as a whole. It increases alertness and muscular strength, counters lethargy, and has been used extensively both in western African and Anglo-American herbal medicine as an antidepres*San*t, particularly during recovery from chronic illness. Like coffee, kola is used to treat headaches and migraine. It is diuretic and astringent, and may be taken for diarrhoea and dysentery.

380. *Colchicum autumnale* *(Liliaceae)*

Vernacular Name: *Eng:* Meadow saffron.

Description: Attractive perennial growing from bulb-like corm to 10cm. Has pointed lance-shaped leaves and tubular 6-petalled pink flowers in autumn.

Habitate: Common in Europe and North Africa, meadow saffron grows wild in woods and damp meadows.

Propagation: By vegetative method.

Parts Used: Corm, Seeds.

Chemical Constituents: Meadow saffron contains alkaloids and flavonoids. Colchicine is anti-inflammatory and is used in conventional medicine for acute attacks of gout. As it affects cell division it can cause foetal abnormality. It has been used in the laboratory to create new genetic strains.

Uses: Despite its toxicity, meadow saffron is considered one of the best remedies for acute gout pain. Leukaemia has been successfully treated with meadow saffron, and the plant has also been used with some success to treat Behcet's syndrome, a chronic disease marked by recurring ulcers and leukaemia. Taken internally, the herb has significant side-effects even at low dosage. Externally, it is applied to relieve neuralgia and itchiness.

381. *Coleus amboinicus* Lour. *(Lamiaceae)*

Synonyms: *Plectranthus amboinicus* (Lour.) Spreng., *Coleus aromaticus* Benth.

Vernacular Name: *Eng*: Countryborage, Indian borage, *Hin*: Patta ajavayin, Patharcur, *Kan*: Karpurahalli, *Mal*: *Kan*nikkurkka, *Kan*nikkurkka, Panikkurkka, *San*: Karpuravalli, Sugandhavalakam, *Tam*: Karpuravalli, *Tel:* Sugandhavalkam.

Description: A large succulent aromatic perennial herb with hispidly villous or tomentose fleshy stem; leaves simple, opposite, broadly ovate, crenate, fleshy, very aromatic; flowers pale purplish indense whorls at distant intervals in a long slender raceme; fruits orbicular or ovoid nutlets.

Habitate: Throughout India, cultivated in gardens.

Propagation: By cutting.

Parts Used: leaves.

Chemical Consistuents: Thymol, carvacrol, comphor.

Uses: The leaves are bitter, acrid, thermogenic, aromatic, anodyne, appetizing, digestive, carminative, stomachic, anthelmintic, constipating, deodorant, expectorant, lithontriptic,diuretic and liver tonic. They are useful in cephalagia, otalgia, anorexia, dyspepsia, flatulence, colic, diarrhoea and cholera especially in children, halitosis, convulsions, epilepsy, cough, chronic asthma, hiccough, bronchitis, renal and vesical calculi, strangury,hepatopathy and malarial fever.

382. *Coleus forskohlii* *(Lamiaceae)*

Synonyms*:* *Plectranthus barbatus.*

Vernacular Name: *Eng:* Coleus.

Description: An aromatic perennial, with tuber-like roots and an erect stem, reaching 60 cm.

Habitate: Native to India, coleus grows on the dry slopes of the Indian plains and in the foothills of the Himalayas.

Propagation: By seeds and vegetative method.

Parts Used: Roots and Leaves.

Chemical Constituents: Volatile oil, Diterpenes.

Uses: Lowers blood pressure, antispasmodic, Dilates the bronchioles, Dilates the blood vessels, Heart tonic.

383. *Collinsonia canadensis* *(Lamiaceae)*

Vernacular Name: *Eng:* Stone root.

Description: Perennial herb growing to 1m. Has a square stem, oval leaves, and clusters of greenish-yellow flowers.

Habitate: This herb is native to moist woodlands of eastern North America. The root is dug up in autumn.

Propagation: By Seeds.

Parts Used: Root, leaves.

Chemical Constituents: Stone root contains a volatile oil, tannins and saponins.

Uses: Stone root has diuretic and tonic properties, and is chiefly employed in the treatment of kidney stones. It is also prescribed to counteract fluid retention. It has been used to reduce back pressure in the veins, which in turn helps prevent the formation or worsening of heamorrhoids and varicose veins. As an astringent, stone root contracts the inner lining of the intestines, and can be helpful in treating disorders of the digestive system such as irritable bowel syndrome and mucous colitis. The fresh leaves or roots of stone root are applied as a poultice to bruises and sores.

384. *Colocasia esculenta* (Linn.) Schott *(Araceae)*

Synonyms: *Colocasia antiauorum* Schott.

Vernacular Name: *San*: Alupam, Alukam, Kachu, *Eng:* Taro, Cocoyam, *Hin:* Arvi, *Kan:* Kaci, Samagoddi, *Mal:* Cempu, *Tam:* Sempu, *Tel:* Cema dumpa, Cema gadda.

Description: A tuberous perennial with a group of underground farinaceous corms consisting of a central large one and surrounding ones of varying sizes; leaves with sheathing leaf base and erect petiole upto 1.2 m long bearing a thinly coriaceous peltate-ovate, cordate lamina; spadix shorter than the petiole and much shorter than the spathe, appendix much shorter than the inflorescence.

Habitate: Cultivated throughout the hotter parts of India.

Propagation: By Rhizomes.

Parts Used: Leaves, corms.

Chemical Constituents: Dihydroxysterols, 14α-methyl-5α-cholesta-9, 24-diene-3β-, 7α-diol and 14α-methyl-24-methylene-5α-cholesta-9, 24-diene-3α, 7 α-diol, besides β-sitosterol and stigmasterol have been isolates. In addition. Five novel compounds, tetracos-20-en-1, 18-diol: 25-methyl triacont-10-one: octacos-10en-l, 12-diol: pentatriacont-1, 7 tien-12-ol and 25-methyl-tritriacont-21-en-1, 9, 11-triol, along with non-acosane and cyaniding-3-glucoside have been reported.

Uses: The leaf juice is styptic, stimulant and rubefacient, and is useful in internal haemorrhages, otalgia, otorrhoea, adenitis and buboes. The juice of the corm is laxative, demulcent and anodyne, and is useful in somatalgia, alopecia areata, haemorrhods and congestion of the portal system.

385. *Commelina diffusa* Burm.F. *(Commelinaceae)*

Description: A sprawling, rhizomatous herb with jointed succulent, ascending stems growing to 75 cm tall. Leaves alternate, mostly without petioles, parallel-veined. Flowers blue, relatively small, zygomorphic, 3-parted, borne in small inflorescences, these subtended by a heart-shaped green bract. Fruit a small dry capsule with minute seeds.

Habitate: Common weed of damp pastures, wet forest, drains, swampy areas and other wet places.

Propagation: By vegetative method.

Part Used: Whole plant.

Chemical Constituents: Acylated anthocyanins, zwitterionic anthocyanins, alkaloids, flavonoid glycoside flavocommelin, saponins, tannins, coumarins, lectin.

Uses: Treatment of fractured bones; as a diuretic and to aid digestion; to treat eye irritation and rashes.

386. *Commersonia bartramia* (L.) Merr. *(Sterculiaceae)*

Description: Shrub to small tree upto 18m tall; young twigs, leaves petioles and buds brown-hairy. Leaves alternate, petiolate, the blades oblong-ovate, acuminate, margins toothed. Flowers borne in many-flowered cymes arising from axils, leaf-opposed, or terminal, flowers 5-parted, small and white. Fruit a bristly capsule with hairs upto 25 mm broad, containing numerous dark brown seeds.

Habitate: Common in secondary and dry forest, edges of forests, and grassland thickets from sea-level to 500 m.

Propagation: By seeds and vegetative method.

Part Used: Gum.

Chemical Constituents: N.A.

Uses: Used for colds and coughs, to treat rheumatism, kidney troubles and dysentery.

387. *Commiphora mukul* (Hook. ex Stocks) Engl. *(Burseraceae)*

Synonyms: *Balsamodendron mukul* Hook. ex Stocks, *Commiphora wightii* (Arn.) Bhandari.

Vernacular Name: *San*: Gugguluh, Mahisaksah, *Eng:* Indian bdellium tree, *Hin:* Gugal, Guggul, *Kan:* Guggulu, *Mal:* Gulgulu, Mahisaksagulgulu, *Tam:* Gukkulu, Mahisaksi, *Tel:* Guggulu.

Description: A small armed tree with spinescent branches and ash-coloured rough bark, peeling off in flakes, young parts glandular, pubescent; leaves alternate, 1-3 foliate obovate, serrate-toothed in the upper parts, lateral leaflets when present only less than half the size of the terminal ones; flowers small, brownish red, polygamous is fascicles; stamens 8-10, alternately long and short; fruits avoid drupes, red when ripe.

Habitate: In arid rocky tracks of Rajputana, Bellari, Mysore, Sindh and Baluchistan.

Propagation: By seeds and vegetative method.

Parts Used: Resinous gum.

Chemical Constituents: Guggulsterone-E, Z, Guggulsterone-I-VI, Cholesterol, seasamin, camphorene, cambrane A-etc.

Uses: The gum is bitter, acrid, astringent, thermogenic, aromatic, expectorant, digestive, anthelmintic, anti-inflammatory, anodyne, depurative vulnerary, antiseptic, nervine tonic, demulcent, aphrodisiac, alterative, stimulant, liver tonic, detergent, antispasmodic, emmenagogue, haematinic, diuretic, lithontriptic, rejuvenating and general tonic, and is useful in vitiated condition of *vata*, gout, scrofula, sciatica, facial paralysis, diplegia, hemiplegia, leprosy, leucoderma, helminthiasis, dyspepsia, cough, asthma, bronchitis, pectoral and hepatic disorders, otorrhoea, epilepsy, fever, strangury, haemorrhodis, dysmenorrhoea, amenorrhoea, wounds and ulcers, cardiac disorders, coronary thrombosis, anaemia, stomatopathy, pharyngopathy, spermatorrhoea, urinary calculus, diabetes, trichosis and skin diseases.

388. *Commiphora myrrha* (Nees) Engl. *(Burseraceae)*

Vernacular Name: *San*: Bolah, Rasagandhah, *Eng:* Myrrh, *Hin:* Bol, Hirabol, *Kan:* Bola, *Mal:* Narumpasamaram, Narumpasa, *Tam:* Vellaippapolam, *Tel:* Balimtra–Polam.

Description: A small tree which is the source of Herabol myrrh. The gum resin exudate from wounds in the stem is pale yellow at first and later solidifies to brown-black.

Habitate: Indigenous to north-east Africa especially Somalia Island. Collected in Saudi Arabia, Abyssinia, Iran, Thailand and sold in India bazaars.

Propagation: By seeds and vegetative method.

Parts Used: Gum.

Chemical Constituents: N.A.

Uses: The gum is bitter, acrid and astringent, acrid after the process of digestion, thermogenic, digestive, carminative, expectorant, intellect promoting, aphrodisiac, anthelmintic, depurative, anti-inflammatory, diuretic, sudorific, deodorant, ophthalmic, antiseptic, stimulant and tonic, and is useful in vitiated conditions of *vata, pitta* and *kapha,* stomatitis, dyspepsia, helminthiasis, amenorrhoea, dysmenorrhoea and other menstrual disorders, bronchitis, asthma, phthisis, ophthalmia, spongy gum, pharyngodynia, rheumatoid arthritis, sciatica, wounds and ulcers, inflammations, strangury and skin diseases.

The Herabol myrrh is also used in perfumery, mouth washes, dentifrices and in religious ceremonies as incense. This is reported to be used by ancients for embalming.

389. *Conium maculatum* *(Apiaceae)*

Vernacular Name: *Eng:* Hemlock.

Description: Graceful biennial growing to a height of 2.5m. Hs slender, rend-speckled stems finely divided leaves, small clusters of white flowers and small seeds that have beaded ridges.

Habitate: Commonly found in Europe, hemlock also grows in temperate regions of Asia and North America.

Propagation: By Seeds.

Parts Used: Leaves, Seeds.

Chemical Constituents: Hemlock contains alkaloids, mainly coniine and a volatile oil. Coniine is extremely toxic and causes congenital deformities.

Uses: In extremely small quantities, hemlock is sedative and analgesic; in larger doses it causes paralysis and death. Rarely used today, it has been prescribed in the past as a treatment for epi9lepsy, Parkinson's disease and Sydenham's chorea. Hemlock has also been used to treat acute cystitis.

390. *Convallaria majalis* L. *(Liliaceae)*

Synonyms: *Convallaria bracteata* Dulac., *Convallaria fragrans* Salisb.

Vernacular Name: *Eng:* May lily, Lily of the valley.

Description: A low, acaulescent perennial herb, its subterranean portion consisting of a branched, creeping, moderately yellow to light brown horizontal rhizome 1-3 mm. in diameter, bearing 3-9 rootlets from its nodes. Each plantlet consists of 2-3 oblong, parallel-veined leaves, with long sheathing petioles. Flowers fragrant, with white, bell-shaped, six, curved perianth lobes, nodding on an angled scape, 15 cm. high, bearing one sided raceme. Stamens 6; ovary superior and trilocular. Flowers in May. Fruits are red berries.

Habitate: Europe, particularly England and South-East United States.

Propagation: By seeds.

Parts Used: Whole plant.

Chemical Constituents: Convallarin, Convallamarin, Convallotoxin, Asparagin, Rutin, Isorhamnetic Kaempferol Gloycoside and Choline.

Uses: It is a great heart remedy. Increases heart tonicity and renders its action regular. Of use when heart ventricles are over distended and dilatation begins and where there is an absence of compensatory hypertrophy, with venous stasis marked. Anascara. Hydora in nose and lips. Epistaxis. See imaginary gray sports about three inches square. Grating of teeth in morning with coppery mouth taste. In females for great soreness in uterus with palpitation of heart, pain in Sacroiliac joints running down legs. Angina pectoris. All complaints better in open air but worse in warm room.

391. *Coptis chinesis* Franch. *(Ranunculaceae)*

Vernacular Name: *Eng:* Chinese goldthread.

Description: A perennial stemless herb, 20-50 cm high. Leaves basal, long-petiolate. Blade triangular-ovate, 3-8 cm long by 2.5-7 cm wide, ternatisect; leaflets pinnatifid, lobes incised, the terminal leaflet longer than the others. Peduncles 1-2, 12-25 cm long, bracts resembling leaves. Inflorescence a terminal cyme with 3-8 flowers. Flowers in spring, whitish-green. Follicles many-seeded. Seeds with a black crustaceous test.

Habitate: Under trees in the mountains, where it is shady and damp, China.

Propagation: By seeds and vegetative method.

Part Used: Rhizomes.

Chemical Constituents: N.A.

Uses: Acute conjunctivitis, mouth ulcers, acute bacillary dysentery; acute gastroenteritis, irritation resulting from heat, haemoptysis; epistaxis, boils, pyogenic infection and ulcerous skin disease, burns.

392. *Coptis teeta* Wall. *(Ranunculaceae)*

Vernacular Name: *San*: Supita, Pita, *Eng:* Gold thread, Coptis, Mouth Root, Vegetable Gold, *Hin:* Mamira, Mamiran, Kan: Vishateetee, *Mal:* Pitarohini, Pitramanikkilannu, *Tam:* Pitarohini, *Tel:* Mismitita.

Description: A rhizomatous, herbaceous perennial with horizontally growing golden yellow woody underground rhizome bearing many fibrous roots; leaves ternatisect, leaflets 5-7.5 cm, ovate-lanceolate, pinnatifid, the terminal largest, the rachis 15-30 cm long; flowers small, white, on slender leafless scapes, fruits many seeded follicles; seeds black, tests crustaceous.

Habitate: Northern frontier of Assam, in damp places.

Propagation: By seeds and vegetative method.

Parts Used: Rhizomes.

Chemical Constituents: Coptine, 0.08; coptisine, 0.02; and jatrorrhizine, 0.01%. berberastine, coptisine, jatrorrhizine, and palmatine.

Uses: The rhizomes are bitter, acrid during the process of digestion, cooling, ophthalmic, expectorant, anthelmintic, diuretic, stomachic, laxative, carminative, depurative, antipyretic and tonic, and are useful in ophthalmopathy, vitiated conditions of *pitta* and *kapha*, cough, bronchitis, atonic dyspepsia, flatulent colic, helminthiasis, diabetes, intermittent fevers, strangury, leprosy, leucoderma, dropsy and general debility.

393. *Coptis trifolia* *(Ranunculaceae)*

Vernacular Name: *Eng:* Goldthread.

Description: Perennial growing to 15 cm. Has a slender golden root, 3-lobed leaves and single small white flowers.

Habitate: Native to eastern North America from Labrador to Tennessee, this herb prefers damp sites.

Propagation: By seeds and vegetative method.

Parts Used: Rhizome.

Chemical Constituents: Goldthread contains isoquiniline alkaloids.

Uses: A strongly bitter tonic, goldthread has been prescribed in the North American tradition principally for indigestion and stomach weakness, though it has also come under consideration as treatment for peptic ulcers, and has been applied as a wash for thrush. Goldthread has been used as a mouthwash, gargle or lotion for mouth ulcers, sore lips and throats. It can help to tighten mucous membranes. The herb's constituents are similar to those of goldenseal and it has been used as a substitute for this herb.

394. *Cordia dichotoma* Forst.f. *(Boraginaceae)*

Synonyms: *Cordia oblique* Willd.

Vernacular Name: *San*: Slesmatakah, Bahuvarah, *Eng:* Sebesten plum, *Hin:* Lasura, Lasora, *Kan:* Cikkacalli, Doducallu, *Mal:* Naruvari, Naruviri, *Tam:* Naruvili, *Tel:* Cinnanakkeru, Botuka.

Description: A medium sized tree with a short crooked trunk; leaves simple, entire or slightly dentate, elliptic-lanceolate to broad-ovate with a rounded or cordate base; flowers white, small in lax terminal or axillary cymes; fruits drupes, yellowish brown, pink or nearly black when ripe with a viscid sweetish transparent pulp surrounding a central stony part.

Habitate: Throughout India in the warmer regions.

Propagation: By seeds.

Parts Used: Bark, leaves, fruits.

Chemical Constituents: N.A.

Uses: The bark is bitter, astringent, acrid after digestion, constipating, anthelmintic, cooling and depurative, and is useful in dyspepsia, fever, diarrhoea, burning sensation, vitiated conditions of *kapha,* and *pitta,* helminthiasis, leprosy and skin diseases. The leaves are aphrodisiac, and are useful in gonorrhoea and ophthalmodynia. The fruits are sweet, cooling, emollient, anthelmintic, purgative, vulnerary, diuretic, expectorant, aphrodisiac, depurative and febrifuge, and are useful in vitiated conditions of *vata* and *pitta,* ulcers, leprosy skin diseases, hyperdipsia, burning sensation, bronchitis, dry cough, pectoral diseases, strangury, urethralgia urethritis, chronic fever, arthralalgia, pharyngopathy, splenopathy and ring worm.

395. *Cordia subcordata* Lam. *(Boraginaceae)*

Vernacular Name: *Eng:* Cordia.

Description: Medium-sized spreading tree to 12 m tall with grayish grooved flaking bark. Leaves alternate, petiolate, the petiole about half as long as blade, broadly ovate and entire, often wavy-margined, the apex obtuse to short-pointed, base rounded, the blade up to 20 cm long. Flowers showy, orange, trumpet-shaped, unscented and borne in small axilary or terminal clusters. Fruit a globose drupe upto 2 cm. Long surrounded by the enlarged calyx, the fruit green, yellowish to black, dry, hard with usually one stony seed inside.

Habitate: The seeds float and are highly resistant to salt water, thus the species is common in coastal areas, especially on atolls where it is both naturally occurring as well as cultivated.

Propagation: By seeds and vegetative method.

Part Used: Stem and leaves.

Uses: A preparation made from the stem is used to promote menstruation. The plant is also used to treat rheumatic aches and swellings of muscles and joints. A preparation made from the leaves is used to treat knee wounds or skin ulcers. The leaves are used in remedies fro bronchitis and asthma where the leaves probably act as a purgative. The plant is also used in the treatment of hepatic infections, cirrhosis of the liver and inflammation of the lymph nodes. It is also used to treat albumin present in the urine. Use the leaves in remedies for abdominal swellings and urinary tract infections.

396. *Cordyline fruticosa* (L.) Chev. *(Agavaceae)*

Synonyms: *Cordyline terminalis* (L.) Kunth.

Description: Sparingly branched shrub arising from subterranean tuber, with slender stem to 5 m tall. Leaves spirally arranged and borne in terminal clusters, elongate-lanceolate, parallel-vened, to 80 cm long. Flowers borne in coupound spikes up to 1 m long, subtended by leafy pinkish bracts, each flower 3-parted, upto 20 cm broad, white to pink coloured. Fruits small red berry with small black seeds.

Habitate: Common in a wide variety of habitats ranging from coastal to over 1000 m elevation.

Propagation: By seeds and vegetative method.

Part Used: Roots and leaves.

Chemical Constituents: Smilagenin, sarsapogenin, imidazole alkaloids, linoleic acid, tyramine, sterol.

Uses: The leaf buds are used to treat lower chest pains. Filariasis is treated with a solution made from the new plant shoots. Liquid from the stem is used to treat sickness after childbirth and also to help expel the afterbirth. The root is used to treat bladness. The juice of the leaves is used to treat earache, infected eyes, colds and coughs, stomachache, eczyma and gastritis. The roots are used in treating toothache and laryngitis. Samoans use an infusion of the leaves as a remedy for swellings, inflammations and for dry fever. The leaves are crushed with oil and applied to abscesses of the gums. The root is used to treat inflammations. The juice of the leaves is used to treat aching limps and fever.

397. *Coriandrum sativum* L. *(Apiaceae)*

Vernacular Name: *San*: Dhanyakam, Dhanaka, *Eng:* Coriander, *Hin:* Dhaniyam, *Kan:* Kottambri, *Mal:* Kottampala, Kottamalli, Malli, Kottampalari, *Tam:* Kottamalli, *Tel:* Daniyalu, Kotimira.

Description: A glabrous, aromatic, herbaceous annual 30-90 cm in height; leaves decompound, lower ones long-petioled and upper ones short petioled or sub-sessile, imparipinnatisect into linear-setaceous lobes; flower small, white or pinkish purple in compound terminal umbels; fruits yellowish brown, globular and ribbed, separating into two halves (mericarps) each containing a seed.

Habitate: Cultivated throughout India.

Propagation: By seeds and vegetative method.

Parts Used: Leaves, fruits.

Chemical Constituents: Linalool, linalyl acetate, thymol, β-caryphyllene, α-pinene, borneol, limonene, β-phellandrene, citranellol, 1, 8-cineole and geranyl acetate.

Uses: The leaves are acrid, astringent, aromatic, analgesic, anti-inflammatory and styptic, and are useful in halitosis, pharyngopathy, epistaxis, ulemorrhagia, chronic conjunctivitis, hiccough, inflammations, suppuration, haemorrhoids, jaundice and odontalgia. The fruits are aromatic, bitter, sweet, acrid, astringent, emollient, thermogenic, anti-inflammatory, anthelmintic, stomachic, carminative, digestive, appetiser, constipating, diuretic, antipyretic, stimulant, expectorant and anodyne, and are useful in vitiated conditions of *pitta*, burning sensation, cough, bronchitis, pharyngopathy, vomiting, dyspepsia, anorexia, colic, flatulence, diarrhoea, dysentery, chronic conjunctivitis, cephalalgia, epistaxis, erysipelas, strangury, dropsy, scrofula, helminthiasis, haemorrhoids, intermittent fevers, hyperdipsia, gout, rheumatism and giddiness. A leaf paste is good for allergic inflammations caused by 'Marking nut' (*bhallatakab*).

398. *Cornus florida* L. *(Cornaceae)*

Synonyms: *Cynoxylon florida* (L.) Raf.

Vernacular Name: *Eng:* Flowering Dogwood.

Description: A shrub or a small tree with spreading branches, 3-4 m. in height rarely up to 12m. Leaves 8-12 cm. long, oval or ovate, acute, dark green, glabrous above, glaucous or pale green or whitish beneath, usually pubescent on the veins, often wavy and curled at edges. Leaves turn deep red before they fall. Covered with 2-armed hairs, encrusted with carbonates. Flowers white or pinkish, 8-10.2 cm. wide, bracts 4, obovate, emarginated. Fruit 1-3 cm. long, scarlet, in dense clusters but individually distinct.

Habitate: United States.

Propagation: By seeds and vegetative method.

Parts Used: Bark.

Chemical Constituents: Glycoside: Cornin, Kaempferol, Quercetin, Scyllitol, Inositol, n-nonacosan. Verbenalide glycoside. Betulinic acid.

Uses: For complaints like Chronic malaria; indigestion; distressing heart-burn; general debility from loss of vital body fluids; neuralgic pain in arms, chest, trunk with sensation as if broken in two; intermittent fever with drowsiness, feels cold but warm to touch. Chill is preceded by drowsiness and heat is associated with drowsiness.

399. *Cornus officinalis* Siebold et Zucc. *(Cornaceae)*

Synonyms: *Macrocarpium officinale.*

Vernacular Name: *Eng:-*Japanese cornelian cherry.

Description: Deciduous shrub to 7 m tall. Branches glabrous, terete. Leaves simple, entire, opposite, ovate, oblong or ovate-laneceolate, 4-12 cm long, 2.5-6 cm wide, acuminate with obtuse tip, rounded at base, with tufts of brown hairs in axils of veins beneath; petioles 5-15 mm long, pubexcent. Inflorescence umbels to 2 cm across, 20-30 flowered, short-pedunculate, involucral bracts 4, falling early, 6-8 mm long, elliptic, acute. Flowers yellow, appearing before leaves, bisexual, 4-merous, small, 4-5 mm across; pedicels about 1 cm long, loosely appressed-pilos. Fruit a 2-celled, 2-seeded drupe, oblong, and 1.5-2 cm long, red.

Habitate: Mainly cultivated for ornamental purposes and for fruit in China and Japan.

Propagation: By seeds and vegetative method.

Parts Used: Pseudocarp.

Chemical Constituents: Iridoids: morronioside, loganin, sweroside. Tannins, lectins.

Uses: Improvement of experimental diabetes, antihistaminic, CNS-depressing, antibacterial, DNA Polymerase inhibition, RNA reverse transcriptase inhibition. Used in spermatorrhoea, impotence, enuresis, liner protection.

400. *Corydalis ternate* Nakai *(Papaveraceae)*

Vernacular Name: *Eng:-*Three-leaf corydalis.

Description: Glabrous, perennial herb with globose tuber. Rhizomes spreading horizontally underground to form small tubers. Stems branched at base, 15 cm tall. Leaves alternate, ternately divided; petioles long, but becoming shorter for upper leaves; leaflets elliptic, ovate or obovate, 8-20 mm long, 3-16 mm wide, incisely serrate, green above, bluishgrey beneath. Inflorescence terminal racemose, bracteate; bracts oblanceolate, 1 cm long, 3 mm wide, leaflike, but entire, becoming smaller as going up. Flowers pedicelled, 15-18 mm long, rose-purple.

Habitate: Fields and low mountain slopes.

Propagation: By seeds and vegetative method.

Parts Used: Tuber.

Chemical Constituents: N. A.

Uses: Antioxytocic, spasmolytic, platelet aggregation inhibition. Used in pains, menorrhalgia, headache, abdominal pain.

401. *Corydalis yanhusuo* W. T. Wang *(Papaveraceae)*

Vernacular Name: *Eng:* Tuber of Yanhusuo.

Description: A perennial herb, 9-20 cm long, glabrous. The stem forms a tuber consisting of small, firm brownish-yellow, flattened pellets. Leaves 2-3 palmatilobed, twice-ternate; the segments wedge-shaped or oblong, more or less lobed. Raceme. Fruit on oblong, linear, capsule.

Habitate: Cultivated in sandy areas in China.

Propagation: By seeds and vegetative method.

Part Used: Tubers.

Chemical Constituents: N.A.

Uses: Headache, abdominal pains, menstrual cramps, stops uterine bleeding; dispels stagnant blood improves blood circulation.

402. *Coscinium fenestratum* (Gaertn.) Colebr. *(Menispermaceae)*

Vernacular Name: *San:* Daru haridra; *Eng:* False calumba, Ceylon calumba root, turmeric tree; *Hin:* Jhari-huldi; *Tel:* Manu pasupu; *Tam:* Mara manial; *Mal:* Mara manial and *Kan:* Marada arashina.

Description: Woody climber, roots and stems yellow inside. Stem-bark longitudinally fluted, whitish-grey in colour. Leaves alternate coriaceous, shining above, minutely whitish tomentose beneathl petiole long, inserted not far from the bae of laminal basal nerves 3-5. Inflorescence in paniculate raceme, borne in the axil of fallen leaves. Flowers unisexual Drupe globose.

Habitate: Grows wild and in indigenous to South viet nam.

Propagation: By seeds and vegetative methods.

Part Used: Stems and roots.

Chemical Constituents: The stems and the roots contain the alkaloid berberine 1.5–3%.

Uses: Berberine is antibacterial. The stem, the roots and the purified berberine are used in treating diarrhoea, bacillary dysentery, enteritis, jaundice, pyrexia and dyspepsia. An eye-lotion berberine chloride is effective for opthalmia.

403. *Costus speciosus* (Koenig ex Retz.) J. E. Smith *(Zingiberaceae)*

Vernacular Name: *San*: Kemuka, *Eng:* Wild Zinzer, Spiral, *Hin:* Kebu, Keyu, Kust, Kenna, *Kan:* Cangalvakostu, *Mal:* Cannakkilannu, Cannakkuvva, Narumcanna, *Tam:* Kostam, *Tel:* Cengalva kostu.

Description: A succulent herb with long leafy spirally twisted stems 2-3 m in height and horizontal rhizomes; leaves simple, spirally arranged, oblanceolate or oblong, glabrous above, silky pubescent beneath with broad leaf sheaths; flowers white, large, fragrant, in dense terminal spikes, bracts bright red, stamen only one, perfect, lip large with incurved margins; fruits globose or ovoid capsules, seeds obovoid or subglobose.

Habitate: Throughout India in moist localities.

Propagation: By vegetative method.

Parts Used: Rhizomes and seeds.

Chemical Constituents: Dioscin, prosapogenins-A and–B of dioscin, protodioscin, methyl protodioscin, gracillin, costusoside-I costusoside-J, 3-0-26-0-22α-methoxy-furost-5-en-3β, 26-diol and β-sitosterol-β-D-glucopyranoside. Dioscin, prosapogenins-A and–B of dioscin, gracillin, and β-sitosterol-β-D-glucoside.

Uses: The rhizomes are bitter, astringent, acrid, cooling, purgative, aphrodisiac, anthelmintic, depurative, febrifuge, expectorant and tonic, and are useful in vitiated conditions of *kapha* and *pitta*, burning sensation, flatulence, constipation, helminthiasis, leprosy, skin diseases, fever, hiccough, asthma, bronchitis, inflammations and anaemia.

404. *Costus specious* (Koenig) Smith *(Zingiberaceae)*

Vernacular Name: *San:* Kemuka; *Eng:* Elegant costus. eylon calumba root, turmeric tree; *Hin:* Keu; *Beng*: Keu; *Tam:* Kuiravam; *Tel:* Chengalvakoshtu and *Kan:* Chengalvakoshtu.

Description: Erect herbaceous plant, attaining 2m. in height, occasionally branched. Rhizome stout, creeping horizontally, leaves alternate, lower part surrounding the stem, tomentose, arranged in a spiral when young. Inflorescence in dense terminal spike; flowers white with yellowish centre; bracts red. Capsule with numerous black seeds.

Habitate: Grows wild in wet places in mountaionous regions.

Propagation: By vegetative method.

Part Used: Stems and rhizomes.

Chemical Constituents: The rhizomes yield steroidal saponins that give diosgenin and tigogenin on hydrolysis.

Uses: The rhizome possesses anti-inflammatory activity. It is indicated in the treatment of feber, urodynia, biliuria, rheumatism, lumbago and neuralgia. The juice of pounded fresh tops of young branches is instilled in the ear of otitis. The plant can be used as raw material for diosgenin extration.

405. *Crataegus oxyacantha* L. *(Rosaceae)*

Synonyms: *Mespilus oxycantha* Crantz., *Crataegus laevigata* D.C.

Vernacular Name: *Eng:* Hawthorn.

Description: An ornamental tree upto 5 m. high, with spreading thorny, glabrous, reddish brown branches and stout spines upto 2.5 cm. long. Leaves glabrous, alternate, with 3-5 lobes. Lobes obtuse, serrate in upper half, bright green above, bluish green underneath, but broadly ovate, cuneate or truncate at base. Flowers white, 15mm. across, in glabrous, 5-12 flowered clusters, characteristically with hairless flower stalks. Sepals entire. Stamens 20, with red anthers; styles 2-3; fruit scarlet, sub-globose to broad ellipsoid, 9-16mm. long with nutlets 2, furrowed on the inner face.

Habitate: North western Himalayas at an altitude of 1800-3000m. in India.

Propagation: By seeds and vegetative method.

Parts Used: Berries.

Chemical Constituents: Cynogenetic glycosides. Crategin. Amines viz. O-methoxy phenethylamine. Tyramine. Rutin, Hyperoside, Vitexin glycosides. Orientin glycosides. Procyanidins. Citric, tartaric and crataegus acids.

Uses: As blood purifier, for high blood pressure, Arteriosclerosis, Cardiac diseases including dyspnoea, its hypertrophy, Valvular insufficiency. Paroxysmal tachycardia. Removes crustaceous and calcareous deposits from inside of arteries. Specific for toning heart muscles, myocarditis, irregular heart beat, painful sensation of pressure in lift side of chest below clavicle and pain in back of h3ad and neck. Cardiac dropsy with fatty degeneration, extreme dyspnoea on least exertion with much increase in pulse. Dialated heart with first sound dull, vulvular murmurs, angina pectoris, skin blueness of fingers and toes. Great insomnia.

406. *Crataegus pinnatifida* Bunge *(Rosaceae)*

Vernacular Name: *Eng:*-Howthorn, thorn, thorn apple.

Description: Thorny, deciduous, small tree, to 6 m tall. Branchlets glabrous, with stout spines. Leaves alternate, triangular-ovate, 5-10 cm long, pinnately 5-9 lobed; the lobes obtuse, slightly toothed on upper margin, dark green above, lustrous on both sides; petiole 2-6 cm long; stipules serrate. Flowers few, white, in corymbs, 5-8 cm across; sepals and petals 5; stamens 20, anthers red. Fruit a small pome with 5 or fewer 1-seeded nutlets, light red, finely dotted, to 2 cm long, ripening in September-October-May.

Habitate: Mountain woods in Korea, China, Siberia and Japan.

Propagation: By seeds and vegetative method.

Parts Used: Fruit.

Chemical Constituents: Amygdalin, quercetin, chlorogenic acid, ursolic acid, arataegalic acid, tartaric acid, citric acid, sexangularetin.

Uses: Digestive, antibacterial, vasodilating, hypotensive, cholesterol level lowering activities, platelet aggregation inhibition. Used in abdominal distension, pain, diarrhoea, induce menstruation.

407. *Crataeva nurvala* Buch.–Ham. *(Capparidaceae)*

Synonyms*: Crataeva religiosa.*

Vernacular Name: *San*: Varuna, Ashmarighna, ashmaghna, *Hin:* Varuna.

Description: A moderate sized deciduous tree. *Bark* grey, smooth horizontally wrinkled. *Leaves* trifoliate. *Flowers* white, or cream in many flowered terminal corymbs. *Fruits* multiple seeded, ovoid berry. Seeds are embedded in yellow fleshy pulp.

Habitate: Evergreen tree growing widely in all parts of India.

Propagation: By seeds and vegetative method.

Parts Used: Roots, stem bark, leaves and flowers.

Chemical Constituents: Triterpenoids lupeol and varunol have been isolated from root and stem bark. The water extract also contains tertiary and quarternery bases including choline. The leaves yield flavonoids including rutin, quercetin and isoquercetin.

Uses: Urolithiasis and crystalluria, Urinary tract infections. In Ayurvedic practice, varuna is used as a litholytic agent, in treating *'Kapha'* and *'Vata'* varieties of ashmari. It also clears crystalluria. It is the drug of choice in all *kapha* disorders of the urinary tract, and in renal and bladder calculi. It is also use as a cholagogue, anti-helmintic and antiameobic in both intestinal and hepatic infestation. Its action as an anti-inflammatory agent is utilized in its used in deep-seated suppurative inflammations, in small joint, diseases and in osteomyelitis. It is also used as an antipyretic.

408. *Cressa cretica* L. (*Convolvulaceae*)

Vernacular Name: *San*: Rudantika, Rudanti, *Hin:* Rudravanti, Lana, *Kan:* Kharda, *Mal:* Alukanni, *Tam:* Uppumarikkoluntu, *Tel:* Uppusanaga.

Description: An erect, small, dwarf shrub upto 38 cm in height with a slender much branched hairy stem; leaves simple, numerous, subsessile, ovate, acute, densely silky hairy; flowers white, in small clusters in the axils of the upper leaves, corolla lobes reflexed, hairy on the back near the tip; fruits ovoid capsules, pointed and pubescent at the apex; seeds usually solitary.

Habitate: Throughout India, along sandy shores.

Propagation: By seeds and vegetative method.

Parts Used: Whole plant.

Chemical Constituents: *n*-octa-cosanol, scopoletin, umbelliferone, isopimpinellin, β-sitosterol and its-D glucoside and quercetin.

Uses: The plant is acrid, bitter, thermogenic, alterant, anthelmintic, expectorant, carminative, digestive, stomachic, aphrodisiac, haematinic and tonic, and is useful in vitiated conditions of *kapha* and *pitta*, consumption, asthma, bronchitis, urethrorrhea, dyspepsia, flatulence, colic, anorexia, helminthiasis, anaemia, diabetes, leprosy and general debility.

409. *Crinum asiaticum* L. (*Amaryllidaceae*)

Vernacular Name: *San:* Nagadamani, nagapatra; *Hin:* Kanwal, pindar; *Beng*: Nagdaun; *Tel:* Kesarchettu, vishamungali; *Tam:* Vishamungil; *Kan:* Vishmungali.

Description: Robust rosette-like herb arising from an underground bulb, upto 2 m high. Leaves linear, parallel veined somewhat fleshy evergreen upto 1 m long, arising from a crown atop a short erect rhizome. Flowers greenish-white, tubular, moderately large, with yellow anthers and purple style, the flowers borne in an inflorescence upto 50 cm long, bearing upto 30 flowers. Fruit yellowish-green with large seeds flowers and fruit available throughout the year.

Habitate: Upper reaches of sandy beaches, coastal areas, and commonly planted in villages or urban areas as an ornamental plants.

Propagation: By vegetative method.

Part Used: Leaves and rhizome.

Chemical Constituents: Lycorine and its glucoside, crinamine, crinine, crinidine, hamayne, stigmasterol, cycloartenol, cyclolaudenol, crinasiadine, phenathridones, palmilycorine, ambeline, hippadine, ungeremine, criasbetaine, flexinine, pratprimine, pratorinine, haemanthamine.

Uses: Leaves are used in the healing of wounds. The leaves are applied to body swellings; and a preparation of the root is given to aid childbirth and for postpartum haemorrhage. The leaves are heated and applied to relieve backaches. The leaves are also used in a preparation to treat permanent retraction of the testes, Blubs are used in an emetic and as a poison antidote.

410. *Crithmum maritimum* (*Apiaceae*)

Vernacular Name: *Eng:* Samphire, Sea fennel.

Description: Maritime herb growing to a height of 60cm. Has long, succulent, bright green leaves and clusters of small yellowish-green flowers.

Habitate: Samphire grows on the Atlantic, Mediterranean and Black Sea coasts of Europe and Asia Minor.

Propagation: By seeds and vegetative method.

Parts Used: Aerial parts.

Chemical Constituents: Samphire contains a volatile oil, pectin, vitamins and minerals.

Uses: Though it is currently little used in herbal medicine, samphire is a good diuretic, and it holds out potential as a treatment for obesity. Samphire has a high vitamin C and mineral content, and is thought to relieve flatulence and to act as a digestive remedy. In this, the plant resembles its inland namesake, fennel.

411. *Crocus sativus* L. *(Iridaceae)*

Vernacular Name: *San:* Keshara; *Eng:* Saffron; *Hin:* Kesar, zafran; *Beng*; jafran; *Tel:* Kunkumapuvu; *Tam:* Kungumapu and *Kan:* Kunkumakesari.

Description: A bulbous, perennial herb with long, linear, channeled leaves; flowers deep violet, funnel shaped, stalkless, and appearing in autumn with the leaves. Petals, narrow elliptic, equal, fused below into long slender corolla tube; styles orange, stima brick red.

Habitate: Cultivated in Jammu & Kashmir.

Propagation: By vegetative method.

Part Used: Stigmas and style tops.

Chemical Constituents: The major volatile components of the oil are safranal, isophorene, glucoside, corcin, crocetin, picro-crocin essential oil, also contain β and R carotene and lycopene.

Uses: Saffron, marketed as a powder or as "hay", performs the function of a spice by adding its faint, delicate and pleasing flavour to foods, such as cream, cottage cheese, bouillabaisse, mayonnaise, rice, cakes, sweetments, chicken, meat, liquerus and cordials. A tincture of saffron oil is used to flavour essence. For complaints including chorea and hysterical affections. Anger with violence followed by repentance. Laughing mania. Vacillating mind with pleasant mania, sings and laughs, behaves happy and affectionate and then angry. With sudden changes from hilarity to melancholy. Wiping of eyes frequently for mucus or water in them. Eyes appear as after weeping and in smoke. Ciliary neuralgia, pain from eyes to top of head. Threatened glaucoma. Epitaxis with dark, stringy, clotted strings of dark blood hanging down the nose. Uterine haemorrhages also with clots with ling strings, with pain in left breast. Crawling sensation in anus, abdomen and stomach.

412. *Crotalaria retusa* L. *(Fabaceae)*

Vernacular Name: *San*: *San*apuspi, *San*aghantika, *Hin:* Khunkhuniyan, *Kan:* Guluguluppahalli, *Mal:* Kilukiluppa, Matrghatini, Tantalakkotti, Cana, *Tam:* Kilukiluppai, *Tel:* Potti giliginca.

Description: An erect, robust undershrub, 60-120 cm high, with glabrous striate branches; leaves oblanceolate-oblong, obtuse or retuse, usually glabrous above and silky pubescent beneath; flowers yellow, numerous, large and showy in erect terminal racemes; fruits stalked pods, slightly broader upwards with 15-20 seeds per pod.

Habitate: Throughout India in fields, waste places and open forest lands, sometimes cultivated.

Propagation: By seeds and vegetative method.

Parts Used: Whole plant.

Chemical Constituents: The seeds contain several pyrrolizidine alkaloids, isatinecine, monocrotaline-N-oxide, retusamine and its N-oxide, retusine and spectabiline. The seeds also contain acyclic-α-amino acids and a flavone, vitexin-4'-O-galactoside.

Uses: The plant is bitter, astringent, expectorant and emetic and is useful in vitiated condition of *kapha* and *vata*, dyspepsia, fever, cardiac disorders and stomatopathy. The leaves are used for curing ptyalism, diarrhoea, scabies and impetigo. The seeds powdered and boiled with milk are said to be very useful for increasing body strength and life span. The seeds are depurative, digestive and febrifuge and are useful in skin diseases, leprosy, flatulence and fever.

413. *Croton tiglium* L. *(Euphorbiaceae)*

Vernacular Name: *San:* Jayapala; *Eng:* Purging croton, purgative croton, true croton, croton-oil plant; *Hin:* Jamalgota; *Beng*: Jayapala; *Kan:* Nepala; *Tam:* Nervalam and *Mal:* Nervalam.

Description: Medium-sized tree, 3-6m. in height leaves alternate, toothed, glabrous, pinkish-violet when young, Inflorescence in terminal raceme; flowers unisexual, monoecious; bemale flowers without petals. Capsule ovoid, obtusely 3-lobed, yellow. Seeds small with hard brownish-yellow shell.

Habitate: Grows wild in hills and damp forests.

Propagation: By seeds and vegetative methods.

Part Used: Seeds.

Chemical Constituents: The seeds yield fatty oil composed principally of stearin, palmitin, glycerides of crotonic and tiglic acids; proteins 18%, the glucoside crotonoside; amino acids; arginine, lysine; alkaloids; the enzyme pipase.

Uses: The processed seeds are used in treating flatulence, dyspepsia, constipation, colic, oedema, dyspnoea and persistent cough. It should be used cautiously because of its high toxicity. Should not be administered to pregnant women. Croton tiglium poisoning is treated with a decoction of cpitis teeta and string beans.

414. *Croton tonkinesis* Gagnep. *(Euphorbiaceae)*

Description: Small plant, 1-1.5m high, Leaves alternate, sometimes clustered, 2-glandular at the base, covered with minute slivery scales on both sides, densely beneath, inflorescence in axillary or terminal raceme; flowers white, unisexual, monoecious. Capsule ovoid, 3-lobed seeds brown.

Habitate: Grows wild and is cultivated every where.

Propagation: By seeds and vegetative methods.

Part Used: Leaves.

Chemical Constituents: N.A.

Uses: The torrefied leaves are employed in the treatment of abscesses, boils, impetigo, rhin it is, dysentery, bloody stools, colic, gastric and duodenal ulcer and dyspepsia. Washing with a concentrated decoction is effective against boils and impetigo.

415. *Cucumis melo* var. *utilissimus* (Roxb.) Duthie & Fuller *(Cucurbitaceae)*

Vernacular Name: *San*: Kharbuja, Eng: Musk Melon, *Hin:* Kharbuja, *Tam:* Mulampazham, *Tel:* Kharbuja dosa.

Description: An annual climbing or creeping herb with angular, scabrous stems; leaves simple, soft hairy, orbicular-reniform in outline, 5-angled or 5-lobed, scabrous on both surfaces; flowers unisexual, yellow.

Habitate: Cultivated throughout north India.

Propagation: By seeds and vegetative method.

Parts Used: Fruits, seeds.

Chemical Constituents: The seeds of melon contain isomultiflorenol, 24-methylenecycloratenol, α-and β-amyrin, lupeol, and cycloartenol. This is supported by evidence on the high enzyme activities of urease, lipase, lipoxygenase, trypsin inhibitor and low activity of β-amylase in musk melon. Volatile compounds of cucumber and musk melon were analysed and methyl-2-methylbutanoate-3 hexanal, 2-hexanal, and ethyl-2 methyl propane were identified as the primary odorants. Ethyl 3-propanate and 3-propyl acetate have been considered to be of importance to the aroma profiles of the fruits. The green notes of musk melon are because of–2 and–3-hexenal, 1,8-cineol and–1,5-octadien-3one.

Uses: The fruits are sweet, acrid, cooling, appetiser, laxative, galactagogue, diuretic, aphrodisiac and tonic, and are useful in vitiated conditions of *pitta*, insanity, ascites, ophthalmia, urethrorrhea, dyspepsia, agalactia and general debility. The seeds are cooling, diuretic, lacrimatory and nutritive and are useful in urodynia, urochesia, ophthalmia, hepatopathy, nephropathy, bronchitis, chronic fever, hyperdipsia and burning sensation.

416. *Cucumis sativus* L. *(Cucurbitaceae)*

Vernacular Name: *San*: Trapusah, *Eng:* Cucumber, Common cucumber, *Hin:* Khira, *Kan:* Mullu savte, *San*tekayi, *Mal:* Vellari, *Tam:* Vellarikkay, Pippinkay, *Tel:* Dosakaya.

Description: A hispidly hairy trailing or climbing annual, leaves simple, alternate, deeply cordate, 3-5 lobed, both surfaces hairy, margin denticulate; flowers yellow, males clustered, bearing anthers cohering, connective crusted or elevated above the cells, females solitary, thickly covered with very bulbous-based hairs; fruits cylindrical pepo of varying sizes and forms; seeds cream or white, testa hard, smooth.

Habitate: Throughout India, cultivated.

Propagation: By seeds and vegetative method.

Parts Used: Fruits, seeds.

Chemical Constituents: The aerial parts of the plant contain a 14 α-methyl-phytosterol.α- and β-amyrin, multiflorenol, isomultiflorenol, 24, methylenecy-cloartenol, cycloartenol, tirucallol. Presence of a cytokinin-binding protein, isopentenyl adenosine trialcolhol is also reported in the cotyledons of var. 'Guntur'.

Uses: The fruits are sweet, refrigerant, haemostatic, diuretic and tonic, and are useful in vitiated conditions of *pitta*, hyperdipsia, burning sensation, thermoplegia, fever, insomnia, cephalalgia, bronchitis, jaundice, haemorrhages, strangury and general debility. The seeds are astringent, sweet, refrigerant, nutritive, purgative, antipyretic, diuretic and tonic, and are useful in vitiated conditions of *pitta*, burning sensation, constipation, intermittent fevers, strangury, renal calculus, urodynia and general debility.

417. *Cucumis trigonus* Roxb. *(Curcurbitaceae)*

Vernacular Name: *San*: Indravaruni, *Eng:* Bitter gourd, *Hin:* Jangal indrayan, Bislambi, *Kan:* Halmekki, Karanti, *Mal:* Kattuvellari (Cerutu),Pekkummatti, *Tam:* Kattutummatti, *Tel:* Adavi pucca.

Description: A perennial scabrid monoecious tendrillar herb with slender angled stem; leaves deeply, palmately five lobed, scabrid on both sides, hispid on the nerves beneath and rounded at the apex; the male flowers yellow in small clusters on slender peduncles; fruits ellipsoid or sub globose, yellow or yellow with green stripes; seeds white, ellipsoid.

Habitate: Throughout India, in dry areas.

Propagation: By seeds and vegetative method.

Parts Used: Roots, fruits, seeds.

Chemical Constituents: N.A.

Uses: The roots are used as a purgative. The fruit pulp is bitter, acrid, thermogenic, anthelmintic, febrifuge, expectorant, liver tonic, stomachic, appetiser, purgative and intellect promoting, and is useful in vitiated condition of *kapha* and *pitta*, helminthiasis, flatulence, leprosy, fever, jaundice, diabetes, cough, bronchitis, ascites, anaemia, constipation, other abdominal disorders and amentia. The seeds are cooling and astringent, and are useful in vitiated conditions of *pitta*.

418. *Cucurbita maxima Duchesne* ex Lam. *(Cucurbitaceae)*

Vernacular Name: *San*: Pitakusmandah, *Eng:* Squash, Red gourd pumpkin, *Hin:* Lalkumra, Kaddu, *Kan:* Kumbalakayi, Gumbaloo, Cinikayi, *Mal:* Mattan, *Tam:* Pusanikkay, *Tel:* Gummadi.

Description: A trailing annual herb with somewhat prickly or hairy stem and axillary tendrils; leaves simple, alternate, nearly orbicular in outline, lobed with deep sinus at the base; flowers large, yellow unisexual, solitary, male flowers with three stamens, anthers one single-celled, two two-celled, conduplicate, female flowers with inferior ovary, short style and three-stigmas; fruits fleshy, indehiscent pepo; seeds ovoid or oblong, compressed.

Habitate: Cultivated throughout India.

Propagation: By seeds and vegetative method.

Parts Used: Fruits, seeds.

Chemical Constituents: Moisture, lipid, protein, and ash. Nonpolar lipids, glycolipids, and phospholipids. The major fatty acid present in the lipids was linolenic. The leaves contain calcium, magnesium, iron, zinc and copper. An esterase was purified from the fruits.

Uses: The fruits are sweet, refrigerant, emollient, diuretic, sedative, and tonic, and are useful in burns, scalds, inflammations, abscesses, boils, migraine and neuralgia, the seeds are anthelmintic, diuretic and nervine tonic, and are useful in taeniasis, strangury and nervous debility.

419. *Cucurbita pepo* *(Cucurbitaceae)*

Vernacular Name: *Eng:* Pumpkin.

Description: Annual plant with twining stems, lobed leaves, yellow flowers and large orange fruit.

Habitate: Probably native to North America, pumpkn is now found worldwide.

Propagation: By seeds and vegetative method.

Parts Used: Seeds, pulp.

Chemical Constituents: Pumpkin seeds contain 30% unsaturated fixed oil. The seeds also contain cucurbitacins, vitamins, and minerals, notably zinc.

Uses: Pumpkin seeds are taken principally as a safe de-worming agent. They are particularly useful against tapeworms in pregnant women and in children, for whom stronger-acting and toxic preparations are unsuitable. The seeds are also mildly diuretic, and have been used in Central America herbal medicine as a treatment for nephritis and other urinary system problems. Varieties of pumpkin that are particularly diuretic, tonic to the bladder and high in zinc have been recommended in the early stages of prostate problems.

420. *Cuminum cyminum* L. *(Apiaceae)*

Vernacular Name: *San:* Jiraka, jira; *Eng:* Cumin; *Hin*: Safed zeera; *Beng*: Jira; *Tam:* Siragam; *Tel:* Jilakara, jiraka; *Kan*: Jeerige and *Mal:* Jorekam.

Description: A slender annual herb, leaves twice or thrice 3-partite segments filiform. Infloscence umbels compound, bracts and bracteoles present, fruit cylindric, tip narrowed primary ridges filiform, distinct, secondary usually hispidulous.

Habitate: Cultivated all over India.

Propagation: By seeds.

Part Used: Fruits.

Chemical Constituents: The characterstic odour of cumin oil is attributed to the presence of sminaldehyde, 1,3-p-menthadien-7-al, and 1,4-p-menthadien-7-al.

Uses: The oil of cumin is used to flavour curries and other culinary preparations, confectionery, beverages, liqueurs and cordials.

421. *Cupressus sempervirens* *(Cupressaceae)*

Vernacular Name: *Eng:* Cypress.

Description: Evergreen tree growing to 30m. Has tiny dark green leaves, and male and female cones.

Habitate: Native to Turkey and cultivated in the Mediterranean.

Propagation: By seeds and vegetative method.

Parts Used: Cones, branches.

Chemical Constituents: Cypress contains a volatile oil and tannins.

Uses: Applied externally as a lotion or as a diluted essential oil, cypress astringes varicose veins and haemorrhoids, tightening up the blood vessels. A footbath of the cones is used to cleanse the feet and counter excessive sweating. Taken internally, cypress acts as an antispasmodic and general tonic, and is prescribed for whooping cough, the spitting up of blood, and spasmodic coughs. Colds, flu and sore throats, and rheumatic aches and pains, also benefit from this remedy.

422. *Curculigo orchioides* Gaertn. *(Amaryllidaceae)*

Vernacular Name: *San*: Musali, *Hin:* Kalimusli, Musli, *Kan:* Nelatali Gaddi, Neladali, *Mal:* Nilappana, Nelppana, *Tam:* Nilappanaikkilanku, *Tel:* Nelatatigadda.

Description: A herbaceous tuberous geophilous perennial with a short or elongate root-stock bearing several fleshy lateral roots; leaves simple, crowded on the short stem, sessile or short petioled with sheathing leaf bases, linear or linear-lanceolate often producing adventitious buds at the tips when in contact with soil; flowers bright yellow, the scape usually very short and hidden among the bases of the leaves underground, the lowest flowers bisexual, the upper male; fruits capsules, derived from inferior tricarpellary syncarpous ovary, 1-4 seeded; seeds black, oblong, deeply grooved in wavy lines.

Habitate: Throughout India, in areas upto 2,250 m elevation.

Propagation: By vegetative method.

Parts Used: Root-stock.

Chemical Constituents: Saponins, curculigo-saponin, sapogenins, curculigenin, phenolic glycosides, corchioside, curculigoside, the chlorophenyl glycosides, curculigines B and C, a triterpene alcohol, curculigol, a pentacyclic triterpene, 31-methyl-3-oxo-20-ursen-28-oic acid, an aliphatic compound, 25-hydroxy-33-methylpentatricontan-6-one, N-acetyl-N-hydroxy-2-carbamic acid methyl ester, 3-acetyl-5-carbomethyoxy-2H-3, 4, 5, 6-tetrahydro-1, 2, 3, 4, 6-oxatetrazine, N,N,N',N'-stigmasterol, cycloartenol, and sucrose.

Uses: The root-stocks are sweet, cooling, bitter, emollient, diuretic, aphrodisiac, depurative, alterant, appetiser, carminative, viriligenic, antipyretic and tonic, and are useful in vitiated conditions of *pitta* and *vata*, leucorrhoea, haemorrhoids, pruritus, skin diseases, asthma, bronchitis, jaundice, diarrhoea, cuts and wounds, dyspepsia, colic, vomiting, ophthalmia, lumbago, and gonorrhoea.

423. *Curcuma amada* Roxb. *(Zingiberaceae)*

Vernacular Name: *San*: Amrardrakam, Karpuraharidra, *Eng:* Mango-ginger, *Hin:* Ama-haldi, *Kan:* Ambarasini, *Mal:* Mannayinci, *Tam:* Mankayyinci, *Tel:* Mamidi Allamu.

Description: A rhizomatous aromatic herb with a leafy tuft, 60-90 cm in height; leaves long, petiolate, oblong-lanceolate, tapering at both ends, glabrous, green on both sides; flowers white or pale yellow in spikes in the centre of the tuft of leaves, lip semi-elliptic yellow 3-lobed, the midlobe emarginated.

Habitate: Cultivated throughout India.

Propagation: By vegetative method.

Parts Used: Rhizomes.

Chemical Constituents: *Cis*-and *trans*-dihydroocimenes, myrcene, ocimene, linalool, nonan-2-one, citronellal, α-and β-terpineol, β-and δ-elemenes, α-and β-curcumenes, β-terpineol, β-co-paene, bisabolene, α-zingiberene, and ar-turmerone. Presende of curzerenone, epicurzerenone, *cis*-ocimene, α-pinene and car-3-ene is also reported in the oil. While *cis*-ocimene is reported to contribute to the green mango aroma, α-pinene and car-3-ene have been repoted to impoart the floral and leafy aroma to the rhizomes.

Uses: The rhizomes are bitter, sweet, sour, aromatic, cooling, appetiser, carminative, digestive, stomachic, demulcent, vulnerary, febrifuge, alexeteric, aphrodisiac, laxative, diuretic, expectorant, anti-inflammatory and antipyretic, and are useful in vitiated conditions of *pitta*, anorexia, dyspepsia, flatulence, colic, bruises, wounds, chronic ulcers, skin diseases, pruritus, fever, constipation, strangury, hiccough, cough, bronchitis, sprains, gout, halitosis, otalgia and inflammations.

424. *Curcuma aromatica* Salisb. *(Zingiberaceae)*

Vernacular Name: *San*: Aranyaharidra, Vanaharidra, *Eng:* Wild turmeric, Cochin turmeric, Yellow zedoary, *Hin:* Ban-haridra, Jangli-haldi, *Kan:* Kasturi-arisina, *Mal:* Kasturimannal, Kattumanna, *Tam:* Kasturimanjal, Kattumanjal, *Tel:* Kasturi Pasupu.

Description: A perennial tuberous herb with annulate aromatic yellow rhizome which is internally orange-red in colour; leaves elliptic or lanceolate-oblong, caudate-acuminate, 30-60 cm long, petioles as long or even longer, bracts ovate, recurved, more or less tinged with red or pink; flowers pink, lip yellow, obovate, deflexed, subentire or obscurely three lobed; fruits dehiscent, globose, three-valved capsules.

Habitate: Wild throughout India, cultivated in Bengal and Kerala.

Propagation: By vegetative method.

Parts Used: Rhizomes.

Chemical Constituents: *d*-camphene, 0.8; *d*-camphor, 2.5; sesquiterpenes, 65.5; sesquiterpene alcohols, 22.0; acids, 0.7; and unidentified residues, 8.5%. A sample from India yielded 9.4% of essential oil, showing high amount of *ar*-curcumene, β-curcumene and xanthorhizol. Presence of 2-4-methylphenol is also reported.

Uses: Rhizomes are bitter, carminative, appetiser and tonic, and are used in combination with astringents and aromatics for bruises, sprains, hiccough, bronchitis, cough, leucoderma and skin eruptions.

425. *Curcuma domestica* Valet. *(Zingiberaceae)*

Synonyms: *Curcuma longa* Linn.

Vernacular Name: *San:* Haridra; *Eng:* Common turmeric, long turmeric; *Hin:* Haldi, halada; *Beng*: Haldi, halada; *Tam:* Manjal; *Tel:* Pasupu and *Kan:* Arishina.

Description: Tufty perennial herb about 1m.high. Rhizome thick much-branched, golden-yellow, Leaves large, entire, long-sheathed, glabrous on both sides. Inflorescence cylindrical, arising from the leaves, on a scape of yellow flowers and greenish or whitish bracts with pink tips.

Habitate: Extensively cultivated as a spice and medicinal plant.

Propagation: By vegetative method.

Part Used: Rhizomes.

Chemical Constituents: The rhizomes contain the pigment curcumin; and essential oil consisting of sesquiterpenes, zingiberene, D-a-phellandrene, turmerone, dehydroturmerone, y and a-alanto lactone, curcumene, cineol.

Uses: The rhizome is well known for its anti-gastric-ulcer, anti-inflammatory and cholagogic properties. It is prescrived in the therapy of gastric and duodenal ulcer, hepatitis, jaundice, menstrual disorders, post-partum or menstrual haematometra, contusions, rheumatism, pain in the extremities, boils and impetigo. It is also used as a pultice for wounds to avoid their cicatrization.

426. *Curcuma pseudomontana* Graham *(Zingiberaceae)*

Synonyms: *C. Montana* sensu Baker non Roscoe.

Vernacular Name: *Mal*: Kattu manjal; *Tam:*-Kattu manjal.

Description: An erect herb, reaching 75 cm tall, with stout rootstock bearing small almond-like sub-globose tubers at the ends of the fibrous roots. The *tubers* are fleshy and white inside, aromatic. *Leaves* 3-5, oblong-lanceolate, 20-30 x 6-9 cm, base acute, apex acuminate, margin entire, hairless, shiny; leaf stalk and the leaf sheath up to 20 cm long. *Flowering spikes* seen in the center of the previously formed tuft of leaves, 10-25 cm long, bearing numerous compactly arranged flowers; flowering *bracts* conspicuous, inverted egg-shaped to lanceolate, 3-5 x 1.5-2cm, apex rounded to acute, hairless, green with a pinktip. Non-flowering bracts (coma) oblong-lanceolate, conspicuous, purple below and pinkish purple above. *Flowers* bisexual, 2-4 in each fertile bract, bright yellow, about 3 cm long and 4 cm broad. *Capsules* globose, splitting by 3-valves, smooth. *Seeds* ovoid or oblong, usually covered with arils.

Habitate: Moist shady areas of wet forests and along sluggish grassy slopes of higher altitude.

Propagation: By vegetative method.

Parts Used: Rhizomes.

Chemical Constituents: N.A.

Uses: The *Savara* tribes in the Eastern Ghats of AndhraPradesh use tuber extracts to cure jaundice. *Jatapu* and *Koya* tribes apply warm tuber paste to treat body swellings. Women of *Jatapu* and *Savara* tribes eat boiled tubers to increase lactation. *Khond* tribes apply tuber paste on the head for cooling effect.

427. Curucma zedoria (Berg.) Rosc. *(Zingiberaceae)*

Vernacular Name: *San:* Sati; *Eng:* Round zedoary, long zedoary, cochin turmeric; *Hin:* Kachura; *Beng*: Kachura; *Kan:* Kachura; *Tam:* Kichili-kizhanghu; *Tel:* Kachoram; *Mal:* Pula-kizhanna.

Description: Perennial herb, 0.5-0.8m. high. Rhizome conical, bearing serveral small tubers with long stalks. Leaves entire largely sheathed, with purple veins along the main nerve on the upper face inflorescence cylindrical, arising from the rhizome before the leaves; flowers yellow; bracts greenish, pink at the tips.

Habitate: Grows wild in damp deciduous forests; is also cultivated for ornament.

Propagation: By vegetative method.

Part Used: Rhizomes.

Chemical Constituents: The rhizomes yield an essential oil consisting principally of a-pinene, D-camphene, cineol, D-camphor, D-borneol, sesquiterpene alcohol, zingiberene.

Uses: The rhizome has stomachic and emmenagogic properties. It is active in dyspepsia, colic, vomiting, cough menstrual haematometra and menstrual disorders. It is also used as a restorative.

428. *Cuscuta chinesis* Lam. *(Convulvulaceae)*

Vernacular Name: *Eng:* Chinese dooder.

Description: Leafless twining parasites Stems filiform, up to 1 m long, much-branched, fleshy, often forming dense yellow masses on some shrubs or herbs amount the compositate or leguminouseae. Flowers in summer, pentamerous, in cymes or dense racemes. Capsule barely 2.5 mm in diameter, glabose or ovoid, hyaline, divided into 2 loves by a deep furrow on tip. 2-4 seeded. Seeds globose, 1-1.5 mm in diameter, with a grayish-brown or yellowish-brown surface.

Habitate: By roadsides, amount grasses or in thickets in China, Japan, Korea.

Propagation: By seeds and vegetative method.

Part Used: Seeds.

Chemical Constituents: N.A.

Uses: Tiredness in lower body and legs, impotence, seminal emissions, frequent micturition, vertigo, dizziness, poor vision, fetal distress.

429. *Cuscuta epithymum* *(Convolvulaceae)*

Vernacular Name: *Eng:* Dodder, Hellweed, Devil's guts.

Description: Leafless parasitic plant. Has thread-like stems, which are usually yellow-red in colour, and small, scented, pale pink flowers.

Habitate: Dodder grows throughout Europe, Asia and southern Africa.

Propagation: By seeds and vegetative method.

Parts Used: Aerial parts.

Chemical Constituents: Dodder contains flavonoids and hydroxycinnamic acid.

Uses: In line with its traditional use to purge black bile, dodder is still considered a valuable, though little-used, herb for problems affecting the liver and gallbladder. It is thought to support liver function and is taken for jaundice. Dodder has a mildly laxative effect, and is also taken for urinary problems.

430. *Cuscuta reflexa* Roxb. *(Convolvulaceae)*

Vernacular Name: *San*:-Akasavalli, Asparsa, Eng:-Dodder, *Hin:*-Akasbela, Amarabela, Kan:-Amaraballi, Akasaballi, Mal: -Akasavalli, Mutillattali, Akasagarudakkoti, *Tam:*-Sadadari, *Tel:* -Sitamma pogunalu.

Description: A slender much branched leafless yellow intertwining parasite on shrubs and trees almost covering them, without contact with the soil; flowers sometimes solitary or in clusters of 2-4; fruits capsules, 6-8 mm diameters, depressed, globose with 2-4 black seeds. The filiform yellowish branches freely swing in the air to and fro. Their broken branches, when they happen to be in contact with a living plant, will soon establish themselves on the host and spread rapidly and will ultimately destroy the host plant.

Habitate: Throughout India.

Propagation: By seeds and vegetative method.

Parts Used: Whole plant.

Chemical Constituents: The fresh plant yields scoparone, melanettin, quercetin, and hyperoside. Field grown plants have shown the ability to synthesize quercetin 3-O-galactoside and 3-O-β-glucoside. Besides, several soluble phenolic compounds, mainly hydroxycinnamic acid derivatives such as 3, 4-dicaffeolyquinic, 3,5-dicaf-feoylquinic, and 3-caffeoylquinic acids have been isolated from the plant. The pattern of phenolics has been found to be stable irrespective of the host plants.

Uses: The plant is bitter, sweet, astringent, expectorant, carminative, tonic, aphrodisiac, diaphoretic, anthelmintic and diuretic, and is useful in jaundice, myalgia, cough, bronchitis, strangury, cephalalgia, fever and paralysis. The seeds are carminative, depurative, and are also applied as an anodyne.

431. *Cyamopsis tetragonoloba* (L.) Taub. *(Fabaceae)*

Synonyms: *Cyamopsis psoralioides* (Linn.) DC.

Vernacular Name: *San*: Ksudrasimbi, Goraksaphalini, *Eng:* Cluster bean, *Hin:* Govar, *Kan:* Gorikayi, Guvarkayi, *Mal:* Kottavara, Kottamara, *Tam:* Kottavarai, *Tel:* Gorucikkudu, Karucikkudu,.

Description: An erect robust annual, 30-60 cm in height, more or less clothed with appressed greyish hairs, stems grooved; leaves 3-foliolate, leaflets elliptic, acute, sharply dentate, hairy on both sides, main nerves prominent; flowers small, purplish in axillary racemes; fruits thick fleshy pods, in clusters, subtetragonal, slightly pubescent, seeds 5-12 per pod, slightly compressed.

Habitate: Throughout India, cultivated.

Propagation: By seeds and vegetative method.

Parts Used: Pods and seeds.

Chemical Constituents: Methionine, globulin, toxic polyphenolic constituents, antitryptic agent. Gallic, chlorogenic, caffeic, and ellagic acids, gallotannins, kaempferol-3-glucoside, kaempferol-7-glucoside-3-glycoside, kaempferol-3-rutinoside, myricetin-7-glucoside-3-glycoside, and 3-O-7-O-β-myricetin.

Uses: The pods are sweet, cooling, laxative, digestive, appetiser, tonic and galactagogue, and are useful in constipation, dyspepsia, anorexia, agalactia, nyctalopia and vitiated conditions of *pitta*.

432. *Cyanopsis tetragonoloba* *(Leguminosae)*

Vernacular Name: *Eng:* Guar gum.

Description: Erect annual growing to 60cm, with hairy 3-lobed leaves, small purple flowers and fleshy seed pods.

Habitate: Native to the Indian sub-continent, guar gum is cultivated extensively in India and Pakistan.

Propagation: By seeds and vegetative method.

Parts Used: Pods, Seeds.

Chemical Constituents: Guar gum contains about 86% water-soluble mucilage, comprising mainly galactomannan.

Uses: Guar gum is an effective bulk laxative, similar in action to psyllium. It delays the emptying of the stomach and thus slows down absorption of carbohydrates. As this appears to help stabilize blood sugar levels, guar gum may prove useful in pre-diabetic conditions and in the early stages of late-onset diabetes. Guar gum also lowers cholesterol levels. In Indian medicine, guar seed is a laxative and a digestive tonic.

433. *Cyathula prostrata* (L.) Blume *(Amaranthaceae)*

Synonyms: *Desmochaeta prostrata* (Linn.) DC.

Vernacular Name: *San*: Raktapamargah, *Eng:* Small prickly chaff-flower plant, *Hin:* Lal circita, Lal cicimda, *Kan:* Uttarani, *Mal:* Cerukatalati, Cuvannakatalati, *Tam:* Cirukatalati, Civappu nayuruvi, *Tel:* Uttareni, Antisa.

Description: A much branched slender prostrate or decumbent herbaceous annual or perennial rooting at the nodes and the ascending branches ending in inflorescence, stems and branches violetish red, leaves simple, opposite, exstipulate, short-petioled, rhomboid or ovate, sub-acute, upto 7 cm long and 3.5 cm broad; flowers reddish violet or violet in terminal spikes or racemes, usually 10-20 cm long; fruits ovoid membranous utricles enclosed in the perianth; seed single, oblong, inverse.

Habitate: Throughout India, in shady, moist localities.

Propagation: By seeds and vegetative method.

Parts Used: Roots.

Chemical Constituents: N.A.

Uses: The roots are acrid, cooling, emetic, alexipharmic, constipating, vulnerary, demulcent and expectorant, and are useful in vitiated conditions of *pitta*, cough, bronchitis, wounds, ulcers, pruritus, skin diseases, abdominal disorders, dyspepsia and diarrhoea.

434. *Cycas circinalis* L. *(Cycadaceae)*

Vernacular Name: *San*: Hintalah, *Eng:* False sago palm, *Hin:* Jangli madan must ka phul, *Kan:* Mund isalu, Goddu eechalu, *Mal:* Eentha pana, Mar: Malabari supari, *Tam:* Madana kama raja, Salaparai, Eentha panai, *Tel:* Rana guvva, Per ita, Madana kamakshi.

Description: A slow-growing palm-like evergreen tree, reaching 5-12 m tall. *Roots* thick, dark brown, coral-like, arranged as a bead. *Trunk* straight, cylindrical, unbranched, brown, with persistent leaf scars. Leaves 1-3 m long, pinnately arranged; *leaflets* opposite, 60-100 pairs, linear, 20-30 cm long, about 1 cm wide, single nerved, apex acuminate, margin entire, shiny, hairless; leaf stalk 40-60 cm long, hairless, stout with few short stout slightly curved spines at base. Male and female *flowers* found in separate plants in the form of 'cones'. *Male cones* consist of numerous compactly arranged fleshy leaf-like structures called as '*microsporophylls*', which produce thousands of powdery male spores. '*Megasporophylls*' are specialized fleshy leaf-like structures, bearing the '*seeds*', which are 2-4 in each megasporophyll, egg-shaped, hard, about 5 x 3 cm, hairless, smooth, brownish yellow.

Habitate: Deciduous to semi-evergreen forests, mostly in tall grasslands and woodland savannahs.

Propagation: By seeds and vegetative method.

Parts Used: Bark, tender leaves, microsporophylls, seeds.

Chemical Constituents: N.A.

Uses: Seeds are used as aphrodisiac as well as to improve the sperm production. Bark and seeds are used as a poultice for sores and swellings. Tender leaves relieve flatulence and vomiting. Powdered endosperm is used to relieve burning sensation and general debility.

435. *Cyclea peltata* (Lam.) Hook. f. &Thoms *(Menispermaceae)*

Synonyms: *Cyclea burmanni* Hook.f. & Thoms., *Cyclea arnottii* Miers.

Vernacular Name: *San*: Patha, *Eng:* Pata root, *Hin:* Path, Pathi, Parvel, Patha, *Kan:* Padvalli, Visapoddi, Vishaddi, *Mal:* atavalli, Patakkilannu, *Tam:* Patakkilanku, *Tel:* Patha.

Description: A slender twining shrub with sparingly pilose stems and branches leaves simple, alternate, petioles long, lamina peltate, glabrous above, pale or glaucous below with the nerves puberulous; flowers small, greenish in axillary panicles, calyx globose or broadly campanulate, petals 4-8, more or less connate, anthers 6-8 celled; fruits ovoid drupes, endocarp horse-shoe shaped, seed curved.

Habitate: Throughout India, upto 900 m.

Propagation: By seeds and vegetative method.

Parts Used: Roots, leaves.

Chemical Constituents: Telradrine, phaeanthine, uronic acid.

Uses: The roots are bitter, acrid, thermogenic, digestive, carminative, anthelmintic, constipating, anti-inflammatory, depurative, febrifuge; diuretic and tonic, and are useful in vitiated conditions of *kapha*, cough, bronchitis, dyspepsia, colic, helminthiasis, diarrhoea, dysentery, dropsy, painful swellings, leprosy, skin diseases, pruritus, fever strangury, metroptosis, spelnomegaly, ulcers, wounds, haemorrhoids, vomiting, hyperdipsia and cardiac disorders. The leaves are cooling and ophthalmic and are useful in dandruff, burning sensation of the eye and fever, and are used in the place of soap.

436. *Cydonia oblonga* *(Rosaceae)*

Vernacular Name: *Eng:* Quince.

Description: Deciduous tree growing to 8m. Has greenO-grey oval leaves, pink or white flowers and yellow, pear-shaped sweet-smelling fruit.

Habitate: Native to south-west and central Asia, quince has become naturalized in Europe, especially in the Mediterranean region.

Propagation: By seeds and vegetative method.

Parts Used: Fruits, Seeds.

Chemical Constituents: The fruit contains tannins, pectin and fruit acids; the seeds contain about 20% mucilage, cyanogenic glycosides fixed oil and tannins.

Uses: The great astringency of the unripe fruit makes it useful as a remedy for diarrhoea, one that is particularly safe for children. The fruit and its juice can also be taken as a mouthwash r gargle to treat mouth ulcers, gum problems and sore throats. When cooked, much of the fruit's astringency is lost; quince syrup is recommended as a plea*San*t, mildly astringent, digestive drink. The seeds contain significant quantities of mucilage and are helpful both in treating bronchitis and as a bulk laxative.

437. *Cymbopogon citratus* (DC.) Stapf *(Poaceae)*

Synonyms: *Andropogon citratus* DC.

Vernacular Name: *San:* Bhustrina; *Eng:* Lemon grass, ginger grass, citronella grass, sere grass; *Hin:* Gandhatrina, agin ghas; *Beng*: Gandhabena; *Tel:* Nimmagaddi; *Tam:* Vasanappillu; *Kan:* Majjigehullu and *Mal:* Vasanappulla.

Description: Perennial, densely tufted, aromatic grass. Stems underground, short, whitish or pale-violet. Leaves in dense clusters, linear amplexicaul, rough-margined, glaucous green on both sides. Inflorescence in many-branched panicles without stalks. All parts of the grass are lemon-flavoured.

Habitate: Spicies cultivated as a culinary herb and for medicinal use.

Propagation: By vegetative method.

Part Used: Whole plant.

Chemical Constituents: The whole plant contains an essential oil consisting of critral, limonene, isopulegol, citronellic acid, geranium acid and a-camphorene.

Uses: The entire plant possesses antiseptic, antifebrile and stomachic properties. It is used in treating coryza, influnza and pyrexia. It is also prescrived agaisnt dyspepsia and vomiting and as a carminative, using three to four drops of the essential oil, diluted in water. Used externally to treat eczema. The essential oil is used as an insecticide against mosquitoes and as a deodorant.

438. *Cymbopogon citratus* (DC.) Stapf *(Poaceae)*

Synonyms: *Andropogon citratus* DC.

Vernacular Name: *San*: Bhustrnah, *Eng:* West Indian lemon grass, *Hin:* Gandhatrn, *Kan:* Majjigahullu, *Mal:* Cennanampullu, Incippullu, Vasanappulu, *Tam:* Vasanapillu, *Tel:* Nimmagaddi.

Description: A tall tufted perennial with a short rhizome, throwing up dense fascicles of leaves; leaf-blades linear, tapering upwards to a long setaceous point, glabrous, margin rough, midrib somewhat stout below, whitish on the upper side, ligules very short, scarious, rounded or truncate, sheath terete; flowers in spikelets, in decompound to sub-decompound loose panicles, fertile spikelets reddish, linear to linear-lanceolate, acuminate, back of the lower glume distinctly concave in the lower half.

Habitate: Cultivated throughout India.

Propagation: By seeds and vegetative method.

Parts Used: Whole plant.

Chemical Constituents: d-Limonene and geraniol, flavones, luteolin and its 7-O-β-glucoside and 7-O-neohesperodoside, iso-orientin and 2″-O-rhamnosyliso-orientin.

Presence of cholrogenic, caffeic and *p*-coumaric acids, fructose, sucrose, octacosanol, triacontanol and dotriacontanol is also reported.

Uses: The plant is aromatic, bitter, acrid, thermogenic, anthelmintic, laxative, appetiser, alexipharmic and anaphrodisiac, and is useful in helminthiasis, flatulence, gastric irritations, anorexia, poisonous bites, bronchitis, epilepsy, leprosy, skin diseases, cholera, neuralgia, sprains, fever and vitiated conditions of *kapha* and *vata*.

439. *Cymbopogon martinii* (Roxb.) Wats *(Poaceae)*

Synonyms: *Andropogon martinii* Roxb.

Vernacular Name: *San*: Dhyamakah, Rohisah, *Eng:* Rosha grass, Rusa grass, Palmarosa, *Hin:* Gandhabel, Rusa ghas, *Kan:* Harehullu, *Mal:* Sambharappullu, *Tam:* Kavattampillu, Munkilpul, Curaippul, *Tel:* Kamakchi-Kassuvu

Description: A perennial, sweet-scented grass, 1.5-2.5 m in height; leaves linear-lanceolate, subcordate or amplexicaul, finely caudate; flowers in spikelets, in panicles, turning reddish brown when mature, the lowest pedicel of the sessile raceme slightly swollen and connate to the base of the rachis, glumes channelled corresponding to a midrib on the inner side, awned.

Habitate: Throughout India, cultivated in dry localities.

Propagation: By seeds and vegetative method.

Parts Used: Whole plant.

Chemical Constituents: Geraniol, geranyl acetate, linalool, geranyl octanoate, geranyl butyrate, dihemiacetal bismonoterpenoid, cymbodiacetal.

Uses: The plant is acrid, bitter, thermogenic, appetiser, carminative, digestive, cardiotonic, depurative, galactagogue, diuretic, sudorific and febrifuge and is useful in vitiated conditions of *kapha* and *vata*, neuralgia, bronchitis, cough, catarrh, helminthiasis, anorexia, dyspepsia, colic, cardiac debility, leprosy, skin diseases, agalactia, strangury, epileptic fits in children, pharyngopathy and fever.

440. *Cynanchum ascyrifolium* Matsumura *(Asclepiadaceae)*

Vernacular Name: *Eng:*-Cruel plant, Mosquito plant.

Description: Erect, crisped-hairy herb, 30-60 cm tall. Leaves opposite, green above, paler beneath, oblong, elliptic, or ovate, 8-15 cm long, 4-8 cm wide, acuminate to short, acuminate; petioles 1-2 cm long. Inflorescence terminal and in upper axils, peunculate, few-branched; pedicels 1-3 cm long. Calyx segments broadly lanceolate; corolla white, 15mm across, the lobes narrowly ovate, 8-10 mm long, glabrous on both surfaces; corona-lobes ovate-deltoid, slightly shorter than the gynostegium. Follicles broadly lanceolate, glabrous, 4-6 cm long, 8 mm wide.

Habitate: Thickets in hills and mountains in Korea, Japan and China.

Propagation: By seeds and vegetative method.

Parts Used: Root.

Chemical Constituents: Related plant, C. atratum Bunge contains: Atratogenin A, B, cynajapogenin A, cynatratosides A, B, C, D, E,glaucogenin A, C, atratosides A, B, C, D.

Uses: Antipyretic, diuretic.

441. *Cynanchum atratum* Bunge. *(Asclepiadaceae)*

Vernacular Name: *Eng:* Blackened swallow-wart.

Description: A perennial, alpine herb, often with milky latex, the stem erect, terete, 30-60 cm high, covered with short grayish-white hairs. Leaves opposite, broadly oval or oblong, 6-15 cm long by 3-10 cm wide; tip acuminate; base rounded or slightly cordate; margin entire, briefly petiolate, pubscent. Inflorescence an axillary, umbellate cyme, sessile. Flowers brownish-red. Fruit an acuminate follicle, fusiform. Seeds numerous, plumose.

Habitate: On mountains, under trees, China, Japan, Korea, Mongolia.

Propagation: By seeds and vegetative method.

Part Used: Roots.

Chemical Constituents: N.A.

Uses: Intermittent fever due to weakness, low fever in late stage of febrile diseases, urinary-tract infection.

442. *Cynanchum wilfordii* (Maxim.) Hemsl. *(Asclepiadaceae)*

Vernacular Name: *Eng:* Wilford's cynanchum.

Description: Glabrous, scandent, perennial herb, 1-3 m tall. Leaves opposite, deltoid, 5-10 cm long, 4-8 cm wide, deeply cordate, entire, petiolate. Inflorescence axillary umbels; peduncles 1-4 cm long; pedicels 5-8 m long. Flowers pale yellow-green; calyx lobes 5, broadly lanceolate, acuminate; corolla 5-lobed, 3 mm long, incurved, puberulent inside. Follicles lanceolate, 8 cm long, 1 cm wide.

Habitate: Open grassy slopes on mountains and hills in Korea, Japan and China.

Propagation: By seeds and vegetative method.

Parts Used: Root.

Chemical Constituents: Sarcostine-, deacylcynanchogenin-, deacylmetaplexigenin-cymarosides, wilforine, cynamoy1 tigloylsarcostine, kidjoranin, caudatin, penupogenin, wilforibose, wilfosides.

Uses: Hepatoprotective activity. Usedin tonic, scrofula, cold knee.

443. *Cynara scolymus* *(Asteraceae)*

Synonyms*: Cynara cardunculus.*

Vernacular Name: *Eng:* Artichoke.

Description: Perennial herb growing to 1.5m. Has large, thistle-like leaves grey-green above and woolly white beneath, and very large purple-green flowerheads.

Habitate: Native to the Mediterranean region, artichoke thrives in rich loam in warm temperate climates.

Propagation: By seeds and vegetative method.

Parts Used: Flowers, leaves root.

Chemical Constituents: All parts of the plant contain the sesquiterpene lactone cynaropicrin and much inulin. The leaves also contain cynarin, which has liver-protective properties.

Uses: Artichoke is a valuable medicinal plant. Like milk thistle it benefits the liver, protecting against toxins and infection. Though the leaves are particularly effective all parts of the plant are bitter and stimulate digestive secretions, especially bile this makes artichoke useful for the treatment of gallbladder problems, nausea, indigestion and abdominal distension, with the added benefit that it lowers blood cholesterol levels.

444. *Cynodon dactylon* (Linn.) Pers. *(Poaceae)*

Vernacular Name: *San*: Niladurva, Durva, *Eng:* Dhub grass, Barmuda or Bahama grass, Conch grass, *Hin:* Dub, Durba, *Kan:* Garika hallu, Kudigarike, *Mal:* Karuka, Karukappullu, *Tam:* Arukampillu, Muyalpul, *Tel:* Garicagaddi, Gerike.

Description: A prostrate extensively creeping glabrous, highly branched perennial grass, rooting at every nods, forming matted tufts; leaves narrow, linear, soft, smooth, distinchous at the base, ligule a very fine ciliate rim; inflorescence terminal spikes. Green or purplish, rachis slender, involucral glumes acute to subulate-mucronulate, floral glume obliquely oblong to semi-ovate; fruits grains, oblong, laterally compressed about 1 mm long.

Habitate: Wild, throughout India, and also cultivated for decorative purposes.

Propagation: By roots and vegetative method.

Parts Used: Whole plant.

Chemical Constituents: β-ionone, 2-propionic , 4-hydroxybenzoic, 2-propionic and 3-methoxy-4-ydroxybenzoic acids, phytol, β-sitosterol-D-glucoside, stigmasterol acetate and a phagostimulant, phytone, glycosides, saponins, tannins, flavonoids and carbohydrates.

Uses: The plant is astringent, sweet, cooling, haemostatic, depurative, vulnerary, constipating, diuretic and tonic, and is useful in vitiated conditions of *pitta* and *kapha*, hyperdipsia, burning sensation, haemoptysis, haematuria, haemorrhages, wounds, haemorrhoids, conjunctivitis, cephalalgia, erysipelas, leprosy, skin diseases, vomiting, diarrhoea, dysentery, strangury, colporrhagia, abortion and general debility.

445. *Cyperus esculentus* Linn. *(Cyperaceae)*

Vernacular Name: *San*: Bhadramusta, Nagaramustakah, *Eng:* Chufa, Rush nut, Tiger nut, *Hin:* Cicoda, Cicada, *Kan:* Konnarigadde, *Mal:* Kalimuttanna, *Tel:* Kalatunga, Musta.

Description: An erect perennial glabrous grass-like sedge, upto 50 cm in height with slender subterranean stolons ending in ovoid or cylindrical brown edible tubers, stems triquetrous, smooth, finely striated, base pale brown; leaf blades shorter than the stems, linear, gradually tapering into a fine acuminate apex; spikelets in umbellate peduncled spikes, spikelets linear, rachis slender with narrow hyaline wing, flowering glumes boat-shaped, with a rounded or slightly emarginated apex and three lateral nerves on each side of the keel nerve; fruit obovoid-ellipsoid nut with 3-sharp angles.

Habitate: In Punjab and Nilgiri hills.

Propagation: By seeds and vegetative method.

Parts Used: Tubers.

Chemical Constituents: Isoleucine, leucine, lysine, methionine, phenylalanine, threonine, tryptophan, valine.

Uses: The tubers are astringent, bitter, acrid, cooling, carminative, digestive, anthelmintic, constipating, galactagogue, aphrodisiac, stimulant, febrifuge and tonic, and are useful in vitiated conditions of *pitta*, dyspepsia, flatulence, colic, helminthiasis, diarrhoea, dysentery, agalactia, bilious and intermittent fevers, hyperdipsia, burning sensation, ophthalmopathy, leprosy, hepatopathy, cephalalgia and general debility.

446. *Cyperus rotundus* L. *(Cyperaceae)*

Vernacular Name: *San:* Mustaka, musta; *Eng:* Nut grass, coco grass; *Hin:* Mutha, motha; *Beng*: Mutha, motha; *Tam:* Korai; *Tel:* Tungamuste and *Kan:* Tungegadde.

Description: Glabrous perennial grass, 20-30 cm. High. Rhizome tuberous, reddish-brown, aromatic, leaves long, very narrow, sheathed and one-nerved, Inflorescence consisting of 4-6 spikes radiating from a slender, tringular stalk, purplish. Fruit angular, greyish.

Habitate: Weed found woild everywhere in Viet Nam.

Propagation: By vegetative method.

Part Used: Rhizomes.

Chemical Constituents: The rhizomes yield an essential oil (0.5-1.25) consisting of cyperene, cyperol, a-cyperone, cineol and L-a-pinene, together with starch.

Uses: The rhizomes give successful resutls in the treatment of irregular meanstruatiiohn, dysmenorrhoea, gastralgia, dyspepsia, diarrhoea and vomiting.

447. *Cypripedium pubescens* *(Orchidaceae)*

Vernacular Name: *Eng:* Lady's slipper, American valerian.

Description: Perennial orchid with several stems sheathed by broad lance-shaped leaves. Has beautiful, complex golden-yellow and purple.

Habitate: This herb is native to eastern North America. Its natural habitat is woods and pastures, but due to overharvesting, it is rarely found in the wild. It is cultivated to a limited degree.

Propagation: By vegetative method.

Parts Used: Rootstock.

Chemical Constituents: Lady's slipper is poorly researched, but it is known to contain a volatile oil, resins, glucosides and tannins.

Uses: Due to its scarcity and cost, lady's slipper is now used on a small scale. A sedative and relaxing herb, it treats anxiety, stress-related disorders such as palpitations, headaches, muscular tension, panic attacks, and neurotic conditions generally. Like valerian, lady's slipper is an effective tranquillizer. It reduces emotional tension and often clams the mind sufficiently to allow sleep. Indeed, its restorative effect appears to be more positive than that of valerian.

448. *Dalbergia sissoo* Roxb. *(Fabaceae)*

Vernacular Name: *San*: Simsapa, *Eng:* Sissoo, *Hin:* Sisam, Sissu, sisam, *Kan:* Agaru, Biridi, *Mal:* Irupul, Sisam, Iruvil, *Tam:* Sisu, Itti, Tesimaram, *Tel:* Errasissu, Simsupa.

Description: A deciduous tree upto 3 m in height with a crooked trunk, light crown and pubescent or tomentose young parts; leaves imparipinnate, alternate, rachis zig-zag, leaflets 3-5, terminal one being the largest and the lowest the smallest, conspicuously and abruptly acuminate; flowers pale yellow, sessile or nearly so in axillary panicles, shorter than the leaves; fruit pods narrowed at the base into a long stalk; seeds 1-4 per pod.

Habitate: Throughout the sub-Himalayan tracts upto 1,500 m, also cultivated in Punjab, U.P. Bengal and Assam.

Propagation: By seeds and vegetative method.

Parts Used: Roots, leaves, bark, heartwood.

Chemical Constituents: Antifungal essential oil. The root contains the isoflavones, biochanin-A, tiobioside. It also contains (S)-4-methoxydalbergione, (R)-latifolin and dalbergin. The fatty acid composition of the seed oil is: palmitic, 16.2; stearic, 7.0; oleic, 14.6; linoleic, 52.5; and linolenie, 8.0%.

Uses: The roots are astringent and constipating, and are useful in diarrhoea and dysentery. The leaves are bitter, ophthalmic, styptic, digestive, constipating, anthelmintic, diuretic and stimulant, and are useful in gonorrhoea, menorrhagia, excoriation, ophthalmopathy, dyspepsia, colic, diarrhoea, dysentery, vomiting, haemorrhoids and burning sensation.

The bark and heartwood are astringent, acrid, bitter, thermogenic, anthelmintic, depurative, vulnearary, anti-inflammatory, emmenagogue, expectorant, aphrodisiac, abortifacient, antipyretic and appetiser, and are useful in hyperdipsia, burning sensation, vomiting, skin diseases, leprosy, leucoderma, scabies, ulcers, dyspepsia, dysentery, scalding of urine, syphilis, gastropathy, helminthiasis, ophthalmopathy, amenorrhoea, dysmenorrhoea, hiccough, bronchitis, sciatica, gout, inflammations, intermittent fevers and vitiated conditions of *vata*.

449. *Daphne mezereum* *(Thymelaeaceae)*

Vernacular Name: *Eng:* Mezereon.

Description: Hardy deciduous shrub growing to 1.2m. Has oval to lance-shaped leaves, clusters of red or pink flowers and small red berries.

Habitate: Mezereon is found in Europe, North Africa and western Asia, in damp mountain woodlands. It is cultivated as a garden plant.

Propagation: By seeds and vegetative method.

Parts Used: Root, root bark, bark.

Chemical Constituents: Mezereon contains diterpenes, and mucilage and tannins. Daphnetoxin and mezerein are highly toxic, but they have anti-leukaemic properties, and have been used in a number of countries in the treatment of cancer.

Uses: Today, mezereon is considered too poisonous to be ingested. It is used occasionally as an external counter-irritant and is effective on rheumatic joints, increasing blood flow to the affected area. It has been considered effective for rheumatic joints, causing inflammation and occasional blistering.

450. *Datura metel* L. *(Solanaceae)*

Vernacular Name: *San:* Dhustura; *Eng:* White datura, white thornapple, downy thornapple, recurved thornapple; *Hin:* Sadahdhatura; *Beng*: Dhatura; *Tam:* Vellum-mattai.

Description: Small herbaceous plant, 1-1.4 m. high Braches pubescent when young, marked with leaf scars, leaves alternate, unequal at the base,minutely pubescent on both surfaces; margins wavy. Flowers large, white, colitary in the leaf axil. Capsule globose, covered with slender spines. Seeds numerous, blackish–brown.

Habitate: Grows wild on waste land;l also cultivated for ornament.

Propagation: By seeds and vegetative method.

Part Used: Leaves and flowers.

Chemical Constituents: The whole plant, especially the leaves and flowers, contain alkaloids. Scopolamine, hyoscyamine, atropine and norhyoscyamine, as well as vitamin C. The total alkaloid content of the roots is 0.10-0.20% leaves 0.1-0.5%; flowers 0.25-0.60% fruits 0.12%,.

Uses: The leaves possess antispasmodic, sedative and anodyne properties. They are used for reating cough, asthma, rheumatism. Chilblains, gastric ulcers, haemorrhoids, sea sickness and air sickness. The dried leaves and flowers are cut into small chips and used in antiasthmatic cigrettes. A poultice of the pounded fresh leaves has an anodyne effect. Warning should be given of their high toxicity.

451. *Datura stramonium* *(Solanaceae)*

Vernacular Name: *Eng:* Thornapple.

Description: Robust annual growing to 1m. Has lobed oval leaves, long white or violet trumpet-shaped flowers, and spiny fruit capsules similar to those of the horse fruit capsules similar to those of the horse chestnut.

Habitate: Thornapple grows in the Americas, Europe, Asia and North Africa. It is cultivated for medicinal use in Hungary, France and Germany.

Propagation: By seeds and vegetative method.

Parts Used: Leaves, flower, Seeds.

Chemical Constituents: Thoranpple contains 0.2-0.45% tropane alkaloids, flavonoids, withanolides, coumarins and tannins. The tropane alkaloids are similar to those found in deadly nightshade acting to reduce secretions and relax smooth muscle.

Uses: At low doses, thornapple is a common remedy for asthma, whooping cough, muscle spasm and the symptoms of Parkinsonism. It relaxes the muscles of the gastro-intestinal, bronchial and urinary tracts, and reduces digestive and mucous secretions. Like deadly nightshade, thornapple may be applied externally to relieve rheumatic pains and neuralgia.

452. *Daucus carota* Linn. Var sativa DC. *(Apiaceae)*

Vernacular Name: *San:* Garjara, Gajara, Narangavarnaka; *Eng:* Cultivated carrot; *Hin:* Gajar; *Beng*: Gajar; *Tam:* Gorjar; *Tel:* Pitakand.

Description: Annual herb, leaves triangular to oblong, 2-3-pinnatisect, inflorescence umbel, fruits, broad, including the prickles, seeds numerous.

Habitate: Cultivated all over India.

Propagation: By seeds and vegetative method.

Part Used: Seeds and roots.

Chemical Constituents: Carrot seed oil contains carotol as the principal constituent. Other components are daucol, bisabolene, daucene oxide and carota-1, 4-oxide. Carrot root oil contains terbinolene, b-and y-bisabolene, y-terpinene, caryophyllene, sabinene, and limonene as the major volatile components, but the flavour is attrivuted to 2-nonenal, octanal, 2-decenal, 2,4Odecadienal, 2-methoxy-3-sec-butylpyrazine and 2-methoxy-3-iso-propylpyrazine. Carrot herb oil contains trans-asarone and b-bisabolene as the major constituents.

Uses: Carrot seed oil with its warm-spicy flavour is used in spice blends, formulation of compound oil for sauces, cured meats, seasonings, etc. and also for flavouring alcoholic beverages. Carrot root oil also has the typical carrot flavour.

453. *Decalepis hamiltonii* Wight & Arn. *(Periplocaceae)*

Vernacular Name: *San*: Sariba, Sveta sariva, *Kan:* Magadi beru, *Mal:* Nannari, *Tam:* Mahali kizhangu, Mavilinga kilangu, Peru nannari, *Tel:* Neemam theega(Chenchu tribes), Maredu geddalu.

Description: A large hairless extensively climbing shrub. *Latex* sticky and milky. Branches jointed, slightly angled and with swollen nodes. Young branchlets, leaves and the leaf nerves are shiny. Distinctly greenish pink and hairless. *Leaves* opposite, egg-shaped to round shaped, about 7 x 5 cm, base gradually tapering to truncate, apex sub-acute to rounded, margin entire to wavy; leaf stalks about 1 cm long. *Flowers* yellow, small mm across, arranged in 3-times branched cymes. *Follicles* cylindrically oblong, about 5 x 3 cm and woody when dry. *Seeds* many, egg-shaped, about 6 x 4 mm, with long white silky hairs.

Habitate: In open rocky slopes and rocky cervices of dry to moist deciduous forests.

Propagation: By seeds, stem cuttings and root suckers.

Parts Used: Roots.

Chemical Constituents: It contains quercetin, kaempferol, coumarin and rutin, lupeol, β-amyrin, 2-hydorxy, 4-methoxy benzaldehyde, and ferulic acid.

Uses: Tuberous roots are used as a cooling agent and blood-purifier. Hence used to prepare refreshing drinks. Roots are used to cure indigestion, deficient digestive power, dysentery, cough, bronchitis, leucorrhoea, uterine haemorrhage, skin diseases, fever, thirst, vomiting, poisoning, chronic rheumatism, anemia, debility, dysuria and blood diseases.

454. *Decaspermum fructicosum* sensu Drake *(Myrtaceae)*

Synonyms: *Decaspermun vitense* (A. Gray) Niederizu.

Vernacular Name: *Eng:* Christmas bush.

Description: A shrub or tree to 14m tall, sometimes with a compacted growth-form, and branchlets often square in cross-section. Leaves opposite and petiolate, blades with small scattered dots (punctuate glands), the blade up to 8 cm. Long, variable in shape but mostly ovate to elliptical with a conspicuous tapering tip. Flowers fragrant, 4 to 5-parted, borne on densely packed inflorescences. Fruit berry-like, roundish, 3-7 mm broad, black when mature, with several small seeds.

Habitate: Very common in dry forests, on ridges, hillside, and secondary forests on dry sides of Fiji's larger islands.

Propagation: By seeds and vegetative method.

Part Used: Fruits.

Chemical Constituents: Essential oils (leaves), coumarins (ellagic acid derivatives).

Uses: Treatment of cancer of the womb (infertile women), wounds (knife, spear, axe), toothache and loss of appetite in children.

455. *Delphinium denudatum* Wall. ex Hook.f.& Thoms.*(Ranunculaceae)*

Vernacular Name: *San*: Nirvisa, Apavisha, Vishalkarani, *Hin:* Nirbisi, Jadvar, *Mal:* Nirvasi, *Tam:* Nirbasi, *Tel:* Nirvisi.

Description: A glabrous branching annual herb, 60-90 cm in height; leaves radical, pinnately lobed or toothed, finely divided to the base, long stalked, stem leaves shortly stalked, uppermost sessile, more or less deeply 3-lobed, lobes narrow, entire; flowers blue to grey, scattered with a straight cylindrical spur; fruits inflated, follicles.

Habitate: In the Himalayas, upto 3,600 m.

Propagation: By seeds and vegetative method.

Parts Used: Roots.

Chemical Constituents: The root contains an oil. The fatty acid composition of the oil is; capric, 2.3; lauric, 1.6; myristic, 3.8; palmitic, 16.0; palmitoleic, 2.5; stearic, 1.3; oleic, 23.0; linoleic, 30.2; and linolenic, 19.30%.

Uses: The roots are acrid, bitter, thermogenic, anodyne, digestive, carminative, anthelmintic, diuretic, lithontriptic, emmenagogue, anti-inflammatory, revulsive, depurative, aphrodisiac, vulnerary, stimulant, alexeteric, alterant, cardiotonic, febrifuge and tonic, and are useful in odontalgia, insanity, haemorrhoids, dyspepsia, flatulence, jaundice, strangury, renal and vesical calculi, dysmenorrhoea, amenorrhoea, inflammations, obesity, leprosy, skin diseases, catarrh, cough, asthma, cardiac debility, fever, ulcers and vitiated conditions of *vata*.

456. *Delphinium staphysagria* Linn. *(Ranunculaceae)*

Vernacular Name: *Eng:* Staqvesacre.

Description: An ornamental, annual herb, with large tapering root. Stem upto 1.3 m. high, stout upright, cylindrical, slightly branched. Leaves 10-12.5 cm. in length, alternate, broad, palmately five to nine cleft, petioled, pubescent or nearly smooth above hairy on the veins beneath. Flowers short spurred, light blue, in lax racemes. Fruit consists of 3 straight, oblong downy capsules, each of which contain about 12 seeds packed in 2 rows. Seeds about 6 mm. long, irregularly 4 sided, pyramidal, sharp-angled, little flattened, rough, testa wrinkled, pitted, blackish-brown, rather brittle, enclosing a soft, whitish, oily endosperm.

Habitate: Native of Italy, Greek islands and Asia minor Mediterranean.

Propagation: By seeds and vegetative method.

Parts Used: Seeds.

Chemical Constituents: Delphinine, Delphisine, Delphinodien, Staphisagroine, Staphisagrine and a resin.

Uses: For complaints of toothache and alveolar periosteum. Effects of anger and insult. Sexual sine and excesses. Pain and neuralgia after extraction of teeth. Neuralgia due to decay in teeth. Sphincters lacerated and stretched. Recurrent styes in eyes. Itches of eye-lids margins. Lacerated and incised wounds of cornea. Stitching pain in throat, pain extending to ears on swallowing especially left. Smarting cutting pain in surgical incised wound of any part. Toothache worse by cold drink and touch.

457. *Dendrocnide harveyi* (Seemann) Chew *(Urticaceae)*

Description: Tree up to 20 m tall with stinging trichomes. Leaves alternate, broadly ovate and with long petioles, the blade to 40 cm long and 15 cm wide. Flowers numerous, small borne on axillary panicles, fruit a small achene.

Habitate: Common in wet primary and secondary forests, edge of forests, and along strems from sea-level to mid-montane.

Propagation: By seeds and vegetative method.

Part Used: Bark and leaves.

Chemical Constituents: N.A.

Uses: A preparation made from scrapings of the bark is used in treating illnesses described as a pain in the lungs with vomiting of blood (tuberculosis)., Liquid squeezed from the leaves is given to cure fits in children, sickness after birth, and to aid expulsion of the afterbirth. Tea made from the leaves of stinging needles is reportedly used in the treatment of venereal diseases. The leaves are used to treat convulsions and releases after child birth and the stems are used to treat the pain in bones or joints, intestinal filariasis and postnatal depression.

458. *Dendrophthoe falcate* (L.f.) Etting. *(Loranthaceae)*

Synonyms: *Loranthus falcatus* Linn.f., *Loranthus longiflorus* Desr.

Vernacular Name: *San*: Vrksadani, *Eng:* Mistletoe, *Hin:* Banda, *Kan:* Badanike, Bandhulu, *Mal:* Ittikkanni, *Tam:* Pulluri, Pulluruvi, *Tel:* Badanika, Jiddu.

Description: A stem parasite with smooth, grey bark; leaves usually opposite, thick, variable in shape from ovate to linear-oblong, mid-rib prominent, secondary nerves obscure; flowers orange-red or scarlet in short spreading, stout, axillary, racemes, calyx present, often as a rim, flowers bisexual; fruits ovoid or oblong berries crowned by cup-shaped calyx.

Habitate: Throughout India, as parasite on trees.

Propagation: By seeds and vegetative method.

Parts Used: Whole plant.

Chemical Constituents: Cytokinins and casein hydrolysate, quercitrin, kaempferol, quercetagetin, quercetin, myricetin, an acylxyloside of quercetin, hyperoside, myricitrin, meratin and rutin.

Uses: The plant is cooling, bitter, astringent, aphrodisiac, narcotic and diuretic, and is useful in pulmonary tuberculosis, asthma, menstrual disorders, swellings, wounds, ulcers, strangury, renal and vesical calculi and vitiated conditions of *kapha* and *pitta.*

459. *Desmodium gangeticum* (L.) DC. *(Fabaceae)*

Vernacular Name: *San*: Prsniparni, Prthakparni, Shalparni; *Hin:* Salpan, Salvan; *Kan:* Nabiyalabune, Nariyalavona; *Mal:* Orila, *Tam:* Orila, *Tel:* Gitanaram.

Description: An erect, diffusely branched undershrub, 90-120 cm in height with a short woody stem and numerous prostrate branches provided with soft grey hairs; leaves unifoliate, ovate to ovate-lanceolate, membranous and mottled with grey patches; flowers white, purple or lilac in elongate lax, terminal or axillary racemes; fruits moniliform, 6-8 jointed glabrescent pods, joints of pods sparsely pubescent with hooked hairs, joints separating when ripe into indehiscent one-seeded segments; seeds compressed reniform.

Habitate: Throughout India in dry forests upto 900 m elevation and as forest undergrowth in low elevations.

Propagation: By seeds and vegetative method.

Parts Used: Roots.

Chemical Constituents: The mineral elements present in the plant are: Ca, 1.84; Cu, 0.002; Fe, 0.2054; K, 1.197; Mg, 0.3155; Mn, 0.007; Na, 0.198; Ba, 0.0048; Al, 0.903; Ce, 0.0381; Sr, 0.02434; V, 0.0008; Hg, 0.00005; Cr, 0.00004; Co, 0.0015; and Zn, 0.0083% (dry wt basis).

Uses: The roots are bitter, sweet, thermogenic, nervine tonic, aphrodisiac, carminative, constipating, diuretic, febrifuge, cardiotohic, anti-inflammatory, expectorant and tonic, and are useful in vitiated conditions of *vata*, anorexia, dyspepsia, haemorrhoids, dysentery, strangury, fever, gout, inflammations, cough, asthma, bronchitis, cardiopathy and debility.

460. *Desmodium triangulare* (Retz.) Merr. *(Fabaceae)*

Synonyms: *Desmodium cephalotes* Wall.

Description: Small tree, 2-3m. high. Branched, Leaves alternate; leaflets 3, ovate to lanceolate, the terminal largest, covered with a dense silvery pubescence beneath. Inflorescence in short axillary raceme; flowers white. Pod minutely constricted between the seeds. Seeds reniform.

Habitate: Grows wild in hilly and mountainous regions.

Propagation: By seeds and vegetative.

Part Used: Leaves.

Chemical Constituents: The leaves contain tannin, flavonoids, organic acids and alkaloids.

Uses: The elaves possess antibacterial and anti-inflammatory properties. They are indicated in the treatment of bacillary dyscentery, dysenteric syndrome and diarrhoea. Snake-bite is treated with finely pounded fresh leaves, the juice being extracted fro oral administration and the residue used for a poultice.

461. *Desmodium triflorum* (L.) DC. *(Fabaceae)*

Vernacular Name: *San*: Tripadi, *Hin:* Kudaliya, Janglimethi, *Kan:* Muntamundu, *Mal:* Nilamparanta, *Tam:* Sirupullati, *Tel:* Muntamandu.

Description: A small perennial much branched prostrate trailing herb with slender stems rooting at the nodes; leaves trifoliate, leaflets membranous, obovate, cuneate, truncate or emarginated or rarely rounded; flowers pink or white, 1-5 fascicled in the axils of leaves; fruits pods, with straight upper edge and indented lower edge, reticulately veined.

Habitate: Throughout India as a weed upto 900 m.

Propagation: By seeds and vegetative method.

Parts Used: Whole plant.

Chemical Constituents: N.A.

Uses: The plant is acrid, sweet, cooling, expectorant and galactagogue, and is useful in vitiated conditions of *pitta,* cough, bronchitis, wounds, abscess, sores, pruritus, erysipelas, dysentery, flatulence and burning sensation.

462. *Desmostachya bipinnata* (L.) Stapf *(Poaceae)*

Synonyms: *Eragrostis cynosuroides* (Retz.) P. Beauv.

Vernacular Name: *San*: Darbhah, Kusah, *Eng:* Sacrificial grass, *Hin:* Dab, Davoli, *Kan:* Darbha, *Mal:* Darbha, Darbhappullu, *Tam:* Darbhaipul, *Tel:* Dharbha, Kusa dharbha.

Description: A tufted perennial grass with a thick scaly root-stock which sends out creeping rhizomes in all directions; leaves many, upto 50 cm long and 1 cm broad at the base with filiform tips and hispid margins, sheaths glabrous; panicle erect, narrowly pyramidal clothed from the base with sessile imbricating spikelets; grains 0.5-0.6 mm long, obliquely ovoid, trigonous and laterally compressed.

Habitate: Throughout India.

Propagation: By vegetative method.

Parts Used: Whole plant.

Chemical Constituents: N.A.

Uses: The roots are bitter, sweet, cooling, diuretic, emollient, astringent and galactagogue, and are useful in asthma, jaundice, vitiated conditions of *pitta,* hyperdipsia and hamopathy. The culms are sweet, diuretic, stimulant, acrid and aphrodisiac, and are useful in dysentery, menorrhagia, jaundice, asthma, strangury, uropathy and skin eruptions.

463. *Dianthus chinensis* L. *(Caryophyllaceae)*

Vernacular Name: *Eng:* Rainbow pink.

Description: Short-lived perennial herb. Stems 30 cm tall, erect, internodes shorter than leaves. Leaves opposite, often united at the base and forming a sheath about the stem; the nodes usually swollen, basal leaves withering early; stem leaves 3-8 cm long, rarely to 0.5 cm wide, cililate, sheath 0.5 cm long. Inflorescence few-15 flowered, loosely clustered, epicalyx scales 4, abruptly contracted into a long point. Flowers solitary at terminals, 2 cm across, not fragrant, rosy-lilac with purplish eye; calyx tubular, 5-toothed, many-nerved, subtended by an epicalyx; petals 5, limb abruptly attenuated into an elongated claw, many-toothed, fimbriate with dark spot close to the tip; stamens 10; ovary 1-celled; styles 2. Fruit a 4-valved capsuile, cylindrical, oblong-ovoid; seeds many.

Habitate: Open grassy places.

Propagation: By seeds and vegetative method.

Parts Used: Whole plant.

Chemical Constituents: Eugenol, phenylethylalcohol, melosides A an L, dianchinenosides A, B, C, D.

Uses: Diuretic, hypotensive, anthlmintic, increasing peristalsis of intestine, antitumour, antioxidant activity. Used in diuretic, menostasis, gonorrhoea, cough, emmenagogue.

464. *Dianthus superbus* L. *(Caryophyllaceae)*

Vernacular Name: *Eng:* Fringed pink; superb pink.

Description: A perennial herb, 50-60 cm tall or more. Stem clustered, erect, glabrous; upper parts branched. Leaves opposite, lanceolate-linear; tip acuminate, margin entire; base amplexicaul; inferior leaves nearly obtuse, 3-veined. Inflorescence a panicled cyme; July-September. Flowers pink or lilac, large, fragrant. Fruit a 4-valved capsule, cylindrical.

Habitate: In tussocks, on hill-sides or in crevices in China, Japan Europe.

Propagation: By seeds and vegetative method.

Part Used: Whole plant.

Chemical Constituents: N.A.

Uses: Genito-urinary tract infection, gravel, oliguria, haematuria, amenorrhoea, eczema.

465. *Dichroa febriguga* Lour. *(Saxifragaceae)*

Vernacular Name: *Hin:* Basak and *Assam*: Basak, bansuk aseru.

Description: Small shrub, 1-2m. high, stems glabrous, greenish or pale–violet. Leaves opposite, oblong, acuminate; margins toothed petiole and main nerve usually violet. Inflorescence in axillary or terminal divarciate cyme: flowers and berriers bluish or lilac, seeds small pear-shaped.

Habitate: Grows wild in wet places or on stream banks.

Propagation: By seeds and vegetative method.

Part Used: Roots and leaves.

Chemical Constituents: The roots contain alkaloids: a-dischronie b-dichroine, y-dischoroine and 4-ketodihydroquinazoline.

Uses: The roots and the leaves possess antifebrile, expectorant and diuretic properties. They are indicated in the tratment of pyrexia, malaria, intermittent feber, cough and oliguria. The raw plant material is vomitive, so the roots and leaves are impregnated with alcohol and torrefied.

466. *Dichrostachys cinerea* (L.) Wight & Arn. *(Araceae)*

Synonyms: *Calliea cinerea* Macb.

Vernacular Name: *San*: Vellantharah, Virataruh, *Hin*: Vurttuli, Kheri, *Kan*: Odatare, *Mal*: Vitattal, Virvarksam, *Tam*: Vitattalai, Vetattala, *Tel:* Veluturu.

Description: A profusely branched thorny shrub or small tree upto 2 m in height, branches and branchlets armed with spiny tips; bark grey or light brown coloured, furrowed; leaves bipinnate, alternate, the main rachis often downy or softly pubescent with a small stipitate erect gland between each pair of pinnae, leaflets numerous, 10-20 pairs, sessile and close-set, linear or strap-shaped, oblique at base, subacute or acute; flowers numerous, minute, pink, yellow or red, sessile, polygamous, dimorphous in dense axillary or extra-axillary spikes, stamens of the perfect flower in the upper half of the spike yellow, the staminoides in the lower half red and much longer than the perfect stamens; fruits glabrous, dark brown, subauriculated, coriaceous pods, twisted when mature; seeds ovoid to obovoid, compressed.

Habitate: Throughout India in dry areas.

Propagation: By seeds and vegetative method.

Parts Used: Roots, tender shoots.

Chemical Constituents: Tannin.

Uses: The roots are bitter, astringent, acrid, thermogenic, anti-inflammatory, anodyne, digestive, constipating, lithontriptic and diuretic, and are useful in vitiated conditions of *kapha* and *vata,* inflammation, arthralgia, elephantiasis, dyspepsia, diarrhoea, vesical calculi, strangury, nephropathy, vaginopathy and metropathy. The tender shoots are useful in opthalmia.

467. *Dictamnus albus* *(Rutaceae)*

Vernacular Name: *Eng:* Dittany, Burning Bush.

Description: Strongly aromatic, bushy and hairy perennial growing to 80cm. Has compound leaves and spikes of 5-petalled white or pink flowers streaked with purple.

Habitate: This herb grows in southern and central Europe and northern Asia, preferring warm, wooded areas.

Propagation: By seeds and vegetative method.

Parts Used: Root, Flowers.

Chemical Constituents: Dittany's potent volatile oil contains estragol and anethole, and a toxic alkaloid, dictamnin.

Uses: Very rarely used by herbalists today, dittany has an action similar to that of rue in that is strongly stimulates the muscles of the uterus, inducing menstruation and sometimes causing abortion. By contract, its effect on the gastro-intestinal tract is antipasmodic. Dittany relaxes the gut and acts as a mild tonic for the stomach.

468. *Dictamnus dasycarpus* Turcz. *(Rutaceae)*

Vernacular Name: *Eng*: Dittany, fraxinella, gas plant, burning bush.

Description: Strong-smelling, hardy perennial herb with thick root, to 90 cm tall. Leaves alternate, pinnate; leaflets 9-11, to 7 cm long, ovate, serrulate, glandular-dotted. Flowers about 2 cm long, 2.5 cm across, light red, in terminal racemes, irregular; pedicel 0.5-2 cm, glandular hairs; sepals and petals 5; stamens 10, curved upward. Fruit a deeply 5-lobed capsule.

Habitate: Mountain slopes of Korea and Japan.

Propagation: By seeds and vegetative method.

Parts Used: Root bark.

Chemical Constituents: Fraxinellone, obaculactone, obacunone, dictamnolides. Alkaloids: dictamnines, skimmianines, isomaculosidine, preskimmianine, robustine, haplopine. Sesquiterpene: dictamnol.

Uses: Mutagenic, Vasorelaxant, plaque formation suppressant effects. Used in carbuncle and rashes.

469. *Digitalis lutea* *(Scrophulariaceae)*

Vernacular Name: *Eng:* Yellow foxglove.

Description: Erect perennial growing to 1m. Has narrow, lance-shaped leaves, and long spikes of yellow, bell-shaped flowers.

Habitate: Native to western and central Europe, this herb grows in woodland areas, hedgerows, and mountainous regions. It is cultivated for medicinal use in Russia.

Propagation: By seeds and vegetative method.

Parts Used: Leaves.

Chemical Constituents: Yellow foxglove contains cardiac glycosides. All act to strengthen the beating of a weakened heart.

Uses: Yellow foxglove is little employed in herbal medicine, but in fact it is a less toxic alternative to purple foxglove and wooly foxglove. It has similar medicinal actions but its alkaloids are more readily metabolized and flushed out by the body. Like other foxgloves, this plant supports and weakened or failing heart, increasing the strength of contraction, slowing and steadying the heart rate, and blowing blood pressure by strongly stimulating the production of urine, which reduces overall blood volume.

470. *Digitalis purpurea* *(Scrophulariaceae)*

Vernacular Name: *Eng:* Common foxglove, Purple foxglove.

Description: Perennial growing to 1.5 m. Has a single erect stem broad lance-shaped leaves and bell-shaped, purple-pink or white flowers in long spikes.

Habitate: This herb is native to western Europe. Though it is also cultivated, the wild plant is considered superior.

Propagation: By seeds and vegetative method.

Parts Used: Leaves.

Chemical Constituents: Foxglove contains cardiac glycosides, anthraquinones, flavonoids and saponins. Digitoxin rapidly strengthens the hearbeat, but is excreted very slowly. Digoxin is therefore preferred as a long-term medication.

Uses: Foxglove has a profound tonic effect on a diseased heart. Heart disease worsens when the heart's ability to maintain normal circulation decreases. Foxglove's cardiac glycosides enable the heart to beat more strongly, slowly and regularly without requiring more oxygen. At the same time it stimulates urine production, which lowers the volume of blood, and thus lessens the load on the heart.

471. *Dioscorea alata* L. *(Dioscoreaceae)*

Synonyms: *Dioscorea atropurpurea, Dioscorea purpurea, Dioscorea rubella* Roxb.

Vernacular Name: *San*: Alukam, Pindelu, *Eng*: Greater yam, Asiatic yam, *Hin*: Chupri alu, Khamalu, *Kan*: Tengugenasu, Heggenasu, *Mal*: Kaccil, Kavuttu, *Tam*: Perumvallikilanku, Kappan kaccil, *Tel:* Pendalamu.

Description: A climber with 4-winged stems twining to the right having scattered broad-based prickles and underground tubers without long stalks and of varying shapes; leaves opposite or rarely alternate, broadly ovate or rounded, cordate, with a broad sinus having five nerves; flowers unisexual, rachis of male spike winged; fruits capsules broadly obcordate, 2.5-4.5 cm wide.

Habitate: Throughout India, cultivated.

Propagation: By vegetative method.

Parts Used: Tubers.

Chemical Constituents: The tubers contain sucrose while leaves contain large quantities of D-fructose, D-glucose and the polyols, 2-deoxyribitol, 6-deoxysorbitol, and glycerol. The stem, roots and tubers contain varying quantities of D-fructose, D-glucose, sucrose and maltose which increase greatly during storage of tubers and decrease during the sprouting period. β-Amylase, peroxidase, pyruvate kinase phosphatase and o-diphenolase activities were observed furing sprouting in minisett yams.

Uses: The tubers are sweet, cooling, aphrodisiac, tonic, diuretic and anthelmintic and are useful in vitiated conditions of *pitta*, haemorrhoids, diabetes, leprosy, gonorrhoea, strangury and helminthiasis.

472. *Dioscorea batatas* Decne. *(Dioscoreaceae)*

Vernacular Name: *Eng:*-Chinese yam, cinnamon vine.

Description: Scandent, perennial, dioecious herb. Tuberous roots to 1 m long, cylindrical or flabellate, deep in ground. Stems long, climbing, twining clockwise, slightly angled, bearing small axillary tubers late in season. Leaves opposite, long-petiolate, deltoid-ovate, acuminiate, broadened into 2 lobes at base, purplish on petioles and nerves; bulbils in axils. Inflorescence in spikes, 1-3 in leaf axils. Flowers small, unisexual, sessile; the staminate erect, many-flowered, stamens 6; the pistillate pendulous, few-flowered. Fruit capsules broad than long; seeds encircled by 3 wings.

Habitate: Woody areas on mountain slopes in Korea, China and Japan.

Propagation: By vegetative method.

Parts Used: Tubers.

Chemical Constituents: Glycoproteins. Saponions, starch, arginine, choline, sterols, allantion, mannan, mucilages Steroids.

Uses: Blood sugar lowering, nutritive, antibacterial. Used in weakness, dyspepsia, furuncle and diarrhoea.

473. *Dioscorea bulbifera* L. *(Dioscoreaceae)*

Vernacular Name: *Eng:* Air potato; aerial yam; bulp-bearing yam.

Description: A perennial herb. Tubers variable, 3-10 cm in diameter. Bulbils numerous, irregular in shape, 1 cm or more across, brown, warty. Stem twining to the left. Leaves alternate, ovate-to-cordate, 7-14 cm long by 6-13 cm wide; apex acuminate, base deeply or broadly cordate; margin entire, 7-11 nerved, glabrous. Flowers in July-October, unisexual, dioecious. Capsule 1.8-2.2 cm long, oblong. Seeds winged at the base.

Habitate: In thickets in China, Japan.

Propagation: By seeds and vegetative method.

Part Used: Tubers.

Chemical Constituents: N.A.

Uses: Haemoptysis, epistaxis, pharyngitis, goiter, pyogenic infections, scrofula, orchitis, sprains and injuries.

474. *Dioscorea villosa* *(Dioscoreaceae)*

Vernacular Name: *Eng:* Wild Yam.

Description: A deciduous perennial vine, climbing to 6m, with heart-shaped leaves and tiny green flowers.

Habitate: Wild yam is native to North and Central America, and has now become naturalized in tropical, semi-tropical and temperate climates around the world.

Propagation: By seeds and vegetative method.

Parts Used: Roots and Tuber.

Chemical Constituents: Steroidal saponins, Phytosterols, Alkaloids, Tannins, Starch.

Uses: Antispasmodic, Anti-inflammatory, Antirheumatic, Increases sweating, Diuretic.

475. *Dioscorea zingiberensis* C.H.Wright *(Dioscoreaceae)*

Description: Glabrous ridig climber 5-10m. long. Rhizome creeping horizontally with rough dark-brown skin. Rootlets rigid. Leaves alternate, base sagittate; apex apiculate. Peptiole long, armed with prickles towards the base, inflorescence in long axillary spike; flowers small, purplish. Fruit 3-winged.

Habitate: Grows wild on the lower slopes of mountains, indigenous in south Viet Nam.

Propagation: By vegetative method.

Part Used: Rhizome.

Chemical Constituents: The rhizome contains diosgenin 2-2.5%.

Uses: Diosgenin is one of the principal materials for the sysnthesis of steriod drugs such as sex hormones, anti-inflammatory corticosteroids, contraceptive drugs and anabolic steriods.

476. *Dioscorea opposita* Thunb. *(Diosocoreaceae)*

Synonyms: *Diosorea batatas* Decaisne.

Vernacular Name: *Eng:* Chinese yam; yam; chinese potato.

Description: A twining perennial herb. Rootstock short, with a vertical thick fleshy cylindrical root, 1 m long by 2-7 cm in diamtter. The root is greyish-brown on the outside with numerous fibrous roots; the cut surface is white and viscid. Stem slender. Riged, usually purplish, glabrous. Leaves opposite or verticillate, petiolate; blades very variable in form, form triangular-ovate to triangular-broadly ovate, 3.5-7 cm long, usually 3-lobed, basal lobes rounded-auriculate, middle lobe acuminate, entire, 7-9 nerved.Flowers dioecious, in axillary spikes, solitary or geminate; June-August. Capsule triquetrous, compressed, winged.

Habitate: On sunny slopes, wild or cultivated in China, Indonesia, Japan, Korea, Malaysia, Philippines and other countries.

Propagation: By seeds and vegetative method.

Part Used: Roots.

Chemical Constituents: N.A.

Uses: Prolonged diarrhoea; chronic enteritis, cough and dyspnaea, seminal emissions; leucorrhoea.

477. *Diospyros candolleana* Wight *(Ebenaceae)*

Vernacular Name: *San*: Nila viruksha, *Kan*: Kare mara, *Mal*: Kari, *Tam*: Kari maram, *Tel:* Jagala ganti.

Description: Medium sized trees, 8-15 m tall, about 90 cm girth. *Bark* about 5 mm thick, surface black, smooth. *Wood* light pink with grey streaks. Branchlets sparsely hairy. *Leaves* alternate, oblong, 6-18 x 3-7 cm, base rounded or sub-truncate, apex shortly acuminate, margin entire, hairless, leathery, shiny; lateral nerves 8-10 pairs, indistinct; leaf stalks about 1 cm long. Flowers unisexual: *male flowers* in dense axillary clusters, pale yellow, about 8 mm across, densely yellowish brown tomentose; *female flowers* stalkless, in axillary clusters, about 1.2 cm long, about 8 mm across; corolla distinctly pot-shaped, greenish yellow. *Berries* conical or ovoid, pointed at apex, about 2.5 cm long, orange-yellow, hairy when young, hairless when ripe, smooth, shiny. *Seeds* 4, oblong, flat, shiny, with wrinkles.

Habitate: Moist deciduous to evergreen forests.

Propagation: By seeds and vegetative method.

Parts Used: Root and root bark.

Chemical Constituents: The bark contains β-sitosterol, 7-methyljuglone, and disopyrin while the wood contains isodiospyrin and a trinaphthaquinone xylopyrin. The roots also contain diospyrin, besides betulin and betulinic acid.

Uses: A decoction of root bark is used to cure joint pain and swelling.

478. *Diospyros malabarica* (Desr.) Kostel. *(Ebenaceae)*

Synonyms: *Disopyros peregrina.*

Vernacular Name: *San*: Tindukah, Tinduki, *Eng*: Gaub persimmon, Indian persimmon, *Hin*: Gabh, Tedu, Kalatendu, *Kan*: Holitupare, Kusarta, Bandadamara, *Mal*: Panacci, Pananci, Panacca, *Tam*: Paniccai, Panicika, *Tel:* Tinduki, Gabu, Tumikiecettu

Description: A medium sized spreading evergreen tree about 15 in height with dark grey or black bark, exfoliating in rectangular scales and young parts clothed with grey or tawny tomentum; leaves simple, alternate or subopposite, oblong, coriaceous, glabrous, main nerves oblique, reticulation prominent, bright red when young; flowers unisexual, males 3-12 together in panicles drooping cymes, females considerably longer than the males, solitary, subsessile; fruits ovoid or globose, yellow when ripe, fruiting calyx thickly coriaceous and flat; seeds compressed, 2-8, oblong, shiny.

Habitate: Throughout India, chiefly along streams, river banks and backwaters extending into the valleys of the Ghats.

Propagation: By seeds and vegetative method.

Parts Used: Bark, leaves, flowers, fruits.

Chemical Constituents: The ethyl acetate extract showed anti-stress and anti-ulcerogenic activity similar to ginseng. It also prevented hepatotoxicity and leucocytosis in experimental animals.

Uses: The bark is astringent, acrid, cooling, anti-inflammatory, constipating, depurative and febrifuge, and is useful in vitiated conditions of *pitta*, burning sensation, inflammations, diarrhoea, dysentery, leprosy, skin diseases, pruritus, dyspepsia, haemorrhags, burns, diabetes, fever, spermatorrhoea and vaginal disorders. The leaves are diuretic and aphrodisiac, and are useful in leucorrhoea, urethrorrhea, splenomegaly, nyctalopia, anaemia, and scabies. The fruits are bitter, acrid, cooling, digestive, carminative and oleaginous, and are useful in aphthae, pharyngodynia and vitiated conditions of *pitta* and *vata*.

479. *Diospyros paniculata* Dalz. *(Ebenaceae)*

Vernacular Name: *San*: Tinduka, *Kan*: Karikoomar, *Mal*: Karivella, Kari, Ilakatta, Kakka kari maram, *Tam*: Karunthovarai, *Tel:* Vasa, Vadaja.

Description: A medium sized tree, 10-18 m tall and 1-1.5 mgirth. *Bark* rough, black, often with grey blotches, about 8 mm thick. *Blaze* dull yellow Branchlets angular, pubescent, drooping. *Leaves* alternate, oblongto lanceolate, 7-20 x 3-7 cm, base rounded or acute, apex bluntly acuminate, margin entire, leathery, hairless; lateral nerves 5-9 pairs, with prominent reticulations; leaf stalks about 1.5 cm long. *Male* and female flowers seen in separate trees. *Male flowers* in branched axillary cymes, shortly stalked, greenish white, about 1 cm across, with a pair of bracts that are egg-shaped-heart-shaped, about 1 cm across, pubescent. *Female flowers* solitary or in 2-3 flowered axillary cymes, about 1.5 cm across, white, on about 2 cm long stalks and having bracts which are larger than that of male flowers. Calyx 5-lobed, each about 1.5 cm long, with reflexed margin. Corolla about 1 cm long, densely white hairy. *Berry* sub-globose to ovoid, about 3 x 2 cm, golden hairy, smooth, green.

Habitate: Moist deciduous to evergreen forests.

Propagation: By seeds and vegetative method.

Parts Used: Fruits.

Chemical Constituents: N.A.

Uses: Dried and powdered fruits are used to heal burns. A decoction of fruits treats gonorrhoea, biliousness. Also used to clean boils.

480. *Diplocyclos palmatus* (L.) Jeffrey *(Cucurbitaceae)*

Synonyms: *Bryonia laciniosa* Linn.

Vernacular Name: *San*: Lingini, *Hin*: Sivalingi, Isvaralingi, *Kan*: Lingatondi, *Mal*: Neyyunni, Sivalingakkaya, Neyyuruni, Aiviralikkova, Sivavalli, *Tam*: Sivalingakkay, Aiviralkkovai, *Tel:* Lingadauda.

Description: A slender much branched tendril climber, from a thick permanent root stock, tendrils 2-fid; leaves simple, alternate, membranous, 5-lobed, scabrid above, pale and smooth beneath deeply cordate at the base, margins sinuate, sometimes subserrate; flowers yellow, unisexual, males in small fascicles of 3-6, females solitary or few; fruits subsessile globose, smooth berry, brick-red when ripe with white vertical lines, seeds yellowish brown.

Habitate: Throughout India, on hedges and bushes upto 1,200 m elevation.

Propagation: By seeds and vegetative method.

Parts Used: Whole plant.

Chemical Constituents: N.A.

Uses: The plant is acrid, thermogenic, anti-inflammatory, foetid, alterant, depurative and tonic, and is useful in vitiated conditions of *pitta*, cough, flatulence, skin diseases, inflammations and general debility.

481. *Dipsacus fullonum* *(Dipsacaceae)*

Vernacular Name: *Eng:* Teasel.

Description: Perennial with a spiny ridged stem growing to 2m. Has lance-shaped leaves and lilac-coloured flowers blooming from hooked heads.

Habitate: Common throughout Europe and western Asia, teasel thrives on wasteground, roadsides and banks. It is cultivated only on a small scale. The root is unearthed in late summer.

Propagation: By seeds and vegetative method.

Parts Used: Root.

Chemical Constituents: Teasel contains inulin, bitter substances and a scabioside.

Uses: Teasel root is little used medicinally today, and it therapeutic applications are disputed. It is thought to have diuretic, sweat-inducing and stomach-soothing properties, cleansing the system and improving digestion. Due to its apparent astringency, teasel is considered helpful in diarrhoea. It is also thought to increase appetite, to tone the stomach, and to act on the liver, helping with jaundice and gallbladder problems.

482. *Dipsacus japonicus* Miq. *(Dipsaceae)*

Description: Annual herbaceous plant 60-90 cm. High roots tuberous, solitary, 10-15cm. Long stems obscurely angular and sparsely spinous. Leaves opposite, margins toothed, the lower deeply loved, the upper entire, inflorescence in dense, long-stalked, cylindrical head, aurrounded by an involucre of strong and wiry bracts; flowers white. Achene 4-angled, glabrous.

Habitate: Common weed of savannas at an altitude of 1000 m. and above.

Propagation: By seeds and vegetative method.

Part Used: Roots.

Chemical Constituents: The roots contain alkaloids, tannins and sugars.

Uses: The roots possess tonic, anodyne and demulcent properties. They are effective in th treatment of lumbago, rheumatism, osteodynia, chilblains, spermatorrhoea, metrorrhoea, colic in pregancy, hepatic and renal hypofunction, ascities, trauma, sprains, closed fractures and furunculosis. They are also galactagogic and haemostatic.

483. *Dipterocarpus indicus* Bedd. *(Dipterocarpaceae)*

Synonyms: *Dipterocarpus turbinatus.*

Vernacular Name: *Hin*: Guya, *Kan*: Yenne mara, Dhuma, Guga, *Mal*: Kal payin, Velayini, *Tam*: Enney.

Description: A lofty evergreen upper canopy tree, reaching to a height of 30 m or even more. Crown round shaped. Trunk pillar-like, straight, undivided, up to 20 m long and about 4 m girth. Bark 8-10 mm thick, surface yellowish brown, mottled with grey and white, smooth, exfoliating into irregular flakes, brittle, exuding resin when cut freshly. Blaze creamy chocolate yellow. Young shoots with fine and short hairs. Leaves alternate, egg-shaped, 15 to 25 cm x 6-17 cm, tip acute or acumiate, base rounded or slightly heart-shaped, margin entire and wavy, hairless; lateral nerves 10-15 pairs, prominent below, parallel. Stipules covering the terminal leaf buds are egg-shaped, acute, softly hair, about 2 cm long; leaf stalk 3-5 cm long, hairy. Flowers white with a pink shade, fragrant, about 5 cm across, in 3 to 8 flowered axillary racemes. Stamens numerous, stalks yellow. Fruit is a non-splitting nut, about 1.5 cm across, brown, sub-globose, hairless, enclosed by two enlarged prominent calyx lobes and three smaller ones known as wings. Wings about 12 cm long and 3 cm across, strongly 3-5 nerved.

Habitate: Tropical semi-evergreen to evergreen forests.

Propagation: By seeds and vegetative method.

Parts Used: Gum.

Chemical Constituents: From the termiticidal fraction of the resin, four sesquiterpenoids were isolated and characterized. The major constituent was α-gurjuene.

Uses: The oleoresin is used for treating rheumatic complaints.

484. Disporopsis aspera (Hua) Engl. ex Krause. *(Liliaceae)*

Description: Perennial herb, 20-50cm. High, withering every year in winter. Rhizome slinder, creeping horizontal, pale-yellow. Leaves alternate, subsessile, coriaceous, dark-green above, pale beneath. Inflorescence in axillary bi-flowered raceme; flowers white, campanulate. Berry globose, dark-violet when ripe.

Habitate: Grows wild in damp places in the highlands.

Propagation: By vegetative method.

Part Used: Rhizomes.

Chemical Constituents: N.A.

Uses: The rhizome is tonic and is ued in general debility, persistent feber, hyperhidrosis, night sweats, polyuria, spermatorrhoea, dry cough and thrist. It is prescribed on its own or in combination with other plants.

485. *Disporopsis longifolia* Caraib *(Liliaceae)*

Description: Perennial herb, about 1 m. high. Stems glabrous, erect, spotted with red. Rhizome stout, horizontal with hollow scar resembling a cup. Leaves alternate, ovate, flowers white, campanulate, axillary. Berry globose, dark-violet when ripe.

Habitate: Grows wild in wet places in mountainous regions.

Propagation: By vegetative method.

Part Used: Rhizomes.

Chemical Constituents: N.A.

Uses: The rhizome has tonic and anodyne properties. It is used in general debility, fatigue, anorezia, lumbago, artharlgia and dry throat. It may be used on its own or in combination with certain other plants.

486. *Dolichos biflorus* L. *(Fabaceae)*

Vernacular Name: *San*: Kulitha, *Hin:* Kulthi.

Description: The plant is common twining creeper, the seeds are small, grayish brown and flattened.

Habitate: Native to most parts of India, and is found upto altitudes of 1000m.

Propagation: By seeds and vegetative method.

Parts Used: Seeds.

Chemical Constituents: The seeds are poor in amino acid content, but rish in urease. A new and nonspecific lectin having the inner carbohydrate moiety as N-acetyl glucosamine, N-β-glycosidically linked to aspargine has been isolated from the seeds of *D. biflorus.* The lectin is not specific for human cells, but agglutinated erythrocytes from other vertebrate species.

Uses: Urolithiasis, dysuria, bleeding piles. In patients with oedema, a diuretic effect has been shown. As a home remedy, kulitha has been used in dysuria, bleeding piles, vaginal bleeding, epistaxis and leucorrhoea. Its use in reducing obesity is also recognized. In dysuria it works due to its diuretic property. It is also used to reduce crystalluria and to lyse stones. The powdered seeds are used as a poultice to induce sweating.

487. *Dolichos lablab* L. *(Fabaceae)*

Vernacular Name: *Eng:* Egyptian kidney bean, purple hyacinth bean, lablab bean, bonavist bean; *Hin:* Sem; *Beng:* Shim; *Tel:* Chikkudu; *Tam:* Avarai; *Kan:* Chapparada avare and *Mal:* Avara.

Description: Perennial twining plant; stems green or pale purple, covered with hairs while uoung. Leaves alternate, grifoliate, slightly hairy. Inflorescence in axillary raceme; flowers white. Pod flat, incurved with remains of persistent style. Seeds reniform, whitish.

Habitate: Cultivated every where for its edible young pods and medically useful fully ripe seeds.

Propagation: By seeds and vegetative method.

Part Used: Seeds.

Chemical Constituents: The seeds contain hydrocarbons, proteins, lipids, amino acids: tryptophan, arginine, tyrosine, tyrosinase; vitamins A,B_1,B_2,C; hydrocyanic acid, and slats of Ca,P,Fe.

Uses: The seeds are considered to be nutritious. They are also angiferile and depurative. They are effective in cases of sunstroke, nausea, vomiting, diarrhoea, enteritis, abdominal pains, alcoholism or aresenism. For sore throat the juice of fresh leaves is administered by mouth.

488. *Dorema ammoniacum* *(Apiaceae)*

Vernacular Name: *Eng:* Ammoniacum.

Description: Very large perennial herb growing to a height of 3 m, with a stout stem, compound leaves and umbels of white flowers.

Habitate: Ammoniacum is native to central Asia, Iran and northern Russia.

Propagation: By seeds and vegetative method.

Parts Used: Oleo-gum-resin.

Chemical Constituents: Ammoniacum contains a resin, gum, volatile oil, free salicylic acid and coumarins.

Uses: Used in both western and Indian medicine, amouniacum is still listed in the *British Pharmacopoeia* as an antispasmodic and as an expectorant that stimulates the coughing up of thick mucus. It is a specific treatment for chronic bronchitis, asthma and persistent coughs. ammoniacum is also occasionally used to induce sweating or menstruation.

489. *Dorstenia contrayerva* *(Urticaceae)*

Vernacular Name: *Eng:* Contrayerva.

Description: Stemless perennial herb growing to 30 cm. Has palm-shaped leaves and long-stalked greenish flowers.

Habitate: Native to Central and South America and the Caribbean island, contrayerva is generally gathered from the wild.

Propagation: By Seeds and vegetative method.

Parts Used: Rhizome.

Chemical Constituents: N.A.

Uses: Contrayerva rhizome is considered aromatic, stimulant and sweat-inducing. Occasionally used in the early stages of serious fevers such as typhoid, it is also given for gastro-intestinal problems such as diarrhoea and dysentery. There is no scientific substantiation of its reputation as an antidote.

490. Dracaena cambodiana Pierr ex Gagnep. *(Liliaceae)*

Vernacular Name: *Eng:* Dragon tree.

Description: Small tree, 2-4m. high. Stems erect, occasionally woody at the base, hollow and brownish-red. Leaves linear with lax sheath and entire margins, crowded in bundles at the end of the branch. Inflorescence in terminal compound raceme; flowers yellowish-green. Berry globose, red when ripe, single-seeded.

Habitate: Grows wild, usually in rocky localities.

Propagation: By seeds and vegetative method.

Part Used: Red wood obtained from the foot of the tree.

Chemical Constituents: N.A.

Uses: The woody part of the stem is a blood circulation stimulant and demulcent remedy. It is used to treat contusions, blood stasis, menstrual haematometra, rheumatism, paresis, lumbago and osteodynia, An alcholic maceration of the mixture with Cinnamomum casia is used externally as a liniment.

491. *Drosera indica* L. *(Droseraceae)*

Vernacular Name: *Kan*: Krimi nashini, *Mal*: Theeppullu, Akara puda, *Tam*: Azhu kanni, Olukanni, Ottunni, Kosu otti,.

Description: A slender erect tuberous herb, 3-15 cm tall, glandular-pubescent throughout, usually unbranched. *Tubers* single, very small. *Leaves* are of two types: the basal leaves are clustered just above the soil surface, deflexed, up to 2.5 cm long; the upper leaves alternate, narrow, linear, 2-3 cm long, with many sticky glandular tentacles above and hairless below. *Flowers* 5-15, arranged in lateral racemes, about 5 mm across, pink to rose. *Capsules* ovoid, minute.

Habitate: Among grasses, in open moist rocky areas from plains to grassy slopes of higher altitudes.

Propagation: By seeds and vegetative method.

Parts Used: Whole plant.

Chemical Constituents: The leaves contain the nephthaquinones, plumbagin, droserone and hydroxdroserone, the flavonoids, quercetin, gossypetin, gosspin and isogossypitin.

Uses: This plant is considered to be a rejuvenating herb and more widely used in Alchemy. Also used to cure corns.

492. *Drosera peltata* J.E.Sm. ex Willd. *(Droseraceae)*

Synonyms: *Drosera lunata* Buch. ham.

Vernacular Name: *Hin*: Mukhajali, chitra, *Mal*: Theeppullu, *Tam*: Kosu otti.

Description: A delicate erect tuberous herb, 10-20 cm tall, occasionally branched near the top. *Tubers* round, smooth, solid, reddish, about 1 cm across. Leaves are of two types: the *lower leaves* are spoon-shaped and arranged in whorls just above the soil surface; the *upper leaves* are alternate, crescent-shaped, peltate, about 5 mm across, with many tentacular projections. *Tentacles* are about 3 mm long, stalked, with sticky glands at tip that secretes sticky glistening liquid and arranged along the leaf margins; leaf stalks very slender, 1-2 cm long, curved. *Flowers* bisexual, about 1 cm across, white, usually 2-8 in terminal and lateral racemes, which are about 5 cm long. *Capsules* globose, about 6 mm across.

Habitate: Along open grassy slopes and moss-clad dripping rocks of higher altitudes.

Propagation: By seeds and vegetative method.

Parts Used: Leaves.

Chemical Constituents: The leaves contain the nephthaquinones, plumbagin, droserone and hydroxdroserone, the flavonoids, quercetin, gossypetin, gosspin and isogossypitin.

Uses: This plant is used in Siddha and Folk medicine. Leaves are used to cure blisters as well as antisyphillitic and tonic.

493. *Drosera rotundifolia* *(Droseraceae)*

Vernacular Name: *Eng:* Sundew.

Description: Evergreen, insectivorous perennial growing to 15 cm. Has small white flowers. The hinged, spoon-shaped leaves edged with spines secrete a sticky fluid which traps insects. They are digested when the leaf closes.

Habitate: Sundew grows in Europe, Asia and North America, and is found in marshy ground at altitudes up to 1,800 m.

Propagation: By seeds and vegetative method.

Parts Used: Arial parts.

Chemical Constituents: Sundew contain naphthaquinones, enzymes, flavonoids and volatile oil. The naphthaquinones are volatile oil. The naphthaquinones are antimicrobial, antispasmodic and also cough-suppressing.

Uses: Sundew is of greatest value in the treatment of spasmodic chest conditions such as whooping cough, bronchial asthma and asthma. In relaxing the muscles of the respiratory tract, the plant eases breathing relieves wheezing and lessens the spasms of the whooping cough. Commonly mixed with thyme in a syrup, sundew is a helpful remedy for coughs in children. The herb is also prescribed for gastric problems.

494. *Dryopteris crassirhizoma* Nakai *(Polypodiaceae)*

Vernacular Name: *Eng*: Crown wood-fern.

Description: Perennial fern, with rhizomes short and stout. Fronds deciduous; blades oblanceolate to broadly oblanceolate, 40-100 cm long, 15-25 cm wide, acuminate, bipinnate; pinnae many, herbaceous, linear-lanceolate, 15-30 mm wide, acuminate, sessile; pinnules narrowly oblong, 2.5-5 mm wide, obtuse, crenate. Sori dorsal on veins, in 2 raws on lower half of pinnules, round; indusia orbicular-reniform, 1.2 mm across, attached by the inner end of the sinus.

Habitate: Shaded and damp places in forests in Korea, China and Japan.

Propagation: By vegetative method.

Parts Used: Rhizome.

Chemical Constituents: Aspidinol, aspidin, albaspidine, filmalone, filicinic acid, filicin, filicic acid. Flavaspidic acid, dryocrassin ABBP, dryocrassin, dryocrassol, diplopterol, norhopane derivatives.

Uses: Anthelmintic action. Parasiticide to tapeworm and hookworm.

495. *Dryopteris filix-mas* (L.) Schoot. *(Polypodiaceae)*

Vernacular Name: *Eng:* Male-fern.

Description: A deciduous perennial herb with stout oblique rhizomes upto 2.5 cm. in diameter appearing much large due to many matted fibres forming a tufty head, blackish and scaly, with numerous long slightly branched, filiform roots. Leaves 30-90 cm. long, bi-pinnate, erect, appearing like a plume, bearing, 20-40 pairs of pinnae, each about 15 cm long having 20-30 pairs of pinnules, which are oblong, incurved serrated towards tips which are blunt. Sori eight to ten, present in the lower 2/3rd of each pinnule; each with a reniform indusia attached by notch to veinlet. Blades glandless and sori glandless.

Habitate: Europe, particularly in U.K. and U.S.A.

Propagation: By vegetative method.

Parts Used: Rhizome.

Chemical Constituents: Filicin; Filmarone; Filicic acid; Aspidinol; Flavaspidic acid; Flavaspidinol; Albaspidin.

Uses: Used as a great vermifuge. For worm symptoms, especially with constipation. Tapeworms. Soporific conditions. Torpid inflammation of lymphatic glands. Blindness. Worm colic with itching of nose, pale face, blue rings around eyes. Gnawing pain in abdomen with diarrhoea and vomiting.

496. *Drypetes roxburghii* (Wall.) Huresawa *(Euphorbiaceae)*

Synonyms: *Putranjiva roxburghii* Wall.

Vernacular Name: *San*: Putrajivah, Putranjivah, *Hin*: Jivputrak, Jiyapota, *Kan*: Aman, Putranjiva, *Mal*: Puttilanni, Putranjivi, Ponkalam, *Tam*: Kattuppacceri maram, Karuvilai, *Tel:* Putrajivika, Kuduru

Description: A moderate–sized evergreen tree upto 12 m in height with pendant branches and dark grey bark having horizontal lenticels; leaves simple, alternate, dark green, shiny, elliptic-oblong, distantly serrulate, main nerves numerous; male flowers very shortly pedicellate in rounded axillary clusters, female flowers 1-3 in an axil, ovary finely silky, 3-celled, styles 3, recurved, stigmas crescent-shaped; fruits ellipsoid or rounded drupes, white tomentose; seed normally one, stone pointed, rugose, very hard.

Habitate: Throughout India, in shandy valleys, in areas upto 900 m elevation.

Propagation: By seeds and vegetative method.

Parts Used: Leaves, seeds.

Chemical Constituents: The oil contain isopropyl and 2-butyl iso-thiocyanates as the main constituents, and 2-methyl-butyl iso-thiocyanate as a minor component; the isothiocyanates are produced on enzymic hydrolysis of glucosidic progenitors present in the kernels, viz. glucoputranjivin,glucocochlearin and glucojiaputin, respectively. An additional glucoside, glucocleomin, has been identified in the seed kernels; on enzymic hydrolysis it affords a non-volatile mustard oil, cleomin. A glucosidic pattern similar to that in the seeds is reported in the shoots and roots.

Uses: The leaves are refrigerant and procreant and are useful in catarrh, fever and sterility.

The seeds are sweet, acrid, procreant, refrigerant, ophthalmic laxative, anti-inflammatory, aphrodisiac and diuretic, and are useful in vitiated conditions of *vata* and *pitta,* burning sensation, hyperdipsia, ophthalmopathy, constipation, elephantiasis, inflammations, strangury, azoospermia, habitual abortion and sterility.

497. *Duboisea myoporoides* R. Br. *(Solanaceae)*

Vernacular Name: *Eng:* Australian Mgmeo.

Description: A tall shrub or small tree, quite glabrous. Leaves alternate, obovate-oblong to oblong-lanceolate, spoon-shaped, obtuse or rarely acute, entire slightly revolute at margins, with petiole 5-10 cm. long. Flowers white or pale arranged in terminal centrifugal panicles, which may become sometimes leafy at base, usually much branched, broadly pyramidal or corymbose. Bracts minute, Calyx 2-lipped campanulate with obtuse teeth. Corolla white or pale, obtuse, short lobed. Stamens 4, didynamous; stamens included in the tube. Fruit an indehiscent black berry, small and nearly globular.

Habitate: New South Wales and Queensland, Australia.

Propagation: By seeds and vegetative method.

Parts Used: Leaf.

Chemical Constituents: Hyoscine, hyoscyamine, Tigloidine, Valeroidine, Poroidine, Isoporoidine, L-anabasine, DL-isopelletierine, Valtropine, Scopolamine, Atropine, Noratropine, Tropine, butropine and Apohyoscine.

Uses: Used as Hypnotic, intoxicant, mydriatic and sedative. For complaints of eye afflictions especially when a red spot interferes with vision, morbid dilation of pupils conjunctivitis, both acute and chronic, paralysis of accommodation of eyes, red fundus, engorgement of eye vessels with dim vision and severe pain. Locomotor ataxia.

498. *Dysoxylum malabaricum* Bedd. ex Hiem *(Meliaceae)*

Vernacular Name: *San*: Agaru, *Kan*: Bile agilu, Bile devadaaru, *Mal*: Vellagil, Akil, *Tam*: Vellaiyagil, Agil.

Description: Large trees, reaching 35 m tall and around 3 m girth, with a straight long cylindrical stem. *Bark* pale grey, rough, fissured, covered with white warty lenticles, exfoliating into large flakes; outer bark grey. *Blaze* creamy to white, fragrant. *Wood* yellow or light orange hard. Leaves alternate, 30-45 cm long, odd-pinnate; rachis angular *leaflets* opposite or alternate, 7-11, elliptic-oblong to inverted egg-shaped or lanceolate, 10-23 x 4-5 cm, base unequal, apex acuminate, margin entire, hairless, with short stalks; lateral nerves 9-20 pairs, prominent beneath. *Flowers* bisexual, in axillary panicles, 5-8 mm long, fragrant white to greenish yellow, distinctly stalked. Panicles 10-20 cm long crowded near the tip of branchlets. *Capsules* pear-shaped, 5-7 cm long, with 4-vertical furrows, bright yellow when ripe, with a brown fleshy rind. *Seeds* 3-4, bluntly 3-angled.

Habitate: Evergreen and semi-evergreen forests.

Propagation: By seeds and vegetative method.

Parts Used: Wood, wood oil.

Chemical Constituents: The stem bark contains an alkaloid, rohitukine possessing anti-inflammatory and immunomodulatory property. The fruits contain a tetranortriterpene, dysobinin showing mild anti-inflammatory acitivty.

Uses: In Siddha this plant is known as *Agil* and used as a substitute for *Aquilaria malaccensis*. The uses are similar to *D. binectariferum*. Wood is used to cure rheumatism; wood oil is used in treating ear and eye diseases.

499. *Echinaceae angustifolia & E. purpurea* *(Asteraceae)*

Vernacular Name: *Eng:* Echinaceae, Purple coneflower.

Description: A perennial growing to 50cm, with daisy-like pruple flowers, and leaves covered in coarse hair.

Habitate: Native to central parts of the US, Echinacea, particularly *E. purpurea,* which is easier to grown, is now commercially cultivated in Europe and the US. Grown from seed in spring or by root division in winter, it thrives best in rich, *San*dy soil.

Propagation: By seeds and vegetative method.

Parts Used: Flower and Roots.

Chemical Constituents: Alkamides, Caffeic acid ester, Polysaccharides, Volatile oil, Echinolone, Betaine.

Uses: Immune stimulant, anti-inflammatory, Antibiotic, Detoxifying, Increases sweating, Heals wounds, Anti-allergenic.

500. *Echinops latifolius* Tausch *(Asteraceae)*

Vernacular Name: *Eng:* Broad-leaved globe-thistle.

Description: A perennial herb with dense white-tomentose foliage. Stem erect, simple up to 1 m high. Leaves alternate, elliptic, 4-10 cm long by 2-6 cm wide, pinnatifid, spinous. Heads in globose involucrate solitary balls, 2-3.5 cm in diameter, blue sessile or shortly stipitate on a common receptacle, 1-flowered; flowers hermaphrodite, all fertile. Involucre oblongl bracts multi-seriate, rigid, pungent, some spinescent, outer shorter, inner spatulat, innermost linear or lanceolate, sometimes all connate into the tube with 1 rigid spine on the outer side. Achenes elongate, subterete or tetragonal, villous.

Habitate: Grows on sunny slopes, at roadsides and in grassland in China, Mongolia.

Propagation: By seeds and vegetative method.

Part Used: Roots.

Chemical Constituents: N.A.

Uses: Acute mastitis; obstruction of milk secretion, skin inflammation, Haemorrhoids.

501. *Echinops setifer* L. *(Asteraceae)*

Vernacular Name: *Eng:* Globe thistle.

Description: Perennial herb, to 1 m tall, branched above; the whole plant covered with whitish hair. Leaves alternate; radical leaves long-petiolate, deeply pinnately dissected, margins prickly; stem leaves sessile, long elliptic, 15-25 cm long, pinnately dissected 5-6 times. Heads of 1 flower within its own involucre; the outer involucral bracts bristlelike; the inner bracts linear; the individual heads aggregated into a dense globose compound head subtended by a small, common, reflexed involucre. Flowers all tubular, bluish purple. Achenes 4-angled, hairy, pappus of many inconspicuous scales.

Habitate: Open grassy areas of Korea.

Propagation: By seeds and vegetative method.

Parts Used: Root.

Chemical Constituents: Echinopsine.

Uses: Weak antitumour, antidote, menostasis, emmenagogue.

502. *Echium vulgare* *(Boraginaceae)*

Vernacular Name: *Eng:* Viper's Bugloss.

Description: Abundantly hairy perennial growing up to 1 m. Has narrow prickly leaves and pink to violet clusters of flowers in dense spikes.

Habitate: Native to Europe, viper's bugloss is commonly found on uncultivated land, by roadsides, and in low-lying and coastal regions.

Propagation: By seeds and vegetative method.

Parts Used: Flowers.

Chemical Constituents: Viper's bugloss contains pyrrolizidine alkaloids, allantoin, alkannins and mucilage. In isolation, pyrrolizidine alkaloids are toxic to the liver. The alkannins are antimicrobial and allntoin helps wounds to heal.

Uses: In many respects, viper's bugloss is similar to borage in that both herbs have a sweat-inducing and diuretic effect if taken internally. Viper's bugloss has also been taken to treat chest conditions, as its mucilage soothes dry coughs and encourages expectoration. The significant mucilage content in viper's bugloss has also proved helpful in treating skin conditions. Prepared in a poultice or plaster, it is an effective balm herb has fallen out of use, due partly to lack of interest in tits medicinal potential, and partly to its pyrrolizidine alkaloids, which is isolation are toxic.

503. *Eclipta alba* *(Asteraceae)*

Vernacular Name: *San*: Bhrangarajah, Tekarajah, *Eng*: Trailing eclipta, *Hin*: Bhamgra, Mocakand, Babri, *Kan*: Garagada soppu, *Mal*: *Kannunni*, Kayyonni, Kayyunni, *Tam*: Kayyantakara, Kaikesi, *Tel:* Galagara, Guntagalijeru.

Description: Perennial herb, erect or prostrate, 30-40 cm. High. Stems green or purple, bristly, thickened at the nodes. Leaves opposite, subsessile, lanceolate-oblong, denticulate, hirsute on both sides. Flowers white in axillary or terminal head; the female radiated, the bisexual in the centre. Achene 3–angled, slightly flattened.

Habitate: Throughout India, at all elevations in waste places and on road sides.

Propagation: By seeds and vegetative method.

Parts Used: Whole plant.

Chemical Constituents: Thiophene derivatives. The co-occurrence of mono-, di-and trithiophene acetylenes together with α-terthienyl in this species is noteworthy. The petroleum ether extract of aerial parts contains a terthienyl aldehyde, ecliptal besides stigmasterol and β-sitosterol, the aerial parts also contain 2-an-geloyloxy methylene-5'-dithiophene, 5'–isovaleryloxy methylene-2-dithiophene. The roots are very rich in thiophene acetylenes. They contain the dithiophene derivatives 5'-seneocioyl oxymehtylene-2-dithiopene, and 5'tigloy-loxymethylene-2-dithiophene in addition to 2-5-thiophene.

Uses: The plant is bitter, acrid, thermogenic, alterative, anti-inflammatory, anthelmintic, anodyne, vulnerary, ophthalmic, digestive, carminative, haematinic, diuretic, aphrodisiac, trichogenous, deobstruant, depurative and febrifuge, and is useful in hepatosplenomeglay, elephantiasis, inflammations, vitiated conditions of *vata*, gastropathy, anorexia, helminthiasis, skin diseases, wounds, ulcers, ophthalmopathy, debility, hypertension, strangury, leprosy, pruritus, fever, jaundice, odontalgia, otalgia and cephalalgia. It is good for blackening and strengthening of the hair, for stopping haemorrhages and fluxes, and for strengthening the gums. The seeds are good for increasing sexual vigour.

504. *Eclipta prostrata* L. *(Asteraceae)*

Vernacular Name: *Eng*: Eclipta.

Description: Erect strigose-pilose annual herb, 10-60 cm tall. Leaves opposite, lanceolate, 3-10 cm long, 5-25 mm wide, acuminate, sessile or short-petiolate, serrulate, densely strigose-pilose on both sides. Heads terminal on stem and branches or axillary, 1 cm across, with pedicel 2-4.5 cm long; involucre companulate, 5 mm long, 6-7 mm across; phyllaries 5-6, green oblong. Ray flowers white, 2.5-3 mm long, 0.4 mm wide, fertile. Disc flowers bisexual, fertile, white, 4-lobed; anthers very shortly bifid at base. Achenes 2.8 mm long, 3-angled in ray flowers, compressed and 4-angled in disc florets.

Habitate: Wet places in fields in Korea, Japan and China.

Propagation: By seeds and vegetative method.

Parts Used: Whole plant.

Chemical Constituents: Eliptine, wedelactones, thiophene-derivatives.

Uses: Antidote for snake venom, antihepatotoxic, anti-inflammatory. Used in eruption, leucorrhoea, enterohaemorrhage.

505. *Elaeocarpus sphaericus* (Gaertn.) K. Schum. *(Elaeocarpaceae)*

Synonyms: *Elaeocarpus ganitrus* Roxb.

Vernacular Name: *San*: Rudraksah, *Eng*: Utrasum-bead tree, *Hin*: Rudraki, Rudraks, *Kan*: Rudraksa, *Mal*: Rudraksam, *Tam*: Ruttiratcam, *Tel:* Rudraksi.

Description: A medium sized evergreen tree with a spreading handsome crown; leaves simple, oblong-lanceolate, sub-entire, or irregularly crenate, decurrent into the petiole, glabrous, acute or acuminate; flowers white, in dense racemes in old leaf axils, stamens about 40 in groups, opposite each petal, anthers linear, one valve tipped at the apex with a small tuft of glistening hairs; fruits globose, or somewhat obovoid purple drupes, stone tubercled, longitudinally grooved, generally 5-celled and 5-seeded.

Habitate: Bihar, Bengal, Assam, Maharashtra and Madhya Pradesh.

Propagation: By seeds and vegetative method.

Parts Used: Fruits, seeds kernel.

Chemical Constituents: N.A.

Uses: The fruits are sour, thermogenic, appetiser and sedative, and are useful in cough, bronchitis, neuralgia, cephalalgia, anorexia, epileptic fits, manic conditions and other brain disorders, and vitiated conditions of *kapha* and *vata*. P.V. Sharma (Darvyagunavijnan, 7th edition-1983) mentions that the fruit stone (seed kernel) is sweet, cooling, emollient, cerebral sedative, expectorant, liver tonic and febrifuge, and is useful in epileptic fits, melancholia, manic conditions, mental disorders, convulsions, insomnia, cephalalgia, hepatopathy, hypertension, bronchitis, fever and vitiated conditions of *kapha* and *vata*.

506. *Elephantopus scaber* L. *(Asteraceae)*

Vernacular Name: *San*: Hastipadi, Gojihva, *Eng*: Prickly leaves elephant's foot, *Hin*: Gobhi, Gojivha, *Kan*: Hakkarike, *Mal*: Anayatiyan, Anaccuvati, *Tam*: Yanaiccuvati, *Tel:* Hastikaraka.

Description: A rigid herb, usually perennial with short root stock; leaves obovate-oblong, mostly radical forming a spreading rosette on the ground, hairy on both surfaces, 12.5-20 cm long and 3.8-5.7 cm broad; flowers purple in heads, heads numerous, closely packed; fruits achenes, pappus of 4-6 bristles dilated at the base.

Habitate: Throughout India, especially in dry localities.

Propagation: By seeds and vegetative method.

Parts Used: Roots, leaves, flowers.

Chemical Constituents: The plant contains hydroxylated germacrianolides, molephantin and molephantinin having cytotoxic and antitumour properties. Phantomolin and its *cis*-epoxide, which exhibit potent inhibitory action on Ehrlich ascitis carcinoma and on Walker 256 carcinosarcoma cells. It also contains elephantin, elephantopin, deoxyelephantopin, iso-deoxyelephantopin and 11,13-dihydrodeoxyelephantopin alongwith α-curcumene, β-amyrin, lupeol, epifriedelanol and stigmasterol.

Uses: The plant is bitter, acrid, astringent, antipyretic constipating, diuretic and tonic. A decoction of the roots and leaves is given dysuria, urethrorrhea, intermittent fevers, diarrhoea and bronchitis. The root decoction is specific for haemorrhoids and a paste made out of leaves is very specific for skin diseases. The flowers are astringent, bitter, sweet, ophthalmic aphrodisiac and expectorant, and are recommended for vitiated conditions of *pitta*, hepatopathy ophthalmopathy, bronchitis, cough and swellings.

507. *Elettaria cardamomum* Maton *(Scitaminaceae)*

Vernacular Name: *San:* Ela-suksmakila-ksudraila; *Eng:* Cardamom, lesser cardamom; *Hin:* Choti Ilayachi; *Beng*: Chot Elach; *Tem*: Illai; *Tel:* Illai.

Description: Rootsock woody or fleshy, branching; stem 1.8-2.7 meters high, clothed below with spongy sheaths. Leaves subsessile, oblong-lanceolate, bracts, linear-oblong, fruits capsules, sub-globose or oblong, marked with many fine vertical ribs.

Habitate: Cultivated in South India.

Propagation: By seeds and vegetative method.

Part Used: Fruits, seeds.

Chemical Constituents: The major components identified in the essential oil are cineole, linalool, terpinayl acetate, d-limonene, a-terpineol, a-and b-pinenes, terpene-4-ol, geranoil and geranyl acetate. In addition, lina lylacetate, sabinene, methyl heptanone, myrcene and a-terpinene are also present.

Uses: Cardamom is used as a culinary flavouring either whole or ground or as seeds. As a spice it is used in a variety of processed foods like spiced rice, meat and vegetable dishes, baked goods including cakes, buns, pastries and bread. As a powder, it is used as an ingredient in curry powder, ausage products, soups, canned fish, etc. It can be sprinkled on fresh fruits like apples, peaches, melons, and bananas. It is used for flavouring coffee, tea and to a small extent tobacco. Cardamom seed oil, as also an oleoresin prepared from the seeds find application in flavouring processed foods generally of intended short shelf-life. It is also used in cordials, bitters and liqueurs.

508. *Elettaria cardamomum* Maton *(Zingiberaceae)*

Vernacular Name: *San*: Sla, Trutih, *Eng*: Cardamom, *Hin*: Elaci, *Kan*: Elakki, *Mal*: Elam, Cittelam, *Tam*: Elam, *Tel:* Elakkayalu.

Description: A tall herbaceous perennial with subterranean branching root stock, 1.5-5 m in height; leaves subsessile, elliptic or lanceolate with sheathing base; flowers in panicles which are many for a plant arising from the base of the vegetative shoots, upright first and becoming prostrate, lip of the corolla white, streaked with violet; fruits trilocular, subglobose capsules, marked with many fine vertical ribs, seeds 15-20 per pod, brownish black covered by a thin mucilaginous membrane.

Habitate: Throughout India, cultivated.

Propagation: By seeds and vegetative method.

Parts Used: Seeds, oil.

Chemical Constituents: The seeds contain palmitic and oleic as dominant fatty acids, besides linoleic and linolenic acids, alongwith α-tocopherol, desmosterol and campesterol. 1,8-Cineole gives a harsh 'eucalyptol' smell to the oil if present in high proportion. α-pinene, β-pinene, α-terpinene, α-terpineol, α-terpinyl acetate, terpinene-4-ol, borneol, nerol, nerolidol, -nerolidol, geraniol, geranyl acetate, linalool and linalyl acetate.

Uses: The seeds are aromatic, acrid, sweet, cooling, stimulant, carminative, digestive, stomachic, diuretic, cardiotonic, abortifacient, alexeteric, expectorant and tonic, and are useful in asthma, bronchitis, haemorrhoids, strangury, renal and vesical calculi, halitosis, cardiac disorders, anorexia, dyspepsia, gastropathy, hyperdipsia, burning sensation, debility and vitiated conditions of *vata*. Cardamom oil is used in several pharmaceutical preparations.

509. *Eleusine indica* (L.) Gaertn. *(Asteraceae)*

Vernacular Name: *Eng:* Crowfoot grass, dog's tail grass, crabgrass, wire grass; *Hin:* Mandla and *Tam:* Thipparagi.

Description: Annual herb; stems erect or ocassionally prostrate in tufts, 30-60cm high leves loricate, narrow, arranged in two rows; the blade glabrous; sheath hairy. Inflorescence in whorl of 5-7 digitate spikes, with single spikelet or two spikelets seperated below. Fruit oblong, nearly trigonal.

Habitate: Common weed on pasture and roadsides.

Propagation: By seeds and vegetative method.

Part Used: Whole plant.

Chemical Constituents: The whole plant contains nitrates.

Uses: It is considered diuretic, laxative, stomachic, depurative and good for the liver. It is used against influenza, hypertension, oliguria and retention of urine.

510. *Eleutherine subaphylla* Gegenep. *(Iridaceae)*

Description: Perennial herb, 30-40 cm. High; usually withered in the dry season. Bulb purplish, leaves lanceolate, acute at both ends, with numerous parallel nerves. Inflorescence in long raceme; flowers white capusule many-seeded.

Habitate: Grows wild but is also cultivated everywhere.

Propagation: By seeds and vegetative method.

Part Used: Bulb.

Chemical Constituents: The bulbs contain quinoid substances, eleutherin, isoeleutherin, eleutherol.

Uses: The bulbs are an antibacterial, demulcent and haemostatic remedy. They are used in treating sore throat, pertussis, boils, impetigo, jaundice, haemopthysis, uterine haemorrhage, trauma, wounds, abortion, anaemia, headache and photopsia and in inserting intra-uterine devices. The external use of an alcholic maceration and ointment is effective for impetigo and boils. The bulbs are also a constituent of composite sedative recipes.

511. *Eleutherococcus senticosus* *(Araliaceae)*

Vernacular Name: *Eng:* Siberian Ginseng.

Description: A deciduous, hardy, shrub, growing to 3m. It has 3-7 toothed leaflets, on each stem.

Habitate: Siberian ginseng is native to eastern Russia, China, Korea and Japan.

Propagation: By seeds and vegetative method.

Parts Used: Root.

Chemical Constituents: Eleutherosides, 0.6-0.9%, Phenylpropanoids, Lignans, Coumarins, Sugars, Polysaccharides, Triterpenoid saponins, Glycans.

Uses: Adaptogenic, Tonic, Stimulant, protects the immune system.

512. *Eleutherococcus sessiliflorus* *(Araliaceae)*

Vernacular Name: *Eng:*-Acanthopanax.

Description: Deciduous shrup, to 3-4 m tall. Stems with gray-brown branchlets, several arising from the base, hardly armed. Leaves alternate, palmately compound; leaflets 3-5, central one largest, to 15 cm long, obovate, acuminatek apices, acute bases, acutely double-toothed, dark-green above, pubescent beneath on veins only; petioles 3-6 cm long. Inflorescence terminal on the new shoots with head like umbels, globose. Flowers purplish, sessile; styles connate the full length, slightly bifid at apex. Fruit ellipsoidal, 10-14 mm long, 3-4 mm in diameter, black.

Habitate: Mountain woods in Korea and China.

Propagation: By seeds and vegetative method.

Parts Used: Bark.

Chemical Constituents: ***Root:*** acanthosides A, B, D (lignan-glycosides), cardiac glycosides, saponins, acidic polysaccharides. Seed; fatty acids, myristic acid, palmitic acid, sterols, stigmasterol, etc.

Uses: Anti-inflammatory and antioedemic, analgesic, antipyretic, hypotensive, adaptogenic, lipid lowering, antimutagenic effects. Used in lumbago, neuralgia, arthritis, oedema.

513. *Elsholtzia ciliata* (Thumb.) Hyland. *(Lamiaceae)*

Description: Small annual plant, with soft pubescence; 40-60 cm. High; stem quadrangular, leaves opposite, margins serrate; nerves apparengly impressed on the lower side. Inflorescence in terminal, unlateral spike; flowers pale-violet or purplish. Achene oblong, glabrous.

Habitate: Extensively cultivted as spice and medicinal plant in India.

Propagation: By seeds and vegetative method.

Part Used: Whole plant.

Chemical Constituents: The whole plant contains an essential oil consisting of Elsholtzia ketones.

Uses: The entire plant is used against influenza, headache, sore throat, measles, ostealgia and furunculosis. It is also haemostatic and is used in menorrhagia, metrorrhagia, haemoptysis and bloody stools. The vapour from the boiling decoction can be inhaled.

514. *Elsholtzia splendens* Nakai et F. Maek. *(Lamiaceae)*

Vernacular Name: *Eng*: Shiny elsholtzia.

Description: Erect annual herb to 60 cm. Stems branched, 4-angled and slightly pubescent. Leaves opposite, membranaceous, ovate, 1-7 cm long, 0.8-4 cm wide, apex acute, base cuneate, attenuate into petiole, acute serrate, pubescent on both sides, especially dense on nerves, lower surface glandular dotted. Spikes terminal and axillary, 2-5 cm long; floral bracts persistent, ovate, dense, purplish. Flowers 6 mm long; calyx 5-lobed; corolla small, tube as long as calyx, pale rose, limb 4-lobed, subbilabiate, the upper lip erect, retuse, the lower lip spreading; stamens 4, exserted, the lower pair longer. Nutlets ovate to oblong.

Habitate: Grassy areas in mountains in Korea and China.

Propagation: By seeds and vegetative method.

Parts Used: Whole plant.

Chemical Constituents: Thymol, a-phellandrene, B-bisabolene, a-trans-bergamotene, monoterpenes and sesquiterpenes.

Uses: Fever, headache, diarrhoea, oedema.

515. *Elusine coracana* (L.) Gaertn. *(Poaceae)*

Synonyms: *Cynosurus coracanus* Linn.

Vernacular Name: *San*: Nrtyakundalah, Narttakah, Ragi; *Eng*: Ragi, Finger millet, African millet; *Hin*: Mandva, Maruva, Kado; *Kan*: Ragi; *Mal*: Muttari, Ragi, Kora, Puncappullu; *Tam*: Ragi, Kelvaragu; *Tel:* Ragulu, Tamidalu

Description: An erect annual grass, 60-120 cm in height with tillering tufted stems which are laterally flattened; leaves 5-7 mm broad with sheath and ligule of hairs far over topping the stem, spikes 4-7, frequently incurved, spikelets awnless, 3-6 flowered, very much congested; each spikelet containing 4-7 seeds; seeds nearly globose or somewhat flattened, varying in colour from dark reddish brown to nearly white.

Habitate: Cultivated throughout south India in areas upto 1,500 m elevation.

Propagation: By seeds and vegetative method.

Parts Used: Grains.

Chemical Constituents: Prolamines, glycemic, glutelins, globulins, albumins, protein, copper, calcium, iron, phosphorus.

Uses: The grains are sweet, astringent, acrid, bitter, cooling, diuretic, depurative and tonic, and are useful in vitiated conditions of *pitta* and *kapha*, burning sensation, hyperdipsia, strangury, reneal and vesical calculi, leprosy, skin diseases and general debility.

516. *Embelia ribes* Burm. f. *(Myrsinaceae)*

Vernacular Name: *San*: Vidangah, Vellah, *Eng*: Embelia, *Hin*: Vayvidamg, Bhabhiramg, *Kan*: Vayuvidanga, *Mal*: Vilal, *Tam*: Vayu-vilamga, *Tel:* Vayuvidangamu, Vidanga.

Description: A large scandent shrub with long, slender, flexible branches and bark studded with lenticels; leaves simple, alternate, elliptic-lanceolate, short and obtusely acuminate, entire, coriaceous, glabrous on both sides, shiny above, silvery beneath gland dotted, glandular pits near the midrib beneath; flowers white or greenish white in terminal and axillary, lax panicled racemes; fruits globular dull red to nearly black berries, longitudinally striated with short slender persistent pedicel and style base; seed single globose, hollowed at the base, white spotted, testa membranous, albumen pitted.

Habitate: Throughout India, in areas upto 1,500 m elevation in hilly regions.

Propagation: By seeds and vegetative method.

Parts Used: Roots, leaves, fruits.

Chemical Constituents: A flatoxin B1, Embelin 2,5-isobutylamine salts.

Uses: The roots are acrid, astringent, thermogenic and stomachic, and are useful in vitiated conditions of *vata*, odontalgia, colic, flatulence and dyspepsia. The leaves are astringent, thermogenic, demulcent and depurative, and are useful in pruritus, skin diseases and leprosy. The fruits are acrid, astringent, bitter, thermogenic, anthelmintic, depurative, brain tonic, digestive, carminative, stomachic, diuretic, contraceptive, rejuvenating, alterant, stimulant, alexeteric, laxative, anodyne, vulnerry, febrifuge and tonic, and are useful in vitiated conditions of *kapha* and *vata*, helminthiasis, skin diseases, leprosy, pruritus, nervous debility, amentia, dyspepsia, flatulence, colic, constipation, strangury, tumours, asthma, bronchitis, dental caries, odontalgia, hemicrania, dyspnoea, cardiopathy psychopathy, ringworm infestation, fever, emaciation and general debility.

517. *Embelia tsjeriam-cottam* (Roem. & Schult.) DC. *(Myrsinaceae)*

Synonyms: *Embelia acutipetalum* (Lam. ex Hassk.) S.M. & M.R. Almeida.

Vernacular Name: *San*: Bidanga, Vidanga, *Hin*: Babrang, Bhingi, *Kan*: Vaivaling, *Mal*: Vilal, Mar: Ambati, Kokla, *Tam*: Vaivilangam, Kakkandankai.

Description: A large woody scandent or straggling shrub (rarely erect shrub). Branchlets densely covered with prominent lenticels, hairless. *Bark* with thin cracks, brown, exuding resin. *Wood* red, exhibiting prominent wheel-like medullary rays when cut. *Leaves* alternate, elliptic, 5-12 x 2-6 cm, papery, base acute, apex acuminate, margin entire or slightly toothed with triangular teeth, hairless, dark green above, often purplish green below; lateral nerves and reticulations prominent; leaf stalks up to 1 cm long. *Flowers* bisexual, greenish white or yellow, about 5 mm across, arranged in 4-7 cm long axillary racemes. *Fruits* globose, about 6 mm across, smooth, red when ripe. *Seeds* 1, round.

Habitate: Deciduous to semi-evergreen forests.

Propagation: By seeds and vegetative method.

Parts Used: Seeds.

Chemical Constituents: N.A.

Uses: Since the seeds have same medicinal properties of *E. ribes*, they are substituted.

518. *Emilia sonchifolia* (L.) DC. *(Asteraceae)*

Vernacular Name: *San*: Sasasrutih, *Hin*: Hirankhuri, *Mal*: Muyalccevi, *Tam*: Muyalccevi.

Description: A soft very variable annual herb, 30-40 cm in height, variously branched, sometimes procumbent and rooting near the nods; leaves simple, both radical and cauline, lyrate-pinnatifid with large terminal lobe, the basal leaf petioled, cauline acutely auricled; flowers purplish in lax corymbose heads, bracts almost equaling the corollas with scarious margins, pappus haris white, soft, nearly equaling the involucral bracts; fruits narrowly oblong, 5-ribbed brown achenes, scabrid on the ribs.

Habitate: Throughout India, as a weed in cultivated fields and waste places.

Propagation: By seeds and vegetative method.

Parts Used: Whole plant.

Chemical Constituents: The aerial parts contain pyrrolizidine alkaloids, senkirkine and doronine. Presence of simiaral, β-sitosterol, stigmasterol, palmitic and triacontannic acids is also reported in the plant.

Uses: The plant is astringent, sweet, thermogenic sudorific, antipyretic, ophthalmic, vulnerary and antiasthmatic, and is useful in vitiated conditions of *vata*, infantile tympanitis, gastropathy, diarrhoea, otalgia, ophthalmia, nyctalopia, cuts and wounds, intermittent fevers, pharyngodynia and asthma.

519. *Enicostemma axillare* (Lam.) Raynal *(Gentianaceae)*

Synonyms: *Enicostemma littorale* auct. Non Blume.

Vernacular Name: *San*: Nagajihva, Mamajjakah, Nahi, *Hin*: Katvinayi, Chota cirayita, Nai, *Kan*: Karibandita, Sogade, *Mal*: Vellaruku, Vallari, *Tam*: Vallari, Vellarugu, *Tel:* Chevvu-kurti.

Description: A glabrous or procumbent perennial herb upto 50 cm in height from a thick root stock, stems and branches sub quadrangular; leaves simple, opposite, sessile, linear, linear-oblong or elliptic-lanceolate, glabrous, 3-nerved marginal nerves often obscure; flowers white, tubular, in whorled axillary clusters; fruits ellipsoid capsules, narrowed at the base and rounded at the apex with the remains of the style.

Habitate: Throughout India in areas upto 450 m elevation, common in coastal areas.

Propagation: By seeds and vegetative method.

Parts Used: Whole plant.

Chemical Constituents: Ophelic acid, chiratin.

Uses: The plant is bitter, acrid, thermogenic, digestive carminative, stomachic, laxative, anthelmintic, anti-inflammatory, liver tonic, urinary astringent, depurative, revulsive and antiperiodic and is useful in dyspepsia, flatulence, colic, helminthiasis, abdominal ulcers, hernia, constipation, dropsy, swellings, vitiated conditions of *kapha* and *vata*, hepatopathy, glycosuria, leprosy, skin diseases, pruritus, intermittent fevers and malaise. The plant is locally applied in snake bite.

520. *Entada phaseoloides* *(Mimosaceae)*

Vernacular Name: *Eng:* Matchbox Bean.

Description: Woody vine with compound leaves and cluster of pea-type flowers hugs, flat brown seedpods, containing black glossy seeds, grow to 1.5 m in length, making them the largest-growing legumes in the world.

Habitate: Matchbox bean is native to Australia and tropical regions of Asia and Africa.

Propagation: By seeds and vegetative method.

Parts Used: Seeds.

Chemical Constituents: Meatchbox bean contains significant amounts of saponins.

Uses: Australia Aboriginals use the sees to treat female sterility and indigestion, and as a painkiller.

521. *Ephedra sinica* Stapf *(Ephedraceae)*

Vernacular Name: *Eng:* Chinese ephedra, ma-huang.

Description: An erect or prostrate undershrub, 20-40 com high. Branches erect, short, gloucous green, somewhat flat, 1.0-1.5 mm thick, with sparse longitudinal striae, fasciated at the nodes; internode 2.5-5.5 cm long by 2 mm in diameter. Leaves opposite, reduced to scales, barely 2 mm, acute-triangular. Flowers in summer, unisexual, dioecious, fruiting with often fleshy red succulent bracts, 2-seeded.

Habitate: On dry slopes or in dried-up riverbeds in China.

Propagation: By seeds and vegetative method.

Part Used: Stems.

Chemical Constituents: N.A.

Uses: Common cold; fever with ahnidrosis, cough and dyspnaea, oedema.

522. *Epimedium koreanum* Nakai *(Berberidaceae)*

Vernacular Name: *Eng*: Korean epimedium.

Description: Low, rhizomatous perennial herb, to 30 cm tall. Rhizome creeping covered with many filiform roots. Base of stems surrounded with scale-like leaves. Leaves alternate, long-petiolate, ternately divided twice; leaflects ovate, acuminate, cordate, 5-13.5 cm long, 1,5-7 cm wide, with margin setose. Flowers small, pale yellowish; sepals 8, the outer 4 unequal, in 2 pairs, soon falling, the inner 4 petaloid, reflexed at flowering time; petals 4, extended into spurs; stamens 4, ovary with several ovules. Follicles 10-13 mm long, 5-6 mm across.

Habitate: Wet areas in forests and mountain valleys.

Propagation: By roots, seeds.

Parts Used: Whole plant.

Chemical Constituents: Icariin, O-methyl-icariin, icaritin-rhamnoside-glucoside and icariresinol Flavonoids; anhydroicarin-3-O-rhamnoside, 2″-O-rhamnosyl ikarisoside A, 2″-O-rhamnosyl icariod II, epimedokoreanin D. Phytosterols: campesterol, campesterol 3-O-Glucopyranoside.

Uses: Aldose reductase inhibition, nerve fibre induction. Used in impotence spermatorrhoea forget fullness.

523. *Epimedium sagittatum* *(Berberidaceae)*

Vernacular Name: *Eng:* Berberidaceae.

Description: An evergreen perennial herb, 10-40 cm high. Rhizome creeping, very slender, covered with long filiform rootlets.Basal leaves 1-3, ternately compound leaflets 3, ovl-lanceolate, 4-9 cm long, apex acute or acuminate, base cordate; lateral leaflets; base sagittate, oblique; margin setosel petiole slender, about 15 cm long. Inflorescence a raceme or panicle, terminal, flowers in spring. Fruit a follicle, ovoid. Few seeds, reniform, black, odourless, taste slightly bitter.

Habitate: Under trees and shrubs and in crevices in the mountains in China, Japan.

Propagation: By seeds and vegetative method.

Part Used: Whole plant.

Chemical Constituents: N.A.

Uses: Imotence; premature ejaculation; incontinence of urine, rheumatic arthritis; chornic pain in the lower body and legs, climacterium hypertension; chronic tracheitis.

524. *Equisetum arvense* *(Equisetaceae)*

Vernacular Name: *Eng:* Horsetail, Bottlebrush.

Description: Perennial plant with a yellowish fruiting stem growing to 35 cm, flowered by a sterile segmented and toothed stem growing to 60 cm. The latter has whorls of needle-shaped leaves.

Habitate: Native to Europe, North Africa, northern Asia and the Americas, horsetail is common plant, preferring damp soil.

Propagation: By seeds and vegetative method.

Parts Used: Aerial parts.

Chemical Constituents: Horsetail contains large amounts of silicic acid and silicates, flavonoids, phenolic acids, alkaloids, and sterols. Much of the therapeutic effectiveness of this herb is due to its high silica content, a large proportion of which is soluble and can be absorbed. Silica supports the regeneration of connective tissue.

Uses: As its traditional usage indicates, horsetail is an excellent clotting agent. It staunches wounds, stops nosebleeds and reduces the coughing up of blood. In addition, horsetail has an astringent effect of the genito-urinary system, proving especially valuable where there is bleeding within the urinary tract, and in cases of cystitis, urethritis and prostate disease. The herb is also prescribed to treat rheumatic and arthritic problems fir chest ailments such as emphysema, for chronic swelling of the legs and for various other conditions.

525. *Equisetum hiemale* L. *(Equisetaceae)*

Vernacular Name: *Eng:* Fern-ally, Polishing rush.

Description: A perennial unbranched, glaucous evergreen herb, upto 3m. high, with creeping rhizome and a tall, stout, rush like, hollow and jointed stem having well defined nodes and longitudinally ribbed internodes; leaves very small simple, scale like, arranged in whorl at the nodes; cone-like strobili at tips of aerial shoots. Stem 11-40 ridged. Stem sheath cylindric, with basal and apical dark bands; teeth lanceolate, connate at base, dark brown with broad scarious margins and subulate tipped.

Habitate: U.S.A.

Propagation: By seeds and vegetative method.

Parts Used: Whole plant.

Chemical Constituents: Silicon oxide 7.5-41.2%; Silicilic Acid, Acotinic Acid, Ferulic acid; Saponins; Flevoglucosides; Alkaloids: Equisetine, Nicotine and Palustrine; Dimethyl sulphone; Enzyme thaiminase.

Uses: Used for Cystitis; Enuresis, Dysuria, Stones and Urethritis, with specific action on urinary bladder. For complaints specifically of frequent intolerable urging to urinate with severe pain at the close of urination. Urinate large quantity without amelioration, but with sharp, burning, cutting pain in urethra. Urine flows drop by drop. Involuntary urination in females. Deep pain in right kidney, extending to lower abdomen with urgent desire to urinate with right lumber pain. Complaints better by lying.

526. *Equisetum hyemale* L. *(Equisetaceae)*

Vernacular Name: *Eng*: Common horsetail, common scouring rush.

Description: Primitive, spore-bearing, vascular perennial, rhizomatous herb, to 1 m tall. Stems slender, hollow, furrowed with 14-40 ridges, rough, jointed, impregnated with silica, branches whorled. Leaves scale like, marginally united into a sheath around each node. Sporophylls in a terminal, spikelike strobilus composed of peltate sporangia-bearing structure.

Habitate: Shaded and wet sandy places in ravines and valleys.

Propagation: By vegetative method.

Parts Used: Whole plant.

Chemical Constituents: Dimethylsulfone, kaempferol-diglucoside, aconitic acid, palustrine (alkaloid), nicotine, caffeic acid, ferulic acid, silicon compound.

Uses: Anticancer, diuretic, apitite stimulation, antihypertensive, toxic effect, anti-inflammatory, antispasmodic.

527. *Erigeron canadensis* *(Asteraceae)*

Synonyms: *Conyza canadensis.*

Vernacular Name: *Eng:* Canadian fleabane.

Description: Erect annual herb growing to 1 m. Has narrow, dark green, lance-shaped leaves and clusters of small white flowerheads that quickly fade into silky white tufts.

Habitate: Native to north America, Canadian fleabane is now common in South America and Europe.

Propagation: By seeds and vegetative metohd.

Parts Used: Aerial parts.

Chemical Constituents: Canadian fleabane contains a volatile oil, flavonoids, terpenes, plant acids and tannins.

Uses: An astringent herb, Canadian fleabane is taken for gastro-intestinal problems such as diarrhoea and dysentery. The herb is occasionally used as a diuretic for bladder problems, to clear toxins in rheumatic conditions and to treat gonorrhoea and other urinogenital disease.

528. *Eriobotrya japonica* (Thumb.) Lindl. *(Rosaceae)*

Vernacular Name: *Eng:* Loquat, Japanese medlar, Japanese plum; *Hin:* Lokat; *Tam:* Ilakotta, nokkottta and *Kan:* Lakkote.

Description: Medium-sized evergreen tree, 5-7 m. high; branches pubescent when young, then glabrous. Leaves alternate, oblong, thick and stiff; velvety pubescent beneath; margins toothed. Inflorescence in terminal raceme, covered with a dense silvery pubescence. Drupe oval or pyriform, yellow when ripe; pulp sweetish, acid and edible 3-5 seeds .

Habitate: Cultivated for its ornamental foliage and edible fruit.

Propagation: By seeds and vegetative method.

Part Used: Leaves and fruit.

Chemical Constituents: The fruit contains sugars: levulose and sucrose; malic, citric, tartaric and succinic acids; cryptoxanthin, B-carotene, neo-B-carotene. The seeds contain amygdalin and a fatty oil. The leaves yield saponins, ursolic acid, oleanolic acid and caryophyllene.

Uses: The leaves possess antitussive and antispasmodic properties. They are prescrived in the treatment of cough, chronic bronchities, excessive exceptoration, feber, coryza, hyperemesis, especially vomiting of pregancy, epistaxis and dyspepsia. The decoction is also to wash wounds.

529. *Eriodictyon californicum* *(Hydrophyllaceae)*

Vernacular Name: *Eng:* Yerba *San*ta.

Description: Sticky evergreen shrub growing to 2.5 m. Its narrow lance-shaped leaves are shiny green on the upper side and hairy white underneath. Trumpet-shaped white or blue flowers grow in clusters.

Habitate: Native to California and Oregon in the US, and northern Mexico, yerba *San*ta flourishes on dry mountain slopes. It grows at altitudes of up to 1,200m.

Propagation: By seeds and vegetative method.

Parts Used: Leaves.

Chemical Constituents: Yerba *San*ta contains a volatile oil, flavonoids and resin.

Uses: An aromatic herb with a plea*San*t sweet taste, yerba *San*ta is a valuable expectorant that can be used to treat tracheitis, bronchitis and asthma and similar respiratory tract ailments.

530. *Ervatamia coronaria* *(Apocynaceae)*

Vernacular Name: *Eng:* Grape jasmine, East Indian Rosebay.

Description: Perennial shrub growing to 2 m. Has dark green, elliptical leaves and strongly perfumed white flowers.

Habitate: Grape jasmine is grown in India, Malaysia and Indonesia.

Propagation: By vegetative method.

Parts Used: Root, leaves, wood, latex.

Chemical Constituents: Grape jasmine contains alkaloids and resins.

Uses: Ayurvedic medicine, the root and the latex are used to expel worms. The root is also chewed to relieve toothache. The latex is used to treat cataracts, eye inflammations and poor eyesight. The leaf juice makes a soothing treatment for skin irritations and wounds. The wood reduces fevers.

531. *Eryngium maritimum* *(Apiaceae)*

Vernacular Name: *Eng:* Sea holly, Eryngo.

Description: Evergreen perennial growing to 60 cm. Has spiny silver leaves, and tiny flowers in summer.

Habitate: Sea holly is found in coastal areas of Europe, preferring *San*dy soils.

Propagation: By seeds and vegetative method.

Parts Used: Root.

Chemical Constituents: Sea holly contains saponins, coumarins, flavonoids and plant acids.

Uses: In contemporary European herbal medicine, sea holly is used as a diuretic. It is prescribed as a treatment for cystitis and urethritis, and taken as a means to alleviate kidney stones. It is unlikely that the herb actually dissolves established stones, but it probably helps retard their formation. Sea holly is also used to treat enlargement or inflammation of the prostate gland, and may be of benefit in treating chest problems.

532. *Erythraea centraurium* *(Gentianaceae)*

Vernacular Name: *Eng:* Centaury.

Description: Biennial herb growing to 24 cm with a basal rosette of leaves and 5-petalled pink flowers in clusters.

Habitate: Native to Europe and south-western Asia, centaury is now found in temperate regions throughout the world.

Propagation: By seeds and vegetative method.

Parts Used: Aerial part.

Chemical Constituents: Centaury contains many bitter constituents, including secoiridoids, also found in gentian.

Uses: One of the most useful bitter herbs, centaury strengthens digestive function, especially within the stomach. By increasing stomach secretions, it hastens the breakdown of food. It also stimulates the appetite and increases bile production. Centaury needs to be taken over some weeks.

533. *Erythrina variegata* L. var. orientalis (L.) *(Fabaceae)*

Synonyms: *Erythrina indica* Lam.

Vernacular Name: *San:* Mandar, parijata; *Eng*: India bean, India coral-bean, mochi wood tree, east indies coral tree; *Hin:* Dadap, mandara; *Beng*: Palita mandar; *Tel:* Badisa, badita, baridamu, modugu; *Tam:* Kaliyanamurukku; *Kan:* Varjipe, harivana and *Mal:* Kalayna-murikku, mandaram.

Description: Tree reaching about 10m in height. Stems branched, smooth, sprasely covered with short prickles. Leaves alternate, trifoliate, the terminal largest; leaflet-stalk glandular, inflorescence in dense axillary and terminal raceme; flowers red, appearing before the leaves. Pod long, black, constricted between the seeds. Seeds reniform, red or brown.

Habitate: Grows wild in deciduous forests and is cultivated in gardens for ornament.

Propagation: By seeds and vegetative method.

Part Used: Leaves.

Chemical Constituents: The leaves and stems contain the alkaloid erythrinaline. The seeds yield the alkaloid hypaphorine and a saponin: migarrhin.

Uses: The leaves are reported to be sedative. It is used for the relief of insomnia and anxiety. It is often associated with other plants such as passiflora hispida and morus alba. Crushed fresh leaves are used externally as poultice in haemorrhoids and metroptosis. Powdered leves are topically applied for wounds and ulcers. The stem bark is used against rheumatism in the form of a decoction.

534. *Erythronium americanum* *(Liliaceae)*

Vernacular Name: *Eng:* Adder's tongue.

Description: Perennial growing to 25 cm from small, bulb-like corm. Has two oblong leaves mottled with purple and a large, bright yellow lily flower.

Habitate: Native to north America, adder's tongue is found mainly in the east, from New Brunswick to Florida.

Propagation: By seeds and vegetative method.

Parts Used: Leaves.

Chemical Constituents: Very little is known about the constituents of this plant. It contains alpha-methylenebutyrolactone.

Uses: An infusion of the leaves is taken for skin problems such as ulcers and tumours, and for enlarged glands. Adder's tongue is often used to treat scrofulous skin arising from tubercular infection. The leaves may also be applied as a poultice for skin conditions. Although the fresh leaves are strongly emetic, they are rarely used to stimulate vomiting.

535. *Erythroxylum coca* *(Erythroxylaceae)*

Vernacular Name: *Eng:* Coca.

Description: Evergreen shrub growing to 3 m. Has alternate oval leaves, small white flowers and small red berries that each contain a single seed.

Habitate: Native to Peru and Bolivia, coca grows in high-rainfall areas of the eastern Andes to altitudes of 1,500 m.

Propagation: By seeds and vegetative method.

Parts Used: Leaves.

Chemical Constituents: Coca contains cocaine and various other alkaloids, a volatile oil, flavonoids, vitamins A and B2, and minerals. The plant's stimulant and anaesthetic action is due largely to cocaine.

Uses: In Bolivia and Peru, coca leaves play an important part in the culture and herbal medicine of the indigenous Aymara and Quechua peoples. High altitudes, cold and an impoverished diet place great physical demands on the population. Coca leaves, chewed with lime or ashes, release small amounts of the active constituents, which act as a tonic and help block the effects of cold, exhaustion and poor nutrition. Coca leaves are also used in South American herbal medicine to treat nausea, vomiting and asthma, and have been used to speed convalescence. Cocaine extracted from coca leaves is used legally in conventional medicine as a local anaesthetic.

536. *Eschscholzia californica* (*Papaveraceae*)

Vernacular Name: *Eng:* Californian poppy.

Description: Annual or perennial growing to 60 cm. Has finely cut leaves and bright orange, yellow, ink or red flowers.

Habitate: Californian poppy is native to western North America. Widely cultivated as a garden plant, it prefers *San*dy soils.

Propagation: By seeds and vegetative method.

Parts Used: Aerial parts.

Chemical Constituents: Californian poppy contains alkaloids and flavone glycosides.

Uses: Though Californian poppy is closely related to the opium poppy, it has a markedly different effect on the central nervous system. Californian poppy is not a narcotic. In fact, rather than disorientating the user, it tends to normalize psychological function. Californian poppy;s gently antispasmodic, sedative and analgesic effects make it a valuable herbal medicine for treating physical and psychological problems in children. Californian poppy may also prove beneficial in attempts to overcome bedwetting, difficulty in sleeping and nervous tension and anxiety.

537. *Eucalyptus globules* Labill (*Myrtaceae*)

Vernacular Name: *San*: Nilaniryasa, Tailaparnah, *Eng*: Blue gum, Eucalypt, *Hin*: Yukeliptas, *Mal*: Yukkalimaram, *Tam*: Yukkalimaram.

Description: A lofty tree about 90 m in height with a clean straight bole and smooth bark, peeling off in long strips; leaves opposite on juvenile shoots, alternate in adult shoots, lanceolate, 20-25 cm long, broad, rather thick and curved; flowers large, white, 1-3 together in axils, operculum thick and warty; fruit a hardened capsule, dehiscing longitudinally at the mouth, seeds very small.

Habitate: Cultivated in various parts of India.

Propagation: By seeds and vegetative method.

Parts Used: Oil.

Chemical Constituents: Eucalyptin, 8-desmethyleucalyptin, sideroxylin, 8-desmethylsideroxylin, quercetin, quercitrin, quercetol and its 3-deglucoside, chrysin, rutin hyperoside, phloroglucin derivatives, EA, to EJ, *n*-tritriacontan-16-18-dione, 4-hydroxytritriaconate-16-18-dione, 16-hydroxy-18-tritriacontanone, 11,12-dehydroursolic lactone acetate, caffeic, ferulic, gallic, gentisic, protocatechuic, maslinic and oleanolic acids.

Uses: The oil is acrid, bitter, astringent, thermogenic, oleaginous, antiseptic, deodorant, stimulant, anodyne, carminative, digestive, anthelmintic, cardiotonic, diuretic, sudorific, expectorant, insect repellent,, rubefacient and antipyretic, and is useful in vitiated conditions of *kapha* and *vata*, halitosis, cephalalgia, tuberculosis, chronic cough, asthma, pneumonosis, bronchitis, pyorrhea, burns, dyspepsia, flatulence, threadworm infestation, cardiac debility, pharyngodynia, hoarseness, strangury, skin diseases and chronic and intermittent fevers.

Internal use of the oil in excess will cause cardiac debility, vomiting and diarrhoea.

538. *Eucalyptus smithii* (*Myrtaceae*)

Vernacular Name: *Eng:* Eucalyptus.

Description: Aromatic evergreen tree growing to 50m.

Habitate: Native to Australia, eucalyptus now grows in temperate and sub-tropical zones around the world.

Propagation: By seeds and vegetative method.

Parts Used: Essential oil.

Chemical Constituents: The volatile oil contains about 70% eucalyptol, as well as pinene, limonene, alpha-terpineol and linalool. While it is similar to the oils of related species, this oil appears to be better tolerated by the skin.

Uses: Eucalyptus essential oil is used in aromatherapy, and also as a disinfectant and antiseptic for the treatment of viral conditions, skin and other infections, and as a decongestant.

539. *Eucommia ulmoides* Olive *(Eucommiaceae)*

Vernacular Name: Tu-chung; gutta-percha tree.

Description: An elm-like tree reaching 20 m in height but generally only 5 m. leaves alternate, petiolate, elliptic or elliptic ovate, 6-13 cm long by 3.5-7 cm wide, tip long-acuminate; base cuneate or wedge-shaped; margin serrate, pinnately nerved. Flowers unisexual, dioecious. Fruit samaroid, indehiscent, 1-seeded, thinly coriaceous, stipitate, oblong-oblanceolate, bifid at the apex. Seed solitary, pendulous from the apex of the loculus, elongate-oblong; endosperm copious.

Habitate: In the mountains; now commonly cultivated in the plains in China.

Propagation: By seeds and vegetative method.

Part Used: Bark.

Chemical Constituents: N.A.

Uses: Tiredness of the lower body and legs; seminal emissions, Dizziness due to hypertension.

540. *Eucommia ulmoides* Olive *(Eucommiaceae)*

Vernacular Name: *Eng:* Gutta-percha tree.

Description: Medium-sized tree, 10m. high or more. Leaves alternate, petiolate, margins toothed. The bark and leaves contain a milky latex which streaches into numerous strands when broken. Flowers unisexual, diocious; perianth none in either sex. Fruit rhomboidal, flat, brown, singhe-seeded.

Habitate: An important plant, cultivated in mountainous regions.

Propagation: By seeds and vegetative method.

Part Used: Bark.

Chemical Constituents: The bark yields gutta-percha, resins, the glucosides aucubin and loganin; lipids, proteins, essential oil and chlorogenic acid.

Uses: Theerapeutic uses: The trunk bark, which possesses antihypertensive and anti-inflammatory properties, is used to rgulate the activity of the sex hormones. It is also used in treating nephrosis, lumbago, arthrodynia, spermatorrhoea, impotence, uterine colic and uterine haemorrhage in pregancy, hypertension, polyuria, rheumatism, inflammation and oedema.

541. *Eugenia aromatica* Kuntze. *(Myrtaceae)*

Synonyms: *Syzigium aromaticum.*

Vernacular Name: *San*: Lavangam, *Hin:* Laung.

Description: *Eugenia aromatica* is a tree reaching a height of 10-15 m, with numerous slender horizontal branches forming a dense pyramidal crown. Bark is pale yellowish grey in colour and smooth. *Leaves* opposite numerous and evergreen, 3-6 inches long. A great profusion of flowers grow in clusters. The *flowers* when gathered are at first of a reddish colour, but on drying they assume a deep brown cast.

Habitate: The clove tree is a native of Malacca islands. The Malaccas, Indonesia, Malaysia and neighbouring areas were the sole areas of clove production till the early modern period.

Propagation: By seeds and vegetative method.

Parts Used: Dried Flowers buds.

Chemical Constituents: Cloves contain about 14-21 per cent of volatile oil, 10 to 13 per cent of tannin and a crystalline substance, caryophyllene, which is white, odourless and is soluble in either and boiling alcohol. Capsaicin is also present in cloves. The oil of clove is prepared by steam distillation and contain 34 to 95% of phenols, sesquiterpenes and small quantity of esters, ketones and alcohols. Medicinal oil has a phenol content of about 82 to 90%. The oils which have relatively low phenol content are mainly used in pharmacy while the strong oils are used in the manufacture of vanillin.

Uses: Toothache. Indigestion/flatulence. Nausea. Halitosis. Hyperacidity. Certain names of this plant like Tikshna-puspha. Ruchiram, Girvana Pushpam suggest of its therapeutic uses as an appetizer, digestive cordial and antitussive. Also as freshner of mouth and throat. Lavangadivati and Avipattikarachurna are widely used preparations.

542. *Eugenia caryophyllata* *(Myrtaceae)*

Vernacular Name: *Eng:* Clove.

Description: An evergreen, pyramid-shaped tree growing to 15m. the tree is strongly aromatic.

Habitate: Originally from the Molucca Islands and the southern Philippines, cloves are now grown extensively in Tanzania and Madagascar, and to a lesser extent in the West Indies and Brazil.

Propagation: By seeds and vegetative method.

Parts Used: Flower buds.

Chemical Constituents: Volatile oil containing eugenol, actely eugenol, methol salicylate, pinene, vanillin, Gum, Tannins.

Uses: Antiseptic, carminative, stimulant, analgesic, prevents vomiting antispasmodic, eliminates parasites.

543. *Euodia hortensis* Forster *(Rutaceae)*

Description: Shrub to small tree to 6 m tall. Leaves opposite, aromatic trifoliate (or simple), if compound, each leaflet oblanceolate, if simple, the blade lanceolate, and up to 30 cm long. Flowers and fruit available throughout the year.

Habitate: Cultivated and naturalized in secondary forest, forest margins and thickets, from sea-level to 500 m.

Propagation: By seeds and vegetative method.

Part Used: Bark, stem and leaves.

Chemical Constituents: Essential oils (caryophyllene, alpha-copaene, arcucumene), menthofuran, evodone, hortensol, berberine, furoquinoline and acridone alkaloids.

Uses: Fluid from the bark is used in jaundice. Liquid from the stem is used in treating children with convulsions. Liquid from the leaves is used as a remedy for swollen testicles. Also used as an emmenagogue. The leaves are used to treat toothache and stomachache.

Use an infusion of the leaves as a laxative, to reduce fevers, to treat swellings and to cure headaches. The leaves are crushed, mixed with oil and applied to sore gums. The leaves are also used to cure headache and earache in Tonga. Since the smell of the leaves is thought to keep away spirits, the plant is used to treat illnesses thought to be brought on by spirits in Tonga, Samoa, Niue and Rotuma. The leaves are heated and rubbed onto bruises. The bark may be chewed with betel nuts and rubbed onto aching body parts.

544. *Euodia officinalis* Dode *(Rutaceae)*

Vernacular Name: *Eng*: Euodia.

Description: Deciduous, tree, to 5 m tall. Young branches pubescent. Leaves opposite, odd-pinnately compound; leaflets 7-15, short-petiolulate, ovate to oblong-obvate or long elliptic, acuminate, 7-8 cm long, granular-dotted, pubescent beneath. Flowers small, in terminal or axillary corymbose, 6-11 cm across, pubescent, unisexual; sepals, petals and stamens 5. Fruit splitting 5, 2-valved, 1-2 seeded sections.

Habitate: Mostly cultivated in Korea and China.

Propagation: By seeds and vegetative method.

Parts Used: Fruits.

Chemical Constituents: Alkaloids: evodiamine, rutaecarpine, higenamine, dehydroevodiamine.

Uses: Analgesis, serotonin antagonism, brain dopamine receptor inhibition, cardiotonic, antihypertensive, MDR-modulating activity, cytotoxicity. Used in gastrointestinal disorder, feeling of chill, pain.

545. *Euonymus alatus* (Thunb.) Siebold *(Celastraceae)*

Vernacular Name: *Eng:*-Winged spindle tree.

Description: Deciduous, horizontally spreading, much-branched shrub, to 3 m tall. Branches glabrous, with 2-4 corky wings. Leaves opposite, simple, short-petiolate, elliptic to obovate, 1.5-7 cm long, 1-4 cm wide, glabrous, acuminate, sharply and finely serrate. Flowers greenish, small, about 6 mm across, in axillary cymes, 1 to few flowered greenish, small, about 2 cm long, the pedicels short; sepals, petals, and stamens, 4. Fruit a capsule, purplish, seed enclosed in a orange aril.

Habitate: Mountain woods of Korea, Japan and China.

Propagation: By seeds and vegetative method.

Parts Used: Twig, bark.

Chemical Constituents: Sesquiterpene-alkaloids: evonine, euonymine, wilfordine, alatamine. Kaempferol-rhamnosyl-xyloside, euolatin, steroids and triterpenes.

Uses: Hypoglycaemic. Used in taenia, cancer, abortifacient, emmenagogue.

546. *Euonymus atropurpureus* *(Celastraceae)*

Vernacular Name: *Eng:* Wahoo bark.

Description: Deciduous tree growing to 8 m. Has smooth branches, serrated elliptical leaves, clusters of purple flowers and 4-lobed scarlet fruit.

Habitate: Native to eastern North America, wahoo bark thrives in damp woods and close to water.

Propagation: By seeds and vegetative method.

Parts Used: Stem bark, root bark.

Chemical Constituents: Wahoo bark contains cardenolides similar to digitoxin, asparagines, sterols and tannins.

Uses: Wahoo bark is considered a gallbladder remedy with laxative and diuretic properties. it is prescribed for biliousness and liver problems, as well as for skin conditions such as eczema and for constipation. In the past, it was often used in combination with herbs such as gentian as a fever remedy, especially if the liver was under stress. Following the discovery that it contains cardiac glycosides, wahoo bark has been given for heart conditions.

547. *Euonymus europaeus* L. *(Celastraceae)*

Synonyms: *Euonymus vulgaris* Mill.

Vernacular Name: *Eng:* Spindle tree.

Description: A much branched, glabrous, deciduous shrub with branches quadrangular and smooth grey bark. Buds 2-4 mm. ovoid. Leaves characteristically glabrous beneath, up to 10 by 3.5 cm., opposite, ovate or lanceolate to elliptical, acute or acuminate. Flowers 3-8 in cymes, tetramerous, yellowish or greenish-white. Fruit a 4-lobed bright pink-capsule, 10-15 mm. wide, smooth angled, with seeds scarlet-orange covered by scarlet or orange aril.

Habitate: Throughout Europe and East Asia.

Propagation: By seeds and vegetative method.

Parts Used: Seed.

Chemical Constituents: Euonymok Euonysterol and Homoeuonysterol.

Uses: For Complaints of liver disorders, biliousness, lumbago, gastric derangements with albuminuria; cutting pains in malar bones, tongue, penis upto bladder better by lying down. Involuntary, profuse diarrhoeia with blood and mucous. Cutting, sticking and drawing pains predominate. Left side is more affected. Violent chill over the whole body.

548. *Eupatorium cannabinum* *(Asteraceae)*

Vernacular Name: *Eng:* Hemp agrimony.

Description: Perennial growing to a height of 1.5 m. Has a red stem, downy leaves and dense bunches of pink to mauve florets.

Habitate: Native to Europe, hemp agrimony is now also found in western Asia and North Africa. It grows in damp woods, ditches, marshes and on wasteground.

Propagation: By seeds and vegetative method.

Parts Used: Root.

Chemical Constituents: Hemp agrimony contains a volatile oil, sesquiterpene lactones, flavonoids, pyrrolizidine alkaloids, and polysaccharides. P-cymene is antiviral, while eupatoriopicrin has anti-cancer properties and inhibits cellular growth. The polysaccharides stimulate the immune system. In isolation, the pyrrolizidine alkaloids are toxic to the liver.

Uses: Hemp agrimony has been employed chiefly as a detoxifying herb for fever, colds, flu and other acute viral conditions. It also stimulates the removal of waste products via the kidneys. The root is laxative, and the whole plant is considered to be tonic. Recently, hemp agrimony has found use as an immune-stimulant, helping to maintain resistance to acute viral and other infections.

549. *Eupatorium perfoliatum* *(Asteraceae)*

Vernacular Name: *Eng:* Boneset.

Description: Erect perennial growing to 1.5 m. Has tapering lance-shpaed leaves and many white or purple florets.

Habitate: Native to eastern North America, boneset is found in meadows and marshland.

Propagation: By seeds and vegetative method.

Parts Used: Aerial parts.

Chemical Constituents: Boneset contains sesquiterpene lactones, polysaccharides, flavonoids, diterpenes, sterols and volatile oil. The sesquiterpene lactones and polysaccharides are significant immune-stimulants.

Uses: A hot infusion of boneset will bring relief to symptoms of the common cold. The plant stimulates resistance to viral and bacterial infections, and reduces fever by encouraging sweating. Boneset also loosens phlegm and promotes its removal through coughing, and it has a tonic and laxative effect. It has been taken for rheumatic illness, skin conditions and worms.

550. *Eupatorium purpureum* L. *(Asteraceae)*

Synonyms: *Eupatorium laevigatum* Torr., *Eupatorium falcatum* Michx., *Eupatorium trifolium* Ell.

Vernacular Name: *Eng:* Queen of the Meadow root

Description: A fibrous rooted perennial, 60 cm. to 2 m. tall, with stem slightly glaucous, usually purple only at nodes, otherwise greenish. Leaves in 3's or 4's lanceolate or ovate to elliptical, mostly 8 to 30 cm. long and 2.5 to 15 cm. wide, gradually or sometimes rather abruptly narrowed to the short petiole pinnately veined, usually sharply or coarsely toothed, loose soft-pubescent to subglabrous beneath; usually minutely atomiferous and glandular. Inflorescence convex with involucre imbricate, 6.5 to 9 mm. high, mostly 4 to 7 flowered, corolla generally very pale-pinkish or purplish, but variable, 4.5 to 7.5 mm. long.

Habitate: Indigenous to North America and common from Canada to Florida.

Propagation: By vegetative method.

Parts Used: Root.

Chemical Constituents: An unsaturated pyrrolizidic alkloid Echinatine. A benzofuran compound Euparin. A flavonoid Eupatorin. Resin and a Volatile oil.

Uses: For complaints specifically of albuminuria, diabetes insipidus, strangury, enlarged prostrates. Excellent in renal dropsy, Chills and pains running upwards. Impotency and Sterility. Left sided headache with vertigo. Pain from left shoulder to occiput. Burning in bladder and urethra on urination. Urine insufficient, milky. No thirst during chill but with much frontal headache. Chill commences in back. Traditionally for gravel stones of bladder, dysuria urethritis and prostatitis.

551. *Eupatorium staechadosmum* Hance *(Asteraceae)*

Description: Perennial herbaceous plant, reaching a height or 1 m. young shoots purplish-violet, longitudinally sulcate. Leaves opposite oblong, acute; margins denticulate; strongly scented when crushed. Inflorescence in dense terminal axillary corymb of many heads; flowers pale-violet. Achene small, black.

Habitate: Cultivated as a vegetable and medicinal plant.

Propagation: By seeds and vegetative method.

Part Used: Whole plant.

Chemical Constituents: The plant contains an essential oil.

Uses: The aerial parts of the plant possess antiseptic, diuretic, stomachic and haemagogic properties. They are used in treating fever, menstrual disorders, dysmenorrhoea, colic following post-partum haematometra, oedema, trauma, vertigo, furnculosis and impetigo. The fresh plant is used as an insecticide for killin lice, bugs, fleas and moths.

552. *Eupatorium triplinerve* Vahl *(Asteraceae)*

Synonyms: *Eupatorium ayapana* Vent.

Vernacular Name: *San*: Ayaparnah, Ajaparnah, *Eng*: Ayapana tea, *Hin*: Ayapana, *Kan*: Ayapanam, *Mal*: Ayyappana, Visappacca, Ayyampana, *Tam*: Ayappani, *Tel:* Ayaparni, Ayappanu.

Description: A profusely branching prostrate undershrub upto 90-120 cm in height with a few ascending branches; leaves simple, opposite, subsessile, lanceolate, 3-nerved, acuminate, subentire, glabrous; flowers slaty blue, all tubular in few headed coryms; fruits achenes, truncate, 5-angled with uniseriate pappus hairs.

Habitate: A native of Brazil, now found throughout India in marshes, also as a weed in plantations.

Propagation: By seeds and vegetative method.

Parts Used: Whole plant.

Chemical Constituents: The plant contains daphnetin dimethyl ether, hydrangetin, daphnetin-7-methyl ether, umbelliferone daphenetin, ayapin and herniarin.

Uses: The plant is bitter, astringent, acrid, thermogenic, stimulant, digestive, carminative, alterant, emetic and purgative in large doses, haemostatic, vulnerary, cardiotonic, antiscorbutic, alexeteric, sudorific, antipyretic, detergent, anti-inflammatory, expectorant and tonic, and is useful in gastropathy, dyspepsia, epistaxis, haematemesis, haemorrhages, haemoptysis, haematuria, menorrhagia, haemorrhoids, wounds, ulcers, ulcerative stomatitis, cardiac debility, skin eruptions, scabies, pruritus, poison bites, intermittent fevers especially yellow fever, inflammations, cough, asthma, vitiated conditions of *kapha* and general debility.

553. *Euphorbia antiquorum* L. *(Euphorbiaceae)*

Vernacular Name: *San*: Vajrakantakah, Tridhara, *Eng*: Triangular spruge, *Hin*: Tidhara, *Kan*: Mudumula, Katakkalli, *Mal*: Caturakkalli, *Tam*: Saturakkalli, Tiruvargalli, *Tel:* Bommajemudu, Bonta kalli, Pedda jemudu.

Description: A small armed tree with whorled fleshy branches, branchlets thick and broad, 3-5 winged, having sharp stipular spines; leaves small, sub-sessile, soon deciduous; involucres 3-nate, the central flower sessile, female, the two laterals on long stout pedicles, glands 5, styles bifid; fruits capsules.

Habitate: Throughout the hotter parts of India in areas upto 600 m elevation.

Propagation: By vegetative method.

Parts Used: Roots, juice.

Chemical Constituents: The stem contains friedelan-3α-ol, and -3β-ol, friedelan-3β, 30-diol diacetate, 30-acetoxyfriedelan-3β-ol, 3β-acetoxyfriedelan-30-ol, friedelan-3β-yl acetate, epi-friedelanol, lupeol cinnamate, mortenone, lupenone, taraxerone, β-amyrin, euphol, β-taraxerol, and ψ-taraxastane-3β, 20-diol. Presence of diterpenoids, antiquorin, and 7-hydroxyingol, 3,12-di-O-acetyl-8-tigiliate is also reported.

Uses: The roots are bitter, acrid, thermogenic, anodyne, purgative, emetic, stomachic, and digestive, and are useful in vitiated conditions of *kapha,* otalgia, flatulence, colic, constipation, dyspepsia, wounds and ulcers. The juice is acrid, anti-inflammatory, deobstruant and purgative, and is useful rheumatism, dropsy, gout, neuropathy, deafness, cough and cutaneous diseaes.

554. *Euphorbia fidjiana* Boiss *(Euphorbiaceae)*

Description: Shrub to 3 m high with white latex and reddish purple stems and leaves. Leaves petiolate, whorled, elliptical upto 9 cm long. Flowers small, borne on terminal cymes. Fruit a capsule with numerous small seeds.

Habitate: Open rocky habitats and cultivated from sea level to 550m.

Propagation: By seeds and vegetative method.

Part Used: Leaves.

Chemical Constituents: 14 ent-atisane diterpenoids, 7 ent-pimarane or ent-abietane diterpenoids, stigmasterol, stigmasterone, 3-beta-hydroxystigmastanone, sitosterone, beta-sitosterol, sycloartane and euphane triterpenoids and homotriterpenoids, octaketides, dihydroisocoumarins, carboaromatic compounds polyols.

Uses: The plant is used to treat constipation. The filtrate of the leaves is used to wean infants from their mothers. Eczyma and headaches are treated with a decoction of the leaves. The plant is also used in treating tuberculosis, stomachache and to protect new born babies from germs.

555. *Euphorbia hirta* *(Euphorbiaceae)*

Synonyms: *Euphorbia hirta.*

Vernacular Name: *Eng:* Pill-bearing spurge, Asthma plant; *Guj*: Dudeli; *Tel:* Reddinanabrolu; *Tam*: Amampatchai arisi; *Mal*: Nela palai; *Hin*: Dudhi; *Beng*: Barokhervie,.

Description: Erect annual or perennial plant growing to 50 cm, with pointed oval leaves and clusters of small flowers.

Habitate: Native to India and Australia, pill-bearing spurge is now widespread throughout the tropics.

Propagation: By seeds and vegetative method.

Parts Used: Aerial parts.

Chemical Constituents: Pill-bearing spurge contains flavonoids, terpenoids, alkanes, phenolic acids, shikimic acid and choline. The latter two constituents may by partly responsible for the antispasmodic action of this plant.

Uses: A specific treatment for bronchial asthma, pill-bearing spurge relaxes the bronchial tubes and eases breathing. Mildly sedative and expectorant, it is also taken for bronchitis and other respiratory tract conditions. It is most often used along with other anti-asthmatic herbs, notably gum plant and lobelia. In the Anglo-American tradition, pill-bearing spurge is taken to treat intestinal amoebiasis.

556. *Euphorbia lathyrus* *(Euphorbiaceae)*

Vernacular Name: *Eng:* Caper spurge.

Description: Vigorous biennial growing to 1 m. Has a hollow stem, heart-shaped leaves, cluster of small green flowers and green fruit.

Habitate: Common throughout much of Europe, Asia and North America, caper spurge grows in low-lying areas.

Propagation: By seeds and vegetative method.

Parts Used: Seeds, latex.

Chemical Constituents: The seeds contain a fixed oil and resin; the latex contain euphorbone and resin.

Uses: Caper spurge is so violent a purgative that it is rarely if ever used in contemporary herbal medicine. This indicates the extent to which medicine as a whole has changed in modern times. Purging was the first resort of many traditional medical systems, and never more enthusiastically so than in Western medicine in the 18th century. Caper spurge seeds were commonly employed, but an oil extracted from them was also used in very small doses. In the past, the milky latex of caper spurge was used as a depilatory and to remove corns, but is too irritant to be used safely.

557. *Euphorbia ligularia* Roxb. *(Euphorbiaceae)*

Synonyms: *Euphorbia neriifolia* sensu. Hook. f.

Vernacular Name: *San*: Snuhi, S undah, *Eng*: Common milk hedge, *Hin*: S hund, Thundar, *Kan*: El kalli, *Mal*: llakkalli, Kalli, *Tam*: llaikkalli, *Tel:* Akujemudu.

Description: A large fleshy, glabrous, branched shrub or a small tree, 1.8-4.5 m high with pairs of stipular spines; leaves fleshy, deciduous, obovate, spathulate, shortly, acute, nerves visible only in transmitted light; involucres usually in threes on a short fleshy peduncle, the glands transversely oblong; fruits tricoccus, seeds greenish brown, about the size of a mustard.

Habitate: Throughout India, often grown as hedge plant.

Propagation: By vegetative method.

Parts Used: Whole plant.

Chemical Constituents: Anti-coagulant activity. The triterpenoids, euphol, 24-methylenecycloartenol, euphorbol hexacosonate, glut-5-en-1-one, glut-5-en-3β-yl-acetate, taraxerol, friedelan-3α-ol, and 3β-ol have been reported from the plant. 12-deoxyphorbol-1β-hydroxyphorbol.

Uses: The plant is bitter, acrid, thermogenic, laxative, abortifacient, digestive, digestive, deobstruant, expectorant, depurative, anti-inflammatory, carminative, febrifuge, stomachic and vermifuge,. It is useful in gastropathy, bronchitis, asthma, inflammations, splenomegaly, cutaneous diseases, dropsy, dyspepsia, flatulence, intermittent fever, jaundice, leprosy, rheumatism and ulcers. The milky juice is acrid, purgative, expectorant and rubefacient and is useful in otalgia and ophthalmia.

558. *Euphorbia longan* (Lour.) steud. *(Sapindaceae)*

Description: Medium-sized tree 5-10 m. high. Leves pinnate, alternate; leaflets 5-9, oblong-lanceolate, glabrous. Inflorescence in terminal paincle; flowers pale-yellow. Fruit globose, skin glabrous or slightly rough, brownish-yellow. Seeds shining black, coated with a fleshy aril.

Habitate: Extensively cultivated for its edible fruit.

Propagation: By seeds and vegetative method.

Part Used: Pulp and seeds.

Chemical Constituents: The arils contain sugars: glucose, saccharose; vitamin A and B; proteins and lipids. The seeds yield saponins, tannin, fatty substances, starch.

Uses: The aril is considered to be nutritious. It is useful for the treatment of neurasthenia, inosmnia, amnesia, mental deficiency, urunculosis and impetigo.

559. *Euphorbia pekinensis* *(Euphorbiaceae)*

Vernacular Name: *Eng:* Da ji.

Description: Erect annual or perennial plant with oblong leaves and dense cluster of small flowers.

Habitate: Native to China, *da ji* is cultivated mainly in the eastern and central provinces.

Propagation: By seeds and vegetative method.

Parts Used: Root.

Chemical Constituents: *Da ji* contains euphorbon.

Uses: *Da ji* is classified as a toxic herb in Chinese herbal medicine, and therefore it is prescribed only for relatively serious illnesses. It is taken as a cathartic to purge excess fluid in conditions such as pleurisy and ascites and for the treatment of kidney problems, especially nephritis. *Da ji* is applied externally to inflamed sores to reduce swelling. The herb is incompatible with liquorice species as it neutralizes their medicinal effects.

560. *Euphorbia thymifolia* L. *(Euphorbiaeae)*

Vernacular Name: *San:* Laghududhika; *Eng:* Thyme-leaved spurge; *Hin:* Choti-dudhi; *Beng*: Shwetheruee; *Tel:* Reddi-vari, manubala and *Tam:* Sittrapaladi.

Description: Small annual herb with milky juice. Stems prostrate, slender, purple and downy, Leaves opposite, oval-shaped, obscurely serrulate, slightly pubescent beneath. Inflorescence in few-flowered axillary cyme. Capsule hairy. Seeds quadrangular, glabrous.

Habitate: Grows wild on pasture land, on railway embankments and in gardens.

Propagation: By seeds and vegetative method.

Part Used: Whole plant.

Chemical Constituents: The whole plant contains 5,7,4-trithydroxy flavone 7-flucoside; essential oil.

Uses: The entire plant possesses antibacterial and galactagogic properties. It is used in treating bacillary dysentery, boils, hypogalactia, galactophoritis, metrorrhagia and infantile lientery. A combination in equal parts with portulaca oleracea is also used for dysentery. A poultice of the pounded leaves is effective against dermatosis and wounds. The plant is also used as an insecticide.

561. *Euphraisa officinalis* L. *(Scrophulariaceae)*

Synonyms:: *Euphrasia latifolia* Pursh., *Euphrasia maculata* Gilib, *Euphrasia minima* Jacq., *Euphrasia pumila* Kern. A., *Euphrasia rostkoviana* Hayna.

Vernacular Name: *Eng:* Eye-bright Euphrasia.

Description: An annual herb, with a white, fibrous root and n erect, opposite, branching, hairy stem upto 2m. in height. Leaves sessile, opposite, ovate or lanceolate, bluntly dentate; the lower ones crenate, the floral briskly toothed. Flowers small, solitary, whitish, yellowish, inodourous and appear in leafy, axillary spikes at tops of the branches with bracts almost equal to the size of leaf having 3-6 teeth. Corolla white with purple veination and a yellow patch on the central lobe with 3-lobed lower lip. Calyx tubular. Stamens 4. Fruit an oblong flattened capsule.

Habitate: Temperate Himalayas, throughout Europe and North America. As a parasite on living plants like Trifolium pretans.

Propagation: By seeds and vegetative method.

Parts Used: Whole plant.

Chemical Constituents: Choline; Phytosterols like β-Sitosterol and Stigmasterol; Ferulic and caffeic acids; Aucubin, Euphroside; Vit. C.

Uses: For complaints of eyes and nose. Severe conjunctivitis producing profuse acrid lachrymation. Eyes water all the time with bland coryzal discharge, thick and excoriating. Burning and swelling of eye-lids with sticky mucus on cornea. Little blisters on cornea. Rheumatic iritis. Profuse, acrid coryza with violent cough and abundant expectoration. In males spasmodic retraction of genitals, condyloma, scycotic excercences and prostatitis. Also stated to be useful in jaundice.

562. *Euryale ferox* Salisb. *(Nymphaeceae)*

Vernacular Name: *Eng*: Fox nut, *Hin*: Makhana, *Tel:* Mellunipadmamu.

Description: Very prickly, aquatic, annual herb with short rhizome. Leaves 30-120 cm across, marginally flat, circular, dark green and reticulate-rugose above, purple and ribbed beneath, spiny on nerves at both sides. Flowers much smaller, 4 cm across, solitary on long, spiny pedicel; sepals green, 4, very prickly outside, reddish inside; petals shorter; ovules 8, 8-celled; ovary inferior. Fruit elliptic or globose, 5-7 cm in diameter, spiny; calyx left at the top.

Habitate: Mountain woods of India, China, Japan and Korea.

Propagation: By seeds and vegetative method.

Parts Used: Twig, bark.

Chemical Constituents: Steryl glycosides, tocopherols. The antioxidants mainly α-, β-, γ- and δ-tocopherol have been extracted with organic solvents from the seed. A cerebroside, N-α-hydroxyl-*cis*-oc-tadecaenoyl-1-O-β-glucopyranosyl-sphingosine.

Uses: Antioxidant, murine retroviral reverse transcriptase inhibition, DNA polymerase α inhibition. Used in weakenss, spermatorrhoea leucorrhoea.

563. *Evodia rutaecarpa* (Juss.) Benth. *(Rutaceae)*

Vernacular Name: *Eng:* Medicinal evodia.

Description: A deciduous small tree, 3-10 m high. Leaves, opposite, imparipinnate compound, 30-40 cm long; leaflets 5-7, winged, nearly sessile, oblng; apex acumiate, generally rounded at the base, entire, the underside villous, dotted with glands. In summer, it bears numerous small white flowers in a corympb on the summer. It bears numerous small white flowers in a corumb on the top of the branches, and in autumn small greenish-red-brown flattish-globular fruit 3-5 mm in diameter, 2-valved, opening at the top and with peculiar aromatic odour.

Habitate: On slopes on the skirts of forests, but mostly cultivated in China, India, Japan.

Propagation: By seeds and vegetative method.

Part Used: Fruit.

Chemical Constituents: N.A.

Uses: Nausea; vomiting; abdominal pain; belching; diarrhoea.

564. *Evolvulus alsinoides* L. *(Convolvulaceae)*

Vernacular Name: *San*: Vishnukranta, Shankhapushpi, *Hin:* Shankhahuli.

Description: A perennial herb with prostrate branches and small elliptic to oblong, lanceolate, obtuse, mucronte *leaves, flowers* mostly solitary in upper axils. Corolla blue rotate and broad funnel shaped, capsule globose.

Habitate: It is a common weed growing wildly in open grassy places throughout India. It is also cultivated.

Propagation: By seeds and vegetative method.

Parts Used: Whole plant.

Chemical Constituents: The plant contains an alkaloid–shankhapushpine. Fresh plant contains volatile oil and potassium chloride. It also contains a yellow neutral fat, an organic, acid and saline substances. Three alkaloids-evolvine, betaine, and an unidentified compound have been isolated.

Uses: Nootropic agent. Chronic bronchitis. General weakness. Used in fever, nervous debility, loss of memory, also in syphilis and scrofula. It is used as Rasayan.

565. *Fagopyrum esculentum* *(Polygonaceae)*

Vernacular Name: *Eng:* Buckwheat; *Hin*: Kotu, phaphra.

Description: An annual herb, 3-5 ft. high with alternate, hastate, acute leaves, flowers in axillary or terminal cymes, pinkish white, fragrant, fruit a 3-cornered achene.

Habitate: Buckwheat is native to central and northern Asia, and is cultivated extensively in temperate regions, of India.

Propagation: By seeds and vegetative method.

Parts Used: Leaves, flowers.

Chemical Constituents: Buckwheat contains bioflavonoids, especially rutin, which is strongly antoxidant. Rutin strengthens the inner lining of blood vessels.

Uses: Used for a wide range of circulatory problems, buckwheat is best taken as a tea or tablet, accompanied by vitamin C or lemon juice to aid absorption. Buckwheat is used particularly to treat fragile capillaries, but also helps strengthen varicose veins and heal chilblains. Often combined with lime flowers, buckwheat is a specific treatm3nt for haemorrhage into the retina. Buckwheat is also commonly taken in combination with other herbs for high blood pressure.

566. *Feronia limonia* *(Rutaceae)*

Synonyms: *Feronia elephantum.*

Vernacular Name: *Eng:* Wood apple; *Hin*: Bilin, kait, kavitha; *Beng*: kati, katbd; *Guj*: Kavti, kotha; *Tel:* Velaga; *Tam*: Vilanga; *Kan*: Bela; *Mal*: Vila, vilatti.

Description: A small deciduous tree with short, erect, cylindrical stem, bearing thorny branches; leaves pinnate, with small ovate or obovate leaflets; flowers in panicles; fruit large, globose; seeds numerous.

Habitate: Native to southern India, wood apple is cultivated in tropical Asia.

Propagation: By seeds and vegetative method.

Parts Used: Fruit and leaves.

Chemical Constituents: The fruit contains fruit acids, vitamins and minerals. The leaves contain tannins and a volatile oil.

Uses: Wood apple fruit is used mainly to stimulate the digestive system. In India, the fruit forms part of a paste applied to tone the breasts. The astringent leaves are used to treat indigestion, flatulence, diarrhoea, dysentery and haemorrhoids.

567. *Ferula asafetida* L. *(Apiaceae)*

Vernacular Name: *San*: *Hingu*, *Eng*: Asafoetida (Asafetida), *Hin*: Himg, *Kan*: *Hingu*, *Mal*: K yam, Karikk yam, Perunk yam, *Tam*: Perunk yam, K yam, *Tel:* Inguva.

Description: A herbaceous perennial with fleshy, massive carrot-shaped root with one or more forks, stem 1.8-3 m high, solid, clothed with membranous leaf sheaths; leaves radical, 45 cm long, shiny, coriaceous with pinnatifid segments and channeled petiode; flowers 10-20 in the main and 5-6 in the partial umbels; fruits flat, thin, reddish brown.

Habitate: Wild in Punjab, Kashmir, Iran and Afghanistan.

Propagation: By seeds and vegetative method.

Parts Used: Resinous exudates of the root.

Chemical Constituents: The gum resin contains the coumarins, 5-hydroxy-umbelliprenin, 8-hydroxyum-belliprenin, 9-hydroxyumbelliprenin, 8-acetoxy-5-hydroxyumbel-liprenin, assafoetidin, ferocolicin, asacoumarin A and B, farnesiferol A, -B and–C and the disulphides, asadisulphide and *sec*-butylpropenyl disulphide.

Uses: The oleo resin is bitter, acrid, carminative, antispasmodic, expectorant, anthelmintic, diuretic, laxative, nervine tonic, digestive, sedative and emmenagogue. It is used in flatulent colic, dyspepsia, asthma, hysteria, constipation, chronic bronchitis, whooping cough, epilepsy, psychopathy, hepatopathy, splnopathy and vitiated conditions of *kapha* and *v ta*.

568. *Ferula gummosa* *(Apiaceae)*

Synonyms*:* *Ferula galbaniflua*.

Vernacular Name: *Eng:* Galbanum.

Description: Perennial with a smooth, hollow stem, finely toothed compound leaves and umbels of small white flowers.

Habitate: Native to central Asia.

Propagation: By seeds and vegetative method.

Parts Used: Oleo-gum-resin.

Chemical Constituents: Galbanum exudate contains a volatile oil, resins gums and a coumarin.

Uses: Galbanum is a digestive stimulant and antispasmodic, reducing flatulence, griping pains and colic. It is also expectorant. Applied as an ointment, the gum may help heal wounds.

569. *Fibraurea recisa* Pierre *(Menispermaceae)*

Description: Woody climbing plant. Roots and old branches yellow inside. Leaves alternate, apex acute, base round or lightly cordate; obviously 3-nerved; petiole long, swollen at both ends. Flowers unisexual, dioecious, greenish-yellow in raceme of old branches. Fruit oval, yellow when ripe;single-seeded.

Habitate: Grows wild in mountainous regions.

Propagation: By seeds and vegetative method.

Part Used: Roots and stems.

Chemical Constituents: The roots yield alkaloids: palmatine, jatrorrhizine, columbamine, and berberine.

Uses: A decoction of the roots is used to treat opthalmia, furunculosis, prurigo, enteritis, gastritis, cystitis, dysentery and feber. In cases of purulent otitis, the powedered roots assiciated with alum are applied topically.

570. *Ficus benghalensis* L. *(Moraceae)*

Vernacular Name: *San*: Nyagr dhah, *Vatah*, *Eng*: Banyan, *Hin*: Bat, Bargad, *Kan*: la, *Mal*: P r l, *Vatavrksam*, *Tam*: lamaram, P r l, *Tel:* Peddamarri.

Description: A very large tree upto 30 m in height with widely spreading branches bearing many aerial roots functioning as prop roots, bark greenish white, leaves simple, alternate, often in clusters at ends of branches, stipulate, 10-20 cm long and 5-12.5 cm broad, broadly elliptic to ovate, entire, coriaceous, strongly 3-7 ribbed from the base; the fruit receptacles are axillary, sessile, in pairs, globose, brick-red when ripe, enclosing male, female and gall flowers; fruits small, crustaceous achenes, enclosed in the common fleshy receptacles.

Habitate: Throughout India, from sea-level to 1,200 m.

Propagation: By seeds and vegetative method.

Parts Used: Aerial root, bark, leaves, buds, fruits, latex.

Chemical Constituents: Bengalenoside and the flavonoid glycosides, leucocyanidin 3-O-β-D-galactosyl cellobioside 5,3'-dimethyl ether and leucopelargonidin-3-O-α-L-rhamnoside 5,7-dimethyl ether, leucopelargonidin glycoside leucocyanidin glycoside.

Uses: All parts of the plant are astringent, acrid, sweet, refrigerant, anodyne, vulnerary, depurative, anti-inflammatory, ophthalmic, styptic, antiarthritic, diaphoretic, antidiarrhoeal, antiemetic and tonic. The aerial roots are useful in obstinate vomiting and leucorrhoea and are said to be used in osteomalacia of the limbs. The bark is useful in burning sensation, haemoptysis, haemorrhages, diarrhoea, dysentery, diabetes, enuresis, ulcers, skin diseases, gonorrhoea, leucorrhoea and hyperdipsia. The leaves are good for ulcers, leprosy, allergic conditions of skin, burning sensation and abscesses. The buds are useful in diarrhoea and dysentery. The fruits are refrigerant and tonic and are useful in vitiated condition of *pitta*. The latex is useful in neuralgia, rheumatism, lumbago, bruises, nasitis, ulorrhagia, ulitis, odontopathy, haemorrhoids, gonorrhoea, inflammations, cracks of the sole and skin diseases.

571. *Ficus carica* *(Moraceae)*

Vernacular Name: *Eng:* Fig; *Hin*: Anjir; *Beng*: Anjir; *Guj*: Anjir; *Tel:* Anjuru manjimedi; *Tam*: Simaiyatti; *Kan*: Anjura; *Mal*: Simayatti.

Description: Deciduous tree growing to 4 m. Has large leaves and fleshy receptacles which ripen into purple-brown, pear-shaped fruit.

Habitate: Native to western Asia, fig now grows wild and is cultivated in many temperate and sub-tropical regions. Fruit harvested in summer.

Propagation: By vegetative method.

Parts Used: Fruit, latex.

Chemical Constituents: Figs contains around 50% fruits sugars, flavonoids, vitamins and enzymes.

Uses: The fruit sugars within the fig have a pronounced but gentle laxative effect; syrup of figs is still a remedy for mild constipation. The fruit's emollient pulp helps relieve pain and inflammation, and it has been used to treat tumours, swellings and gum abscesses-the fruit often being roasted before application. Figs are also mildly expectorant and, when used with herbs such as elecampane are helpful in treating dry and irritable coughs and bronchitis. The milky latex from leaves and stems is reputed to be analgesic, and has long been used to treat warts, insect bites and stings.

572. *Ficus pumlia* L. *(Moraceae)*

Vernacular Name: *Eng:* Creeping fig. Climbing fig.

Description: Climbing shrub, stems rooting at the nodes. Leves alternate, glabrous, of two kinds, one kind shaped like scales and the other obovate. Inflorescence in the axil of the leaves, bearing male flowers above and female below. Solitary, pyriform, glabrous, brownish-violet when ripe.

Habitate: Grows wild on rocks and tree trunks and is cultivated for covering walls.

Propagation: By seeds and vegetative method.

Part Used: Fruit and leafy branches.

Chemical Constituents: The gum obtained from the plant yields glucose, fructose and arabinose on hydrolysis. The fruit contains proteins and latex.

Uses: The aerial parts constitute a systemic remedy and blood reconstituent. They are used in treasting chronic dysentery, haemorrhoids, galactophoritis, spermatorrhoea, impotence, menstrual disorders, dysuria, dyschezia, rheumatism, lumbago, osteodynia, boils and impetigo.

573. *Ficus racemosa* L. *(Moraceae)*

Synonyms*: Ficus glomerata.*

Vernacular Name: *San*: Udmbar; *Hin:* Gular.

Description: The tree is medium tall with quite rich green foliage that provides good shade. The *fruits* resemble figs and are obovate in shape with innumerable tiny grain-like seeds.

Habitate: It is cultivated all over India. It also grows wild in many forests and hills.

Propagation: By seeds and vegetative method.

Parts Used: Bark, fruit, latex, root.

Chemical Constituents: Glycosides are present in the plant. β-sitosterol and lupeol have been isolated from the petroleum ether extract of the root-bark of the plant. Tannins are also present. Psoralens have also been detected.

Uses: Excessive appetite. External burning. Skin inflammation. Diarrhoea/Dysentery. Leucoderma. It is astringent, carminative, vermifuge and an anti-dysentery drug. It is a good remedy for excessive appetite. The extract of fruit is used in diabetes, leucoderma and menorrhagia. It is used locally to relieve inflammation of skin wounds, lymphadenitis, in sprains and fibrousitis.

574. *Ficus religiosa* L. *(Moraceae)*

Vernacular Name: *San*: Pippalah, Asvatthah, *Eng*: Peepal tree, Sacred fig, *Hin*: Pippal, Pipli, Pipar, *Kan*: aswaththa, *Mal*: Arayal, *Tam*: Arasu, asvattam, *Tel:* Ravi.

Description: A large deciduous tree with few or no aerial roots, often epiphytic, the dropping branchlets bear long-petioled ovate, cordate, shiny leaves which produce a characteristic rustling sound when the wind blows; leaves bright green, the apex produced into a linear-lanceolate tail about half long as the main portion of the blade; the receptacles occurring in pairs, axillary, depressed globose, smooth, purplish when ripe.

Habitate: Throughout India, wild as well as cultivated.

Propagation: By seeds and vegetative method.

Parts Used: Bark, leaves, tender shoots, fruits, seeds, latex.

Chemical Consistuents: Arabinose, mannose, glucose, phenolic glucoside ester, flacourtin. Steroid, ramontoside, β-sitosterol and its β-Dglucopyranoside.

Uses: The bark is astringent, sweet, cooling and aphrodisiac, and an aqueous extract of it has an antibacterial activity against *Staphylococcus aureus* and *Escherichia coli.* It is used in the treatment of paste of the powdered bark is a good absorbent for inflammatory swellings and good for burns. Leaves and tender shoots have purgative properties and are also recommended for wounds and skin diseases. Fruits are laxative and digestive; the dried fruit pulverized and taken in water cures asthma; seeds refrigerant and laxative. The latex is good for neuralgia, inflammations and haemorrhages.

575. *Filipendula ulmaria* *(Rosaceae)*

Vernacular Name: *Eng:* Meadowsweet, queen of the Meadow.

Description: A perennial reaching 1.5m, with toothed leaves and clusters of creamy, scented flowers.

Habitate: Native to Europe, meadowsweet grows easily in damp places, preferring ditches and the banks of streams and rivers.

Propagation: By vegetative method.

Parts Used: Flowers and Leaves.

Chemical Constituents: Flavonol glycosides, mainly glycosides of quercetin, phenolic glycosides, volatile oil, polyphenols.

Uses: Anti-inflammatory, antirheumatic, astringent, diuretic, eases stomach pain.

576. *Flacourtia indica* (Burm. F.) Merr. *(Flacourtiaceae)*

Synonyms: *Flacourtia ramontchi* L' Herit.

Vernacular NameS: *San*: Aghori, *Eng*: Governor's plum, Madagascar plum, *Hin*: *Kan*cu, Bilangra, Kataiya, *Kan*: Nakkeharagu, *Mal*: Aghori, Mullullakatta, *Tam*: Sottaikala, *Ma*lukkarai, *Tel:* Putikatada.

Description: A small deciduous thorny shrub; leaves simple, elliptic, acute or acuminate, coarsely crenate or serrate, glabrous; flowers greenish yellow, in short simple or branched tomentose racemes; fruits globose, dark purple drupes with juicy pulp and hard endocarp, seeds 8-16.

Habitate: Throughout India, in scrub forests and rocky hills upto 900 m.

Propagation: By seeds and vegetative method.

Parts Used: Roots, leaves fruits.

Chemical Consistuents: Arabinose, mannose, glucose, phenolic glucoside ester, flacourtin. Steroid, ramontoside, β-sitosterol and its β-Dglucopyranoside.

Uses: The roots are sweet, refrigerant, depurative alexipharmic and diuretic. They are useful in vitiated conditions of *pitta* and v ta aphthae, poisonous bites, skin diseases. Pruritus, erysipelas, strangury, nephropathy and psychopathy. The leaves are useful in pruritus and scabies. The fruits are sweet, appetizer, digestive and diuretic, and are useful in strangury, jaundice, gastropathy and splenomegaly.

577. *Focus vesiculosus* *(Fucacee)*

Vernacular Name: *Eng:* Bladderwrack, Kelp.

Description: Brownish-green alga growing to 1 m in length. Has flat, usually forked, fronds containing air bladders.

Habitate: Bladderwrack is native to the shores of the North Atlantic and western Mediterranean, and is harvested throughout the year.

Propagation: By seeds and vegetative method.

Parts Used: Whole plant.

Chemical Constituents: Bladderwrack contains phenols, polysaccharides and minerals, especially iodine. The polysaccharides are immune-stimulant. The iodine may stimulate the thyroid gland.

Uses: Due to its iodine content, bladderwrack is taken as an anti-goitre remedy. The plant appears to raise the metabolic rate by increasing hormone production by the thyroid gland, but this increase may be limited to poorly functioning thyroids. Bladderwrack is reputedly helpful in rheumatic conditions.

578. *Foeniculum vulgare* Mill. *(Apiaceae)*

Synonyms: *Forniculum capillaceum* Gilib.; *Forniculum officinale* All.

Vernacular Name: *Eng:* Fennel; *Hin:* Saunf; *Beng*: Panmuhori; *Kan:* Badisepu; *Tam:* Shombu; *Tel:* Sopu.

Description: An aromatic, perennial herb 1-2 m high. Leaves alternate, 3 or 4 times pinnate, the ultimate leaflets very numerous, filiform, very elongated, the superior leaves with sheaths longer than the blade. Umbels compound, large, long-pedunculate, nearly, regular. Flowers yellow, not involucrate, July-October, calyx with 5 very slight teeth. Petals 5, entire; tips involute. Stamens 5, ovary 2-celled; stylopodium large, conical. Fruit avoid, 6 mm long by 2 mm in diameter, greenish; glabrous mericarp compressed dorsally, semicylindrical, with 5 prominent, nearly regular ribs. Seeds somewhat concave with longitudinal furrows. The fruit tastes sweet and pungent and smells of anis seed.

Habitate: Commonly cultivated in fields.

Propagation: By seeds and vegetative method.

Part Used: Fruit.

Chemical Constituents: Major components of fennel oil are *trans*-anethole, fenchone, limonene, methyl chavicol, and α-pinene, besides α-phellandrene, myrecene, and *cis*-ocimene.

Uses: Feeling of cold and pains in stomach and lower abdomen, 2-dysmenorrhoea, hernia pain. Fennel is used to confer flavour and aroma to soups, meat dishes, sauces, bakery and confectionery products, liqueurs, and pickles. Fennel oil is used to flavour seasonings, confectionery, culinary preparations, tobacco, cordials and liqueurs.

579. *Forsythia suspensa* *(Oleaceae)*

Vernacular Name: *Eng:* Lain qiao, Weeping forsythia.

Description: Deciduous shrub growing to 3 m. Has toothed leaves, bright yellow flowers and woody fruit.

Habitate: Native to china and Japan, *lian qiao* is cultivated in the northern and central areas of China and in other temperate regions.

Propagation: By seeds and vegetative method.

Parts Used: Fruit.

Chemical Constituents: The fruit contains forsythin.

Uses: A bitter-tasting, pungent herb with an antiseptic effect, *lian qiao* is chiefly used to treat boils, carbuncles, mumps and infected neck glands. It is also a remedy for colds, flu, sore throats and tonsillitis, and for the early stages of fevers. It is given in combination with other herbs for dysentery and skin infections. *Kian qiao* has been used for 'cold" swellings of the neck. In Chinese folk medicine, it is a treatment for breast cancer. The herb is sometimes taken to induce menstruation.

580. *Fragaria vesca* *(Rosaceae)*

Vernacular Name: *Eng:* Wild strawberry.

Description: Low-growing perennial herb spread by runners. Has 3-lobed leaves, white flowers and small red berries.

Habitate: Wild strawberry is native to Europe and temperate regions of Asia.

Propagation: By vegetative method.

Parts Used: Leaves, fruit.

Chemical Constituents: The leaves contains flavonoids, tannins and a volatile oil. The fruit contains fruit acids and a volatile oil with methyl salicylate and borneol.

Uses: Wild strawberry leaves are mildly astringent and diuretic. The plant is little used medicinally today, but it can be taken to treat diarrhoea and dysentery. The leaves were used as a gargle for sore throats, and in a lotion for minor burns and grazes. In Europe, the fruit is considered to have cooling and diuretic properties, and has been prescribed as part of a diet in cases of tuberculosis, gout, arthritis and rheumatism.

581. *Fraxinus Americana* L. *(Oleaceae)*

Synonyms: *Fraxinus Novae-angliae* Mill., *Fraxinus alba* Marsh., *Fraxinus canadensis* Gaertn.

Vernacular Name: *Eng:* White ash.

Description: A tall tree up to 40 m. in height, with branchlet and petiole glabrous. Calys 4, corolla none. Stamens 2. Leaflets 5 to 9, usually 7, oblong to ovate or obovate, usually abruptly acuminate, entire or serrulate towards the summit, rounded to broadly acute at base, paler beneath, 7.6 to 12.7 cm. Fruit a winged samara, 1-seeded, 3 to 5 cm. long, obtuse or retuse at the summit, winged, wings not decurrent, wing extending about a third of the length of terete body, free portion above the apex of the body, longer than the body itself subtending calyx 1 to 1.3 rarely 2 mm. long, seldom cleft on one side only.

Habitate: U.S.A. (Chicoga, Florida) and Canada.

Propagation: By seeds and vegetative method.

Parts Used: Inner bark.

Chemical Constituents: Fraxin; Fraxetin and Quercetin.

Uses: For complaints specifically of uterus. Enlargement of uterus. Uterine fibroids with bearing down sensation, cramps in feet, unirritating leucorrhoeia. Prolaps uteri. Throbbing pain in back and head. Nervous restlessness. Hot spots on top of head. Tenderness in left inguinal region.

582. *Fraxinus excelsior* *(Oleaceae)*

Vernacular Name: *Eng:* Ash.

Description: Deciduous tree growing to 40 m. Has pale grey bark, black conical leaf buds and bright green leaves with 7-13 oval leaflets.

Habitate: Common in Europe, ash thrives in lowland and moorland.

Propagation: By vegetative method.

Parts Used: Leaves, bark.

Chemical Constituents: Ash leaves and bark contain coumarins, flavonoids, tannins, sugars and a volatile oil.

Uses: Ash bark is tonic and astringent. Little used in herbal medicine today, it is occasionally taken for fever. The leaves are also astringent, and they have a laxative and diuretic effect. They have been used as a mild substitute for senna.

583. *Fraxinus rhynchophylla* Hance *(Oleaceae)*

Vernacular Name: *Eng*: Chinese ash.

Description: Deciduous tree, to 10 m tall, but usually much smaller. Leaves opposite, odd-pinnate; leaflet 5-7, wide ovate or wide lanceolate, 6-15 cm long, green, glabrous above, pubescent on mid-vein beneath, crenate or smooth. Flowers small, in axillary panicles, with or after leaves, unisexual; calyx small, 4-lobed; petals none in male flowers, 2-4 in female flowers. Fruit a l-seeded, winged samara, to 5 cm long.

Habitate: Mountain woods in Korea and China.

Propagation: By seeds and vegetative method.

Parts Used: Bark.

Chemical Constituents: Related species, F. japonicum, contains: Lignans. Coumarins: scopoletin, isofraxidin, esculetin, fraxetin, esculin, fraxin, fraxidin, fraxinol.

Uses: Related species, F. japonicum, shows platelet antiaggregatory, antibacterial, and lipoxygenase inhibition, HMG-Co A reductase inhibition activities. Used in eye diseases, apoplexy, liner diseases.

584. *Fritillaria thunbergii* *(Liliaceae)*

Vernacular Name: *Eng:* Zhe bei mu.

Description: Bulbous perennial with erect stems, long narrow leaves and hanging bell-shaped flowers.

Habitate: Native to China and Siberia, *zhe bei mu* is cultivated in eastern China.

Propagation: By vegetative method.

Parts Used: Bulb.

Chemical Constituents: The bulb contains alkaloids, including peimine, which affects the parasympathetic nervous system.

Uses: *Zhe bei mu* increases the coughing up to mucus and relieves irritability in the respiratory tract. It is given for bronchitis and tonsillitis, and for fever and respiratory symptoms accompanying other acute infections such as flu. *Xhe bei mu* is through to act specifically on tumours and swelling of the throat, neck and chest, and is taken for thyroid gland nodules, scrofula, abscesses and boils, and breast cancer. It has also been used to treat dysentery, and to increase breast-milk production.

585. *Fumaria officinalis*

Fumariaceae

Vernacular Name: *Eng:* Fumitory

Description: Climbing annual growing to 30 cm. Has compound leaves and maroon-tipped pink tubular flowers.

Habitate: Native to Europe and North Africa, fumitory also grows in Asia, North America and Australia.

Propagation: By seeds and vegetative method

Parts Used: Flower

Chemical Constituents: Fumitory contains isoquinoline alkaloids.

Uses: The herb has a stimulant action on the liver and gallbladder and is chiefly used to treat skin conditions such as eczema. It is also diuretic and mildly laxative.

586. *Fumaria officinalis* L. *(Fumariaceae)*

Vernacular Name: *San*: Parpata, *Hin:* Pitapapra.

Description: The plant is of a grayish yellow colour. *Leaves* greenish, thick and narrow, stems grayish yellow, one or two inches long, furrowed and rather quadrangular. *Fruit* capsules are very small grayish green, slightly compressed and with a transverse ridge scar to the apex. *Flowers* are irregular, asymmetrical and either violet or white, *seeds* small and consist of fleshy albumin.

Habitate: The plant is found in many parts of India, Nepal and in the Nilgiri mountains.

Propagation: By seeds and vegetative method.

Parts Used: Whole plant.

Chemical Constituents: The plant contsins fumaric acid and fumarine. Fumarine exists in irregular 6-sided crystals or in monochlonic prisms, insoluble in alcohol, chloroform, benzol and amyl alcohol sparingly soluble in water and soluble in either. Seven alkaloids have been isolated from the alcoholic extract of whole plant.

Uses: Common cold and fever. Intestinal colic. Hyperacidity. Jaundice. It is often used in common cold and fever and also in certain skin disorders. With black pepper it is given in jaundice. It is given to relieve vomiting and thirst in febrile conditions.

587. *Galega officinalis* *(Leguminosae)*

Vernacular Name: *Eng:* Goat's rue.

Description: Bushy perennial growing to about 1 m. Has compound leaves with lance-shaped leaflets, delicate pink pea-type flowers on terminal spikes, and red-brown seedpods in autumn.

Habitate: Native to Asia and continental Europe, and naturalized in Britain, goat's rue grows in damp and low-lying areas.

Propagation: By seeds and vegetative method.

Parts Used: Aerial parts.

Chemical Constituents: Goat's rue contains alkaloids, saponins, flavonoids and tannins. Galegine strongly reduces blood sugar levels.

Uses: Today, goat's rue is chiefly used as an anti-diabetic herb, having the ability to reduce blood sugar levels. It is not a substitute for conventional treatments but can be valuable in the early stages of late-onset diabetes and is best used as an infusion. The herb has the effect of increasing breast-milk production. It is also a useful diuretic.

588. *Galipea officinalis* *(Rutaceae)*

Synonyms: *Galipea cusparia.*

Vernacular Name: *Eng:* Angostura.

Description: Evergreen tree growing to 15 m with grey bark, shiny bright green leaflets and foul-smelling flowers.

Habitate: Angostura is native to some Caribbean island and to tropical South America. The bark is gathered throughout the year.

Propagation: By seeds and vegetative method.

Parts Used: Bark.

Chemical Constituents: Angostura bark contains bitter principles, alkaloids, including cusparine, and 1-2% volatile oil.

Uses: A strong bitter with tonic properties angostura stimulates the stomach and digestive tracts as a whole. It is antispasmodic and is reported to act on the spinal nerves, helping in paralytic conditions. Angostura is typically given for weak digestion, and is considered valuable as a remedy for diarrhoea and dysentery. In south America, it is sometimes used as a substitute for cinchona to control fevers.

589. *Galium aparine* *(Rubiaceae)*

Vernacular Name: *Eng:* Cleavers, Goose grass.

Description: Straggling, square-stemmed annual growing to a height of 1.2 m with whorls of lance-shaped leaves, clusters of small white flowers and small, round, green fruit with hooked prickles.

Habitate: Common throughout Europe and North America, cleavers is found in many other temperate regions, including in Australia.

Propagation: By seeds and vegetative method.

Parts Used: Aerial parts.

Chemical Constituents: Cleavers contains iridoids, polyphenolic acids, anthraquinones, alkanes, flavonoids and tannins. asperuloside is a mild laxative.

Uses: A valuable diuretic, cleavers is often taken for skin diseases such as seborrhea, eczema and psoriasis; for swollen lymph glands; and as a general detoxifying agent in serious illnesses such as cancer. The plant is commonly prepared in the form of an infusion, but for conditions such as cancer, it is best taken as a juice, which is strongly diuretic. The juice and the infusion are also taken for kidney stones and other urinary problems.

590. *Gallium verum* *(Rubiaceae)*

Vernacular Name: *Eng:* Lady's bedstraw.

Description: Short, sprawling perennial growing to 80 cm. Has whorls of narrow dark green leaves and tufts of very small bright yellow flowers.

Habitate: Found throughout Europe and western Asia, and naturalized in North America.

Propagation: By seeds and vegetative method.

Parts Used: Aerial parts.

Chemical Constituents: Lady's bedstraw contains iridoids, flavonoids, anthraquinones and alkanes.

Uses: A slightly bitter-tasting remedy, lady's bedstraw is used mainly as a diuretic and for skin problems. Like its close relative, cleavers the herb is given for kidney stones, bladder stones and other urinary conditions, including cystitis. It is occasionally used as a means to relieve chronic skin problems such as psoriasis, but, in general, cleavers is preferred as a treatment for this condition. Lady's bedstraw has had a long-standing reputation, especially in France, of being a valuable remedy for epilepsy, though it is rarely used for this purpose today.

591. *Garcinia gummi-gutta* (L.) Robson *(Clusiaceae)*

Synonyms: *Garcinia cambogia* (Gaertn.) Desr.

Vernacular Name: *Hin*: Bilatti-amli, *Kan*: Upagi mara, Simai hunase, *Mal*: Kodam puli, Meen puli, Perum puli, Mar: Dharambe, *Tam*: Penam puli, Kodakka puli, *Tel:* Sima chinta.

Description: Medium sized trees, 5-15 m tall. *Bark* about 5 mm thick, brown, smooth, exudes yellow gum when cut freshly. *Blaze* deep yellow. Mature branches horizontal or drooping. *Leaves* opposite, 7-15 x 2-7 cm, oblong, elliptic or lanceolate, base wedge-shaped, apex acute to rounded, margin entire, hairless, glossy, dark green; lateral nerves 10-20 pairs, parallel, slender, prominent; leaf stalks about 1.2 cm long, stout, centrally grooved. *Male*, female & bisexual flowers are separately seen in same or different plants, sub-fleshy, distinctly stalked; *male flowers* in a group of 5-10 seen in leaf axils of on branches, about 1.5 cm long, 1 cm across, orange-yellow. *Female* and *bisexual flowers* solitary or in clusters of 2-3 in terminal and axillary fascicles, orange, slightly larger than male flowers. *Berries* 3-7 cm across, pome-shaped, fleshy, sub-globose to globose, shiny, hairless, with 4-10 vertical grooves, ripening yellow, with a distinct persistent projection at tip. *Seeds* 4-10, egg-shaped, about 3 cm long, flat, brown, smooth, shiny, covered with fleshy, white or red aril.

Habitate: Semi-evergreen to evergreen forests.

Propagation: By seeds and vegetative method.

Parts Used: Seeds.

Chemical Constituents: The plant contains cambogin and camboginol. The fruit contains about 30% acid, which is essentially-hydroxy-citric acid.

Uses: The leaves, fruits and seed oil are reported to be purgative, hydragogue and emetic. Useful in curing ulcers, inflammations, bleeding piles, diarrhoea, dysentery, indigestion, hyperdipsia and particularly in dropsy and worm cases. Citrin is extracted from the fruits and is reportedly used for treating obesity.

592. *Garcinia indica* (Thouars) Choisy *(Clusiaceae)*

Vernacular Name: *San*: Amlavetasa, Tintidika, Vrksamla, *Hin*: Kokam, *Kan*: Murgina huli mara, Murgal, *Mal*: Punam puli, *Mar*: Katambi, Kokam, Ratamba, *Tam*: Murgal.

Description: Slender trees, 4-10 m tall, with drooping branches. *Wood* greyish white. *Bark* light brown, thin and smooth. *Blaze* bright yellow. Branchlets sub-cylindrical, slender, hairless. *Leaves* opposite, 5-10 x 2-5 cm, inverted egg-shaped-oblong to elliptic-lanceolate, narrowed at base, rounded or shortly acuminate at apex, shiny, dark green; lateral nerves 7-18 pairs, prominent. *Male* and female flowers are separated, fleshy, stalked, orange-yellow. *Male flowers* 4-8 in a cluster, about 1.2 cm long; *female flowers* solitary, terminal. *Berries* spherical, 3-4 cm across, wine brown or purple or pinkish orange, with persistent calyx lobes; fruit pulp white with red tinge, acidic, fleshy. *Seeds* 5-8, flat, smooth, shiny and brown.

Habitate: Coastal to evergreen forests.

Propagation: By seeds and vegetative method.

Parts Used: Fruits.

Chemical Constituents: The fruit rind contains a polyisoprenylated phenolic pigment, garcinol and its isomer isogarcinol, along with hjydroxycitric acid, cyaniding-3-glucoside and cyaniding-3-sambubioside. L-Leucine and DNP-L-leucine hydrochloride have been reported from the leaves.

Uses: The seed butter is used as a remedy in scrofulous diseases, dysentery, mucous diarrhoea and externally applied for excoriations, chaps, fissures of lips and as a substitute for spermaceti. The ripe fruit is anthelmintic and cardiotonic. Root bark, fruit and seed oil are used to cure piles, sprue, abdominal disorders, mouth diseases, cardiac diseases plus worm infestation.

593. *Garcinia morella* (Gaertn.) Desr. *(Clusiaceae)*

Vernacular Name: *San*: *Kan*kustha, *Tam*ala, *Hin*: *Tam*al, *Kan*: Devana huli, Pon puli, Arsina gurgi, *Mal*: Chigiri, Karukam puli, Pinnar puli, Mar: *Tam*ala, Mahabala, *Tam*: Makki, Solai puli, *Tel:* Reval chinni, Pasupuvarne.

Description: Trees, 7-15 m tall, with spreading branches and dense crown. *Wood* yellow mottled, hard. *Bark* brownish grey, thin, about 5 mm thick, smooth, exuding brilliant, dark yellow, sticky, thick latex. *Blaze* yellow. Branchlets 4-angled, hairless, horizontal. *Leaves* opposite, elliptic-egg-shaped, about 7-15 x 4-8 cm, base acute, apex rounded to shortly acuminate, margin entire, hairless, shiny; lateral nerves 8-15 pairs, unequally parallel, obscure; leaf stalks up to 1 cm long, stout, thickened at base. *Mal*e, female and bisexual flowers are separated, succulent, stalked, pinkish red. *Male flowers* 2-3 together in leaf axils and on old branches, about 8 mm long, faintly fragrant; *female flowers* axillary, solitary, equal to or larger than male flowers. *Berries* 1.5-2.5 cm across, globose or rarely ovoid, hairless, shiny, smooth, stalkless, pinkish brown when ripe; pulp sweet, acidic. *Seeds* 1-4, kidney-shaped to ovoid, laterally compressed, brown.

Habitate: Moist deciduous to evergreen forests.

Propagation: By seeds and vegetative method.

Parts Used: Fruits.

Chemical Constituents: It contains morellin, neo-morellin, β-guttiferin and α-l-guttiferin.

Uses: Commonly called *Svarnaksiri* indicating the golden yellow juice. It is light bitter tonic, astringent and anthelmintic. Cures dropsy, hydragogue, drastic cathartic, rheumatism, constipation, dysentery, colic and other intestinal affections. The golden yellow exudates is used for treating blisters, indolent ulcers, leprosy and other skin infections. Seeds are used to relieve cough, catarrh affections of the throat, pulmonary mucous membrane and asthma. Seed oil is applied externally to ulcers, herpetic eruptions and other skin diseases. All parts of the plant reportedly posses antibacterial activity.

594. *Garcinia sessilis* (Forster) Seemann *(Clusiaceae)*

Description: Tree upto 20 m high with yellow latex. Leaves opposite, petiolate, simple, ovate to elliptical, upto 10 cm long. Flowers unisexual (Plants dioecious), 4-parted, pale pink, borne in axillary clusters of 3-9 flowers. Fruit a red drupe, obovoid, upto 4 cm long.

Habitate: Common forest tree occurring in both wet and ry forest.

Propagation: By seeds and vegetative method.

Part Used: Leaves.

Chemical Constituents: N.A.

Uses: Crushed leaves in water commonly used as an eyewash for eye problems.

595. *Garcinia travancorica* Bedd. *(Clusiaceae)*

Vernacular Name: *Mal*: *Mal*a pongu, *Tam*: *Mal*am punku.

Description: A medium sized tree, 7-15 m tall. *Wood* yellowish white, hard, heavy with small brown-streaked heartwood. *Bark* 5-6 mm thick, surface brown, rough, exudes yellow sticky latex when cut. *Blaze* yellow. Branchlets bluntly 4-angled, shiny. *Leaves* opposite, linear-oblong or slightly spoon-shaped with backward folded margins, 8-10 x 1.5-2.5 cm, acute, at base, rounded at apex, hairless, leathery, dark green above, pale beneath; lateral nerves slender, many, horizontal, closely arranged; leaf stalks 6-18 mm long. *Male*, female & bisexual flowers are separately seen in the same plant, orange-yellow, fleshy. *Male flowers* 2-6, in terminal cymes, about 1 cm across, white with numerous stamens. *Female flowers* terminal and axillary, slightly larger than male flowers. *Berries* 3-5 x 1.5-2.5 cm, oblong, flattened, purplish brown when ripe, ending into a short, thick style with a broad, imbricate stigma which is about 8 mm across. *Seeds* 1-2, about 3 x 1.5 cm, brown, smooth, shiny.

Habitate: In evergreen and shola forests.

Propagation: By seeds and vegetative method.

Parts Used: Stem bark.

Chemical Constituents: N.A.

Uses: Stem bark and fruitsare reportedly used asmedicine by the members of *Kani* tribe.

596. *Gardenia gummifera* L.f. *(Rubiaceae)*

Vernacular Name: *San*: Nadihingu, Gandharaj, *Hin*: Dikamali, *Kan*: Kal kambi, Kambi pisin, Bikki gida, *Mal*: Gandharajan, Somanadikayam, Mar: Dekamali, Karmarri, *Tam*: Kambi, Vella pavetta, Thikka malli, *Tel:* Bikki, Sirubikki, Manchibikki, *Tel*lamanga.

Description: A small tree or large shrub, 3-7 m tall. Branchlets twisted, crooked, brittle. Bark thin, smooth, greyish brown. *Wood* yellowish white, hard and close-grained. *Leaves* opposite, inverted egg-shaped to oblong, 4-8 x 2-4 cm, base rounded to slightly heart-shaped, apex abtusely acute, margin entire, leathery, nearly stalkless; lateral nerves 10-16 pairs, distinct, with a dot-like gland known as 'domatia' at the axil of each nerve. *Flowers* bisexual, solitary, axillary; corolla-tube 3-5 cm long with 5 spreading lobes at apex which is about 5 cm across, white turning yellow, fragrant. *Berries* ellipsoid to oblong, about 4 x 3 cm, smooth, not prominently ribbed. *Seeds* many, minute.

Habitate: In degraded slopes and thickets of dry forests.

Propagation: By seeds and vegetative method.

Parts Used: Resin.

Chemical Constituents: Resin, vol-oil, colouring matter: gardenin.

Uses: Resin from leaf buds is used in curing wounds, indigestion, gas trouble, piles, chronic coughs, neuropathy, anorexia, colic, foul ulcers, intestinal worms (especially round worms), cardiac debility, leprosy, skin diseases, intermittent fever, enlargement of the spleen and obesity. The plant is one of the ingredients of a veterinary herbal antiseptic ointement MELICON V, which is effective in healing wounds, fungal infections and other skin lesions in cattle. The ointment showed prominent antimicrobial effect.

597. *Gardenia jasminoides* Ellis. *(Rubiaceae)*

Synonyms: *Gardenia florida* Linn.; *Gardenia augusta* Merrill.

Vernacular Name: *San:* Gandharaj; *Eng:* Cape jasmine; *Hin:* Gandharaj and *Beng*: Gandharaj.

Description: Small evergreen tree, 1-2 m.high. leaves opposite or in whorl of 3, shining, glabrous on the upper side; stipule large, amplexicaul. Flowers yellowish-white, fragrant, solitary at the end of branchlets. Fruit ovoid, angular, tripped with remains of calyx, pulp yellowish-orange. Seeds numerous.

Habitate: Grows wild in wet places and is cultivated for ornament.

Propagation: By seeds and vegetative method.

Part Used: Leaves and fruit.

Chemical Constituents: The leves and fruit contain flucosides (gardenoside, gentiobioside, geniposide, crocin, gardenin); tanin essential oil; pectin: B-sitosterol; d-mannitol; nonacosane.

Uses: The leves and fruit possess antibacterial, antifebrile, demulcent, cholagogic and diuretic properties. They are used in treating feber, jaundice, epistaxis, sore throat, haemoptysis, bloody stools, dysuria, burns, boils and impetigo. A poultice of pounded fresh leaves is effective for wounds, phlegmon and acute conjunctivitis.

598. *Gardenia taitensis* DC. *(Rubiaceae)*

Vernacular Name: *Eng:* Tahitian gardenia, tiare.

Description: Shrub or small tree to 6 m high with conspcious stipules. Leaves opposite, petiolate, broadly elliptical, upto 15 cm long. Flowers showy, white, fragrant, borne singly on stems arising from upper leaf axils. Fruit a yellowish-green sub-globose to ellipsoid capsule 5 cm long containing numerous whitish seeds surrounded by an orangish pulp.

Habitate: Coastal limestone rock and occasionally in coastal forest near the shore.

Propagation: By seeds and vegetative method.

Part Used: Flowers and leaves.

Chemical Constituents: 9,19-cyclollanostane-3, 23-dione.

Uses: Merely smell the flowers to relieve headaches. Migriane headaches may be cured by immersing the head in a solution with the crushed flowers. The flowers are also used to treat childhood diseases. In American Samoa, A medicine including the leaves of this plant is used to purify the blood in prenatal care and diabetes treatment. The plant is also used in treating inflammations in children. In futuna, however, it is thought that an infusion of the bark can be used to induce an abortion. Vaginal bleeding is treated with an infusion of the leaves.

599. *Gastrodia elata* Blume *(Orchidaceae)*

Vernacular Name: *Eng*: Tall gastrodia.

Description: Saprophytic, leafless, perennial herb with thickened rhizome, 60-100 cm tall. Rhizomes oblong, fleshy, 10-18 cm long, 3.5 cm in diameter. Stems yellowish brown, simple, erect, loosely scaly. Inflorescence loose racemes, erect, bracteate, 10-30 cm long, many-flowered; bracts lanceolate to linear-oblong, 7-12 mm long, 2 mm wide. Flowers yellowish brown; sepals and petals connate; perianth tube broadly ovoid, oblique at mouth, 7-8 mm long, inflated at base.

Habitate: Mountain woods in Korea, Japan and China.

Propagation: By vegetative method.

Parts Used: Tuber.

Chemical Constituents: Phenolic compounds; vanillin, gastrodin, p-hydroxybenzy1 alcohol, p-hydroxy-benzaldehyde, 4,4'-dihydroxy dibenzylether.

Uses: Sedative, anticonvulsive, anti-inflammatory, antiepileptic, hypnotic, analgesic, antithrombotic, anti-platelet aggregation, antioxytocic. Used in headache, infantile, convulsion, neurasthenia.

600. *Gaultheria procumbens* L. *(Ericaceae)*

Synonyms: *Gaultheria humilis* Salisb.

Vernacular Name: *Eng:* Checker berry-winter green.

Description: A small, procumbent, evergreen shrub, with slender creeping stem giving rise to erect branches, upto 15 cm. high, bearing towards their ends 3-8 leaves; leaves alternate, dark green, oval or ovate, almost glabrous, 2.5-5 cm. long with mucronate apex and slightly revolute margins having serration or ciliate teeth. Flowers white, solitary, pentamerous, nodding in the leaf axil. Corolla white, ovate; calyx saucer shaped. Anthers with 4 awns, filaments pubescent. Fruit a berry, bright red, enclosed within bright red calyx.

Habitate: North United Stated and Canada.

Propagation: By seeds and vegetative method.

Parts Used: Leaf.

Chemical Constituents: Important of them include: Volatile oil; Benzoic acid; Gaultherine, Gaultherilene. Arbutin. Salicylic acid.

Uses: For complaints of inflammatory rheumatism, sciatica and neuralgia. Neuralgia of head and face. Skin smarting and burning with intense erythema which is worse by cold washing. Cystic and prostatic irritation. Acute gastritis with severe epigastric pain and prolonged vomiting.

601. *Gelidium amansii* *(Rhodopyceae)*

Vernacular Name: *Eng:* Agar.

Description: Seaweed with red-brown, translucent, multi-branched ribbons and found growing to about 1 m in length. It has spherical fruit that appears in late autumn and winter.

Habitate: Agar is native to the Pacific coasts of china and Japan, and the coast of South Africa.

Propagation: By seeds and vegetative method.

Parts Used: Seaweed extract.

Chemical Constituents: Agar contains polysaccharides, mainly agarose and agaropectin, which are very mucilaginous.

Uses: Like most seaweeds and their derivatives, agar is nutritious and contains large amounts of mucilage. Its chief medicinal use is as a bulk laxative. In the intestines, agar absorbs water and swells, stimulating bowel activity and the subsequent elimination of faeces.

602. *Gelsemium sempervirens* (L.) Ait. *(Loganiaceae)*

Synonyms: *Bignonia sempervirens* Linn., *Gelsemium lucidum* Poir., *Gelsemium nitidum* Michx.

Vernacular Name: *Eng:* Carolina-Yellow-Jasmine, Italian gelsomino.

Description: An evergreen vine, some times climbing upto 8 m. with leaves opposite, lanceolate to ovate-lanceolate, 2.5-10 cm. long, entire, short petioled acute or acuminate, shining above. Flowers showy, bracteate with bracts 2 or more pairs, scale like, very fragrant, dimorphous, in 1-6 fid cymes, bright yellow, 2.5-4 cm. long; blooming throughout the season. Corolla funnel form, 5 lobed, each lobe with a notch at the top; style slender. Fruit a capsule, flat, 2.5-9 summit. Seeds flattened and winged.

Habitate: Found in Virgina, Carolina, Georgia, Guatemala and Mexico in rich moist soil along the sea coas.

Propagation: By seeds and vegetative method.

Parts Used: Rhizomatous root-stocks and roots.

Chemical Constituents: Gelsemine, Gelsemidine, Gelsemicine, Sempervirine, Gelsevirine, β-methylaesculetin, n-pentatri acontane, emodin, phytosterol and Ipuranol.

Uses: For complaints of muscular paralysis and disorders due to nerve disorders, causing motor paralysis. Paralysis of muscles about eyes, throat, chest, Larynx, sphincters and extremities. Complete relaxation and prostration of muscles. Fear of heart may not stop and therefore keeps one moving. Pulse slow but increases on motion. Vertigo spreading from occiput, with a band feeling around the head, pain in temple extending in ears. Double vision with disturbed eye muscular coordination. Blurred vision. Orbital neuralgia. Fever with chilliness moving up and down along spine. Bad effect of fright, fear and exciting news and sudden emotions.

603. *Geniostoma rupestre* S.L. Forst. *(Longaniaceae)*

Synonyms: *Geniostoma insulare* A.C.Sm.

Description: Shrub or slender tree to 10 m tall. Leaves opposite, petiolate, ovate to elliptical up to 20 cm long. Flowers white, small 5-parted, borne in axilalry cluster of 3 to numerous flowers. Fruit an elliptical dehiscent capsule upto 10 cm long which contains numerous small seeds. Flowers in late summer and fruit follows later in the year.

Habitate: Common in both primary and secondary forests, thickets and open rocky areas (including limestone), from sea-level to montane.

Propagation: By seeds and vegetative method.

Part Used: Bark.

Chemical Constituents: N.A.

Uses: An infusion of the bark as a purgative to treat stomachache and other internal ailments. The plant is used to treat diarrhoea, the ailments involving the kidney or bladder.

604. *Gentiana litea* L. *(Gentianaceae)*

Vernacular Name: *Eng:* Great yellow Gentian.

Description: An ornamental plant with smooth stem up to 1 m. in height with long thick tap root. Leaves opposite; lower leaves petiolate, upper sessile, their bases embrcing the stem, yellowish-green, oblong, pointed with five prominent veins on underside. Flowers yellow, large, in racemes, heads or paniculated cymes in axil of leaves. Calyx tubular, 5, persistent. Corolla tube nearly cylindrical, lobes 5. Stamens as many as corolla lobes, included. Ovary 1-celled with stigma 2-lobed; ovules several or many. Capsule sessile or stalked.

Habitate: Europe and Spain.

Propagation: By seeds and vegetative method.

Parts Used: Rhizomes and roots.

Chemical Constituents: Gentiopicrin, Gentiamarin, Gentiin, Gentianine and Gentianin. No. Starch.

Uses: Used to improve appetite, stimulate gastric secretions. For Atonic dyspepsia and Gastro-marked. Acidity, nausea and aching in stomach with distention and extreme sensitivity of umbilicus. Frontal headache, worse on motion but better by eating.

605. *Gentiana macrophylla* *(Gentianaceae)*

Vernacular Name: *Eng:* Qin jiao.

Description: Perennial herb growing to 70 cm. Has opposite lance-shaped leaves, and bell-shaped violet flowers emerging from the leaf axils.

Habitate: *Qin jiao* is native to Mongolia and north-eastern provinces of China.

Propagation: By seeds and vegetative method.

Parts Used: Root.

Chemical Constituents: *Qin jiao* contains alkaloids such as gentianine and gentianindine, and bitter principles.

Uses: Like its European cousin, gentian, *qin jiao* is a strongly bitter herb. It is commonly taken in the form of a tincture in order to stimulate the digestion and "cool" the body in general. Unlike gentian, however, *qin jiao* is also mildly pungent, and is therefore appropriate for a somewhat different range of illnesses. In Chinese herbal medicine, it is prescribed for the treatment of "wind-damp" conditions such as fever, jaundice and "dry" constipation and is used generally to help support the function of the liver and digestive system. As it is anti-inflammatory and mildly sedative, *qin jiao* is also prescribed as a treatment for various rheumatic and arthritic conditions.

606. *Gentiana scabra* L. *(Gentianaceae)*

Vernacular Name: *Eng:*-Gentain.

Description: Perennial herb. Stems more or less erect, leafy, 20-60 cm tall, 4-striate, with short rhizome. Leaves opposite, sessile, lanceolate, margins and midrib rough, 4-8 cm long, 1-3cm wide, with 3 veins, green above, pale-green beneath. Flowers several in terminal clusters; calyx tubular, to 1.5 cm long; corolla dark-blue, campanulate, to 3 cm long; stamens 5, united to corollar tube; style 1. Fruit capsule with withered corolla and calyx; seeds many, broad lanceolate, winged.

Habitate: Grassy places and wet meadows in low mountain elevation in Korea, China and Japan.

Propagation: By seeds and vegetative method.

Parts Used: Root.

Chemical Constituents: Gentiopicroside, swertiamarin, gentisin, gentisis acid.

Uses: Stimulation of gastric secretion and motility, choleretic activity, stimulation of bowel movement. Used in stomatics, anorexia, dyspepsia, inflammation, liver diseases.

607. *Geranium maculatum* *(Geraniaceae)*

Vernacular Name: *Eng:* American cranesbill.

Description: Perennial growing to 60 cm. Has deeply cleft leaves, pink-purple flowers and beak-shaped fruit.

Habitate: Native to woodlands of eastern and central North America.

Propagation: By vegetative method.

Parts Used: Root.

Chemical Constituents: American cranesbill contains up to 30% tannins.

Uses: An astringent and clotting agent, American cransebill is used today much as in earlier times. The herb is often prescribed for irritable bowel syndrome and haemorrhoids, and it is used to staunch wounds. It may also be used to treat heavy menstrual bleeding and excessive vaginal discharge.

608. *Geranium robertianum* *(Geraniaceae)*

Vernacular Name: *Eng:* Herb Robert.

Description: Strong-smelling annual or biennial herb growing to 50 cm. Has deeply cleft red-green leaves, bright pink flowers and pointed seed capsules.

Habitate: Native to Europe and Asia, herb Robert is naturalized in North America.

Propagation: By vegetative method.

Parts Used: Root.

Chemical Constituents: Herb Robert contains tannins, a bitter principle, traces of volatile oil and citric acid.

Uses: Herb Robert is little used in contemporary European herbal medicine. It is occasionally employed in much the same way as American cranesbill as an astringent and wound healer. The herb bears closer investigation as a remedy. According to one authority it is also effective against stomach ulcers and inflammation of the uterus, and it holds out potential as a treatment for cancer.

609. *Geum urbanum* *(Rosaceae)*

Vernacular Name: *Eng:* Avens.

Description: Downy perennial growing to 60 cm. Has wiry stems, compound leaves, small, yellow 5-petalled flowers, and fruit covered with hooks.

Habitate: Native to Europe and central Asia, avens is a common wayside plant.

Propagation: By seeds and vegetative method.

Parts Used: Root.

Chemical Constituents: Avens contains phenolic glycosides, tannins a volatile oil and possibly a sesquiterpene lactone.

Uses: Avens is an astringent herb, used principally for problems affecting the mouth, throat, and gastrointestinal tract. It tightens up soft gums, heals mouth ulcers, makes a good gargle for infections of the pharynx and larynx, and reduces irritation of the stomach and gut. It may be taken for peptic ulcers, irritable bowel syndrome, diarrhoea and dysentery.

610. *Ginkgo biloba* L. *(Ginkgoaceae)*

Vernacular Name: *Eng*: Maidenhair tree.

Description: Deciduous, resinous, dioecious tree, to 60 m or more tall. Branches stiff, with both elongated and spur shoots. Leaves alternately clustered, fan-shaped, cut in middle dichotomously veined, long-petioled. The female reproductive structures consisting of 2 ovules, rarely more, on a long peduncle, usually only 1 maturing . Seeds plum-like in appearance, yellowish, drupelike, to 2.5 cm long, long peduncled, outer coat fleshy, inner coat stony.

Habitate: Widely planted in Korea and China.

Propagation: By seeds and vegetative method.

Parts Used: Seed and leaf.

Chemical Constituents: Phenolic acids; ginkgolic acid, hydroginkgolic acid, ginkgolides. Flavonoids. Biflavonoids; sciadopitysin, ginkgetin, bilobetin.

Uses: Antibacterial and antifungal, PAF-receptor binding antagonistic, many other activities. Used in asthma, sputum and cough, leucorrhoea.

611. *Glechnia littoralis* Fr. Schm. Ex Miq. *(Apiaceae)*

Vernacular Name: *Eng:* Coastal glehnia.

Description: A perennial herb 7-35 cm. High. The rhizome is somewhat thick and the greater part of the stout stem is buried in sand. The leaves are few, alternate, pinnate-compound, thick and very lustrous and yellowish-green. The pedicles are light-red. Umbels compound, terminal, no bracts, rays 10-14, bracteoles 8-12, linear-lanceolate; flowers 15-20, small, white, bloom in short umbels in summer. Fruit dividing into 2 elliptical mericarps,.

Habitate: In sandy soil along the sea coast; also cultivated in China.

Propagation: By seeds and vegetative method.

Part Used: Roots.

Chemical Constituents: N.A.

Uses: Dry cough, bronchitis.

612. *Glechoma hederacea* *(Lamiaceae)*

Vernacular Name: *Eng:* Ground ivy.

Description: Creeping perennial herb growing to 15 cm. Has long rooting runners, notched kidney-shaped leaves and purple-blue flowers in whorls.

Habitate: Native to Europe and western Asia, ground ivy is now naturalized in other temperate regions, including North America. It thrives on the outskirts of woods and alongside paths and hedges. It is gathered in summer.

Propagation: By seeds and vegetative method.

Parts Used: Aerial parts.

Chemical Constituents: Ground ivy contains sesquiterpenes, flavonoids, a volatile oil, a bitter principle, saponin, resin and tannins.

Uses: Ground ivy is tonic, diuretic and anticatarrhal, and is used to treat many problems involving the mucous membranes of the ear, nose, throat and digestive system.

613. *Gleditsia japonica* Nakai *(Caesalpiniaceae)*

Vernacular Name: *Eng*: Korean honey locust.

Description: Deciduous tree, to 20 m tall, armed with stout spines. Young branches green, with many lenticels on the surface. Leaves alternate, odd-pinnate, 1-or 2-pinnate, 12-22 cm long; leaflets 11-17, obtuse or emarginated, cremulate, 3-3.5 cm long. Flowers small, greenish, 6 mm across, in spikelike racemes, unisexual or bisexual; sepals and petals 5; stamens 9-10, 4-5 mm long, green, filaments hairly. Fruit a large flat legume, 23 cm long, 3 cm wide, twisted.

Habitate: Near streams in low mountain elevations of Korea.

Propagation: By seeds and vegetative method.

Parts Used: Spine and fruit.

Chemical Constituents: Gleditsia saponins. Falvonoids and phenylpropanoids.

Uses: Anti-inflammatory and antiulcer activities, anti-HIV activity. Used in cough, expectorant constipation, abortifacient, liver diseases.

614. *Glehnia littoralis* F. Schmidt *(Apiaceae)*

Vernacular Name: *Eng:*-Glehnia.

Description: Pubescent perennial herb with thick, elongated rhizomes, to 5-23 cm tall. Leaves twice ternately pinnate, long-petioled, deltoid 10-20 cm long; leaflets elliptic, dentate, 2-5 cm long, 1-3 cm wide, irregularly dentate. Umbels 1-3 compound, terminala dn axillary at upper part, densely pubescent, without an involucre; involucels 10, 4-6 cm long; umbellets 20-40 flowered; bract of involucels few, linear, calyx teeth evident, linear-deltoid, acute, petals white, obovate, emarginated ellipsoidal, densely pubescent, carpels with thick, winglike prominent ribs; lateral ribs broader than dorsal ones; the vittae numerous, pericap corky.

Habitate: *San*dy beaches of Korea, China, Japan, and North America.

Propagation: By seeds and vegetative method.

Parts Used: Root.

Chemical Constituents: Coumarins: psoralen, bergapten, marmesin, osthenol-7-O-gentiobioside.

Uses: Korea, China, Japan, Pacific coast of North America antibacterial, Antiulcer. Used as antipyretic, analgesic and in migrane headache.

615. *Gloriosa superba* L. *(Liliaceae)*

Vernacular Name: *San*: Langali, Agnisikha, *Eng*: Supper Lilly, Tiger Lilly, *Hin*: Karihari, Languli, *Kan*: Karadi kannina gadde, Huliyuguru, Sivasakthi balli, *Mal*: Mentonni, Ventoni, Mar: Karianag, Nagkaria, *Tam*: *Kan*vali poo, Kaandal, Kalappai kizhangu, *Tel:* Kalappa gadda, Potti dumpa, Adavi nabhi.

Description: A herbaceous climber. *Root* stock tuberous, cylindrical, 15-25 x 2.5-4 cm, pointed at both ends, 'V' or 'L'-shaped, fleshy, white; roots fibrous. Branchlets hairless, cylindrical, weak. *Leaves* alternate, rarely opposite or in whorls, egg-shaped-lanceolate, stalkless, about 5-15 x 2-4 cm, base heart-shaped, apex produced into a coiled tendril, margin entire, hairless, papery; lateral nerves parallel. *Flowers* bisexual, axillary, solitary or somewhat sub-corymobose at the ends of branches, 8-10 cm across. Floral stalk 6-14 cm long with reflexled apex. *Perianth* lobes 6, oblong-lanceolate, about 6 x 1 cm,with crisply wavy margins, greenish at first, then yellow, passing through orange and scarlet to crimson colour. *Capsules* ellipsoid-oblong, 3-5 x 1-2.5 cm, splitting by 3-valves. *Seeds* numerous, globose, dorsally compressed, with warty projections, straw-coloured.

Habitate: Sea level to semi-evergreen forest in a wide range of habitats except desert.

Propagation: By seeds and vegetative method.

Parts Used: Seeds and tubers.

Chemical Constituents: The tubers contain colchicines, benzoic and salicylic acid, sterols and resinous substances. Colchicines, 3-demethylcolchicine, 1,2-didemethylcolchicine, 2,3-didemethylcolchicine, N-for-myl-N-deacetylcolchicine and colchicocide. The seeds also contain gloriosine. In the world market, they are considered a rich source of colchicines and gloriosine.

Uses: The tuberous roots are useful in curing inflammations, ulcers, scrofula, bleeding piles, white discharge, skin diseases, leprosy, indigestion, helminthiasis, snake bites, baldness, intermittent fever and debility. Roots aregiven internallyas an antidote for snake poison. Considered useful in promoting labour and expulsion of the placenta. If consumed in large doses, it is highly poisonous, it causes vomiting, purging, stomachache and burning sensation. Seeds are used for relieving rheumatic pain and as a muscle relaxant.

616. *Glycine max* Merr. *(Fabaceae)*

Vernacular Name: *Eng*: Soybean, soja bean, soya bean.

Description: Hairy erect annual, to 60 cm tall, with brown hairs. Leaves alternate, long petiolate; leaflets 3, ovate or elliptic, acuminate or rounded, stipules linear. Flowers small, papilionaceous, in axillary racemes, pink or white; calyx campanulate, 5-toothed, with upper 2 lobes partly united. Fruit a linear legume, to 7.5 cm long, brown and hairy, pendant, constricted between seeds, valves spiral after dehiscence.

Habitate: Widely cultivated in India.

Propagation: By seeds and vegetative method.

Parts Used: Fruits and seeds.

Chemical Constituents: Large amount of protein, carbohydrate, vitamin B, carotenoids amino acids, soyasaponins, fatty acids, flavones, sojagol, glyceollin IV, agmatine, flazin.

Uses: Soybean sprout shows estrogen-like activity and antispasmodic activity. Reduced ovulation rate (coumestrol), wound healing (allantion), haemolytic, insecticidal (soyasaponins).

617. *Glycosmis macrocarpa* Wight *(Rutaceae)*

Synonyms: *G. pentaphylla* Hook. f. var. macrocarpa (Wight) Hook.f.

Vernacular Name: *San*: Ashvashakota, Pathalgurudi, *Hin*: Ban-nimbu, *Kan*: Manikyan, *Mal*: Panal, Panchi, Mar: Kirmira, *Tam*: Anam, *Tel:* Golugu.

Description: Shrubs, 1-3 m tall. Branchlets without hairs. *Leaves* alternate, odd-pinnate; leaflets 3-5, alternate, oblong-elliptic or egg-shaped-oblanceolate, 7-23 x 4-9 cm, base wedge-shaped, apex acuminate, margin entire, hairless, with short prominent stalk; lateral nerves 5-7 pairs, prominent below, faint above with fine reticulations. *Flowers* bisexual, arranged in axillary or terminal short panicles, white or pale yellow, about 5 mm long. *Berries* sub-globose, constricted below and depressed above, about 2 x 1.5 cm, smooth, shiny with gland dots, rosy when ripe. *Seeds* single.

Habitate: Evergreen forests.

Propagation: By seeds and vegetative method.

Parts Used: Leaves.

Chemical Constituents: Arborine, skimmianine and arborinine, carbazole, 3-methylcarbazole, homoglycosolone, homoglycolone, glycolone, glycozoline and glycozolidine, the roots contains glycozolicine, 3-formyl carbazole and glycosinine.

Uses: Leaf juice is used for the treatment of fever, liver complaints, vermifuge, eczema and other skin troubles.

618. *Glycyrrhiza uralinsis* *(Fabaceae)*

Synonyms*:* *Glyeyrrhiza viscida.*

Vernacular Name: *Eng:* Gan cao.

Description: Perennial herb growing to 1 m. Has fibrous roots, a hairy stem, clusters of purplish flowers and flat pods.

Habitate: *Gan cao* grows in China, Mongolia and eastern Russia. The root is unearthed in spring or autumn.

Propagation: By Root.

Parts Used: Root and rhizome.

Chemical Constituents: *Gan cao* contains triterpene saponins, flavonoids and isoflavonoids and chalcones.

Uses: *Gan cao* is one of the most important medicinal herbs in China. It is used to "harmonize" different herbs prescribed together, but it is also valuable in its own right. A sweet-tasting tonic with therapeutic properties similar to those of liquorice, *gan cao* is prescribed for sore throats, wheeziness, coughs, mouth ulcers, peptic ulcers and gastritis.

619. *Glycyrrhize glabra* L. *(Fabaceae)*

Vernacular Name: *San:* Madhuka, yashti-madhu; *Eng:* Liquorice; *Hin:* Mulhatti, jethi-madh; *Beng*: Jashtimadhu, jaishbomodhu; *Tel:* Yashtimadhukam, atimadhuramu; *Tam:* Atimaduram; *Kan:* Yashti madhuka atimad-hura and *Mal:* Iratimadhuram.

Description: A hardy herb or undershrub; rootstock thick with many branched stems or roots; leaves pinnate; flowers lavender or violet in axillary spikes; pods compressed.

Habitate: Cultivated in India.

Propagation: By vegetative method.

Part Used: Roots and underground stems.

Chemical Constituents: The characteristic aroma of the volatile oil of liquorice is due to the presence of a mixture of estragole, anethole, eugenol, indole, y-nonalactone and cumic alcohol.

Uses: Liquorice extracts are mainly used as a condiment or as a flvouring for tobacco, confectionery, beverages, jams and marmalades. Ammoniated glycyrrhizin, a product of liquorice extract is used as a flavorant in sweet auces, reconstituted vegetable proteins, chocolates, chewing gum and diet colas.

620. *Gnaphalium uliginosum* *(Asteraceae)*

Vernacular Name: *Eng:* Marsh cudweed.

Description: Annual plant growing to 20 cm. Has narrow silver-grey leaves and tiny yellow flowerheads.

Habitate: Marsh cudweed is native to Europe, the Caucasus and western Asia, and is naturalized in North America. It prefers damp areas, and is gathered in summer when in flower.

Propagation: By Seeds.

Parts Used: Aerial parts.

Chemical Constituents: Marsh cudweed contains a volatile oil and tannins.

Uses: While little used medicinally today, marsh cudweed has astringent, antiseptic and anticatarrhal properties. In British herbal medicine, it is occasionally taken for tonsillitis, sore throat and hoarseness, and for catarrh in the throat, nasal passages and sinuses. Marsh cudweed is used in Russia to reduce high blood pressure. It is thought to be antidepres*San*t and aphrodisiac.

621. *Grewia tiliifolia* Vahl *(Tiliaceae)*

Vernacular Name: *Eng*: Dhaman, Hun: Dhamni, Dhaman, *Kan*: Dadasalu, *Mal*: Catacci, Dhanvanavrksam, *San*: Dhanvangah, Dhanurvrksah, *Tam*: Catacci, Unnu, *Tel:* Peddatena.

Description: A medium sized tree upto 20 m in height, with a clear bole of 8 m and 65 cm in diameter and grey to blackish brown rough fibrous bark peeling off in thin flakes leaves simple, alternate, ovate with obilique base, surface hoary-tomentose; flowers yellow, small on thick axillary peduncles; fruits globose drupes of the size of a pea, 2-4 lobed, black when ripe, seeds 1-2.

Habitate: Throughout India, in deciduous and semi-evergreen forests upto 1,200 m.

Propagation: By seeds and vegetative method.

Parts Used: Bark, fruits.

Chemical Consistuents: N.A.

Uses: The bark is astringent, sweet, acrid, refrigerant, oleaginous, expectorant, antipruritic, vulnerary, constipating, emetic, styptic, aphrodisiace and tonic. It is useful in vitiated conditions of *pitta* and *kapha*, burning sensation, hyperdipsia, rhinopathy, pharyngopathy, cough, skin diseases, pruritus, wounds, ulcers, diarrhoea, haematemesis, epistaxis, haemorrhages, seminal weakness and general debility. The fruits are sweet, sour, cooling and edible, and are useful in vitiated conditions of *vata* and *kapha*.

622. *Grindelia camporum* *(Asteraceae)*

Synonyms: *Grindelia robusta* var. *rigida*.

Vernacular Name: *Eng:* Gumplant.

Description: Perennial herb growing to 1 m. Has triangular leaves and yellow-orange daisy-type flowers.

Habitate: Native to south-western US and Mexico, gumplant grows in arid and saline soil.

Propagation: By Seeds and vegetative method.

Parts Used: Leaves, flowers.

Chemical Constituents: Gumplant contains diterpenes, resins and flavonoids.

Uses: Gumplant is a valuable remedy for bronchial asthma, and for states where phlegm in the airways impedes respiration. Both antispasmodic and expectorant, gumplant helps to relax the muscles of the smaller bronchial passages and to clear congested mucus. Additionally, it is thought to desensitize the nerve endings in the bronchial tree and to slow the heart rate, both leading to easier breathing. Gumplant is also taken for bronchitis and employsema, and to clear catarrh in the throat and nose. It has been employed in the treatment of whooping cough, hay fever and cystitis, and externally to help speed the healing of skin irritation and bums.

623. *Guaiacum officinale* *(Zygophyllaceae)*

Vernacular Name: *Eng:* Lignum Vitae.

Description: Evergreen tree growing to 10 m. Has compound oval leaves, small, deep blue star-shaped flowers, and heart-shaped seed capsules.

Habitate: Lignum vitae is native to South America and the Caribbean islands. It grows in tropical rainforests.

Propagation: By seeds and vegetative method.

Parts Used: Wood and resin.

Chemical Constituents: Lignum vitae continas lignuns, 18-25% resin, vanillin and terpenes.

Uses: Used in Europe, especially in Britain, as a remedy for arthritic and rheumatic conditions, lignum vitae has anti-inflammatory properties that help to reduce joint pain and swelling. It is also diuretic, laxative and sweat-including and speeds the elimination of toxins, which makes it valuable for treating gout. Tincture of lignum vitae is commonly used a s a friction rub on rheumatic areas. Cottonwool moistened with the resin may be applied to aching teeth.

624. *Guarea rusbyi* *(Meliaceae)*

Vernacular Name: *Eng:* Cocillana.

Description: Evergreen tree with pale grey bark, compound lance-shaped leaves and green-white flowers.

Habitate: Cocillana is native to the eastern Andes. The bark is gathered throughout the year.

Propagation: By seeds and vegetative method.

Parts Used: Bark.

Chemical Constituents: Cocillana contains beta-sitosterol, and probably also resins, a fixed oil, tannin, an alkaloid and a glycoside.

Uses: Cocillana is used in cough mixtures, being an even more powerful expectorant than ipecacuanha. Cocillana is taken as a treatment for coughs, excessive mucus production in the throat and chest, and bronchitis. At a high dosage, the plant induces vomiting.

625. *Guettarda speciosa* L. *(Rubiaceae)*

Vernacular Name: *Tel:* Pnniru chettu; *Tam:* Pannir; *Kan:* Bilihuvinalakki and *Mal:* Ravupu.

Description: Spreading and much branched tree upto 20 m high. Leaves opposite, petiolate, leathery, oval with conspicuous striate veins, relatively large (to 20 cm long). Flowers white, tubular, fragrant, borne in terminal clusters. Fruit a round and green syncarp with one seed per locule.

Habitate: Common along the seashore, sea cliffs, beach thickets, and lowland forest.

Propagation: By seeds and vegetative method.

Part Used: Stem, leaves and bark.

Chemical Constituents: Loganic acid and secologanin.

Uses: The stem is used in preparation utilised to promote menstruation. The plant is used to treat maternal postpartum infections. A decoction of the leaves is used to treat coughs, colds and sore throats. The inner bark is used in a treatment for conjiunctivities. The leaves are used for poultices. A tea made from inner bark is used to treat epilepsy. Menorrhagia is treated with decoction of the bark. Infusion of the bark is used in treating postpartum discharges. A decoction of the bark or an infustion of the leaves is drunk daily treat secondary amenorrhoea. A decoction of the bark is drunk daily as a treatment for vaginal bleading. The plant has antidiarrhoetic, febrigugal and anticholinergic application. A preparation of the bark is drunk to cure dysentery. The bark is applied to wounds and sore. Itchy skin rashes are treated with fluid from the leaves. The shoots are washed in oil and used in treating ulcerated sores of the anus. Liquid from the bark is drunk to treat oedema.

626. *Gymnema khandalense* Santapau *(Asclepiadaceae)*

Synonyms: *Bidaria khandalense* (*Sant.*) Jagtap & Singh.

Description: Large woody elegant climbers. The basal stems about 30 cm girth, cylindrical. *Bark* ashy brown, distinctly marked with wing-like ridges of cork. Young branchlets yellowish green, densely pubescent, older ones with many lenticels. Stems and branchlets with plenty of white sticky latex. *Leaves* opposite, broadly egg-shaped to elliptic-oblong, 7-15 x 6-10 cm, base truncate to rounded, apex acute to acuminate, margin entire, slightly leathery, densely orange-yellow pubescent on nerves beneath, becoming hairless when mature; lateral nerves 5-6 pairs; leaf stalks 1-4 cm long, densely hairy. *Flowers* bisexual about 5 mm across, yellow, shortly stalked, arranged in axillary umbellate cymes. *Follicles* cylindrical, 7-10 cm long, 0.3-0.6 cm across, gradually tapering towards apex, straight or curved, greenish-brown, pubescent. *Seeds* about 12, ovoid, about 12 x 4 mm, flat, winged along margin, with about 4 cm long white silky hairs at apex.

Habitate: Deciduous to moist deciduous forests.

Propagation: By seeds and vegetative method.

Parts Used: Leaves.

Chemical Constituents: N.A.

Uses: Leaves may possess the same medicinal properties as that of *Gymnema sylvestre,* which is widely used for the treatment of diabetes and poisonous bites.

627. *Gymnema sylvestre* (Retz.) R. Br. *(Asclepiadaceae)*

Vernacular Name: *San*: Mesasrngi, Madhunasini, *Eng*: Periploca of the woods, *Hin*: Gudmar, Merasimgi, *Kan*: Kadhasige, *Mal*: Cakkarakkolli, Madhunasini, *Tam*: Sirukurumkay, Sakkaraikkolli, *Tel:* Podapatra.

Description: A large, woody, much branched climber with pubescent young parts; leaves simple, opposite, elliptic or ovate, more or less pubescent on both sides, base rounded or cordata; flowers small, yellow in umbellate cymes; fruits slender, follicles upto 7.5 cm long.

Habitate: Throughout India, in dry forests upto 600 m.

Propagation: By seeds and vegetative method.

Parts Used: Whole plant/ leaves.

Chemical Consistuents: Anti-sweet principles, gymnema saponins I-V were isolated from the plant. An aqueous extract of the leaves contained the saponins gymnemic acid III, IV,V VIII and IX. Four additional saponins, gymnemic acid XV-VVIII, with anti-sweet property, have been isolated from the leaves. They have been characterized as 21-0-2-methylbutyryl-22-0-2-methylbutyryl-22-0-2-methylcrotonyl, 16-22-0-bis-2-methylcrotonyl, 21-0-benzoyl, and 28-0-benzoyl gymnemagenin 3-0-glucuronides, respectively. Gymnemic acid VIII and IX have been renamed as gymnemic acid XV and XVI, respectively. The leaves also contain dammarane-type saponins, gymnemasides I-VII and gypenoside XXVII, XXXVIII, LV, LXII and LXIII. Gymnema extracts are useful as pharmaceuticals and as low-calorie foods. The bitterness of the extracts can be reduced by mixing them with five-flod starch followed by treatment with cyclodextrin glucosyltransferase and γ-cyclodextrin.

Uses: The plant is bitter, astringent, acrid, thermogenic, anti-inflammatory, anodyne, digestive, liver tonic, emetic, diuretic, stomachic, stimulant, anthelmintic, alexipharmic laxative, cardiotonic, expectorant, antipyretic, and uterine, tonic. It is useful in inflammations, hepatosplenomegaly, dyspepsia, constipation, jaundice, halminthiasis, cardiopathy, cough, asthma, bronchitis, intermittent fever, amenorrhoea, vitiated conditions of *vata*, conjunctivitis and leucoderma. The fresh leaves when chewed have the remarkable property of paralyzing the sense of taste for sweet and bitter substances for sometime.

628. *Gyrocarpus americanus* Jacq. *(Gyrocarpaceae)*

Synonyms: *Gyrocarpus jacquinii* Gaertn.

Vernacular Name: *Hin:* Zaitun; *Beng*: Zaitun; *Tel:* Tanuku, nallaponaku; *Tam:* Tanakku, kadavai, karamanikka, teppum, munuvu and *Kan:* Kadubende, pollika.

Description: Tree to 2o m high. Leaves mostly croseded towards ends of branches, alternate, pitiolate, the blades broadly ovate, deeply 3-loved on younger trees, smaller and almost entire on older trees. Flowers very small, borne on axillary inflorescence arising on the upper parts of the branches. Fruit an ovoid drupe with two long wings arising from the apex, about 1.5 cm long. Flowers mostly available April to July and fruit available July to January.

Habitate: Common along beaches, dry coastlines and open coastal woodlands.

Propagation: By seeds and vegetative method.

Part Used: Bark and leaves.

Chemical Constituents: Auroramine, maroumine, aporphines, benzylisoq-uinolines, bisbezylisoquinolines, O-methyl limacusine, gyrocarpusine, gyroamericine, gylidine, gyrocarpine, phaenthine, magnocurine, O-desmethyl phaeanthine, ferulic and sinapic acids, and the flavonoids kaempferol and quercetin.

Uses: To treat relapsed illness, childbirth swellings, stomachache, and intestinal filariasis. In Tonga, an infusion of the bark or leaves is taken internally or applied to the skin to treat skin inflammations. Used to heal wounds.

629. *Habenaria edgeworthii* Hook. F. ex Collett. *(Orchidaceae)*

Vernacular Name: *San*: Rddhi, *Hin*: Rddhi, *Kan*: Rddhi, *Mal*: Rddhi, *Tam*: Rddhi, *Tel:* Rddhi.

Description: A tuberous terrestrial herb upto 75 cm in height with somewhat flexuous leafy stem covered with hairs; leaves sheathing, 2-4, the second largest, ovate-lanceolate; flowers yellowish green deflexed in buds in cylindrical inflorescence, lip bright yellow, entire, strap-shaped, base forming slightly channeled claw, spur longer than ovary, spreading and directed upwards usually hooked downwards towards the tip, column 2-3 mm in height, anther canals and stigmatic processes short, ovary glabrous, twisted.

Habitate: In Simla, Garhwal and Uttar Pradesh, at about 2,500 m.

Propagation: By vegetative method.

Parts Used: Tubers.

Chemical Consistuents: N.A.

Uses: The tubers are sweet, refrigerant, emollient, intellect promoting, aphrodisiac, depurative, appetizer, anthelmintic, rejuvenating and tonic. They are useful in vitiated conditions of *pitta* and *vata*, burning sensation, hyperdipsia, fever, cough, asthma, insanity, cataplexy, leprosy, skin diseases, anorexia, helminthiasis, emaciation, haematemesis, gout and general debility.

630. *Habenaria intermedia* D. Don *(Orchidaceae)*

Vernacular Name; *Hin*: Vrddhi, *Kan*: Vrddhi, *Mal*: Vrddhi, *San*: Vrddhi, *Tam*: vrddhi, *Tel:* Vrddhi.

Description: A terrestrial plant upto 50 cm in height with oblong, sessile tuberoides; leaves 3-5, ovate-oblong, acuminate with sheathing leaf bases; flowers large, greenish white, 1-6 in an inflorescence, petals white, crescent-shaped, recurved and adherent to the dorsal sepal, lip pale yellowish green, 3-lobed, midlobe linear-acuminate, straight or slightly turned upwards, fringed on the outer margin, spur green, column about 7 mm in height, stigmatic processes green, slender and incurved, ovary slightly twisted.

Habitate: In the Himalayas.

Propagation: By vegetative method.

Parts Used: Tubers.

Chemical Consistuents: N.A.

Uses: Same as that of *raddhi.*

631. *Haldina cordifolia* (Roxb.) Ridsdale *(Rubiaceae)*

Synonyms *Adina cordifolia* (Roxb.) Hook. F. ex Brandis.

Vernacular Name: *San*: Dharakadambah, Girikadambah, *Eng*: Haldu, *Hin*: Haldu, Kadami, *Kan*: Anavu, *Mal*: Mannakkatampu, *Mal*ankatampu, *Tam*: Mannakkatampu, *Tel:* Pasupukadamba.

Description: A tall deciduous tree, 15-35 m in height, with a large crown and buttressed at the base; leaves large, orbicular-cordate, abruptly acuminate; flowers yellow in globose pedunculate heads; fruits capsules, splitting into two dehiscent cocci, seeds many, narrow, small, tailed above.

Habitate: Throughout India, in deciduous and semi-evergreen forests, especially in the Eastern Ghats, Karnataka and Kerala.

Propagation: By seeds and vegetative method.

Parts Used: Bark and roots.

Chemical Consistuents: The orange-coloured oleoresin, obtained by incision of the trunk, and also extracted from its sawdust, has the following properties: $d^{25°}$, 0.9358-0.9429; $n^{25°}_{D}$, 1.5058-1.5138; $^{25°}_{D}$, -3°7′ to 14°2′; acid val, 5.6-9.2; sap val, 12.6-16.8; and sap val after acetylation, 31.8-52.6. it yields an essential oil. Analysis of the wood gave α-cellulose, 70.0; β-cellulose, 0.95; γ-cellulose, 2.26; lignin, 21.8; hemicllulose A, 8.02; and hemicellulose B, 3.0%. destructive distillation of the heartwood gave: moisture, 9.3; charcoal, 32.1; total distillate, 48.1; pyroligneous acid, 47.3 (wet), 38.0(dry) and tar, 10.2%. the heartwood contained adifoline, cordifoline, 10-deoxyadifoline. 10-deoxycordifoline, benzoic acid, umbelliferone, and β-sitosterol. It also contained a yellow pigment. Adinin.

Uses: The roots are astringent and constipating, and are useful in diarrhoea and dysentery. The bark is acrid, bitter astringent, refrigerant, vulnerary, diuretic, demulcent, aphrodisiac and tonic. It is useful in vitiated conditions of *pitta*, wounds and ulcers, strangury, skin diseases, gastropathy, fever and burning sensation.

632. *Hamamelis virginiana* *(Hamamelidaceae)*

Vernacular Name: *Eng:* Witch Hazel.

Description: A small deciduous tree growing to 5m, with coarsely toothed, broadly oval leaves.

Habitate: Witch hazel is a woodland tree, indigenous to Canada and eastern parts of the US. Commonly cultivated in Europe. The trees are grown from hardwood cuttings or from seed, both of which are planted in autumn. The leaves are gathered in summer and dried. The bark is harvested dried as quickly as possible in the shade.

Propagation: By seeds and vegetative method.

Parts Used: Leaves and Barks.

Chemical Constituents: Tannins, flavonoids, bitter principle, volatile oil.

Uses: Astringent, anti-inflammatory, stops external and internal, bleeding.

633. *Harapagophytum procumbens* *(Pedaliaceae)*

Vernacular Name: *Eng:* Devil's Claw.

Description: A trailing perennial, reaching 1.4m, in length, with fleshy lobed leaves and barbed, woody fruit.

Habitate: Devil's claw is native to southern and eastern Africa, and is found most commonly on the veldt in the Transvaal. It thrives in clay or *San*dy soils, preferring roadsides and wasterground, especially places where natural vegetation has been cleared. Propagated from seed in spring, the young tubers are unearthed in autumn and cut into pieces about 1 cm long. Care is taken not to mix the tubers, which contain the active constituent, whit the roots, as this can render the herb ineffective.

Propagation: By seeds and vegetative method.

Parts Used: Tubers.

Chemical Constituents: Irodoid glycosides, sugars, phytosterols, flavonoids harpagoquinone.

Uses: Anti-inflammatory, analgesic, digestive stimulant.

634. *Haronga madagascariensis* *(Guttiferae)*

Vernacular Name: *Eng:* Haronga.

Description: Small evergreen tree growing to 8 m. Has black-doted leaves with a dark green upper surface and red-brown hairs underneath, and clusters of rust-coloured flowers.

Habitate: Haronga is native to Madagascar and East Africa, and grows in tropical areas.

Propagation: By seeds and vegetative method.

Parts Used: Leaves, bark.

Chemical Constituents: Horonga bark contains phenolic pigments, triterpenes, anthraquinones and tannins. The leaves contain phenolic pigments, hypericin, flavonoids and tannins.

Uses: Thought to stimulate bile secretion, haronga is used in European herbal medicine to treat indigestion and poor pancreatic function. In African herbal medicine, haronga is chiefly employed as an astringent and mild laxative, and is also given for digestive system ailments such as diarrhoea and dysentery.

635. *Hedychium coronarium* Koenig *(Zingiberaceae)*

Vernacular Name: *Eng*: Common Zinzer Lilly, Garland Flower, *Tam*: Seemai kitchili kizhangu, Karppura ver, Cantira mooligal.

Description: A robust, rhizomatous, tall, herbaceous plant, growing 1-3 m height. *Rootstock* horizontal, 2-5 cm diameter, fleshy, jointed, white, faintly fragrant. *Leaves* arranged in two rows, lanceolate to oblong-elliptic, 20-40 x 5-10 cm, base wedge-shaped to sub-acute, apex gradually tapering into acuminate with a tail-like lip, margin entire, hairless, papery, sheathing at base, distinctly stalked. *Flowering spikes* 10-18 cm long; floral bract 5-8 cm long, conspicuous, greenish, consisting 3-4 flowers in each. *Flowers* bisexual, about 10 cm long, pure-white or tinged with yellow, fragrant, with broad round to inverted heart-shaped lip that is 2-lobed at apex. *Capsules* globose to oblong, about 2 cm across, hairless, dehiscing by 3-valves, red when ripe. *Seeds* many, small, black, covered with crimson red-coloured aril.

Habitate: Along streamside and marshy areas in higher altitudes.

Propagation: By seeds and vegetative method.

Parts Used: Flowers and rhizomes.

Chemical Constituents: The flowers yield a concrete having the following main constituents; linalool, 29.3; methyl benzoate, 5.7; *cis*-jasmone, 1.2; eugenol, 1.4; -isoeugenol, 18.4; jasmin lactone, 3.5; methyl jasmonate, 1.8; methyl eip-jasmonate, 1.6; and indole, 7.0%. the rhizome conatins cytotoxic principles as labdane-type diterpenes, coronarin, A, B, C, D and labda-8, 12-diene-15, 16-dial, besides coronarin E and F, methyl and ethyl ethers of coronarin-D, isocoronarin-D and 14, 15, 16-trinorlabda-8, 11-dien-13-al.

Uses: Rhizomes are used as carminative and stimulant. Rhizome paste is applied to bruises and sprains.

636. *Hedychium spicatum* Ham. ex. Smith. *(Zingiberaceae)*

Vernacular Name: *San*: Shathi, *Hin:* Kapurkachali.

Description: It is an annual herb, with a horizontal *root-stock,* and tubesous *root fibres, leaves* are 30 cms or more in length. *Inflorescence* is spiked. *Flowers* ascending and dense yellow coloured. *Capsule* is globose.

Habitate: It grows in subtropical Himalayas, and also abundantly in Punjab and Nepal.

Propagation: By seeds and vegetative method.

Parts Used: Rhizomes.

Chemical Constituents: The dried rhizome of the plant contains essential oil, starch, resins, organic acids and a glycoside; albumen and saccharine are also present. The essential oil has ethyl ester of p-methoxy cinnamic acid, d-sabirene cineole, sesquiterpenes and pentadecane methyl paracumarine acetate. It contain β-sitosterol and its β-D-glycoside.

Uses: Nausea, vomiting. Bronchial asthma. Halitosis. Diminished appetite. Hiccups. Local inflammation. The rootstalk is useful in local inflammatory, nauseas, asthma, bronchitis, hiccups, and in pain. The rhizome of the plant is said to be carminative, stimulant and a tonic. It has been described as useful, specially as an antiasthmatic agent. Clinical trials have been conducted in tropical eosinophilia, with promising results. It counteracts bad mouth taste and smell.

637. *Hedyotis capitellata* wall ex G. don *(Rubiaceae)*

Synonyms: *Hedyotis Scandens* Roxb.

Vernacular Name: *Assami*: Bhedeli, lot.

Description: Twining suffrutescent climber. Stems cylindrical, swollen at the nodes. Leavees opposite, dark-green above, pale below; stipule ciliate. Inflorescence in axillary or terminal paniculate cyme; flowers white or yellowish-white. Capsule small, many-seeded, crowned by segments of the persistent calyx.

Habitate: Grows wild in the hills and mountains.

Propagation: By seeds and vegetative method.

Part Used: Whole plant.

Chemical Constituents: The whole plant contains alkaloids, saponins and tannin.

Uses: The stem offers an effective remedy for gastralgia, gastric ulcer, heartburn, during the colic pains or before meals, A mouth-wash prepared with Hedyotis stem liquid extract and honey is used for ulcerous stomatitis. A poultice made or pounded fresh leaves acts as a vulnerary, promoting tissue regeneration in wounds.

638. *Hedyotis corymbosa* (L.) Lam. *(Rubiaceae)*

Synonyms *Oldenlandia corymbosa* Linn.

Vernacular Name: *San*: Parpatah, Parpatakah, *Hin*: Daman pappar, Pitapra, *Kan*: Parpata hullu, *Mal*: Parppatakappullu, Parppatakam, *Tam*: Parpatagam, *Tel:* vermela-vemu.

Description: A much spreading suffruticose annual, upto 38 cm in height with erect ascending or spreading slender stems; leaves simple, opposite, sub-sessile, linear, narrow with recurved margins, stipules short, membranous, with a few short bristle; flowers white in pairs or in threes, pedicelled on a very slender axillary solitary peduncle; fruits loculicidal capsules.

Habitate: Throughout India, both on dry and wet lands as a weed.

Propagation: By seeds and vegetative method.

Parts Used: Whole plant.

Chemical Consistuents: Caffeine and fumaric acid, the air-dried plant contains 0.12% alkaloids, biflorone and biflorone; the alkaloids are interconvertible. In stored plants, the concentration of biflorone increases at the cost of biflorine.

Uses: The plant is bitter, acrid, refrigerant, febrifuge, pectoral, digestive, stomachic, aperient, anthelmintic, diuretic, depurative, diaphoretic, expectorant and liver tonic. It is useful in fevers, depression, jaundice, heat eruptions, vitiated conditions of *pitta*, hyperdipsia, giddiness, dyspepsia, flatulence, colic, constipation, helminthiasis, strangury, leprosy, skin diseases, cough, catarrh, bronchitis and hepatopathy.

639. *Hedyotis herbacea* L. *(Rubiaceae)*

Synonyms *Oldenlandia herbacea* (Linn.) Roxb.

Vernacular Name: *San*: Chayaparpatika, *Hin*: Paper-bhed, *Mal*: Nonnanampullu, *Tam*: Nonnanampullu, *Tel:* Chiriveru.

Description: An erect much branched glabrous bushy annual or biennial, branches slender, 4-gonous, divaricate; leaves simple, opposite, sessile, linear–lanceolate, usually with recurved margins, lower broader than the upper ones; flowers small, white, solitary or in paniculate axillary cymes, corolla tube slender; fruits subglobose capsules, capsule valves elongate, seeds ellipsoid.

Habitate: Throughout India, in open waste places upto 1,650 m.

Propagation: By seeds and vegetative method.

Parts Used: Whole plant.

Chemical Consistuents: N.A.

Uses: The plant is bitter, sweet, cooling, febrifuge, anthelmintic, anti-inflammatory, expectorant, stomachic and tonic. It is useful in elephantiasis, fever, verminosis, dyspepsia, flatulence, colic, inflammations, asthma, bronchitis, consumption, ulcers and hydrocele.

640. *Helianthus annus* L. *(Asteraceae)*

Vernacular Name: *Eng*: Common sunflower, *Hin*: Surajmukhi, *Kan*: Adityabhakti, *Mal*: Suryakanti, Suryappu, *San*: Adityabhakta, Suryamukhi, *Tam*: Curiyakanti, *Tel:* Aditya-bhakti, Suryakanti.

Description: An annual herb upto 5 m in height with erect rough hispid or hirsute stem and few branches at the top; leaves simple, alternate, long-stalked, broadly ovate to cordate, coarsely toothed, rough pubescent on both sides; flowers bright yellow, in heads, terminal on the main axis and branches; fruits slightly compressed cypsela, pappus falling off early.

Habitate: Throughout India, cultivated.

Propagation: By seeds and vegetative method.

Parts Used: Roots, leaves, flowers, seeds.

Chemical Consistuents: The seed kernel contains albumin, globulin, glutelin and insoluble protein; no alcohol-soluble protein has been reported. The distribution of total nitrogen in the seed is as follows: humin N, cystine N, arginine N, lysine N, histidine N, mono-amino N, non-amino N, and amide N. approximate amino acid composition of the total protein is as follows: arginine, histidine, lysine, tyrosine, tryptophan, phenyl-alanine, cystine; methionine, threonine, leucine, isoleucine, and valine, N. the globulin contain: glycocoll, alanine, valine, leucine, serine, aspartic acid, glutamic acid, tyrosine, phenyl-alanine, proline, cystine, tryptophan, arginine, histidine, and lysine.

Uses: The roots are anodyne, and are useful in odontalgia and for strengthening the teeth. The leaves are emetic, and are useful in lumbago, malarial fever, ulcers, wounds, cephalalgia and burning sensation. The flowers are acrid, bitter, refrigerant, anthelmintic, antiperiodic, emmenagogue and aphrodisiac. They are useful in inflammations, leprosy, skin diseases, pruritus, ulcers, hysteria, bronchitis, asthma, urethrorrhea, anaemia, burning sensation, pectoralgia, hepatopathy, pneumonosis, haemorrhoids, ophthalmia, ascites, nephropathy, helminthiasis, intermittent, fevers, amenorrhoea, dysmenorrhoea and vitiated conditions of *pitta*. The seeds are expectorant and diuretic, and are useful in cough, pneumonosis and strangury.

641. *Helicteres isora* L. *(Sterculiaceae)*

Vernacular Name: *San*: Avarttani, Mrgasrngi, *Eng*: East-Indian screw tree, *Hin*: Marodphali, *Kan*: Kempukaveri, *Mal*: Itampirivalampiri, *Tam*: Valampiri, *Tel:* Adavi-camanti.

Description: A large shrub or small tree upto 5 m in height with grey bark and young shoots clothed with stellate hairs; leaves simple, alternate, bifarious, obovate, obliquely cordate, serrate, scabrous above, pubescent beneath; flowers red, fading to lead colour, distinctly bilabiate, in axillary clusters of 2-6 together, staminal column fused with the gynophore, much exserted, suddenly deflexed; fruits greenish brown beaked, cork screw like 5-folicles, seeds numerous, angular testa wrinkled.

Habitate: Throughout India, in forests as undergrowth.

Propagation: By seeds and vegetative method.

Parts Used: Roots, bark, fruits.

Chemical Consistuents: Chemical examination of the bark showed the presence of chloroplast pigments, phytosterol, a hydroxy-carboxylic acid, an orange-yellow crystalline coloruing matter, saponins, sugars, phlobotannins and lignin.

Uses: The roots and bark are expectorant, demulcent, constipating and lactifuge, and are useful in colic, scabies, empyema, gastropathy, diabetes, diarrhoea and dysentery. The fruits are astringent acid, refrigerant, demulcent, constipating, stomachic, vermifuge, vulnerary, haemostatic and urinary astringent. These are useful in vitiated conditions of *pitta*, ophthalmitis, colic flatulence diarrhoea, dysentery, verminosis, wounds ulcers, haemorrhages, epistaxis and diabetes.

642. *Heliotropium indicum* L. *(Boraginaceae)*

Vernacular Name: *San*: Vrscikali, Hathi-sunda, *Eng*: Indian turnsole, *Hin*: Siriyari, Hattasura, Hatta-juri, *Kan*: Calubaldagidha, *Mal*: telkkata, Terkkata, Tekkata, Tekkita, *Tam*: *Tel*kodukkai, *Tel:* Kodikki, Nagadanti.

Description: A coarse, somewhat succulent foetid herbaceous annual, 15-60 cm height with densely hirsute ascending branches; leaves simple, alternate or subopposite, ovate, obtuse, narrowed or cordate at base, often unequal upto 10 cm long and 7.5-10 cm broad, hispid-pubescent, veins and veinlets conspicuous on the lower side; flowers pale violet, many, 2-ranked, in extra axillary, bristly scorpiod cymes; fruits nutlets combined in pairs, separating later, beaked, each lobe 4-ribbed.

Habitate: Throughout India, on roadsides and waste places.

Propagation: By seeds and vegetative method.

Parts Used: Whole plant.

Chemical Consisituents: Tannin and alkaloids.

Uses: The plant is bitter, astringent, thermogenic, emollient, vulnerary and diuretic, It is useful for local application for ulcers, sores, wound, skin affections, stings of insects, ulitis and rheumatism. The roots are bitter, astringent, aphrodisiac, expectorant, febrifuge and ophthalmic, and are useful in cough, bronchitis, fever, ringworm, rheumatism and ophthalmopathy. The leaves are useful in fever, urticaria, ulcers, wounds, localized inflammation, gonorrhoea, ringworm, rheumatism, erysipelas and pharyngodynai. The flowers are emmenagogue in small doses and abortifacient in large doses. The seeds are stomachic.

643. *Heliotropium keralense* Sivar. & Manilal *(Boraginaceae)*

Vernacular Name: *Mal*: Telkkatta.

Description: An erect sub-succulent herb, up to 30 cm tall. branchlets profusely hairy throughout. *Leaves* alternate or sub-opposite, egg-shaped, up to 10 x 6 cm, base wedge-shaped and decurrent on leaf stalk, apex rounded or acute, margin sub-entire, hairless above, sparsely strigose hairy below on nerves, membranous; lateral nerves 4-6 pairs, forking near margins; leaf stalks up to 9 cm long. *Flowers* bisexual, arranged in 12-18 cm long terminal or leaf opposed scorpioid cymes, 3-4 mm long, 2-3 mm across, white, wheel-shaped, villous hairy. *Fruits* consist of 4-nutlets combined in 2 pairs, ribbed, about 4 mm across, sparsely hairy, with a distinct beak at apex.

Habitate: Moist localities in fields, open wet places, disturbed forests and along the banks of water-bodies.

Propagation: By seeds and vegetative method.

Parts Used: Seeds.

Chemical Constituents: N.A.

Uses: This species may possess medicinal properties similar to *Heliotropium indicum* which is used to treat ulcers, sores, wounds, skin diseases, insect stings, rheumatism, cough, bronchitis, fever, ringworm, eye diseases, gonorrhoea and as abortifacient.

644. *Helleborus niger* L. *(Ranunculaceae)*

Synonyms: *Helleborus grandiflorus* Salisb.

Vernacular Name: *Eng:* black hellebore.

Description: A perennial having brownish-black, knotted, brittle, fleshy rhizome, 2.5-7.5 cm. long, 6-12 mm. thick. Leaves on long stalks, which spring directly from the root. Stalks are cylindrical, tapering, smooth, shining and pale green tapering, smooth, shining and pale green, mottled with red. Leaves 7-9 palmately lobed with lateral segments again deeply divided into several nearly separate lobes, coarsely serrate in the upper part, dark green above, paler in the upper part, dark green above, paler beneath. Flowers first pinkish-white becoming green, on a red spotted scape bearing several serrated bracts.

Habitate: Found in alpine regions.

Propagation: By vegetative method.

Parts Used: Rhizome.

Chemical Constituents: Helleborine, Helleborein, Hellebrin, Aconitic acid and Kaempferol glucosides.

Uses: Great hydrogogue. Cathartic. Emmenagogue. Heart stimulent. Used predominantly for mental symptoms. Brain troubles with serous effusion. Acute idiocy. Acute cerebro-spinal meningitis and tubercular meningitis with exudation and paralysis, more or less complete.

Hydrocephalus. Convulsion s with extreme coldness of body, except head or occiput which may be hot. Constant boring of head into pillow, rolling from side to side, beating head with hands. Thoughtless open staring eyes, insensible to light. Diarrhoea associated with all mental symptoms. General dropsy of brain, chest and abdomen. Falling of lower jaw.

645. *Helminthostachys zeylanica* (L.) Hook. *(Ophioglossaceae)*

Synonyms: *Osmunda zeylanica* L.

Description: A creeping rhizomatous herb. Rhizomes up to 1 cm diameter, cylindrical, tuberous, covered with small pale brown rounded scales and with thick fleshy roots; leaf stalk single, cylindrical, hairless, pale brown below, greenish above, about 30 cm long, 5-8 mm width, produced every year from the same rhizome. Leaf blade (lamina) round-shaped in outline, up to 30 cm in diameter, ternately divided, each branch 3-lobed, with short stalks. Each lobe oblong-lanceolate, about 13 x 3 cm, base wedge-shaped, apex acute, margin slightly wavy with narrow pale brown membranous border, pale green, hairless, papery; main nerve (costa) shallowly grooved above and raised below; lateral nerves forked once or twice, free, parallel, ending at the margin. Fertile branch solitary, arising from the base of the leaf blade bearing about 7 cm long spike, which contains many crested clusters of sporangia. Sporangia (reproductive organs contain spores) are seen in groups of 4, minute, green.

Habitate: Swamps and marshy areas, rarely on tree trunks and moist rocks.

Propagation: By vegetative method.

Parts Used: Leaves.

Chemical Constituents: They contain: moisture, nitrogen fat, crude fibre and ash, calcium, riboflavin, niacin, and ascorbic acid.

Uses: Leaves are aperients, intoxicant, anodyne and used to relieve sciatica. Rhizomes used to cure dysentery, catarrh, malaria, as an antidote for snake poison and as a tonic. Decoction of the rhizome is used to treat impotency. Leaf juice reportedly relieves blisters on the tongue.

646. *Hemerocallis fulva* L. *(Liliaceae)*

Vernacular Name: *Eng:* Yellow day-lily, orange day-lily, tawny day-lily.

Description: Perennial herbaceous plant with tuberous roots. Leaves linear, arranged in two rows. Flowers funnel-shaped, orange-yellow 6-10 on a forked scape. Fruit triangular. Seeds shining black.

Habitate: Cultivated for ornament and medicinal use.

Propagation: By vegetative method.

Part Used: Turbers, leaves and flowers.

Chemical Constituents: The flowers yield proteins, fatty substances, sugars, vitamin A and C; amino acids; adenin, choline, arginine and iodine.

Uses: The roots, the leaves and the flowers possess anti-inflammatory and heamostatic properties. They are used in treating feber, colitis, dysentery, oedema, dysuria, urinary lithiasis, heamorrhage, haemoptysis, epistaxis, mastitis and rheumatism. The external application of pounded fresh roots and leaves in a poultice is effective against inflammation.

647. *Hemidesmus indicus* (L.) R. Br. *(Asclepiadaceae)*

Vernacular Name: *San*: Anantamulah, Sariba, *Eng*: Indian sarasaparilla, Country sarasaparilla, *Hin*: Anantamul, Magrabu, *Kan*: Namadaballi, *Mal*: Nannari, Naruninti, Narunenti, *Tam*: Nannari, Saribam, *Tel:* Sugandipala.

Description: A perennial, slender, laticiferous, twining or prostrate, wiry shrub with woody root-stock and numerous slender, terete stems having thickened nodes; leaves simple, opposite, very variable from elliptic-oblong to linear-lanceolate, variegated with white above, silvery white and pubescent beneath; flowers greenish purple crowded in subsessile cymes in the opposite leaf axils; fruits slender follicles, cylindrical, 10 cm long, tapering to a point at the apex, seeds flattened, black, ovate-oblong, coma silvery white. The tuberous root is dark-brown, coma silvery white, tortuous with transversely cracked and longitudinally fissured bark. It has a strong central vasculature and a pleasant smell and taste.

Habitate: Throughout India.

Propagation: By seeds and vegetative method.

Parts Used: Roots, leaves, stem.

Chemical Consistuents: Air-dried roots yield essential oil containing *p*-methoxy salicylic aldehyde as the major constituent. The aroma of the drug is attributed to this aldehyde. Other constituents present in the roots are: β-sitosterol, α-and β-amyrins, lupeol, tetracyclic triterpene alcohols, small amounts of resin acids, fatty acids, tannins, saponins, a glycoside and a ketone.

Uses: The roots are bitter, sweet, astringent, aromatic, refrigerant, emollient, depurative, aphrodisiac, carminative, appetizer, anthelmintic, alterant, demulcent, diaphoretic, febrifuge, expectorant and tonic. They are useful in vitiated conditions of *pitta*, burning sensation, leucoderma, leprosy, skin diseases, pruritus, asthma, bronchitis, hyperdipsia, ophthalmopathy, hemicrania, epileptic fits, dyspepsia, helminthiasis, diarrhoea, dysentery, haemorrhoids, strangury, leucorrhoea, syphilis, abscess, arthralgia, fever and general debility. The leaves are useful in vomiting, wounds and leucoderma. The stems are bitter, diaphoretic and laxative, and are useful in inflammations, cerebropathy, hepatopathy, nephropathy, syphilis, metropathy, leucoderma, odontalgi, cough and asthma. The latex is good for conjunctivitis.

648. *Heracleum candolleanum* (Wight & Arn.) Gamble *(Apiaceae)*

Synonyms: *H. rigens* Wall. ex DC. var. candolleanum (Wight & Arn.) C.B. Clarke.

Description: A perennial stout hairy herb, up to 2 m tall, with woody reddish brown rootstock. Stems many, radiating from the rootstock, with many vertical parallel lines. Leaves are alternately arranged and are of two different types. The *lower leaves* two times pinnate, egg-shaped in outline, about 35 x 25 cm; *upper leaves* gradually becoming smaller towards the apex, 3-5 or often irregularly lobed, egg-shaped to oblong about 10 x 5 cm, base clasping the stem, apex acute or acuminate, margin shallowly or deeply toothed with saw-like teeth, pubescent; leaf stalks up to 15 cm long, with a broad sheath at base. *Flowers* polygamous, arranged in multi-branched compound umbels, yellow, minute, about 1.5 mm across, faintly fragrant. *Fruits* are called as mericarps (one-seeded unit of a compound fruit), elliptic to inverted egg-shaped, about 1 x 0.8 cm, dorsally compressed and laterally winged with prominent 3-ribs, hairless.

Habitate: Exposed montane grassland slopes.

Propagation: By seeds and vegetative method.

Parts Used: Whole plant.

Chemical Constituents: N.A.

Uses: In Kerala the tubers are reportedly used by Folk proactitioners. The fruits and seeds of its related species, *H. rigens,* are reportedly used in treating abdominal pain, cardiac diseases, constipation, cough, diarrhoea, gastritis, headache, hyperacidity, indigestion and wounds.

649. *Hernandia nymphaeifolia* (Presl.) Kubitzki (*Hernandiaceae*)

Synonyms: *Hernandia peltata* Meissn.

Description: Large, spreading tree, upto 20 m high, with robust trunk and grey to whitish bark. Leaves alternate, petiolate, the blades mostly peltate, dark green, shiny above, 10-30 cm long, 7-20 cm. Wide, with 7-9 conspicuous veins radiating palmately from point of attachment to petiole. Flowers relatively small and unisexual, white or greenish-white, fragrant, tubular, and borne in dense panicles. Fruit a brown drupe, completely enclosed in a whitish to reddish cupule, about 2.5 cm across, clearly marked with 8 broad, raised longitudinal ribs, enclosing a single hard seed.

Habitate: Common along the upper edge of beaches and in coastal woodlands.

Propagation: By seeds and vegetative method.

Part Used: Leaves.

Chemical Constituents: Isoquinoline alkaloids and bisbenzylalkaloids, ambrimine, afatine, hebridamine, malekulatine, thalicarpine 2-N-oxide, thalicarpine, vilaportine, and lignans, Essential oil, flavonoids.

Uses: To treat child birth illnesses (speed placenta expulsion, general weakness), relapsed illness and to treat post-natal depression.

650. *Herniaria glabra* (*Caryophyllaceae)*

Vernacular Name: *Eng:* Rupturewort.

Description: Prostrate annual or perennial with bright green oval leaves and clusters of green flowers.

Habitate: Rupturewort is found throughout Europe and western Asia. It thrives in barren areas, in lime and *San*dy soils.

Propagation: By seeds and vegetative method.

Parts Used: Aerial part.

Chemical Constituents: Rupturewort contains coumarins, flavonoids, phenolic acids and saponins.

Uses: Rupturewort of value chiefly as a diuretic herb. The fresh plant treats urinary problems such as cystitis, irritable bladder and kidney stones. It is also astringent, and has been applied as a poultice to speed the healing of ulcers. The whole plant appears to have an antispasmodic effect on the bladder.

651. *Heterosmilax erythrantha* Baill. (*Liliaceae*)

Description: Glabrous climber, unarmed, Leaves alternate, ovate, base subcordate; petiole long, with tendrils, Inflorescence in long-stalked axillary umbel; flowers pink or spotted with red, the male and female on different plants. Fruit globose, 8-10 mm. In diameter, black when ripe seeds 2-4 ovate.

Habitate: Grows wild in the mountains and the midlands.

Propagation: By seeds and vegetative method.

Part Used: Tuber.

Chemical Constituents: The tuberous roots contain saponins, tannin and resins.

Uses: The tuberous roots possess anti-inflammatory and antiallergic properties and are used in treating rheumatism, arthralgia, osteodynia, lumbago, boils, impetigo and prurigo.

652. *Hibiscus aculeatus* Roxb. *(Malvaceae)*

Synonyms *Hibiscus furcatus* Roxb.

Vernacular Name: *San*: Sathambasthi, *Kan*: Bendhegida, *Mal*: Paniccakam, Pariccakam, Naranampuli, *Tam*: Kontagomgura, *Tel:* Bendakaya.

Description: A suffrutescent trailing prickly herb, 60-150 cm in height; leaves simple, alternate, entire in early stages, 3-7 lobed in later stages clothed with appressed hairs, cordate or truncate at the base, prickly on the nerves beneath, crenate-serrate; flowers large, yellow with purple center; fruits ovoid pointed capsules enclosed in the enlarged calyx, seeds somewhat triangular, striated.

Habitate: Throughout India, as undergrowths in forests upto 900 m.

Propagation: By seeds and vegetative method.

Parts Used: Roots, leaves.

Chemical Consistuents: N.A.

Uses: The roots are refrigerant, anti-inflammatory and diuretic, and are useful in hyperdipsia, burning sensation, inflammations and nephropathy. The leaves are sour, astringent, anti-inflammatory, anthelmintic and ophthalmic, and are useful in all types of inflammations, helminthiasis dyspepsia and ophthalmopathy.

653. *Hibiscus mutabilis* L. *(Malvaceae)*

Vernacular Name: *Eng:* Chinese rose, changeable rose, rose-mallow, cotton-rose; *Hin:* Shalapara, sthal kamal; *Beng*: Sthalpadama; *Tam:* Irratai-vellaichembarattam, sembarattai; *Kan:* Bettada tavare, neladavare, surgakanti and *Mal*: Chinapparatti, hinaparutti.

Description: Plant growing several metres high; young twig tomentose. Leaves alternate, long-petioled, palmatilobed, hairy on the lower side, margins toothed. Flowers large, simple or compound, solitary in the axil of the leaves, first white then pink capsule globose, covered with haris seeds ovate and silky-villous.

Habitate: Cultivated every where for ornament.

Propagation: By seeds and vegetative method.

Part Used: Leaves and flowers.

Chemical Constituents: The flowers contain anthocyanosides.

Uses: The leaves and the flowers possess antibacterial. Demulcent and diuretic properties. They are used in treating boils, particularly on the chin, in the form of poultice made or powdered dried leaves and flowers mixed with concentrated tea infusion, which makes the boils burst earlier and leass painfully. Also used in treating impetigo, prurigo, metritis, leucorrhoea, mastitis, nephritis, cytitis, dysuria and infections.

654. *Hibiscus sigittifolius* Kurz var. *quinquelobus* Ganep. *(Malvaceae)*

Description: Herbaceous plant about 50cm. High. Tuberous roots fleshy. Leaves alternate, long-petioled, serrate, polymorphous, the lower entire, the upper palmaterly 5-lobed. Flowers large, red, solitary in the leaf-axils. Capsul ovate-acuminate, loculicidally 5-valved when ripe. Seeds numerous, brown all parts of the plant are hirsute.

Habitate: Grows wild in mountainous regiuons and is cultivated fro medicinal use.

Propagation: By seeds and vegetative method.

Part Used: Roots.

Chemical Constituents: The roots yioeld starch and mucilaginous substances.

Uses: The roots, which possess reconstituent, antitussive and emmengotgic properties. Are used in trating genral debility, insomnia, pulmonary turbeculosis, anorexia, infantile stomatitis, rachitis, persistent feber and cough, sore throat, bronchitis, menstrual disorders, lumbago, body pains, photopsia, vertigo and leucorrhoea.

655. *Hibiscus syriacus* L. (Mal*vaceae*)

Vernacular Name: *Eng:*-Rose-of Sharon, althaea, shrub althaea.

Description: Erect, nearly glabrous shrub or small tree, 2-3 m tall. Leaves mostly less than 8 cm long, triangular to rhombic ovate in outline, mostly deeply and narrowly 3-lobed, coarsely toothed. Flowers on short pedicels, in upper leaf axils; involucral bracts 6-8, mostly lanceolate, less than 2 cm long and 0.5 cm wide; calyx slightly longer than bracts; corolla single; petals 5, longer than calyx, 3-8 cm long, whitish purple, with crimsom base; stamens united n a tubular column, included; style 5-branched at the apex. Fruit a 5-celled capsule, each cell with 3 or more seeds.

Habitate: Commonly planted in gardens and roadsides of China and Korea.

Propagation: By seeds and vegetative method.

Parts Used: Bark.

Chemical Constituents: Mucilages, carotenoids, anthocyanidins, alkanes, aromatics, sesquiterpenes.

Uses: Antipyretic, anthelmintic, antifungal, anticomplementary, hypoglycaemic, antiulcer. Used in dysentery, abdominal pain, leucorrhoea, omalgia.

656. *Hibscus rosa-sinensis* L. *(Malvaceae)*

Vernacular Name: *San:* Japa, java, rudra pushpam; *Eng:* Red hibiscus, rose of china, Chinese hibiscus; *Hin:* Jasut, jasum; Beng: Joba; *Tel:* Java pushpamu dasana; *Tam:* Semparuthi; *Kan:* Dasavala and *Mal:* Chembarathi.

Description: An evergreen woody, glabrous, showy shrub, 5-8 ft. high; leaves bright green, ovate, entire below, coarsely toothed above; flowers solitary, axillary, bellshaped, with pistil and stamens projecting from the centre; capsules roundish, many seeded.

Habitate: Commonly cultivated as a garden ornamental shrub from sea-level to 500 m.

Propagation: By seeds and vegetative method.

Part Used: Leaves and flowers.

Chemical Constituents: Taraxeryl acetate, beta-sitosterol, campesterol, stigmasterol, cholesterol, erogosterol, lipids, citric, tartaric and oxalic acids, fructose, glucose, sucrose, flavonoids and flavonoid glycosides. Hibiscetin, cyaniding and cyanin glucosides. Alkanes.

Uses: To induce abortion, ease menstrual cramps and to help in childbirth. To treat headaches. A preparation from the leaves is used to treat postpartum relapse sickness, to treat boils, sores and inflammations. Good for hairs.

657. *Hibscus tiliaceus* L. *(Malvaceae)*

Vernacular Name: *Eng:* Beach hibiscus; *Hin:* Bola, chelwa; *Beng*: Bola, chelwa; *Tel:* Etagogu; *Tam:* Nirparathi, attuparathi and *Mal:* Nirparathi, attuparathi.

Description: Spreading medium-sized tree upto 15 m tall. Leaves alternate, petiolate, broadly ovate to cordate and palmately veined. Flowers large and showy, yellow with deep maroon center and conspicuous staminal column arising from base of ovary. Fruit a subglobose capsule upto 25 cm long with numerous small seeds.

Habitate: Common on beaches, in thickets, weedy forest margins, disturbed areas, margins of swamps and rivers.

Propagation: By seeds and vegetative method.

Part Used: Leaves, fruits and bark.

Chemical Constituents: Gemlofuran, hibiscolactone, hibiscones, hibiscoquinones, lapachol, gossypol, gossypetin, mansonnes, hyperoside, kaempferol, quercetin and 3-O-galactosides of quercetin and kaempferol, gossypetin glucosides, gossypitrin and gossytrin, cyaniding-2-sophoroside, beta-sitosterol, para-coumaric and fumaric acids.

Uses: The leaves are wrapped around fractured bones and sprained muscles. Juice from the leaves is used in treating gonorrhoea. The fluid from the bark is used to promote menstruation. The flowers are used in making a salve. The bark and the young leaves are used to treat skin diseases.

658. *Hieracium pilosella* *(Asteraceae)*

Synonyms: *Pilosella officinarum.*

Vernacular Name: *Eng:* Mouse-ear Hawkweed.

Description: Perennial herb growing to a height of 20 cm from a rosette of basal leaves. Stems bear single bright yellow flowerheads.

Habitate: Mouse-ear hawkweed is common throughout much of Europe and temperate regions of Asia. It is naturalized in North America.

Propagation: By seeds and vegetative method.

Parts Used: Aerial parts.

Chemical Constituents: Mouse-ear-hawkweed contains a coumarin, flavonoids and caffeic acid. It is thought to be mildly antifungal.

Uses: Mouse-ear hawkweed relaxes the muscles of the bronchial tubes, stimulates the cough reflex and reduces the production of catarrh. This combination of actions makes the herb effective against all manner of respiratory problems, including asthma and wheeziness, whooping cough, bronchitis and other chronic and congested coughs. mouse-ear hawkweed's astringency and its diuretic action also help to counter the production of catarrh, sometimes throughout the respiratory system. The herb is used to control heavy menstrual bleeding, and to ease the coughing up of blood. It may be applied as a poultice to heal wounds.

659. *Hippophae rhamnoides* *(Elaegnaceae)*

Vernacular Name: *Eng:* Sea buckthorn.

Description: Thorny deciduous shrub growing to 5 m. Has narrow silvery leaves, male or female flowers and clusters of brownish-orange berries.

Habitate: Native to Europe and Asia, sea buckthorn grows mainly in *San*dy coastal areas and in dry riverbeds in mountainous regions. The berries are harvested in autumn.

Propagation: By seeds and vegetative method.

Parts Used: Berries.

Chemical Constituents: The fruit contains flavonoids, fruit acids and vitamin C.

Uses: Sea buckthorn berries are very high in vitamin C. They have principally been used to help improve resistance to infection.

660. *Hiptage benghalensis* (L.) Kurz *(Malpighiaceae)*

Synonyms: *Hiptage madablota* Gaertn.

Vernacular Name: *San*: Madhavi, Atimukha; *Eng*: Clustered hiptage; *Hin*: Madhavilata, Madhumalati; *Kan*: Madhavivasantadhuti; *Mal*: Sitampu, Sitampu; *Tam*: Madhavi, Vasantagalamalligai; *Tel:* Madavi Tige.

Description: A large, handsome, woody much-branched evergreen climbing shrub with silky young parts; leaves simple, opposite, coriaceous, elliptic-oblong, ovate-lanceolate, 10-23 cm long; flowers yellowish white, fragrant, in erect finely tomentose recemes, petals twice as long as the sepals, the uppermost petal broader than the rest, fringed on the margin; fruits 2-3 winged samara, seed globose, solitary.

Habitate: Throughout India, in forests upto 1,800 m.

Propagation: By seeds and vegetative method.

Parts Used: Bark, leaves, flowers.

Chemical Consistuents: The bark is an aromatic bitter. It contains a crystalline glucoside, hiptagin. The bark also contains tannin.

Uses: The bark, leaves and flowers are aromatic, bitter acrid, astringent, refrigerant, vulnerary, expectorant, cardiotonic, anti-inflammatory and insecticidal. They are useful in vitiated conditions of *pitta,* burning sensation, wounds ulcers, cough, asthma, cardiac debility, inflammations, skin diseases leprosy, scabies, rheumatism and hyperdipsia.

661. *Holarrhena antidysenterica* *(Apocynaceae)*

Vernacular Name: *San:* Kutaja, kalinga; *Eng:* Conessi bark, kurchi bark, bitter oleander, dysentery rose-bay, Tellicherry bark; *Hin:* Kurchi, karchi, karra, kora, kuar kureya, kura; *Beng*: Kurchi; *Tel:* Pala kodaga; *Tam:* Veppalei, kodagapalei, indrabam; *Kan:* Beppale, koodsaloo, korchie and *Mal:* Kodagapala.

Description: A tree reaching about 10m. in height or more. Bark pale-brown, lenticellate. Yong twigs tomentose. Leaves opposite, oval, subsessile. Flowers white in axillary or terminal corymbiferous cyme. Follicles cylindrical in pairs. Long, narrow, incurved. Seeds numerous, brownish, crowned with a tuft of long haris one end.

Habitate: Grows wild in the mountains and the midlands.

Propagation: By seeds and vegetative method.

Part Used: Bark and seeds.

Chemical Constituents: The trunk bark contains alkaloids: conessine, nor-conessine, conessimine, isoconessimine, curchine, conimine, conamine, conkurchine, holarrhine, holarrhenine and holarrhimine; gum, resins, tannin, triterpene alcohol, lupeol, b-sitosterol.

Uses: The trunk bark possesses amoebicidal properties. It is effective against amoebiasis. The sum of the alkaloids and conessine are also used. A bath containing a decoction of bark or leaves cures scabies. An alcoholic maceration of pounded roots is also used topically against scabies. Bark, is astringent, anthelmintic, stomachic, antipyretic, tonic and antidysenteric, used in amoebie dysentery and diarrhoea. Contains alkaloid conessine, a gum-resin, and tannin.

662. *Holoptelea integrifolia* (Roxb.) Planch. *(Ulmaceae)*

Vernacular Name: *San*: Cirabilvah, Putikaranhah; *Eng*: Indian elm, Kanju; *Hin*: Cilbil, *Kanju*; *Kan*: Tapasigida; *Mal*: Avil, Aval, Nattavil, Nettaval; *Tam*: Avali, Kanji; *Tel:* Tapasi.

Description: A medium sized to large glabrous deciduous tree, 15-25 m in height with whitish or yellowish grey bark exfoliating in irregular flakes and with an offensive smell when freshly cut; leaves simple, alternate, distichous, elliptic, entire, glabrous with rounded or cordate base and 5-7 pairs of main nerves; flowers greenish yellow, male and hermaphrodite mixed in short racemes of fascicles near the leaf scars; fruits suborbicular samara with membranous reticulately veined wings.

Habitate: Throughout India, in deciduous forests.

Propagation: By seeds and vegetative method.

Parts Used: Bark, leaves.

Chemical Consistuents: The seed cake contains N, 10.3; lysine, 3.3; glutamic acid, 13.0; and histidine, 1.3%.

Uses: The bark and leaves are bitter, astringent, acrid, thermogenic, anti-inflammatory, digestive, carminative, laxative, anthelmintic, depurative, revulsive and urinary astringent. They are useful in vitiated conditions of *kapha* and *pitta*, inflammations, dyspepsia, flatulence, colic, helminthiasis, vomiting, skin diseases, leprosy, diabetes, haemorrhoids and rheumatism.

663. *Holostemma ada-kodien* Schultes *(Asclepiadaceae)*

Synonyms: *Holostemma annulare* (Roxb.) K. Schumn.), *Holostemma rheedei* Wall.

Vernacular Name: *San*: Jivanti, Arkapushpi, *Hin*: Chirvel,Charivel, *Mal*: Atapatiyan, Atapotiyan, Atakotiyan, *Tam*: Palaikkirai, *Tel:* Palagurugu.

Description: A handsome, laticiferous twining shrub with large conspicuous flowers; leaves simple, opposite, codate; flowers purple in axillary umbellate cymes; fruits thick follicles, 9 cm long, cylindrical, bluntly pointed. The roots are pretty long upto a meter or more, irregularly twisted, thick and cylindrical.

Habitate: Throughout India, in hedges and open forests.

Propagation: By seeds and vegetative method.

Parts Used: Tubers.

Chemical Consistuents: Analysis of the root powder gave; moisture, protein, sugar, starch, fibre, and ash. The ash contained; calcium and phosphate.

Uses: The roots are sweet, refrigerant, ophthalmic, emollient, alterant, tonic, stimulant, aphrodisiac, expectorant and galactagogue. They are useful in ophthalmopathy, orchids, cough, burning sensation, stomachalgia, consumption, fever and *tridosa*. The leaves, flowers and fruits are eaten as a vegetable.

664. *Homalonema occulta* (Lour.) Schott *(Araceae)*

Description: Perennial herb. Rhizome long, tubular, with hard fibres. Leaves large, sagittate-cordate with tightly clasping sheath. Inflorescence in axillary spadixl the male flowers above, the female below perianth absent in both sexes. Berry red when ripe.

Habitate: Grows wild along stream banks and on the sides of rocky ravines in mountainous regions.

Propagation: By vegetative method.

Part Used: Rhizome.

Chemical Constituents: The rhizome contains an essential oil consisting or linalool, a-terpineol, linalyl acetate, sabinene, limonene, propionic aldehyde and acetic acid.

Uses: The rhizome possesses anti-inflammatory, anodyne and stopachic properties. It is used in treating rheumatism. Arthralgia, paresis, gastralgia, dymenorrhoea, osteodynia of the aged and dyspespsia. Massage with a fresh rhizome maceration has an anodyne effect.

A poulitic of pounded fresh leaves in active on boils. The rhizome is also an insecticide against moth.

665. *Homonoia riparia* Lour. *(Euphorbiaceae)*

Vernacular Name: *San*: Jalavetasah, vetasah, Pashanbedaka, *Hin*: Jalbent, *Kan*: *San*napasanabheda, *Mal*: Attuvanni, Pulavanni, Nirvanni, Katallari, *Tam*: Kattuarali, *Tel:* Siridamanu.

Description: Rigid evergreen willow-like dioecious shrub with dark grey or brown bark and grayish brown moderately hardwood and pubescent young parts; leaves linear or linear-oblong, entire or more or less serrulate towards the apex, glabrous above and glandular scaly beneath, main nerves 10-30 pairs; flowers sessile in axillary, elongated, pubescent spikes, stamens in male flowers papillose; fruits globose capsules, seeds yellowish brown, smooth, slightly angular on the inner surface and rounded on the back.

Habitate: Throughout India, at lower elevations on the banks of rivers and streams especially among rocks.

Propagation: By seeds and vegetative method.

Parts Used: Roots, leaves, fruits.

Chemical Consistuents: N.A.

Uses: The roots are laxative, diuretic, refrigerant, depurative and emetic. They are useful in haemorrhoids, vesical calculi, strangury, urethrorrhea, gonorrhoea. Syphilis and odontalgia. Leaves and fruits are depurative and antiseptic, and are useful for ulcers, wounds and skin diseases.

666. *Hordeum distichon* *(Poaceae)*

Vernacular Name: *Eng:* Barley.

Description: Annual grass growing to about 1 m. Has an erect hollow stem, lance-shaped leaves, and ears bearing twin rows of seeds and long bristle.

Habitate: Barley is cultivated in temperate regions worldwide.

Propagation: By seeds and vegetative method.

Parts Used: Seeds.

Chemical Constituents: Barley contains proteins, sugars, starch, fats and B vitamins. The young seedlings also contains the alkaloids hordenine and gramine.

Uses: An excellent food for convalescence in the form of porridge or barley water, barley is soothing to the throat and provides easily assimilated nutrients. It can also be taken to clear catarrh. Its demulcent quality soothes inflammation of the gut and urinary tract. Barley aids in the digestion of milk and is given to babies to prevent the development of curds within the stomach. It is commonly given to children suffering from minor infections or diarrhoea, and it is particularly recommended as a treatment for feverish states. Made into a poultice, barley is an effective remedy for soothing and reducing inflammation in sores and swellings.

667. *Hordeum vulgare* L. *(Poaceae)*

Synonyms: *Hordeum sativum* Jessen.

Vernacular Name: *San*: Yavah, *Eng*: Barley, *Hin*: Jav, Jau, *Kan*: Yava, Jave-godhi, *Mal*: Yavam, Barli, *Tam*: Barliarisi, *Tel:* Yava.

Description: An erect, stout, tufted annual herb upto 100 cm in height; leaves few, flaccid, linear upper ones close to the spike, sheath smooth, ligule short, membranous, spike flattened, 2-ranked, 20-30 cm long, terminal spikelets sessile, arranged in threes on two sides of the rachis, all fertile or lateral ones barren; fruit an elliptic short pointed grooved caryopsis.

Habitate: Throughout north India, cultivated.

Propagation: By seeds and vegetative method.

Parts Used: Grains.

Chemical Consistuents: Arginine, Histidine, Lysine, Tyrosine, Tryptophan, Phenylalanine, Cystine, Methionine, Threonine, Leucine, Isoleucine, Valine, Glycine.

Uses: The grains are astringent, sweet, acrid, refrigerant, emollient, diuretic, intellect promoting, aphrodisiac, mucilaginous, digestive and tonic. They are useful in vitiated conditions of *kapha* and *pitta*, cough, asthma, strangury, amentia, fever, bronchiotitis, urocystitis urethjritis, dyspepsia, gastropathy, ulcers, burns cephalalgia, anaemia and in the diet of invalids.

668. *Houttuynia cardata* Thunb. *(Saururaceae)*

Vernacular Name: *Eng*: Houttuynia, stink grass.

Description: Glabrous perennial herb with creeping rhizome, 20-50 cm tall. Leaves alternate, ovate, 3-8 cm long, 3-6 cm wide, cordate, stipules oblong, obtuse, united to petioles. Inflorescence dense lateral spike subtended by 4 involucral bracts; spikes 1-3 cm long, cylindric, densely many-flowered; peduncles 2-3 cm long. Flowers small, bracted, perianth none; stamens 3, united at base to 1-celled ovary; stigma 3. Fruit dry opening at top.

Habitate: Wet places in lowlands of Himalayas, Korea, Japan and China.

Propagation: By seeds and vegetative method.

Parts Used: Whole plant.

Chemical Constituents: Flavonoids: querctrin, isoquercitrin. Benzamide: cis and trans-N-(4-hydroxystyryl)-benzamide. Fatty aldehydes: decanoylacetaldehyde, lauryladehyde, methy1 nonylketone, Monoterpenes and sesquiterpenes.

Uses: Anti-inflammatory, antiviral, vitamin P-like, anifungal, antimicrobial, platelet coagulation depressing, plaque formation suppressant, hypoglycaemic activities. Used in suppuration and poisoning.

669. *Houttuynia cordata* Thunb. *(Saururaceae)*

Vernacular Name: *Eng:* Tsi.

Description: Perennial herbaceous plant, 20-40cm. High. Stems greenish or reddish-purple. Leaves alternate, heart-shaped with stalk sheathing the stems, emitting a fishy smell when crushed. Inflorescence in axillary or terminal spike; flowers small, pale-yellow; bracts white seeds oval, glabrous.

Habitate: Grows wild in rice-fields and on stream banks.

Propagation: By seeds and vegetative method.

Part Used: Whole plant.

Chemical Constituents: The whole plant yields and essential oil consisting of methyl-nonyl ketone, myrcene, DOlimonene, a-pinene, p-cymene, linalool and geraniol; the alkaloid cordiline; the flavone quercitrinl lipidsl hexadecanoic and decanoic acids.

Uses: The whole plant has a beneficial effect in the treatment of haemorrhoids, acute conjunctivitis and ocular infections due to Bacillus pyocyaneus. It is also used in treating measles, enteritis and irregular menstruation. The juice of the crushed fresh plant is also administered orally. In case of contusions and ophthalmia, crushed fresh leaves are applied externally in a poultice.

670. *Hovenia dulcis* Thunb. *(Rhamnaceae)*

Vernacular Name: *Eng:* Japanese raisin tree, coral tree; *Hin:* Sicka and *Assam*: Chetia-bola.

Description: Evergreen tree about 7-10m. in height. Young twigs lenticellate and pubescent. Leaves alternate, long-petioled, with 3 nerves from the basel margins sharply denticulate. Inflorescence in axillary or terminal cymel flowers pale-green. Fruit globose, borne on pinkish-brown swollen peduncles, sweetish and edible. Seeds round, slightly compressed.

Habitate: Grows wild and is cultivated in the mountains.

Propagation: By seeds and vegetative method.

Part Used: Fruit and fruit-bearing branches.

Chemical Constituents: The fruit contains sugars; flucose, fructose and sucrose; salts: potassium nitrate, potassium malate.

Uses: The ripe fruit and the small twigs bearing ripe fruit are a reconstituent and depurative remedy. The are used for the treatment of alcoholic intoxication, dysuria, general debility and dry throat.

671. *Hoya australis* R. Br. *(Asclepiadaceae)*

Vernacular Name: *Eng:* Wax Plant.

Description: Climbing semi-woody vine with latex. Leaves opposite, petiolate, fleshy, broadly ellipitic up to 15 cm long. Flowers small but showy, fragrant, borne in an umbel-like head containing numerous flowers. Fruit a thin cylindric follicle up to 15 cm long containing numerous plumed seeds.

Habitate: Common as a vine or epiphyte in beach thickets, sea cliffs, edges of mangroves and in primary forest to over 1000 m elevation.

Propagation: By seeds and vegetative method.

Part Used: Leaves.

Chemical Constituents: Amyrins, apigenin glucoside, australinals, australinoic acid, australinols, benzoic acid, chorogenic acid, chrysoeriol glycoside, cosmosin, lupeol, lipids, nyctanthic acid derivatives, 3,4-seco-3-nor-oelenenol.

Uses: The plant is used to treat swollen testicles. The leaves are used to make lotion for body rashes. An infusion of the leaves is applied as a lotion and taken internally for skin inflammations. The juice from the plant is applied to body burns. An infusion of the leaves is taken for many types of swellings and inflammations. It is also used to treat stomach ailments in Samoa, as well as in Futuna.

672. *Hugonia mystax* Linn. *(Linaceae)*

Vernacular Name: *San*: Kamsamarah, *Eng*: Climbing flax, *Kan*: Mrema, *Mal*: Karttotti, Motirakkanni, *Tam*: Motirakkanni, *Tel:* Kakibira.

Description: A rambling scandent shrub with yellow tomentose twigs; branchlets horizontal provided with a pair of strong circinate hooks; leaves simple, alternate, elliptic-obovate glabrous and penninerved; flowers yellow at the ends of the branchlets, pedicels short, clothed with soft yellow hairs, petals many times longer than the sepals; fruits globose fleshy drupes, seeds 2 or 3 compressed.

Habitate: Throughout India, in dry forest areas.

Propagation: By seeds and vegetative method.

Parts Used: Roots.

Chemical Consistuents: N.A.

Uses: The roots are astringent, bitter, sweet, febrifuge and anthelmintic. They are useful in fevers, verminosis, and vitiated conditions of *vata*, externally as a paste for inflammations.

673. *Humboldtia vahliana* Wight *(Caesalpiniaceae)*

Vernacular Name: *San*: Jelavedesa, *Mal*: Korathi, Karappongu, *Tam*: Neer vanchi, Athu vanji.

Description: Medium sized trees, 7-15 m tall, about 1.2 m girth. *Bark* smooth, about 5 mm thick, dark brown mottled with white. *Blaze* whitish. *Wood* lightbrown, moderately hard. Branchlets hairless, drooping. *Stipules* egg-shaped, 1.5-2.5 x 0.7 cm long, apex acute, with a kidney-shaped appendage, green. Rachis 1-1.5 cm long, cylindrical. Leaves alternate, pinnately compound; *leaflets* 6-10, opposite, distinctly stalked, oblong-lanceolate, leathery, 10-25 x 4-6 cm, base rounded, apex acuminate, margin entire, hairless. *Flowers* bisexual, in axillary racemes. 2.5-3 cm long, white, stalked. Peduncle of racemes about 15 cm long, velvety. *Pods* flat, oblong, leathery, 15-20 x 3.5-5 cm, dull brown, tapering at both ends, yellowish brown pubescent. *Seeds* 3-4, compressed.

Habitate: Along watercourses of semi-evergreen to evergreen forests.

Propagation: By seeds and vegetative method.

Parts Used: Bark.

Chemical Constituents: N.A.

Uses: Bark is used for treating ulcers, biliousness, leprosy and epilepsy.

674. *Humulus lupulus* *(Cannabinaceae)*

Vernacular Name: *Eng:* Hops.

Description: A perennial, twining, scaabrid herb, dioecious, monoecious plants are also found. Aerial stem oppositely branched, angular, flexible; leaves opposite, stipulate; lower longer, 3-5 lobed; upper smaller, ovates or cordate, serraates minutely prickly; petioles long male flowers small, greenish yellow, arranged in paniculate cymes; female flowers in cone-like inflorescences; fruit an achene.

Habitate: Indigenous to Europe and Asia, hops flourish in hedgerows and on wasteground.

Propagation: By seeds and vegetative method.

Parts Used: Strobiles.

Chemical Constituents: Bitter principles, volatile oil, humulene, flavonoids, polyphenolic tannins, oestrogenic substances, asparagin.

Uses: Sedative, soporific, antispasmodic, aromatic bitter.

675. *Hydnocarpus alpina* Wight *(Flacourtiaceae)*

Vernacular Name: *Kan*: Torathi, *San*usotti, *Mal*: *Mal*a maravetti, Pinervetty, Mar: Kastel, *Tam*: Athu chankalai, *Mal*ai vattai, Oily maram.

Description: Medium sized trees, 10-20 m tall. *Outer bark* about 5 mm thick, smooth, black, mottled with grey; *inner bark* pinkish cream. Young branchlets hairless, drooping. *Leaves* alternate, entire, elliptic-oblong to oblong-lanceolate, 6-25 x 2-9 cm, base acute, apex acuminate, hairless; lateral nerves 7-10 pairs, prominent; leaf stalks 7-15 mm long.

Male and female flowers are separately seen in the same plant. *Male flowers* are clustered in the leaf axils, about 2 cm across, 2-4 in a group, borne on a golden-hairy stalk, greenish white; *female flowers* usually single in leaf axils, around 2 cm across, dull yellow. *Berries* globose, 5-7 cm across, smooth, brownish hairy, with a woody rind. *Seeds* 10-12 embedded in white pulp.

Habitate: Semi-evergreen to evergreen forests especially along stream banks and in moist valleys.

Propagation: By seeds and vegetative method.

Parts Used: Seeds and seed oil.

Chemical Constituents: Chaulmoogric, Hydnocarpic, Alepric, Aleprylic, Aleprestic, Aleprolic, Gorlic.

Uses: The fruits and seeds are used as a substitute for *H. pentandra*. These are heavily traded for oil extraction. The seed oil is used in the treatment of leprosy.

676. *Hydnocarpus anthelmintica* pierre *(Flacourtiaceae)*

Vernacular Name: *Eng*: Sponge-berry, common chaulmongra tree.

Description: Tall tree, 10m. high or more Bark whitish grey. Leaves alternate, coriaceous, shining greenl entirely pinkish when young. Flowers unisexual or polygamous, in axillary raceme, both sexes on the same plant. Fruit large, globose. Seeds numerous, angular, embedded in the pulp.

Habitate: Grows wild but is commonly cultivated for shade and ornament.

Propagation: By seeds and vegetative method.

Part Used: Seeds.

Chemical Constituents: The seed kernels contains lipids 40-55%, a glucoside that yields glucose and hydrocyanic acid on hydrolysis; a fatty oil consisting or glycerides of chaulmoogric, hydnocarpic and gorlic acids.

Uses: The seeds kernels are used in treating leprosy, scabies, impetigo and some other dermatitides. They are applied externally in the form of medicinal oil or ointment. An emulsion of the seed kernel oil is exceptionally administered orally in the form of drops, but caution must be exercised because of its very high toxicity.

677. *Hydnocarpus laurifolia* (Dennst.) Sleumer *(Flacourtiaceae)*

Synonyms: *Hydnocarpus wightiana* Bl., *Hydnocarpus pentandre*.

Vernacular Name: *San*: Tuvarakah, Garudaphala; *Eng*: Marothi tree, Chaulmugra; *Hin*: Calmogara; *Kan*: Toratti, Surti, Suranti; *Mal*: Marotti, Niratti, Maravatti, Nivatti, Niralam; *Tam*: Maravattai, Maravetti; *Tel:* Adisadamu, Niradi.

Description: A medium sized to large dioecious evergreen tree, 15-30 m in height with pale brown somewhat rough bark mottled with white; leaves simple, alternate, ovate, oblong, lanceolate or elliptic more or less serrate; flowers small, greenish white, solitary or in fascicles or in small racemes, unisexual; fruits globose or obovoid tomentose berries, seeds 15-20 per fruit, obtusely angular, yellowish.

Habitate: In the forests of the Western Ghats, upto 600 m.

Propagation: By seeds and vegetative method.

Parts Used: Seeds, oil.

Chemical Consistuents: Chaulmoogric, hydnocarpic, gorlic, lower homologues of chaulmoogric.

Uses: The seeds and oil are acrid, astringent, bitter thermogenic, emollient, depurative, vermifuge, anodyne, purgative, emetic, carminative, stomachic, suppurative, alterant, haematinic and tonic. They are useful in leprosy, skin diseases, pruritus, leucoderma, dermatitis, bronchopathy, eczema, phthisis, vitiated conditions of *vata* and *kapha*, scrofula, sprains, bruises, tubercular laryngitis, chronic ulcers, dyspepsia colic, flatulence, verminosis, diabetes, wounds, ulcers and scald-head.

678. *Hydnocarpus macrocarpa* (Bedd.) Warb. *(Flacourtiaceae)*

Synonyms: *Taraktogenos macrocarpa* (Bedd.) Balakr., *Asteriastigma macrocarpa* Bedd.

Vernacular Name: *Mal*: Mala kummatti, *Tam*: *Mal*ai maravattai.

Description: A medium sized tree, 6-15 m tall. *Outer bark* dull brown, *inner bark* pale-purplish brown. Branchlets minutely yellow hairy. *Leaves* alternate, oblong to elliptic-lanceolate, 15-30 x 6-10 cm, apex abruptly acuminate, base rounded and unequal, margin entire, shiny and dark green; lateral nerves about 7 pairs, prominently raised below; leaf stalks 1-2 cm long, hairy. *Mal*e, female and bisexual flowers are separated, foul smelling; *male flowers* about 2.5 cm across, white, clustered on old stems; *female flowers* few, borne on a short stalk of older stems. *Fruits* spherical, about 15 cm across, dark brown, densely velvety hairy with woody rind. *Seeds* about 50, egg-shaped, dark brown.

Habitate: Semi-evergreen to evergreen forests.

Propagation: By seeds and vegetative method.

Parts Used: Seeds and seed oil.

Chemical Constituents: Chaulmoogric, hydnocarpic, gorlic, lower homologues of hydnocarpic, palmitic, and oleic.

Uses: The seed oil is used to cure skin diseases and leprosy.

679. *Hydrangea arborescens* L. *(Saxifragaceae)*

Synonyms: *Hydrangea cordata* Pursh., *Hydrangea glauca* Rafin., *Hydrangea Vulgaris* Michx.

Vernacular Name: *Eng:* Seven bark hydrangea.

Description: An erect smooth shrub, upto 3 m. in height. Leaves long petioled, ovate, acute or acuminate, rounded or cordate at base, serrate, green and nearly glabrous on both sides, sometimes somewhat pubescent or glaucous beneath, 7-15 cm. long. Flowers: in cymes up to 12 cm. broad with none or few sterile flowers. Fertile flowers with petals white 2 mm. long, with minute sepals. Sterile flowers only with sepals, 1 cm. long, reticulately veined.

Habitate: United States, Virginia, Carolina, Michigan.

Propagation: By vegetative method.

Parts Used: Rhizome.

Chemical Constituents: Hydrangin; Hydrangenol; flavonoids like Kaempferol, Quercetin, Rutin. Tanins absent.

Uses: Used for Renal Calculi expulsion. Bladder stones. Prostatic ailments, cystitis and urethritis. Used for complaints predominantly of stones, profuse deposit of white amorphous salts in urine. Renal Calculi, renal colic, blood in urine. Uterine complaints, pain in lumbar region. Burning in urethra with frequent desire. Heavy deposits of mucus in urine. Sharp pain in loins, especially left. Enlarge prostates. All complaints with great thirst.

680. *Hydrastis Canadensis* L. *(Ranunculaceae)*

Synonyms: *Warnera Canadensis* Mill., *Warnera tinctoria* Rafin.

Vernacular Name: *Eng:* Golden seal.

Description: A deciduous perennial herb, having a thick, longitudinally wrinkled, knotted, horizontal, bright yellow rhizome, with slender roots beneath and encircled by scale leaf scars. Stem simple, erect, 15-30 cm. high, sub-cylindrical, with downward-pointed hairs. Leaves two typed; stem leaves sessile, two alternate, near the top; basal leaf, one and petiolate. Leaves palmate, broad, 5 lobed; lobes incised, doubly serrate, acuminate flowers, solitary, small, terminal, greenish white, apetatlous.

Habitate: Canada and the United States, North Carolina, Oregan.

Propagation: By vegetative method.

Parts Used: Rhizome.

Chemical Constituents: Isoquinoline alkaloids viz. Hydrastine 1.5-4.0%, Berberine 0.5-6.0%, Berberastine, Canadine; Candaline, Canadaline; Chlorogenic acid. Resins. Meconic acid. Lactone.

Uses: For complaints like catarrhal thick, yellowish, ropy secretions from throat, stomach, uterus and urethra. Weak muscles, poor digestion and obstinate constipation. Lumbago, emaciation and prostration. Cancer and cancerous conditions. In small pox, in mitigating its bad effects. Thick, yellowish tenacious nasal discharge falling in nasopharyngeal region. Eustachian catarrh causing deafness. Follicular pharyngitis with smarting, excoriating pain Tender liver, Jaundice. Dull, dragging pain in the bark with stiffness, particularly across the lumbar and must use arm-support to rise. Gonorrhea. Erosion of cervix.

681. *Hygrophila angustifolia* auct. *(Acanthaceae)*

Synonyms: *Asteracantha longifolia* (Linn.) Nees, *Hygrophila salicifolia.*

Vernacular Name: *San*: Kokilaksah, Iksurah, *Eng*: Long-leaves barleria, *Hin*: Talmakhana, Kamtakaliya, *Kan*: Kolavalike, *Mal*: Vayalcculli, Culli, *Tam*: Nirmulli, *Tel:* Kokilaksamu.

Description: An erect, hispid, semiwoody, annual with numerous fasciculate sub-quadrangular stems; leaves in verticels of six at a node, 2 very large, upto 18 cm long, bearing three straight, sharp yellow spines in each axil, hispid on both sides, lanceolate or oblanceolate, tapering at both ends, margins slightly serrulate, flowers bluish purple or rose tint or whitish in axils of leaves, amidst spines, bracts and bracteoles, corolla bilipped, the upper 2-lobed and the lower 3-lobed; fruits linear oblong compressed capsules with 4-8 seeds on hard small retinacula, seeds flat or compressed, smooth with mucilaginous coating.

Habitate: Throughout India, in plains.

Propagation: By seeds and vegetative method.

Parts Used: Roots, leaves, seeds.

Chemical Constituents: They yield 25% of a fatty oil and contain traces of an unidentified alkaloid, a bitter substance, and 4% ash consisting chiefly of calcium phosphate and potassium chloride.

Uses: The roots are sweet, sour, bitter, refrigerant, diuretic, anti-inflammatory, aphrodisiac and tonic. They are useful in dropsy of chronic Bright's disease, inflammation, ascites, hyperdipsia, vesical calculi, strangury, jaundice, flatulence, dysentery and vitiated conditions of *vata*. The leaves are sweet, sour, bitter, oleaginous, aphrodisiac, anti-inflammatory, stomachic, ophthalmic and tonic. They are useful in jaundice, dropsy, rheumatism, lumbago, arthralgia, anasarca, diseases of the urogenital tract, arthritis, cough, vitiated conditions of *pitta*, gastropathy, anaemia and ophthalmopathy. The seeds are acrid, bitter, refrigerant, liver tonic aphrodisiac, diuretic, rejuvenating, lithontriptic, nervine tonic, constipating and tonic. They are useful in gonorrhoea, promoting sexual vigour and strength, arresting abortion, burning sensation, anaemia, vitiated conditions of *pitta*, diarrhoea, dysentery, strangury, renal and vesical calculi, gout rheumatism and general debility.

682. *Hygrophila spinosa* *(Acanthaceae)*

Vernacular Name: *Eng:* Gokulakanta.

Description: Thorny, red-stemmed annual growing to 60 cm. Has bright blue flowers and small, flat, dark red seeds.

Habitate: Native to India, gokulakanta is now widely distributed throughout tropical regions. It is gathered when in flower.

Propagation: By seeds and vegetative method.

Parts Used: Root.

Chemical Constituents: Gokulakanta contains mucilage, fixed and volatile oils and an alkaloid.

Uses: Commonly used as a remedy in India, gokulakanta is taken chiefly for its reputed aphrodisiac properties. Both the aerial parts and ash of the burned plant are strongly diuretic, and are used to flush water from the body in cases of excess fluid retention. Gokulakanta root is demulcent, and is used to alleviate the inflammation produced by urinary tract support the liver in conditions such as jaundice and hepatitis.

683. *Hygroryza aristata* (Retz.) Nees ex Wight & Arn. *(Poaceae)*

Synonyms: *Pharus aristatus* Retz.

Vernacular Name: *San*: Nivarah, Aranyadhanya, Aranyajali, *Eng*: Bengal wild rice, *Hin*: Jungali-dal, *Mal*: Varinellu, Nirvallippullu, *Tam*: Vallippul.

Description: A floating glabrous aquatic grass with culms 30–45 cm long.

Habitate: Throughout India, in tanks, ponds and wet grounds.

Propagation: By seeds and vegetative method.

Parts Used: Roots, seeds.

Chemical Consistuents: N.A.

Uses: The roots and seeds are sweet, acrid, cooling, diuretic, emollient, galactagogue, constipating, and tonic. They are useful in strangury, diarrhoea, otopathy, vitiated conditions of *pitta*, burning sensation, hyperdipsia, fatigue and general debility.

684. *Hyoscyamus niger* L. *(Solanaceae)*

Vernacular Name: *San:* Dipya, parasikaya; *Eng:* Black henbane; common henbane; *Hin:* Khurasaniajavayan; *Beng*: Khora-saniajowan; *Tel:* Khurashanivamam; *Tam:* Kurasaniyomam and *Kan:* Khurasanivadaki.

Description: An erect, beinnial or annual herb 30-80 cm high, villous, viscid and with a disagreeable,heavy odour. Stem robust, 0.3-0.9 m. Basal leaves spreading, petiolate, oblong-ovate, 15-20 cm coarsely sinuate-toothed. The cauline leaves smaller, sessile, clasping, oval-oblong, sinuate, pinnatifid; lobes irregular, triangular, lanceolate. Flowers in terminal, scorpioid cymes, or axillary, nearly entirely sessile; june. Calyx tubular-campanulate, segments 5, mucronate, persistent, accrete, Corolla infundibular, 5-lobed, irregular, dirty-yellow veined with violet, the throat purplish-black. Stamens 5, barely exserted; ovary 2-celled. Fruit a capsule, enclosed in the persistent and enlarged calyx. Seeds small, compressed nearly ovoid, slightly reniform, 1 mm in diameter, brownish-gray, surface reticulate.

Habitate: On the outskirts of villages; mostly cultivated in Asia, Europe, North Africa, England, Germany and Soviet Union.

Propagation: By seeds and vegetative method.

Part Used: Seeds.

Chemical Constituents: Alkaloids hyoscyamine and hyoscine or scopolamine.

Uses: Gastric or intestinal cramps, diarrohea; prolapse of the rectum, neuralgia, cough, hysteria; manis, skin inflammation and boils; pain due to dental caries. Hyoscyamus has anodyne, narcotic, and mydriatic properties; employed as a sedative in nervous affections and irritable conditions, such as asthma and whooping cough, and is substituted for opium in cases where the latter is inadmissible. In veterinary practice used as a urnary sedative. Plant, especially the seeds, in large doses, produce poisonous effects similar to those of Datura poisoning, such as dryness of tongue and mouth, giddiness, and delirium.

685. *Hypericum perforatum* *(Hypericaceae)*

Vernacular Name: *Eng:* St John's Wort, Y Fendigedig (Walsh).

Description: A rhizomatous perennial herb up to 3 ft. high; stem 2-edged; leaves opposite, sessile, oblong, ovate or linear, black dotted; flowers yellow, in terminal corymbose cymes; capsule ovoid; seeds many small.

Habitate: Native to Britain and Europe, St John's wort now grows wild throughout much of the world. In India, found in Himalayas.

Propagation: By seeds and vegetative method.

Parts Used: Flowers.

Chemical Constituents: Volatile oil, Hypericin & pseudohypericin, Flavonoids.

Uses: AntidepresSant, antispasmodic, stimulates bile flow, astingent, sedative, relieves pain, antiviral.

686. *Hyptis pectinata* (L.) poit. *(Lamiaceae)*

Vernacular Name: *Eng:* mint weed, oregano.

Description: Perennial, erect aromatic herb to small shrub upto 4 m high with distinct, 4-angled stems. Leaves opposite, petiolate, the blade ovate to nearly triangular with serrate margins, pubescent, 1.5 to 7 cm long, 1 to 2.5 cm wide. Flowers small, strongly zygomorphic, white or pink tinged, borne in dense cyme-like clusters arising from spike-like inflorescences 30-60 cm long. Fruit a nutlet. Flowers and fruits throughout the year.

Habitate: A common weed of cultivated land, pastures, plantations, road and trialsides, and waste places.

Propagation: By seeds and vegetative method.

Part Used: Leaves.

Chemical Constituents: Monoterpenes, p-cymene, thymol (more than 60%), gamma-terpinene, alpha-thujene, mycrene, hyptolide (a lactone), essential oils, ursolic acid.

Uses: Leaves have wound-healing qualities and are especially usefl in treating cuts in the case of diabetics; leaves are also used to treat cough, chest pains and painful breathing.

687. *Hyssopus officinalis* L. *(Lamiaceae)*

Vernacular Name: *Eng:* Hyssop.

Description: Aromatic shrubby perennial; leaves linear-oblong or lanceolate; flowers bluish purple in unilateral tufts; nutlets dark brown, trigonous.

Habitate: Throughout in India.

Propagation: By seeds and vegetative method.

Part Used: Aerial parts.

Chemical Constituents: Major components of the oil are pinocamphone, a-and b-pinenes, camphene, a-terpinene and pinocampheol.

Uses: The leaves and flowering tops are employed as flavouring for salads and soups, and in the preparation of liqueurs. Hyssop oil with its warm, slightly burning flavour is used to replace the herb in pickles, meat sauces and seasonings, and to give bouquet to alcoholic beverages.

688. *Iberis amara* *(Cruciferae)*

Vernacular Name: *Eng:* Wild candytuft.

Description: Downy annual growing to 30 cm. Has deeply toothed leaves, and clusters of white or mauve flowers.

Habitate: Wild candytuft is native to Europe and North Africa, growing on wasteground, in arable fields and vineyards. The aerial parts are gathered in summer; the seeds are gathered after they have matured in autumn.

Propagation: By seeds and vegetative method.

Parts Used: Seeds.

Chemical Constituents: Contains mustard seed oil glycosides and vitamin C.

Uses: Little used in herbal medicine today, wild candytuft is a bitter-tasting tonic, aiding digestion and relieving wind and bloating. It is traditionally taken to treat gout, rheumatism and arthritis. It also has a high vitamin C content.

689. *Ichnocarpus frutescens* (L.) R. Br. *(Apocynaceae)*

Vernacular Name: *San*: Ulpalasariba, Palindi, Shyamlata, Sariva, *Hin*: Kalidudhi, Dudhi, *Kan*: Kappunamadaberu, *Mal*: Parvalli, Palvalli, *Tam*: Udarkkoti, Paravalli, *Tel:* Nallatiga.

Description: A much branched extensively climbing rusty-villous evergreen, laticiferous woody climber; leaves simple, opposite, elliptic-oblong to broadly lanceolate, acute or acuminate, main nerves 5-7 pairs; flowers greenish white, fragrant, numerous in axillary or terminal panicles of cymose clusters; fruits straight or slightly curved, cylindrical follicles, usually 2, divaricate, seeds black, comose, coma white.

Habitate: Throughout India, in the plains and lower hills upto 1,200 m.

Propagation: By seeds and vegetative method.

Parts Used: Roots.

Chemical Consistuents: N.A.

Uses: The roots are sweet, refrigerant, febrifuge, aphrodisiac, alterant, diaphoretic, diuretic, depurative, demulcent and tonic. They are useful in vitiated conditions of *pitta*, burning sensation hyperdipsia, fever, seminal weakness, nephrolithiasis, strangury, skin diseases, leprosy, pruritus, dyspepsia, vomiting, diabetes, cephalalgia and general weakness.

690. *Ilex aquifolium* *(Aquifoliaceae)*

Vernacular Name: *Eng:* Holly.

Description: Evergreen bush or tree growing to about 5 m with shiny, deep green leaves edged with spines, clusters of small white flowers and round red berries.

Habitate: Holly grows throughout much of Europe, western and central Asia and North Africa. It is found in woods and hedges, and thrives in gravelly soil or loam. It is also grown as a garden plant.

Propagation: By seeds and vegetative method.

Parts Used: Leaves, berries.

Chemical Constituents: Holly contains ilicin, ilexanthin, theobromine and caffeic acid. Theobromine is a caffeine-type alkaloid, used to treat asthma.

Uses: Holly is little used today. Its leaves are diuretic, fever-reducing and laxative, and they have been employed to treat fever jaundice and rheumatism. Holly berries purge the bowels and cause vomiting if taken in large doses.

691. *Ilex paraguariensis* *(Aquifoliaceae)*

Synonyms: *Ilex paraguensis.*

Vernacular Name: *Eng:* Mate.

Description: Evergreen shrub or small tree growing to 6 m. Has large leaves, white flowers and small reddish fruit.

Habitate: Mate grows wild in northern Argentina, Paraguay, Uruguay and southern Brazil, and is widely cultivated in Argentina, Spain and Portugal.

Propagation: By seeds and vegetative method.

Parts Used: Leaves.

Chemical Constituents: Mate contains xanthine derivatives, including about 1.5% caffeine, about 0.2% theobromine, theophylline, and up to 16% tannins. The high tannins content means that mate should not be consumed with meals, as tannins impair the absorption of nutrients.

Uses: Mate is a traditional South American tea that increases short-tem physical and mental energy levels. It is taken as a fortifying beverage in much the same way as tea is consumed throughout Asia and Europe. Mate has properties similar to those of tea and coffee. It stimulates the nervous system, is mildly analgesic and diuretic. As a medicinal herb. Mate is used to treat headaches, migraine, neuralgic and rheumatic pain, fatigue and mild depression. It has also been used in the treatment of diabetes.

692. *Illicium verum* Hook.f. *(Magnoliaceae)*

Vernacular Name: Eng: True star-anise, Chinese anise; *Hin:* Anaspbhal; *Tel:* Anaspuvu and *Tam:* Anashuppu, anasi-pu.

Description: Medium-sized tree, 6-10m. high, branches erect, glabrous and brittle. Leaves entire, thick and shining glabrous, usually crowded in bundles at the end of the branches. Flowers pink, solitary in the leaf-axil. Fruit of 8 follicles, radiating, compressed; each follicle contains one seed.

Habitate: Cultivated in mountainous regions, especially in Lang Son province.

Propagation: By seeds and vegetative method.

Part Used: Fruit.

Chemical Constituents: The fruit contains an essential oil (9-10%) consisting of anethol (85-90%), a-pinene, limonene, b-phellandrene, a-terpineol, farnesol and safrol.

Uses: The fruit is considered to be carminative stomachic and glactagogic. It is also used in treating vomiting, dyspepsia, abdominal pains and food poisoning. An alcoholic maceration is prescrived for massage in rheumatism and ostealgia.

693. *Impatiens balsamina* L. *(Balsaminaceae)*

Vernacular Name: *San:* Dushpatrijati; *Eng:* Garden balsam; *Hin:* Gulmendhi; *Beng*: Dupati; *Tam:* Kasittumbai; *Mal:* Mecchingom.

Description: An annual herb, erect 30-90 cm high, Stem fleshy, cylindrical, glabrous or pubscent, slightly branched. Leaves alternate 5-15 cm long by 1.2-2.5 cm wide, lanceolate, apex longacuminate, base cuneate and decurrent, margin serrate, petiolate. Flowers in summer, pink or white in colour, showy, pedicels 1-3, axillary, slender, pubescent, shorter than the leaves.Sepals minute, ovte. Standard small, orbicular, retuse, horned. Wings broad, lateral lobes rounded, terminal sessile, very large. Lip small, boatshaped, mucronate. Spur short or long, incurved. Capsules tomentose. Seed reticulate.

Habitate: Along watercourses and in damp ground on field margins; commonly cultivated in China, India, Japan and Malaysia.

Propagation: By seeds and vegetative method.

Part Used: Seeds.

Chemical Constituents: β-amyrin, ∝-spinasterol, balsamin asterol, linoleic, parinaric, oleic, arachidic.

Uses: Amenorrhoea; dystocia, dysphagia. Leaves and seeds edible. Flowers and leaves are at times used as a substitute for henna. Flowers mucilaginous and cooling used for lumbago and intercostals neuralgia; they improve circulation and relievestasis. Seeds contain a fatty oil used for cooking and as an illuminant; also suitable for use in the surface-coating industry.

694. *Imperata cylindrical* (L.) P. Beauv. *(Poaceae)*

Synonyms: *Imperata arundinacea* Cyr.

Vernacular Name: *San:* Darbha; Eng: Lalang-grass,alang-alang, bedding grass; *Hin:* Dabh, siru, ulu; *Beng*: Ooloo, ulu; *Tel:* Balbajamu, barhisan, darbha gaddi; *Tam:* Dharbai pul, inankapillu, nanal, varli-pillu; *Kan:* Sanna dabbai hullu and *Mal:* Vidulam.

Description: Perennial herb, 0.60-1.50m. high, Rhizome hard coriaceous, descending deeply into the soil. Clums erect, with wiry hairs. Leaves narrow and long, prominently nerved; scabrous on the upper surfacel margins sharp-edged. Inflorescence of many spikes, silver-white, densely silky.

Habitate: A common weed everywhere, specially in hilly regions.

Propagation: By seeds and vegetative method.

Part Used: Rhizomes.

Chemical Constituents: The rhizomes contain glucose, fructose and organic acids.

Uses: The rhizome, a diuretic and febrifuge, is used in the treatment of urodynia, pollakiuria, haematuria and feber. It is available in the form of a decoction for oral administration. The drug is often combined with corn silk, which enhances its diuretic action.

695. *Imperatorial ostruthium* *(Apiaceae)*

Vernacular Name: *Eng:* Masterwort.

Description: Perennial growing to 60 cm with green leaves divided into 3 leaflets with 3 lobes each, white flowers on large umbels, and winged seeds.

Habitate: Native to central and southern Europe, and Asia, masterwort is most often found in the wild. The root is unearthed in autumn or spring.

Propagation: By seeds and vegetative method.

Parts Used: Root.

Chemical Constituents: Masterwort contains a camphoraceous volatile oil, peucadanin, oxipeucadanin and oxtrutol.

Uses: Masterwort is little used today, but it may well be a herb that bears further investigation. The root is aromatic, warms central areas of the body and is a bitter tonic. It has a strong action within the stomach and gut, settling indigestion and relieving wind and griping. Masterwort is also beneficial for chest conditions, and is used for colds, asthma and bronchitis. It can also be helpful for menstrual problems.

696. *Impmoea purga* *(Convolvulaceae)*

Synonyms: *Convolvulus jalapa.*

Vernacular Name: *Eng:* Jalap.

Description: Evergreen vine reaching about 4 m. Has heart-shaped leaves and trumpet-like purple flowers.

Habitate: Native to Mexico, jalap is cultivated in Central America, the West Indies and South-East Asia. The root is unearthed in summer.

Propagation: By seeds and vegetative method.

Parts Used: Root.

Chemical Constituents: Jalap contains the resin convolvulin.

Uses: Jalap is such a powerful cathartic that its medicinal value is questionable. Even in moderate doses it stimulates the elimination of profuse watery stools and in larger doses it causes vomiting.

697. *Impomoea digitata* L. *(Convolvulaceae)*

Vernacular Name: *San*: Vidari, *Hin:* Bilaikand.

Description: It is a perennial, with large ovoid or elongated tuberous roots. *Stems*-long, thick, twining, tough and glabrous. *Leaves* are often broader than its length, deeply palmately divided. *Flowers* in many-flowered corymbosely paniculate cymes. *Seeds* are clothed with brownish detachable hairs.

Habitate: The plant grows throughout the warm and moist regions of India.

Propagation: By seeds and vegetative method.

Parts Used: Roots.

Chemical Constituents: In preliminary studies the plant root is found to contain steroids, sugars, and amino acids. Sterols, coumarin glycosides of the tubers were investigated. An ether insoluble, alcohol soluble fraction D has been studies.

Uses: General weakness. Diminished lactation. Sore. Throat. It is commonly used as a general tonic and in hoarseness of voice, hepatosplenomegaly, cough, diminished lactation etc.

698. *Indigofera tinctoria* L. *(Fabaceae)*

Vernacular Name *San*: Nilini, *Eng*: Indian indigo, *Hin*: Nil, *Kan*: Nili, *Mal*: Nilamari, Amari, *Tam*: Avari, Nili, *Tel:* Nili.

Description: A branching shrub upto 2 m high, leaves with 7-13 leaflets, green when fresh and grayish back on drying, tender branches bluish red in colour, flowers many in nearly sessile lax spicate racemes which are much shorter than the leaves, red or pink; fruits cylindric pods, pale greenish grey when young and dark brown on ripening with 10-12 seeds.

Habitate: Throughout India, mainly as an escape from cultivation.

Propagation: By seeds and vegetative method.

Parts Used: Whole plant.

Chemical Consistuents: Nitrogen, phosphoric acid, potash, and lime. It is a rich source of potash, the ash containing as much as 9.5% of soluble potassium salts.

Uses: The roots, stems and leaves are biter, thermogenic, laxative, trichogenous, expectorant, anthelmintic, tonic and diuretic, and are useful for promoting the growth of hair and in gastropathy, splenomegaly, cephalalgia, cardiopathy, chronic bronchitis, asthma, ulcers and skin diseases. The juice expressed from the leaves is useful in the treatment of hydrophobia. An extract of the plant is good for epilepsy and neuropathy. The plant possesses anti-toxic property.

699. *Inula helenium* L. *(Asteraceae)*

Vernacular Name: *Eng:*-Elecampane.

Description: Robust perennial herb, to 1.5 m tall. Stems furrowed, with spreading hairs. Leaves alternate, irregularly toothed, nearly glabrous above, velvety-tomentose beneathe beneath; basal leaves elliptic, to 40 cm long on petioles; stem leaves ovate-cordate, successively reduced upward, sessile, clasping. Heads to 5-10cm across, solitary or 2-3 in a cluster; involucre hemisphere; phyllaries imbricate in several raws; the outer herbaceous, the inner usually narrow and scarious; receptacle flat, naked. Ray flowers female, yellow. Disk flowers tubular, bisexual, yellow, anthers sagittate-tailed. Achenes nearly cylindrical to 4-5 ribbed; pappus of 1 row of many capillary bristles.

Habitate: Cultivated in Korea and Central Asia.

Propagation: By seeds and vegetative method.

Parts Used: Root.

Chemical Constituents: Sesquiterpenes: alatolactone, helenine, isoalantolactone, dihydroisoalantolactone, alantic acid, alantol, dammaradienyl acetate, alantopicrin, inunolide, tomentosin, costunolide.

Uses: Clonorchicidal, antibacterial, increase peristalsis of large intestine, hypotensive, anthelmintic, smooth muscle relaxant, platelet aggregation inhibition, allergenic. Used in bronchitis, whooping cough and diarrhoea.

700. *Inula japonica* Regal *(Asteraceae)*

Vernacular Name: *Eng*: Japanese inula.

Description: Perennial herb, 20-60 cm tall. Basal and lower leaves smaller than middle ones; middle leaves lanceolate to long-elliptic, slightly acute, 5-10 cm long, 1-3 cm wide, sessile, partially grasping stems, appressed-pilose on both sides. Heads solitary or few, 3-4 cm across; involucre hemisphere, 7-8 mm long, 15-17 mm across; phyllaries 5-seriate, nearly equal, the outer lanceolate, the inner narrow, both cililolate. Ray flowers 16-19 mm long, 1.5-2 mm wide, yellow. Achenes 10-ribbed, pilose; pappus 5 mm long, bristles minutely scabrous.

Habitate: Wet areas in lowlands in Korea, Japan and China.

Propagation: By seeds and vegetative method.

Parts Used: Flowers heads.

Chemical Constituents: Inusterol A, B, C. Inulicin, secoeudesmanolides, quercetin, isoquercetin.

Uses: Used in wheezing, copious sputum, vomiting. Antibacterial increases intestinal motility.

701. *Inula racemosa* Hook. f. *(Asteraceae)*

Vernacular Name: *San*: Pauskaram, Puskaram; *Hin*: Pohakarmul, Puskarmul; *Kan*: Rasnabheda; *Mal*: Puskkaramulam; *Tam*: Puskkaramulam; *Tel:* Puskaramu.

Description: A stout herb upto 1.5 m in height with rough grooved sterm; leaves simple, alternate radical or cauline, crenate, leathery, rough above, densely hairy beneath; flowers yellow, many in heads, outer bracts broad, tips triangular, recurved, inner bracts linear, sharp pointed; fruits slender achenes with reddish pappus. The fresh root is brownish externally and white internally.

Habitate: In the Western Himalayas from 1,500 m to 4,200 m.

Propagation: By seeds and vegetative method.

Parts Used: Roots.

Chemical Consistuents: They contain inulin and an essential oil containing alantolactone. Alantolactone is the chief constituent of the oil obtained from the European species *I. helenium* Linn.

Uses: The roots are biter, acrid, thermogenic, aromatic stimulant, antiseptic, alexipharmic deodorant, anodyne, anti-inflammatory, digestive, carminative, stomachic, cardiotonic expectorant, bronchodilator, diuretic, uterine stimulant, aphrodisiac, sudorific, emmenagogue, resolvent, febrifuge and tonic. They are useful in vitiated conditions of *kapha* and *vata*, foul ulcers and wounds, hemicrania, cardiodynia, hepatalgia, splenalgia, arthralgia, inflammations, anorexia, dyspepsia, flatulence, colic, cardiac debility, hiccough, cough, cardiac and bronchial asthma, bronchitis, strangury, nephropathy, amenorrhoea, dysmenorrhoea, skin diseases, cerebropathy, pneumonosis, emaciation, anaemia, fever and general debility.

702. *Ipomoea batatas* (L.) Lam. *(Convolvulaceae)*

Vernacular Name: *San*: Pindaluh, Raktaluh; *Eng*: Sweet potato; *Hin*: Mitha alu, Sakkarkand; *Kan*: Sihigenasu; *Mal*: Madhurakkilannu, Sarkkarakkilannu; *Tam*: Cakkaravallikkilanku; *Tel:* Genusu.

Description: A slender prostrate vine with tuberous roots which may be red or white in colour, leaves simple, alternate, ovate-cordate, entire, angular or deeply lobed; flowers purple, solitary or in cymose clusters, corolla widely tubular, funnel-shaped; fruits globose or ovoid capsules, seeds 2-4, flat, black and small.

Habitate: Throughout India, cultivated.

Propagation: By vegetative method.

Parts Used: Tuberous roots.

Chemical Consistuents: Amylase, protease, invertase, catalase, laccase, arabinase, galactanase, polygalacturonase, peroxidases, monophenolase, catecholase, cytochrome c-oxidase, phosphorylase and phosphatases.

Uses: The roots are sweet, refrigerant, laxative, aphrodisiac, diuretic and tonic. They are useful in vitiated conditions of *pitta*, burning sensation, hyperdipsia, constipation, strangury, renal and vesical calculi, diabetes and general weakness.

703. *Ipomoea indica* (Burm.) Merr. *(Convolvulaceae.)*

Vernacular Name: *Eng:* morning-glory.

Description: Herbaceous twining sprawling vine. Leaves alternate, long-petiolate, cordate with acuminate apex and rounded base, upto 17 cm long. Flowers large and showy, trumpet-shaped, white to purple or blue, borne in small axillary clusters. Fruit a subglobose capsule about 1 cm in diameter, usually with 4 large smooth brown seed.

Habitate: Common climbing over low vegetations along roadsides, forest margins, disturbed forests, waste places and gardens.

Propagation: By seeds and vegetative method.

Part Used: Roots and leaves.

Chemical Constituents: N.A.

Uses: The plant is used as a laxative. A paste made from the roots is applied as a poultice to backaches and sore muscles.

704. *Ipomoea mauritiana* Jacq. *(Convolvulaceae)*

Synonyms *Ipomoea paniculata* R. Br.

Vernacular Name: *Eng*: Giant potato, *Hin*: Bhilaykand, Bhuyikohada, *Kan*: Nadakumbala, *Mal*: Palmutuku, Mutalakklannu, Ancilattali, *San*: Ksiravidari, *Tam*: Palmudamgi, Palmodikkay, *Tel:* Nelagummudu.

Description: A much branched perennial climber with large tuberous roots and glabrous tough stems and branches; leaves palmately 5-7 lobed, ovate-lanceolate, acute or acuminate, glabrous, nerves prominent beneath; flowers purple, in pedunculate corymbose axillary panicles, lobes of the limb emarginated; fruits ovoid, 4-celled and 4-valved capsules, surrounded by enlarged fleshy sepals, seeds clothed with many long tawny cottony hairs.

Habitate: Throughout India, in deciduous and evergreen forests and coastal tracts.

Propagation: By vegetative method.

Parts Used: Tuberous roots.

Chemical Consistuents: N.A.

Uses: The roots are sweet, sour, acrid, astringent, cooling, emollient, aphrodisiac, galactagogue, rejuvenating, diuretic, depurative, stimulant, appetizer, carminative, stomachic, anthelmintic, expectorant and tonic. They are useful in vitiated conditions of *pitta* and *vata*, agalactia, emaciation in children, consumption, strangury, leprosy, skin diseases, anorexia, dyspepsia, colic, flatulence, helminthiasis, bronchitis, fever, burning sensation, nausea, vomiting, pharyngodynia, syphilis, gonorrhoea, inflammation, splenopathy, hepatopathy, menorrhagia and general debility.

705. *Ipomoea nil* (L.) Roth *(Convolvulaceae)*

Synonyms *Ipomoea hederaceae* auct. Non (Linn.) Jacq.

Vernacular Name: *San*: Krsnabijah; *Eng*: Morning glory, Pharbitis seeds; *Hin*: Kaladana, Jharmaric; *Kan*: Gouribija; *Mal*: Taliyari; *Tam*: Kakkattan, Sirikki, Kotikkakkattan; *Tel:* Kollivittulu.

Description: An extensively twining hairy herbaceous annual or perennial; leaves simple, ovate, cordate, more or less deeply 3-lobed, lobes ovate-acuminate, sparsely hairy; flowers large, funnel shaped, blue tinged with pink, turning to red on aging, in umbellate cymes; fruits subglobose or ovoid smooth capsules, seeds black, 4-6, nearly triquetrous, glabrous.

Habitate: Throughout India, wild, upto 1,800 m, also cultivated.

Propagation: By seeds and vegetative method.

Parts Used: Seeds.

Chemical Consistuents: Palmitic, stearic, arachidic, behenic, linolenic, linoleic, oleic, coprosterol, deep violer and red violet flowers contain peonin chloride 3.5-diglucoside of peonidin chloride.

Uses: The seeds are acrid, sweet, thermogenic, purgative, vermifuge, depurative, anti-inflammatory, carminative and behic. They are useful in vitiated conditions of *kapha* and *vata*, inflammations, constipation, verminosis, skin diseases, leucoderma, scabies, dyspepsia, flatulence bronchitis, gout, arthralgia, cephalalgia, hepatopathy, splenopathy and fever.

706. *Ipomoea pes-caprae* (L.) R. Br. *(Convolvulaceae)*

Synonyms *Ipomoea biloba* Forssk., *Ipomoea maritime* R. Br.

Vernacular Name: *San*: Maryadavalli, Sagaramekhala, *Eng*: Goat's foot creeper, *Hin*: Dopatilata, *Kan*: Bangadivalli, *Mal*: Atampuvalli, Atampu, *Tam*: atampu, Atappan koti, *Tel:* Balabantatige.

Description: An extensively trailing sand binding perennial herb with long tap root; leaves deeply two-lobed, alternate, glabrous, parallel veined; flowers large, purple red, usually solitary, corolla tubular-infundibuliform; fruits ovoid, glabrous capsules, seeds-4, dark brown tomentose.

Habitate: Throughout India, especially along sandy shores.

Propagation: By seeds and vegetative method.

Parts Used: Whole plant.

Chemical Consistuents: The plant contains a mucilage, a volatile oil, resins, bitter substances, red colouring matter, pentatriacontane, triacontane, a sterol and behenic, melissic, butyric and myristic acids. The volatile oil has the following constants.

Uses: The plant is astringent, acrid, refrigerant, mucilaginous, stomachic, laxative, diuretic, and tonic. It is useful in skin diseases, boils, swellings, wounds ulcers, carbuncle, dropsy, menorrhagia, haemorrhoids, proctitis, proctoptosis, vomiting, colic, flatulence, dyspepsia, cramp, strangury, vitiated conditions of *pitta* and burning sensation.

707. *Ipomoea sepiaria* Roxb. *(Convolvulaceae)*

Synonyms: *Ipomoea maxima* acut. non (Linn.f.) Sweet.

Vernacular Name: *San*: Laksmana, *Hin*: Bankalmi, *Kan*: Laksmana, *Mal*: Tirutali, *Tam*: Talikkirai, Talikkoti, *Tel:* Laksmana.

Description: A slender twining perennial with usually villous stems and slightly tuberous roots; leaves simple, alternate, petiolate, ovate-cordate with a wide sinus and rounded basal lobes, bloched with brownish or purplish patches towards the center; flowers pale purple or pink, large, funnel shaped in umbellate or subumbellate axillary cymes; fruits ovoid capsules, 8 mm long, 4 or 2-seeded, seeds grey covered with silky pubescence.

Habitate: Throughout India, in hedges near streams and tanks upto an elevation of 150 m.

Propagation: By seeds and vegetative method.

Parts Used: Whole plant.

Chemical Consistuents: N.A.

Uses: The plant is sweet, cooling, rejuvenating, diuretic, aphrodisiac, laxative, deobstruant, uterotonic and tonic. It is useful in vitiated conditions of *pitta,* burning sensation, strangury, hyperdipsia, general debility and sterility in women.

708. *Iris versicolor* *(Iridaceae)*

Vernacular Name: *Eng:* Blue flag, Wild Iris.

Description: Perennial growing to about 1 m. Has erect stems, sword-shaped leaves and 2-3 resplendent blue to violet flowers per stem.

Habitate: Blue flag is native to North America. Preferring damp and marshy areas in the wild.

Propagation: By seeds and vegetative method.

Parts Used: Rhizome.

Chemical Constituents: Blue flag contains triterpenoids, salicylic and isophthalic acids, a very small amount of volatile oil, starch, resin, an oleo-resin and tannins.

Uses: Blue flag is currently used mainly to detoxify the body. It increases urination and bile production, and has a mild laxative effect. This combination of cleansing actions makes it a useful herb for chronic skin diseases such as acne and eczema, especially where gallbladder problems or constipation contribute to the condition. Blue flag is also given for biliousness and indigestion. In small doses, it relieves nausea and vomiting. However, in large doses blue flag will itself cause vomiting. The traditional use of blue flag for gland problems persists. It is also believed by some to aid weight loss.

709. *Ixora coccinea* Linn. *(Rubiaceae)*

Vernacular Name: *San*: Paranti, Raktaka, Bandhuka, *Eng*: Jungle-flame ixora, Sacred ixora, *Hin*: Rangan, Rukmini, Rajana, *Kan*: Kiskara, Keppulagida, *Mal*: Tacci, Cetti, Tetti, *Tam*: Cetti, Vedcci, *Tel:* Manmadibanum.

Description: A large glabrous shrub with few branches; leaves simple, opposite decussate, elliptic, ovate or obovate sessile or nearly so, main nerves 8-12 pairs, coriaceous, olive green when dry; flowers scarlet, in dense sessile or short peduncled corymbiform cymes; fruits globose, fleshy, smooth, crowned with the persistent calyx, purple when ripe, seeds concave on the ventral surface.

Habitate: Throughout the West Coast, in forest lands and road cutting, also cultivated as ornamental plants.

Propagation: By seeds and vegetative method.

Parts Used: Roots, leaves, flowers.

Chemical Consistuents: The roots are reported to contain an acrid aromatic oil, tannin, fatty acids and a white crystalline substance. The root bark contains, II-octadecadienoic acid, mannitol and myristic acid. A yellow colouring matter related to quercitrin, an astringent principle, a wax and a neutral crystalline substance have been isolated from the flowers.

Uses: The roots are astringent, acrid, febrifuge, sedative, stomachic and antiseptic. They are useful in hiccough, fever, gonorrhoea, anorexia, diarrhoea, dysentery, cephalalgia, sores, chronic ulcers and skin diseases. The leaves are useful in diarrhoea. The flowers are astringent bitter, sweet, carminative, digestive and constipating. They are useful in dysentery, dysmenorrhoea, leucorrhoea, haemoptysis, catarrhal bronchitis, ophthalmopathy, sores and ulcers.

710. *Jasminum angustifolium* (L.) Willd. *(Oleaceae)*

Vernacular Name: *San*: Asphoa, Vanamallika, *Eng*: Wild jasmine, *Hin*: Banmallika, *Kan*: Adavimallige, *Mal*: Kattumulla, Kattumallika, *Tam*: Kattumalligai, Kattumullai, *Tel:* Advaimalli.

Description: A wiry small scandent shrub with glabrous stems, pubescent branches; leaves simple, small, ovate, acute rounded at base, glabrous; flowers on long slender pedicles, more often in threes at the ends of short lateral twigs, white, corolla tube about 1.6 cm, lobes 7 or 8, equaling the tube; fruits, didymous berries, ripe carpels broadly ovoid, seed one in each carpel.

Habitate: In Karnataka and Kerala, on the hills of lower elevations.

Propagation: By vegetative method.

Parts Used: Roots, leaves.

Chemical Consistuents: N.A.

Uses: The roots are bitter, acrid, and are useful for external application in ringworm and herpes, and are recommended for ophthalmopathy, ulcerative stomatitis, leprosy, pruritus and wounds. The leaves are used as an emetic in cases of poisoning.

711. *Jasminum arborescens* Roxb. *(Oleaceae)*

Synonyms: *Jasminum roxburghianum* Wall.

Vernacular Name: *San*: Nagamalli, *Eng*: Tree jasmine, *Hin*: Bela, Cameli, *Kan*: Visamallige, *Mal*: Nagamallika, *Tam*: Nagamalli, *Tel:* Adavimalli.

Description: A large suberect shrub with hairy climbing branchlets; leaves simple opposite, ovate or ovate-oblong, acuminate, grey-tomentose on both surfaces; flowers white, fragrant, in lax trichotomous pubescent panicles; fruit single, ellipsoid, black, often curved berry.

Habitate: Throughout India, in forests upto 1,200 m.

Propagation: By vegetative method.

Parts Used: Leaves.

Chemical Consistuents: N.A.

Uses: The leaves are bitter, astringent, sweet, refrigerant, stomachic, emetic and tonic. They are useful in obstruction of the bronchial tubes, menstrual disorders, vitiated conditions of *pitta*, colic, flatulence, cough and general debility.

712. *Jasminum auriculatum* Vahl *(Oleaceae)*

Vernacular Name: *San*: Yuthika, Magadhi, Sucimallika; *Eng*: Needle flower jasmine; *Hin*: Juhi, Juyi; *Kan*: Kadaramallige; *Mal*: Tusimulla, Sucimulla; *Tam*: Usimalligai; *Tel:* Adavimulla.

Description: A scandent, pubescent or velvety shrub with grey-pubescent branchlets; leaves trifoliate with two lower leaflets very small and frequently wanting, central leaflets broadly ovate, acuminate or rounded, main nerves few inconspicuous, petioles very short; flowers white, sweet scented, many in trichotomous paniculate cymes, corolla lobes 5-8; fruits globose, black.

Habitate: Throughout south India, on the dry slopes of the Western Ghats.

Propagation: By vegetative method.

Parts Used: Roots, flowers.

Chemical Consistuents: It contains esters alcohols, indole, and methyl anthranilate.

Uses: The roots are useful in skin diseases especially for ring-worm. The flowers are fragrant, bitter, acrid, sweet, refrigerant, astringent, cardiotonic, diuretic and depurative. They are useful in burning sensation, hyperdipsia, ulcers odontalgia, stomatopathy, ophthalmpathy, cardiopathy, urolithiasis, nephrolithiasis, strangury and dermatopahty.

713. *Jasminum grandiflorum* L. *(Oleaceae)*

Synonyms: *Jasminum officinale* (Linn.) forma grandiflorum (Linn.) Kobuski.

Vernacular Name: *San*: Jati, *Mal*ati, *Eng*: Spanish jasmine, Common jasmine, Catalonian jasmine, *Hin*: Jati, Chameli, *Kan*: *Mal*lige, *Mal*: Piccakam, Piccakamulla, *Tam*: Kotimalligai, Picci, *Tel:* Jaji, *Mal*ati.

Description: A large nearly glabrous, suberect, twining evergreen shrub; leaves imparipinnately compound, opposite, terminal leaflets larger than the laterals, ovate, lanceolate, acute or acuminate, laterals ovate; flowers very fragrant, white tinged with pink outside in lax terminal and axillary cymes, calyx lobes long and linear; fruits elliptic, globose berries, black when ripe.

Habitate: Throughout India, in forests upto 2,500 m, also extensively cultivated.

Propagation: By vegetative method.

Parts Used: Whole plant.

Chemical Consistuents: Linalyl acetate, benzyl benzoate, benzyl alcohol, geraniol, nerol, l-α-terpineol, d-and di-linalool, and alcohol with an odour reminiscent of β, γ-hexenol, farnesol, nerolidol, an unidentified alcohol, which plays an important role in the fixation of odorous principles, eugenol, p-cresol, creosol, lactones with lasting and fruity odour, benzaldehyde, jasmone, an unidentified ketone, benzoic acid, methyl anthranilate and indole.

Uses: The plant is bitter, astringent, acrid, thermogenic, aphrodisiac, antiseptic, anodyne, depurative, emenagogue, emollient, diuretic, anthelmintic, deobstruant, dentifrice, suppurative and tonic. The roots are useful in cephalalgia, vitiated conditions of *vata*, paralysis, facial paralysis, mental debility, chronic constipation, flatulence, strangury sterility, dysmenorrhoea, amenorrhoea, ringworm, leprosy, skin diseases and giddiness.

The leaves are useful in odontalgia, fixing loose teeth, ulcerative stomatitis, leprosy, skin diseases, ottorrhoea, otalgia, strangury, dysmenorrhoea, ulcers, wounds and corns. The flowers are refrigerant and ophthalmic. They are useful in stomatopathy, cephalopathy, odontopathy, opthalmopathy, leprosy, skin diseases, pruritus, strangury, dysmenorrhoea, ulcers and vitiated conditions of *pitta*.

714. *Jasminum multiflorum* (Burm. f.) Andr. *(Oleaceae)*

Synonyms *Jasminum pubescens* Willd.

Vernacular Name: *San*: Kundah, *Eng*: Downy jasmine, *Hin*: Kundphul, *Kan*: Magimallige, *Mal*: Kurukkuttimulla, *Tam*: Makarandam, *Mal*ligai, *Tel:* Gajari, Kundamu.

Description: A large scandent tomentose shrub with young branches clothed with velvety pubescence; leaves simple, opposite, ovate, more or less pubescent beneath, base rounded or often cordate main nerves 4-6 pairs, petioles densely villous; flowers white, slightly fragrant, sessile in dense terminal capitate cymes at the extremities of short axillary branches; fruits black, globose berries surrounded by suberect calyx teeth.

Habitate: Throughout India, in the forests of Western Ghats and sub-Himalayan tracts upto 1,500 m.

Propagation: By vegetative method.

Parts Used: Leaves, flowers.

Chemical Consisituents: N.A.

Uses: Dried leaves are good for indolent ulcers. The flowers are sweet, bitter, acrid, refrigerant, laxative, cardiotonic, alexipharmic depurative and digestive. They are useful in vitiated conditions of pita, inflammations, rheumatism and cephalalgia.

715. *Jasminum sambac* (L.) Ait *(Oleaceae)*

Vernacular Name: *San*: *Mallika*; *Eng*: Arabian jasmine, Tuscan jasmine, Sambac jasmine; *Hin*: Bel, Moghra; *Kan*: Dundumallige; *Mal*: Mulla; *Tam*: Kundumalligai Malligai; *Tel:* Malli.

Description: A suberect or sometimes climbing shrub with pubescent branchlets; leaves simple, opposite, variable in shape, usually broadly ovate or elliptic, acute, entire, nearly glabrous, main nerves 4-6 pairs; flowers white, very fragrant, solitary or in 3-flowered terminal cymes, calyx lobes curled especially in fruits; fruits berries, black when ripe.

Habitate: Throughout India, cultivated.

Propagation: By vegetative method.

Parts Used: Roots, leaves, flowers.

Chemical Consisituents: Esters, alcohols methyl anthranilate and indole.

Uses: The roots along with leaves are useful in ophthalmopathy. The leaves are useful in skin diseases, ulcers and fever. The flowers are bitter, acrid, refrigerant, alexipharmic, ophthalmic, purgative and lactigue. They are useful in vitiated conditions of *pitta,* ophthalmopathy, pruritus, cephalalgia, otopathy, stomatopathy, leprosy, ulcers, fever, vomiting, hiccough, insanity and galactorrhoea.

716. *Jasminum subtriplinerve* Blume *(Oleaceae)*

Description: Small trailing shrub. Branches glabrous. Leaves opposite, glabrous and shining on both surfaces, 3 nerves from the base. Inflorescence in axillary or terminal raceme; flowers 2-3, white, fragrant. Berry globose with remains of persistent calyx, black when ripe.

Habitate: Grows wild in the mountains and the midlands.

Propagation: By seeds and vegetative method.

Part Used: Leaf-bearing twigs.

Chemical Constituents: The leaves contain alkaloids, resins and flavonoids.

Uses: The branches and the leaves possess antibacterial and anti-inflammatory properties. They are used in treating post-partum hyperthemic infection, lymphadentis, metritis, glactophoritis, leucorrhoea, rheumatism, ostealgia, impetigo, pruigo, dysmenorrhoea and haematometra. They are also effective as a bitter tonic for parturients. A decoction of the fresh leaves is used for washing and bathing in the case of wounds and impetigo and a fresh-leaf poultice is used for abscesses and mastitis.

717. *Jateorhiza palmate* *(Menispermaceae)*

Synonyms: *Jateorhiza calumba.*

Vernacular Name: *Eng:* Calumba.

Description: A dioecious twiher; Rhizome short, rounded, irregular; leaves alternate, palmately 3-7 lobed, deeply cordate at the base; petioles long; flowers in conspicuous, in large dropping, axillary panicles; fruit a fleshy drup, ovoid.

Habitate: Calumba is a creeping vine, native to the rainforests of east Africa, especially Mozambique and Madagascar. It grows to a great height, often reaching the tops of trees. Calumba is cultivated in other tropical regions and also in Europe.

Propagation: By seeds and vegetative method.

Parts Used: Root.

Chemical Constituents: Isoquinoline alkaloids, Bitter principles, Volatile oil, Mucilage.

Uses: Bitter, eases stomach pain, Tonic Reduces fever, expels worms.

718. *Jatropha curcas* L. *(Euphorbiaceae)*

Vernacular Name: *San*: Dravanti, *Eng*: Purging nut, Physic nut, *Hin*: Jungli, errand, Pahari errand, Ratanjot, *Kan*: Belioudalu Doddaharalu, *Mal*: Katalavanakku, Kammatti, Kattavanakku, *Tam*: Katalamanakku, Kattamanakku, Kattukkottai, *Tel:* Adavi-amudamu.

Description: A large deciduous soft wooded shrub, 3-4 m in height with sticky juice; leaves alternate, broadly ovate, cordate, 3-5 lobed, glabrous, base seven nerved, stipules zero, flowers yellowish green in loose panicles of cymes; fruits ovoid, black, splitting into three, 2-valved cocci, seeds dull brownish black.

Habitate: Throughout India, in plains and in hedges.

Propagation: By seeds and vegetative method.

Parts Used: Leaves, seeds, oil.

Chemical Consistuents: It has the following range of constins: acid val., sap. Val., iod. Val., hydroxyl val., R.M. val.; Polenske val., centipoises; and unsapon. Matter. The fatty acid composition of the oil is as follows; myristic, palmitic, stearic, arachidic, oleic, and linoleic acid.

Uses: The leaves are galactagogue, rubefacient, suppurative and have insecticidal properties, and are useful in foul ulcers, tumours and scabies. The latex is stypic, purgative and haemostatic, and is good for wounds and ulcers. The seeds are powerful purgative, acrid, sweet, aphrodisiac, thermogenic, digestive tonic, anthelmintic and depurative. They are useful in haemorrhoids, wounds, splenomegaly and skin diseases. The yellow oil obtained from roots has a strong anthelmintic action. The oil from the seeds possesses purgative properties and is used externally in rhumatism and paralytic affections.

719. *Juglans cinerea* *(Juglandaceae)*

Vernacular Name: *Eng:* Butternut.

Description: Deciduous tree growing to 30 m. Has grey bark, long leaves with many leaflets, male catkins and female flowers, and an oval-shaped fruit containing a hard dark-coloured nut.

Habitate: Native to North American forests, butternut is cultivated for its timber in other temperate regions.

Propagation: By seeds and vegetative method.

Parts Used: Inner bark.

Chemical Constituents: Contains naphthaquinones, a fixed and a volatile oil, and tannins. The naphthaquinones have an approximately similar laxative effect to the anthraquinones found in plants such as senna and Chinese rhubarb. Juglone is purgative, anthimicrobial, antiparasitic and cancer-inhibiting.

Uses: Used to this day as a laxative and tonic, butternut is a valuable remedy for chronic constipation, gently encouraging regular bowel movements. It is especially beneficial if combined with a carminative herb, such as ginger or agnelica. Butternut also lower cholesterol levels, and promotes the clearance of waste products by the liver. It has a positive reputation in treating intestinal worms and being antimicrobial and astringent, it has been prescribed as a treatment for dysentery.

720. *Juglans regia* L. Var. kumaonia DC. *(Juglandaceae)*

Vernacular Name: *San*: Aksotah, *Eng*: Common walnut, Persian walnut, European walnut, *Hin*: Akhor, Akhrot, *Kan*: Akrodu, *Mal*: Akrottu, *Tam*: Akrottu, *Tel:* Akrotu.

Description: A large deciduous monoecious tree with tomentose shoots; bark grey, longitudinally fissured; leaves alternate, imparipinnate; leaflets entire, aromatic; flowers small, yellowish green, male in pendulous slender catkins, female in 1-3 flowered terminal catkins; fruits drupes, 5 cm long with leathery exocarp, woody wrinkled, hard endocarp enclosing 4-lobed, corrugated, oily, edible seed.

Habitate: Cultivated in the Himalayas and the Khasia hills.

Propagation: By seeds and vegetative method.

Parts Used: Leaves, bark, fruits.

Chemical Consistuents: A globulin, juglansin, has been isolated from the edible kernel. The nitrogen distribution of the globulin is as follows; basic N, 5.41; non-basic N, 11.51; humin N, 0.15; and amide N, 1.78. The globulin contains cystine and tryptophane.

Uses: Leaves are astringent, tonic and anthelmintic. The leaves and bark are antiscorbutic and detergent, and are useful in herpes, eczema, scrofula and syphilis. The fruits are sweet, emollient, thermogenic, aphrodisiac, tonic and carminative. They are useful as alternant in rheumatism. The expressed oil of the fruit is considered useful against tapeworm and is used to strengthen and lubricate the muscles. The kernels are said to posses aphrodisiac properties and are recommended in colic and dysentery.

721. *Juglans sinensis* Dode *(Juglandaceae)*

Vernacular Name: *Eng*: *Eng* walnut, Persian walnut, Madeira walnut.

Description: Deciduous, monoecious tree, to 30 m tall, with silvery-gray bark. Pith in the twigs with minute cross-partitions. Leaves large aromatic, odd-pinnate; leaflets usually 7-9, obtuse, to 15 cm long, entire except in young tree. *Mal*e flowers in drooping catkins borne on the previous year's wood. Female flowers on wood of current year. Fruit a drupelike furrowed nut enclosed within a thick, indehiscent husk.

Habitate: Mostly cutivated in Korea.

Propagation: By seeds and vegetative method.

Parts Used: Seed.

Chemical Constituents: Gangliosides.

Uses: Spermatorrhoea, frequent urination, dermititis.

722. *Juncus effusus* var. decipiens Buchenau *(Juncaceae)*

Vernacular Name: *Eng:*-Soft rush, Japanese-mat rush.

Description: Glabrous, stiffish, perennial herb. Stems 30-90 cm tall, arching, ascending, in dense tussocks, striated and ridged. Leaves reduced to basal sheaths. Inflorescence pseudolateral, the lowest bract growing to 10-20 cm, appearing like the continuation of stem, many-flowered, open, the branches many. Flowers yellowish-green to pale brown, 2-2.5 mm long; perianth segments 2-3 mm long, lanceolate; sepals and petals 3, scalelike; stamens 3; ovary 3-celled. Fruit a capsule; seeds many, 0.5 cm long.

Habitate: Wet areas in lowlands and mountains in Korea, Japan and China.

Propagation: By seeds and vegetative method.

Parts Used: Whole plant.

Chemical Constituents: Undecan-2-one, tridecanone, ionoes, bisabolene, lutiolion and its glycoside, ρ-coumaroyl glyceride, effusol, dehydroefusol, juncanol, juncunone, micrandol B, a-tocopherol, alkanes, phenylpropanoids.

Uses: Used in urethritis, fracture, lumbago, diuretic and toothache. Antitumour, cytotoxic, antioxidant, antimicrobial.

723. *Juniperus communis* L. *(Pinaceae)*

Synonyms: *Juniperus argaea* Bal ex. Parl., *Juniperus borealis* Salisb., *Juniperus combrassa* Hort ex. Car.

Vernacular Name: *Eng:* Common Juniper.

Description: A dense shrub, more or less procumbent. Leaves 5-13 mm. long, in whorls of 3, linear, sharply pointed, spreading nearly at right angles from the branchlets, convex on the back, concave and glaucous, bluish-whish on upper surface with a pale line running the whole surface, jointed at the base and continued down the stem with a large gland on the decurrent portion. Cones unisexual, axillary. Fruit 7.5-10 mm. long, subglobose, fleshy, blue-black, glaucous; seeds 1-3.

Habitate: North-West Himalayas of India.

Propagation: By seeds and vegetative method.

Parts Used: Ripe Berries.

Chemical Constituents: Geijerone C_{12} Terpenoid; Junionone; Desoxypodophyllotoxin; α-pinene, Myrcene, cineole; p-cymene, α-and γ-cadinene; Limonene, β-pinene, y-terpinene; terpinene-4-ol; α-Thujene Borneol; Sesquiterpenes viz. caryophyllene, epoxydihydrocaryophyllene and β-elemem-7-α-ol. Querceting, Amentoflavone, isoquercitrin.

Uses: For complaints specially of catarrhal inflammation or kidneys, dropsy & suppression of urine. Chronic pyelitis, strangury. Bloody scanty urine with prostatic discharge & renal hyperaemia. Urogenital irriation.

724. *Juniperus Sabina* L. *(Pinaceae)*

Synonyms: *Juniperus humilis* Salisb., *Juniperus prostrata* Pers.

Vernacular Name: *Eng:* Savin.

Description: An evergreen shrub, spreading horizontally or rising erect to the height of 1-5 m. The trunk has pale, reddish brown, scaly bark. Leaves scale-like, imbricate, rhomboidal each with an oil gland under its dorsal surface, opposite, in 4 rows, decussate, in overlapping pairs, firm smooth, pointed, dark-green, bitter and have a strong disagreeable smell. Flowers unisexual, dioecious, small; the males in catkins, each with a bract, the females in cones at the extremeties of lateral branches. Berry, bluish, black, small with 2 seeds.

Habitate: U.S.A., Southern & Central Europe.

Propagation: By seeds and vegetative method.

Parts Used: Stem & leaves.

Chemical Constituents: A volatile oil, consisting chiefly alcohol Sabinol and its acetic ester, Cadinene, Pinene, Sabinene, Pinipicrin, α-thujene, Thujone. Geraniol & Cetronellol.

Uses: For complaints predominantly of uterine disorders. Drawing pain in small of back moving from sacrum to pubes. Uterine haemorrhages with pain extending from secrum paroxysms with colic & labour like pain extending from secrum to pubes. Retained placenta from atony of uterus. Inflammation of ovary and uterus after abortion, promotes expulsion of moles or foreign bodies from uterus. Music intolerable.

725. *Justicia beddomei* (Clarke) Bennet *(Acanthaceae)*

Synonyms *Adhatoda beddomei* C. B. Clarke.

Vernacular Name: *Hin*: Adusa, Arusa, *Kan*: *San*na-adusoga, *Mal*: Atalotakam, Cittatalotakam, *San*: Vasa, *Tam*: Adutota, Cittadalodakam, *Tel:* Addasaramu.

Description: A large glabrous shrub; leaves opposite, short-petioled upto 15 cm long, 3.75 cm broad, main nerves about 8 pairs; flower heads short, dense or condensed spikes; fruits capsules with a long solid base.

Habitate: In Kerala, in the hilly regions.

Propagation: By seeds and vegetative method.

Parts Used: All parts of the plant.

Chemical Consistuents: N.A.

Uses: The plant is bitter, astringent, refrigerant, expectorant, diuretic, antispasmodic, febrifuge, depurative, styptic and tonic. Leaves are good for irritable cough and for bleeding in diarrhoea and espeaially in haemoptysis. Flowers are used in ophthalmia. The roots along with the leaf-juice are used in phthisis, cough, haemoptysis and asthma.

726. *Justicia gendarussa* Burm. f. *(Acanthaceae)*

Synonyms: *Gendarussa vulgaris* Nees.

Vernacular Name: *San*: *Vata*ghni; *Hin*: Nilinirgundi, Udisambhalu, Kala adusa; *Kan*: Karinekki; *Mal*: *Vatam*kolli; *Tam*: *Vata*ikkutti; *Tel:* Addasaramu.

Description: An erect undershrub, 0.6 to 1.2 m in height with profuse subterete branches, stems and branches dark violet; leaves simple, opposite, lanceolate, or linear-lanceolate, 7.5 to 12.5 cm long, short-petioled, glabrous, dark violet green above and pale green beneath, main nerves about 8 pairs, mid rib and main nerves prominent, on the under surface; flowers white, spotted purple within, clustered in the interrupted spikes; fruits glabrous capsules.

Habitate: Throughout India, also cultivated as a hedge plant.

Propagation: By vegetative method.

Parts Used: Roots, leaves.

Chemical Consistuents: N.A.

Uses: The roots and leaves are acrid, bitter, thermogenic, anodyne, emetic, expectorant, anti-inflammatory, diaphoretic, emmenagogue, antiperiodic and insecticidal. They are useful in chronic rheumatism, cephalalgia, hemiplegia, facial paralysis, otalgia, hemicrania, cough, bronchitis, arthritis, dysmenorrhoea, amenorrhoea, internal haemorrhages, intermittent fevers, ascites and debility.

727. *Kaempferia galanga* L. *(Zingiberaceae)*

Vernacular Name: *San:* Chandramulika, sugandhavacha; *Eng:* East Indies galingale; *Hin:* Chandramula; *Beng*: Chandumula; *Tel:* Kachoram; *Tam:* Kacholam, kacholakilangu; *Kan:* Kachchura; *Mal:* Katjulam, kacholam.

Description: Perennial herbaceous plant. Rhizome includes little ovate tubers. ***Leaves:*** 2-3 with broad blade, spreading flat on the ground, appearing annually in rainy season, hairy beneath. Flowers white tinged with violet, sessile, arising from the axil.

Habitate: Grows wild in the mountains and is cultivated in some places for medicinal use.

Propagation: By vegetative method.

Part Used: Rhizomes.

Chemical Constituents: The rhizomes contain an essential oil (2.4-3.9%), coinsisting of p-methoxy transcinnamate ethyl, p-methoxy transcinnamic acid, transcinnamic acid, p-methoxystrene, p-coumaric acid, n-pentadecane, 3, careen, borneol and camphene.

Uses: The rhizome is recommended for dyspepsia and is very useful for the treatment of pectoral and abdominal pains, headache, toothache and cold. It is prescrived in deciction, powder or pill form for oral administration. And alcoholic maceration is employed externally in massage for the treatment of rheumatism.

728. *Kaempferia rotunda* L. *(Zingiberaceae)*

Vernacular Name: *San*: Bhumicampaka, Bhucampaka, Hallakah, *Eng*: Indian crocus, *Hin*: Bhuyicampa, Bhumichampa, *Kan*: Nelasampige, *Mal*: Cennalinirkkilannu, Cennalinirkuva, *Tam*: Nerppicin, *Tel:* Bhucampakamu.

Description: A handsome aromatic herb with tuberous root-stalk and very short stem; leaves simple, few, erect, oblong or ovate-lanceolate, acuminate, 30 cm long, 10 cm wide, variegated green above, tinged with purple below; flowers fragrant, white, lip purple or lilac in crowded spikes. Opening successively.

Habitate: Throughout India, in moist soil, also cultivated.

Propagation: By vegetative method.

Parts Used: Tubers.

Chemical Consistuents: The oil contains cineol and probably methyl chavicol. The rhizomes and young leaves are conmetics.

Uses: The tubers are acrid, thermogenic, aromatic, stomachic, anti-inflammatory, sialagogue, emetic and vulnerary. They are useful in vitiated conditions of *vata* and *kapha*, gastropathy, dropsy inflammations, wound, ulcers, blood clots, tumours and cancerous swellings.

729. *Kalanchoe pinnata* (Lam.) Pers. *(Crassulaceae)*

Description: Perennial succulent herb, 40-60cm. High. Stems tubular and glabrous, mottled with purple. Leaves opposite, entire or 3-lobed, rarely 5-7 lobed; blade thick and fleshy; margins cerenate. Inflorescence in terminal paniculate cyme with long stalk; flowers pendulous, red or orange-red. Fruit of 4 follicles.

Habitate: Commonly found in arid soil and cultivate for ornament.

Propagation: By seeds and vegetative method.

Part Used: Whole plant.

Chemical Constituents: The whole plant contains bryophyllin and organic acids: citric, isocitric and malic.

Uses: The fresh leaves, which possess antibacterial and demulcent properties, are used in the treatment of burns, wounds, impetigo, ulcer, phlegmon and congestive ophthalmial they are also haemostatic and depurative. Poultices and ointments are prepared with fresh leaves for external application.

730. *Kalopanax pictus* (Thunb.) Nakai *(Araliaceae)*

Vernacular Name: *Eng*: Tree aralia.

Description: Prickly, deciduous tree, to 30 m tall. Leaves alternate, palmately compound, to 30 cm across 5-7 lobed, lobes toothed, dark green above, light green beneath, usually glabrous but somewhat pubescent when young; petioles 10-30 cm long. Flowers in umbels forming large, terminal panicles; main branch short, obsolete; the branches to more than 10, 8-15 cm long, spreading, with few umbels at the apex; bracts 1-2 cm long; pedicels 7-10 mm long; petals 5, white, valvate; stamens 5; ovary inferior, 2-celled; style bifid. Fruit globose drupe.

Habitate: Mountain woods in Japan, Korea and China.

Propagation: By seeds and vegetative method.

Parts Used: Bark.

Chemical Constituents: Saponins: hederagenin glycosides. Lignans: syringin, liriodendrin, glucosyringic acid. Kalopanaxins A, B, C, D. Fatty acids: arachidic acid, etc. Phenols: coniferin, protocatechuic acid, chlorogenic acid. Flavonol glycosides: hyperin, quercitrin.

Uses: Antifungal, antihepatotoxic DNA polymerase a inhibition, RNA reverse transcriptase inhibition. Used in contusion, beri-beri, lumbago, neuralgia, pleurisy.

731. *Kingiodendron pinnatum* (Roxb. ex DC.) Harms*(Caesalpiniaceae)*

Synonyms: *Hardwickia pinnata* Roxb.

Vernacular Name: *Kan*: Yenna mara, Chou-paini; *Mal*: Kiyavu, Shurali; *Tam*: Madayan sambrani, Koda palai.

Description: A lofty evergreen tree, reaching a height of 40 m and a girth of 3 m. Trunk straight, unbranched up to 15 m tall. Bark about 5 mm thick, rough, surface dark brown mottled with green, dull red inside, exuding dark sticky resin when cut. Branchlets cylindrical, lenticellate, hairless. Leaves alternate, odd-pinnate, up to 30 cm long; rachis 10-15 cm long, swollen at base; leaflets 3-7, alternate, elliptic or elliptic-oblong to egg-shaped-lanceolate, 5-15 x 2.5-7 cm, base rounded, apex acute or bluntly long acuminate, margin entire, shiny, hairless, distinctly stalked; lateral nerves 4-6 pairs, prominently joining along the margin. Flowers bisexual, small, about 5 mm across, dull yellow, mildly fragrant, densely arranged in axillary cylindrical paniculate racemes; racemes 10-15 cm long; petals absent. Pods obovoid-oblong, 3-5 x 2-3 cm, turgid, woody, compressed, brown, lenticellate, hairless, apex shortly beaked. Seeds 1, brown, ellipsoid, flat, hard, about 3 x 1.5 cm.

Habitate: Semi-evergreen to evergreen forests.

Propagation: By seeds and vegetative method.

Parts Used: Resin.

Chemical Constituents: Trace, nil; sap. Val., nil; acetyl val., 12.6, 1.4, nil; and solubility in 95% alcohol, I in 5 vol., or more. The main constituent of the oil is β-caryophyllene; α-caryophyllene and a cadinene sesquiterpene are also present. The oil may be used as a substitute for imported clove oil.

Uses: The oleoresin is reportedly used for treating gonorrhea, rheumatism and as a dressing for sores of elephants.

732. *Knema attenuata* (Wall. ex Hook. f. & Thoms.) Warb.*(Myristicaceae)*

Synonyms: *Myristica attenuata* Wall. ex Hook. f. & Thoms.

Vernacular Name: *Kan*: Ratha mara; *Mal*: Chora pathri, Chennelli, Chora payin; *Mar*: Rakt mara; *Tam*: Chorappattiri, Suriya pathri, Kariyan.

Description: Medium sized trees, 10-18 m tall, about 1.5 m girth. *Bark* 5-8 mm thick, smooth, greenish black to grey-brown mottled with green and white, with irregular exfoliation, exuding watery reddish latex when cut freshly. *Blaze* pinkish red. Branches from the main stem in whorls, horizontal drooping; branchlets with yellowish brown tomentose hairs. *Leaves* alternate, elliptic-lanceolate to oblong-lanceolate, 10-25 x 4-7 cm, base rounded, apex acuminate, margin entire, hairless above, brown tomentose and blue-green tinged along the nerves below, distinctly stalked; lateral nerves 10-20 pairs, joining along the margin. Flowers unisexual, male and female flowers seen in separate trees, distinctly stalked, urn-shaped, brown tomentose hairs outside, hairless and pink inside. *Male flowers* arise in axillary clusters on stout and short stalks, 5-6 mm long. *Female flowers* 1-3 in leaf axils. *Drupes* ovoid, 2.5-4 x 1.5-2 cm, densely brown tomentose. *Seeds* solitary, egg-shaped and enclosed within a crimson red-coloured fleshy aril.

Habitate: Semi-evergreen to evergreen forests.

Propagation: By seeds and vegetative method.

Parts Used: Seeds and seed oil.

Chemical Constituents: A fixed oil is obtained from crushed seeds of the plant by extraction with petroleum ether. On cooling the extract to room temperature, a phytosterol settles out; a second crystalling substance probably a phenolic acid separates on cooling the petroleum ether extract to o°. The seed fat, free from solvent, has m.p., 34°.

Uses: It is one of the ingrediant of *'Ashwagandhadhi nei'* (medicated ghee) used for treatment of spleen disorders, breathing disorders and tastelessness.

733. *Kochia scoparia* Schrad. *(Chenopodiaceae)*

Vernacular Name: *Eng*: Summer cypress, belvedere.

Description: Annual herb, to 1 m tall, usually much-branched, if columnar or pyramidal to globular habit, more or less hairy. Leaves alternate, lanceolate to harrow-linear, entire, to 8 cm long, ciliate. Flowers inconspicuous, axillary, leaves at the terminal reduced to bracts resembling spike superficially, bisexual or female; calyx 5-lobed; corolla none; stamens 5, exerted; ovary 1-celled; stigmas mostly 2. Fruit a utricle enveloped by the calyx, which develops transverse wings in age. July-August.

Habitate: Naturalized in fields and mountains.

Propagation: By seeds and vegetative method.

Parts Used: Fruit.

Chemical Constituents: Triterpenoid saponins. Phytoecdysterols, betanin, phyllocatin, isophyllocatin, isobetanin Harman, harmine.

Uses: Cytotoxic, intercalating agent (Harman), adverse GI and CNS effects in humans (harmine). Used in uretic, eczema, scabies.

734. *Krameria triandra* *(Krameriaceae)*

Vernacular Name: *Eng:* Rhatany.

Description: Dense evergreen shrub growing to 90 cm. Has a deep root, oblong leaves and large red flowers.

Habitate: Rhatany is found in Ecuador, Peru and Bolivia on western slopes of the Andes at altitudes of 900 to 3,000 m. The root is unearthed throughout the year.

Propagation: By seeds and vegetative method.

Parts Used: Root.

Chemical Constituents: Rhatany contains 10-20% tannins, including phlobaphene, benzofurans and n-methyltyrosine.

Uses: Rhatany is astringent and antimicrobial. It is a useful remedy taken principally for problems affecting the gastro-intestinal tract. It is most commonly used for diarrhoea and dysentery. In addition, rhatany makes a good mouthwash and gargle for bleeding and infected gums, moth ulcers and sore throats. The plant's astringency makes it useful in the form of an ointment, suppository or wash for treating haemorrhoids. Rhatany may also be applied to wounds to help staunch blood flow, to varicose vines and over areas of capillary fragility that may be prone to easy bruising.

735. *Kyllinga brevifolia* Rottb. *(Cyperaceae)*

Synonyms: *Cyperus brevifolium* (Rottb.) Hassk.

Vernacular Name: Kyllinga.

Description: Perennial sedge arising from a thin creeping rhizome bearing three-angled stems up to 30 cm high. Leaves basal, in three ranks, long-linear (grassOlike), about the same length as stems. Flowers minute, borne in a terminal white globose head (occasionally two smaller lateral heads may also be present), subtended by three spreading leaf-like bracts up to 15 cm long. Fruit a minute achene up to 1.5 mm. Long. Flowers and fruit usually available throughout the year.

Habitate: Common in damp, disturbed places such as pastures, cane fields, stream sides, etc. from near sea-level up to over 1000 m elevation.

Propagation: By seeds and vegetative method.

Part Used: Whole plant.

Chemical Constituents: Okanin and vitexin.

Uses: Used for liver disease.

736. *Kyllinga nemoralis* (forster) Dandy *(Cyperaceae)*

Vernacular Name: *Eng:* kyllinga.

Description: Loosely tufted perennial sedge from a long creeping rhizome bearing three-angled stems up to 45 cm high. Leaves basal, long-linear (grass-like), usually shorter than stems and relatively soft. Flowrs minute, borne in a terminal solitary white globose head, subtended by three or sometimes four spreading leaf-like bracts upto 30 cm long. Fruit achene, up to 1.5 mm. Long. Flowers and fruit usually available throughout the year.

Habitate: Common along beaches, roadsides, trails, forest margins, pastures, gardens and disturbed places from sea-level to over 850 m elevation.

Propagation: By seeds and vegetative method.

Part Used: Whole plant.

Uses: The plant is used in remedies for treating sprains and contusions.

737. *Labalb purpureus* L. (*Fabaceae*)

Synonyms: *Dolichos lablab* Linn.

Vernacular Name: *San*: Nispavah, *Eng*: Lablab bean, Bonavist bean, Indian butter bean, *Hin*: Sem, Bhatvas, *Kan*: Capparada-avare, *Mal*: Amara, Avara, *Tam*: Avarai, *Tel:* Cikkudu.

Description: A tall, nearly glabrous twining perennial herb; leaves 10-20 cm long; flowers in racemes, white or pink, fruits white pods, green or purple margined; seeds white, yellow, purple or black.

Habitate: Throughout India, cultivated.

Propagation: By seeds and vegetative method.

Parts Used: Leaves, seeds.

Chemical Consisuents: The plant contains alkaloid, trigonelline, known for its hypoglycaemic activity.

Uses: Leaves are alexipharmic and emmenagogue, and are given in colic. Seeds are sweet, astringent, sour laxative, diuretic, galactagogue, anaphrodisiac, stomachic and anti-spasmdic. They are useful in inflammations, strangury, agalactia and vitiated conditions of *kapha.*

738. *Lactuca indica* L. (*Asteraceae*)

Synonyms: *Lactuca brevirostris* Champ.

Vernacular Name: *Eng:* Indian lettuce.

Description: Annual herbaceous plant, 0.5–1m. high; rarely branched. Leaves alternate, sessile; the lower deeply lobed; the upper occasionally entire; margins toothed. Influrenscence in terminal head; flowers yellow. Achene small, tipped with a tuft of hairs.

Habitate: Grows wild in waste places.

Propagation: By seeds and vegetative method.

Part Used: Whole plant.

Chemical Constituents: N.A.

Uses: The entire plant, and especially the leaves, is employed as a depurative and demulcent. The leaves are used in treating mastitis, galactophoritis, furunculosis and abscesses. They are also effective for gastralgia and dyspepsia. A mixture with some other plants is used externally in the form of a poultice of pounded fresh leaves.

739. *Lactuca virosa* (*Asteraceae*)

Vernacular Name: *Eng:* Wild lettuce.

Description: Hollow-stemmed biennial growing to about 1.2 m. Has broad spiny leaves and clusters of pale yellow composite flowers. All parts of the plant exude a white milky latex.

Habitate: Common throughout Europe, wild lettuce grows on wasteground, roadsides and in hedgerows.

Propagation: By seeds and vegetative method.

Parts Used: Leaves, latex.

Chemical Constituents: The latex contains sesquiterpene lactones the leaves also contains flavonoids and coumarins. The sesquiterpene lactones have a sedative effect.

Uses: Wild lettuce is a safe sedative that can be given to adults and children to encourage a sound night's sleep or to calm overactivity or overstimulation. Most commonly, it is recommended for excitability in children. It is also taken to treat coughs, often in combination with herbs such as liquorice thought to lower the libido. It may also be used to relieve pain.

740. *Lagenaria siceraria* (Mol.) Standley *(Cucurbitaceae)*

Synonyms: *Lagenaria leucantha* (Duchesne) Rusby, *Lagenaria vulgaris* Ser.

Vernacular Name: *San*: Katutumbi, Tiktalabu; *Eng*: Bitter bottle gourd, Bitter calbash gourd; *Hin*: Titalauki, Kadvilauki; *Kan*: Kadusore; *Mal*: Peccura, Kattucura, Kaippan cura; *Tam*: Sorakkai; *Tel:* Sorakkaya.

Description: A large softly pubescent, climbing or training herb with 5-angled hispid stems and 2-fid long tendrils; leaves simple, long-petioled with two glands at the apex, 5-lobed, cordate, dentate, hairy on both surfaces; flowers large, white, solitary, the males long-stalked and the females short-stalked; fruits large, spherical, bottle or dumb-bell shaped, rind woody when ripe enclosing soft juicy flesh; seeds many, white, compressed smooth with a marginal groove.

Habitate: Throughout India, wild or cultivated.

Propagation: By seeds and vegetative method.

Parts Used: Whole Plant.

Chemical Consistuents: Bitter fruits yield 0.013% of a solid foam containing cucurbitacins B, D, G and H, mainly cucurbitacin B; these bitter principles are present in the fruit as aglycones. Leaves contain traces of E the fruit juice contains β-glycosidase, opt. *p*H in phosphate buffer, 4.0-5.5; opt. temp., 50°.

Uses: The roots are emetic, purgative and anti-inflammatory and are useful in vitiated conditions of *kapha,* constipation and inflammations. The leaves are bitter, refrigerant, emetic, purgative, anodyne, expectorant, diuretic and febrifuge. They are useful in vitiated conditions of *pitta,* burning of the feet, cough, bronchitis, inflammation, skin diseases, leprosy, fainting and fever. The seeds are purgative, diuretic, cooling and brain tonic, and are useful in cough, fever, scalding of urine, otalgia, inflammations and dropsy.

741. *Lamium album* *(Lamiaceae)*

Vernacular Name: *Eng:* White deadnettle.

Description: An ascending or decumbent, glabrous or hispidly hairy perennial herb, 25-50 cm. high, with a creeping root stock; leaves ovate-cordate, crenate or serrate; flowers white or pale pink, in axillary whorls; nutlets long, smooth, black or dark brown.

Habitate: White deadnettle is native to and widespread in Europe and central and northern Asia. It thrives in fields and on wasteground.

Propagation: By seeds and vegetative method.

Parts Used: Flowers.

Chemical Constituents: White deadnettle contains a saponin, flavones, mucilage and tannins.

Uses: White deadnettle is astringent and demulcent. It is chiefly used as a uterine tonic, to arrest intermenstrual bleeding and to reduce excessive menstrual flow. It is also a traditional treatment for abnormal vaginal discharge. The herb is sometimes taken to relieve painful periods. Its astringency helps treat diarrhoea, and used externally, it can relieve haemorrhoids and varicose veins.

742. *Lamprachaenium microcephalum* Benth. *(Asteraceae)*

Vernacular Name: *San*: Brahmadandi, Ajadandi; *Mar*: Brahmadandi.

Description: An erect branched long-hairy herb, reaching 30-60 cm tall. Stems with vertical striations, densely hairy. *Leaves* alternate, elliptic, 3-9 x 1.5-4 cm, base tapering, apex acuminate, margin distantly toothed, sparsely with bristly hairs above and woolly tomentose beneath, dotted with minute glands, distinctly stalked. *Flowers* minute, purplish pink, aggregated in about 5 mm across conical-shaped heads. The *heads* are arranged in axillary and terminal corymbs. Bracts arranged in many rows, hairy outside with fringed-hairy margins. *Achenes* obovoid, slightly compressed, about 2 mm long, shiny, smooth, with red pappus hairs at apex.

Habitate: Open grasslands at higher altitudes.

Propagation: By seeds.

Parts Used: Whole plant.

Chemical Constituents: N.A.

Uses: This plant is reportedly used for treatment of skin diseases like leucoderma and in *vata* and *kapha* inflammations.

743. *Lannea coromandelica* (Houtt.) Merr. *(Anacardiaceae)*

Synonyms: *Odina wodier* Roxb., *Lamea grandis Eng*l.

Vernacular Name: *San*: Jhingini, Jingini; *Eng*: Wodie,r Jhingam; *Hin*: Jhingan, Mohin; *Kan*: Manjistha; *Mal*: Karasu, Kalasu, Udi, Karayam, Otiyamaram; *Tam*: Oti, Udi, Vodiyar; *Tel:* Oddimanu.

Description: A medium sized to large tree 12-28 m in height with grayish bark rough, exfoliating in thin irregular flakes; leaves imparipinnately compound, crowded at the ends of branches, leaflets membranous, 7-9, oblong-ovate, green above, brown beneath, glabrous, base acute or rounded, often oblique, main nerves 6-8 pairs; flowers small, yellowish or purplish, the male racemes compound, the female simple; fruits reniform, compressed, 1-seeded red drupes.

Habitate: Throughout India, in deciduous forests upto 1,500 m also cultivated.

Propagation: By seeds and vegetative method.

Parts Used: Bark, leaves.

Chemical Consistuents: Hydrolysis, *l*-arabinose, *d*-galactose and a complex monobasic acid, named jeolic acid, the bar contain *c*-8% phlobatannin and may be used for tanning and dyeing purposes and as a preservative for fishing nets.

Uses: The bark is acrid, astringent, sweet, thermogenic, stomachic, and anodyne. It is useful in cuts, wounds, bruises, ulcers, ophthalmia, gout, ulcerative stomatitis, odontalgia, sprains, diarrhoea, and dysentery. The leaves are useful in elephantiasis, inflammations, neuralgia, sprains and bruises.

744. *Lantana camara* L. Moldenke *(Verbenaceae)*

Synonyms: *L aculeate* Linn, *L camara* auct. Non Linn.

Vernacular Name: *San*: Caturangi, Vanacchedi; *Eng*: Wild sage, Lantana weed; *Hin*: Caturang, Ghaneri; *Kan*: Kadugulabi, Lantavanigidda; *Mal*: Arippu, Pucceti; *Tam*: Arisimalar, Unnicceti; *Tel:* Pulikampa.

Description: A large scrambling evergreen, strong smelling shrub with stout recurved prickles; leaves opposite, often rugose, scabrid on both sides; flowers small, normally orange but often white to dark red, in heads which are prominently capitate; bracts conspicuous, persistent; fruits fleshy drupes, 5 mm in diameter, endocarp hard green when young and blue or black on ripening.

Habitate: A native of tropical America, but now naturalized in many parts of India as a troublesome prickly weed.

Propagation: By seeds and vegetative method.

Parts Used: All parts of the plant.

Chemical Consistuents: Catalase, amylase, invertase, lipase, tannase and glucosidase. Appreciable amounts of tannins and sugar, crystalline glucoside has been separated from the resin by ether extraction, caryophyllene, l-α-phellandrene small amounts of aldehydes alcohols are present lantadene A, lantadene B which is inactive and a steroid, lancamarone quinine-like alkaloid, lantanine.

Uses: The plant is vulnerary, diaphoretic, carminative, antispasmodic and tonic. It is useful in tetanus, vitiated conditions of *vata* malaria epilepsy and gastropathy. A decoction of fresh roots is a good gargle for odontalgia and this is used by hill tribes for all types of dysentery. Powdered leaves are used for cuts, wounds, ulcers and swellings. An infusion of the leaves is good for bilious fever, vitiated conditions of *vata* and *kapha*, eczema and eruptions. The fruits are useful in fistula, pustules, tumours and rheumatism.

745. *Larix decidua* *(Pinaceae)*

Synonyms: *Larix europeae.*

Vernacular Name: *Eng:* Larch.

Description: Deciduous conifer growing to 50 m. Has clusters of needle-like leaves, male and female flowers and small, light brown cones.

Habitate: Native to the alps and the Carpathian mountains of eastern Europe, larch grows to altitudes of 2,000 m. It is widely cultivated for its timber.

Propagation: By seeds and vegetative method.

Parts Used: Inner bark and resin.

Chemical Constituents: Larch contains lignans, resins and volatile oil.

Uses: Larch has astringent, diuretic and antiseptic properties. the bark may be used to treat bladder and urinary tubule infections such as cystitis and urethritis, and respiratory problems, wounds, where it protects and counters infection.

746. *Larrea tridentate* *(Zygophyllaceae)*

Vernacular Name: *Eng:* Chaparral, Creosote Bush.

Description: Thorny shrub growing to 2 m, with small finely divided leaves.

Habitate: Chaparral is found in large numbers in the deserts of south-western US and Mexico.

Propagation: By seeds and vegetative method.

Parts Used: Aerial parts.

Chemical Constituents: Chaparral contains about 12% resin and nordihydroguaiaretic acid. The latter is reportedly harmful to the lymph glands and the kidneys.

Uses: Until recently, chaparral remained in wide use in the US, with an average of 9.07 tonnes consumed there each year. It was thought to be a beneficial remedy for rheumatic disease, venereal infections, urinary infections and certain types of cancer, especially leukaemia. Chaparral was also taken internally for skin afflictions such as acne and eczema, and applied as a lotion to sores, wounds and rashes. Recently, however, its sale was banned in the US, due to concern over its potential toxic effect on the liver.

747. *Laurus nobilis* *(Lauraceae)*

Vernacular Name: *Eng:* Bay laurel.

Description: Aromatic evergreen shrub or tree growing to 20 m. Has leathery, dark green leaves, small yellow male and female flowers and shiny black berries.

Habitate: Native to Mediterranean countries, bay laurel prefers damp and shady sites. It is also a popular garden herb, cultivated largely for culinary use. The leaves are picked all year round.

Propagation: By seeds and vegetative method.

Parts Used: Leaves.

Chemical Constituents: Bay laurel contains up to 3% volatile oil.

Uses: Bay laurel is used mainly to treat upper digestive tract disorders and to ease arthritic aches and pains. It is settling to the stomach and has a tonic effect, stimulating the appetite and the secretion of digestive juices. When used as an ingredient in cooking, bay laurel leaves promote the digestion and absorption of food. The leaves have mush the same kind of positive effect as spearmint and rosemary in assisting the breakdown of heavy food, especially meat. Bay laurel has also been used to promote the onset of menstrual periods. The essential oil is chiefly employed as a friction rub, being well diluted in a carrier oil and massaged into aching muscles and joints.

748. *Lavandula officinalis* *(Lamiaceae)*

Synonyms*:* *Lavandula angustifolia.*

Vernacular Name: *Eng:* Lavender.

Description: A perennial shrub growing to 1m, with spikes of violet-blue flowers extending above the foliage.

Habitate: Native to France and the western Mediterranean, lavender is cultivated worldwide for its volatile oil, and is grown as a garden plant as far north as Norway.

Propagation: By seeds and vegetative method.

Parts Used: Flowers.

Chemical Constituents: Volatile oil containing over 40 constituents, including linalyl acetate, cineole, linalool, nerol, borneol, Flavonoids, Tannins, Coumarins.

Uses: Carminative, Relieves muscle spasms, antidepres*San*t, Antiseptic & antibacterial, Stimulates blood flow.

749. *Lawsonia inermis* L. *(Lythraceae)*

Synonyms *Lawsonia alba* Lam.

Vernacular Name: *San*: Medhini, Madayantika, Nakharanjani; *Eng*: Henna, Egyptian priven, Cypress shrub; *Hin*: Mehandi; *Kan*: Madurangi; *Mal*: Mailanci, Mayilanci; *Tam*: Mailenanti, Marutani; *Tel:* Goranta.

Description: A glabrous much-branched deciduous shrub with 4-gonous lateral branches often ending in spines; leaves simple, opposite, entire, lanceolate, petioles very short or absent; flowers white, or rose-coloured, fragrant, in large terminal pyramidal panicled cymes, stamens 8, in 4 pairs inserted on the calyx tube; fruits globose capsules, tipped with the style and supported by the persistent calyx, seeds numerous, smooth, pyramidal.

Habitate: Scarcely in dry deciduous forests, widely cultivated as a hedge plant.

Propagation: By seeds and vegetative method.

Parts Used: Roots, leaves, flowers, seeds.

Chemical Consistuents: Henna contains 25-33% water-soluble matter; aqueous solutions are orange in colour and show a green fluorescence. The principal colouring mater is lawsone, 2-hydroxy-I: 4-naphthaquinone which is present in dried leaves in a concentration of I-0-I-4%. Behenic, arachidic, stearic, palmitic, oleic.

Uses: The roots are bitter, refrigerant, depurative, diuretic, emmenagogue, abortifacient and trichogenous, and are useful in burning sensation, dipsia, leprosy, skin disease, strangury, amenorrhoea, dysmenorrhoea, and premature graying of hair. The leaves are bitter, astringent, acrid, refrigerant vulnerary, diuretic, emetic, expectorant, anodyne, anti-inflammatory, constipating, depurative, liver tonic, haematinic, styptic febrifuge and trichogenous. They are useful in wounds, ulcers strangury cough, bronchitis, vitiated conditions of *kapha* and *pitta,* burning sensation, cephalalgia, hemicrania, lumbago, rheumatalgia, inflammations, diarrhoea, dysentery, leprosy, leucoderma, scabies, boils, hepatopathy, splenopathy, anaemia, haemorrhages, haemoptysis, fever, ophthalmia, amenorrhoea, dysmenorrhoea, falling of hair, greyness of hair and jaundice. The flowers are intellect promoting, cardiotonic, refrigerant, soporific, febrifuge and tonic. They are useful in cephalalgia, burning sensation, sardiopathy, amentia, insomnia, and fever.

750. *Ledum palustre* L. *(Ericaceae)*

Synonyms: *Ledum decumbens* Lodd ex. steud., *Ledum graveolens* Gilib.

Vernacular Name: *Eng:* Wild Rosemary.

Description: An evergreen shrub, upto 1m. in height with several clustering round branches covered with a rust coloured fur; stem-bark ash coloured. Leaves 5 cm. long, 8-12 mm. broad, entire, linear, alternate, short petioled, lanceolate, rolled back on edges; glabrous, green and shining above; red, rust-coloured and downy below. Flowers in dense terminal corymbs, with filiform, pubescent pedicels, white or pale rose red colour. Stamens usually 10, petals 5, sepals 5.

Habitate: Swamp and wet places in Northern & Central Europe.

Propagation: By seeds and vegetative method.

Parts Used: Whole plant.

Chemical Constituents: Volatile oil containing; Ledum camphor; palustrol; Stearopten; valeric acid; Ericolin & Ericinol. Leditannic acid. Quercetin. Hyperoside.

Uses: For complaints of contusion of eyes & eyelids, ecchymosis of lids & conjunctiva. Eheumatism or gout beginning in lower limbs ascending upwards with joints becoming the seat of nodosities, involving particularly left shoulder & right hip joints. Punctured wounds produced by sharp-pointed instruments or bites, particularly if wounded parts are cold. Twisting of muscles near wounds. Red pimples on forehead & cheeks. All complaints associated with great chill. Bronchitis with emphysema.

751. *Leea indica* (Burm. f.) Merr. *(Vitacecae)*

Synonyms: *Leea sambucina* (Linn.) Willd.

Vernacular Name: *San*: Chatri, Kukkurajihva; *Hin*: Kurkurjihava; *Kan*: Gadhapatri, Andilu; *Mal*: Kutanaluku, Naluku, Nallu, Nakku, Erattayani, Maniperanti; *Tam*: Naikki, Ottanali; *Tel:* Ankadora.

Description: A large shrub with numerous tough branches, the young ones green, glabrous, very large, much divided, leaflets oblong or elliptic-oblong, chartaceous, coarsely and irregularly serrate, dark brown when dry, petiole dilated at the base into sheathing stipules; flowers white in large branched corymbose cymes; fruits purple, depressed globular berries.

Habitate: Throughout India, in evergreen forests upto 1,200 m.

Propagation: By seeds and vegetative method.

Parts Used: Roots, leaves.

Chemical Consistuents: N.A.

Uses: The roots are astringent, acrid, cooling anthelmintic and sudorific. They are useful in diarrhoea, dysentery, colic, hyperdipsia, ulcers and skin diseases. The young leaves are digestive and are applied to the head in vertigo.

752. *Lens culinaris* Medikus *(Fabaceae)*

Synonyms: *Lens esculenta* Moench.

Vernacular Name: *San*: Masurah; *Eng*: Lentil; *Hin*: Masur, Masuri; *Kan*: Kesaribele; *Mal*: Canampayar, Vattupparippu, Athanapparippu; *Tam*: Misur parupu, Atanapparuppu; *Tel:* Misuripappu.

Description: A small erect softly pubescent herb, branching from the base, 15-75 cm in height; leaves compound, leaflets 4-6 pairs, sessile; flowers white, rose, red or violet; solitary or in 2-4 flowered racemes; fruits smooth, compressed, oblong or rhomboid pods, seeds usually two, smooth, compressed with minute spots.

Habitate: Throughout the colder parts of India, cultivated.

Propagation: By seeds and vegetative method.

Parts Used: Seeds.

Chemical Consistuents: Calcium, phosphorus, iron, sodium, potassium, magnesium, sulphur and chlorine, iodine, bromine, managanese, aluminium, copper, zinc and arsenic are also present lipoidal, nuclein, phytin and mineral. Calcium magnesium inositol phosphates are present to the extent of 0.52% in fat-free lentils amylase, proteo-lytic enzymes, phosphatase and phytase.

Uses: The seeds are sweet, refrigerant, astringent constipating, diuretic and tonic. They are useful in ophthalmopathy, mammillitis, vitiated conditions of *pitta*, diarrhoea, dysentery, strangury, tumours, cardiopathy, foul and indolent ulcers, skin diseases, anaemia and general debility.

753. *Leonurus artemisa* (Lour.) S.Y. Hu *(Lamiaceae)*

Vernacular Name: *Eng:* Siberian motherwort, lion's tail.

Description: Annual herbaceous plant, 0.5–1m. high. Stems quadrangular. Leaves opposite, the basal nearly round, long-petioled, dentate-crenate; the middle long, pinnatipartite; the upper short, usually entire, Flowers white or pink in axillary whorls. Nutlet small, glabrous.

Habitate: Grows wild in we places and is also cultivated.

Propagation: By seeds and vegetative method.

Part Used: Whole plant.

Chemical Constituents: The whole plant contains a flavonoid (rutin), leucoanthocyanoglucosides, steroids, alkaloids, choline, amino acids and tannin.

Uses: The drug enjoys a long-standing reputation in the treatment of irregular menstruation, sysmenoorrhoea, polymenorrhoea and post-partum haematometra. It is also used for hypertension and heart disease.

754. *Leonurus cardiaca* *(Lamiaceae)*

Vernacular Name: *Eng:* Motherwort.

Description: A perennial pubescent herb, up to 1-2 m in height. Rootstock stout; lower leaes ovate-cordate or ovate-lanceolate, deeply & irregularly lobed, upper leaves lanceolate, lobed or entire; flowers pink or white; nutlets smooth.

Habitate: Native to central Asia, motherwort is now naturalized in much of Europe and North America. India, it is found in himalay region.

Propagation: By seeds and vegetative method.

Parts Used: Aerial parts.

Chemical Constituents: Motherwort contains alkaloids an iridoid, diterpenes, flavonoids, caffeic acid and tannins.

Uses: A remedy for the heart and nerves and often prescribed for palpitations, motherwort strengthens heart function, especially where it is weak. Antispasmodic and sedative, the herb promotes relaxation rather the drowsiness. However, motherwort stimulates the muscles of the uterus, and is particularly suitable for delayed periods, period pain and premenstrual tension. It should not be used if menstrual bleeding is heavy.

755. *Leonurus japoncus* Houtt. *(Lamiaceae)*

Synonyms: *Leonurus artemisi* (Loureiro) S.Y. Hu.

Vernacular Name: *Eng:* Wormwoodlike motherwort.

Description: An annual or biennial herb, 60-100 cm high. Stem erect; simple or branched, tetragonal, pubescent. Leaves opposite, long-petioled, palmate-tripartite, the lobes themselves coarsely divided into 3-4 parts, 7 cm long by 4 cm wide. Inflorescence a compact, axillary verticil,June-August. Flowers 2-lipped. Calyx campanulate, teeth 5. Corolla exserted, 10-15 mm long, red tube equalling the limb in length, straight, superior lip oboval, curved, concave, inferior lip equally long, expanded-trilobate; median lobe truncate, broad, obcordate; lateral lobes smaller, rounded. Stamens 4. Fruit a collection of smooth, triquetrous nutlets.

Habitate: On the outskirts of villages, on the banks of streams and on damp soil in China, Japan, Korea.

Propagation: By seeds and vegetative method.

Part Used: Whole plant.

Chemical Constituents: Contain alkaloid leonurine. Seeds contain fatty and volatile oils.

Uses: Whole plant used in Amenorrhoea dystocia and dysphagia.

756. *Leonurus sibiricus* L. *(Lamiaceae)*

Vernacular Name: *Eng*: Motherwort; *Hin*: Guma.

Description: Biannual herb upto 1-1.5 m tall, gray-green, white-pubscent. Stems square in cross section. Basal leaves ovate-cordate, toothed and incised, long-petiolate, withering before flowers appear; stem leaves 5-10 cm long, pinnately dissected, long-petioled; uppermost leaves often entire, linear-lanceolate. Flowers in many-flowered verticillasters, 2 cm long; bractlets shorter than calyx; calyx companulate, 5-nerved, 5-toothed, teeth spiny; corollar tube shorter than calyx, rose-pink, limb 2-lipped; upper lip erect, entire; lower lip spreading, 3-lobed; stamens 4, in 2 pairs; anther cells opposite, opening by a common slit. Fruit of 4 glabrous, 3-angled, nutlets.

Habitate: Grassy areas in lowlands of Asia, China, Korea Japan and India.

Propagation: By seeds and vegetative method.

Parts Used: Whole plant.

Chemical Constituents: Alkaloids: leonurinine, leonuridine, stachydrin, leuronurine. Prehispanolone, cycloleonurinine, leoheterin, preleoheterin.

Uses: Uterotonic, hypotensive, anticancer, antibacterial, platelet activating factor antagonistic, anticoagulant activities. Used in malaria and amenorrhoea.

757. *Lepidium opetalum* Willd. *(Cruciferae)*

Vernacular Name: *Eng:* Pepperweed, peppergras.

Description: An annual biennial herb. Stem erect or diffuse, 5-35 cm high, densely covered with small capitate glandular hairs. Basal leaves pinnatisect 3-5 cm long by 1-1.5 cm wide, petiole 1-2 cm long; cauline leaves sessile, lower leaves narrowly elongated-elliptic, dentate, upper linear, nearly entire or repand. Racemes elongated, terminal. Flowers small, pedicels slender. Short pods oval-elliptic, 2.5 mm long, compressed, flat, slightly emarginate, winged above. Seeds very small, 1.5 mm long by 0.75 mm wide, oboval, light reddish-brown or yellowish-brown.

Habitate: By roadsides and among grasses in China, Europe and Soviet Union.

Propagation: By seeds and vegetative method.

Part Used: Whole plant.

Chemical Constituents: N.A.

Uses: Abundant expectoration with cough and dyspnaea, distension in the chest and hypochondrium, Oedema, oliguria.

758. *Lepidium sativum* L. *(Cruciferae)*

Vernacular Name: *San*: Asalika, Asalic; *Eng*: Garden cress, Water cress; *Hin*: Chandrasur, Halim, Halo; *Kan*: Alavibija; *Mal*: Asali; *Tam*: Alivirai; *Tel:* Aditya.

Description: An erect herbaceous glabrous annual upto 45 cm in height; leaves entire or variously lobed or pinnatisect, the lower petiolate, the upper sessile; flowers white, small, in long racemes; fruits obovate, small pods, notched at the apex with two seeds per pod.

Habitate: Cultivated throughout India as a culinary vegetable.

Propagation: By seeds and vegetative method.

Parts Used: Roots, leaves, seeds.

Chemical Consistuents: Analysis of leaves gave the following values; water, protein, fat, carbohydrate, mineral matter, calcium and phosphorus, trace elements: iron nickel cobalt and iodine; vitamins; vitamin A, thiamine, riboflavin, niacin and ascorbic acid. Cooked leaves contain vitamin A, thiamine, riboflavin, niacin, and ascorbic acid, moisture, protein, fat, ashand sulphur. The seeds contain an alkaloid, glucotropaeloin, sinapin, sinapic acid, mucilaginous matter and uric acid. The percentages of saturated and unsaturated acids in the oil are as follows; palmitic, stearic, arachidic behenic lignoceric, loeic, and linolenic. The usaponifiable mater contains β-sitosterol and α-tocopherol. The oil possesses anti-oxidant properties; the optimum stabilizing concentration when used as an additive for linseed oil is 10%.

Uses: The roots are bitter and acrid, and are useful in secondary syphilis and tenesmus. The leaves are stimulant, diuretic and antibacterial and are useful in scorbutic diseases and hepatopathy. The seeds are bitter, thermogenic, depurative, rubefacient, galactagogue, emmenagogue, tonic, aphrodisiac, ophthalmic and diuretic. They are useful as poultices for sprains and in leprosy, skin diseases, dysentery, diarrhoea, splenomegaly, dyspepsia, lumbago, ophthalmopathy, leucorrhoea, scurvy, seminal weakness, asthma, cough, hiccough, haemorrhoids and vitiated conditions of *vata*. It can be administered to cause abortion.

759. *Lepidium virginicum* *(Cruciferae)*

Vernacular Name: *Eng:* Virginia peppergrass.

Description: Annual herb growing to about 60 cm. Has slender lance-shaped leaves and small white flowers.

Habitate: Virginia peppergrass is native to eastern North America and the Caribbean, and is naturalized in Australia.

Propagation: By seeds and vegetative method.

Parts Used: Leaves, root.

Chemical Constituents: Virginia peppergrass contains high levels of vitamin C.

Uses: Virginia peppergrass is nutritious and generally detoxifying. It has been used to treat vitamin C deficiency and diabetes, and to expel intestinal worms. The herb is also diuretic and benefit in easing rheumatic pain. The root is taken to treat excess catarrh within the respiratory tract.

760. *Leptadenia reticulata* W. & A. *(Asclepiadaceae)*

Vernacular Name: *San*: Jivanti; *Hin:* Dori; *Guj*: Dodi, nahanidodi, khirkhodi; *Tel:* Kalasa, mukkutummudu; *Tam*: Palaikkodi.

Description: A twining shrub, *stems* with cork-like deeply cracked bark, branches numerous, younger ones glabrous. *Leaves* coriaceous, ovate, acute, glabrous above finely pubescent. *Flowers* greenish-yellow, in lateral or subaxillary cymes. Often with small hairs. *Fruit* follicles sub-woody, 6.3-9cm tapering *seeds* 6mm.

Habitate: Distributed in India in Punjab, Konkan, Poona and Gujarat, also in the Western peninsula.

Propagation: By seeds and vegetative method.

Parts Used: Roots.

Chemical Constituents: Stigmasterol and tocopherols were isolated from the plant and from the stem and leaves hentriacontanol α-amyrin, α-amyrin, stigmasterol and β-sitosterol were isolated and identified. Two flavonoids, diosmetin and luteolin were also isolated.

Uses: Diminished lactation. Skin infections. The plant is a stimulant and a tonic. The leaves and roots are useful in various skin diseases, inflammation of the skin and on wounds.

761. *Leptandra virginica* *(Scrophulariaceae)*

Synonyms: *Veronicastrum virginicum.*

Vernacular Name: *Eng:* Black root.

Description: Perennial herb growing to 1 m. Has an erect stem, lance-shaped leaves and white flowers.

Habitate: Black root grows across North America in meadows and woodlands.

Propagation: By seeds and vegetative method.

Parts Used: Root.

Chemical Constituents: Black root contains a volatile oil, saponins, sugars and tannins.

Uses: Black root is used in small doses today as a laxative and a remedy for liver and gallbladder disorders. The herb also treats flatulence and bloating, and eases the discomfort of haemorrhoids, chronic constipation and rectal prolapse. It may be given for skin problems if poor liver function is a factor.

762. *Leucaena leucocephala* (Lam.) De Wit. *(Mimosaceae)*

Vernacular Name: *Eng:* Lead tree, white popinac, jumpy bean.

Description: Small evergreen tree, several metres in height. Leaves bipinnate, leaflets small. Flowers white in axillary panicle. Pod thin and flat, brownish when ripe. Seeds glabrous, dark-brown.

Habitate: Grows wild and is cultivated as a shade tree in coffee plantations.

Propagation: By seeds and vegetative method.

Part Used: Seeds.

Chemical Constituents: The seeds contain a fatty oil. Consisting of plamitic, stearic, oleic, linoleic, behenic and lignoceric acids and the alkaloid leucenine (leucenol) 3-5%. The leaves yield tannin, quercitrin and alkaloids.

Uses: The seeds have a beneficial effect in ascariasis. The torrefied seeds are prescribed in the form of a powder or sugared cake. They are occasionally used fres.

763. *Leucas aspera* Spreng *(Lamiaceae)*

Vernacular Name: *San*: Dronapuspi; *Eng*: Thumbe; *Hin*: Chota halkkusa; *Kan*: Tumbe; *Mal*: Tumpa; *Tam*: Tumbai; *Tel:* Tummacettu.

Description: An erect or diffuse much branched herbaceous annual, 15-20 cm in height with hispid or scabrid quadrangular stems and branches; leaves sub-sessile, linear or linear-oblong or linear-lanceolate, obtuse, entire or crenate, pubescent upto 7.5 cm long and 1.25 cm broad; flowers pure white, small, in dense terminal or axillary whorls; fruits nutlets, 2.5 mm long, oblong,, brown, smooth, inner face angular and outer face rounded.

Habitate: Throughout India, as a weed on waste land and road sides upto 900 m.

Propagation: By seeds and vegetative method.

Parts Used: Leaves, flowers.

Chemical Consistuents: Alkaloid & Glucoside.

Uses: The leaves and flowers are acrid, thermogenic, carminative, digestive anthelmintic, anti-inflammatory, emmenagogue, sudorific antipyretic, expectorant, antibacterial and depurative. They are useful in colic, dyspepsia, verminosis, arthralgia, chronic skin eruption psoriasis, cough, dyspepsia, verminosis, arthralgia, chronic skin eruptions, psoriasis, cough and catarrh in children, amenorrhoea, dysmenorrhoea, intermittent fevers and ulcers.

The juice of the leaves is highly recommendable as an eyedrop in encephalopathy due to worm infestation in children and is useful as a nasa drop in catarrh and cephalalgia.

764. *Levisticum officinale* *(Apiaceae)*

Synonyms*: Ligusticum levisticum.*

Vernacular Name: *Eng:* Lovage.

Description: Perennial growing to 2 m. Has glossy, toothed compound leaves, greenish-yellow flowers, and tiny oval seeds.

Habitate: Lovage is found in southern Europe and south-western Asia. I thrives on sunny mountain slopes.

Propagation: By seeds and vegetative method.

Parts Used: Root, seeds and leaves.

Chemical Constituents: Lovage contains a volatile oil, coumarins, plant acids, beta-sitosterol, resins and gums. The phthalides are sedative and anticonvul*San*t.

Uses: Lovage is a warming and tonic herb for the digestive and respiratory systems. It treats indigestion, poor appetite, wind and colic, and bronchitis. Lovage is significantly diuretic and antimicrobial and is commonly taken for urinary tracts complaints. It also promotes menstruation and relieves period pain. Its warming nature improves poor circulation.

765. *Ligustrum lucidum* Ait. *(Oleaceae)*

Synonyms: *Ligustrum spicatum.* Hort.

Vernacular Name: *Eng:* Glossy privet, Chinese privet, white was tree, chinese was tree, shiny-leaved privet.

Khasi Hills: soh-pah-iet, dieng-soh-la-paier.

Description: An evergreen large shrub or tree, up to 10 m high; branchlets often lenticellate, glabrous. Leaves opposite, petioles 1-2 cm long, blade ovate to oval-lanceolate 6-12 cm long by 4-6 cm wide; apex acuminate or acute; base broadly coneate or rounded. Flowers in summer. Panicles terminal. Flowers white, fragrant, sessile. Calyx small, 4-toothed. Corolla campanulate, lobes 4. Stamens 2 on the corolla-tube; ovary superior, 2-celled, style longish, stigma bifid. Drupe 1 cm long, becomes black at mathrity, one-seeded. The crude drug is ovate, ellipsoidal or reniform, 6-8.5 mm long and 3.5-5.5 mm in diameter. The surface is dark-purple or greyish black, with many wrinkles. The drupe tastes bitter-sweet and slightly astringent.

Habitate: Mostly cultivated in China.

Propagation: By seeds and vegetative method.

Part Used: Fruit.

Chemical Constituents: N.A.

Uses: Vertigo; dizziness; tinnitus, premature greying of hair, tirendness in thinghs and knees. Decoction of bark and leaves prescribed as a sudorific. Berries used in rheumatism.

766. *Lilium brpwnii* F.E. Brown var. colchesteri Wilson *(Liliaceae)*

Vernacular Name: *Eng*: Brown's lily.

Description: Perennial herbaceouse plant, 0.5-1m high Bulb stout, white, leaves alternate, oblong-lanceolate, subsessile; margins entire. Flowers 3-5, funnel-shaped, white in terminal raceme. Capsule 3-celled. Seeds numerous, small.

Flowering period: May-July.

Habitate: Grows wild in savannas at an altitude of 1000m. or above.

Propagation: By vegetative method.

Part Used: Bulb.

Chemical Constituents: The bulbs contain proteins 4%, lipids 0.1% glucides 30%, vitamin C and colchiceine.

Uses: The bulbs are an effective remedy for dry cough or cough with consistent phlegm, haemoptysis, bronchitis, fever and neurasthenia. They are also diuretic and useful in oedema. In case of cough with ches pains and haemoptysis, they are commonly used fresh, in the form of expressed juice.

767. *Lilium lancifolium* Thunb. *(Liliaceae)*

Vernacular Name: *Eng*: Tiger lily.

Description: Perennial herb, with the bulb scaly. Stems unbranched, to 1-2 m, purplish, scabrous, cobwebby-hairy, with bulbils in leaf axils. Leaves alternate, many, broadly linear to laceolate, 5-18 cm long, 5-15 cm wide. Flowers 1-25 in a raceme, nodding, to 12 cm across, orange-red, spotted inside with purple-black; perianth funnelform, segments 6, strongly reflexed, each with a vassal nectar-bearing gland; stamens 6, anthers versatile. Fruit a 3-valved, loculicidal capsule, the margins of valves flat; seeds many, flat, in 2 rows in each cell.

Habitate: Woods in lowlands and mountains of Korea, Japan and China.

Propagation: By seeds and vegetative method.

Parts Used: Tuber.

Chemical Constituents: Liliumla-glucomannan, lilioside C, phenylpropanoids.

Uses: Anti-inflammatory. Used in cough, sore throat, palpitation & boils.

768. *Lilium polyphyllum* D. Don *(Liliaceae)*

Vernacular Name: *San*: Ksirakakoli; *Eng*: Ksheerakakoli; *Hin*: Ksirakakoli; *Kan*: Ksirakakoli; *Mal*: Ksirakakoli; *Tam*: Ksirakakoli; *Tel:* Ksirakakoli.

Description: A narrow bulbous herb upto a metre in height with few narrow subequal fleshy scales; leaves in whorls many nerved, narrowly lanceolate or linear, margins papilose; flowers 4-10, pendulous, fragrant, dull yellowish or greenish outside; white within, speckled with long purple streaks, in racemes, raised on the naked top of the stem; perianth recurved when fully expanded; fruit a capsule.

Habitate: Western temperate Himalayas, upto 3,600 m.

Propagation: By seeds and vegetative method.

Parts Used: Bulb.

Chemical Consistuents: Linalool, a-terpineol.

Uses: The bulbs are sweet, bitter, refrigerant, galactagogue, expectorant, aphrodisiac, diuretic, antipyretic, and tonic. They are useful in agalactia, cough, bronchitis, vitiated conditions of *pitta*, seminal weakness, strangury, burning sensation, hyperdipsia, intermittent fevers, haematemesis, rheumatalgia and general debility.

769. *Limnophila aromatica* (L.) Merr. *(Scrophulariaceae)*

Synonyms *Limnophila gratissima* Blume.

Vernacular Name: *San*: Amragandhah; *Hin*: Kutra; *Kan*: Mangannari; *Mal*: Mannanari; *Tam*: Mankainari.

Description: A much branched decumbent aromatic (odour of turpentine) herb, 30-50 cm in height, copiously rooting at the lower nodes; leaves sessile, opposite or in whorls of 3, linear-oblong or lanceolate sharply serrate; flowers purplish in axillary and terminal racemes, pedicels long slender and glandular, fruits small obovoid-oblong capsules covered by the striate calyx.

Habitate: Throughout India, upto 600 m in marshes, margins of ponds and back waters.

Propagation: By seeds and vegetative method.

Parts Used: Whole plant.

Chemical Consistuents: d-limonene, d-perillaldehyde.

Uses: The plant is sour, slight, bitter refrigerant emollient antiseptic, galactagogue, aperient, appetizer, digestive, carminative, anthelmintic, anti-inflammatory, diuretic, and febrifuge. It is useful in vitiated conditions of *pitta*, foul ulcers, agalactia, galactic impurities, anorexia, dyspepsia, helminthiasis, constipation, inflammations, strangury, fever and pharyngitis.

770. *Limonia acidissima* L. *(Rutaceae)*

Synonyms: *Feronia elephantum* Corr., *Feronia limonia*.

Vernacular Name: *San*: Kapitthah; *Eng*: Elephant, apple, Wood apple; *Hin*: Katbel, Kaith, Kavita; *Kan*: Bela; *Mal*: Vilarmaram, Vilavu; *Tam*: Vilankay maram; *Tel:* Velagapandu.

Description: A moderate sized to fairly large glabrous deciduous tree, armed with strong, straight, axillary spines, having a much branched dense crown of dark foliage and dark grey longitudinally furrowed rough wrinkled bark; leaves compound, imparipinnate, alternate, raachis narrowly winged, leaflets 3-7, obovate, crenulate, tip often notched, gland dotted; flowers small, frangrant, dull red, polygamous in lateral and terminal pubescent panicles; fruits globose, woody, rough, grey-coloured berries, seeds oblong, compressed, embedded in the pulp.

Habitate: Throughout India, in the hotter and drier parts upto 450 m.

Propagation: By seeds and vegetative method.

Parts Used: Bark, leaves, fruits, gum.

Chemical Consistuents: Moisture, protein, ether extr., mineral matter, fibre, carbohydrate, calcium and phosphorus, iron, riboflavin, vitamin C. wood apple is rich in mineral constituents especially calcium and phosphorus. It contains 3-5% pectin and forms an excellent materials for making jelly.

Uses: The bark is aromatic and cooling, and is useful in vitiated conditions of *pitta*. The leaves are aromatic, astringent, carminative, constipating, antiemetic, expectorant and cardiotonic. They are useful in gastropathy, anorexia, diarrhoea, vomiting, cough, bronchitis, hiccough, cardiac debility and vitiated conditions of *vata*. The unripe fruits are sour, aromatic, astringent, bitter, refrigerant, aromatic, anodyne, constipating, aphrodisiac, antiscorbutic, alexipharmic, cardiotonic, diuretic, vulnerary, expectorant, stomachic and antiemetic. They are useful in diarrhoea, dysentery, vomiting, hyperdipsia, hiccough, pharyngodynai, stomatitis, gingivitis, tumours, cough, asthma, consumption, ophthalmia, otalgia, cephalalgia, leucorrhoea, wounds and ulcers, anorexia, dyspepsia, cardiac debility, strangury and vitiated conditions of *vata* and *pitta*. The gum is demulcent and constipating, and is useful in diarrhoea, dysentery, gastropathy, haemorrhoids and diabetes.

771. *Linaria vulgaris* *(Scrophulariaceae)*

Vernacular Name: *Eng:* Common Toadflax.

Description: Upright perennial growing to about 50 cm. Has linear leaves and yellow double-lipped flowers with long spurs.

Habitate: Common toadflax is native to Europe and Asia, and is naturalized in North America. It flourishes along roadsides and on wasteground.

Propagation: By seeds and vegetative method.

Parts Used: Aerial parts.

Chemical Constituents: Common toadflax contains linarin, sterols, sugars, tannins and mucilage.

Uses: Rarely used today, common toadflax is primarily a herb for the liver and digestion. It is helpful in treating jaundice, chronic constipation and skin diseases. It may be applied externally to soothe sores, skin ulcers and haemorrhoids. It can also relieve inflammation of the eyes.

772. *Lindera strychnifolia* (sieb. Et Zucc.) Vill. *(Lauraceae)*

Vernacular Name: *Eng:* Combined spicebush.

Description: An aromatic evergreen shrub or small tree up to 5 m high. Root robust, ligneous, fusiform, dilated in parts, and with a light purplish-red external layer. Young branches covered with brownish pubescence. Leaves alternate, petiolate, oval-elliptical, often orbicular 3-7 cm long by 1.5-4 cm wide. Abruptly acuminate, coriaceous, 3-veined. Glossy above, glaucous and puberulous beneath. Flowers dioecious or polygamous. Fruit a black drupe.

Habitate: In thickets on exposed slopes in Japan China, Philippines.

Propagation: By seeds and vegetative method.

Part Used: Root tubers.

Chemical Constituents: N.A.

Uses: Chest, gastric or abdominal pains, dysmennorrhea, hernia pain, rheumatic bone and joint pains; pain from external injuries.

773. *Linum usitatissimum* L. *(Linaceae)*

Vernacular Name: *San*: Atasi, *Eng*: Linsed, Flax plant, *Hin*: Alsi, Tisi, *Kan*: Alasibija, *Mal*: Akasi, Cerucana, Kayavu, *Tam*: Alivirai, *Tel:* Avisi.

Description: An annual herb, 60-120 cm high; stems solitary of few, corymbosely branched; branches ascending towards the apex; leaves upto 3.8 cm long, linear-lanceolate, flowers small, blue, bluish violet or white in terminal panicles; fruits capsular with 5-cells; seeds compressed, ellipsoid, smooth, dark brown, shiny.

Habitate: Cultivated throughout India, occasionally found run wild.

Propagation: By seeds and vegetative method.

Parts Used: Flowers, seeds, oil.

Chemical Consistuents: Analysis of a cample of Indian linseed gave the following values; moisture, protein, fatty oil, carbohydrates, fibre, mineral mater, calcium and phosphorus, iron the seeds caontin; carotene, thiamine, riboflavin, niacin, pantothenic acid choline and vitamin E.

Uses: The flowers are considered as cardiotonic. The seeds are sweet, bitter, acrid, emollient, thermogenic, expectorant and diuretic. It is astringent after roasting. The whoel seed is prescribed as a laxative. The mucilaginous infusion–'Linseed tea'–is used internally as a demulcent in coughs, catarrh and bronchial affections, ureteritis, gonorrhoea and diarrhoea. The mucilage is dropped into the eye in irritable conditions of the conjunctiva. Crushed linseed is applied in the form of poultice for the relief of local inflammations, ulcers, boils and carbuncles. In veterinary practice linseed infusion is used as a demulcent drink for horses, cattle and occasionally for small animals. Crushed linseed is used as a poultice. The surface of the poultice is smeared with oil to prevent its adhering to the skin. Linseed oil is recommended mainly for external application. It is a common base for embrocations and liniments. Linseed oil has laxative properties but is seldom employed due to its unpleasant taste. In veterinary practice linseed oil is employed as a laxative for horses and cattle.

774. *Lippia citriodora* *(Verbenaceae)*

Synonyms: *Aloysia triphylla.*

Vernacular Name: *Eng:* Lemon Verbena.

Description: Deciduous shrub growing to 2 m. Has strongly scented lance-shaped leaves and clusters of tubular, pale green to mauve flowers.

Habitate: Lemon verbena is native to South America. It is cultivated in temperate climates as an aromatic, ornamental plant and for its leaves, which are used to make herbal tea.

Propagation: By seeds and vegetative method.

Parts Used: Leaves.

Chemical Constituents: Lemon verbena contains a volatile oil, mucilage, tannins and flavonoids.

Uses: An undervalued medicinal herb, lemon verbena shares qualities with lemon balm. Both herbs contain a strong lemon-scented volatile oil that has claming and digestive properties. Lemon verbena has a gentle sedative action and has a reputation for soothing abdominal discomfort. Its tonic effect on the nervous system is less pronounced than that of lemon balm, but it nonetheless helps to lift the spirits and counter depression.

775. *Liquidambar formosana* Hance *(Hamamelidaceae)*

Vernacular Name: *Eng:* Gragrant maple.

Description: A tree 40 m high. Leaves alternate, palmate; lobes 3-5, acuminate, base cordate or truncate, 8-12 wide; petiole lengthy. Inflorescence monoecious; March. Fruit spherical, 3 cm in diameter hispid and with numerous holes; August-September. Surface of the dried fruit is brownish.

Habitate: At forest edges, on hillsides or in spares woods and shrubby areas near villages; mostly cultivated in gardens in South China, Japan, Laos and Viet Nam.

Propagation: By seeds and vegetative method.

Part Used: Fruit.

Chemical Constituents: N.A.

Uses: Deficient lactation, Irregular menstruation, rheumatic joint pains, Lumbago, dysuria, urticaria.

776. *Liquidamber orientalis* Mill. *(Hamamelidaceae)*

Vernacular Name: *San*: Sihlakah, Turuskah; *Eng*: Oriental sweet-gum, Liquid amber, Asiatic storax; *Hin*: Silaras; *Kan*: Kundurka; *Mal*: Arabikkunturukkam, Turuskam; *Tam*: Neri–arisippal; *Tel:* Silarasu.

Description: A medium sized much branched tree, 6-12 m or more in height; leaves palmately 5-lobed; flowers yellow, monoecious in globular heads. The 'balsam' exuded from the inner bark is purified by boiling with water. It is dark brown in colour and is of semi-solid consistency. It is transparent in thin layers and possesses an agreeable balsamic odour and taste.

Habitate: In Asia Minor.

Propagation: By seeds and vegetative method.

Parts Used: Balsam.

Chemical Consistuents: Alcoholic resin, named storesin occurring free and as cinnamic ester; it contains also free cinnamic acid, cinnamyl cinnamate or styracine, phenylpropyl cinnamate and small amounts of ethyl cinnamate, benzyl cinnamate, styrene, a pleasant smelling liquid probably styrocamphene, and traces of vanillin. Phenylpropyl cinnamyl alcohols and cinnamic acid.

Uses: The balsam is bitter, acrid, sweet, aromatic, thermogenic, emollient, deodorant, antibacterial, vulnerary, expectorant, depurative, anodyne, diuretic, aphrodisiac, emmenagogue, constipating, febrifuge and tonic. It is useful in foul ulcers and wounds, leprosy, skin diseases, pruritus, vitiated conditions of *vata*, inflammations, chronic cough, bronchitis, consumption, strangury, anenorrhoea, diarrhoea, fever and general debility.

777. *Liriope platyphylla* Wang et Tang *(Liliaceae)*

Vernacular Name: *Eng*: Lilyturf.

Description: Evergreen, perennial herb. Plants tufted with thick, fasciculate rhizomes; leaves grasslike, deep-green, clustered from the base, 30-50 cm long, 8-12 mm wide, 11-15 nerved; scape 30-50 cm long; flowers pale violet, in axillary fascicles arranged in terminal spikes, few to several in a group, pedicels 2-5 mm long, perianth-segments 6, separate, stamens 6, ovary superior; fruit berrylike, black, seed 1 or 2, fleshy.

Habitate: Shaded areas in mountains woods.

Propagation: By Seeds.

Parts Used: Tuber.

Chemical Constituents: Saponins: ophiogonins A, B, C, D, etc. Monoterpenoids: borneol derivative.

Uses: Anti-inflammatory, antiallergic. Used as tonic, sputum remedy, strengthening stamina.

778. *Liriosma ovata* *(Oleaceae)*

Vernacular Name: *Eng:* Muira puama.

Description: Tree growing to 15 m with a grey trunk, dark brown leaves, white flowers and orange-yellow fruits.

Habitate: Muira puama is native to Brazilian rainforests, especially the Rao Negro and Amazonas regions.

Propagation: By seeds and vegetative method.

Parts Used: Root, bark, wood.

Chemical Constituents: Muria puama contains esters and plant sterols.

Uses: Muira puama has long been used by indigenous Amazonians as a tonic and aphrodisiac. It is still considered a valuable remedy for impotence. The bark is strongly astringent and may be employed as a gargle for sore throats and taken in the form of an infusion in order to treat diarrhoea and dysentery.

779. *Lobelia chinensis* Lour. *(Lobeliaceae)*

Vernacular Name: *Eng:* Chinese lobelia.

Description: A perennial procumbent herb, 5-15 cm high, glabrous, with milky latex, leaves alternate, linear or lanceolate, 1.2-2.5 cm long by 2.5-6 mm side, remotely toothed or sub-entire, sessile, often bifarous. Flowers in summer, pedicels axillary, as long as or longer than the leaves; one-flowered. Capsule 4-6 mm long, base acute. Seeds numerous, minute, ellipsoidal, slightly compressed.

Habitate: On damp fields and on the edge of ditches in China.

Propagation: By seeds and vegetative method.

Part Used: Whole plant.

Chemical Constituents: N.A.

Uses: Snake bites; boils, ascites from cirrhosis and schistosomiasis; nephritic oedema, purulent infections, enteritis; diarrhoea.

780. *Lobelia inflata* L. *(Lobeliaceae)*

Vernacular Name: *Eng:* Indian Wild tobacco, Bladder podded lobelia.

Description: An annual or biennial herb up to 60 cm. high. Stem winged, irregularly furrowed yellowish-green pubescent, branched. Leaves alternate, ovate or oblong with serrate denticulate margin, each tooth with a yellowish brown glandular projection with water pores; the lower short petioled, the upper sessile. Inflorescence is a terminal raceme of small pale-blue, short pedicelled flowers. Calyx tube with 5-subulate teeth; corolla, bluish tubular, 5 parted, upper 2-lobed portion cleft near the base; Stamens with anthers united above into a curved tube. Pedicels bracteolate at the base. Fruit a bladdery, ovoid or ellipsoidal, 2-celled capsule containing numerous small oblong coarsely reticulate, brown seeds.

Habitate: U.S.A. & Canada.

Propagation: By seeds and vegetative method.

Parts Used: Whole plant excluding roots.

Chemical Constituents: Alkaloids viz. Lobeline, Lobelanine, Lobelanidine, Norlobelanine, Lelobanidine, Lobinine, Lobelanin, Norlobelanidine, Norlelobanidine; Glycosidelobelacrin, Chelidonic acid, Isolobenine, Lobinanidine, di-lelobanidine, l-lelobanidine I & II.

Uses: For complaints of gastric derangement, extreme nausea, vomiting, morning sickness, spasmodic asthma, pertussis, dyspnoea, threatening suffocation. Dyspnoea with constriction of middle of chest, worse by exertion. Deep seated pain at the base of heart. Nausea. With profuse cold sweet and marked prostration, but with profuse salivation and good appetitie. Extreme sensitiveness of sacrum which cannot bear slightest touch even of soft pillow & therefore avoids touch with clothes. Bad effect of excessive tea & tobacco. Catarrhal jaundice. Urine deep red coloured with sediments.

781. *Lobelia syphilitica* L. *(Lobeliaceae)*

Synonyms: *Labelia glandulosa* Dennis., *Lobelia reflexa* Stokes., *Lobelia speciosa* Sweet.

Vernacular Name: *Eng:* Blue cardinal flower.

Description: A deciduous, perennial herb with stem stout, up to 1.5 m. in height, angular, glabrous or sparsely hirsuite, leaves finely serrate, alternate, unequally serrate, thin, narrowly oblong or elliptic, lanceolate or oblancealate, usually 8-12 cm. long, acuminate to obtuse, narrowed to a sessile base, glabrous to hirsutus. Flower light blue, solitary, axillary, crowded in a dense raceme or a long spike, bracteolate above the middle of pedicel. Lower bracts lanceolate foliaceous, up to 5 cm. long, upper ones reduced, sepals entire lanceolate to ovate, 8-12 mm. long with foliaceous auricle; pedicels ascending, 4-12 mm. long, smooth to hirsute.

Habitate: Western U.S.A. and Canada. Common in low grounds and marshy areas.

Propagation: By seeds and vegetative method.

Parts Used: Whole plant.

Chemical Constituents: Lobeline, Lobelanidine, Lobelamine.

Uses: For complaints of excessive sneezing influenza, involving posterior nares, palate & fauces. Great depression. Great oppression in lower part of the chest because of suffocation feeling. Pain in chest under short ribs of left side. Hecking dry cough with aching pain at the root of nose. Eustachian catarrh. Pain over eyes. Pain and flatulence in bowels followed by copious watery stool with tenesmus & soreness of anus.

782. *Lodoicea maldivica* (Poir.) Pers. *(Arecaceae)*

Synonyms: *Lodoicea seychellarum.*

Vernacular Name: *San*: Arkaragah, Agnijarah, abdhinarikelah; *Eng*: Double coconut palm, Sea coconut palm; *Hin*: Darya-ka-nariyal, Dariya-I-nariyal; *Kan*: Kadalutengu; *Mal*: Aklarittenna, Katalttenna; *Tam*: Kadalttengai; *Tel:* Samudraputenkaya.

Description: A tall palm, 12-30 m high, with smooth annulated trunk bearing a crown of large fan-shaped leaves. The palm is dioecious and its fruits are large weighing 11-27 kg, one seeded, deeply bilobed and bony. The shell is thick and black.

Habitate: In Seychelles Islands.

Propagation: By seeds and vegetative method.

Parts Used: Husk, endosperm.

Chemical Consistuents: N.A.

Uses: A decoction of the fibrous husk as well as the kernel is reported to reduce the quantity of sugar in urine in diabetes mellitus. The kernel is sweet, acrid, refrigerant, digestive, carminative, febrifuge and tonic. It is useful in vitiated conditions of *vata* and *kapha*, cholera, hyperdipsia, oedema, acute diarrhoea, colic and also as an antidote in opium and aconite poisoning. It is a good cardiotonic. The water of the green fruit and its kernel are antacid and are useful in vitiated conditions of *pitta.*

783. *Lonicera japonca* Thunb. *(Caprifoliaceae)*

Vernacular Name: *Eng:* Japanese honeysuckle.

Description: A twining evergreen plant, pubescent. Stems brownish-red. Leaves opposite, tomentose. Flowers in axillary pedunculate pairs, often crosded at the end of branchlets, fragrant, white when blooming, then changing to yellow. Berry globose, black when ripe.

Habitate: Grows wild in the mountains and is cultivated for ornament.

Propagation: By seeds and vegetative method.

Part Used: Whole plant.

Chemical Constituents: The whole plant contains tannins, saponins, luteolin, inositol and carotenoid: cryptoxanthin.

Uses: The leaf-bearing stem is antibacterial and antiallergic. It is recommended in the treatment of boils, impetigo, urticaria, allergic rhinitis, feber, malaria, erythema, measles, diarrhoea, dysentery, syphilis, rheumatism and lichen tropicus.

784. *Lophatherum gracile* Brongn. *(Poaceae)*

Vernacular Name: *Eng:* Common lophaterum.

Description: A perennial herb. Stem 40-100 cm. High. Ascending from a branched woody rootstock. Leaves alternate, petioled or sessile, broadly lanceolate, 5-30 cm long by 2-35 cm wide, apex acuminate, base subrounded or cuneate, margin entire, nerves tessellate. Spikelets about 1 cm long, including the short awns of the colsely imbricate upper empty glumes, which form the apex of the tightly rolled flowering glumes.

Habitate: Grows plentifully on waste land and slopes, usually in shady and damp places in China.

Propagation: By seeds and vegetative method.

Part Used: Whole plant.

Chemical Constituents: N.A.

Uses: Hyperpyrezia; anexiety; thirst, aphathae; swelling of the gums; yellowish or reddish urine, Urethritis; ardour urinae.

785. *Lophophora williamsii* *(Cactaceae)*

Vernacular Name: *Eng:* Peyote, Mescal.

Description: Cactus growing to 5 cm. Has a squat grey-green body with tufted hairs, and pink or white flowers.

Habitate: Peyote is native to northern Mexico and the south-western US.

Propagation: By Root suckers.

Parts Used: Whole plant.

Chemical Constituents: Peyote contains alkaloids, principally mescaline, which is a powerful hallucinogen.

Uses: Peyote is a shamanistic plant, taken in Native American rituals to deepen spiritual understanding. It plays an important part in the emotional and mental state of the community. It is also used to treat fevers, as a painkiller for rheumatism and to treat paralysis. It is applied as a poultice for fractures, wounds and snake bite. Peyote is also used induce vomiting.

786. *Ludwigia adscendens* (L.) Hara *(Onagraceae)*

Vernacular Name: *Eng:* Floating Malayan willow-herb.

Description: Aquatic herb, creeping by means of ovate, white, porous floats, stems slender, rooting at the nodes. Leaves alternate, oval, base long, apex round, flowers white, solitary in the axil of the leaves. Capsule long, villous. Seeds numerous.

Habitate: A common weed found everywhere in rice-fields, ponds and swamps.

Propagation: By seeds and vegetative method.

Part Used: Whole plant.

Chemical Constituents: N.A.

Uses: The entire plant, except the roots, is recommended as an antibacterial and diuretic in cases of feber, cystitis, dysuria, oliguria, haematuria, chyluria, haematochyluria and haemorrhagic dysentery. External application of po9ultices made of pounded fresh plant matter is prescribed against snake-bite, burns, impetigo and diseases of the scalp.

787. *Ludwigia octovalvis* (Jacq.) Raven *(Onagraceae)*

Synonyms: *Sessiliflora* (Michli) Raven, *Jussiaea suffruticosa* Linn.

Vernacular Name: *Eng*: Primrose willow, *Hin*: Banlumga, *Kan*: Bavakula, Kauakula, *Mal*: Kattukarayampu, *San*: Bhulavangah, *Tam*: Kattukkirampu, *Tel:* Nirubaccala.

Description: An erect much branched perennial suffrutiocose under shrub upto 1.2 m in height with stiff, terete, striate branches; leaves alternate, nearly sessile, broadly elliptic to lanceolate, acute or more or less woolly, main nerves numerous, flowers yellow, tetramerous, axillary and solitary; fruits subquadrangular, truncate, 8-ribbed capsules, breaking up between the ribs clove-like in appearance, seeds numerous, minute, ovoid.

Habitate: Throughout India, in moist localities in the palms.

Propagation: By seeds and vegetative method.

Parts Used: Whole plant.

Chemical Consistuents: N.A.

Uses: The plant is astringent, carminative, vermifuge, laxative, diuretic, anti-inflammatory, expectorant and febrifuge. It is useful in dyspepsia, verminosis, flatulence, strangury, dropsy, cough, asthma, vitiated conditions of *vata*, neuropathy, diarrhoea, dysentery, cephalalgia, orchitis, leucorrhoea, cervical adenitis, and fever.

788. *Luffa acutangula* (L.) Roxb. *(Cucurbitaceae)*

Vernacular Name: *San*: Dhamargavah, Svadukosataki, *Eng*: Ridged gourd, Ribbed gourd, *Hin*: Tori, Kali tori, *Kan*: Kadupadagila, *Mal*: Piccil, Piccinna, *Tam*: Pikangai, Pirkkangai, *Tel:* Birakaya.

Description: A large monoecious climber with 5-angled glabrous stems and 3-fid tendrils; leaves orbicular-cordate palmately 5-7 lobed, scabrid on both sides, veins and veinlets prominent beneath; flowers yellow, males in 12-20 flowered axillary racemes, female flowers solitary, in the axils as the males, ovary strongly ribbed; fruits oblong-clavate with 10-sharp oblong, much compressed, not winged.

Habitate: Cultivated throughout India.

Propagation: By seeds and vegetative method.

Parts Used: Leaves, fruits, seeds.

Chemical Consistuents: Arginine, glycine, threonine, glutamic acid, leucines, serine, alanine, γ-amino butyric acid and pipecolic acid, saturated, oleic, linoleic.

Uses: The leaves are used in splenitis, haemorrhoids, leprosy, granular-conjunctivitis and ringworm. Fruits are demulcent, diuretic, tonic and nutritive, and are used as excellent vegetable. The seeds are bitter, emetic, expectorant and purgative, and are useful in dematopathy.

789. *Luffa cylindrica* (L.) M. Roem. *(Cucurbitaceae)*

Synonyms: *Luffa aegyptiaca* Mill.

Vernacular Name: *San*: Mahakosataki; *Eng*: Sponge gourd, Vegetable sponge, Wash sponge; *Hin*: Ghiya tori; *Kan*: Tuppahire; *Mal*: Kattupiccil, Puttilpiram, Kattupiram, Perumpiram; *Tam*: Mulukkupperakkai; *Tel:* Netibirakaya.

Description: A large monoecious number climber with stout 5-angled twisted nearly glabrous stems; leaves orbicular-reniform, palmately 5-lobed, scabrous and punctate, glabrous except the pubescent nerves beneath; male flowers in axillary racemes, crowded at the top, female flowers solitary, usually from the same axils as the lames; fruits large, cylindric, smooth, 12.5-30 cm long, 10-ribbed, seeds black or grey, much compressed, narrowly winged smooth on sides.

Habitate: Throughout India, wild in waste lands especially along the coastal areas and also cultivated.

Propagation: By seeds and vegetative method.

Parts Used: Fruits, seeds.

Chemical Consistuents: Lysine, arginine, aspartic acid, glycine, threonine, glutaqmic acid, alanine, tryptophan, phenylalnine and leucines palmitic, stearic, oleic, linoleic.

Uses: The fruits are diuretic, emollient, depurative, laxative, expectorant, tonic, carminative, anthelmintic and galactagogue. They are useful in vitiated conditions of *pitta*, splenopathy, leprosy, haemorrhoids, fever, haematuria, syphilis, bronchitis, and tumours. The seeds are bitter, emetic and cathartic, and are useful in dermatopathy.

790. *Lycium barbarum* L. *(Solanaceae)*

Vernacular Name: *Eng:* Barbary boxthorn, common matrimoney-vine, duke of argyll's tea-tree.

Description: A spinous shrub up to 3 m high, branches white or grey, armed with sharp conical spines which sometimes lengthen and bear leaves an flowers. Leaves berry variable, sometimes solitary, oblong-lanceolate, reaching 4.5 cm by 6 mm. More commonly in fascicles and oblong spatulate or linear, obtuse, attenuated into a short petiole, glabrous or nearly so. Flowers solitary or in fascicles of 2-5; pedicels filiform, 6-13 mm long. Berry bright red, 1-2 cm long and 6 m in diameter, seated on the slightly enlarged and often deformed calyx. Seeds 2.5 mm in diameter, discoid or subreniform, embedded in a soft glutinous viscid pulp very minutely pitted, orange-yellow.

Habitate: On slopes, cultivated or wild in China, Japan and Soviet Union.

Propagation: By seeds and vegetative method.

Part Used: Fruit and root bark.

Chemical Constituents: N.A.

Uses: Seminal emissions, sores on the lower part of the body due to kidney deficiency, vertigo; emblyopia, root bark, low fever due to pulmonary tuberculosis. Cough.

791. *Lycium Chinese* Mill. *(Solanaceae)*

Vernacular Name: *Eng:* Chinese box-thorn, Chinese desert thorn, Chinese wolfberry, Chinese matrimony vine.

Description: Small shrub, 0.5–am. High; branches spinulous. Leaves alternate or in fascicles of 3-5, short-petioledl margins entire. Flowers small, pale-violet, solitary or fascicled in the axil of the leaves. Berry ovoid, bright red when ripe. Seeds numerous, small.

Habitate: Largely cultivated fro its leaves, eeaten as a begetable; the roots and seeds are medicinal.

Propagation: By seeds and vegetative method.

Part Used: Ripe fruit and root-bark.

Chemical Constituents: The berries contains salts of Ca, Fe, NH4; P vitamin C, nicotinic acid, carotene; amino acids (lysine, choline, betaine); lapids, proteins and hycrocyanic acid. The root-bark yields saponins 1.07%, alkaloids 0.08%.

Uses: The fruit is used in treating general debility, impotence, serrmatorrhoea, lumbago, amblyopia, vertigo and diabetes mellitus. It also has rejuvenating proterties. The root-bark is effective for haemoptysis, night sweats and haematuria.

792. *Lycopersicon esculentum* Mill. *(Solanaceae)*

Synonyms: *Lycopersicon lycopersicum* (Linn.) Karsten.

Vernacular Name: *San*: Raktamaci; *Eng*: Tomato; *Hin*: *Tam*atar; *Kan*: Capparabadane; *Mal*: Takkali; *Tam*: Takkali; *Tel:* Simavanga.

Description: An unarmed herbaceous spreading pubescent annual; leaves unevenly pinnate, curled, pubescent throughout, lobes acute or acuminate, veins prominent below; flowers yellow in extra axillary cymes; fruits globose, villous when young, glabrous and shining when mature, red or yellowish red on ripening seeds many on fleshy palcentum, flat, kidney shaped.

Habitate: Throughout India, cultivated.

Propagation: By seeds and vegetative method.

Parts Used: Fruits.

Chemical Consisituents: Carotenoids, Lycopene, Carotene, Xanthophylls, Xanthophylls Etser.

Uses: The fruits are sweet, emollient, carminative, digestive, aperient, haematinic, depurative, intestinal antiseptic, liver and kidney stimulant and tonic. They are useful in atomic dyspepsia, anorexia, flatulence, constipation, asthma, bronchitis, dermatopathy, ulcerative stomatitis, hepatopathy, nephropathy and general debility.

793. *Lycopodium clavatum* *(Lycopodiaceae)*

Vernacular Name: *Eng:* Club moss.

Description: Creeping evergreen moss growing to 12 cm. Has numerous straggling branchlets covered with bright green linear leaves, and scaly spikes bearing yellow spores.

Habitate: Club moss is found throughout regions of the northern hemisphere. It is common on mountains and in moorland. The plant is gathered in summer.

Propagation: By Seeds and vegetative method.

Parts Used: Moss, spores.

Chemical Constituents: Club moss contains about 0.1-0.2% alkaloids, polyphenols, flavonoids and triterpenes.

Uses: Club moss is diuretic, sedative and antispasmodic, and it is particularly useful for treating chronic urinary complaints. The herb may also be taken for indigestion and gastritis. The spores may be applied to the skin to relieve and protect itchy or irritated areas.

794. *Lycopus lucidus* Turcz *(Lamiaceae)*

Vernacular Name: *Eng:* Shiny bugleweed; wastern water-hourhound.

Description: An erect perennial herb, 40-100 cm high. Rhizome horizontal, thick fleshy, white. Stem usually simple, 4-sided, green or purplish; hairy clusters often grow on the nodes. Leaves oppositel subsessile; blade lanceolate, 4.5-11 cm long by 8-35 mm wide; tip acuminate; margin coarsely toothed, densely puncuate underneath, July-august. Flowers small, in dense axillary whorls. Nutlets 4, smooth, compressed, dull-brown.

Habitate: Grows in damp places on wasteground or in tussocks along streams in East Asia, Northwest America.

Propagation: By seeds and vegetative method.

Part Used: Aerial parts.

Chemical Constituents: N.A.

Uses: Amenorrhoea; irregular menstruation, postpartum haematoma, oedema, injuries.

795. *Lycopus virginicus* *(Lamiaceae)*

Vernacular Name: *Eng:* Bugleweed.

Description: Perennial herb growing to 60 cm. Has a square stem, lance-shaped leaves and whorls of whitish flowers.

Habitate: Bugleweed is common throughout most of North America, thriving close to water. It is harvested in summer when in flower.

Propagation: By seeds and vegetative method.

Parts Used: Aerial parts.

Chemical Constituents: Bugleweed contains phenolic acids.

Uses: Bugleweed has sedative properties and today the herb is principally prescribed to treat an overactive thyroid gland and the racing heartbeat that often accompanies this condition. Bugleweed is also considered an aromatic and tonic astringent that reduces the production of catarrh.

796. *Lysimachia vulgaris* *(Primulaceae)*

Vernacular Name: *Eng:* Yellow loosestrife.

Description: Attractive perennial growing to 1 m with whorls of broadly lance-shaped leaves and bright yellow flowers.

Habitate: Native to Europe, yellow loosestrife commonly grows in damp hedgerows and near water. It is also cultivated as a garden plant. It is gathered when in flower in summer.

Propagation: By seeds and vegetative method.

Parts Used: Aerial part.

Chemical Constituents: Yellow loosestrife contains a benzoquinone, saponins, flavonoids and tannisn.

Uses: An astringent herb, yellow loosestrife is principally used to treat gastro-intestinal conditions such as diarrhoea and dysentery, to stop internal and external bleeding, and to cleanse wounds. It makes a serviceable mouthwash for sore gums and mouth ulcers, and may be used to treat nosebleeds. Yellow loosestrife has also been taken as an expectorant.

797. *Lythrum salicaria* *(Lythraceae)*

Vernacular Name: *Eng:* Purple loosestrife.

Description: Attractive perennial growing to about 1.5 m. Has straight red stems, pointed lance-shaped leaves and spikes of brilliant purple flowers.

Habitate: Purple loosestrife is native to Europe but well established in the wild in North America. It thrives in marshes and along rivers and streams, to altitudes of 1,000 m. It is gathered when in flower in summer.

Propagation: By seeds and vegetative method.

Parts Used: Aerial parts.

Chemical Constituents: Purple loosestrife contains salicarin, a glycoside, tannins, a volatile oil, mucilage and plant sterols.

Uses: The astringent purple loosestrife is mainly employed as a treatment for diarrhoea and dysentery. It can be safely taken by people of all ages; some herbalists recommend it to help arrest diarrhoea in breast-feeding babies. The herb may also be used to treat heavy periods and for inter-menstrual bleeding. Externally, it is applied as poultice or lotion to wounds, leg ulcers and eczema, and used to treat excess vaginal discharge and vaginal itching. Purple loosestrife is now little used to treat eye problems, but, as Culpeper's experience suggests, the herb could be worth further investigation as a remedy for disorders of the eyes and vision.

798. *Maclura cochinchinesis* (Lour.) Corner *(Moraceae)*

Description: Spreading shrub; bark grey, spotted with white, Stems and branches with incurved spines. Leaves alternate, shining green above. Flowers dioecious, pale-yellow; the male long-pedicelled in a short raceme, the female sessile in a dense axillary head. **Fruit:** a syncarp.

Habitate: Grows wild in the hills and mountains and on roadsides.

Propagation: By seeds and vegetative method.

Part Used: Roots and leaves.

Chemical Constituents: The roots and leaves contain flabonoids.

Uses: The fresh leaves, stripped of their petioles and finely pounded, or a decoction of leaves, are used in poultices for the healing of wounds of the soft parts. For penetrating wounds, poultices are applied on both sides and coverd with a dressing. Poultices and dressings are changed once a day. The roots are effective in rheumatism, oedema, blood stasis, dysmenorrhoea and contusions.

799. *Macrotyloma uniflorum* (Lam.) Verdc. *(Fabaceae)*

Synonyms: *Dolichos biflorus* Linn.

Vernacular Name: *San*: Kulatthah, *Eng*: Horse gram, *Hin*: Kultthi, *Kan*: Huruli, *Mal*: Mutira, *Tam*: Kollu, *Tel:* Ulavalu.

Description: A much branched suberect or trailing annual, leaves trifoliate, leaflets lanceolate or oblong, entire, membranous; flowers yellow, 1-3 in the axils of the leaves, one at the base and two placed laterally; fruits sword-shaped, compressed pods about 5 cm long, tipped with the persistent style, seeds 5-6 compressed reniform, usually reddish brown.

Habitate: Cultivated throughout India.

Propagation: By seeds and vegetative method.

Parts Used: Seeds.

Chemical Consistuents: The seeds contain several common phytosterols including 24-methylene-25methylcholesterol and 24α-ethyl-5α-cholest-9-en-3β-ol.

Uses: The seeds are bitter, acrid, thermogenic, anthelmintic, astringent, diaphoretic, diuretic, emmenagogue, expectorant, febrifuge, ophthalmic and tonic. They are useful in haemorrhoids tumours, bronchitis, cardiopathy, nephrolithiasis, urolithiasis, splenomegaly, asthma, strangury, hiccough, ophthalmopathy, verminosis and vitiated conditions of *vata*.

800. *Madhuca indica* (Koenig) Macbride *(Sapotaceae)*

Synonyms: *Madhuca longifolia* Koenig,.

Vernacular Name: *San*: Madhukah; *Eng*: Butter tree, Mahuva; *Hin*: Mahva, Mohva; *Kan*: Erappe; *Mal*: lippa, lrippa; *Tam*: lluppai; *Tel:* lppa.

Description: A large evergreen tree with a dense spreading crown with dark grey or brownish scaly bark leaves thin, clustered near the ends of branches upto 18 cm long, 4 cm broad with slender petioles and 12-15 pairs of main nerves; flowers pale yellow and fleshy appearing in dense clusters near the ends of branches, corolla tubular, fleshy, pale yellow, aromatic and caduceus; fruits ovoid berries, yellow when ripe.

Habitate: In the forests of Karnataka and Kerala, M.P and Rajasthan.

Propagation: By seeds and vegetative method.

Parts Used: Bark, heart-wood, flowers, fruits, seeds.

Chemical Consistuents: Myristic, Palmitic, Stearic, Arachidic, Oleic, Linoleic.

Uses: The bark is sweet, bitter astringent and emollient, and is good for inflammations, sprains and pruritus. The heart-wood is recommended for epilepsy and alleviates *vata* and *pitta*. Flowers are stimulant, diuretic, sweet, refrigerant and anthelmintic, and are useful in strangury, verminosis, haemoptysis and hepatopathy and gastropathy especially in children. The fruits are sweet, refrigerant, aphrodisiac and tonic, and are useful in dipsia, bronchitis, consumption. The oil obtained from the seed-Mahua oil-is emollient and laxative, and is useful in dermatopathy, rheumatism, cephalagia, and haemorrhoids.

801. *Madhuca neriifolia* (Moon) H. J. Lam *(Sapotaceae)*

Synonyms: *Bassia malabarica* Bedd.

Vernacular Name: *Kan*: Hole hippe, Neeru hippe, *Mal*: Attu illuppa, *Tam*: Aathu ilupai.

Description: A medium sized evergreen tree, 7-20 m tall and about 1 m girth. *Bark* dark brown, about 8 mm thick, rough, knotty, oozing milky and sticky juice when bruised. *Blaze* pinkish white. *Wood* dark red, hard. *Leaves* alternate, crowded at the end of angular branchlets, linear-oblong or oblanceolate, 8-22 x 3-6 cm, base wedge-shaped, apex acute to rounded, margin entire, leathery, hairless, shining, with distinct stalk; lateral nerves 15-25 pairs. *Flowers* bisexual, in axillary clusters, dull white, fragrant, about 1.5 cm across, with distinct stalks. *Berries* egg-shaped, fleshy, about 3 x 1.5 cm, smooth, hairless. *Seeds* 1-2, ellipsoid, compressed, shiny, brown.

Habitate: Frequent in the evergreen and semi-evergreen forests, along the streams and banks of rivers.

Propagation: By seeds and vegetative method.

Parts Used: Seeds, Flowers.

Chemical Constituents: N.A.

Uses: Heartwood decoction is used for the treatment of ulcers. Flowers soaked in water used for treatment of kidney complaints.

802. *Magnolia officinalis* Rehd et wills. *(Magnoliaceae)*

Vernacular Name: *Eng:* Officinal magnolia.

Description: A deciduous tree, large, upto 22 m high. Bark smooth, light rusty-ash colour and aromatic. Branchlets light-free or yellowish. Leaves very large, elliptic-obovate, up to 35 cm long and 17-18 cm wide. Flowers large, fragrant, in may; creamy-white. Fruit cones 10-12 cm in length. Seeds single.

Habitate: In mountains in China.

Propagation: By seeds and vegetative method.

Part Used: Bark.

Chemical Constituents: N.A.

Uses: Sensation of fullness in the chest and abdomen; indigestion, diarrhoea, cough and sputum.

803. *Majorana hortensis* Moench. *(Lamiaceae)*

Synonyms: *Origanum majorana* Linn.

Vernacular Name: *Eng:* Sweet majoram; *Hin:* Murwa; *Beng*: Murru; *Tam:* Marru, maruvu; *Kan:* Maruga; *Mal:* Maruvamu.

Description: An aromatic, branched perennial, 30-60 cm. high; leaves oblong-ovate; flowers small, whitish or purplish, in terminal clusters; seeds minute, oval, dark brown.

Habitate: Commonly grown in Indian gardens.

Propagation: By seeds and vegetative method.

Part Used: Leaves.

Chemical Constituents: The major constituents of the oil are carvacol, a-terpinene, linalool, geraniol, p-cymene and thymol.

Uses: Marjoram leaves are used for flavouring processed meat products, soups, salads, dressings for stews, vegetables, cheese and poultry dishes. Sweet marjoram oil is used in high-grade flavour preparations and in liqueur industries.

804. *Malaxis acuminata* D. Don *(Orchidaceae)*

Synonyms: *Microstylis wallichi* Lindl.

Vernacular Name: *San*: Jivakah, *Eng*: Jeevak, *Hin*: Jivak, *Kan*: Jivaka, *Mal*: Jivakam, *Tam*: Jivakam, *Tel:* Jivakamu.

Description: A short stemmed terrestrial herb upto 30 cm in height with more or less pseudo bulb at the base and fibrous roots, new plant arising from the side of the mother plant which is decaying; leaves simple, 3 or 4, alternate, sheathing, ovate or lanceolate, acute, 5-15 cm long; flowers minute, pale yellowish green tinged with purple in terminal racemes, sides of the lip produced upwards into auricles, apex notched.

Habitate: Throughout India, on hills upto 3,000 m.

Propagation: By vegetative method.

Parts Used: Green swollen stem base covered by brown scales.

Chemical Consistuents: N.A.

Uses: The stem base is sweet, refrigerant, aphrodisiac, febrifuge, and tonic. It is useful in haematemesis, vitiated conditions of *pitta* and *vata* fever, seminal weakness, burning sensation, dipsia, emaciation, tuberculosis and general debility.

805. *Malaxis muscifera* (Lindley) Kuntze *(Orchidaceae)*

Synonyms: *Microstylis muscifera* (Lindley) Ridley.

Vernacular Name: *San*: Rsabhakah, *Eng*: Risabak, *Hin*: Rsabhak, *Kan*: Rsabaka, *Mal*: Itavakam, *Tam*: Itavagam, Rsabakam, *Tel:* Rsabaka.

Description: A terrestrial herb upto 40 cm in height with small ovoid pseudo-bulb and fibrous roots; leaves 3-5, unequal, short-petioled, oblong or ovate; flowers pale yellowish green in terminal racemes, lip fleshy, broadly ovate, 2 mm long, basal portion excavated, obscurely angled on either side of the base, apex acuminate.

Habitate: Throughout India, in hills upto 4,000 m.

Propagation: By stems.

Parts Used: Green swollen stem base covered with brown scales.

Chemical Consistuents: N.A.

Uses: The swollen stem is sweet, refrigerant, aphrodisiac, styptic, antidysenteric, febrifuge and tonic. It is useful in sterility, vitiated conditions of *pitta* and *vata*, seminal weakness, internal and external haemorrhages, dysentery, fever, emaciation, burning sensation general debility.

806. *Mallotus philippensis* (Lam.) Muell.-Arg. *(Euphorbiaceae)*

Vernacular Name: *San*: Recanakah, Kampillakah, *Eng*: Kamala tree, *Hin*: Sindur, Kamala, Rohini, *Kan*: Kampillaka, *Mal*: Sinduri, Manjana, Kuramatakku, Kampipala, *Tam*: Manjanai, Kunkumam, Kamala, *Tel:* Sundari, Vasanta, Kumkumamu.

Description: A small tree about 10 m in height with grey or pale brown rough bark with irregular fissures; leaves alternate, longer than broad, three ribbed at the base ovate or ovate-lanceolate, entire or shortly serrate, red glandular beneath, the transverse nervules prominent; flowers dioecious, small in spikes, the males clustered sessile or very shortly pedicellate in erect long terminal spikes usually several together, the females nearly sessile in short spikes; fruits globose, three-lobed capsules covered over with dense reddish brown glandular pubescence, seeds black, smooth, sub-globose.

Habitate: Throughout India, in evergreen and deciduous forests upto 1,500 m.

Propagation: By seeds and vegetative method.

Parts Used: The glandular hairs of the fruit.

Chemical Consistuents: Kamlolenic, conjugated dienoic, linoleic, oleic, lauric, myristic, plmitic and stearic.

Uses: The glandular hairs, which are reddish brown in colour, are acrid, thermogenic, purgative, digestive, lithontriptic, styptic, vermifuge, alexipharmic and depurative. They are useful in vitiated conditions of *kapha* and *vata*, verminosis, constipation, flatulence, wounds ulcers, cough, renal and vesical calculi, haemorrhages, poisonous affections, scabies, ringworm herpes and other parasitic skin affections.

807. *Malus doumeri* (Bois.) A. Chev. *(Rosaceae)*

Synonyms: *Malus sylvestris.*

Description: Evergreen tree, up to 15m. high. Young stems spinous and pubescent. Leaves alternate, ovate, base round, apex pointed; margins toothed; pubescent when young, then glabrous. Inflorescence in axillary cluster; flowers 3-5 white. Drupe globose, slightly compressed, greenish-yellow when ripe, edible.

Habitate: Grows wild and is cultivated in mountainous regions.

Propagation: By seeds and vegetative method.

Part Used: Fruits.

Chemical Constituents: The fruit, contains tannin, sugars, and tartaric and citric acids.

Uses: The fruit possesses stomachic properties. It is used in traating dyspepsia, colic, flatulence, diarrhoea and colic consequent upon post-partum haematometra. It is also antihypertensive and anodyne. Bathing and washing with a decoction of the fruit are effective against impetigo and lqcquer allergic dermatitis.

808. *Malva sylvestris* *(Malvaceae)*

Vernacular Name: *Eng:* Common Mallow.

Description: An erect, branched, woody biennial or perennial 30-120 cm. high, leaves 3-7 lobed, on long stalked; flowers purple; fruit smooth; seeds reniform.

Habitate: Common mallow is native to Europe and Asia. It is naturalized in the Americas and Australia, growing on waste ground and on hedges and fences.

Propagation: By seeds and vegetative method.

Parts Used: Leaves, root, flowers.

Chemical Constituents: Common mallow contains flavonol glycosides, mucilage and tannins. The flowers also contain malvin.

Uses: Though less useful than marshmallow common mallow is an effective demulcent. The flowers and leaves are emollient. The flowers and leaves are emollient and good for sensitive areas of the skin. It is applied as a poultice to reduce swelling and draw out toxins. Taken internally, the leaves reduce gut irritation and have a laxative effect. When common mallow is combined with eucalyptus, it makes a good remedy for coughs and other chest ailments. As with marshmallow, the root may be given children to ease teething.

809. *Malva verticillata* L. *(Malvaceae)*

Vernacular Name: *Eng:* Cluster mallow; curly-leaved mallow.

Description: A biennial herb, 30-90 cm high. Stem erect, branched, glabrous, covered with stellate hairs, green. Leaves alternate, simple, reniform or rounded, palmately lobed. Petioles 2-8 cm long. Cyme axillary, each cluster consisting of 4-5 flowers borne on a short peduncle. Flowers reddish. Capsule splitting into many one-seeded mericarps. Seeds flattened, with a V-shaped slit on one side.

Habitate: Along roadsides and near villages, mostly cultivated in China, Europe and India.

Propagation: By seeds and vegetative method.

Part Used: Cluster mallow; curly-leaved mallow.

Chemical Constituents: N.A.

Uses: Infection of urinary system, lithiasis, obstruction of milk secretion, coproma. Stems and leaves, icteric type of hepatitis. Roots, tiredness of the lower limbs and body, perspiration caused by weakness or of unknown origin, rectocele, chronic nephritis.

810. *Mandragora officinarum* *(Solanaceae)*

Vernacular Name: *Eng:* Mandrake.

Description: Perennial growing to 5 cm. Has a deep branching root, a rosette of broad floppy leaves, funnel-shaped white to purple flowers and yellow fruit.

Habitate: Native to the Mediterranean region of Europe, mandrake grows on dry riverbeds.

Propagation: By seeds and vegetative method.

Parts Used: Root.

Chemical Constituents: Mandrake contains 0.4% tropane alkaloids.

Uses: Mandrake has now largely fallen out of use. The herb is sometimes applied as a poultice or plaster for rheumatic and arthritic pains, ulcers and similar kinds of skin disorders.

811. *Mangifera indica* L. *(Anacardiaceae)*

Vernacular Name: *San*: Amrah, Chuta, *Eng*: Mango tree, Spring tree, *Hin*: Am, Amb, *Kan*: Mavu, *Mal*: Mavu, *Tam*: Mamaram, Mankai, *Tel:* Mamidi.

Description: A large spreading evergreen tree upto 45 m in height with a heavy doom shaped crown, straight, stout bole and thick rough dark grey bark; leaves simple, crowded at the ends of branches, linear-oblong, or elliptic-lanceolate, acute, acuminate or sub-obtuse; flowers small, pungently odorous, reddish white or yellowish green in large many-flowered pubescent panicles, longer than the leaves; fruits large, fleshy drupes, green, orange, yellow or red in colour, seed solitary, encased in a hard compressed fibrous endocarp.

Habitate: Throughout India, in forests upto 1,200 m also widely cultivated.

Propagation: By seeds and vegetative method.

Parts Used: Roots, bark, leaves, flowers, fruits, seed kernel.

Chemical Consisuents: β-Carotene and xanthophylls are the principal pigments present in ripe mango; neo-β-cartoene U and neo-β-carotene B are present only in a few varieties. Xanthophylls, 42.1; β-carotene, 96.3; noe-β-carotene U, 7.3; and neo-β-carotene B, 19.2. It contsins 2-octene, α-and β-pinene, α-phellandrene, limonene, dipentene, nerol, geraniol, neryl acetate, citronellal, a sesquiterpene alcohol named mangiferol and a sesquiterpene ketone.

Uses: The roots and bark are astringent, acrid, refrigerant, styptic, antisyphilitic, vulnerary, antiemetic, anti-inflammatory and constipating. They are useful in vitiated conditions of *pitta*, metrorrhagia, colonorrhagia, pneumorrhagia, leucorrhoea, syphilis, wounds, ulcers, vomiting, uteritis, diarrhoea, dysentery, diphtheria and rheumatism. The leaves are astringent, refrigerant, styptic, vulnerary and constipating. They are useful in vitiated conditions of *kapha* and *pitta* hiccough, hyperdipsia, burning sensation, haemorrhages, haemoptysis, haemorrhoids, wounds, ulcers, diarrhoea, dysentery, pharyngopath and stomatopathy. The ash of the burnt leaves are useful in burns and scalds. The flowers are astringent, refrigerant, styptic, vulnerary, constipating and haematinic. They are useful in vitiated conditions of *pitta*, haemorrhages, haemoptysis, wounds, ulcers, anorexia, dyspepsia.

812. *Mangonolia denudata* Desr. *(Mangnoliaceae)*

Synonyms: *Magnolia yuln* Desf.

Vernacular Name: *Eng:* Yuland magnolia, lily tree, yulan tree.

Description: A deciduous tree 3-10 m high, branching widely, flowering in march and early April. Branch lets slender, brown-grey in winter, glabrous. Leaves obovate-elliptic of obovate-oblong, 8-18 cm long by 3-10 cm wide; tip acute or acuminate; base cuneate, entire. Flower buds 2.5 cm long by 1.2 cm in diameter, enclosed in few bracts, usually three; apex bluntly acuminate, rounded at base, densely covered with silver-grey hairs. The bud which has an aromatic odour and pungent taste in cup-shaped when upright, opening to horizontal. Fruit cones about 15 cm in length, oblong or spindle-shaped. The ripening cones turn a rather faded pink colour and the seeds when fully developed are a bright red.

Habitate: In mountains China and Japan.

Propagation: By seeds and vegetative method.

Part Used: Spores, whole plant.

Chemical Constituents: N.A.

Uses: Headache, nasal obstruction, nasal discharge; acute and chronic rhinitis.

813. *Manihot esculenta* Crantz *(Euphorbiaceae)*

Synonyms: *M. utilissima* Pohl.

Vernacular Name: *San*: Darukandah, Kalpakandah, *Eng*: Cassava, Manioc, Tapioca, *Hin*: Sakkarkand, *Kan*: *Ma*ragenasu, *Mal*: *Ma*raccini, *Ma*rakkilannu, Kollikkilannu, Pulakkilannu, Kappa, *Tam*: *Ma*ravallikkilanku, *Tel:* Karrapendalamu.

Description: A shrub 2-5 m in height with stems and branches of varying colour, marked by leaf scars and clusters of tuberous roots; leaves palmate, pale green, 5-9 lobed, lobes lanceolate, acuminate, entire; flowers yellow or greenish white, unisexual, in terminal cymes; fruits capsules containing 3 seeds.

Habitate: Cultivated widely in Kerala, *Tam*il Nadu and Gujarat.

Propagation: By roots.

Parts Used: Tuberous roots.

Chemical Consistuents: The tuber contains small quantities of albumin, globulin and glutelin; prolamine is present in negligible amounts. The essential amino acids present in the total proteins, arginine, histidine, isoleucine, leucine, lysine, methionine, phenylalanine, threonine, tryptophan, and valine.

Uses: The juice of the grated tubers to treat constipation and indigestion. Diarrhoea is treated by eating the boiled tubers. The fresh tubers are grated and used as a poultice on sores and boils. The leaves are infused in the bath water to treat fever. The stem is folded and rubbed across the eyes of people suffering from glucome. The bark of the plant together with that of Cordyline terminalis, is thought to prolong life Tthe leaves are heated and rubbed across sore eyes.

814. *Manilkara hexandar* (Roxb.) Dubard *(Sapotaceae)*

Synonyms: *Mimusops hexandra* Roxb.

Vernacular Name: *San*: Rajadanah, *Eng*: Obtuse leaved mimusops, *Hin*: Khirni, *Kan*: Hale Hannu, *Mal*: Palamunpala, Palamunnippala, *Tam*: Ulakkaippalai, Palai, *Tel:* Patla, Pola, Kirni.

Description: A small to medium sized glabrous evergreen tree, 15-18 m in height with smooth grey bark and conical hard degenerate branchlets; leaves simple, alternate, elliptic-obovate or oblong, coriaceous, rounded or emarginated at the apex, glabrous on both sides, main nerves 12-20 pairs; flowers white or pale yellow, axillary, solitary or in fascicles; fruits one seeded reddish yellow berries, ovoid or ellipsoid, seeds ovoid, reddish brown with shining testa.

Habitate: Throughout India, in evergreen forests, also cultivated.

Propagation: By seeds and vegetative method.

Parts Used: Bark, fruits.

Chemical Consistuents: Moisture, protein, fat, carbohydrates and mineral matter, calcium, phosphorus, iron carotene, thiamine, riboflavin, nicotinic acid and ascorbic acid.

Uses: The bark is astringent, sweet, refrigerant, aphrodisiac, alexipharmic, stomachic, and anthelmintic. It is useful in ulorrhagia, ulitis, odontopathy, fever, flatulence, colic, dyspepsia, helminthiasis, hyperdipsia, burning sensation and vitiated conditions of *pitta*. It retards the fermentation process in toddy. The fruits are milky, sweet, sour, cooling, aphrodisiac, appetizer, emollient and tonic. They are useful in consumption, hallucinations loss of consciousness, anorexia, dipsia, bronchitis, urethrorrhea, leprosy and vitiated conditions of *pitta*. The seeds are useful in ulcers and the opacity of the cornea.

815. *Maranta arundinacea* L. *(Marantaceae)*

Vernacular Name: *San*: Tavaksiri, Tugaksiri; *Eng*: Arrowroot, West Indian arrowroot; *Kan*: Alasibija Kuvehitt, Tavaksiri; *Hin*: Tikhor; *Mal*: Kuvva; *Tam*: Kuvai, Araruttukkilangu; *Tel:* Palagunta.

Description: An erect slender branched herb, 90-180 cm high with fleshy cylindrical obovoid rhizome covered with pale scales leaving scars on falling; leaves ovate-oblong to ovate-lanceolate, base rounded or cuneate, tip acute; flowers white in clusters on diverging inflorescence branches, fertile stamen with appendage, ovary one-celled, one-ovuled.

Habitate: Cultivated throughout India.

Propagation: By vegetative methods.

Parts Used: Underground rhizome.

Chemical Consistuents: Moisture, crude protein, fat, starch, dextrin and sugars, crude fibre and ash.

Uses: Starch obtained from rhizome is astringent, sweet, refrigerant, tonic aphrodisiac, emollient, expectorant, febrifuge and rubefacient. It is useful in dysentery, diarrhoea, dyspepsia, bronchitis, cough and also as a nourishing food for infants, invalids and convalescents. It is the main ingredient in biscuits, cakes puddings, jellies and face powders.

816. *Marrubium vulgare* *(Lameaceae)*

Vernacular Name: *Eng:* White horehound.

Description: A tall, robust hearbaceous perennial, 40-120 cm. high; leaves leathery or thick, orbicular or elliptic-ovate, villous, rugose or wrinkled; flowers small, white, in dense axillary whorls; nutlets very small; faintly rugose.

Habitate: Native to Europe, white horehound is naturalized in North and South America. It flourishes on wasteground and in dry, bare areas and is gathered in spring.

Propagation: By seeds and vegetative method.

Parts Used: Leaves.

Chemical Constituents: White horehound contains the diterpenes marrubiin and marrubenol, flavonoids, alkaloids and 0.6% voltile oil. Marrubiin is strongly expectorant and bitter.

Uses: White horehound is helpful for wheeziness, bronchitis, bronchiectasis, bronchial asthma, non-productive coughs and whooping cough. The herb apparently causes the secretion of a more fluid mucus, readily cleared by coughing. As a bitter tonic, white horehound increases the appetite and supports the function of the stomach. The herb may also act to normalize heart rhythm, improving its regularity.

817. *Marsdenia condurango* *(Asclepiadaceae)*

Synonyms*:* *Gonolobus condurango.*

Vernacular Name: *Eng:* Condurango.

Description: Climbing vine growing to 10m. Has heart-shaped leaves and funnel-shaped, white-green flowers.

Habitate: Condurango is native to deciduous forests of the Andes in Peru and Ecuador. It generally grows at altitudes between 1,000-2,000 m.

Propagation: By seeds and vegetative method.

Parts Used: Bark, latex.

Chemical Constituents: Condurango bark contains glycosides a volatile oil and phytosterols.

Uses: The bark's main effect is to stimulate stomach secretions. It is often used in South American folk medicine as a bitter and digestive tonic. Condurago is a specific treatment for nervous indigestion and anorexia nervosa, since its bitterness slowly increases the appetite as well as the stomach's ability to process more food. The herb is also thought to stimulate the liver and pancreas, and may be taken for liver disorders. Condurango also encourages menstruation. The caustic white latex is applied to remove warts.

818. *Marsilea quadrifolia* L. (*Marsileaceae)*

Synonyms: *Marsilea minuta.*

Vernacular Name: *San*: Sunisannah, Catuspatri; *Hin*: Caupatiya, Sunsuniya; *Kan*: Citiginasoppu; *Mal*: Niraral; *Tam*: Nirarai; *Tel:* Ciklintakura.

Description: A creeping herbaceous perennial with slender long dichotomously branching rhizome rooting at the nodes; leaves quadrifoliolate, circinate when young, petioles long, slender, flexible, lamina divided into four leaflets, sporocarps bean-like borne on short or long stalks inserted a short distance above the base of the petiole.

Habitat: Throughout India, in marshy places and along the banks of canals and rivers.

Propagation: By seeds and vegetative method.

Parts Used: Whole plant.

Chemical Constituents: N.A.

Uses: The plant is sweet, astringent, refrigerant, acrid, emillent, anodyne, hypnotic, ophthalmic diuretic, constipating, expectorant, aphrodisiac, depurative and febrifuge. It is useful in psychopathy, ophthalmia, strangury, diarrhoea, cough, bronchitis, leprosy, skin diseases, haemorrhoids, dyspepsia, fever and insomnia.

819. *Melaleuca leucadendra* (L.) *(Myrtaceae)*

Vernacular Name: *Eng:* Cajeput tree, paper bark tree.

Description: Erect evergreen tree, up to 10m. high. Bark white, soft, peeling off in rough flakes. Leaves alternate, entire, thick incurvedly nerved with whitish willi when young. Inflorescence in more or less interrupted elongate terminal spike; flowers small, creamy white. Capsule subglobose, many-seeds.

Habitate: Grows wild int eh jhills and in salt-marshes.

Propagation: By seeds and vegetative method.

Part Used: Leaves.

Chemical Constituents: The leaves yield and essentiual oil consisisting of cineol 50-60%. A-terpineol and its esters, L-a-pinene, L-limonene, dipenetene, sesquiterpene, azulene, sesquiterpene alcohol, valerianic aldehyde and benzaldehyde.

Uses: The leaves possess antibacterial, anti-inflammatory and anodyne properties. They are effective for coryza, influenza, cough, asthma, dyspepsia, earache, toothache, rheumatism, osteodynia, neuralgia, wounds, burns and post-partum haematometra. An essential oil solution is prescribed for massage and for oral administration, parenteral injection or nasal instillation.

820. *Medicago sativa* *(Fabaceae)*

Vernacular Name: *Eng:* Alfalfa, Lugerne.

Description: Perennial herb growing to 80 cm. Has 3-lobed leaves, flowers theat range in colour from yellow to violet-blue, and spiraling seed pods.

Habitate: Native to Europe, Asia and North Africa, alfalfa is found in meadows, on wasteground and in cultivated areas.

Propagation: By seeds and vegetative method.

Parts Used: Seeds.

Chemical Constituents: Alfalfa contains isoflavones, coumarins, alkaloids, vitamins and prophyrins. The isoflavones and coumarins are oestrogenic.

Uses: Alfalfa is perhaps more therapeutically useful as a food than a medicine. It is given to convalescents who require easily assimilated nutrients. In view of alfalfa's oestrogenic activity, it could prove useful in treating problems relating to menstruation and the menopause.

821. *Melaleuca alternifolia* *(Myrtaceae)*

Vernacular Name: *Eng:* Tea Tree.

Description: An evergreen reaching 7m, with layers of papery bark, pointed leaves and white flower spikes.

Habitate: Tea tree is native to Australia, flourishing in moist soils in northern New South Wales and Queensland. It is now cultivated extensively, especially in New South Wales.

Propagation: By vegetative method.

Parts Used: Leaves.

Chemical Constituents: Volatile oil, terpinen-4-ol-40%, gamma-terpinene 24%, alphaterpinene 10%, cineol 5%.

Uses: Antiseptic, Antibacterial, Antifungal, Antiviral, Immune stimulant.

822. *Melandrium firmum* (Siebold et Zucc.) Rohrb. *(Caryophyllaceae)*

Vernacular Name: *Eng*: Catchfly, cockle.

Description: Biennial, erect herb, to 30-80 cm tall. Stems glabrous, green, but dark purple at nodes. Leaves opposite, ovate-elliptic or ovate-lanceolate, 3-10 cm long, hairy at edges and on both sides; stipules absent. Flowers white; calyx tubular, 5-toothed, 10-veined; petals 5, 2-lobed; coronal scales present at juncture of blade and claw; stamens 10; ovary 1-celled above but 3-5 celled at base; styles 3, alternate with calyx teeth, Fruit a capsule, dehiscent, dehiscent by teeth twice as many as the styles; seeds many, reniform.

Habitate: Open areas in lowlands and mountains.

Propagation: By seeds and vegetative method.

Parts Used: Whole plant.

Chemical Constituents: Flavonoids; linarin, schaftoside, 3-B-D-Glucuronopyranosylmelandrigenin methyl ester, saponins.

Uses: Induction of drug metabolizing enzymes in liver, aldose reductase inhibition. Used in gonorrhoea, galactagogue, emmenagogue and cantra ception.

823. *Melia azedarach* L. *(Meliaceae)*

Vernacular Name: *San:* Mahanimba; *Eng:* Margosa tree, China berry, Barbados lialac, pride of India, Persian lialc, bead tree, hoop tree; *Hin:* Drek, bakain; *Beng*: Mahanim, ghora nim; *Tel:* Turaka vepa; *Tam:* Malai vembu; *Mal:* Karin vembu, sima veppu and *Kan:* Arebevu.

Description: A tree 10m. high or more. Bark pale-brown, lenticellate, longitudinally furrowed. Leaves alternate, odd-pinnate; leaflets opposite, serrate, glabrous on both sides. Influrescence in axillary or terminal biparous cyme; flowers white-lilac. Drupe ovate or ellipsoid-globose with 4 seeds, yellow when ripe.

Habitate: Cultivated every where for wood.

Propagation: By seeds and vegetative method.

Part Used: Bark.

Chemical Constituents: The stem-bark and root-bark contain the alkaloid azaridine (margosine), sterols and tannins. The leaves yield the alkaloid paraisine and the flavonoid rutin. The seeds are rich in fatty oil consisting o stearic, palmitic, oleic and linoleic acids.

Uses: Thje internal silky layer of the torrefied root-bark is ued in treating ascariasis and oxyuriasis; it is less toxic then the trunk bark. Vaginal injection of the decoction is effective for trichomonas infections. Precautions must be taken because of the drug's high toxicity.

824. *Melilotus officinalis* *(Fabaceae)*

Synonyms: Melilotus arvensis.

Vernacular Name: *Eng:* Melilot.

Description: A tall robust biennial herb, 1.0 m or more in height; leaves trifoliolate; leaflets obovate, oblong or oblanceolate; flowers in lax racemes, yellowish; pods ovoid, transversely rugose, compressed, brown when ripe; seeds oval, yellowish green smooth.

Habitate: Melilot is native to Europe, North Africa and temperate regions of Asia, and is naturalized in North America.

Propagation: By seeds and vegetative method.

Parts Used: Aerial parts.

Chemical Constituents: Melilot contains flavonoids, coumarins, resin, tannins and volatile oil. If allowed to spoil, the plant produces dicoumarol, a powerful anticoagulant.

Uses: As with horse chestnut, long-term use of melilot-internally or externally-can help varicose veins and hemorrhoids. Melilot also helps reduce the risk of phlebitis and thrombosis. The plant is mildly sedative and antispasmodic, and is given for insomnia and anxiety. It has been used to treat flatulence, indigestion, bronchitis, associated with the menopause, and rheumatic pains.

825. *Melissa officinalis* *(Lamiaceae)*

Vernacular Name: *Eng:* Lemon Balm, Balm.

Description: A perennial growing up to 1.5m, with tiny white flowers and deeply veined, toothed leaves.

Habitate: Native to southern Europe, western Asia and northern Africa, lemon balm now grows throughout the world. The plant is propagated from seed or cuttings in spring. The aerial parts are picked from early summer onwards and are best harvested just before the flowers open, when the concentration of volatile oil is at its highest.

Propagation: By seeds and vegetative method.

Parts Used: Leaves.

Chemical Constituents: Volatile oil up to 0.2%, Flavonoids, Triterpenes, Polyphenols, Tannins.

Uses: Relaxant, Antispasmodic, Increases sweating, Carminative, Antiviral, Nerve tonic.

826. *Melothria maderaspatana* (L.) Cogn. *(Cucurbitaceae)*

Synonyms: *Mukia maderaspatana* (Linn.) Roem.

Vernacular Name: *Hin*: Agumaki, Bilari; *Mal*: Mukkappiram, Mukkalpiram; *San*: Trikosaki, Krtarandhrah; *Tam*: Musumusukkai; *Tel:* Pottibudamu.

Description: A scabrous scandent or prostrate much branched climbing annual with very hispid angular stem and simple tendrils; leaves simple, alternate ovate or subdeltoid, entire or 3-5 lobed, minutely denticulate, very scabrid above, cordate at the base with a wide sinus; flowers small, yellow, male in small fascicles on very short peduncles, females almost sessile solitary or subfasciculate; fruits globose, brownish yellow, finally turning red, seeds ovoid-oblong, compressed.

Habitate: Throughout India, upto 1,800 m.

Propagation: By seeds and vegetative method.

Parts Used: Whole plant.

Chemical Consistuents: N.A.

Uses: The plant is bitter, sweet, refrigerant, carminative, aperient, vulnerary, sudorific expectorant, anodyne and tonic. It is useful in vitiated conditions of *pitta,* burning sensation, dipsia, flatulence, colic, constipation, ulcers, cough, asthma, neuralgia, notalgia, odontalgia and vertigo.

827. *Mentha arvensis* L. *(Lamiaceae)*

Vernacular Name: *Eng:* Field mint, corn ming, Japanese mint, Japanese pepperming; *Hin:* Podina, pudina; *Kan:* Chetni; *Beng*: Podina, pudina; *Tel:* Podina, pudina.

Description: Perennial herb, 30-50 cm. High; Stems quadrangular, erect or prostrate, rooting at the nodes. Leaves opposite, ovate, softly tomentose on both sides; margins serrate, Inflorescence in axillary capitate whorl; flowers small, white or lilac.

Habitate: Grows wild in the mountains and is cultivated every where.

Propagation: By vegetative method.

Part Used: Whole plant.

Chemical Constituents: The whole plant yields an essential oil consisting of L-menthol 65-85%, menthhyl acetate, L-menthone, L-a-pinene,: -limonene.

Uses: The entire plant, apart from the roods, is antibacterial and antifbrile. It yields an essential oil and menthol which exert, through their rapid evaporation, aslightly anaesthetic and anodyne local effect. It is effective in coryza, adiaphoretic fever, headache, rhinitis, cough sore throat, arthralgia, neuralgia, colic, vomiting, dyspepsia, diarrhoea and prurigo. The essential oil and menthol are the constituents of several balsams. Poultices of fresh leves and the inhalation of essential oil and menthol are also prescribed.

828. *Mentha haplocalyz* *(Lamiaceae)*

Vernacular Name: *Eng:* Bo he, Corn mint.

Description: Perennial herb growing to 60 cm. Has a square stem, oval toothed leaves, and whorls of pale lilac flowers growing from the leaf axils.

Habitate: *Bo he* is native to temperate regions of the northern hemisphere, and is widely cultivated in China.

Propagation: By Root.

Parts Used: Aerial parts.

Chemical Constituents: *Bo he* contains a volatile oil comprising mainly methol with methone, menthyl acetate, camphene, limonene and other terpenoids.

Uses: In Chinese herbal medicine *bo he* is a popular treatment for colds, sore throats, sore mouth and tongue, and a host of other conditions ranging from toothache to measles. Like peppermint, it helps to lower the temperature, has anticatarrhal properties, and may be taken for dysentery and diarrhoea. The juice has also been used to treat earache. *Bo he* is often combined with *ju hua* to treat headaches and bloodshot or sore eyes.

829. *Mentha pipertia* L. Emend. Huds. *(Lamiaceae)*

Vernacular Name: *Eng:* Peppermingl, Gamathi phudina and *Hin:* Paparaminta, gamathi, phudina.

Description: A strongly sc\ented, perennial herb;;eaves ovate or oblong-lanceolate, serrate; flowers ligh purple, in thick terminal spikes.

Habitate: Cultivated in Kashmir, dehra dun, delhi, nilgiris, and mysore.

Propagation: By seeds and vegetative method.

Part Used: Leaves.

Chemical Constituents: Major components of pepperming oil are menthol besides menthone, menthyl acetate, isomenthone, neomenthol, cineole, limonene, pipertione, and pulegone.

Uses: The dried flowering tops are used to prepare beverages like peppermint tea and in the formulation of liqueurs and bitters. Peppermint oil is used to flavour non-alcoholic beverages, ice-creams, candies, baked goods, gelatins and puddings, chewing gum and some ment preparations.

830. *Mentha pulegium* *(Lameaceae)*

Vernacular Name: *Eng:* Pennyroyal.

Description: A perennial, glabrous, strongly scented herb; stem erect, 30-90 cm. high, purplish or green; Leaves ovateor oblong-lanceolate. Petioled long, acute or obtuse at the base, coarsely serrate, smooth and dark green above, pale or sparingly hairy below; flowers purplish, in thick terminal spikes.

Habitate: Pennyroyal is native to Europe and western Asia, and has become naturalized in the Americas.

Propagation: By Root.

Parts Used: Aerial parts.

Chemical Constituents: Pynnyroyal's volatile oil contains pulegone, isopulegone, menthol and other terpenoids. Pennyroyal also contains bitter and tannins.

Uses: Similar in many respects to peppermint, pennyroyal is a good digestive tonic. It increases the secretion of digestive juices, relieves flatulence and colic, and occasionally is used as a treatment for intestinal worms. It makes a good remedy for headaches and for minor respiratory infections, helping to check fever and reduce catarrh. Pennyroyal powerfully stimulates the uterine muscles and encourages menstruation. An infusion of pennyroyal is used externally to treat itchiness and formication, inflamed skin disorders such as eczema, and rheumatic conditions including gout.

831. *Mentha spicata* L. Emend. Nathh. *(Lamiaceae)*

Vernacular Name: *Eng:* Spearming, garden mint, lamb mint; *Hin:* Pahari, Pudina, Pudina and *Beng*: Pahari, Pudina, Pudina.

Description: A glabrous perennial, 30-90 cm. high, with creeping rhizomes; leaves smooth or nearly so, sessile, lanceolate to ovate, acute, coarsely, dentate, smooth above, glandular below; flowers lilac, in loose, cylindrical, slender, interrupted spikes.

Habitate: Throughout in India, under cultivation.

Propagation: By seeds and vegetative method.

Part Used: Whole plant.

Chemical Constituents: Major components in the spearming oil are carvone, dipentent, dihydrocarveol, dihydrocarveol acetate, and limonene.

Uses: The green leaves of the plant are used for flavouring culinary preparations, vinegar, jellies and iced drinks. The oil is used to flavour chewing gum and candy, non-alcoholic beverages, baked goods, gelatin and puddings, ice-creams. Etc.

832. *Menyanthes trifoliate* L. *(Gentianaceae)*

Synonyms: *Menyanthes palustris* Gray, S.F., *Menyanthes verna* Rafin.

Vernacular Name: *Eng:* Bitter worm, Bogbean.

Description: A perennial herb, with a thick, horizontal rhizome. Leaves alternate, trifoliolate–each with 3 obovate leaflets, arise from rhizome on long, broad, flattened and striated petiole, 16 cm. in length with broad, sheathing stipules at the base. Leaflets, ash-green, glabrous somewhat flesh, obtuse or acute at apex, with margins entire or coarsely undulate, base cuneate, 3-8 cm. long with prominent midrib. Flowers white or pink, in 7.5 cm. long conical raceme, on stout, glabrous pedicels. Calyx 5-cleft, calyx lobes somewhat re-curved and ovate. Corolla pink outside, pale or white within, funnel-shaped, much fimbriate on its upper surface. Stamens-5. Bicarpellary pistil with slender style and 2-lobed stigma. Fruits, many seeded unilocular capsule.

Habitate: Europe & U.S.A.

Propagation: By seeds and vegetative method.

Parts Used: Whole plant.

Chemical Constituents: Pyridine type Gentianidine, Gentianin; choline; Scopoletin; Menyantin, Meliantin; Chlorogenic acid, caffeic acid, ferulic acid, Salicyclic acid; Hyperin, Quercetin, Rutin, Kaempferol; Loganin; α-spinasterol.

Uses: For complaints predominantly of headache. Pressing headache in vertex from above downwards, better by hard pressure with hand, but pain if pressed by two hands together. Pressing headache as if a heavy weight presses upon the head at every step when ascending a staircase, often associated with icy coldness of hands & feet. Headache better stooping. Cramp like pain in extremeties with jerks and twitches as he lies down. Fever but with predominating coldness.

833. *Merremia emarginata* (Burm. f.) Hall. f. *(Convolvulaceae)*

Synonyms: *Merremia gangetica* (Linn.) Cuf., *Ipomoea reniformis* Choisy.

Vernacular Name: *San*: Akhukarni, *Hin*: Musakani, Musakari, *Mal*: Eliccevi, *Tam*: Eikkatukkirai, Perattaikkirai, *Tel:* Elika jimudu.

Description: A creeping perennial herb rooting at the nodes; leaves simple, long stalked reniform or ovate-cordate; flowers yellow, axillary on 1-3 flowered, very short peduncles which are shorter than the petioles; fruits subglobose capsules with 2-4 glabrous light brown seeds.

Habitate: Throughout India, in plains and hills upto 900 m.

Propagation: By seeds and vegetative method.

Parts Used: Whole plant.

Chemical Consistuents: N.A.

Uses: The plant is bitter, acrid, refrigerant, deobstruant, diuretic, alterant, anthelmintic, carminative and digestive. It is useful in nephropathy, uropathy, pneumonosis, cardiac diseases, gastropathy, metropathy, fever, anaemia, leucoderma, strangury, otalgia, cephalalgia and rat bite.

834. *Merremia tridentate* (L.) *Hallier f. ssp tridentate(Convolvulaceae)*

Synonyms: *Ipomoea tridentate* (Linn.) Roth.

Vernacular Name: *Mal*: Prasarini, Talanili, *San*: Prasarani, *Tam*: Mutiyakuntal, Trippanpul, Savolikkoti, *Tel:* Sitasavaram.

Description: A perennial wiry herb with woody root-stock and slender glabrous angular elongate stems; leaves simple, alternate, variable, linear-hastate or oblong-obovate, the linear leaves usually acute, the obovate ones obtuse deeply emarginate and 3-toothed, all auricled at the base and toothed; flowers pale yellow, funnel-shaped, 1-3 together or axillary peduncles; fruits globose capsules, seeds 2-4, trigonus, glabrous with a longitudinal ridge on the back.

Habitate: Throughout India, on hedges and open waste lands.

Propagation: By seeds and vegetative method.

Parts Used: Whole plant.

Chemical Consistuents: N.A.

Uses: The plant s bitter, astringent, thermogenic, calefacient, aphrodisiac, laxative anodyne and tonic. It is useful in vitiated conditions of *vata*, hemiplegia, haemorrhoids, uropathy, inflammations and general debility.

835. *Mesua ferrea* L. *(Guttiferae)*

Synonyms: *Mesua nagassarium* (Burm. f.) Kosterm.

Vernacular Name: *San*: Nagapuspah, Nagakesarah, *Eng*: Mesua, Iron-wood tree, *Hin*: Nagakesar, *Kan*: Nagasampige, *Mal*: Nagappuvu, Nagacampakam, Nanku, Vayanavu, Curuli, Eliponku, *Tam*: Nagapppu, Nanku, *Tel:* Nagakesaramu, Gajapuspam.

Description: A medium sized to large handsome, glabrous, evergreen tree, 18-30 m in height and reddish brown bark which peels off in thin flakes; leaves simple, opposite, thick lanceolate, coriaceous, covered with waxy bloom underneath, red when young, acute or acuminate, nerves.

Habitate: Throughout India, in evergreen forests upto 1,500 m.

Propagation: By seeds and vegetative method.

Parts Used: Flowers, oil.

Chemical Consistuents: Polenske val Hehner val., palmitic, stearic, oleic, and linoleic, palmitostearo-olein, dipalmito-olein distearo-olein, stearo diolein, palmito-diolein, linoleodiolein, triolein.

Uses: The flowers are astringent, bitter, acrid, mildly heating, anodyne, sudorific, digestive, carminative, constipating, anthelmintic, diuretic, alexipharmic, expectorant, stomachic, haemostatic, aphrodisiac, febrifuge and cardiotonic. They are useful in vitiated conditions of *patta* and *vata*, asthma, cough, hiccough, halitosis, leprosy, scabies, dermatopathy, pruritus, pharyngodynia, vomiting, dysentery, haemorrhoids, ulcers burning sensation of the feet, dipsia, impotency, leucorrhoea, haemoptysis, strangury, cephalagia, fever and cardiac debility.

The seed oil is used in vitiated conditions of *vata* and skin diseases.

836. *Michelia champaca* L. *(Magnoliaceae)*

Vernacular Name: *San*: Campakah; *Eng*: Champak, Golden champa; *Hin*: Campa, Campaka; *Kan*: Sampige; *Mal*: Campakam, Cempakam; *Tam*: Sempakam, Sempuga; *Tel:* Campangi, Campangipuvvu.

Description: A tall handsome evergreen tree upto 30 m in height and 50-80 cm in diameter with straight stem and smooth grey or brown black; leaves simple, alternate, oblong-lanceolate or lanceolate, subcoriaceious, entire, glabrous above; flowers yellowish to orange, very fragrant, solitary and axillary; fruits 5-10 cm long, ovoid or ellipsoid capsules, dark brown opening on the back by two valves, valves wood, covered with white warty excrescences, seeds 1-12, brown rounded on the back with pink fleshy aril.

Habitate: Throughout India, in evergreen forests, also cultivated.

Propagation: By seeds and vegetative method.

Parts Used: Whole plant.

Chemical Consistuents: Palmitic, Oleic, Carbonyl, Val, ester Val.

Uses: The root and root bark are purgative and emmenagogue and are useful in the treatment of abscesses, inflammation, constipation, amenorhoea, and dysmenorhoea. The stem bark is astringent, febrifuge, diuretic, stimulant and expectorant and is useful in chronic gastritis, fever, strangury, cough, bronchitis and cardiac debility. Flowers, flower buds and fruits are bitter, astringent, acrid, refrigerant haemostatic, digestive, carminative, depurative, vulnerary, anthelmintic, diuretic, diaphoretic, expectorant, emmenagogue, cardiotonic, stimulant, antispasmodic, stomachic and antipyretic. They are useful in dyspepsia, nausea, vitiated conditions of *pitta* and *vata*, burning sensation, haemoptysis, pruritus, skin diseases, leprosy, wounds and ulcers, anorexia, colic, flatulence, helminthiasis, vertigo, cephalalgia, ophthalmia, nephropathy, gout, cough, bronchitis, amenorrhoea, dysmenorrhoea, strangury, malarial fever, cardiac debility and general debility. The seeds and fruits are useful in the treatment of psoriasis plantaris.

837. *Michelia nilagirica* Zenk. *(Magnoliaceae)*

Vernacular Name: *Hin*: Pila champa; *Kan*: Dodda sampige; *Mal*: Kattu chempakam, Vella chempakam; *Mar*: Pilachampa; *Tam*: Kattu shenbagam, Nilagiri chempakam, Sappa maram; *Tel:* Tella sampanga.

Description: Trees, up to 15 m tall. The *heartwood* is yellow. Young branches are densely matted with woolly hairs and become dark when dry. *Leaves* inverted egg-shaped, 5-10 x 3-7 cm, hairless, base acute, apex sub-acuminate, margin entire. *Stipules* about 3 cm long, sericeous; leaf stalks up to 2 cm long. *Flowers* bisexual, arise singly in leaf axils, less than 6 cm across, fragrant, white to cream, distinctly stalked. *Fruits* found in clusters, pendulous. Each fruitlet is egg-shaped, about 2 cm long. *Seeds* 1-2.

Habitate: Evergreen to shola forests.

Propagation: By seeds and vegetative method.

Parts Used: Seeds, flowers, bark, root and leaves.

Chemical Constituents: Volatile oil, acrid resins, tannin.

Uses: The bark and leaves are considered febrifuge.

838. *Micromelum minutum* (Forster f.) Seemann. *(Rutaceae)*

Description: Shrub or small slender tree up to 15m high. Leaves alternate, pinnately compound with 7-12 unequal-sides leaflets, each with a short petiole, the entire leaf up to 50 cm long. Flowers white, 5-parted, fragrant, borne in many-flowered terminal or axillary panicles. Fruit an elongated red drupe with small puncate dots (glands) on the surface, the fruit up to 1 cm long.

Habitate: Common in thickets, dense, dry or open forest, disturbed areas, and rocky coasts.

Propagation: By seeds and vegetative method.

Part Used: Leaves and bark.

Chemical Constituents: Angelical, butyl-7-methoxyfindersine, imperatorin, limettin, micromelin, dihydromicrmelin A, micromeliunin microminutin, microminutinin, minumicrolin, micropubescin, murralongin, and murrangatin derivative,s scopoletin, phebalosin.

Uses: The juice from the leaves is used to treat white scum on the tongue, bad breath and haemorrhoids. Fluid from the bark is used to treat headaches and sore throats. Parts of the plant is used to treat swellings. Use the plant to cure headache. Tongans use an infusion of the leaves to treat toothache and teething problems in babies. An infusion of the bark is ingested to cure stomachache.

839. *Mikania micrantha* HBK. *(Asteraceae)*

Vernacular Name: *Eng:* mile-a-minute.

Description: Perennial scrambling or climbing vine. Leaves opposite, petiolate, the blade up to 19 cm long, cordate to triangular with a broad cordate base. Flowers minute, white or cream coloured, borne in small densely packed heads which superficially resemble a single large flower. Fruit a small achene with white bristles which aid in wind dispersal of the seeds.

Habitate: A common weed of pastures, roadsides, fences, forest edges and clearings, secondary forests, and tree crops.

Propagation: By seeds and vegetative method.

Part Used: Whole plant.

Chemical Constituents: Twenty-seven terpenoid constituents, kaur-16-en-19-oic acid, kauren-16-beta-ol, taraxasterol, essential oils, coumarin, betaOsitosterol, stigmasterol.

Uses: To stop bleeding. To treat gastritis, insect bites and various skin irrigations.

840. *Millettia reticulata* *(Fabaceae)*

Vernacular Name: *Eng:* Ji xue teng.

Description: Low—growing plant with compound leaves and clusters of pea-type flowers producing large beanpods.

Habitate: Native to China, *ji xue teng* cultivated in the south-east of that country.

Propagation: By seeds and vegetative method.

Parts Used: Root, vine.

Chemical Constituents: Little is known about the active constituents.

Uses: In Chinese herbal medicine, pain is often thought to be due to poor or obstructed blood flow. In this tradition, *ji xue teng* is classified as a herb that invigorates the blood, and is mainly used to treat menstrual problems. *Ji xue teng* is used to relieve period pain or normalize an irregular or absent cycle, especially where this may be due to anaemia. This herb is also prescribed for certain types of arthiritc pain, as well as for numbness of the hands and feet.

841. *Millettia speciosa* Champ. *(Fabaceae)*

Description: Woody climber, reacing 5-6m. Roots fleshy. Young shoots hoary. Leaves odd-pinnate, alternate, pubescent, especially when young. Inflorescence in axillary or terminal raceme; flowers white or pale-yellow. Pod compressed, pubescent. Seeds 2-5, subquadrangular.

Habitate: Grows wild in forests and in the hills.

Propagation: By seeds and vegetative method.

Part Used: Whole plant and Tuberous roots.

Chemical Constituents: The whole plant yields an essential oil consisting of L-menthol 65-85%, menthhyl acetate, L-menthone, L-a-pinene,: -limonene.

Uses: The tuberous roots posess reconstituent and antitussive properties. They are utilized in the treatment of general debility, anorexia, phlegmy cough (soaked in ginger juice and torrefied), and headache, dry cough, thirsty evening feber, dysuria (soaked in honey and torrefied).

842. *Mimosa pudica* L. *(Mimosaceae)*

Vernacular Name: *San:* Lajja; *Eng:* sensitive plant; *Hin:* Lajwanti, chui-mui; *Beng*: Lajjabati; *Tel:* Attapatti, peddanidrakanni; *Tam:* Tottaladi, thottalchinungi; *Kan:* Lajja, nachike, mudugu-davare and *Mal:* Tintarmani.

Description: Semi-prostrate, prickly course herb or subshrub up to 0.5m tall. Leaves alternate, bipinnately compound which fold up when disturbed. Flowers pink with several stamens up to 8 mm. Long, borne on globose heads. Fruit a flat, hairy legume (pod) breaking into 2-4 one-seeded segments.

Habitate: Common in disturbed open places, especially roadsides, cultivated land, and waste areas.

Propagation: By seeds and vegetative method.

Part Used: Whole plant.

Chemical Constituents: Amino acid (mimosine), norepinephrine, gentisic acid, jasmonic acid and D-panitol.

Uses: The leaves together with the leaves from other plants are used in treating haemorrhoids and urinary infections. A decoction of the roots is also used in treating urinary infections. Treat dysentery, fever, syphilis, leprosy, stomach worms, veneral diseas, insect bite, insomnia, nervouness and piles.

843. *Mimusops elengi* L. *(Sapotaceae)*

Vernacular Name: *San*: Bakulah; *Eng*: Bullet-wood tree; *Hin*: Bakul Maulsiri; *Kan*: Pagademara; *Mal*: llanni, Elanni; *Tam*: Magilam, llanci; *Tel:* Pogada.

Description: A large evergreen tree with dark grey fissured bark and dense spreading crown; leaves oblong, glabrous leathery with way margins; flowers white, fragrant, axillary, solitary of fascicled; fruits ovoid or ellipsoid berries, seeds 1-2 per fruit, ovoid, compressed grayish brown, shiny.

Habitate: Throughout south India and Andman Islands in evergreen forests and grown as avenue tree.

Propagation: By seeds and vegetative method.

Parts Used: Bark, flowers, fruits seeds.

Chemical Consistuents: Saponin, rhamnose, arabinose, glucose, tannin, palmitic, linoleic, oleic.

Uses: The bark, flowers and fruits are acrid, astringent, cooling and anthelmintic. Bark is tonic and febrifuge, and is used as a gargle for odontopathy, ulitis and ulemorrhagia. Tender stems are used as toothbrushes. It is also useful in urethrorrhoea, cystorrhoea, diarhoea and dysentery. Flowers are sued for preparing a lotion for wounds and ulcers; powder of dried flowers is a brain tonic, and is useful as a snuff to relieve cephalagia. Unripe fruit is used as a masticatory and will help to fix loose teeth. Seeds are used for preparing suppositories in cases of constipation especially in children.

844. *Mitchella repens* *(Rubiaceae)*

Vernacular Name: *Eng:* Squaw vine.

Description: Evergreen herb growing to 30 cm and forming mats on the ground. Has rounded shiny leaves, a flowering stem gearing fragrant white flowers and small, bright red berries.

Habitate: Squaw vine is native to eastern and central US. It grows in dry sites in woodlands, and is harvested in late summer.

Propagation: By seeds and vegetative method.

Parts Used: Aerial parts and berries.

Chemical Constituents: Squaw vine is believed to contain tannins, glycosides and saponins.

Uses: Squaw vine is still extensively used to aid labour and childbirth, and is also considered to have a tonic action on the uterus and the ovaries. It is taken to normalize menstruation and to relieve heavy periods and period pain. This herb has also been recommended for stimulating breast-milk production, but other herbs with a similar action, such as fennel, are preferred. The berries, crushed and mixed with tincture of myrrh are helpful for sore nipples. An astringent herb, squaw vine has also been prescribed for diarrhoea and colitis.

845. *Mitragyna parvifolia* (Roxb.) Korth. *(Rubiaceae)*

Synonyms: *Stephegyne parvifolia* Roxb.

Vernacular Name: *Eng*: Kaim; *Hin*: Kayim; Kaddam Kamgi; *Kan*: Kongu, Kadaga; *Mal*: Vimpu, Nirkkatampu, Rosu, katampu; *San*: Vitanah; *Tam*: Katampai, Nirkkatampu, Sinnakkatampu; *Tel:* Nerkadamba.

Description: A medium sized to large deciduous tree with rounded crown and light grey smooth bark exfoliating in small scales; leaves simple, opposite, very variable, elliptic, suborbicular or obovate, rounded, acute or bluntly acuminate, glabrous on both sides, main nerves 6-8 pairs, stipules 13 by 5.8 mm; flowers greenish yellow, fragrant, in globose heads; fruits oblong capsules with blunt rounded tops and blunt ribs.

Habitate: Throughout India, in deciduous and evergreen forests upto 1,200 m.

Propagation: By seeds and vegetative method.

Parts Used: Roots, bark, leaves.

Chemical Consistuents: Pyroligneous acid, methyl acetate, ketones and aldehydes methanol, tar, pitch and losses.

Uses: The roots and bark are acrid, bitter, stomachic and febrifuge, and are useful in gastropathy, colic and fever. The leaves are acrid, bitter, sweet, styptic, vulnerary, stomachic, anti-inflammatory, anodyne depurative and febrifuge. They are useful in vitiated conditions of *vata* and *kapha*, internal and external haemorrhages, wounds, colic, flatulence, dyspepsia, inflammations, myalgia, skin diseases, leprosy, erysipelas and fever.

846. *Momordica charanita* L. *(Cucurbitaceae)*

Vernacular Name: *San:* Sushavi; *Eng:* bitter gourd; balsam pear; balsam apple; *Hin:* Karela, kareli; *Beng*: Karela; *Tam:* Pakal, pavakka; *Kan:* Hagal and *Mal:* Kaippa kaippavalli.

Description: Climbing or scrambling hebaceous vine with tendrils. Leaves alternate, petiolate, the blade with 5-7 deep palmate lobes and quite variable in size. Flowers unisexual, tubular, 5-lobed, moderate sized, pale yellow to orangish. Fruit a pepo with black seeds embedded in a reddish pulp.

Habitate: Common in coastal thickets, along creeks and streams, and lowland forest margins Also occasionally cultivated.

Propagation: By seeds and vegetative method.

Part Used: Fruits.

Chemical Constituents: Vicine, mycose, steroidal glucoside, momorcharaside A,B, cucubitane triterpenoids, momordicines I and II, cycloeucalenol, spinasterol, stigmasterol, taraxerol, lophenol, momordicosides, diosgenin, thiocyanogen, 24-methylencycloartenol, phenyl propanoids, carotenoids, squalene (seed essential oil), stigmastadien-3-beta-ol and glucoside.

Uses: Fruit used to treat leprosy and malignant ulcers to treat stomach worms, fever and phlegm, hypertension, dysentery and diabetes.

847. *Momordica cochinchinesis* (Lour.) *(Cucurbitaceae)*

Vernacular Name: *San:* Karkataka; *Hin:* Gulkakra, gangerua; *Beng*: Go-ka-kara, kakrol; *Tel:* Adavi kakara.

Description: Twining perennial with tendrils. Leaves alternate, deeply 3-5 lobed; margins toothed; leaf-stalk glandular. Flowers unisexual, monoecious, pale-yellow, solitary in the axil of the leaves. Fruit big, oval-shaped, densely aculeate, red when ripe. Seeds round, compressed, the margins sculputured.

Habitate: Cultivated everywhere for its edible fruit.

Propagation: By seeds and vegetative method.

Part Used: Seed membranes, kernels & roots.

Chemical Constituents: The seed membranes contains b-carotene and lycopene. The seed kernels yield a fatty oil. The roots contain triterperiod saponins.

Uses: The seed membrane is rich in b-carotene and is used in treating infantile rickets, xerophthalmia and nyctalopia. The juice of kernels triturated in alcohol or venegar is applied locally for furunculosis and phelegmon. In cases of rheumatism the roots are prescribed in the form of a decoction.

848. *Monarda punctata* *(Lamiaceae)*

Vernacular Name: *Eng:* Horsemint.

Description: Strongly aromatic perennial growing to 90 cm. Has downy lance-shaped leaves, and double-lipped, red-spotted yellow flowers growing in whorls from the leaf axils.

Habitate: Native to eastern and central US, horsemint is found in dry and *San*dy areas. It is gathered when in flower in summer and autumn.

Propagation: By seeds and vegetative method.

Parts Used: Aerial parts.

Chemical Constituents: Horsemint's volatile oil has thymol as the main constituent.

Uses: Having a strong volatile oil, horsemint is primarily used for digestive and upper respiratory problems. It is taken as an infusion to relieve nausea, indigestion, flatulence and colic. It is also employed to reduce fevers and upper respiratory catarrh. The herb has an antiseptic action within the chest. Taken internally or applied externally, horsemint reduces fever by encouraging seating. It also strongly stimulates menstruation. Applied externally, the plant is a counter-irritant. It helps to lessen the pain in arthritic and rheumatic joints by increasing the flow of blood in the affected area, and thereby hastening the flushing out of toxins.

849. *Monochoria vaginalis* Presl *(Pontederiaceae)*

Vernacular Name: *San*: Indivarah; *Mal*: Karinkuvvalam, Kakapola; *Tam*: Karimkuvalam; *Tel:* Nirkanca.

Description: A perennial aquatic herb with suberect spongy root-stock; leaves long-petioled, linear to ovate or subreniform, nerves very close and numerous, 7.5-20 cm long,

2-15 cm wide, petioles of the floral leave embracing the short stout peduncle; flowers blue usually spotted with red in subspicate racemes; fruits ellipsoid capsules.

Habitate: Throughout India, in ponds and marshes upto 1,500 m.

Propagation: By Rhizomes.

Parts Used: Root-stock, leaves.

Chemical Consisituents: N.A.

Uses: The root-stock and leaves are cooling, bitter, sweet, aromatic, alterant, diuretic and tonic. They are useful in burning sensation of the body, vitiated conditions of *pitta*, dipsia, strangury, gastropathy, hepatopathy, cough, asthma, odontalgia, scurvy, boils and haemorrhages.

850. *Monsonia ovata* *(Geraniaceae)*

Vernacular Name: *Eng:* Monsonia.

Description: Small herbaceous plant with mulit-branched stems, very small oblong leaves and white solitary or paired geranium-like flowers.

Habitate: Native to south Africa and Namibia, monsonia is found growing in arid conditions.

Propagation: By seeds and vegetative method.

Parts Used: Aerial parts.

Chemical Constituents: N.A.

Uses: Monsonia is used throughout south-western Africa as a treatment for diarrhoea, acute and chronic dysentery, and ulcerative colitis. The plant's astringent properties act to tighten and protect the inner linings of the intestinal tract. Given monosnia's long traditional use for intestinal disorders and infections, it is possible-but as yet unsubstantiated by research-that the plant has a direct antimicrobial effect.

851. *Montia perfoliata* *(Portulacaceae)*

Vernacular Name: *Eng:* Miner's lettuce.

Description: Annual growing to 10 cm with pointed oval leaves and white 5-petalled flowers.

Habitate: Miner's lettuce is native to western North America, and has become naturalized in temperate regions around the world, especially in Australia.

Propagation: By seeds and vegetative method.

Parts Used: Aerial parts.

Chemical Constituents: Miner's lettuce is rich in vitamin C.

Uses: Apart from its value as a nourishing vegetable, miner's lettuce, like its relative purslane, may also be taken as an invigoration spring tonic and an effective diuretic.

852. *Morinda citrifolia* L. *(Rubiaceae)*

Vernacular Name: *San:* Ashyuka; *Eng:* Indian mulverry, East Indian mulberry, awl tree; *Hin*: Al, ach, surangi, bartundi; *Beng*: Al, ach, surangi, bartundi; *Tel:* Maddi, togaru; *Tam:* Nuna, togaru; *Kan:* Ainshi, tagase and *Mal:* Kattapitalavam.

Description: Medium-sized tree, 6-8m. in height. Yoiung twigs angular, slightly compressed and grooved, leaves opposite, stipuliferous; shining green agove, pale belowl margins undulate. Inflorescence in dense ovoid head, opposite to the leaf; flowers white, then yellow. Fruit ovoid including many drupelets, yellow when ripe. Seeds numerous, embedded in the pulp.

Habitate: Grows wild and is externsively cultivated in the south of Viet Nam.

Propagation: By seeds and vegetative method.

Part Used: Roots, fruit and leaves.

Chemical Constituents: The root-bark contains morindon, morindin morindadiol, soranjidiol, rubichloric acid, alizarin a-methyl ether, and rubiadin 1-methyl ether.

Uses: The root-bark has a beneficial effect in hypertension, osteodynia and lumbago. A decoction of the leaves taken by mouth in effective for fever, dysentery and diarrhoea. A poultice of pounded fresh leaves cures furunculosis. The fruit, taken together with a little salt, is stomachic, aperient, and active on dysentery, uterine haemorrhage, metrorrhoea, cough, coryza, oedema and neuralgia.

853. *Morinda officinalis* How. *(Rubiaceae)*

Description: Perennial slender climbing shrub. Young shoots violet, hairy. Leaves opposite, oblong, hairy on both sides. Stipule tubular, Inflorescence in axilary panicle; flowers small, white, fruit globose, scarlet wen ripe, 2-seeded.

Habitate: Indigenous to noth VietNam, commonly found wild in hilly and mountainous regions.

Propagation: By seeds and vegetative method.

Part Used: Roots.

Chemical Constituents: The roots contain organic acids, sugars, resins, vitamin C, an essential oil, anthraglucosides and phytosterols.

Uses: The roots are reported to exert a tonic effect. They are useful in treationg impotence, spermatorrhoea, delayed menstruation, hypertension and rheumatism.

854. *Morinda pubescens* J. E. Smith *(Rubiaceae)*

Synonyms: *Morinda coreia* Buch.-Hom, *Morinda tinctoria* Roxb.

Vernacular Name: *San*: Paphanah, *Eng*: Morinda tree, *Hin*: Acc, Al, *Kan*: Haladipavete, Tagatemara, *Mal*: Pavitta, Mannappavitta, *Tam*: Mannanatti, Mannanunai, *Tel:* Maddicettu.

Description: A moderate sized deciduous tree, upto 4.5 m in height with spongy deeply cracked grayish yellow bark; leaves simple, opposite, elliptic-ovate or lanceolate; flowers white, scented, in dense ovoid leaf opposed heads; fruits multiple globose drupes about 2 cm in diameter.

Habitate: Bengal, Central Provinces and south India.

Propagation: By seeds and vegetative method.

Parts Used: Root, leaves.

Chemical Consistuents: The root bark of *M. coreia* contains morindone and its glucoside morindin. The heartwood contains three anthraquinone pigments, namely, morindone, damnacanthal and *nor*-damnacanthal.

Uses: The roots are styptic, constipating, anti-inflammatory, alexeteric and tonic, and are useful in haemorrhages, dysentery, inflammations, boils and general debility. The leaves are digestive, carminative, febrifuge and tonic. They are useful in gastropathy, dyspepsia, diarrhoea, ulcerative stomatitis, wounds, gout, inflammation, hernia, sarcocele and fever.

855. *Moringa concanensis* Nimmo ex Dalz. & Gibson *(Moringaceae)*

Vernacular Name: *San*: Sigru, Madhusigru; *Hin*: Sajana; *Kan*: Nugge; *Mal*: Murinna; *Mar*: Sajana, Muwa; *Tam*: Kattu murungai, Kari murungai; *Tel:* Adavi munaga, Konda munaga.

Description: Deciduous trees, 8-20 m tall, about 2 m girth. *Woodsoft,* white. *Bark* about 1.5 cm thick, rough, corky, vertically irregularly fissured, cement-white, easily brittle, exuding colourless, watery juice becoming jelly-like and turning yellowish brown and hard on exposure. *Blaze* whitish, smooth, and fibrous. Branches cylindrical, warty, easily broken and densely minutely tomentose. *Leaves* about 100 x 80 cm, doubly pinnate; rachis jointed; primary pinnae 5-8 pairs, opposite; secondary pinnae 4-6 pairs, opposite; leaflets opposite, egg-shaped to elliptic, 1-3 x 1-2 cm, papery, shortly stalked, base rounded, apex rounded or deeply notched, margin entire, pale green above, blue-green below. *Flowers* bisexual, irregular, about 0.5 cm across, white with purple streaks, arranged in axillary divaricate tomentose about 30 cm wide panicles, mildly fragrant; floral stalks up to 1 cm long, distinctly jointed. *Capsules* elongated, slightly 3-angled, woody when mature, about 60 cm long and about 2 cm wide, splitting by 3-valves. *Seeds* numerous, 3-angled, about 2 x 1.5 cm, with white papery marginal wings.

Habitate: Hills of deciduous belt.

Propagation: By seeds and vegetative method.

Parts Used: Fruits, Root, Root bark.

Chemical Constituents: N.A.

Uses: The medicinal properties of *M. concanensis* and the commonly cultivated *M. oleifera* (drumstick) are considered similar. Root and root bark of *M. olifera* is considered useful for the treatment of paralysis, intermittent fever, abscess, epilepsy, rheumatism, fainting and giddiness. Stem bark is abortifacient and fruits are used for curing liver & spleen diseases, joint pains and paralysis. Flowers are used as aphrodisiac. Seed oil is used for treatment of rheumatism. Gum is used for treating dental and ear problems.

856. *Moringa oleifera* Lam. *(Moringaceae)*

Synonyms: *Moringa* pterygosperma Gaertn.

Vernacular Name: *San*: Sigruh, Sobhanjanah, *Eng*: Horse-radish tree, Drumstick tree, *Hin*: Sahijan, Mungana, *Kan*: Nuggi, Murunga, *Mal*: Murinna, *Tam*: Murunkai, *Tel:* Munaga, Mulaga.

Description: An unarmed middle sized graceful tree with corky grey bark and easily breakable branches; leaves usually tripinnate, rachis slender, thickened and articulated at the base, leaflets elliptic or obovate, rounded at the apex, nerves obscures; flowers white in large puberuous axillary panicles; fruits pods, upto 45 cm long, pendulous, greenish, triangular, 9-ribbed, seeds trigonous, the angles winged.

Habitate: Throughout India, also cultivated.

Propagation: By seeds and vegetative method.

Parts Used: Roots, bark, leaves, seeds.

Chemical Consistuents: Carotene, nicotinic acid and ascorbic acid ascorbic acid oxidase sulphur, and a prolamin. The essential amino acids present in the total proteins are arginine, histidine, lysine, tryptophan, phenylalanine, methionine, threonine, leucine, isoleucine, and valine, No.-protein nitrogen histidine, arginine, threonine, valine, methionine, phenylalanine, isoleucine, leucine, and tyrosine, lysine and tryptophan traces and cystine nil. The essential amino acids present in the leaf proteins are arginine histidine lysine tryptophan, phenylalanine, methionine, threonine, leucine, isoleucine, and valine.

Uses: The roots are bitter, acrid thermogenic, digestive, carminative, anthelmintic, constipating, anodyne, anti-inflammtory, emmenagogue, sudorific diuretic, ophthalmic, rubefacient, expectorant, haematinic, antilithic, alexipharmic stimulant and vesicant. They are useful in vitiated conditions of *vata* and *kapha*, dyspepsia, anorexia, verminosis, diarrhoea, colic flatulence, otalgia, paralysis, inflammations, amenorrhoea, dysmenorrhoea, fever, strnagury, vesical and renal calculi, ascites, ophthalmopathy, cough, asthma bronchitis, pectoral diseases, splenomegaly, epilepsy, hysteria, cardiopathy, abscess and pharyngodynia. The bark is acrid, bitter, thermogenic, abortifacient, antifungal and cardiac and circulatory stimulant. It is useful in ascites, vitiated conditions of *vata* and *kapha* and ringworm. The leaves are anti-inflammatory, anodyne, anthelmintic, ophthalmic and rich in vitamins A and C. They are useful in scurvy, vitiated conditions of *kapha* and *vata*, wounds tumours, inflammations and helminthasis. The seeds are acrid, bitter, anodyne, anti-inflammatory, purgative, antipyretic and ophthalmic. They are useful in neuralgia, inflammations, intermittent fevers and ophthalmopathy.

857. *Morus acidosa* Griff. *(Moraceae)*

Description: Small plant 2-3m. high, occasionally reaching 5-6m. when old. Leaves alternate, entire or trilobed; margins toothed; 3 nerves from the base. Flowers unisexual, monoecious, in axillary spike (catkin). **Fruit:** syncarp of many drupes, initially red then dark purple to black.

Habitate: Cultivated for its leaves, used as food for silk-worms, and its edible fruit.

Propagation: By seeds and vegetative method.

Part Used: Leaves, fruit and root-bark.

Chemical Constituents: The leaves contain amino acids: phenylalanine, leucine, alanine, arginine, sarcosine; pipercholic acid; proteins; vitamins C,B_1,D; organic aacids; succinic, propionic and isobutyric; tannin.

Uses: The leaves are used in treating coryza, cough and insomnia. The root bark is employed in the treatment of asthma, oliguria, rheumatism and osteodynia. The fruit in elixir and syrup form is prescribed for anaemia and dysopia. Syrup made of the ripe fruit serves as a mouth-wash in cases of sore throat and ulcerous stomatitis.

858. *Morus alba* L. *(Moraceae)*

Vernacular Name: *Eng:* white mulverry, white-fruited mulberry; *Hin*: Tut, tutri, chinni; *Beng*: Tut; *Guj*: Shetur; *Tel:* Reshme, chattu; *Tam*; Musukette, kambli; *Kan*: Hipnerle.

Description: A deciduous tree, 3-15 m high, bark or large stems brown, rough; fissures mostly vertical. Leaves alternate, very variable in size and shape, usually broadly oval, 6-18 m long by 2.0-4.5 cm wide, apex acuminate; base rounded or cordate; margin irregularly dentate or incised-lobate, glabrous or slightly purescent along the nerves beneath, in young plants and on vigourous shoots usually lobed; basal nerve 3, lateral nerves forked near the margin; petiole usually 1.8-2.5 cm long. Flower monoecious or dioecious, greenish, frouped in stalked, hanging catkins, may. Fruit aggregate, consisting of all the ovaries of the catkin forming a crustaceous achene.

Habitate: Mostly cultivated; also grows in the wild in China, India, Japan, Pakistan, Philippines, Sri Lanka, Viet Nam.

Propagation: By vegetative method.

Part Used: Root bark.

Chemical Constituents: N.A.

Uses: Cough, dyspnaea, facial dropsy, oedema, oliguria, injury.

859. *Mucuna pruriens* (L.) DC. *(Fabaceae)*

Synonyms: *Mucuna prurita* Hook.

Vernacular Name: *San*: Atmagupta, Kapikacchuh; *Eng*: Common cowitch, Cowhage; *Hin*: Gonca, Kaunc, Kivacc; *Kan*: Nasuganni, Nayisonanguballi; *Mal*: Naykkorana, Naykkurana, Corivalli; *Tam*: Punaikkali, Punaippidukkan; *Tel:* Pilliadugu.

Description: A slender climbing annual with hairy branches; leaves trifoliate, leaflets broadly ovate, elliptic or rhomboid ovate, membranous, unequal at base, pubescent above and densely clothed with silvery grey hairs beneath; flowers purple, in axillary pendulous, 6-30 flowered racemes; fruits turgid pods, longitudinally ribbed, curved, densely clothed with persistent pale brown or grey irritant bristles, seeds black, 4-6 per pod, ovoid.

Habitate: Throughout India among hedges and bushes.

Propagation: By seeds and vegetative method.

Parts Used: Roots, leaves, seeds, hairs.

Chemical Consistuents: Moisture, protein ether extr fibre and mineral matter, calcium, phosphorus, and iron sulphur and manganese are present. The seeds contain dihydroxyphenylalanine or dopa glutathione, lecithin, galic acid and a glucoside are present. They contain also a number of alkaloids including nicoting, prurieninine, pruienidine, and five other base designeated base.

Uses: The roots are bitter, sweet thermogenic emollient, stimulant, purgative, aphrodisiac, diuretic, emmenagogue, anthelmintic, febrifuge, diuretic and tonic. They are useful in vitiated conditions of *vata* and *pitta*, constipation, nephroathy, strangury, dysmenorrhoea, amenorrhoea, elephantiasis, dropsy, neuropathy, consumption, ulcers, helminthiasis, fever and delirium. The leaves are aphrodisiac, anthelmintic and tonic, and are useful in ulcers, inflammation, helminthiasis, cephalalgia and general debility. The seeds are astringent, laxative, anthelmintic, aphrodisiac, alexipharmic and tonic. They are useful in gonorrhoea, consumption, sterility, vitiated conditions of *vata* and general debility. The hairs and flowers are vermifuge.

860. *Murraya glabra* Guill. *(Rutaceae)*

Description: Medium-sized bush, 3-7 m. high. Young shoots reddish-purple. Leaves alternate, imparipinnate, including 4-7 leaflets, thick, entire or minutely dentate. Inflorescence in terminal corymbiferous cyme; flowers white, fragrant, berry subglobose, rough, with glands, red when ripe.

Habitate: Common wild plant among limestone rocks.

Propagation: By seeds and vegetative method.

Part Used: Leaves and roots.

Chemical Constituents: The whole plant, especially the leaves and fruit, yield and essential oil containing isomenthone and menthone.

Uses: The leaves and roots give beneficial results in the treatment of influenza, headache and abdominal pains. They are also useful for the treatment of rheumatism and arthralgia. The essential oil from the leaves is used externally as a liniment. In cases oif luxation or closed ffacture the leaves are crushed and employed locally as a poultice.

861. *Murraya koenigii* (L.) Spreng. *(Rutaceae)*

Vernacular Name: *San:* Surabhininiba; *Eng:* Curry lea tree; *Hin:* Kathnim, mitha neem, kurry patta, gandhela, barsanga; *Beng*: Barsanga, kariaphulli; *Tel:* karepaku; *Tam:* Karivempu, karuveppilei, kattuveppilei; *Kan:* Karibevu and *Mal:* Kariveppilei.

Description: An aromatic shrub or small tree; leaves pinnate, leaflets mostly ovate, crenate-dentate; flowers white in corymbose cymes; berries purplish black.

Habitate: Throughout India.

Propagation: By seeds and vegetative method.

Part Used: Leaves.

Chemical Constituents: The major aroma constituents in the oil are b-caryophyllene, b-gurjunene, b-elemene, and b-phellandrene.

Uses: The leaves are extensively used for flavouring curries, chuntneys, soups, pickles, etc.

862. *Musa nana* Lour. *(Musaceae)*

Synonyms: *Musa acuminata* Colla.

Vernacular Name: *Eng:* Chinese or dwarf Cavendish banana.

Description: Herb with pseudostems up to 2 m high arising from fleshy corms. Leaves spirally arranged with overlapping bases that form a pseudostem, petiolate, relatively large. Flowers strongly zygomorphic, unisexual, borne on a terminal inflorescence which arises from the center of the pseudostem. Fruit a slightly shortened banana (moderately long yellow berry with fleshy mesocarp and seedless).

Habitate: Cultivated only, probably native to Cambodia, Laos and Viet nam, and now widely cultivated in the tropics.

Propagation: By vegetative method.

Part Used: Leaves and roots.

Chemical Constituents: Serotonin, norepinephrine; the banana peel contains beta-carotene, alpha and delta-tropherol, riboflavin, niacin, ascorbic acid, carbohydrates, proteins, iron, and vitamins A,B, and C.

Uses: A decoction of the leaves is drunk to treat consumption, Painful urination is treated with juice form the leaves, and dysentery is treated with the leaves. The leaves, together with the leaves of some other species, are used to treat navel pains and filarial fever in males. The roots are used to treat convulsions, and the pith of the suckers is used to treat burns. The stem is used to treat swellings of the armpit and groin and to treat haemorrhoids.

863. *Musa paradisiaca* L. *(Musaceae)*

Synonyms: *Musa sapientum* Linn.

Vernacular Name: *San*: Kadali, *Eng*: Kadali, Plantain, *Hin*: Kela, *Kan*: Balehannu, *Mal*: Kadalivala, Ksetrakadali, *Tam*: Kadali valai, *Tel:* Ariti, Kadalamu.

Description: A tall herb with aerial pseudo stem dying after flowering, leaves oblong, narrowed to base; flowers unisexual in spikes, dropping, females at the bottom and males at the top, bracts conspicuous, dull brown, falling off in succession; fruits berries in several clusters, golden yellow colour on ripening.

Habitate: Cultivated throughout India.

Propagation: By vegetative method.

Parts Used: Roots, leaves, fruits, stem.

Chemical Consistuents: The principal proteins of the banana are an albumin and a globulin; glutelin, prolamines and proteoses are also present. Cystine, lysine, histidine, arginine, serine, glycine & aspartic acid, threonine, glutamic acid, alanine, γ-Amino butyric acid, tyrosine, methionine & valine, phenylalanine, leucine, isoleucine,.

Uses: The roots are anthelmintic, antiscorbutic, depurative and tonic, and are useful in venereal diseases, helminthiasis, scabies, leprosy, skin diseases and debility. The tender leaves are useful in scabies, inflammations, ophthalmopathy, blisters and burns. The fruits are sweet, astringent, emollient, cooling, anthelmintic, aphrodisiac, antiscorbutic, demulcent and tonic. They are useful in vitiated conditions of *pitta*, dipsia, helminthiasis, scabies, pruritus, bronchitis, pharyngodynia, nephropathy, strangury and general debility. The ashes obtained by burning the plant are antiscorbutic, anthelmintic and stomachic, and are useful in hyperacidity, heartburn, colic and verminosis. The flowers are good for dysentery, diabetes, ascites and dropsy. The inflorescence axis (stem) is very specific for renal and vesical calculi.

864. *Mussaenda frondosa* L. *(Rubiaceae)*

Vernacular Name: *San*: Sriparnah, Rajatarih; *Hin*: Bedina, Bedina; *Kan*: Bellotigida Belloti; *Mal*: Vellila, Vellilam, Vellilattali; *Tam*: Vellai ilai, velli matantai; *Tel:* Nagavalli, Sribati.

Description: A handsome erect or scandent shrub with grey bark; leaves simple, opposite, ovate, acuminate at apex, densely soft white tomentose beneath, transverse nervules obscure; flowers yellowish green outside and orange green within, in terminal cymes, one of the calyx lobes becomes enlarged into white foliaceous structure; fruits subglobose or ovoid green berries.

Habitate: Throughout India in forests, also cultivated.

Propagation: By seeds and vegetative method.

Parts Used: Whole plant.

Chemical Consistuents: N.A.

Uses: The plant is astringent, sweet, expectorant, febrifuge, anti-inflammatory, vulnerary, alterant, demulcent, ophthalmic and cardiotonic. It is useful in cough, bronchitis, fever, inflammation, wounds and ulcers, leucoderma, pruritus, ophthalmopathy, jaundice, metropathy and uropathy.

865. *Mussaenda raiateenisis* J. W. More. *(Rubiaceae)*

Description: Shrub to small tree up to 10 m tall. Leaves opposite, short-petiolate, ovate, 8-25 cm. long and hairy. Flowers tubular, usually yellowish-orange, subtended by 1 white or yellowish conspicuous leaf like sepal, the flowers borne in dense terminal clusters. Fruit a green berry up to 20 mm long. Flowers and fruit available throughout the year.

Habitate: Common in forest clearings, secondary forests, open ridges from sea-level to mid-montane.

Propagation: By seeds and vegetative method.

Part Used: Leaves and bark.

Chemical Constituents: Quercetin, rutin, hyerin, ferulic acid, sinapic acid, bets-sitosterol glucoside, oligosaccharides, saponin.

Uses: To improve fertility and to relieve vaginal pain to treat respiration illness, severe pain (during pregnancy), rheumatic aches, sore throat, toothache, diarrhoea, and liver truble. The leaves are used in a remedy for treating hernia. The liquid from the stem bark is drunk for sharp pain in the eye sockets (especially during pregnancy). The bark in the treatment of the cancer of the uterus and to treat high fever. An infusion of the bark is given to infants who are ill or undernourished especially when breastfed by the mother who is pregnant again. An infusion of the leaves or bark is applied as poultice where children's skin becomes black, beginning form the buttocks.

866. *Myrica cerifera* (*Myricaceae*)

Vernacular Name: *Eng:* Bayberry.

Description: Evergreen shrub or small tree growing to 10 m. Has narrow leaves, small yellow flowers in catkins and waxy grey berries.

Habitate: Bayberry is found in coastal regions of the eastern and southern US, as far west as Texas.

Propagation: By seeds and vegetative method.

Parts Used: Root bark.

Chemical Constituents: Bayberry contains triterpenes, flavonoids, tannins, phenols, resins and gums. Myricadiol has a mild effect on potassium and sodium levels. Myrictrin is antibacterial.

Uses: Bayberry is used to increase circulation, stimulated perspiration and keep bacterial infections in check. Colds, flu, coughs and sore throats benefit from treatment with this herb. It helps to strengthen resistance to infection and to tighten and dry mucous membranes. An infusion is helpful for spongy gums, and a gargle is sued for sore throats. Bayberry's astringency is beneficial of irritable bowel syndrome and mucous colitis. An infusion can help treat excess vaginal discharge. A paste of the powdered root bark may be used externally on ulcers and sores.

867. *Myristica beddomei* King. (*Myristicaceae*)

Synonyms: *Myristica dactyloides* Gaertn., *Myristica contorta* Warb.

Vernacular Name: *Hin*: Jayaphal; *Kan*: Kadu jaapatre, Kadu jajikai; *Mal*: Panthappayin, Adakkappayin, Kattu jathi; *Mar*: Jayaphal; *San*: Jatiphala; *Tam*: Kattu jathikaa, Kakkai moonji, Perumpattai.

Description: A large evergreen dioecious tree, reaching 30 m height and about 2 m girth. *Bark* smooth, surface blackish green, with small exfoliation; *outer bark* 1-2 mm thick, dead; *inner bark* 1-1.3 cm thick, fibrous, striate, deep red, exuding reddish watery juice when cut freshly. *Wood* yellowish brown, moderately hard. Branchlets robust, hairless, the terminal bud velvety. *Leaves* alternate, simple, elliptic to oblong-lanceolate, 10-25 x 5-10 cm, base rounded, apex acute, margin entire, hairless, leathery, shining above, bluish grey beneath; lateral nerves 16-18 pairs, prominent. Flowers unisexual, male and female flowers seen in separate trees. *Male flowers* 5-6 long, white, stalkless or shortly stalked, 10-20 together arising on short woody structures, hairy, brown tomentose, thin fleshy. *Female flowers* usually solitary, rarely 3-4 together, more or less stalkless, slightly bigger than male flowers, white. *Drupes* 1-3 together, broadly ovoid to ellipsoid, 4-8 x 3-6 cm, powdery-pubescent, with fleshy outer rind. *Seeds* ovoid, 2-4 x 1.5-3 cm, smooth, covered with fleshy dissected orange-red to creamy white aril.

Habitate: Evergreen forests.

Propagation: By seeds and vegetative method.

Parts Used: Seeds.

Chemical Constituents: Triglycerides, palmitic, stearic oleic and linoleic, glyceride trisaturated, trace; di-saturated mono-unsaturated, mono-saturated di-unsaturated and tri-unsaturated.

Uses: Aril with dried ginger is rubbed in cold water and given to check diarrhoea. Aril is also used in treating cough, bronchitis, fever, burning sensation, inflammation of joints, skin disorders, wounds, sleeplessness, indigestion, liver disorders and worms.

868. *Myristica fragrans* Houtt. *(Myristicaceae)*

Vernacular Name: *San:* Jatiphala; *Eng:* Nutmeg tree; *Hin:* Jaiphal, japatri, jotri, jayapatri; *Beng*: Jaiphal, japatri, jotri, jayapatri; *Tel:* Jajikai, jadikai, jadipattiri, japatri; *Tam:* Jajikai, jadikai, jadipattiri, japatri; *Kan:* Jajikai, jadikai, jadipattiri, japatri; *Mal:* Jajikai, jadikai, jadipattiri, japatri.

Description: A lofty tree with branches slender. Leaves 7-10 cm., coriaceous, dark green, entire, elliptic-oblong or lanceolate, acuminate both at apex and base, glauxous beneath, nerves about 8 pairs, slender; petiole 6-12 mm. flowers dioecious. Male flowers 3-5 in racemes, 2.5-5 cm. flowers 6 mm. long ellipsoid nodding, with a scale like bracteole under the glabrate perianth; anthers 9-12, connate in a cylindric stipilate column. Pistillate flowers yellow, small axillary, often solitary. Fruit ovoid, sub-globose or pyriform, 4-5 cm. long, valved. Seed one, almost completely surrounded by a fleshy, irregularly slit or holed arillode.

Habitate: Grown in southern state of India, particularly Tamil Nadu.

Propagation: By seeds and vegetative method.

Part Used: Fruit.

Chemical Constituents: Major constituents of nutmeg oil are d-b-pinene, myristicin, linalool, safrole, dl-a-pinene, dipentene, and linalyl acetate.

Uses: The kernel as well as the aril are used whole or ground as culinary spice, in spice and in bakery and confectionery items. Nutmeg is used in flavouring desserts and in meat seasoning. Mace is used in meat seasoning, sausage fillings, sauces, pickles, soups and curries. Solvent extracted oleoresin as such and in encapsulated form is used as substitute for the whole or ground spice. Nutmeg oil is used to flavour liqueurs, canned soups, cooked cabbage, and other food products.

869. *Myristica malabarica* Lam. *(Myristicaceae)*

Vernacular Name: *San*: Gostani, Vanyajati; *Eng*: Bombay mace, False nutmeg; *Hin*: Bambay-jayphal, Van-jayphal; *Kan*: *Kan*agi; *Mal*: Pasupasi, Kattujati Patri; *Tam*: Pattiri, Kattu, jatikkai; *Tel:* Rampatri, Vanajati.

Description: A moderate sized evergreen tree with grayish black smooth bark and whorls of branches; leaves simple, alternate, elliptic-oblong, subobtuse, thinly coriaceous, shiny above, dull beneath, nerves about 10 pairs; flowers small in dichasial cymes, unisexual, male flowers in slender cymes, females more globose and larger than the males; fruits elongate, densely rugose-tomentose, seeds arillate, aril reddish yellow, irregularly lobed, extending upto the apex of the seed.

Habitate: Throughout south India, in evergreen forests of low elevations upto 300 m.

Propagation: By seeds A lofty tree with branches slender. Leaves 7-10 cm., coriaceous, dark green, entire, elliptic-oblong or lanceolate, acuminate both at apex and base, glauxous beneath, nerves about 8 pairs, slender; petiole 6-12 mm. flowers dioecious. Male flowers 3-5 in racemes, 2.5-5 cm. flowers 6 mm. long ellipsoid nodding, with a scale like bracteole under the glabrate perianth; anthers 9-12, connate in a cylindric stipilate column. Pistillate flowers yellow, small axillary, often solitary. Fruit ovoid, sub-globose or pyriform, 4-5 cm. long, valved. Seed one, almost completely surrounded by a fleshy, irregularly slit or holed arillode.

Parts Used: Seed and aril.

Chemical Consistuents: Myristic, palmitic and oleic. The glyceride composition of the fat was as follows; tri-saturated, di-saturated mono-unsaturated, mono-saturated di-unsaturated, and tri-unsaturated, amylodextrin, glucose, starch, a volatile oil.

Uses: The aril of the seeds is cooling, febrifuge and expectorant, and is useful in vitiated conditions of *vata*, cough, bronchitis, fever and burning sensation. The fat obtained from the seeds is good for vitiated conditions of *vata*, myalgia, sprains and sores.

870. *Myroxylon pereirae* (*Fabaceae*)

Synonyms: *Myroxylon balsamum var. pereirae.*

Vernacular Name: *Eng:* Peruvian balsam.

Description: A tall tree, 12-30 m. high, with a spreading crown. Leaves imparipinnate; leaflets oblong; flowers yellowish, in small axillary racemes; pod yellow.

Habitate: Native to central America, Peruvian balsam grows wild in tropical forests.

Propagation: By seeds and vegetative method.

Parts Used: Oleo-resin.

Chemical Constituents: The oleo-resin contains 50-65% volatile oil and resins.

Uses: Peruvian balsam is strongly antiseptic and stimulates repair of damaged tissue. It is most commonly taken internally as an expectorant and anticatarrhal remedy to treat bronchitis, emphysema and bronchial asthma. It may also be taken to treat sore throats and diarrhoea. Externally, the balsam is applied to skin afflictions.

871. *Myrtus communis* L. (*Myrtaceae*)

Synonyms: *Myrtus acuta* Mill, *Myrtus media* Molina., *Myrtus minima* Mill.

Vernacular Name: *Eng:* common myrtle.

Description: An evergreen shrub, 1-3 m. or more high, leaves sessile or short petioled, gland dotted, strongly scented, small, ovate or lanceolate, entire, smooth, shining, coriaceous; peduncles solitary; flowers in leaf axils, white and reddish with reddish brown pedicels with two aixllary linear bractlets; stamens numerous larger than petals; berries ellipsoid, blue black; seeds white, kidney shaped.

Habitate: U.S.A., Europe. Cultivated in North West Himalayas.

Propagation: By seeds and vegetative method.

Parts Used: Whole plant excluding roots.

Chemical Constituents: Myrtle oil containing cineole, Myrtenole. Oleic, linoleic, Myristic & palmitic acids.

Uses: For complaints of incipient phthisis, bronchitis, cystitis and pyelitis. Stiching pain in left breast, running through to shoulder blade. Dry cough with burning sensation in left chest. Traditionally used for cerebral affections, dyspepsia and scorpion bite.

872. *Myxopyrum serratulum* A. W. Hill (*Oleaceae*)

Synonyms: *Myxopyrum smilacifalium.*

Vernacular Name: *San*: Hemamalati, Caturdharalata; *Hin*: Pilacameli; *Mal*: Caturamulla, Caturavalli; *Tam*: Caturamullai; *Tel:* Caturdharalata.

Description: A large scandent shrub with 4-angled branches; leaves simple, opposite obovate, elliptic, serrulate, triplicostate; flowers small, yellowish in axillary or terminal trichotomous panicles stamens 2, attached to the base of the corolla tube; fruits obovoid berries with one or two seeds, seeds erect, testa membranous.

Habitate: Throughout Kerala, in evergreen forest sat altitudes of 600 to 900 m.

Propagation: By stem cutting.

Parts Used: Roots, leaves.

Chemical Consistuents: N.A.

Uses: The roots are useful in scabies and prurigo in children. The leaves are astringent, acrid, sweet, thermogenic, anodyne, febrifuge and tonic. They are useful in vitiated conditions of *kapha* and *vata*, cough, asthma, rheumatism, cephalalgia, notalgia, consumption, fever, otopathy, neuropathy and cuts and wounds.

873. *Naravelia zeylanica* (L.) DC. *(Ranunculaceae)*

Vernacular Name: *San*: Dhanavalli; *Kan*: Neendamalli; *Mal*: Poytalacci, Polutalacci, Karuppakkoti, Talavedana valli, *Vatakkoti*; *Tam*: *Vatamkolli*, Nintavalli.

Description: A scandent or climbing shrub with tuberous roots, wiry stem and strong tendrils; leaves 3-foliate, opposite, terminal leaflet modified into a 3-branched tendril, leaflets ovate-lanceolate, serrate or crenate, prominently nerved; flowers yellow, fragrant in axillary and terminal panicles, sepals downy, petals linear-clavate, elongate; fruits aggregate of achenes, ending in twisted feather tails.

Habitate: Throughout India, common in hedges and thickets.

Propagation: By seeds and vegetative method.

Parts Used: Whole plant.

Chemical Consistuents: N.A.

Uses: The plant is astringent, bitter, sweet, anthelmintic, depurative, anodyne, anti-inflammatory and vulnerary. It is useful in vitiated conditions of *pitta*, helminthiasis, dermatopathy, leprosy, rheumatalgia, odontalgia, cephalalgia, colic, inflammations, wounds and ulcers. The roots and stems have a strong penetrating smell, and are used by tribes for cephalalgia.

874. *Nardostachys jatamansi* DC. *(Valerianaceae)*

Vernacular Name: *San*; Jatamasni; *Hin:* Jatamansi; *Beng*: Jatamansi; *Guj*: Jatamasi, kalichhad; *Tel:* Jatamamshi; *Tam*: Jatamashi; *Kan*: Jatamamshi; *Mal*: Jatamashi.

Description: Erect herb, *rhizome* thick covered with a bundle of fine, reddish brown fibres, fragrant. *Leaves* radical, 15-20 cm narrowed into the petiole, entire *flowers* capitate, pinkish white.

Habitate: The herb grows at heights upto 5000 m in the Easter Himalayas, in Nepal, Bhutan and Sikkim.

Propagation: By vegetative method.

Parts Used: Rhizome, oil from rhizome.

Chemical Constituents: A volatile essential oil 0.5% resin, sugar, starch bitter extractive matter and gum are obtained from the rhizomes. The oil contains a ketone, jatamansone which is the same as valeranone. It also contains jatamansic acid. Jatamansone semi-carbazone is a sesquiterpenic ketone isolated from the rhizomes.

Uses: Hysteria and convulsion syndromes. Hair loss and greying of hair. Dysmenorrhoea. Insomnia and agitation. The rhizome is used in Ayurveda for the treatment of hysteria and other neurological disorders. It is very interesting to note that in conditions of insomnia and restlessness this drug was used by Sushruta to produce tranquility and sedation. It promotes the growth and blackness of hair. Infusion prepared from the fresh roots is employed in the treatment of spasmodic hysterical states, palpitations and tension headache. It is also said to be useful in menopausal disturbances. Clinical trials were carried out with jatamansone in essential hypertension. Jatamansone has been used in febrile delirium and also in delirium tremens. In dysmenorrhoea, it is used for pain relief and a smooth menstrual flow.

875. *Naregamia alata* Wight & Arn. *(Malliaceae)*

Vernacular Name: *Eng*: Goanese Ipecacuanha; *San*: Amlavalli, Triparnika; *Hin*: Tinparni; *Kan*: Nelanaringa, Nepanaringa; *Mal*: Nilanarakam; *Tam*: Nilanaragam; *Tel:* Pagapapu.

Description: A small handsome undershrub upto 30 cm in height with pungent aromatic root; leaves trifoliate, alternate, petioles winged, leaflets small, cuneate-obovate; flowers large, white, solitary or 2 together in axils, staminal tube long, cylindric below, inflated near the top, obscurely 10-crenate at the mouth; fruits ovoid globose capsules, loculicidally 3-valved, seeds curved, truncate at both ends.

Habitate: Throughout south India, in all districts upto 900 m.

Propagation: By seeds and vegetative method.

Parts Used: Whole plant.

Chemical Consistuents: Aromatic odour.

Uses: The plant is acrid, sweet, cooling, aromatic, alexeteric, vulnerary, emetic, cholagogue, expectorant, depurative and antipyretic. It is useful in wounds, ulcers, vitiated conditions of *pitta* and *vata*, halitosis, cough, asthma, bronchitis, splenomegaly, scabies, pruritus, dysentery, dyspepsia, catarrh, anaemia and malarial fevers.

876. *Nasturtium officinale* *(Cruciferae)*

Vernacular Name: *Eng:* Watercress.

Description: A perennial much-branched, aquatic herb with creeping or floating stem; Leaves pinnate, leaflets 7-11, sessile, ovate-oblong or sinuately lobed, obtuse; flowers white, in short racemes; fruita siliqua, shortly cylindric; seeds minute, ovoid, muriculate.

Habitate: Found in temperate regions throughout the world, watercress thrives alongside or in fresh running water. While commonly fund in the wild.

Propagation: By seeds and vegetative method.

Parts Used: Aerial parts.

Chemical Constituents: Watercress contains vitamin A, B^1, B^2, C and E and minerals.

Uses: Watercress is a valuable source of vitamins and a good detoxifying herb. Its high content of vitamin C and mineral make sit a remedy that is particularly valuable for chronic illnesses. The plant is thought to stimulate the appetite and to relieve indigestion, to help in cases of chronic bronchitis to be generally stimulating, and to act as a powerful diuretic.

877. *Neisosperma oppositifolium* (Lam.) Fosb. & sachet *(Apocynaceae)*

Description: Small to medium sized tree to 15 m high with latex. Leaves whorled, petiolate, oblong to 30 cm long, upper surface glossy, flowers white, tubular, 5-parted, borne on several-flowered cymes which arise from the axils or are terminal cymes. Fruit is green drupaceous mericarp up to 10 cm long with fragrant mescocarp surrounding a fibrous endocarp with large single seed within.

Habitate: Common in littoral forest as an understory tree, edges of mangrove swamps, and on limestone.

Propagation: By seeds and vegetative method.

Part Used: Bark.

Chemical Constituents: Indole Alkaloids: bleekerine, ochropposinine, 3-epirivuvanine, isoreserpline.

Uses: An infusion of the bark is used to treat diabetes, high blood pressure and even serious illnesses such as cancer.

878. *Nelumbo nucifera* Gaertn. *(Nymphaeaceae)*

Synonyms: *Nelumbium nelumbo* Druce.

Vernacular Name: *San:* Ambuja, padma, pankaja, kamala; *Hin:* Kanwal, kamal; *Beng*: Padma; *Tel:* Kalung, erra-tamara; *Tam:* Ambal, thamarai; *Kan:* Kamala, tavaregadde; *Mal:* Thamara, senthamara.

Description: Perennial aquatic herb. Root-stock stout, cylindrical, embedded in the mud. Leaves peltate, radiately nerved; margins wavy; petiole long, aculeate, inserted in the middle of the leaf. Flowers large, solitary, handsome and fragrant, rosy or white, carpels numerous, ovoid, fleshy, sunk separately in cavities of receptacle, maturing into nut-like achenes; skin hard and blackish-brown when ripe.

Habitate: Common, cultivated in ponds and swamps.

Propagation: By rhizome.

Part Used: Leaves, seeds, receptacles, filaments and plumules. The leaves can be harvested in autumnl the flowers in summer. The seeds are collected with fully ripe.

Chemical Constituents: The leaves contain alkaloids: nuciferine, roemerine, nor-nuciferine and the flabonoid: quercetin. The plumules yield proteins, sugars and vitamins. The receptacles contain quercetin.

Uses: The ripe seeds produce a wholesome effect in cases of neurasthenia, spermatorrhea and metrorrhoea. The leaves and the seed cores in decoction are effective for insomnia, haemorrhage and haematemesis. The plumules, the filaments or the receptacles in the form of a decoction are used in treating bloody stools, haematuria, uterine haemorrhage and haematemesis.

879. *Nepeta cataria* *(Lamiaceae)*

Vernacular Name: *Eng:* Catnip.

Description: Downy, aromatic perennial growing to 1 m. Has heart-shaped, grey-green leaves and whorls of white flowers with purple spots.

Habitate: Catnip is native to Europe and naturalized in North America. It grows in dry wayside places and in mountainous regions up to altitudes of 1,500 m.

Propagation: By seeds and vegetative method.

Parts Used: Aerial parts.

Chemical Constituents: Catnip contains iridoids, tannins and volatile oil.

Uses: Catnip settles the stomach, is sedative and, as it stimulates sweating, reduces fever. The herb's plea*San*t taste and gentle action make it suitable for colds, flue and fever in children, especially when mixed with elderflower and sweetened with honey. Catnip is markedly antiflatulent, helping to settle indigestion ad colic. The herb is also useful in treating headaches related to digestive problems a tincture is beneficial as a friction rub for rheumatism and arthritis., and it can be made into an ointment for treating haemorrhoids.

880. *Neptunia oleracea* Lour. *(Mimosaceae)*

Vernacular Name: *San*: Alambusa, *Eng*: Sensitive water plant, *Hin*: Lajjalu, *Kan*: Nidrayam, *Mal*: Nirtottavati, Nittitottavati, *Tam*: Suntaikkirai, *Tel:* Nirutalavapu.

Description: A floating aquatic annual herb with fibrous rooted nodes and soft elongate internodes bearing spongy floats; leaves bipinnate, leaflets 8-15 pairs, small, sensitive, narrow-oblong, obtuse, glabrous, flowers minute, yellow, in axillary oblong heads; fruits stalked, deflexed, oblique oblong pods seeds 6 to 9 slightly compressed obvoid-oblong brown.

Habitate: Throughout India is tanks lakes and other stagnant waters.

Propagation: By seeds and vegetative method.

Parts Used: Whole plant.

Chemical Consistuents: N.A.

Uses: The plant is astringent, sweet, refrigerant, diuretic, antidiarrhoeal, anthelmintic and anodyne. It is useful in vitiated conditions of *pitta*, otalgia, cephalalgia, syphilis, burning sensation, dipsia, diarrhoea, strangury and helminthiasis.

881. *Nerium indicum* Mill. *(Apocynaceae)*

Synonyms: *Nerium oleander* Linn., *Nerium odorum* Soland.

Vernacular Name: *San*: Karavirah, *Eng*: Indian oleander, Sweet-scented oleander, *Hin*: *Kan*er, Karber, Karuvira, *Kan*: *Kan*agilu, Paddale, Dhavekaneri, *Mal*: Arali, *Kan*aviram, Karaviram, *Tam*: Arali, lrattai sivapparali, Vellai arali, *Tel:* Ganneru, Karaviramu, Kasturipattu.

Description: A large glabrous evergreen shrub with milky latex; leaves three in a whorl, shortly stalked, linear, dark green and shiny above; flowers red, rose-coloured or white, fragrant; fruits follicles, at length separating.

Habitate: Cultivated throughout India.

Propagation: By cutting.

Parts Used: Roots, leaves.

Chemical Consistuents: All parts of the plant are poisonous. Roots, bark and seeds contain cardio-active glycosides, formerly adesignated as neriodorin, neriodorein and karabin; neriodorin and karabin were reported to have a paralyzing action on the heart, like digitalin, and a stimulating action on the spinal cord, like strychnine; neriodorein was less active. Digitosigenin-β-D-diginoside, Uzarigenin-β-D-diginoside, Digitoxigenin-β-D-glucosido-β-D-diginoside, Digitoxigenin-β-D-glucosido-β-D-digitaloside, Digitoxigenin-β-D-glucosido-β-D-glucosido-monoacetyl--β-D-digitaloside, Digitoxigenin-β-D-digitaloside, Uzarigenin-β-D-glucoside-β-D-glucoside-β-D-diginoside, Uzarigenin-β-D-glucosido-β-D-diginoside, Uzarigenin-β-D-glucosido--β-D-diginoside, Decomposes to D-digitalose and a derivative of 16-anhydrodigitoxigenin, an isomer of L.

Uses: The roots are bitter, acrid, astringent, anthelmintic, thermogenic, aphrodisiac stomachic, febrifuge and diuretic. They are useful in cardiac asthma, srngury, renal and vesical calculi, chronic stomachalgia, arthralgia, leprosy, pruritus and ulcers. The root bark is very specific for ringworm. The leaves are a powerful repellent and are used for scabies, haemorrhoids and vitiated conditions of *vata*. The juice of the tender leaves is good for ophthalmia with copious lacrimation. The flowers are reported to have the property of purifying the air.

882. *Nervilia aragoana* Gaud. *(Orchidaceae)*

Synonyms: *Pogonia flabelliformis* Lindl., *Pogonia carinata* Wt.

Vernacular Name: *San*: Padmacarini, *Hin*: Sthalapadma, Sthalakamal, *Mal*: Orilattamara, Kalttamara, Nilattamara, *Tam*: Orilaittamarai.

Description: A terrestrial orchid with a single lotus-like leaf raised on a long stalk with subglobose white fleshy tubers; leaves single, simple, orbicular or subreniform, base cordate, 13 or more ribbed, margin wavy, almost coarsely dentate, 10-25 cm diameter, petiole 10-20 cm long, sepals and petals pale green veined with purple, lip white 3-lobed about the middle, veined with purple, tinged with yellow near the base, mid lobe ovate, acute, crisped hariy.

Habitate: In the Travancore and Pulney hills at all elevations.

Propagation: By rhizomes.

Parts Used: Whole plant.

Chemical Consistuents: N.A.

Uses: The plant is bitter, acrid, cooling, galactagogue, diuretic and tonic. It is useful in uropathy, lithiasis, colic, agalactia, mental instability, epileptic fits, haemoptysis, diarrhoea, asthma,cough, vomiting and vitiated of *pitta*.

883. *Nicotiana tabacum* L. *(Solanaceae)*

Vernacular Name: *San*: *Tam*akhuh; *Eng*: Tobacco; *Hin*: *Tam*aku, *Tam*paku; *Kan*: Hogesoppu, Tambaku; *Mal*: Pukayila Pokala; *Tam*: Pugaiyilai; *Tel:* Pogaku.

Description: A glandular pubescent erect herb with few branches; leaves simple, ovate, oblong-lanceolate or elliptic upto 100 cm or more in length, the lower ones semi-amplexicaul and decurrent; flowers light red, white or pink in many flowered panicled racemes; fruits narrowly elliptic, ovoid capsules, seeds many, brown, with fluted ridges.

Habitate: Cultivated in the hotter parts of India.

Propagation: By seeds and vegetative method.

Parts Used: Leaves.

Chemical Consistuents: Nicotine, nornicotine, Anabasine, *l*-Nicotine, Nicotyrine, Nicotimine, *l*-Noricotine, *d*-Nornicotine, Piperidine, Pyrrolidine, N-Methylpyrroline, 2,3'-Dipyridyl, *l*-Anabasine, N-Methyl-*l*-anabasine, *l*-Anatabine, N-Methyl-*l*-anatabine, Nicotoine, Necotelline, Myosmine.

Uses: The leaves are bitter, acrid thermogenic, sedative, narcotic, anodyne anti-inflammatory, anthelmintic, carminative, laxative, emetic, abortifacient, styptic, mental stimulant and tonic. They are useful in odontalgia, dental caries, inflammations, helminthiasis, dyspepsia, flatulence, haemorrhages, bronchitis, asthma, scabies skin diseases, ulcers, painful tumours, strangulated hernia, purulent discharge from the nose, tubercular glands of the neck, vitiated condition of *vata* and otalgia.

884. *Nigella sativa* L. *(Ranunculaceae)*

Vernacular Name: *San*: Upakuncika, Karavi, Krsnajiraka; *Eng*: Small fennel, Black cumin; *Hin*: Kalajira, Kalomji; *Kan*: Karijirigae; *Mal*: Karincirakam; *Tam*: Karum ciragam; *Tel:* Nallajilakarra.

Description: A pretty small herb, 30-60 cm in height; leaves compound 2-3 pinnatisect cut into linear or linear-lanceolate segments; flowers pale blue, solitary, long peduncles without an involucre, seeds trigonous, black, rugulose-tubercular.

Habitate: In Punjab, Bihar; often cultivated.

Propagation: By seeds and vegetative method.

Parts Used: Seeds.

Chemical Consistuents: The fatty acids of the oil are as follows: myristic, plmitic, stearic, oleic, and linoleic. The component glycerides of the oil are the following: trilinolein, oleodilinolein, dioleolinolein, palmito-oleo-linolein, and stearo-oleolinolein, glycerides of some volatile acids are also present in the oil in small quantities tannins, resins, proteins, reducing sugars, cystine, lysine, aspartic, acid, leucine; asparagines is not present.

Uses: The seeds are acrid, bitter, thermogenic, aromatic, carminative, diuretic, emmenagogue, anodyne, antibacterial, anti-inflammatory, deodorant, appetizing, digestive, anthelmintic, constipating, sudorific, febrifuge, stimlant, galactagogue and expectorant. They are useful in skin diseases, haemorrhoids, cephalalgia, jaundice, inflammation, fever, paralysis, ophthalmia, halitosis, anorexia, dyspepsia, flatulence, diarrhoea, dysentery, cough, amenorrhoea, dysmenorrhoea, helminthiasis especially tapeworm, strangury, intermittent fevers, agalactia and vitiated conditions of *vata* and *kapha.*

885. *Nothapodytes nimmoniana* (Graham) Mabb. *(Icacinaceae)*

Synonyms: *Mappia foetida* Miers.

Vernacular Name: *Kan*: Durvasane mara; *Mar*: Kalgur, Kalagaura, Ghanera; *Tam*: Arali, Perum pulagi, Kal kurinji.

Description: Small stress, 3-8 m tall. *Bark* smooth, grey, wrinkled, about 5 mm thick. Branchlets slightly angled, corky, with prominent leaf scars. *Leaves* alternate, slightly leathery, broadly egg-shaped to elliptic-oblong, 7-25 x 4-12 cm, base often unequal, apex acute to acuminate, margin entire, hairless above, thinly hairy beneath, crowded at the ends of branchlets; lateral nerves 8-10 pairs; leaf stalks 3-6 cm long. *Flowers* bisexual, creamy yellow, foul smelling, about 5 mm across, in terminal corymbose cymes; petals hairy inside. *Drupes* oblong to ellipsoid, about 2 x 1 cm, smooth, purplish black when ripe. *Seeds* single.

Habitate: Moist deciduous to evergreen and shola forests.

Propagation: By seeds and vegetative method.

Parts Used: Seeds.

Chemical Constituents: Palmitic, stearic, oleic, linolenic acid.

Uses: Medicinal use is not reported in any of the codified systems of Indian medicine or in the Folk traditions. Modern usage is reportedly for obtaining CAMPTOTHECIN which is being employed for the treatment of tumours.

886. *Nuphar luteum* Sibth & Smith. *(Nymphaeaceae)*

Synonyms: *Nuphar systylum* Wallr., *Nuphar tenellum* Reichb.

Vernacular Name: *Eng:* European yellow pond lily.

Description: A perennial aquatic plant with stout root-stock, creeping in the mud. Submerged leaves very thin and roundish; floating leaves oval, generally with narrow or closed sinus, usually without stomata. Petiole triangular. Flowers yellow, about 6 cm. across, somewhat fragrant; sepals 5, nearly equal; petals 5, longer than sepals and dilated upwards; stigmas 10 to 30 rayed with characteristic entire margin. Fruit globular, with a short narrow neck.

Habitate: North America, Europe particularly U.K.

Propagation: By vegetative method.

Parts Used: Rhizome.

Chemical Constituents: Nupharidine.

Uses: For complaints mainly of male sex organs, which includes complete absence of sexual desire with parts relaxed, penis retracted; desire with parts relaxed, penis retracted; impotence with involuntary emissions during stool or when urinating. Spermatorrhoea. Pain in testicles & penis. Entero-colitis with yellow diarrhoea which is worse in morning.

887. *Nyctanthes arbor-tristis* L. *(Oleaceae)*

Vernacular Name: *San*: Parijatah, Sephalika; *Eng*: Night jasmine, Coral jasmine; *Hin*: Harsimgar, Parja; *Kan*: Parijata; *Mal*: Pavilamalli, Parijatam; *Tam*: Pavilamalligai; *Tel:* Pagadamalli, Swetasarasa.

Description: A hardy large shrub or small tree upto 10 m in height with grey or greenish white rough bark and sharply quadrangular strigose young branches; leaves simple opposite, ovate, acute or acumiante, scabrous above with short bulbous hairs, densely pubescent beneath with appressed hairs, main nerves few, conspicuous beneath; flowers small, white with bright orange corolla tubes, 3-7 in each head, in trichotomous cymes; fruits capsules, compressed, separating into two one-seeded segments.

Habitate: Throughout India upto 1,500 m, also cultivated in gardens.

Propagation: By seeds and vegetative method.

Parts Used: Leaves, flowers, seeds.

Chemical Consistuents: The flowers contain *d*-mannitol, tannin and glucose. The oil consists of the glycerides of linoleic, oleic, lignoceric, stearic, palmitic and probably myristic acids. β-Stiosterol is the main component of the un-saponifiable matter. The leaves of the plant contain tannic acid, methyl salicylate, an amorphous glycoside, mannitol, an amorphous resin and a trace of volatile oil.

Uses: The leaves are bitter, acrid, thermogenic, antibacterial, anodyne, anti-inflammatory, digestive, cholagogue, anthelmintic, depurative, sudorific, febrifuge, expectorant, diuretic, laxative, trichogenous and tonic. They are useful in vitiated conditions of *kapha* and *vata*, obstinate sciatica, inflammations, dyspepsia, helminthiasis, pruritus, dermatopathy, chronic fever, bronchitis, asthma, cough strangury, constipation, hepatopathy, haemorrhoids, greyness of hair and bladness. The flowers are bitter, astringent, ophthalmic, stomachic, carminative and trichogenous, and are useful in inflammations, ophthalmopathy, flatulence, colic, dyspepsia, splenomegaly, greyness of hair and baldness. The seeds are very useful in baldness, scurvy and affections of the scalp.

888. *Nymphaea alba* *(Nymphaceae)*

Vernacular Name: *Eng:* White water lily.

Description: Perennial aquatic plant with deep roots, plate-shaped leaves on long cylindrical stems, and large-petalled white flowers occasionally tinged with pink.

Habitate: Native to Europe, white water lily is found in ponds and in still water in lakes, rivers and canals.

Propagation: By seeds and vegetative method.

Parts Used: Rhizomes and flowers.

Chemical Constituents: The rhizome contains alkaloids, resin, glycosides and tannins.

Uses: The rhizome of the white water lily is astringent and antiseptic. White water lily has also been employed to treat bronchial catarrh and kidney pain, and taken as a gargle for sore throats. The rhizome may be used to make a douche for vaginal soreness and discharge, or to make a poultice-often in combination with slippery elm or linseed for boils and abscesses. White water lily flowers have long been reputed to reduce sexual drive. Their generally calming and sedative effect on the nervous system makes them useful in the treatment of insomnia, anxiety and similar disorders.

889. *Nymphaea nouchali* Burm. f. *(Nymphaeaceae)*

Synonyms: *Nymphaea pubescens* Wild, *Nymphaea lotus* Hooks.

Vernacular Name: *San*: Kumudam; *Eng*: Indian water-lily; *Hin*: *Kan*val, Kokka; *Kan*: Bilenaydile, Biletavare; *Mal*: Ampal; *Tam*: Vellampal, Allittamarai; *Tel:* Allikada, *Tel*lakaluva.

Description: A large perennial aquatic herb with short, erect, roundish, tuberous rhizomes; leaves floating, peltate, sharply sinuate-toothed, flowers large, floating, solitary, variable in colour from pure white to deep red; fruits spongy many seeded berries, seeds minute, grayish black when dry with longitudinal striations.

Habitate: Throughout the warmer parts of India, in tanks, ponds and ditches.

Propagation: By rhizomes.

Parts Used: Rhizomes, flowers, seeds.

Chemical Consistuents: Nymphaeine, Nymphalin.

Uses: The rhizome is cooling, sweet, bitter and tonic, and is useful in diarrhoea, dysentery, dipsia, and general debility. The flowers are astringent and cardiotonic. The seeds are sweet, cooling, constipating, aphrodisiac, stomachic and restorative. They are useful in vitiated conditions of *pitta*, dipsia, diarrhoea and dermatopathy.

890. *Ochreinauclea missionis* (Wall. ex G. Don) Ridsdale *(Rubiaceae)*

Synonyms: *Nauclea missionis* Wall. ex Don.

Vernacular Name: *Hin*: Phuga; *Kan*: Anavu; *Mal*: Attu vanji, Neer vanji; *Tam*: Athu vanji, Neer vanji.

Description: Trees, 8-20 m tall. *Bark* smooth, brown, with vertical irregular indistinct cracks, about 8 mm thick. *Wood* dark yellow, moderately hard. *Balze* white. *Leaves* opposite, elliptic-oblong to lanceolate, 10-18 x 4-6 cm, base acute, apex rounded to acute, hairless, glossy, leathery; lateral nerves 10-15 pairs; leaf stalks 4-7 mm long. *Flowers* bisexual, numerous, about 5 mm long, greenish yellow, fragrant, aggregated in 2-4 cm across axillary globose heads. Peduncles about 2 cm long with 4 minute leaf-like structures called 'bracts' near the base. *Fruits* fused into a fleshy globose mass, small.

Habitate: Along the banks of streams and rivers of moist forests.

Propagation: By stem cuttings and air-layers.

Parts Used: Bark.

Chemical Constituents: N.A.

Uses: Stem bark is reportedly used in the treatment of constipation, leprosy, rheumatism and ulcers. Root and root bark are employed to treat rheumatic and paralytic affections, general anasarca, skin diseases, dropsy, eye diseases, constipation, piles, jaundice, fever, oedema and hepatic and haemophiic disorders.

891. *Ocimum americanum* L. *(Lamiaceae)*

Synonyms: *Ocimum canum* Sims.

Vernacular Name: *San*: Vanabarbarika, Aranyatulasi; *Eng*: Hoary basil; *Hin*: Vantulsi; *Kan*: Nayitulasi; *Mal*: Kattutulasi, Kattutrttavu, Katturamattulasi; *Tam*: Nayttulac; *Tel:* Kuppatulasi, Kukkatulasi.

Description: A pubescent erect much branched herb, 15-60 cm high with sub-quadrangular striate branches; leaves elliptic-lanceolate, entire or faintly toothed, glabrous and gland dotted; flowers white, pink or purplish in elongate racemes with more or less closely set whorls fruits small, nutlets pitted, mucilaginous when wetted.

Habitate: Throughout India, in fields and waste lands.

Propagation: By seeds and vegetative method.

Parts Used: Leaves, seeds.

Chemical Consistuents: Citral, linalool, geraniol, citronellol.

Uses: The leaves are aromatic, acrid, bitter, thermogenic, appetizing, digestive, carminative, depurative, expectorant, anthelmintic, cardiotonic, febrifuge, alexeteric and tonic. They are useful in vitiated conditions of *vata* and *kapha*, helminthiasis, anorexia, dyspepsia, flatulence, dysentery, leprosy, pruritus, parasitic, affections, vomiting, poisonous affections, haemoptysis, strangury, migraine, malaria and fever. The seeds are useful in hyderdipsia, malaria, migraine and emaciation.

892. *Ocimum basilicum* L. *(Lamiaceae)*

Vernacular Name: *San:* Munjariki, surasa, varvara; *Eng:* Sweet basil, common basil; *Hin:* Babui tulsi, gulal tulsi, kali tulsi, marua; *Tel:* Bhutulasi, rudrajada, vepudupachha; *Tam:* Tirnirupachal, karpura tulasi and *Kan:* Kama kasturi, sajjagida.

Description: An erect, almost glabrous herb, 30-90 cm high, leaves ovate-lanceolate, acuminate, toothed or entire, glabrous on both surfaces, glandular; flowers white or pale purple, in simple or much-branched racemes, often thysoid; nutlets ellipsoid, black, pitted.

Habitate: Throughout India.

Propagation: By seeds and vegetative method.

Part Used: Leaves.

Chemical Constituents: The major component of the essential oil is either methyl cinnamate, linalool, or methyl chaviocol in different samples. Other major components include ocimene, linalyl acetate, eugenol and trans-anethole.

Uses: Oil of basi is used as a flavouring agent in confectionery, baked goods, sauces, ketchups, tomato pastes, pickles, fancy vinegars, spiced meats, sausages, and beverages. A tincture of the herb finds use in liqueurs, as a flavour modifier. An oleoresin extracted from the leaves is used as a flavour ingredient in all major food products.

893. *Ocimum gratissimum* L. *(Lamiaceae)*

Vernacular Name: *San:* Vriddhutulsi; *Eng:* Lemon basil, large basil, shrubby basil; *Hin:* Ban tulsi, ram tulsi; *Beng*: Ban tulsi, ram tulsi; *Tel:* Nimma tulasi, rama tulasi; *Kan:* Nimma tulasi, rama tulasi; *Tam:* Elumicham tulasi.

Description: Much-branched perennial shrub, 1-1.5m. high stems quadrangular, pubescent, woody at the base. Leaves opposite, apiculate, pubescent on both surfaces; margins coarsely toothed. Inflorescence axillary or terminal in simple or branched whorled raceme; flowers white, Nutlets subglobose, rugose.

Habitate: Grows wild but is cultivated for its essential oil.

Propagation: By seeds and vegetative method.

Part Used: Whole plant.

Chemical Constituents: The whole plant contains an essential oil (0.6-0.8%), consisting of eugenol 45-70%, methyl eugenol 20% carbacrol, ocimene, p-cymene, camphene, limonene, a-pinene and b-pinene.

Uses: The whole plant is used in treating sunstroke, headache and influenza. It is considered to be diaphoretic. It serves also as material for the extraction of essential oil and qugenol. Eugenol is used widely in odontology and for the synthesis of vanillin.

894. Ocinum *sanctum* L. *(Lamiaceae)*

Vernacular Name: *San*: Surasah, Tulasi; *Eng*: Holy basil, Sacred basil; *Hin*: Kalatulsi, Tulsi; *Kan*: Karitulasi; *Mal*: Krsnattulasi, tulasi, Trttavu, Karuttatrttavu; *Tam*: Karuttulaci, Tulaci; *Tel:* Tulasi.

Description: An erect much branched softly pubescent undershrub, 30-60 cm high with red or purple subquadrangular branches; leaves simple, opposite, elliptic, oblong, obtuse or acute, entire, serrate or dentate, pubescent on both sides, minutely gland dotted, petioles slender, hairy; flowers purplish in elongate racemes in close whorls, stamens exserted, upper pair with a small bearded appendage at the base; fruits nutlets, smooth, not mucilaginous when wetted.

Habitate: Throughout India as well as cultivated.

Propagation: By seeds and vegetative method.

Parts Used: Whole plant.

Chemical Consistuents: Eugenol, eugenol methol ether and carvacrol, methyl chavicol cineole and linalool.

Uses: The plant is bitter, acrid, aromatic, stomachic, demulcent, diaphoretic, digestive, diuretic, expectorant, febrifuge, vermifuge and alexeteric. It is useful in cardiopathy, haemopathy, leucoderma, asthma, bronchitis, catarrhal fever, otalgia, hepatopathy, vomiting, lumbago, hiccough, ophthalmia, gastropathy in children, genito-urinary disorders, ringworm, verminosis and skin diseases.

895. *Oenanthe phellandrium* Lanks. *(Apiaceae)*

Synonyms: *Phellandrium aquaticum* Linn., *Oenanthe aquatica* (L.) Poir., *Phellandrium consioides* Nolite ex. Nym., *Phellandrium divaricatum* Gilib.

Vernacular Name: *Eng:* Water Hamlock

Description: A biennial herb with root spindle shaped, thick, horizontal, crooked, oblique resembling a turnip; stem 60 to 90 cm. high, very stout at the base, hollow, furrowed, very bushy, with numerous spreading leafy branches. Leaves shining; petionlate, spreading, tripinnate with innumerable fine acute segments. Flowers in innumerable fine acute segments. Flowers in umbel and all fertile, white, upper ones largest. Brats absent. Bracteoles bristle like.

Habitate: Northern Asia and Europe.

Propagation: By vegetative method.

Parts Used: Fruit.

Chemical Constituents: Essential oil containing 80% phelandrene (α-and β-phelandrene); Resin and Mucilage.

Uses: For complaints predominantly of respiratory system. Offensive expectoration and cough in phthisis, bronchitis and emphysema. Tuberculosis of middle lobes. Haemoptysis. Everything tasting sweet. Aching and burning in temples and above eyes. Crushing feeling & heaviness in vertex, ciliary neuralgia of eyes with aversion to light. Stitching pain through right breast near sternum, extending to back near shoulders.

896. *Oenothera biennis* *(Onagraceae)*

Vernacular Name: *Eng:* Evening primrose.

Description: Biennial herb growing to 20 cm. Has red blotches on stem, crinkled lance-shaped leaves, 4-petalled yellow flowers and elongated seed capsules.

Habitate: Native to North America, evening primrose is now commonly found in many temperate zones around the world. It thrives on wasteground, especially in dunes and *San*dy soil. Evening primrose is grown commercially for its seeds oil.

Propagation: By seeds and vegetative method.

Parts Used: Leaves, stem bark, flowers, seed oil.

Chemical Constituents: Eveing primrose oil is rich in essential fatty acids–cis-linoleic and cis-gammalinolenic acid in particular. Is action mostly depends on the gammalinolenic acid, a precursor of prostaglandin E1. The oil is often combined with vitamin E to prevent oxidation.

Uses: The flowers, leaves and stem bark of evening primrose have astringent and sedative properties. All three parts have been employed in the treatment of whooping for digestive problems and asthma, and used as a poultice to ease the discomfort of rheumatic disorders. The oil, applied externally, is beneficial in the treatment of eczema, certain other itchy skin conditions and breast tenderness. Taken internally, the oil has an effect in lowering blood pressure, and in preventing the clumping of platelets. The oil is now commonly taken for premenstrual problems, including tension and abdominal bloating. Multiple sclerosis may benefit from internal treatment with the oil, as may rheumatoid arthritis, intermittent claudication and other problems relating to the circulation.

897. *Olea europeae* *(Oleaceae)*

Vernacular Name: *Eng:* Olive.

Description: Evergreen tree growing to 10 m. Has a deeply grooved grey trunk, small leathery leaves, cluster of small greenish-white flowers and a green fruit ripening to black.

Habitate: Olive trees grow wild in the Mediterranean region and are cultivated in Mediterranean countries and in regions with a similar climate in the Americas.

Propagation: By seeds and vegetative method.

Parts Used: Leaves, oil.

Chemical Constituents: Olive leaves contain oleoropine, oleasterol and leine. Olive oil contains about 75% oleic acid, a mono-unsaturated fatty acid.

Uses: Olive leaves lower blood pressure and help to improve the function of the circulatory system. They are also mildly diuretic and may be used to treat conditions such as cystitis. Possessing some ability to lower blood sugar levels, the leaves have been taken for diabetes. The oil is nourishing and improves the balance of fats within the blood. It is traditionally taken with lemon juice in teaspoonful doses to treat gallstones. The oil has a generally protective action on the digestive tract and is useful for dry skin. Externally, it is a good, although sticky, carrier oil for essential oils.

898. Omalanthus nutans (Forst f.) Guillemin. *(Euphorbiaceae)*

Description: Shrub or small tree upto 10 m high with white latex leaves alternate, petiolate (elongate), rhomboidal, paler underneath. Flowers tiny, unisexual, borne on terminal racemes. Fruit small, pinkish to red containing a single seed. Flowers and fruit available throughout the years.

Habitate: Common in forests, thickets, hillsides, and forest clearings.

Propagation: By seeds and vegetative method.

Part Used: Leaves, bark roots, stem and fruits.

Chemical Constituents: Anti HIV (prostratin).

Uses: The leaves are used to treat elephantiasis and circumcision wounds and sores. The root bark is used to treat whooping cough. The stem bark is used for stomachache. A decoction of the fruit is used to relieve painful urination.

899. *Ononis spinosa* *(Leguminosae)*

Vernacular Name: *Eng:* Spiny restharrow.

Description: Spiny perennial with 3 small leaflets per leaf, bright pink, pea-like flowers and small seedpods.

Habitate: A relatively common European plant, spiny restharrow thrives in dry grassland and along roadsides.

Propagation: By seeds and vegetative method.

Parts Used: Root.

Chemical Constituents: Spiny restharrow root contains phenols, lectins, triterpenoids and a volatile oil. The volatile oil in the root is diuretic the non-volatile oil content is anti-diuretic. If a diuretic is desired, the root is made into an infusion.

Uses: The root is used as a diuretic and to prevent kidney and bladder stones. It is of value in a range of urinary system problems including stones, gout and cystitis. For excess fluid retention, spiny restharrow is best taken as a short-term treatment, in the form of an infusion.

900. *Operculina turpethum* (L.) Silva Manso *(Convolvulaceae)*

Synonyms: *Merremia turpethum* (Linn.) G. L. Shah & R. G. Bhat), *Ipomoca turpethum* R. Br.

Vernacular Name: *San*: Trivrt; *Eng*: Indian jalap, Turpeth; *Hin*: Nisoth, Nisotar, Pitohri; *Kan*: Sigade; *Mal*: Trikolpakkonna, Triputa, Sivata; *Tam*: *Sivatai*, Kumbham; *Tel:* Tegada.

Description: A large stout perennial twiner with milky juice, winged, twisted, pubescent, twining stems and long slender fleshy much branched roots; leaves simple, large, very variable in shape, subacute, mucronate, more or less pubescent on both sides especially when young, base cordate or truncate; flowers white, tubular-campanulate in few flowered cymes; fruits globose capsules, enclosed in enlarged brittle imbricate sepals, seeds 4 or less, glabrous dull black.

Habitate: Throughout India upto 900 m, occasionally cultivated.

Propagation: By seeds and vegetative method.

Parts Used: Roots.

Chemical Consistuents: Glycosidic resin, turpethin, α-turpethein and β-turpethein.

Uses: The roots are bitter, acrid, sweet, thermogenic, purgative, carminative, anthelmintic, expectorant, antipyretic, hepatic, stimulant and hydragogue. They are useful in colic, constipation, dropsy, vitiated conditions of *vita*, paralysis, myalgia, arthralgia, pectoralgia, bronchitis, obesity, helminthiasis, gastropathy, ascites, inflammations, intermittent fever, leucoderma, pruritus, ulcers, erysipelas, haemorrhoids, tumours, jaundice, consumpation and ophthalmia.

901. *Ophiopogon japonicus* (L.f.) ker.-Gawl. *(Liliaceae)*

Description: Astoloniferous perennial herb, growing intufts with tuberous roots, fleshy. Leaves linear, long, dark-green above, pale below, with numerous parallel nerves. Inflorescence in axillary apike with long stalk; flowers small, pale-green, Berry globose, violet then silvery grey.

Habitate: Grows wild among limestone rocks and is also cultivated in gardens for ornament and medicinal use.

Propagation: By vegetative method.

Part Used: Tuberous roots.

Chemical Constituents: The tuberous roots contain mucilage and sugars (glucose, fucose, rhmnose, xylose); b-sitosterol; ophiopogenins A,B,C,d; ruscogenin.

Uses: The ruberous roots possess expectorant and antitussive properties. They have a beneficial effect in sore throat, bronchitis, tuberculosis, haeemoptysis, haematemesis, evening fever with thrist, epistaxis, oliguria, hypogalactia, galactophoritis and constipation.

902. *Ophiorrhiza mungos* L. *(Rubiaceae)*

Vernacular Name: *San*: Sarpaksi, Sarpari; *Eng*: Mongoose plant, Indian snake root; *Hin*: Sarahati; *Kan*: Patalagaruda; *Mal*: Avilpori; *Tam*: Krippuntu, Kirippurantan; *Tel:* Sarpasicettu.

Description: A herbaceous undershrub upto 60 cm in height; leaves simple, opposite, 5-15 cm long, lanceolate, much tapering at the base and decurrent on short petiole, glabrous above, finely puberulous on veins beneath, thin, lateral veins very numerous, prominent beneath; flowers white, in minutely rusty-puberulous spreading subumbellate cymes; fruits glabrous, coriaceous capsules, very much compressed, protruding beyond the calyx, seeds numerous, angular pale brown.

Habitate: Throughout India, in shady places on plains and hills of low elevations.

Propagation: By seeds and vegetative method.

Parts Used: Roots.

Chemical Consistuents: They contain starch, a light brown resin and small amounts of a bitter amorphous alkaloid. β-Stiosterol, 5α-ergost-7-en-3β-ol and 5α-ergost-8-en-3β-ol have been identified in root extracts. Leaves and stems contain traces of hydrocyanic acid.

Uses: The roots are acrid, bitter, thermogenic, vulnerary, anthelmintic, alexeteric, stomachic, laxative, sedative and tonic. They are useful in vitiated conditions of *kapha*, wounds, ulcers, helminthiasis, snake poison, poisonous wounds, gastropathy, eclampsia, leprosy, hydrophobia and cancer.

903. *Opuntia ficus-indica* *(Cactaceae)*

Vernacular Name: *Eng:* Prickly pear.

Description: Perennial cactus growing to 3 m. Has large spatula-shaped stems covered in clusters of spines, brilliant yellow flowers and roundish purple fruit.

Habitate: Prickly pear is native to Mexico and naturalized in semi-tropical regions around the world.

Propagation: By stem cutting.

Parts Used: Flowers, fruit, stems.

Chemical Constituents: The fruit of prickly pear contains mucilage, sugars, vitamin C and other fruit acids. The flowers contain a flavonoid.

Uses: Prickly pear flowers are astringent and reduce bleeding, and are used for problems of the gastro-intestinal tract-particularly diarrhoea, colitis and irritable bowel syndrome. The flowers are also taken to treat an enlarged prostate gland. The fruit is nutritious.

904. *Orchis latifolia* Linn. *(Orchidaceae)*

Vernacular Name: *San*: Salampamisri, Munjatakah; *Eng*: *Mar*sh orchid, Salep; *Hin*: Salampanja, Salam; *Kan*: Salamisri; *Mal*: Salamisri; *Tam*: Salamisri; *Tel:* Salamisri.

Description: A tuberous terrestrial orchid with stems 30-90 cm in height, leaves many, erect, oblong, linear-oblong or lanceolate; flowers dull purple in cylindric spikes, sepals and petals acute or obtuse, lip oblong or rhomboid, entire, or 3-lobed spotted with dark purple, spur straight or curved.

Habitate: Throughout India is tanks lakes and other stagnant waters.

Propagation: By vegetative method.

Parts Used: Whole plant.

Chemical Consistuents: Volatile oil, loroglossin.

Uses: The plant is astringent, sweet, refrigerant, diuretic, antidiarrhoeal, anthelmintic and anodyne. It is useful in vitiated conditions of *pitta*, otalgia, cephalalgia, syphilis, burning sensation, dipsia, diarrhoea, strangury and helminthiasis.

905. *Orchis mascula* *(Orchidaceae)*

Vernacular Name: *Eng:* Purple Orchid, Salep.

Description: Perennial herb growing to 60cm. Narrow leaves often have purple-black blotches. Flowering stem bears purple or purple-pink flowers. Has two tuberous roots, one larger than the other.

Habitate: Purple orchid is native to Europe, the Middle East and North Africa. It is commonly found in clearings in woodland, scrubland and grassland.

Propagation: By vegetative method.

Parts Used: Tuber.

Chemical Constituents: Purple orchid contains about 48% mucilage.

Uses: Once believed to have aphrodisiac powers, salep is now seen as a nourishing vegetable somewhat similar to the potato. Its current medicinal used is generally confined to the treatment of diarrhoea and irritated gastro-intestinal tracts in children.

906. *Origanum majorana* *(Lamiaceae)*

Synonyms*:* *Majorana hortensis.*

Vernacular Name: *Eng:* Sweet marjoram.

Description: Woody perennial herb growing to 50 cm. Has aromatic oval leaves and pinkish-white flowers emerging from the upper leaf axils.

Habitate: Sweet marjoram is native to countries bordering the Mediterranean. It is much cultivated as a culinary herb, and for its essential oil.

Propagation: By seeds and cutting.

Parts Used: Aerial parts, essential oil.

Chemical Constituents: Sweet marjoram contains about 3% volatile oil, flavonoids, caffeic and rosmarinic acid and triterpenoids.

Uses: While mainly used as a culinary herb, sweet marjoram is also medicinally valuable due to its stimulant and antispasmodic properties. Like wild marjoram, it treats flatulence, colic and respiratory problems, but it appears to have a stronger effect on the nervous system then its wild cousin. Sweet marjoram is a good general tonic, helping to relieve anxiety, headaches and insomnia. The herb is also thought to lower the sexual drive.

907. *Origanum vulgare* *(Lamiaceae)*

Vernacular Name: *Eng:* Wild marjoram; *Hin*: Sathra; *Tel:* Mridu-maruvamu; *Kan*: Maruga.

Description: An aromatic, branched perennial herb, 30-90 cm. high, leaves broadly ovate, entire or rarely toothed; flowers purple or pink, in corymbose cymes; nut lets smooth, brown.

Habitate: Wild marjoram is native to Europe and naturalized in the Middle East. The plant thrives in chalky soils close to the sea.

Propagation: By seeds and vegetative method.

Parts Used: Aerial parts, essential oil.

Chemical Constituents: Wild marjoram contains a volatile oil, tannins, resin, sterols and flavonoids. Both carvacrol and thymol are antibacterial and antifungal.

Uses: Wild marjoram helps settle flatulence and stimulates the flow of bile. Strongly antiseptic, it may be taken to treat respiratory conditions such as coughs, tonsillitis, bronchitis and asthma. It is also considered to be a useful promoter of menstruation. The diluted oil can be applied to toothache or painful joints.

908. *Ornithogalum umbellatum* L. *(Liliaceae)*

Synonyms: *Ornithogalum hortense* Jord & Fourr., *Ornithogalum minus* Linn., *Ornithogalum rusticum* Jord & Fourr.

Vernacular Name: *Eng:* Star of Bethlehem.

Description: A perennial herb with subglobose bulbs, bearing numerous bulbils. Leaves 6-9, narrow, linear, elongated, cylindrical, sometimes flat or deeply channeled on dorsal aspect, upto 6 mm. wide, dark green and distinctly white spotted. Inflorescence a raceme of 3-7 flowers, sometimes 12-20 flowers, with pedicels of lower flowers 2-6 cm. long. Flowers usually erect with perianth segments 6, wide spreading, oblong-lanceolate, 15-20 mm. long, brilliant white above, with a broad green median stripe beneath. Stamens 6 with filaments tapering at apex; ovary superior, 3–celled. Fruit a capsule.

Habitate: Europe, particularly U.K.

Propagation: By seeds and vegetative method.

Parts Used: Whole plant.

Chemical Constituents: Colchicines, Convallotoxin, Convalloside, Strophanthindin, Rhodexin-A, Rodexoside, Unsaturated Phospholipids and Mucilage.

Uses: For complaints specifically chronic gastric indurations. Ulcerative or cancer conditions of intesting, stomach, pylorus and duodenum. Painful soreness & contraction in pylorus and duodenum with flatus. Gastric ulceration with haemorrhages. Increase in pain in intestine when food passes pyloric outlet.

909. *Orostachys japonicus* A. Berger. *(Crassulaceae)*

Vernacular Name: *Eng*: Rock pine.

Description: Glabrous, succulent perennial herb. Rosettes flowering and dying, but often offsets, withering in autumn, leaving compact winter bud of mostly callus leaves that grow basally in spring to form callus-tipped foliage leaves. Stems leaves sessile, dense on stem, subulate as tip, lanceolate, green, sometimes purplish or powdery white. Lnflorescence a terminal, pyramidal thyrse 6-15 cm long. Flowers white, 5-merous; sepals nearly equal, lanceolate, pale green; petals spreading, nearly separate, lanceolate, 6 mm long; stamens 10.

Habitate: Surface of mountain rocks in Korea, Japan and China.

Propagation: By seeds and vegetative method.

Parts Used: Whole plant.

Chemical Constituents: Fatty acid esters: friedelin, glutinone, glutinol, l-hexatriacokntanol, etc., taraxerone, stigmast-4-en-3-one, ergost-4-en-3-one. Flavonoids.

Uses: Cytotoxic, pyruvate-orthophosphate dikinase, antispasmodic activities.

910. *Oroxylum indicum* (L.) Benth. Ex Kurz *(Bignoniaceae)*

Vernacular Name: *San*: Syonakah, Tuntukah, *Eng*: Indian trumpet tree, *Hin*: Sonapatha, Syona, Arlu, Pharkhat, *Kan*: Tattuna, *Mal*: Palakappayyani, Palakappayyana, Payyalanta, *Tam*: Palaiyudaycci, Paiyaralantai, *Tel:* Dundillum, Pampana.

Description: A small to medium sized deciduous tree upto 12 m in height with soft light brown bark with corky lenticels; leaves very large, 90-180 cm long, 2-3 pinnate with 5 or more pairs of primary pinnate, rachis very soft, cylindri,c swollen at the junction of the branches, leaflets 2-4 pairs ovate or elliptic, acuminate, glabrous; flowers lurid to reddish purple outside, dull or pale pinkish yellow within, numerous in large erect racemes; fruits flat capsules, upto 1 m long tapering to both ends.

Habitate: Throughout India in deciduous forests, in moist areas.

Propagation: By seeds and vegetative method.

Parts Used: Roots, leaves, fruits, seeds.

Chemical Consistuents: The stem and root barks contain three flavone colouring matters, viz. oroxylin-A, baicalein and chrysin. Oroxylin-A is the 6-methyl ether of baicalein and has been synthesized. The bark contains also traces of an alkaloid, charya. The seeds contain a yellow crystalline principle and baicalein and its glucoside named tetuin.

Uses: The roots are sweet, astringent, bitter, acrid, refrigerant, anti-inflammatory, anodyne, aphrodisiac, expectorant, appetizing, carminative, digestive anthelmintic, constipating, diaphoretic, diuretic, antiarthritic, febrifuge, and tonic. They are useful in vitiated conditions of *vata* and *kapha*, inflammations, dropsy, sprains, neuralgia, hiccough, cough, asthma, bronchitis, anorexia, dyspepsia, flatulence, colic, helminthiasis, diarrhoea, dysentery, strangury, gout, vomiting, leucoderma, wounds rheumatoid arthritis and fever. The leaves are stomachic and anodyne, and are useful in stomachalgia, flatulence, cephalalgia, ulcers, splenomegaly and vitiated conditions of *vata*. The tender fruits are expectorant, carminative and stomachic, and are useful in cough, bronchitis, dyspepsia, flatulence, colic and leucoderma. The mature fruits are acrid, sweet, anthelmintic and stomachic. They are useful in pharyngodynia, cardiac disorders, helminthiasis, gastropathy, bronchitis and haemorrhoids. The seeds are purgative.

911. *Orthosiphon aristatus* (Blume) Miq. *(Lamiaceae)*

Vernacular Name: *Eng:* Java tea, kidney tea plant.

Description: Perennial herb, 0.5-1. high Stems erect quadrangular, usually tinged violet-brown. Leaves opposite, short petioled, coarsely toothed; apex acute. Inflorescence in a close-whorled raceme at the end of the branches; flowers white, stamens and pistil exserted. Nutlets oblong, compressed, rugulose.

Habitate: A rare wild plant, in mountainous regions but cultivated in some places.

Propagation: By seeds and vegetative method.

Part Used: Whole plant.

Chemical Constituents: The whole plant contains a bitter glucoside: orthosiphonin, saponins, alkaloids, tannin, essential oil, flavonoids, treaterperiod alcohol, choline, betaine, organic acids (tartaric, citric and glycolic), and potassium salts.

Uses: The entire plant, except for the roots, possesses diuretic properties and is used in treating urinary lithiasis, oedema, eruptive fever influenza, rheumatism, hepatitis, jaundice and biliary lithiasis.

912. *Orthosiphon thymiflorus* (Roth) Sleasen *(Lamiaceae)*

Synonyms: *Orthosiphon glabratus* Benth., *Orthosiphon tomentous* Benth. Var. glabrous Hook. f.

Vernacular Name: *San*: Pratanika, *Mal*: Cilannippatam, *Tam*: Cliantippatam.

Description: An erect herb about 60 cm in height with a woody root-stock; leaves simple, opposite, decussate, broadly ovate, acute, obtuse or subcordate at base, coarsely crenate or serrate, nearly glabrous, leaf petioles upto 6.5 cm long; flowers in whorls in terminal racemes, calyx-throat not villous within, corolla tube longer than the calyx, slender, pubescent without; fruits 4, dry ellipsoid smooth nutlets.

Habitate: Throughout south India, upto 900 m in dry open forests.

Propagation: By seeds and vegetative method.

Parts Used: Whole plant.

Chemical Consistuents: N.A.

Uses: The plant is bitter, acrid, depurative, antidiarrhoeal, alexeteric, vulnerary and febrifuge. It is useful in erysipelas, leprosy, dermatopathy such as scabies, dermatitis and pruritus, diarrhoea, haemorrhoids, wounds, ulcers and fever.

913. *Oryza sativa* Linn. *(Poaceae)*

Synonyms: *Oryza plena* (Prain) Chowdhuryi.

Vernacular Name: *San*: Dhanyah, Vrihi, Sali; *Eng*: Paddy, Rice; *Hin*: Dhan, Caval; *Kan*: Akki, Bhatta; *Mal*: Nellu, Navaranellu, Ari; *Tam*: Nellu, Arisi; *Tel:* Biyyam, Vari.

Description: An annual or perennial grass with tuft of fibrous roots and swollen nodes; leaves simple with sheathing bases, long and narrow, slightly pubescent with spiny hairs on the margins; flowers spikelets in terminal compound panicles, lamma punctate or granulate without wing on the back, lemma and palea surrounding the kernel, golden yellow, reddish purple, brown or smoky black becoming straw-coloured on ripening, grains narrowly oblong, free within the lemma and palea.

Habitate: Throughout India, cultivated.

Propagation: By seeds and vegetative method.

Parts Used: Roots, grains.

Chemical Consistuents: Protein, Fat, Carbohydrates, Fibre, Ash, Thiamine, Riboflavin, Nicotinic Acid, Pantothenic Acid, Pyridoxine, Choline Choloride.

Uses: The roots are cooling, diuretic and febrifuge, and are useful in burning sensation, dipsia, bilious fever, strangury and diabetes. The grains are sweet, acrid, oleaginous, aphrodisiac, diuretic, carminative, antidysenteric and tonic. They are useful in vitiated conditions of *pitta*, pneumonosis especially pulmonary consumption, diarrhoea and colonopathy.

914. *Ougeinia oojeinensis* (Roxb.) Hochr. *(Fabaceae)*

Synonyms: *Ougeinia dalbergioides* Benth.

Vernacular Name: *San*: Tinisah, Syandanah; *Eng*: Sandan; *Hin*: Sandan, Tinnas, panjan, panan; *Kan*: Karimutale; *Mal*: Totukara, Malavenna; *Tam*: Narivengai; *Tel:* Tellamotuku.

Description: A medium sized deciduous pretty tree, 6-12 m in height with a short crooked trunk and dark brown deeply cracked bark; leaves pinnately 3-foliate, leaflets large, rigidly coriaceous, the terminal broadly elliptic or roundish, sometimes trapezoidal, main nerves 4-8 pairs, prominent; flowers numerous, white or pink in short fascicled racemes from the nodes of old branches; fruits linear, elongate, flat pods, light brown in colour, seeds 2-5 per pod.

Habitate: Throughout India, in deciduous forests.

Propagation: By seeds and vegetative method.

Parts Used: Bark.

Chemical Consistuents: The heartwood contains a dimethoxy isoflavone, homoferreirin, and an isoflavone, ougenin.

Uses: The bark is astringent acrid, cooling, stimulant, anti-inflammatory, constipating, urinary astringent, anthelmintic, sudorific, depurative, styptic, febrifuge and rejuvenating. It is useful in vitiated conditions of *pitta*, burning sensation, inflammations, diarrhoea, dysentery, urorrhagia, diabetes, verminosis, leprosy, leucoderma, haemorrhages, fevers, ulcers, gonorrhoea, anaemia and general debility.

915. *Oxalis corniculata* L. *(Oxialidaceae)*

Vernacular Name: *San:* Amilika; *Eng:* wood sorrel or yellow sorrel; *Hin:* Amrul sak, chukka tripati; *Beng*: Amrul sak, chukka tripati; *Tel:* Pulichinta; Tam Puliyarai; *Kan:* Hulichikkai, pullam purachi, uppinasoppu; *Mal:* puliyarel.

Description: Small creeping perennial herb which forms roots at nodes. Leaves alternate, long-petiolate, trifoliate (clover-like in appearance), the leaflets obcordate with a conspicuous notched apex, each leaflet up to 2 cm long. Flowers yellow, 5-merous, borne in axillary few-flowered inflorescences. Fruit a sub-cylindrical capsule up to 20 cm long containing numerous tiny black seeds.

Habitate: Common in damp shady places, roadsides, pastures, plantation, lawns etc.

Propagation: By seeds and vegetative method.

Part Used: Whole plant.

Chemical Constituents: Glyxylic acid, oxalic acid, vitexin and isovitexin, vitexin-2-o-beta-d-glucopyranoside, neutral lipids, glycolipids; vitamin c; phospholipids; fatty acids, 1: 2, 18: 3, a6: 01 saturated acids alpha and beta tocopherols; 2-heptenal 2-pentylfurn; trans-phyto.

Uses: The plant is used as a remedy for convulsions in children and for healing fractured bones. The ground leaves are eaten as a chutney to help purify the blood. Ground leaves are also used in treating dizziness, diarrhoea and dysentery. The juice from the leaves is applied to open wounds. The plant is used to treat burns, wounds and body sores. An infusion of the leaves is used to cure convulsions in infants. The crushed leaves are used to treat children with mouth infections as well as to treat infected navels of babies. The crushed leaves are also applied to the heads of babies having symptoms though to be caused by the delayed closing of their fontanelles. An infusion of the leaves is used to treat induration of the breasts, and watery vaginal discharges. It is used to treat wounds and sores and swelling beneath tongue. Use the leaves to treat body pains and internal bleeding It is also used as a remedy for thrush.

916. *Paederia foetida* L. *(Rubiaceae)*

Vernacular Name: *San:* Prasarani; *Eng:* Chinese moon-creeper, king's tonic, strinking opalberry; *Hin:* Gandhali, somaraji; *Beng*: Gandha bhadulia; *Tel:* Savirela; *Tam:* Penarisangai; *Kan:* Hesarane; *Mal*: Talanili.

Description: Perennial climbing plant. Leaves opposite, margins entire, purple beneath, Inflorescence in axillary cyme; flowers small white with pale-violet spots. Fruit sub-ovoid, slightly compressed glabrous. The whole plant is covered with pubescence; it has a fetid smell when crushed.

Habitate: Grows wild and is also cultivated as a spice and medicinal plant.

Propagation: By seeds and vegetative method.

Part Used: Fresh leaves.

Chemical Constituents: The leaves contain an essential oil and alkaloids a-paederine and b-paederine.

Uses: The leaves are well known for their antidysenteric properties and are indicated in the treatment of bacillary dysentery. Fresh leaves, which are fine-cut and mixed with a hen egg, then covered with bananan leaves and grilled, or fried (without fat) in a frying-pan, a decoction of the leaves is also used in teating urinary lithiasis, dysuria, rheumatism, dyspepsia, gastritis and enteritis.

917. *Paeonia lactiflora* Pall. *(Paeoniaceae)*

Synonyms: *Paeonia albiflora* Pall.

Vernacular Name: *Eng:* White-flowered peony.

Description: A perennial herb, 50-80 cm high, with a stout branched root. Leaves alternate, biternate, the ultimate segments red-veined, oblong-elliptical. Flowers large, solitary, white red or purple. Fruit of 3-5 coriaceous few-seeded folicles. Seeds large, subglobose; test thick.

Habitate: Wild and cultivated in China, India, Japan.

Propagation: By seeds and vegetative method.

Part Used: Roots.

Chemical Constituents: N.A.

Uses: Anemic condition, Irregular menstruation, metrorrhagia, diarrhoea, perspiration from no apparent causal night sweats.

918. *Paeonia officinalis* L. *(Paeoniaceae)*

Synonyms: *Paeonia femina* Linn., *Paeonia foemina* Gars ault., *Paeonia elegans* Sabine ex. salm., *Paeonia rubra* Hort. ex. steud., *Paeonia fulgida* Sabine.

Vernacular Name: *Eng:* Peony.

Description: A perennial herb up to 1 m. high. Stem stout, 1-headed. Leaves dark above, pale beneath, the lower divided in 3 leaflets, each of which again divides to form 15 to 20 oblong-lanceolate lobes, 2.5 cm. or more broad; sepals outer leaflike; petals dark crimson 3-5 cm. long, roots composed of several round, oblong knob like tubers which hang below each other, connected by strings.

Habitate: Europe & West Asia.

Propagation: By stem cutting.

Parts Used: Roots.

Chemical Constituents: Paeonin containing Paeondin and glucose; Metarabinic acid, Peonol, paeoniafloureszine, Peoniide, Peregrinine.

Uses: Rectal and anal are most important complaints covered by this drug for which it is used. It is used for complaints of biting itching in anus with anal orifice swollen, burning in anus after stool with internal chilliness. Fistula ani with anal burning and internal chilliness. Painful rectal ulcers, oozing offensive moisture on perineum. Haemorrhoids, fissures, ulceration of anus and perineum, purple covered with crust. Chronic ulcers on lower parts of body, leg, foot, toe & breast. Skin sensitive, painful with ulcers below coccyx, around sacrum.

919. *Paeonia suffruticosa* Andrews (*Paeoniaceae*)

Vernacular Name: *Eng*: Tree peony.

Description: Coarsely branched, small shrub, 1-1.5 m tall. Leaves alternate, 2-pinnate; leaflets deeply and incisively divided, 3-5 clefted, acute, whitish beneath, with a few hairs along midrib. Flowers large and showy, 10-15 cm across, rose-pink to white; stamens many; carpels 2-6, densely brown-pubescent, at first enveloped by a thin, white lobe of the disc that splits as the follicles develop. Fruit a cluster of horizontally spreading follicles.

Habitate: Mostly cultivated in Korea.

Propagation: By Roots.

Parts Used Root bark.

Chemical Constituents: Phenolic compounds: paeonol, paeonolide, paeonoside. Monoterpene glycosides: paeoniflorin, oxypaeoniflorin derivatives. Flavonoids.

Uses: Diuretic, antiviral, anticoagulant, antiulcer, anti-inflammatory, antispasmodic, aldose-reductase inhibition. Used in headache, stomachic, cough, cold, lumbago.

920. *Panax bipinnatifidus* Seem. (*Araliaceae*)

Vernacular Name: *Eng:* Wild false-ginseng.

Description: Perennial herb. Tuberous roots, long and many-noded. Stems erect, 30-50 cm. High, usually withered in the dry season. Leaves palmate, with 2-3 in a whorl; leaflets 5-7, long, irregularly lobed; margins toothed and ciliated. Inflorescence in terminal simple umbel; flowers small, greenish-white, Berry scarlet when ripe, 1-2 seeded.

Habitate: Grows wild in the mountains at an altitude of about 1600m. and above.

Propagation: By seeds and vegetative method.

Part Used: Tuberous roots.

Chemical Constituents: N.A.

Uses: The roots, which possess tonic and antianaemic properties, are used in treating anaemia and general debility and are especially valuable in treating parturients for those conditions. They are also aphrodisiac and have salutary effect in the treatment of sterility.

921. *Panax notoginseng* (*Araliaceae*)

Vernacular Name: *Eng: San* qi.

Description: Deciduous perennial with an erect stem growing upto 1m, compound leaves, small greenish flowers and small, berry-like fruit.

Habitate: Native to China.

Propagation: By roots and cutting.

Parts Used: Root.

Chemical Constituents: *San qi* contains steroidal saponins and a flavonoid.

Uses: Like ginseng, *San qi* is a tonic the supports the function of the adrenal glands, in particular the production of corticosteroids and male sex hormones. *San qi* also helps to improve blood flow through the coronary arteries, thus finding use as a treatment for arteriosclerosis, high blood pressure and angina. *San qi* treats internal bleeding of almost any kind. The herb may also be applied externally as a poultice as a means to help speed the healing of wounds and bruises.

922. *Panax pseudo-ginseng* Wall. *(Araliaceae)*

Vernacular Name: *Eng:* false ginseng.

Description: Perennial herb. Tuberous roots, short and fleshy. Stems erect, 30-50 cm. High, usually withered in the dry season. Eleaves palmate, long-petioled in whorl; leaflets 5-7, margins dentate, hairy on both sides. Inflorescence in terminal simple umbel; flowers small, yellowish-green. Berry globose, slightly compressed, red when ripe, 2-seeded.

Habitate: Cultivated in cold, climatic regions.

Propagation: By seeds and vegetative method.

Part Used: Tuberous roots.

Chemical Constituents: The tuberous roots contain triterpenoid saponins (saponins A,B,C,D), oleanolic acid, amino acids: leucine, valine, proline, oxyproline, histidine, lysine and cysteine; Fe, Ca.

Uses: The roots possess well known haemostatic, tonic, hormonal and circulation-promotion properties and have a beneficial effect in haematemesis, metrorrhagia, menorrhagia, post-partum haematometra, ocular congestion, bloody stools, epistaxis, rheumatism, phelegmon and contusions. They are also effective in case of anaemia and general debility, especially in parturients, and sterility.

923. *Panax quinquefolium* L. *(Araliaceae)*

Synonyms: *Ginseng quinquefolia* Linn., *Aralia quinquefolia* Decne and Planch., *Panax ginseng* Mey, C.A.

Vernacular Name: *Eng:* Ginseng.

O**Description**: A perennial herb with fleshy often forked roots, up to 30 cm. in height. Stem bearing a single whorl of ternatelly compound leaves. Leaflets 3-7, usually 5 on each branch, stalked, the basal pair much smaller than the others, all lanceolate, dentate, acuminate; peduncle upto 50 cm. bearing a 6-20 flowered umbel. Flowers greenish white, all or mostly perfect. Styles usually 2. Berry bright red about 1 cm. in diameter.

Habitate: China, Japan, Korea, Eastern North America.

Propagation: By seeds and vegetative method.

Parts Used: Root.

Chemical Constituents: Choline; Ginsenosides viz. $Rb\text{-}_1$, R_c and $R_{g\text{-}1}$; Sesquiterpenes viz. Panacene, Limonene, Terpineol, eucalyptol, Citral, α-phellandrene; Sesquiterpene alcohols viz. Pnasinsanol A and B and Ginsenol, Polyacetylene: Panquillon; Vitamins B_1, B_2, B_{12}; Panthotenic acid.

Uses: For Restoring exhausted power. As stimulant. Stomachic. For Neurasthenia, Neuralgia, Insomnia, Hypotonia. Depression with sexual inadequacy. General vitality. For complaints of lower parts of spinal cord, lumbago, sciatica, rheumatism, paralytic weakness, itching pimples on neck and chest. Diminutive vitality. Vertigo with gray spots before eyes, dubbling of vision. Abdominal pain in right side with loud gurgling in Ileo-caecal region. Testicular rheumatic pain after emission.

924. *Pandanus fascicularis* Lamk. *(Pandanaceae)*

Synonyms: *Pandanus odoratissimus* Linn.

Vernacular Name: *San:* Ketaki; *Eng:* Screw pine; *Hin:* Keura, kewda, ketki, gagandhul; *Beng*: Keya, kedki-keya, keori; *Tel:* Mugali, ketaki, gajangi; *Tam:* Tazhai, thalay; *Kan:* Tale mara, kyad-agegida; *Mal:* Kaida, thala.

Description: A branched palm-like shrub; leaves ensiform, spinescent; male flowers in spikes enclosed in large, white, fragrant spathes; female flowers in solitary spadix; syncarpium yellow or red, drupes numerous.

Habitate: Coastal regions of India and the Andaman Islands.

Propagation: By seeds and vegetative method.

Part Used: Spadices, spathes.

Chemical Constituents: The principal constituent of kewda oil, responsible for the characteristic aroma of spadices is b-phenyl ethyl methyl ether. 2-acetyl-1pyrroline is a major volatile component in the tender floral leaves or spathes.

Uses: The tender floral leaves are used to flavour cream, rice (giving a flavour similar to basmati rice), sherbets, jellies and sometimes curries. Kewda attar or water, prepared by distillation of spadices, is similarly used to flavour various goods, sweets, syrups and soft drinks.

925. *Pandanus odoratissimus* L. F. *(Pandanaceae)*

Synonyms: *Pandanus tectorius* auct.non Soland. Ex. Parkinson.

Vernacular Name: *San*: Ketaki; *Eng*: Screw pine, Umbrella tree; *Hin*: Kedgi, Kevda; *Kan*: Kedage, Mundige; *Mal*: Pukkaita, Kaita, Kainari, Talampu; *Tam*: Talai, Talai; *Tel:* Mogali, Ketaki, Gajangi.

Description: A tortuous small tree or shrub, rarely erect with many aerial roots; leaves glaucous-green, 90-150 cm long, coriaceous, marginal spines pointing forward and those of the midrib forward and backward; male flowers in numerous subsessile cylindric spikes with fragrant caudate-acuminate spathes, female flowers in solitary spadix; fruits oblong or globose syncarps, yellow or red when ripe.

Habitate: Throughout India, along the sea coast and water courses.

Propagation: By root suckers.

Parts Used: Roots, leaves, flowers.

Chemical Consistuents: The chief constituent of *kewda* oil is methyl ether of–phenylethyl alcohol to which is due the characteristic aroma of the spadices. The oil also contains dipentene, *d*-linalool, phenylethyl acetate, citral, phenylethyl alcohol, ester of phthalic acid, fatty acids and stearoptene.

Uses: The roots are bitter, sweet, acrid, thermogenic, emollient, depurative, procreant, antiseptic, cephalic, aphrodisiac, carminative, stomachic, suppurative, anodyne, deodorant, urinary astringent, vulnerary, sudorific, febrifuge and tonic. They are useful in vitiated conditions of *kapha* and *pitta*, skin diseases, leprosy, cephalalgia, coxalgia, otalgia, wounds, ulcers, dyspepsia, flatulence, colic, fever, diabetes, sterility, spontaneous, abortion and general debility. The leaves are acrid, bitter, alexeteric aphrodisiac, depurative and sommiferous. They are useful in tumorus, leprosy, smallpox, syphilis, scabies, leucoderma and cardiopathy and cerebropathy due to insomnia. The flowers are acrid, bitter, aphrodisiac, anodyne and demulcent, and are useful in pruritus, otalgia, cephallgia, leucoderma, and skin eruptions. The oil obtained from the bracts is stimulant and antispasmodic, and is useful in cephalalgia, rheumatoid arthritis and coxalgia.

926. *Pandanus pyriformis* (Martelli) St. John. *(Pandanaceae)*

Description: Simple to sparsely branched palm-like tree with conspicuous prop and aerial roots up to 12 m high. Leaves spiraled and confined to apices of stems and branches, long upto 180 cm and linear with sharp-toothed margins. Flowers unisexual and borne in large male or female heads. Fruit a syncarp up to or exceeding 25 cm pyriform fruit (phalanges), each up to 8 cm long and containing a single seed.

Habitate: Common in coastal areas especially along beaches and among lowland vegetation from near sea-level to 400 m elevation.

Propagation: By seeds and vegetative method.

Part Used: Leaves, aerial roots and bark.

Chemical Constituents: The volatile oil of the male flowers contain methyl beta-phenylethyl ether, dipentene, linalool, phenylethyl acetate, citral phenylethyl alcohol, and an ester of phtyalic acid.

Uses: Diarrhoea is treated with a tea made from the leaves. A filtrate of the aerial roots is used to treat asthama and back pains. Liquid from the aerial roots and inner bark is used to treat heart attacks. Internal fractures are treated with the juice from the root and bark. The root is used in a treatment for fish poisoning.

927. *Panicum sumatrense* Roth ex Roem. Et Schult. *(Poaceae)*

Synonyms: *Panicum* miliare Lam.

Vernacular Name: *San*: Syamakah, *Eng*: Little millet, *Hin*: Savan, Kumku, Kutki, *Kan*: Save, Baragu, Navanikki, *Mal*: Cama, *Tam*: Camai, *Tel:* Korralu.

Description: A slender erect branched annual, 30-90 cm in height, usually leafy upto the panicle; leaves linear, tapering from a broad base, upto 60 cm long, glabrous or finely hairy; panicles very compound, contracted, often nodding; spikelets glabrous, not gaping lower floral glume 9-nerved, upper floral glume 3-5 streaked; fruits caryopsis, glabrous, striated, brown.

Habitate: Cultivated throughout India upto an elevation of 2,100 m.

Propagation: By seeds and vegetative method.

Parts Used: Grains.

Chemical Consistuents: Arginine, lysine, methionine, phenylalanine, threonine, tryptophan and valine.

Uses: The grains are astringent, sweet, emollient, cooling, desiccating constipating, alexeteric, and digestive. They are useful in vitiated conditions of *kapha* and *pitta*, burning sensation, diarrhoea, dysentery, dyspepsia, wounds, ulcers and gonorrhoea.

928. *Papaver rhoeas* *(Papaveraceae)*

Vernacular Name: *Eng:* Red poppy; *Hin*: Lalpost, Post, Posteke bija; *Beng*: Lal posht; *Guj*: Lala, Lalkhaskhas; *Tel:* Erragassagassala, errapostakaya; *Tam*: Siguppuppostaka, Sivappugashagasha; *Kan*: Kempu gasgase, Kempukhasakhasi; *Mal*: Shivappupostakachedi, Chovannakashakasha,.

Description: Delicate hairy-stemmed annual growing to 90 cm. Has basal rosette of lance-shaped leaves and deeply incised stem leaves, four-petalled red flowers with black anthers and small rounded seed capsules.

Habitate: Red poppy is native to Europe, North Africa and temperate regions of Asia, and is naturalized in North and South America. It thrives on cultivated land and on road verges. The flowers are picked in summer.

Propagation: By seeds and vegetative method.

Parts Used: Flowers.

Chemical Constituents: Red poppy contains alkaloids, meconic acid, mekocyanin, mucilage and tannins. the alkaloids are similar to those in the opium poppy, but are much milder.

Uses: Red poppy flowers are mildly analgesic and sedative, and have long been used in European herbal medicine, particularly for ailments in children and the elderly. Chiefly employed as a mild pain reliever and as a treatment for irritable coughs, red poppy also helps reduce nervous overactivity. The herb may be used in the treatment of insomnia, general irritability, coughs-especially paroxysmal coughs-and asthma, and is generally given as a syrup.

929. *Papaver somniferum* L. *(Papaveraceae)*

Vernacular Name: *San:* Ahifen, chosa, khasa; *Eng:* Opium poppy, white poppy; *Hin*: Afim, afyun, kashkash, post; *Beng*: Pasto; *Tel:* Abhini, gasalu, kasakasa; *Tam:* abini, gashagasha, kasakasa, postaka; *Kan:* Afim, biligasgase, khasakhasi; *Mal:* Afium, kashakhasa.

Description: Erect annual herb, about 1m. hign. Stems slender, glabrous Leaves alternate, sessile, amplexicaual, irregularly lobed and toothed. Flowers large, handsome, of various shades: white, scarlet or lilac, solitary ath the top, with long stalk, Capsule globular, longitudinally goooved, Seeds numerous, small and black.

Habitate: Cultivated in the highlands.

Propagation: By seeds and vegetative method.

Part Used: Latex obtained by incising unripe capsules and seeds.

Chemical Constituents: The latex is rich in alkaloids: morphine, codeine, thebaine, nacrocotine, narceine and papaverine; organic acids: meconic, lactic, malic, tartaric, citric, acetic and succinic; it contains in addition proteins, dextrose and pectin.

Uses: The latex possesses hypnotic, analgesic, antitussive and antidiarrhoeal properties. It is also effective in dyspnoea consequent upon heart failure. It is prescribed daily in a dose of 0.005-0.02g according to the amount of morphine. The cure is limited to 7 days. The capsules from which the latex has been drawn off are used in treating chronic cough, pertussi, and diarrhoea.

930. *Parietaria officinalis* *(Urticaceae)*

Synonyms*:* *Parietaria diffusa.*

Vernacular Name: *Eng:* Pellitory of the wall.

Description: Annual growing to 70cm. Has deep green leaves, greenish flowers and small dark seeds.

Habitate: Native to Europe, this plant is commonplace in southern countries, where it is found on walls and in dry stony sties.

Propagation: By seeds and vegetative method.

Parts Used: Aerial parts.

Chemical Constituents: Pellitory of the wall contains flavonoids and tannins.

Uses: Pellitory of the wall is chiefly employed as a diuretic, demulcent and stone-preventing herb. In European herbal medicine, it is regarded as having a restorative action on the kidneys, supporting and strengthening their function. It has been prescribed for conditions such as nephritis, pyelitis of the kidney stones, renal colic, cystitis and oedema. It is also occasionally taken as a laxative.

931. *Paris quadrifolia* L. *(Liliaceae)*

Synonyms: *Paris pentafolia* Renault.

Vernacular Name: *Eng:* Herb, Herba peridis, Crow's eye, Uva lupina, Uva vulpine.

Description: Perennial herb with creeping fleshy, root stock. Root vertical rampant, rounded, jointed, fleshy, whitish. Stem erect, single, round, unifloral and smooth. Leaves, all cauline with short petioles, broad-elliptical or oval, pointed, entire, glabrous, disposed as a cross, shining beneath, glabrous, disposed as a cross, shining beneath, with reticulate venation being exceptional among monocotyledons. Flowers with a perianth of 8 lobes, yellowish green, in 2 whorls. Lobes of outer whorl broad, oval, larger, while that of inner whorl, more yellowish, much narrower, thin, tapering at apex, alternating with outer perianth lobes. Stamens 8, in two whorls, alternating perianth. Peduncles 2.5-5 cm. above leaves, furrowed. Fruit bluish-black berry, shining, slightly quadrangular.

Habitate: North & Central Europe and Russia.

Propagation: By stem cutting.

Parts Used: Whole plant.

Chemical Constituents: Strychinen, Glaycosides: Paradine and Paridol: Glycosides: α-paristyphin, Paristyphinen.

Uses: For complaints of aches and soreness of head, occiput and eyes. Apprehension of head becoming large. Coldness of right side and hotness of left side of the body. Soreness of top of head & therefore cannot brush hairs. String pull like aches from eyes to occiput. Occipital headache with numbness of left side. Sensation of a sting pull in eye balls. Dryness of mouth, without thirst. Neuralgia of face & coccyx. Traditionally, it is used for neuralgic, headache, bronchitis and cramps.

932. *Paspalum scrobiculatum* L. *(Poaceae)*

Synonyms: *Paspalum scrobiculatum* Lam.

Vernacular Name: *San*: Kodravah, *Eng*: Kodo millet, *Hin*: Kodo, Kodra, *Kan*: Harike, *Mal*: Varaku, *Tam*: Varagu, *Tel:* Kiraruga.

Description: An annual grass, culms upto 90 cm in height, tufted on a very short rhizome, leafy from the base upwards; leaves 2-ranked, 15-45 cm long, glabrous or sometimes softly hairy, ligule short, membranous, spikelets suborbicular normally 2-ranked, glumes glabrous, upper lemma and palea crustaceous, palea with wide membranous auricles at the base, grain biconvex, shining, deep purple with a conspicuous ridge along the margin, tightly enclosed in the hardened lemma and palea.

Habitate: Throughout India, wild, also cultivated.

Propagation: By seeds and vegetative method.

Parts Used: Grains.

Chemical Consistuents: The essential amino acids present in the proteins are; arginine, histidine, isoleucine, leucine, lysine, methionine, phenylalanine, threonine, tryptophan, and valine, N. Lysine is the limiting amino acid.

Uses: The grains are sweet, bitter, astringent, cooling, constipating, diuretic, sedative, alexeteric, styptic and tonic. They are useful in ulcers, flatulence strangury, diarrhoea hallucination, inflammation, hepatopathy, haemorrhages, vitiated conditions of *pitta* burning sensation and general debility.

The stem is useful for corneal opacity.

933. *Passiflora edulis* Sims *(Passifloraceae)*

Vernacular Name: *Eng:* Passion fruit, purple granadilla.

Description: A woody climber; leaves deeply 3-lobed, serrate; flowers white with purple; fruit globose or avoid, rind hard, pulp purple or yellow, edible.

Habitate: Hilly areas of Tamilnadu, Andhra Pradesh, West Bengal and Assam.

Propagation: By seeds and vegetative method.

Part Used: Fruit.

Chemical Constituents: The flavour component s of passion fruit juice of purple variety are edulan I, Edulan II.

Uses: Passion fruit juice is used for flavouring candy, ice-cream, cake-fillings, frostings, carbonated beverages and cordials.

934. *Passiflora foetida* L. *(Passifloraceae)*

Vernacular Name: ***Eng*: Stinking passion flower, tagua passion floer, hispid granadilla; *Tel:* Tellajumiki; *Tam*: Mupparisavalli, siruppunaikkalli; *Kan*: Kukkiballi; *Mal*: Chadayan, Poochapazham.**

Description: Perennial climber with tendrils. Stems hollow, tubular, Leaves alternate, trilobed, flowers white, solitary in the axil of leaves; coronal violet. Fruit globose, enveloped by remains of pinnatifid bracts, yellow when ripe, edible; seeds numerous. The whole plant is densely hirsute.

Habitate: Found wild among shrubs.

Propagation: By seeds and vegetative method.

Part Used: Whole plant.

Chemical Constituents: The fruit, seeds and leaves contain an unstable substance that yields hydrocyanic acid and acetone. The ripe fruit yields Ca, P, Fe.

Uses: The whole plant is considered to have sedative properties and is used in the treatment of neurasthenia, insomnia, nightmares and anxiety. It is also indicated for hypertension in the form of decoction, fluid extract or syrup.

935. *Passiflora incarnata* L. *(Passifloraceae)*

Vernacular Name: *Eng:* Maypop.

Description: A perennial twining herb with longitudinally striated stem. Leaves petiolate, alternate, palmately 3-5 lobed, with margins serrate, base cordate, apex acute, glands on the under surface; stipules present. Petioles, upto 5 cm. long with two nectar-glands near the summit. Tendrils, numerous and closely coiled. Flowers, large, solitary, on jointed, axillary peduncles, 5 cm. broad, whitish, with a triple purple and flesh coloured corona. Bracts usually 3. Calyx 5-lobed and cup-shaped. Corolla 5, springing from throat of the calyx. Coralla, with one or more rows of fine threads of corona springing from corolla tube and one or more membranous folds arising lower-down. Gynophore, surrounded at base by a shallow membranous cup. Stamen 5, monoadulphous, anthers oblong, 2-celled, dorsi-fixed; pollen grains reticulate on the surface. Ovary, externally green or yellow, somewhat shriveled.

Habitate: U.S.A. & Europe.

Propagation: By seeds and vegetative method.

Parts Used: Leaves.

Chemical Constituents: Alkaloids viz. Harman, Harmaline, Harmalol, Harmine, Harmol; Vitexin, Isovitexin, Apigenin, Orientin, Homoorientin, Lucenin, Maltol, Ethylmaltol, Passicol, Myristic acid, Oleic acid, Formic acid, Scopoletin & Umbelliferone.

Uses: For complaints, mainly of neuralgia and insomnia both associated. Tetanus. Hysteria. Violent headache as if top of head would brust. Insomnia due to worries, overwork & exhaustion. Noctural cough. Traditionally it is used for neuralgia, insomnia, dysmenorrhoea, used as sedative, hypnotic, antispasmodic and anodyne.

936. *Patrinia scabiosaefolia* Fisch. *(Vlerianaceae)*

Vernacular Name: *Eng:* Dahurian patrinia.

Description: A perennial herb. Rhizome horizontal, stout. The root of this plant smell like spoiled soy-paste, especially when dry. The stem stands upright and grows to a height of 60-150 cm. Basal leaves in rosettes, long-petiolate, long-ovate, acuminate, marginscoarsely serrate; cauline leaf opposite, short-petiolate or subsessile, pinnately parted or divided; segments 3-11; the terminal segment is larger than the other, elliptic-lanceolate; the lateral segments lanceolate to linear, margins corasely serrate, both surfaces hispid. Cymes terminal or axillary, corymb-like panicles with small yellow flowers 2-4 mm in diameter; bracts small, linear. Fruit elliptic, triangular.

Habitate: On slopes, in grasslands and on the skirts of forests in China, Japan, Korea,.

Propagation: By seeds and vegetative method.

Part Used: Whole plant.

Chemical Constituents: N.A.

Uses: Fever, abscesses.

937. *Paullinia cupana* *(Sapindaceae)*

Synonyms*:* *Paullinia sorbilis.*

Vernacular Name: *Eng:* Guarana.

Description: Woody vine growing to height of 10m. Has divided compound leaves, cluster of inconspicuous yellow flowers and pear-shaped fruit that contains small shiny brown seeds.

Habitate: Guarana is native to tropical forests of the Brazilian Amazon, and is also cultivated in Brazil.

Propagation: By seeds and vegetative method.

Parts Used: Seeds.

Chemical Constituents: Guarana contains xanthine derivatives, tannins and saponins. The xanthines are stimulant, diuretic and reduce fatigue over the short term.

Uses: Guarana's medicinal uses are similar to those of coffee-it is taken for headache and migraine, for mild depression and to boost energy levels. The problems that apply to long-term or excessive coffee consumption also apply to guarana-both stimulate over the short term but tend to inhibit the body's restorative processes over the longer term. In view of guarana's high tannin content, long-term use is even less advisable, because tannins impair the intestines' ability to absorb nutrients. Nevertheless, guarana is a useful short-term remedy for boosting energy, or for treating a tension headache that cannot be treated with rest. Guarana's astringency also treats chronic diarrhoea.

938. *Pedalium murex* L. *(Pedaliaceae)*

Vernacular Name: *San*: Sthulagoksurah, Tiktagoksurah, *Hin*: Bara gokhru, Bada gokhru, *Kan*: Aneneggilu, doddaneggili, Anenegaligida, *Mal*: Kattunerinnil, Ananerinnil, *Tam*: Yanai nerunci, Perunerunci, *Tel:* Pedda palleru.

Description: A much branched foetid smelling succulent herb upto 38 cm in height with rough slime secreting glands; leaves simple, opposite, somewhat fleshly, broadly ovate-oblong, coarsely crenate-serrate or sublobate, glabrous above, provided with minute scales on the lower side; flowers bright yellow, axillary and solitary; fruits bluntly 4-angled with stout, sharp, conical horizontal spines from the angles.

Habitate: Throughout India, especially in the coastal areas of south India.

Propagation: By seeds and vegetative method.

Parts Used: Seeds, leaves.

Chemical Consistuents: Alkaloid, Greenish fatty oil, resin.

Uses: The plant is sweet, cooling, mucilaginous, diuretic, lithontriptic aphrodisiac, antispasmodic, emmenagogue, anti-inflammatory, digestive carminative, tonic, and rejuvenating. It is useful in strangyr, renal and vesical calculi, aphthae, puerperal diseases, spermatorrhoea, spasmodic affections, amenorrhoea, dysmenorrhoea, vitiated conditions of *pitta*, inflammation splenomegaly dyspepsia, flatulence ulcers, fever and general debility.

939. *Peganum harmala* *(Zygophyllaceae)*

Vernacular Name: *Eng:* Harmala, African rue; *Hin*: Harmal, isband-lahouri; *Beng*: Isband; *Guj*: Harmal, ispun; *Tel:* Sima-goranta; *Kan*: Sima-goranta; *Tam*: Simaiyaravandi, simaiyalavinall,.

Description: Multi-branched shrubby perennial growing to 50cm. Has deeply cleft linear leaves, white 5-petalled flowers and rounded 3-celled seed capsules.

Habitate: Native to the Middle East, North Africa and southern Europe, harmala is naturalized in other sub-tropical regions, including Australia.

Propagation: By seeds and vegetative method.

Parts Used: Seeds, root.

Chemical Constituents: Harmala contains up to 4% indole alkaloids, which are similar in action to the alkaloids found in ayahuasca, yohimbe and passion flower. Harmine has been used to help alleviate the tremors of Parkinsonism.

Uses: Despite its long history as a euphoric and purportedly aphrodisiac herb, harmula is little used in contemporary Western herbal medicine due to its potential toxicity. The seeds have been taken to treat eye disorders and to increase the volume of breast-milk production. In central Asia, the root is a popular medicinal remedy, used to treat rheumatism and nervous conditions.

940. *Pentapetes phoenicea* L. *(Sterculiaceae)*

Vernacular Name: *San*: Bandhukah, arkavallabhah; *Eng*: Noon plant; *Hin*: Dopahariya; *Kan*: Bandure; *Mal*: Uccamalari; *Tam*: Uccittilakam; *Tel:* Makinacettu.

Description: A branched herb, 60-150 cm high, leaves lanceolate, crenate-serrate; flowers red or scarlet, solitary or in pairs on short peduncles; capsules sub-globose, bristly, seeds 8-12, sub-globose, dotted.

Habitate: Throughout India as well as cultivated.

Propagation: By seeds and vegetative method.

Parts Used: Whole plant.

Chemical Consistuents: N.A.

Uses: The plant is bitter, acrid, aromatic, stomachic, demulcent, diaphoretic, digestive, diuretic, expectorant, febrifuge, vermifuge and alexeteric. It is useful in cardiopathy, haemopathy, leucoderma, asthma, bronchitis, catarrhal fever, otalgia, hepatopathy, vomiting, lumbago, hiccough, ophthalmia, gastropathy in children, genito-urinary disorders, ringworm, verminosis and skin diseases.

941. *Pergularia daemia* (Forssk.) Chiov. *(Asclepiadaceae)*

Synonyms: *Pertularia extensa* (Jacq.) N.E. Br., *Daemia extensa* (Jacq.) R. Br.

Vernacular Name: *San*: Kurutakah, Uttamarani; *Hin*: Utaran, Sagovani, Jutak; *Kan*: Talavaranaballi, Juttuve, Halokoratige; *Mal*: Velipparutti; *Tam*: Velipparutti; *Tel:* Gurticettu, Jittupaku, Dustapucettu.

Description: A slender foul smelling perennial milky twining herb with hispid stems; leaves simple, opposite, suborbicular, cordate, acuminate, velvety pubescent beneath, margins ciliate; flowers greenish yellow or dull white tinged with purple, in axillary long peduncled umbellate or corymbose clusters; fruits relfexed follicles with long beak and soft spines, seeds many, ovate, truncate at the apex, densely velvety-pubescent on both sides.

Habitate: Throughout the hotter parts of India, upto 900 m.

Propagation: By seeds and vegetative method.

Parts Used: Whole plant.

Chemical Consistuents: The musculotropic activity of the plant extract, formerly attributed to a bitter glucodisic principle, is due to the presence of a polypeptide in combination with betaine. The plant also contains hentriacontane, lupeol, α-and β-amyrins, β-sitosterol, two new sterols, viz., 5β-stigmast-7en-3α-ol and 5β-stigmast-8-en-3α-ol and three unidentified sterols. A more recent examination of the plant showed the presence of several cardenolides in the seeds and stems; calctin, calotropin and calotropagenin were identified in the seeds, and uzarigenin and coroglaucigenin in the stems.

Uses: The plant is astringent, acrid, thermogenic, emetic, expectorant, emenagogue, anthelmintic, antipyretic and laxative. It is useful in urethororrhoea, strangury, metropathy, inflammations, vitiated conditions of *vata* and *kapha*, cough, asthma, amenorrhoea, dysmenorrhoea, intermittent fevers and leucoderma.

The leaves are bitter, thermogenic, anthelmintic and depurative. They are useful in vitiated conditions of *kapha*, helminthiasis, haemorrhoids and laprosy. The fruits are acrid, thermogenic and digestive, and are useful in vitiated conditions of *kapha* and dyspepsia.

The plant extract is useful in uterine and menstrual disorders and in facilitating parturition.

942. *Perilla frutescens* (L.) Britton. *(Lameaceae)*

Synonyms: *Perilla ocimoides* Linn.

Vernacular Name: *Eng:* Perilla; *Hin:* Bhanjira; *Beng*: Ban tulsi; *Assam*: Arim, angami, kenia.

Description: Small aromatic plant, 0.5–1m. high. Stems 4–angled, striate. Leaves opposite, long-petioled, coarsely settate, pale-green or purplish-violet above, purplish-violet beneath. Inflorescence in terminal whorled spike; flowers white. Achene of 4 nutlets. All parts of the plant are covered with a dense pubescence.

Habitate: Cultivated in gardens as a spice and medicinal plant.

Propagation: By seeds and vegetative method.

Part Used: Whole plant.

Chemical Constituents: The whole plant contains an essential oil consisting of perilla-aldehyde (4-isopropenyl 1-cyclohexen7-al); limonene, a-pinene, and dihydrocumine. The seeds yield a fatty oil, containing oleic, linoleic and linolenic acids; and amino acids: arginine, histidine, leucine, lysine and valine.

Uses: In the therapy of influenza, coryza and headache, the plant is recommended in the form of decoction. The drug is also useful in caes of threatened abortion. The fruit is effective against cough.

943. *Perilla grutescen* Britton *(Lamiaceae)*

Synonyms: *Perilla ocimoides* Linn.

Vernacular Name: *Eng:* Beng-ban tulsi; *Hindi*: Bhanjira.

Description: An aromatic bushy annual leaves broadly ovate, serrate; flowers white, in racemes; nutlets pale brown.

Habitate: The Himalayas and hills of Assam and Bihar.

Propagation: By seeds and vegetative method.

Part Used: Leaves and inflorescence.

Chemical Constituents: Major compounds in the essential oil are rosfuran, b-caryophyllene, perilla ketone, perillene, germacrene-D, a-phellan drene, a-humbulene, a-cadinene and a-terpineol.

Uses: The leaves and flowering tops are used as flovouring. The oil is used to a small extent for flavouing table-sauces and confectionery. The seeds are used in meat, fish and vegetable preparations.

944. *Persea americana* *(Lauraceae)*

Vernacular Name: *Eng:* Avocado.

Description: A large tree, 15-18 m high; leaves oblong or elliptic-lanceolate, upto 40 cm long; flowers small, greenish, in compact panicles; fruit baccate, large 5-20 cm long, pear shaped, ovate or spherical, yellow-green to maroon and purple, skin thin or woody; seed single, large, globe or pointed.

Habitate: Indigenous to Central America, avocado is widely cultivated for its fruit in tropical and sub-tropical areas, including Israel, Spain and South Africa.

Propagation: By seeds and vegetative method.

Parts Used: Fruit, Seed and Leaves.

Chemical Constituents: ***Leaves & Bark:*** volatile oil, Flavonoids, Tannins. Fruit pulp: Unsaturated fats, Protein, Sesquiterpenes, Vitamins A, B^1 and B^2.

Uses: ***Leaves & bark:*** Astringent, Carminative, Relieve coughs, Promote menstrual flow. Fruits pulp: Emollient, carminative. Rind: Eliminates worms.

945. *Petasites hybridus* *(Compsitae)*

Vernacular Name: *Eng:* Butterbur.

Description: Downy perennial growing to 1m. Has very large heart-shaped leaves, and lilac-pink flowers growing in large spikes.

Habitate: Butterbur flourishes throughout Europe. It prefers damp or moist sites.

Propagation: By seeds and cutting.

Parts Used: Root.

Chemical Constituents: Butterbur contains pyrrolizidine alkaloids, sesquiterpene lactones, a volatile oil, pectin, mucilage and inulin. Pyrrolizidine alkaloids in isolation are toxic to the liver.

Uses: Butterbur has tonic and expectorant properties, and is antispasmodic and analgesic, acting specifically on the stomach, bile ducts and duodenum. It has been used mainly to treat chest problems such as bronchitis, asthma and whooping cough. Butterbur helps to and whooping cough. Butterbur helps to strengthen the digestion, and is particularly effective where indigestion results from obstructed bile flow. Butterbur has also been given for inflammation of the urinary tract, and it has been used externally as a poultice to speed the healing of wounds and skin eruptions.

946. *Petroselinum crispum* *(Apiaceae)*

Synonyms: *Petroselinum sativum* Hoffm. P.

Vernacular Name: *Eng:* Parsley.

Description: A hardy, aromatic, biennial herb, sometimes lasting upto 4 years, producing a rosette of finely divided redical leaves in the first year and a flowering stack up to 100 cm high in the second, leaves 2 or 3 pinnate, ultimate segments cuneate-ovate or some times linear, oblong, incised, dentate or entire, often much crisped, upper cauline leaves often ternate; flower yellow or yellowish-green in compound umbels fruit 2-3 mm long, crescent shaped, conspicuously ridge. Consisting of two mericarp.

Habitate: Cultivted in kitchen gardens.

Propagation: By seeds and vegetative method.

Part Used: Leaves.

Chemical Constituents: Major constituents of leaf oil are 1,3,8-p-menthatriene, b-phellandrene, myristicin and myrcene. Those of the seed oil are myristicin, a-and b-pinens, m-metntha-1-8-diene, elemecin, b-farnesene, and sabinene.

Uses: Fresh and dried leaves are used for garnishing and seasoning in sours, sews, salads, sauces, meat, and poultry. Parsley herb oil is used as an exclusive flavouring in sauces, pickles, meat additives, and various spaces. Blends. The seed oil is blended with sweeter spice oils and used as a substitute for hers oil in meat sauces, seasonings, spice blends, canned foods. Pickles etc.

947. *Peucedanum decursivum* maxim. *(Apiaceae)*

Vernacular Name: *Eng:* Common hog-fennel.

Description: A perennial herb, 70-140 cm high. Stem erect, simple, purplish. Leaves 1-2 pinnate, ultimate leaflets long-ovate, toothed, petiole expanded, clasping the stem. Umbels compound, rays 10-20. Flowers dark purple. Fruit dividing into 2 mericarps, compressed, oblong carpels ribbed and with vittae.

Habitate: On slopes and in shrubland in China, Japan, Korea.

Propagation: By seeds and vegetative method.

Part Used: Roots.

Chemical Constituents: N.A.

Uses: Common cold, upper respiratory tract infection, cough, abundant expectoration.

948. *Peucedanum japonicum* Thunb. *(Apiaceae)*

Vernacular Name: *Eng*: Japanese peucedanum.

Description: Glaucous perennial herb, glabrous in lower part, short pubescent in upper part, to 60-100 cm tall. Leaves alternate, long, often 3-lobed, irregularly deeply dentate; upper leaves reduced, with a membraneous, uninflated sheath. Umbels many, on short peduncles; peduncles 10-20, 2-3.5 cm long, densely pubescent; involucre abscetn; involucels 5-10, deltoid or lanceolate; pedicels 20-30. Fruit elliptic, puberulent, 4-5 mm long; the dorsal ribs slender and filiform; the lateral narrowly winged.

Habitate: *San*dy places near seashores.

Propagation: By seeds and vegetative method.

Parts Used Root.

Chemical Constituents: Coumarins and dihydrocoumarins.

Uses: Platelet aggregation ihnibiton, cytotoxicity.

949. *Peumus boldus* *(Apiaceae)*

Vernacular Name: *Eng:* Boldo.

Description: Strongly aromatic multi-branched evergreen shrub or tree growing to 6m. Has egg-shaped leathery leaves with a lemony scent, cluster of white or yellow bell-shaped flowers and small yellow berries.

Habitate: It is native to Chile and Peru, and has become naturalized in the Mediterranean region and the west coast of North America.

Propagation: By seeds and vegetative method.

Parts Used: Leaves.

Chemical Constituents: It contains 0.7% isoquinoline alkaloids, as well as a volatile oil and flavonoids.

Uses: Boldo stimulates liver activity and bile flow and is chiefly valued as a remedy for gallstones and liver or gallbladder pain. It is normally taken for a few weeks at a time, either as a tincture or infusion. Boldo is also a mild urinary antiseptic and demulcent and may be taken for infections such as cystitis. In the Anglo-American tradition, boldo is combined with barberry and fringe tree in the treatment of gallastones.

950. *Pharbitis nil* (L.) Choosy *(Convolvulaceae)*

Synonyms: *Convulvulus nil* L.; *Ipomaea nil* (L.) Roth.

Vernacular Name: *Eng:* Smaller morning-glory.

Description: An annual herb. Stems and branches twining, terete, hairy. Leaves petiolate, cordate-ovate, 2-lobed, downy; 3-6 cm long apex acute, base cordate, peduncles axillary, hairy, from 2 to 3 flowered in summer. Bracts and sepals linear. Flowers large, of a beautiful light bright blue. Stigma subglobose, large, glandular, 3-lobed. The capsule is triocular, each loculus containing two seeds 6 mm long by 4 mm wide, triangular, smooth, black or light-brown.

Habitate: Commonly cultivated in China, India and other tropical and subtropical regions.

Propagation: By seeds and vegetative method.

Part Used: Smaller morning-glory.

Chemical Constituents: N.A.

Uses: Oedema ascitis due to liver cirrhosis, constipation, abdominal pain due to parastic infection.

951. *Phaseolus vulgaris* *(Fabaceae)*

Vernacular Name: *Eng:* French bean, Haricot bean.

Description: Slender-stemmed, annual climber growing to 4m. Has pointed oval leaflets, curly tendrils, clusters of white or lilac flowers and a beanpod containing kidney-shaped seeds.

Habitate: French beans are thought to have originated from South America.

Propagation: By seeds and vegetative method.

Parts Used: Beanpods, beans.

Chemical Constituents: French beans contain alllantoin, sugars, leucine, tyrosine, arginine and inositol.

Uses: In addition to being an important food in many parts of the world, French beans have two principal medicinal uses. The pods are a medium-strength diuretic, stimulating urine flow and the flushing of toxins from the body. Powdered or infused, they are also hypoglycaemic, reducing blood glucose levels in the treatment of diabetes. Powdered beans may be dusted on to eczema to ease itching and dry the skin.

952. *Phellodendron amurense* Rupr. *(Rutaceae)*

Vernacular Name: *Eng:* Amur cork-treel siberian cork-tree.

Description: A deciduous tree 10-15 m high, with grey, deeply fissured, corky bark. Leaves opposite, compound imparipinnate, reaching a length of 30 cm; leaflets 5-13, oval-lanceolate or nearly ovate, 5-11 cm long by 2-3.8 cm wide, tip acuminate, base broadly cuneate or rounded, margin obscurely serrate, the underside greyish-green, glabrous, inflorescence a some what contracted panicle 6-8 cm long, pubescent, flowers 1-sexual, dioecious,4 mm in diameter, yellowish-green. Fruit an oval drupe 1 cm in diameter becoming black when ripe and containing 5 seeds.

Habitate: Grows in mountainous districts in China, Japan, Korea and Soviet Union.

Propagation: By seeds and vegetative method.

Part Used: Bark.

Chemical Constituents: The trunk bark contains 0.6% berberine, palmatine, obakunone, obakulactone and sterols.

Uses: Genito-urinary tract infectin, diarrhoea, flaccidity and arthralgia, leucorrhoea, haemorrhoids, complicated by anal fistula. Inflammatory skin disease; sphthae; eczemal pustules; scalds and burns.

953. *Phoenix pusilla* Gaertn. *(Arecaceae)*

Synonyms: *Phoenix farinifera* Roxb.

Vernacular Name: *Eng*: Small wild date-palm, *Hin*: Palavat, *Kan*: Indu, Eechakeya, *Mal*: Cittintal, *San*: Parusakah, *Tam*: Siruintu, Cittintu, *Tel:* Cinna, Eechala.

Description: A shrubby stoloniferous palm with a very short stem enveloped in the sheaths of the leaves; leaves pinnate, rachis with one or more pairs of spines, leaflets subopposite, 4-farious, sword-shaped, rigid, pale grey with an orange-red pulvinus at the junction with the rachis; flowers in much branched spadix enclosed in spathes, male flowers white, female flowers greenish, not on the same plant; fruits berries, dull purple, black when ripe, seeds cartilaginous, grooved longitudinally with a small elevation on the middle of the back.

Habitate: In the dry forests of Kerala, Karnataka and *Tam*ilnadu at low elevations.

Propagation: By seeds and suckers.

Parts Used: Fruits.

Chemical Consistuents: Galactose, galacturonic acid.

Uses: The fruits are sweet, sour, cooling, laxative, cardiotonic, aphrodisiac, carminative and roborant. They are useful in vitiated conditions of *vata* and *pitta*, hyperdipsia, burning sensation, fever, consumption, cardiac debility, seminal weakness, gastropathy and general debility.

954. *Pholomis umbrosa* Turcz. *(Lamiaceae)*

Vernacular Name: *Eng*: Phlomis.

Description: Pubescent perennial herb up to 1 m tall. Some roots thickened to spindle shape. Leaves opposite, long-petiolate, suborbiculate to cordate, 13 cm long, 10 cm wide; the upper leaves smaller, pubescent beneath, margins crenate. Flowers in axillary verticillasters; calyx tubular 8 mm long, 5-toothed; corolla purple, 2-lipped; upper lip hooded; lower 3-lobed, spreading.

Habitate: Mountains and hills.

Propagation: By seeds and vegetative method.

Parts Used Root.

Chemical Constituents: Shanzhiside methylester, succinic acid, bentonicine, umbroside.

Uses: Antihepatotoxic. Uued in haemostatic and tineapedis.

955. *Phyla nodiflora* L. *(Verbenaceae)*

Synonyms: *Lippa nodiflora* (Linn.) A. Rich.

Vernacular Name: *Eng*: Purple lippia; *Hin*: Jalpapli; *Kan*: Nelahippali; *Mal*: Nirtippali; *San*: Jalapippali, Toyavallari; *Tam*: Potuttalai; *Tel:* Bokkena.

Description: A creeping much branched perennial herb rooting at the nodes and with subquadrangular stems and branches; leaves simple, opposite, subsessile, cuneate-spathulate or obovate, sharply serrate towards the apex; flowers white or pale pink, sessile, densely packed in axillary spikes, globose at first, afterwards elongating, peduncles usually single; fruits globose, oblong, dry, splitting into one-seeded pyrenes.

Habitate: Throughout India, upto 900 m in wet places along bunds of irrigation channels, canal edges and river banks.

Propagation: By seeds and vegetative method.

Parts Used: Whole plant.

Chemical Consistuents: N.A.

Uses: The plant is acrid, astringent, cooling, appetizing, stomachic, constipating, anthelmintic, digestive, vulnerary, aprhdisiac, aphrodisiac, ophthalmic, diuretic, alexeteric and febrifuge. It is useful in vitiated conditions of *pitta*, burning sensation, anorexia, flatulence, colic, dyspepsia, helminthiasis, diarrhoea, ulcers, ophthalmopathy, strangury, asthma, bronchitis, knee joint pain, gonorrhoea, irritation of internal haemorrhoids, cardiopathy, lymphadenitis, erysipelas and fever.

956. *Phyllanthus emblica* L. *(Euphorbiaceae)*

Synonyms: *Emblica officinalis* Gaertn.

Vernacular Name: *San*: Amalaki, Dhatri; *Eng*: Emblic myrobalan, Indian gooseberry; *Hin*: Amlika Amalak, Amvala; *Kan*: Nellka; *Mal*: Nellimaram, Nellikka; *Tam*: Nelli; *Tel:* Usirikaya, Amalakamu.

Description: A small to medium sized deciduous tree, 8-18 m in height with thin light grey bark exfoliating in small thin irregular flakes; leaves simple, very many, subsessile, closely set along the branchlets, distichous, light green having the appearance of pinnate leaves; flowers greenish yellow, in axillary fascicles, unisexual, males numerous on short slender pedicels, females few, subsessile, ovary 3-celled; fruits globose, fleshy, pale yellow with six obscure vertical furrows enclosing 6 trigonous seeds in 2-seeded 3 crustaceous cocci.

Habitate: Throughout India, in deciduous forests and on hill slopes upto 200 m, also cultivated in plains.

Propagation: By seeds and vegetative method.

Parts Used: Root bark, bark, leaves, fruits.

Chemical Consistuents: The major amino acids present are; alanine, aspartic acid, glutamic acid, lysine, and proline, analysis of fresh fruit pulp gave moisture, protein, fat carbohydrates fibre, minerals, iron, niacin, and vitamin fruit ash contains; chromium and copper.

Uses: The root bark is astringent, and is useful in ulcerative stomatitis and gastrohelcosis. The bark is useful in gonorrhoea, jaundice, diarrhoea and myalgia. The leaves are useful in conjunctivitis, inflammation, dyspepsia, diarrhoea and dysentery. The fruits are sour, astringent, bitter, acrid, sweet, cooling, anodyne, ophthalmic, carminative, digestive, stomachic, laxative, alterant, alexeteric, aphrodisiac, diuretic, antipyretic, tonic and trichogenous. They are useful in vitiated conditions of tridosa; diabetes, cough, asthma, bronchitis, cephalalgia, ophthalmopathy, dyspepsia, colic, flatulence, hyperacidity, peptic ulcer, erysipelas, skin diseases, leprosy, haematemesis, inflammations, anaemia, emaciation, hepatopathy, jaundice, strangury, diarrhoea, dysentery, haemorrhages, leucorrhoea, menorrhagia, cardiac disorders, intermittent fevers and greyness of hair.

957. *Phyllanthus niruri* L. *(Euphorbiaceae)*

Vernacular Name: *San*: Bahupatra; *Hin:* Bhuiamla.

Description: The annual herb, is 30-60 cm high, quite glabrous, *stem* often branched at the base, angular. *Leaves* numerous, subsessile distichous often imbricating, elliptic oblong obtuse. Stipules present, very acute. *Flowers* yellowish, very numerous, axillary, the male flowers 1-3, female flowers solitary. *Capsules* 2.5 mm diameter depressed globose, smooth scarcely lobed.

Habitate: Common in Central and Southern India extending to Sri Lanka.

Propagation: By seeds and vegetative method.

Parts Used: Whole plant.

Chemical Constituents: In the aerial part, three crystalline lignans including phyllanthine and hypophyllanthine have been found. Five flavonoids have been identified, quercetin, astralgin, quercitrin, isoquercitrin and rutin. Four leucodelphinidine alkaloids were separated from the leaves and stems, one of them being an enantiomorph of securinine.

Uses: Viral hepatitis. Oedema. Anorexia. The fresh root is used for the treatment of viral hepatitis. The plant is also used as a diuretic in oedema. It is also used to increase appetite and locally to relieve inflammations.

958. *Phyllanthus reticulates* Poir. *(Euphorbiaceae)*

Synonyms: *Kirganelia reticulata* (Poir.) Ball.

Vernacular Name: *Hin*: Pancoli, Makhi; *Kan*: Pulaveri, Puttae; *Mal*: Niruri, Niroli; *San*: Pulika, Krsnakamboji; *Tam*: Karinelli, Kattukilanelli; *Tel:* Pulaguvva.

Description: A large glabrous or pubescent subscandent shrub, 1.5-4.5 m in height with smooth or lenticellate branches; leaves elliptic to oblong or obovate, obtuse or acute, thin, main nerves few; flowers unisexual, axillary, male in fascicles of 2-6, female solitary; fruit a purplish black berry, globose, smooth and shining, seeds irregularly 3-gonous, finely granulate.

Habitate: Throughout India, in hedges or waste places near villages and in thickets along streams and canals.

Propagation: By seeds and vegetative method.

Parts Used: Whole plant.

Chemical Consistuents: Tannic acid.

Uses: The plant is astringent, sweet, cooling, diuretic, alterant, stomachic, constipating and attenuant. It is useful in vitiated conditions of *pitta*, burning sensation, strangury, gastropathy, ulemorrhagia, ophthalmodynia, sores, burns, suppuration, diarrhoea, skin eruptions and obesity. Used in bleeding gums, smallpox, asthama and syphilis.

959. *Phyllanthus urinaria* L. *(Euphorbiaceae)*

Vernacular Name: *Hin:* Lal-bhuin anvalah, hazar mani; *Beng*: Hazar mani; *Tel:* Erra uririka; *Tam:* Shivappu keela melli; *Kan:* Kempu nela nelli; *Mal:* Chirukizhuka nelli, chuvannakizha nelli.

Description: Diffuse annual or perennial herb, 20-30cm.high.stems glabrous, usually purplish. Leaves alternate, very short-petioled, prominently arranged in two rows, resembling a pinnate leaf. Flowers minute, yellowish, unisexual, solitary in the axils; both sexes on the same plant. Capsule without stalk, globose, slightly compressed, echinate.

Habitate: Common weed everywhere.

Propagation: By seeds and vegetative method.

Part Used: Whole plant.

Chemical Constituents: The whole plant contains bitter substances, alkaloids.

Uses: The whole plant, which possesses antibacterial and demulcent properties, is useful in the treatment of sore throat, boils, especially on the chin, impetigo, infantile cheek eczema, tongue thrush, arthralgia, snake and centipede bites, post-partum haematometra, feber, opthalmia and hepato-biliary diseases.

960. *Physalis alkekengi* *(Solanaceae)*

Synonyms*:* *Physalis franchetti.*

Vernacular Name: *Eng:* Winter Cherry, Cape gooseberry.

Description: Perennailherb growing to 80 cm. Has oval-to diamond-shaped leaves, long-stemmed white flowers and a transluscent papery sheath surrounding an orange-red fruit.

Habitate: Winter cherry is native to central and southern Europe and China.

Propagation: By seeds and vegetative method.

Parts Used: Fruit.

Chemical Constituents: Winter cherry contains flavonoids, plant sterols, vitamins A and C, and in the roots, tropane-type alkaloids.

Uses: Though commonly eastern as a fruit, winter cherry is also a useful diuretic. The fruit is traditionally used within European herbal medicine to treat kidney and bladder stones, fluid retention and gout. It has also been taken to reduce fever.

961. *Physalis angulata* L. *(Solanaceae)*

Vernacular Name: *Eng:* cape gooseberry; wild tomato.

Description: Annual heary herb upto 1 m high with hollow stems. Leaves alternate, petiolate, ovate to oblong-lanceolate, the blade 5-10 cm long and 2-8 cm broad, with irregular sparsely-toothed margins, with rounded base and an acuminate apex. Flowers pale yellow or whitish, 5-parted, about 3 cm broad, solitary and pedicilate in leaf axils. Fruit a green to yellowish globose berry up to 12 mm broad with numerous small seeds.

Habitate: Common weed of waste, places, roadsides, gardens, villages, agricultural fields, secondary forest margins, plantations. Also found on dry slope and along creeks.

Propagation: By seeds and vegetative method.

Part Used: Whole plant.

Chemical Constituents: Vitasteroids, selenium, zinc, copper and steroidal lactones, acetylcholine, glcoalkaloids, ayanin (flavonoid), 14-alpha hydroxyixocarpanolide, phygrine, phenyl propanoids, vitanolides, physagulide, physagulins, physalins, funiferine, beta-sitosterol, vamonolide, withanolides.

Uses: Anti-inflammatory, antibacterial, antitumour, cytotoxic, hypontensive, antibody enhancement, protein synthesis inhibition, anticoagulant, antiviral, lymphocyte, blastogenesis stimulant, immunosuppressant. To facilitate childbirth to treat infertility in women and dengue fever.

962. *Physalis minima* L. *(Solanaceae)*

Vernacular Name: *Eng*: Country gooseberry, *Hin*: Bandhapariya, Cirpoti, Tulati pati, *Kan*: Guddehannu, *Mal*: Nottanotiyan, Notinotta, *San*: Mrdukuncika, Cirapotha, *Tam*: Tottakkali, *Tel:* Kuppante.

Description: A herbaceous annual 15-30 cm in height; leaves simple, alternate, ovate, shallowly toothed or lobed, more or less pubescent; flowers yellow, solitary, nodding, fruits green, many seeded round berry, enclosed in enlarged calyx which is 5-10 ribbed, seeds many, discoid, orange yellow.

Habitate: Throughout India, upto 2,300 m as a weed on cultivated land.

Propagation: By seeds and vegetative method.

Parts Used: Whole plant.

Chemical Consistuents: Alkaloids.

Uses: The plant is bitter, sweet, cooling, diuetic laxative, expectorant, appetizing and tonic. It is useful in vitiated conditions of *pitta*, burning sensation, strangury, splenomegaly, ascites, gastropathy, colic, ulcers, cough, bronchitis, pruritus and erysipelas.

963. *Phytolacca acinosa* Roxb. *(Phytolaccaceae)*

Synonyms: *Phytolacca Americana* L.

Vernacular Name: *Eng:* Indian pokeweed; *Hin:* Matazor, sarangum.

Description: A perennial herb, up to 1.5 m high. Root robust, cylindrical, fleshy, yellowish on the outside with many long transverse lenticels. Stem erect, slightly ligneous at the vase, green or purplish. The whole plant is glabrous. Leaves alternate, elliptic or elliptic-ovate, 12-15 cm long by 5-8 cm wide; apex acuminate; margin entire; base narrowed into the stout petiole. Inflorescence a briefly pedunculate raceme. Greenish white flowers in terminal or axial spikes. Calyx with 5 nearly regular lobes, corolla-like. Petals none. Stamens 8-10. Carples 8-10. The fruits are black and contain deep purple juice when they ripen in the autumn.

Habitate: In fields or cultivated in China, Japan and India.

Propagation: By seeds and vegetative method.

Part Used: Roots.

Chemical Constituents: Unsaturated acids, Phytolacca toxin, Picro toxin,.

Uses: Oedema, ascites, difficulty in micturition, erosion of the cervix uteri, malignant boils. Tender leaves and twings cooked as a vegetable. Herb has narcotic effect, but it is destroyed on boiling. Fruit occasionally used as a flavouring. It is not uncommon for the local people to mistake *Atropa acuminate* Royle for *P. acinosa*, resulting in serious food poisoning; for the same reason roots and leaves of *P. acinosa* have been found mixed in belladonna consignments exported from India. Seeds yield a fatty oil.

964. *Phytolacca americana* L. *(Phytolaccaceae)*

Synonyms: *Phytolacca decandra* Linn., *Phytolacca vulgaris* Crantz.

Vernacular Name: *Eng:* American night shade.

Description: A strong smelling herb, 1-4m. in height. Leaves oblong or ovate-lanceolate, 10-30 cm. long; acute, or acuminate. Flowers small, about 2.5 cm. across; in peduncled racemes, 5-20 cm. long which are nodding in fruits; pedicels bracted at bae; stamens many in 2 series; ovary subglobose; fruit a fleshy berry, dark purple, about 12 mm. across, containing 10 fruitlets, each containing a black shining, oval flattened seed.

Habitate: U.S.A., Canada.

Propagation: By Rhizomes.

Parts Used: Roots.

Chemical Constituents: Betanidine, Betanine, Isobetanine; isobetanidine, Isoprebetanine, Phytolaccine; Prebetanine. Phytolaccosides A-1, D2 & O; Phytolaccagenin, Jaligonic acid, phytolaccagenic acid, Aesculentic acid and Acinosilic acid methyl ester.

Uses: For complaints mainly aching, soreness, associated with restlessness & prostration due to glandular affections. Glandular swellings with heat & inflammation. Sore throat, quinsy & diphtheria in eyes. Fistula lachrymalis of eyes. Throat dark red or bluish red, with roughness & soreness in throat, tonsils, especially rightside tonsils swollen aching with pin shooting into ears on swallowing. Ulva large, dropsical. Tonsils & fauces swollen with burning pain and therefore cannot swallow even water. Follicular mumps. Throat complaints associated with heat. Shooting pain in right shoulder causing stiffness, with pain flying like electric shock, laciniating & shifting. In females mastitis. Mammae hard & very sensitive. Nipples cracked, ulcerated & sensitive. Right side ovarion neuralgia.

965. *Phytolacca decandra* *(Phytolaccaceae)*

Vernacular Name: *Eng:* Poke root.

Description: Herbaceous perennial growing up to 3m. Has alternate lance-shaped leaves, spikes of greenish-white flower and clusters of fleshy, purple berries.

Habitate: Native to North America, and now naturalized in the Mediterranean region.

Propagation: By seeds and vegetative method.

Parts Used: Root.

Chemical Constituents: Poke root contains triterpenoid saponins, lectins, proteins, resin and mucilage. The triterpenoid saponins are strongly anti-inflammatory, the proteins are antiviral and the lectins are mitogenic.

Uses: Poke root is taken internally as a tincture in small amounts to treat rheumatic and arthritic conditions. The root has also been used to treat respiratory tract infections, such as sore throats and tonsillitis, as well as swollen glands and chronic infections. The herb is sometimes prescribed for pain and infection of the ovaries or testes, and as a lymphatic "decongestant", stimulating the clearance of waste products. As a poultice or ointment, it is applied to sore and infected nipples and breasts, acne, folliculitis, fungal infections and scabies.

966. *Phytolacca esculenta* Van Houtte *(Phytolaccaceae)*

Vernacular Name: *Eng*: Pokeweed, pokeberry.

Description: Perennial herb, to 1 m tall, slightly woody at base. Leaves margins entire; petioles 1.5-2.5 cm long. Inflorescence racemes, 10-12 cm long. Flowers small, bisexual, white; sepals 5, ovate, obtuse; petals none; stamens 8, anther pale pink; carpels 8; style 1, curved outwards. Fruit a depressed-globose berry; each carpel 1-seeded.

Habitate: Abandoned or open fields near residences.

Parts Used: Root.

Propagation: By seeds and vegetative method.

Chemical Constituents: Saponions; many oleanane-derived phytolaccosides, 3-acetylmyricadiol.

Uses: Anti-inflammatory, hypotensive, purgative, diuretic, toxic (convulsive) activities. Used in oedema, beri-beri, tineapedis, lumbago and rheumatism.

967. *Picrasma excelsa* *(Simaroubaceae)*

Synonyms: *Picraenia excelsa.*

Vernacular Name: *Eng:* Quassia.

Description: Deciduous tree growing to 30m. Has smooth grey bark, compound leaves, small yellow flowers and pea-sized black fruit.

Habitate: Native to tropical America and the Caribbean, quassia grows in forests and near water.

Propagation: By seeds and vegetative method.

Parts Used: Bark.

Chemical Constituents: Quassia contains quassinoid bitter principles, alkaloids, a coumrin and vitamin B^1. Some of the quassinoids have been shown to have cytotoxic and anti-leukaemic actions.

Uses: The strongly bitter quassia supports and strengthens weak digestive systems. It increases bile flow, the secretion of salivary juices and stomach acid, and improves the digestive process as a whole. Quassia is commonly used to stimulate the appetite, especially in the treatment of anorexia. Its bitterness has led to its being used for malaria and other fevers, and it is given in the Caribbean for dysentery. The bark has been used in the form of an enema to expel threadworms and other parasites.

968. *Picrorhiza kurroa* Pennell *(Scrophulariaceae)*

Synonyms: *Picrorhiza scrophulariiflora* auct. Non Royle.

Vernacular Name: *Eng*: Picrorhiza; *Hin*: Katuka, Kuru, Kutki; *Kan*: Katukarohini; *Mal*: Katukurohini, Katurohini; *San*: Katvi, Katurohini, Katuka; *Tam*: Katugurohini; *Tel:* Katki.

Description: A small nearly hairy perennial herb with a woody elongate creeping root stock; leaves spathulate, serrate; flowers white or bluish in dense terminal spicate raceme; fruits ovoid capsules.

Habitate: In the Himalayas, from Kashmir to Sikkim at an elevation of 2,700-4,500m.

Propagation: By Rhizomes.

Parts Used: Dried rhizomes.

Chemical Consistuents: Glucosidal bitter principle named kutkin, non-bitter product named kurrin and later identified as D-mannitol, vanillic acid, alcohol kutkiol, sterol kutki-sterol.

Uses: The rhizomes are bitter, acrid, cooling, laxative, carminative, digestive, stomachic, anthelmintic, anti-inflammatory, depurative, cardiotonic, galactopurifier, expectorant, antipyreticand antiperiodic, and purgativein large doses. They are useful in vitiated conditions of *kapha* and *pitta*, burning sensation, constipation. Gastropathy, flatulence, colic, anorexia, verminosis, inflammations, leucoderma, leprosy, skin diseases, cardiac disorders, hypotension, cough, asthma, bronchitis, hiccough, fever, bilious fever, intermittent fever, diabetes, jaundice, haemorrhoids, impurity of breast milk and general debility.

969. Pimenta dioica (L.) Merril *(Myrtaceae)*

Synonyms: *Pimenta officinalis.*

Vernacular Name: *Eng:* Jamaiaca pepper tree, pimento tree.

Description: A bushy, evergreen tree; leaves oblong to oblong lanceolate, leathery; flowers white in trichotomous, paniculate cymes; berries black or purple, globose, 2-seeded.

Habitate: Grown in gardens, throughout in India.

Propagation: By seeds and vegetative method.

Part Used: Fruits, leaves.

Chemical Constituents: Eugenol is the principal consituent of the berry oil, besides methyl eugenol, limonene, b-caryophyllene, 1-8-cineole, a-phelandrene, terpinolene, b-selinene, a-humulene, and p-cymene. The leaf oil contains mainly eugenol, b-caryophyllene, 1,8-cineole, a-humulene, and caryophyllene oxide.

Uses: Allspice berries are dried and used whole or grounds as a flavouring in ketchiups, soups, sauces, pickles, canned meat, fish, poultry, etc. fast foods like hamburgers, sausages, grankfurters, and in the liqueur industry particularly in mulled wines. Pimenta berry oil replaces the ground spice to great advantage. Pimenta leaf oil is slightly inferior to bery oil and is used to flavour meat products and confectionery. Besides, an oleoresin prepared from pimenta berries with a flavour superior to that of the oil, is used in spice blends for the canning and meat processing industry.

970. *Pimenta officinalis* *(Myrtaceae)*

Vernacular Name: *Eng:* Allspice.

Description: Aromatic evergreen tree growing up to 12m. Has leathery oblong leaves, clusters of small white flowers and tiny green berries that turn brown as they become ripe.

Habitate: Allspice is native to the Caribbean and to Central and South America, and is extensively cultivated in Jamaica and other parts of the region.

Propagation: By seeds and vegetative method.

Parts Used: Berries, essential oil.

Chemical Constituents: Allspice contains about 4% volatile oil, proteins, lipids, the vitamins A, C B^1 and B^2, and minerals.

Uses: A digestive stimulant, allspice is taken to relieve flatulence and indigestion. It may also be used to treat diarrhoea. Allspice is often combined with herbs that have a tonic or laxative effect. The herb has an action that is similar to that of cloves; both are stimulant, stomach-settling and antiseptic. Allspice essential oil is also stomach-settling.

971. *Pimpinella anisum* *(Apiaceae)*

Vernacular Name: *Eng:* Anise; *Hin*: Saunf, sawolf, badian; *Beng*: Muhuri, mitha-jira; *Guj*: Anisa; *Tel:* Kuppi, sopu; *Tam*: Shomba; *Kan*: Shomba.

Description: An annual herb, 30-60 cm high, leaves pinnatifid or ternately pinnate, flowers small, white in compound umbels; fruit avoid or pyriform, laterally compressed, broad, greyish green to greyish brown; mericarp broadly ovoid, 5 ridged with short hairs and numerous vittae.

Habitate: Anise is native to the eastern Mediterranean, western Asia and North Africa.

Propagation: By seeds and vegetative method.

Parts Used: Seeds.

Chemical Constituents: Anise contains a volatile oil, furanocoumarins, flavonoids, fatty acids, phenylpropanoids, sterols and proteins. Anethole has an observed oestrogenic effect, and the seeds as a whole are mildly oestrogenic. The effect any substantiate the herb's use as a stimulant of sexual drive and of breast-milk production.

Uses: Anise seeds are known for their ability to reduce wind and bloating, and to settle the digestion. They are commonly given to infants and children to relieve colic, and to people of all ages to ease nausea and indigestion. Anise seeds' antispasmodic properties make them helpful in countering period pain, asthma, whooping cough and bronchitis. The seeds' expectorant action justifies their use for these respiratory ailments. Anise seeds are thought to increase breast-milk production and may be beneficial in treating impotence and frigidity. Anise essential oil is used for similar complaints, and is also used externally to treat lice and scabies.

972. *Pinellia pedatisecta* schott. *(Araceae)*

Vernacular Name: *Eng:* Pedatisect pinellia.

Description: A perennial herb, with a strong pungent taste. The tuber has 1-4 leaves on the top and the small tubes on the sides look like a tiger's pad in shape and grow up to 4 cm in diameter. The pedatisect segments, from 6 to 11 in number are lanceolate, acuminate, the one in the middle being the largest, 15-18 cm long by about 3 cm wide. The spadix is composed of a peduncle, greenish, 15-50 cm long; a spathe which has a tube 2-4 cm long and 1-1.5 cm in diameter and a lamina 8-15 cm long, lanceolate and acuminate; female and male flowers on the axis, with an appendix about 10 cm long. The berry in the spathe is ovoid, about 1 mm in diameter.

Habitate: On damp, shady slopes and under trees in China, Japan and Korea.

Propagation: By seeds and vegetative method.

Part Used: Tubers.

Chemical Constituents: N.A.

Uses: Apoplexy, infantile convulsions; tetanus, Rheumatic disease, swelling, snake bite.

973. *Pinellia ternate* (Thunb.) Breitenb. *(Araceae)*

Vernacular Name: *Eng*: Three-leaf pinellia.

Description: Perennial herb with corm. Corm 1 cm in diameter. Leaves 1-2, directly from the corm, ternate; petiole 10-20 cm long, with bulbils borne on the petiole; leaflets 3, sessile, entire, 3-12 cm long, 1-5 cm wide, ovate-elliptical to oblong, glabrous. Scape olitary, 20-40 cm long; spathe green, 6-7 cm long; the tubular part 1.5-2 cm long; the blade lanceolate, rounded at apex, puberulent inside; spadix with appendage filiform, erect, 6-10 cm long. Fruit berry, small, green.

Habitate: Common in cultivated fields and roadsides Korea, China and Japan.

Propagation: By seeds and vegetative method.

Parts Used: Corm.

Chemical Constituents: Amino acids, polysaccharides, homogentisic acid, ephedrine, 3,4-dihydroxybenzaldehyde-diglucoside, pinellin (low molecular weight crystalline protein), phytosterols.

Uses: Anti-emetic, sedative, antitussive, expectorant activities by boiled extract, emetic action by unprocessed extract. Mitogenic, haemagglutinating activities by pinellin. Aldose reductase inhibition. Used in vomiting damp and phlegm.

974. *Pinguicula vulgaris* *(Lentibulariaceae)*

Vernacular Name: *Eng:* Butterwrot.

Description: Insectivorous perennial growing to 10 cm. has fleshy leaves in a basal rosette and double-lipped, purple-blue flowers.

Habitate: Native to northern and western Europe, butterwort grows in moorland and on mountains.

Propagation: By seeds and vegetative method.

Parts Used: Leaves.

Chemical Constituents: Butterwort contains mucilage, tannins, benzoic acid, cinnamic acid and valeric acid. Cinnamic acid has antispasmodic properties.

Uses: Butterwort is little employed in European herbal medicine today. Its main use is as a cough remedy, with properties similar to those of sundew, another insect-eating plant. Butterwort may be used to treat chronic and convulsive coughs.

975. *Pinus koraiensis* Siebold et Zucc. *(Pinaceae)*

Vernacular Name: *Eng*: Korean pine.

Description: Tall, coniferous, evergreen, monoecious tree, up to 30 m tall or more. Branchlets yellow-brown-tomentose. Leaves of two kinds; the scalelike ones soon dediduous; the needle-shaped ones long, in fascicles of 5, to 10 cm long, dark green. *Mal*e cones catkinlike, clustered. Female cones conic-oblong, to 15 cm long; scales woody, persistent, thickened at the end, with a terminal projection; seeds 2 to each scale, without wing.

Habitate: Mountain woods at high elevation Japan, Korea and China.

Propagation: By seeds and vegetative method.

Parts Used: Seed.

Chemical Constituents: Oleic acid ester, linoleic acid ester, essential oil, various monoterpene, sesquiterpene and diterpene derivatives.

Uses: Inhibition of TXB2 formation (piceid), hypolipidaemic (piceid) , analgesic, anti-inflammatory, antibacterial. Used in tonic, earache, galactagogue and epistaxis.

976. *Pinus roxburghii* Sarg. *(Pinaceae)*

Synonyms: *Pinus longifolia* Roxb.

Vernacular Name: *Eng*: Chir pine,Himalayan long-leaved pine, Three-leaved pine, *Hin*: Cid, Cil, Sarala, *Kan*: Sarala, *Mal*: Caralam, Saralam, *San*: Saralah, *Tam*: Caraladevataru, *Tel:* Sarala.

Description: A tall coniferous tree with whorled branches and dark grey or reddish deeply fissured, rough, exfoliating bark; leaves in bundles of three, 20-30 cm long, triquetrous, bright green, each bundle surrounded at base by a persistent sheath; male cones about 13 mm long, ripe female cones 10-20cm long on short stiff stalks; seeds winged, wings membranous.

Habitate: Throughout the Himalayas from Kashmir to Bhutan, Siwalik hills, Ooty, Kodaikanal at altitudes of 450-2,400 m.

Propagation: By seeds and vegetative method.

Parts Used: Wood, oleoresin, oil.

Chemical Consistuents: α-pinene, β-pinene, careen and longifolene and other terpenes. The presence of β-carene, β-longifolene and longicyclene has also been reported.

Uses: The wood is acrid, bitter, sweet, thermogenic, emollient, aromatic antiseptic, deodrant, haemostatic, stimulant, anthelmintic, digestive, liver tonic, diaphoretic, rubefacient and diuretic. It is useful in ophthalmopathy, otopathy, pharyngopathy, vitiated conditions of *vata*, halitosis, foul ulcers, haemorrhages, haemoptysis, helminthiasis, dyspepsia,flatulence, hepatopathy, strangury, bronchitis, inflammations, skin diseases,pruritus and giddiness. The oleoresin is acrid, bitter, thermogenic, expectorant, anodyne, anti-inflammatory, purgative and demulcent. It is useful in vitiated conditions of *vata*, asthma,chronic bronchitis, otalgia,odontalgia,inflammations, hepatopathy, splenopathy, urethrorrhea, gonorrhoea, scabies, epilepsy, lumbago, haemorrhoids and tuberculous glands.

977. *Pinus sylvestris* *(Pinaceae)*

Vernacular Name: *Eng:* Scots pine.

Description: Coniferous tree growing up to 30m. Has reddish-brown bark, pairs of fine, needle-like leaves, yellowish buds in winter and oval to conical cones.

Habitate: Native to mountainous regions of Europe and north and west Asia.

Propagation: By seeds and vegetative method.

Parts Used: Leaves, Branches, Stems, Seeds, essential oil.

Chemical Constituents: The leaves of Scots pine contain a volatile oil.

Uses: Scots pine leaves, taken internally, have a mildly antiseptic effect within the chest, and may also be used for arthritic and rheumatic problems. Essential oil from the leaves may be taken for asthma, bronchitis and other respiratory infections, and for digestive disorders such as wind. Scots pine branches and stems yield a thick resin, which is also antiseptic within the respiratory tract. The seeds yield an essential oil with diuretic and respiratory-stimulant properties. The seeds are used for bronchitis, tuberculosis and bladder infections.

978. *Piper angustifolia* *(Piperaceae)*

Vernacular Name: *Eng:* Matico.

Description: Perennial shrub reaching 3m. Has deeply veined aromatic lance-shaped leaves, spikes of tiny yellow flowers and small black fruit.

Habitate: It is native to mountainous regions of Bolivia, Peru and Ecuador. It is found in the wild and is widely cultivated in these and other countries in tropical South America.

Propagation: By vegetative methods.

Parts Used: Leaves.

Chemical Constituents: Matico contains a volatile oil, tannins, mucilage and resins.

Uses: Matico is an aromatic stimulant, diuretic and astringent used extensively for gastric and intestinal problems including peptic ulcers, diarrhoea and dysentery. It is commonly used in South American herbal medicine for internal bleeding, particularly within the digestive tract-for example, rectal bleeding and haemorrhoids. It is also taken for bleeding in the urinary tract. Applied externally.

979. *Piper betle* L. *(Piperaceae)*

Vernacular Name: *San:* Nagavalli, tambula; *Eng:* Betel leaf vine, betel leaf pepper, betel pepper; *Hin:* Pan, tambuli; *Beng*: Pan; *Tel:* Tamalapaku, nagavalli; *Tam:* Vettilai; *Kan:* Villayadele and *Mal:* Vettila.

Description: A slender creeper with adventitious roots. Setms glabrous, sulcate, thickened at the nodes, Leaves alternate, heart-shaped, palmately nerved, glabrous and shining on both sides. Inflorescence in drooping, dense axillary spike, consisting of male and female flowers Berry globose, hairy at the apex (rarely produced). All parts of the plant have a special aroma.

Habitate: Cultivated in many areas, especially in the south India.

Propagation: By seeds and vegetative method.

Part Used: Leaves and roots.

Chemical Constituents: The whole plant yields and essential oil containing eugenol, carvacrol, chavicol, allyl catechol, chavibetol, cineol, estragole, methyl eugenol, p-cymene, caryophyllene and cadinene; tannins; sugars; carotene, thiamine, riboflavin, nicotinic acid, vitamin C and amino acids.

Uses: The leaves possess antibacterial properties and are beneficial in the treatment of purulent parodontosis in the form of a collutory made of the juice or extract. A poultice of the leaves and a wash with the decoction are used in treating wounds, burns, impetigo, furunculosis, eczema and lymphangitis. The leaves if topically applied to the chest cure cough and asthma, and if applied to the breast arrest lactation. Frection of the spinal column with the leaves in recommended for treating colds. The roots are used in treating rheumatism.

980. *Piper brachystachyum* Wall. *(Piperaceae)*

Synonyms: *Chavica sphaerostachya* Miq.

Vernacular Name: *Eng*: Wild pepper, *Hin*: Cab, *Kan*: Cavya, *Mal*: Kattumulaku, Kattukurumulaku, *San*: Cavyah, *Tam*: Kattumilagu, *Tel:* Caikama, Sevasu.

Description: A much branched woody climber trailing up the branches of trees and rocks rooting like ivy; leaves elliptic-ovate or lanceolate; obtusely caudate-acuminate, acute at base, 3-5 ribbed with another pair a little higher up, shortly petioled; fruiting spikes globose, male spikes very slender 5-7.5 cm long; fruits small ovoid or globose 1-seeded berries, seeds globose.

Habitate: In the Western Ghats, Nilgiris, Anamalais, Pulneys and hills of southern Kerala, in Shola forests above 1,500 m.

Propagation: By vegetative methods.

Parts Used: Roots.

Chemical Consistuents: N.A.

Uses: The roots have the same properties as that of Piper longum roots. The roots are bitter, acrid, alexeteric, thermogenic, aromatic, appetizing, digestive, carminative, anthelmintic, expectorant and stomachic. They are useful in asthma, bronchitis, dyspepsia, anorexia and vitiated conditions of *kapha* and *pitta*.

981. *Piper cubeba* L.f. *(Piperaceae)*

Vernacular Name: *Eng*: Cubebs, Tailed pepper, Tailed cubebs, Java pepper; *Hin*: Kababcini; *Kan*: Gandhamenasu; *Mal*: Valmulaku; *San*: *Kan*kolam; *Tam*: Valmilagu; *Tel:* Calavamiriyalu, Tokamiriyalu.

Description: A perennial woody climber with ash grey climbing stems and branches, rooted at the joints; leaves simple, ovate-oblong, smooth, base cordate or rounded, tip pointed, lower surface densely provided with minute sunken glands; flowers small, unisexual, in smooth scaly spikes, female spikes often curved; fruits subglobose berries, stalked, somewhat apiculate.

Habitate: Native of Indonesia, cultivated in Karnataka.

Propagation: By vegetative methods.

Parts Used: Dried unripe berries.

Chemical Consistuents: Including cubebin having a bitter taste, cubebol and cubebic acid. The therapeutic value of the drug is said to be largely due to cubebic acid.

Uses: The berries are acrid, bitter, thermogenic, aromatic, stimulant, anodyne, dentifrice, anti-inflammatory, anthelmintic, deobstruant, vulnerary, appetizing, carminative, digestive, stomachic, cardiotonic, expectorant, rejuvenating, emmenagogue, diuretic, sedative and antiseptic. They are useful in somatalgia, odontalgia, cephalalgia, halitosis,inflammation, helminthiasis, wounds and ulcers, catarrh, anorexia, dyspepsia, flatulence, haemorrhoids, cardiac debility, cough, asthma, bronchitis, amenorrhoea, dysmenorrhoea, strangury, genito-urinary diseases like gonorrhoea, cystitis and gleet, rheumatism and hay fever.

982. *Piper lolot* C. DC. *(Piperaceae)*

Vernacular Name: *Eng:* Lolot pepper.

Description: Perennial creeper. Stems swollen at the nodes, downy while young, 30-40 cm. High. Leaves alternate, broadly cordate, amplexically petioled, glabrous above, downy on the nerves benethl margins wavy. Inflorescence in erect axillary spike of unisexual flowes. Berry single-seeded.

Habitate: Found wild in damp forests, along stream banks.

Propagation: By seeds and vegetative method.

Part Used: Whole plant.

Chemical Constituents: The whole plant contains an essential oil.

Uses: The entire plant possesses anti-inflammatory and anodyne properties. It is utilized in the treatment of rheumatism, Ostealgia, lumbago, headache, paresis, hypehidrosis of the extremities, dyspepsia, vomiting, flatulence, colic, diarrhoea, toothache, chronic catarrhal rhinitis and oedema. It is used in combination with other plants for treating mushroom poisoning and snake-bite. It is administered perlingually for toothache.

983. *Piper longum* L. *(Piperaceae)*

Vernacular Name: *Eng*: Idnian Long Papper; *Hin*: Pipli; *Kan*: Hippali; *Mal*: Thippali; *Mar*: Pimpli; *San*: Pippali, Kana; *Tam*: Thippili; *Tel:* Pippallu.

Description: A slender sub-scandent herb, branchlets erect, straggling or sometimes climbing, hairless, with swollen nodes and those of creeping branches with roots at lower nodes. *Leaves* alternate, variable in shape, usually egg-shaped-heart-shaped, 7-15 x 4-6 cm, base heart-shaped and unequal, apex acute to acuminate, margin entire, hairless, lower leaves with long stalks and upper ones without stalk; lateral nerves 5-7 arising from the base. *Male spikes* erect, 2-7 cm long, greenish yellow, fleshy, cylindrical, with minute male flowers. *Female spikes* erect, 1-3 cm long, yellow. Fruiting spikes cylindrically oblong, about 4 x 1 cm. Berries globose, about 2 mm across, partly sunken in the rachis, compactly arranged, red turning black when ripe.

Habitate: Moist deciduous to evergreen forests.

Propagation: By seeds and vegetative methods.

Parts Used: Fruits and roots.

Chemical Constituents: *n*-hexadecane, *n*-heptade-cane, *n*-octadecane, *n*-nonadecane, *n*-eicosane, *n*-heneicosane, α-thujene, terpinolene, zingiberene, *p*-cymene, *p*-methoxy acetophenone, trace; dihydrocarveol, phenethyl alcohol and new monocyclic sesquiterpenes piperine piplartine traces of a yellow crystalline pungent alkaloid triacontane dihydrostigmasterol and unidentified steroid reducing sugars and glycosides. Tow new alkaloids, named piperlongumine and piperlonguminine.

Uses: Roots and fruiting spikes are used in treating diarrhoea, indigestion, jaundice, urticaria, abdominal disorders, hoarseness of voice, asthma, hiccough, cough, piles, malarial fever, flatulence, vomiting, thirst, oedema, earache, wheezing, chest conjestion, throat infections, worms and sinusitis. This is one of the ingredients in the Siddha medicine '*trikadugu*'. Also considered a rejuvenating plant.

984. *Piper methysticum* Forster f. *(Piperaceae)*

Description: Woody aromatic shrub to 4 m high, often with green zig-zag stems bearing conspicuous enlarged nodes. Leaves alternate, petiolate, heart-shaped, up 30 cm long with palmate veins and cordate base. Flowers minute, borne in erect greenish-white spikes up to 6 cm long, each spike arising from an axil opposite a leaf. Fruit not known.

Habitate: Commonly cultivated in native gardens and damp areas such as near streams from enar sea-leel to 800 m elevation.

Propagation: By vegetative method.

Part Used: Whole plant.

Chemical Constituents: Several alpha-pyrone derivatives (e.g.kawain, yangonin, methysticin, dihydrokwain, dihydro-methysticin), flavokawains, alkaloids (pipermethysticine and epharadione A), campesterol, cholesterol, bets-sitosterol, stigmasterol.

Uses: Convulsions and stiffness in children are treated with liquid pressed from the leaves. The branches are used in remedy for sore throats. The black stem is used to prepare various medicines and the plant is also used in treating filariasis which is caused by interstinal parasites. The leaves are chewed as a treatment for bronchitis. The root bark scrapings are chewed to soothe sore throats and toothaches. The leaves are rubbed onto centipede bites, insects stings and stings from poisonous fish. An infusion of the leaves is spread onto a certain type of inflammation and is used to treat watery vaginal discharges. The plant was used to treat rheumatism, bronchitis and gonorrhoes. The shrub is used in treatments for stomachache, backache and inflammations.

985. *Piper mullesua* Buch.-Ham. ex D. Don *(Piperaceae)*

Synonyms: *Piper brachystachyum* Wall. ex Hook. f.

Vernacular Name: *Hin*: Cab, Pahari papal, Pahari pan; *Kan*: Cavya; *Mal*: Kattu kuru mulagu; *San*: Gaja pippali, Cavyah; *Tam*: Kattu thippilli; *Tel:* Sevasu.

Description: A much-branched woody climber, trailing on trees and rocks. Lower branchlets tomentose, corky, rooting at nodes and have white small egg-shaped leaves; upper branches have larger leaves. *Leaves* alternate, usually egg-shaped-elliptic to lanceolate, 3-10 x 2-4 cm, base acute, apex bluntly acuminate, margin entire, hairless, shortly stalked, 3-5 nerved from base. *Male* and female *flowers* in separate spikes, minute, greenish yellow. *Male spikes* 3-6 cm long, erect, slender and cylindrical. *Female spikes* globose-oblong, erect, about 1 x 0.5 cm. *Fruiting spikes* globose-ovoid, about 2 x 1 cm. *Berries* ovoid, about 2 mm across, smooth, green turning orange-red when ripe.

Habitate: Specific to higher altitudes of evergreen to shola forests.

Propagation: By stem cuttings, seeds, suckers and offshoots.

Parts Used: Roots & Fruits.

Chemical Constituents: N.A.

Uses: Roots and fruiting spikes are used in the Ayurvedic system of medicine similar to *Piper longum.*

986. *Piper nigrum* L. *(Piperaceae)*

Vernacular Name: *San:* Maricha, ushana, hapusha; *Eng:* Black pepper common pepper, white pepper; *Hin:* Kalimirch, kalamorich, golmorich; *Beng*: Kalimirch, kalamorich, golmorich; *Tel:* Miriyala tige; *Tam:* Milagu; *Kan:* Kare menasu and *Mal:* Kurumulaku, nallamulaku.

Description: Climbing perennial plant, stems glabrous, rooting at the nodes. Leaves alternate, coriaceous, rounded at the base; apex pointed; recurved nerves prominent beneath. Inflorescence in drooping spike of dioecious flowers, opposite to and shorter than the leaf. Berry globular, red when ripe, turning black after drying, 3-4 mm. In diameter, strongly scented and bitter to the taste.

Flowering period: May-August.

Habitate: Extensively cultivated in hotter and moist parts of India.

Propagation: By seeds and vegetative method.

Part Used: The fruit, picked when fully ripe, is dried in the sun or in ovens. After drying, the pericarp may be removed.

Chemical Constituents: The seeds contain alkaloids: piperine, piperetine, chavicine and an essential oil, consisting of terpene, phellandrene, caryophyllene, piperonal-dihydrocarbeol and caryophyllene oxide. The major components of the oil are sabinene, myrcene, limonene, α-and β-pinenes, caryophyllene, αbergamotene, α-humulene, *p*-cymene, and α-selinene.

Uses: The berries, well known for their stomachic, anodyne and antibacterial properties, are prescribed for treating dyspepsia, vomiting, diarrhoea and colic resulting from cold. The powdered berries, applied topically, cure toothache. They can also be used as an insecticide against clothes moths.

987. *Piper puberulum* Benth. ex Seemann *(Piperaceae)*

Description: Shrub to 4 m tall with soft wood. Leaves alternate, petiolate and subtended by conspicuous stipules, the blade ovate to cordate up to 20 cm long with palmate veins.

Flowers minute, unisexual borne in erect greenish-white spikes as long or longer than the leaves (up to 25 cm long). Fruiting spikes are aggregates of red fleshy druplets, each with a single small seed.

Habitate: Very common in disturbed forests, along streams, beach thickets, forest margins, plantations and waste areas from sea-level to over 1000 m elevation.

Propagation: By vegetative method.

Part Used: Whole plant.

Chemical Constituents: Piperine S, piperlactam S, neolignans (puberulins A, B, and C).

Uses: Liquid from the leaves is used to treat influenza. Convulsions in children are treated with a preparation made from the leaves and stems. Swelling of the testicles originating through a cold, and swollen breasts, especially after childbirth, are treated with the leaves of the plant, Juice of the leaves is used to treat toothache. The leaves are crushed with coconut oil to give a paste used to treat peeling skin and scabies. An infusion of the inner bark is drunk to treat inflammation. The leaves are pounded and applied to boils. A decoction of the leaves is taken as a tonic after childbirth and is also used to treat blood in the stool. An infustion of the bark is used to treat fever.

988. *Piscidia erythrina* *(Fabaceae)*

Vernacular Name: *Eng:* Jamaica Dogwood.

Description: Deciduous tree or shrub growing to 15m. Has compound leaves, blue to white flowers with red stripes, and winged seedpods.

Habitate: Jamaica dogwood is native to the southern US, Central America, northern South America and the Caribbean.

Propagation: By seeds and vegetative method.

Parts Used: Root bark.

Chemical Constituents: Jamaica dogwood contains isoflavones, organic acids, beta-sitosterol and tannins.

Uses: Jamaica dogwood is a useful and undervalued remedy that acts both as a sedative and as a painkiller. It is chiefly employed in the treatment of insomnia and overexcitability, as it calms mental activity. It is also prescribed for nerve pain, toothache and period pain. As an antispasmodic, it is useful for treating muscle spasms, especially in the back, and spasmodic respiratory ailments such as asthma and whooping cough.

989. *Pistacia integerrima* Stewart ex Brandis *(Anacardiaceae)*

Synonyms: *Pistacia chinensis* Bunge ssp. integerrima (Stewart) Rich.f.

Vernacular Name: *Hin*: Kakkatasimgi, Kakra; *Kan*: Karkatakasrngi; *Mal*: Karkkatakasrmgi, Karkkatasrmgi; *San*: Karkatasrngi, Karkata; *Tam*: Kakkatasrngi; *Tel:* Kakarasrnga.

Description: A moderate sized deciduous tree upto 18 m high with dark grey or blackish bark; leaves pinnately compound, leaflets lanceolate; flowers small, reddish in lateral panicles; fruits globose drupes, grey when ripe. Galls produced on the leaves are used commercially as *karkkatasrngi.* The galls are pale greenish brown or pinkish, elongate, horn-shaped, hollow, twisted, curved or straight. When young they are coriaceous, but later become hard. They persist for long periods on branches after the escape of the aphids. This gall is caused by the insect *Dasia aedifactor* (Homoptera).

Habitate: Himalayas, Garhwal, Kumaon, Bengal and Assam.

Propagation: By seeds and vegetative method.

Parts Used: Galls.

Chemical Consisuents: The galls contains tannins an essential oil, and a resin which is identical with gum mastic from *P. lentiscus*. The following compounds have been isolated from petroleum ether extract of the galls; two isomeric triterpenic acids designated pistacienoic acid B a triterpene alcohol probably tirucallol β-sitosterol and a waxy compound. The two triterpenic acids are ketocarboxylic and appear to be identical with the α-and β-acids.

Uses: The galls are bitter, acrid, astringent, thermogenic, anti-inflammatory, depurative, digestive, constipating, febrifuge, tonic, aromatic and expectorant with terebinthine odour. They are useful in asthma, cough, hiccough, dysentery, diarrhoea, ulcers,bronchitis, fever, consumption, irritability of stomach, psoriasis, leprosy, skin diseases, vitiated conditions of *tridosa*, dyspepsia, inflammations, fever, dipsia, anorexia, pharyngitis, leucorrhoea and general debility. It is also very effective in children for diseases at the time of teething.

990. *Pistacia lentiscus* *(Anacardiaceae)*

Vernacular Name: *Eng:* Mastic tree.

Description: Multi-branched perennial growing to 3m. Has small elliptical leathery leaves, clusters of reddish flowers and round scarlet fruit that ripens to black.

Habitate: Mastic tree is native to the Mediterranean region. It grows wild in scrub and on wasteground. Besides growing wild, it is also cultivated for its resin, which is collected from incisions made in the bark in summer and autumn.

Propagation: By seeds and vegetative method.

Parts Used: Resin.

Chemical Constituents: The resin contain alpha and beta-masticoresins, a volatile oil, tannins masticin and mastic acid. Pinenes are strongly antiseptic.

Uses: Mastic resin is little used today, though it could be employed as an expectorant for bronchial troubles and coughs, and as a treatment for diarrhoea. It has also been used to treat boils, ulcers and similar skin conditions. The resin has been missed with other compounds as a temporary filling for decayed teeth.

991. *Plantago asiatica* L. *(Plantaginaceae)*

Vernacular Name: *Eng*: Asian plantain.

Description: Perennial herb with radical leaves. Leaves all basal, cauline, ovate, 5-15 cm long, 3-8 cm wide, obtuse, with several parallel nerves; petioles as long as leaves, dilated at base. Scapes 10-50 cm long. Spike solitary, densely many-flowered, glabrous. Flowers bisexual, small, not showy, calyx 4-parted; corolla 4-lobed, scarious; stamens 4, exerted; ovary superior. Fruit a capsule enclosed by calyx.

Habitate: Roadsides, fallow fields.

Propagation: By seeds and vegetative method.

Parts Used Seed.

Chemical Constituents: Polysaccharides: plantasan, plantago-mucilage A. Flavonoids: plantagoside, plantaginin, homoplantaginin, aucubin. Monoterpenes, phenylpropanoids.

Uses: Choleretic, blood sugar lowering, inhibition of complement activation by plantago-mucilage A. Used in cough, diarrhoea & inflammation of eyes.

992. *Plantago depressa* Willd. *(Plantaginaceae)*

Vernacular Name: *Eng:* Depressed plantain.

Description: A perennial. Herb 10-15 cm high, glabrous or slightly pubescent. Rootstalk short with a main root. Leaves basal, in rosettes, blade long-elliptic or elliptic-lanceolate, 4-11 cm long by 2-4 cm wide; apex acute; margin irregular, toothed; base tapering and decurrent into the petiole 5-7 nerved; petioles usually longer than the leaf-blade, somewhat winged, sheathing at the base. Inflorescence an erect spike, elongated, cylindrical, somewhat loose at the base; May-June. Flowers small. Calyx in 4 segments. Corolla grayish, 2-lobed. Ovary 2-celled. Fruit a membranous pyxidium, opening circularly toward the base. Seeds 4-5, small, angled, dull black. The taste of the whole plant is slightly bitter.

Habitate: In villages and fields, on waste ground and in damp soil in Asia.

Propagation: By seeds and vegetative method.

Part Used: Whole plant and seeds.

Uses: Urinary stones and infections; nephritic oedema, iarrhoea, cold;cough;bronchitis, acute conjuncitivitis, skin inflammation and boils.

993. *Plantago major* L. *(Plantaginaceae)*

Synonyms: *Plantago officinarum* Crantz., *Plantago maxima* Ruching.

Vernacular Name: *Eng:* Great plantain.

Description: A perennial herb with an erect stout root stock. Leaves alternate, radical 2.5-12.5 cm. long, ovate or ovate-oblong, obtuse or sub-acute, entire or toothed, nearly glabrous, base tapering and decurrent into the petiole, commonly 7 nerved; petioles usually longer than lade, broad sheathing at base. Flowers scattered or crowded in long slender rather lax spikes 5-15 cm. long; spikes seldom less than 3; bracts 1.5-2 mm. long, shorter than the calyx, broadly ovate-oblong, obtuse, with scarious margins. Calyx, 3 mm. long, glabrous, oblong, obtuse or subacute, outusely keeled on the back and with broad scabrous margins. Corolla, 4 mm. long, glabrous; lobes lanceolate, acute, reflexed. Capsule ovoid, lobes lanceolate, acute, reflexed. Capsule ovoid, 3-4 mm. long, glabrous. Seeds 4-8 angled, rugulose, dull black, 0.85 mm. long usually 8-16 seeds in a capsule.

Habitate: All over temperate Himalayas in India.

Propagation: By seeds and vegetative method.

Parts Used: Whole plant, seeds.

Chemical Constituents: Alkaloids: Boschinakine and methyl esters of Boschniakinic acid; Choline: Steroids: Thioglucosides: Aucubin, Plantaenaloside, Acuboside; Melitoside; Flavonoids viz. Scutellarein, Homoplantaginin, Hispidulin, Plantagoside; Caffeix acid, cinnamic acid, Ferulic acid, Fumaric acid, Salicylic acid, Syringic acid Aucubin, Holoside Planteose.

Uses: For complaints specifically of toothache, earache and enuresis. Sharp pain in eyes due to toothache and inflammatory erache. Eyeball, very tender to touch. Earache due to toothache. Pyorrhea alveolaris. Depression and insomnia due to chronic tobacco addiction. Periodic Noctural enuresis. Itching & burning urticaria. Chilbains. Pruritis. Traditionally used for Bee sting, incised wounds and bleeding piles.

994. *Plantago ovata* Forssk. *(Plantaginaceae)*

Vernacular Name: *Eng*: Ispaghula, Blond psyllium, Spogel seeds; *Hin*: Isabgol, Isabgul; *Kan*: Issabagolu; *Mal*: Snigddhajirakam, Ispaghal; *San*: Snigdhabijah, Snigdhajirakah; *Tam*: Iskol, Isphogol; *Tel:* Isapgaluvittulu.

Description: A very short-stemmed softy hairy annual herb; leaves simple, narrowly linear or filiform, finely acuminate, entire or distantly toothed, usually 3-nerved; flowers small, in cylindric or ovoid spikes; fruits ellipsoid obtuse capsules, the upper half coming off as a blunt conical lid, seeds smooth, yellowish brown, ovoid-oblong, boat-shaped.

Habitate: Cultivated in Punjab, Gujarat and Haryana.

Propagation: By seeds and vegetative method.

Parts Used: Seeds.

Chemical Consistuents: Linolenic linoleic oleic, palmitic, stearic, lignoceric. The embryo yields 14.7 per cent of a linoleic acid-rich oil.

Uses: The seeds are sweet, astringent, refrigerant, emollient, mucilaginous, diuretic, laxative, anti-inflammatory, antidysenteric, expectorant, aphrodisiac, roborant and tonic. They are useful in vitiated conditions of *tridosa*, burning sensation, habitual constipation, strangury, gastritis, chronic diarrhoea, dysentery, colonalgia, dry cough, erysipelas, gout, gonorrhoea, bilious fever, nephropathy, duodenal ulcers, haemorrhoids, emaciation and general debility.

995. *Platycodon grandiflorum* (Jacq.) DC. *(Campanulaceae)*

Synonyms: *Campanula grandiflora* Jacq.

Vernacular Name: *Eng:* Ballon flower; Chinese bellflower; Japanese bellflower.

Description: An erect perennial herb, 30-100 cm high, more or less glaucous, glabrous, containing an abundant milky latex. Leaves alternate, opposite or verticillate, nearly sessile, ovoid or oval-lanceolate, 3-6 cm long by 1-2.5 cm wide, acuminate, coarsely dentate. Flowers solitary, long-pedunculate, broadly campanulate or deeply saucer-shaped. Clayx in 5 segmens 5. Ovary 5-celled. Fruit an ovoid capsule, dehiscent at the top. Seeds ovoid, compressed, obtuse, first violet then brown. The root is cylindrical, sometimes branched, more or less twisted. 7-29 cm long and 1-1.5 cm in diameter. The surface is yellowish-white, with rather deep longitudinal furrows, the leaf-scars visible in the short rootstock.

Habitate: At the edges of ponds or streams or in swamps in China, India, Japan, Korea and Soviet Union.

Propagation: By seeds and vegetative method.

Part Used: Rhizomes.

Chemical Constituents: Roots possess hemolytic action due to the presence of a saponin, platycodin.

Uses: Polydipsia due to stomach heat, vomiting, fever due to measles. Roots tonic, astringent, carminative, and expectorant, used in cough and for throat ailments.

996. *Plectranthus vettiveroides* (Jacob) Singh & Sharma *(Lamiaceae)*

Synonyms: *Coleus vettiveroides* K. C. Jacob.

Vernacular Name: *San*: Valakam, Hriberam; *Hin*: Valak, *Kan*: Muchivala, Lavanchi; *Mal*: Iruveli; *Tam*: Kuruver, Vettiver; *Tel:* Vettiveru, Kuriveru.

Description: A small profusely branched, succulent, aromatic herb with quadrangular stems and branches and deep straw-coloured aromatic roots; leaves glandular hairy, broadly ovate with dentate margins and prominent veins on the back; flowers blue in terminal racemes; fruits nutlets.

Habitate: Cultivated in south India through vegetative.

Propagation: By cuttings.

Parts Used: Whole plant.

Chemical Consisstuents: N.A.

Uses: The plant is bitter, cooling, diuretic, trichogenous and antipyretic. It is useful inhyperdipsia, vitiated conditions of *pitta*, burning sensation, strangury, leprosy, skin diseases, leucoderma, fever, vomiting, diarrhoea and ulcers. It promotes the growth of hair.

997. *Pluchea indica* (L.) Less. *(Asteraceae)*

Vernacular Name: *Beng*: Kukronda, munjhu rukha.

Description: Slender shrub 1-2m. tall. Branches pubscent and then glabrous. Leaves alternate, subsessile, glaucos-green on both sides; margins serrate. Inflorescence in terminal corymb of many heads; flowers lilac. Fruit small, angular.

Habitate: Grows wild in marshes or swamps but is usually cultivated for quickest hedges.

Propagation: By seeds and vegetative method.

Part Used: Roots and leaves.

Chemical Constituents: The leaves contain proteins 2.9%. The whole plant contains chlorogenic acid and an essential oil.

Uses: The roogs, which possess antifebrile, demulcent and anodyne properties, are recommended for treating adiaphoretic feber, headache, rheumatism, lumbago, osteodynia, sprain, dysentery and dyspepsia. A decoction of the fresh leaves is used in an inhalation for cold and a wash for scabies, while a mixture with alcohol is applied topically as an anodyne. The powdered leaves misxed with beeswax and castor oil are used in bandaging closed fractures.

998. *Pluchea lanceolata* B.C. Clarke & Olive. *(Asteraceae)*

Vernacular Name: *San*: Raasna, Yuktaa, Elaparnee; *Hin:* Rasna.

Description: Erect undershrub, 30-60 cm. high, stem and branches terete, ashy and pubescent. *Leaves*-sessile, very coriaceous, 25-27 by 0.6-1.6 cm. oblong or lanceolate, obtuse apiculate narrowed at the base, finely ashy, pubescent on both sides, entire or toothed round the apex main nerves prominent, *Inflorescence*-heads in compound corymbs, involucre contracted at the mount. Outer bracts 2-3 seriate, oblong, very botuse, pubescent, usually tinged with purple, the innermost bracts linear, sub-acute, few pappus hairs distinctly connate at the base.

Habitate: Grows in the upper Gangetic plain, Punjab, Rajasthan, Sind, Afghanistan, Baluchistan and N. Africa.

Propagation: By vegetative methods.

Parts Used: Whole plant.

Chemical Constituents: The petroleum ether extract of the plant on saponification with strong alkali, ether treatment, chromatographic analysis on aluminium hydroxide by elution with differentsolvents give different fractions-compound A Compound B probably taraxosterol and Compound C. The same author reported the isolation of tertiary bases and a large number of water soluble quarternary bases, incljuding pluchine, which has been indentified with betaine hydrochloride. Quercetin and isorhamentin are present as aglacones in the leaves. Glycosides and tannins were absent.

Uses: Arthritis. Constipation. Respiratory diseases. The decoction of the plant has been used traditionally in arthritis. The leaves are aperient and used as a laxative, analgesic and antipyretic.

999. *Plumbago indica* L. *(Plumbaginaceae)*

Synonyms: *Plumbago rosea* Linn.

Vernacular Name: *Eng*: Rosy-flowered leadwort, Fire plant; *Hin*: Lalcitra, Raktacitra; *Kan*: Kempucitramula; *Mal*: Kotuveli, Cettikkotuveli, Cuvannakotuveli; *San*: Citrakah, Dahanah; *Tam*: Cenkotiveli, Cittiramulam; *Tel:* Yerracitramulam.

Description: A pretty subscandent perennial shrub with semi-woody striate stems and flexible branches; leaves simple, alternate, oblong, short-cuneate at the base passing into a very short amplexicaul, exauriculate, reddish petiole; flowers bright red, in long terminal spikes, the calyx ribs covered with stipitate, bifarious and subsessile glands, corolla tube slender, 4 times as long as the calyx. The stout roots are cylindrical, irregularly bent, light yellowish brown with smooth surface having short transverse shallow fissures at the regions of the bents.

Habitate: Throughout India, in moist situations, as well as cultivated.

Propagation: By seeds and vegetative method.

Parts Used: Roots.

Chemical Consistuents: *P. indica* contains an orange yellow pigment named plumbagin a sitosterol, a fatty alcohol probably arachidly alcohol, tannin and an amorphous brown pigment. The flowers contains 3-rhamnosides of pelargonidin, cyaniding delphinidin and kaempferol.

Uses: The roots are acrid, astringent, thermogenic, anthelmintic, constipating, expectorant, anti-inflammatory, abortifacient, alterant, antiperiodic, carminative, digestive, sudorific, narcotic, gastric and nervous stimulant and rejuvenating. They are useful indyspepsia, colic, inflammations, cough, bronchitis, helminthiasis, haemorrhoids, elephantiasis, chronic and intermittent fever,leprosy, leucoderma, ring-worm, scabies, hepatosplenomegaly, amenorrhoea, odontalgia, vitiated conditions of *vata* and *kapha* and anaemia.

1000. *Plumbago zeylanica* *(Plumbaginaceae)*

Vernacular Name: *Eng:* Ceylong Leadwort; *Hin*: Chita, Chitarak, Chitra; *Beng*: Chita, Chitarak, Chitra; *Guj*: Chitaro, Chitrak; *Tel:* Agnimata, Chitramoolam; *Tam*: Cithiramulana; *Kan*: Chitramula, Vahni; *Mal*: Tumba koduveli, Vellakoduveli,.

Description: A perennial, sub-scandent shrubs; glabrous; flowers white, in elongated spikes; capsule oblong, pointed contained in viscid glandular persistent calyx.

Habitate: Ceylong leadwort is native to southern India and Malaysia, and is now naturalized in much of South-East Asia and in Africa. The leaves and root are gathered throughout the year.

Propagation: By seeds and vegetative method.

Parts Used: Leaves, Root.

Chemical Constituents: Ceylong leadwort contains plumbagin, which stimulates sweating.

Uses: Ceylong leadwort root is acrid and stimulates sweating. In West Africa, the root is traditionally mixed with okra to treat leprosy. In Indian herbal medicine, the leaves and root are used to treat infections and digestive problems such as dysentery. Externally, a paste of the leaves and root is applied to painful rheumatic areas or to chronic and itchy skin problems. The paste acts as a counter-irritant. By raising blisters and increasing circulation, it speeds the clearing of toxins from the affected area.

1001. *Plumeria rubra* L. *(Apocynaceae)*

Synonyms: *Plumeria acuminata* Ait, *Plumeria acutifolia* Poir,.

Vernacular Name: *Eng:* Temple tree, pagoa tree, frangipani plant; *Tam:* Segappu arali; *San*: Kshirachampa; *Hin*: Golainchi; *Beng*: Dalan phul; *Guj*: Rhada champo; *Tel:* Nuru varahaalu; *Kan*: Devaganigile; *Mal*: Ezha-champakam,.

Description: Medium-sized tree, 5-6m. high. Brancehes fleshy, brittle. Leaves alternate, usually crosded in thick terminal cluster, entire and attenuate at both ends. Inflorescence in terminal cyme; flowers white with a yellow center, or reddish-pink, fragrant. Follicles divaricate, with numerous winged seeds. All parts of the plant yield a milky latex.

Habitate: Cultivated for ornament, particularly in the vicinity of religiouys shrines and burial grounds.

Propagation: By seeds and vegetative method.

Part Used: Bark, latex and flowers.

Chemical Constituents: The stem-bark contains plumierides and fulvoplumierin.

Uses: The flowers are used in treating cough, constipation, acute enteritis, dysentery and haemophilia. A decoction of the stem-bark is administered by mouth for hydropsia and purgative; an alcoholic maceration is used as a gargle to cure paradontosis. The latex is used in the same way as the stem-bark, but in lower doses. The plant is proscribed for pregnant women.

1002. *Podophyllum peltatum* L. *(Berberidaceae)*

Synonyms: *Podophyllum montanum* Rafin.

Vernacular Name: *Eng:* May-apple

Description: An erect herb upto 1 m. in height; leaves large green, upto 30 cm. across, 5 lobed, the lobes oblong and usually 2-cleft and denate at apex; flowering stems with usually similar leaves; flowers white solitary, nodding, borne on the fork between the 2 leaves; sepals-6 petaloid, shed early; petals 6-9, longer than the sepals; stamens twice as many as pistils; fruit ovoid, yellowish, 2.5-5 cm. long, edible.

Habitate: Throughout U.S.A. in shady woods & marshy grounds.

Propagation: By seeds and vegetative method.

Parts Used: Rhizome.

Chemical Constituents: Pdophyllo-resin (Podophyllin), Podophyllotoxin, Quercetin. α-and β-peltatin.

Uses: For complaints mainly of rectum & liver. Gastro-enteritis with colicky pain and bilious vomiting. Stool watery with jelly like mucous, painless, profuse, gushing, involuntary type and offensive. Cholera infantum and morbus. Prolapsus rectum due to diarrhoea. Liver region painful. Diarrhoea after acid fruit, during dentition. Above symptoms associated with grinding of teeth at night, intense desire to press the gum together, burning sensation of tongue, delirium. In females pain in uterus and right ovary with shifting noises along ascending colon.

1003. *Pogostemon cablin* (Blanco) Benth. *(Lameaceae)*

Synonyms: *Pogostemon patchouli* Pellet.

Vernacular Name: *Eng:* Patchouli; *Hin:* Pacholi, peholi; *Beng*: Pachapat; *Tam:* kadirpachai; *Kan:* Patche tene and *Mal:* Pachila.

Description: A fragrant perennial herb, 30-100 cm high. Stem erect and thick, the upper parts branched and covered densely with dull-yellow tomena. The lower parts, terete, ligneous. Leaves opposite, petiole 2-5 cm long, also with tomenta. Blade broadly ovate or ovate, 5-10 cm long by 2.5-7 cm wide tip sub-acutue, base cuneate or lightly cordate. Margin obtusely dentate or incised, both surfaces covered with dense hairs and oil glands. Summer. Flowers small in terminal or axillary spikes. Calyx tubular, 6 mm long 5-lobed. Corolla bilabiate, 8 mm long, light reddish-purple. Stamens 4, extending from the corolla-tube. Nutlets smooth.

Habitate: Mostly cultivated in warm and moist regions in China, India, Malaysia and Philippines.

Propagation: By stem cutting.

Part Used: Stems and leaves.

Chemical Constituents: Patchoulol.

Uses: Fever caused heat stroke; headache, poor appetite; nausea; vomiting; diarrhoea. Leaves yield an essential oil known as Patchouli Oil much used in perfumery industry for scenting soaps and other cosmetics, tobacco and incenses; an excellent masking agent in depilatory creams. It yields an excellent attar on blending with sandalwood oil. Infusion of fresh leaves is given in menstrual troubles. Dried leaves used for scenting wardrobes.

1004. *Polyalthia longifolia* (Sonn.) Thwaites *(Annonaceae)*

Vernacular Name: *Eng*: Mast tree, Cemetery tree; *Hin*: Debdari, Asoka; *Kan*: Assoti; *Mal*: Aranamaram; *San*: Ulkatah, Kastadaruh; *Tam*: Asogu, Nettilingam; *Tel:* Asokamu.

Description: A tall handsome evergreen tree, bark smooth, greyish brown, thick; leaves simple, green, shining with undulate margins; flowers yellowish green in fascicles; fruits a bunch of small ovoid one-seeded berries.

Habitate: Cultivated all over India.

Propagation: By seeds and vegetative method.

Parts Used: Bark.

Chemical Consistuents: N.A.

Uses: The bark is bitter, acrid, cooling, febrifuge and anthelmintic. It is useful in fever, skin diseases, diabetes, hypertension, helminthiasis and vitiated conditions of *vata* and *pitta*.

1005. *Polygala senega* *(Polygalaceae)*

Vernacular Name: *Eng:* Seneca Snakeroot.

Description: A pluircaulous, perennial haerb, 20-30 cm . high; leaves mostly linear-lanceolate to elliptic or ovate, flowers white, in terminal racemes, fruits 2-celled capsules.

Habitate: Seneca snakeroot is native to North America, and found in dry stony open ground and woodland.

Propagation: By seeds and vegetative method.

Parts Used: Root.

Chemical Constituents: Seneca snakeroot contains triterpenoid saponins, phenolic acids, emthyl salicylate, polygalitol, and plant sterols. The triterpenoid saponins promote the clearing of phlegm from the bronchial tubes.

Uses: In North American and European herbal medicine, Seneca snakeroot is used as an expectorant to treat bronchial asthma, chronic bronchitis and whooping cough. The root has a stimulant action on the bronchial mucous membranes, promoting the coughing up of phlegm from the chest and thereby easing wheeziness. In large doses, the root is emetic.

Seneca snakeroot is also thought to encourage sweating and to stimulate the secretion of saliva.

1006. *Polygala vulgairs* *(Polygalaceae)*

Vernacular Name: *Eng:* Milkwort.

Description: Short perennial with pointed lance-shaped leaves and spikes of small blue, mauve or white flowers.

Habitate: Milkwort is common in grassy and moorland areas in much of western and northern Europe.

Propagation: By seeds and vegetative method.

Parts Used: Root.

Chemical Constituents: Milkwort contains triterpenoid saponins, a volatile oil, gaultherin and mucilage.

Uses: The bitter tasting milkwort still has a reputation for increasing milk production in nursing mothers, but this attribute is in fact unfounded. While milkwort is infrequently used in European herbal medicine today, it–like Seneca snakeroot is a valuable herb for the treatment of respiratory troubles such as chronic bronchitis, bronchial asthma and convulsive coughs, including whooping cough. Milkwort is also thought to have sweat-inducing and diuretic properties.

1007. *Polygonatum cirrhifolium* (Wall.) Royle *(Liliaceae)*

Vernacular Name: *Eng*: Meda; *Hin*: Meda; *Kan*: Medha; *Mal*: Meda; *San*: Meda; *Tam*: Meda; *Tel:* Meda.

Description: A herb upto 120 cm in height with thick root-stock, upper part of the stem creeping, leafy and grooved; leaves in whorls of 4, sessile, linear, acute; flowers purplish tinged with white and green, 2-3 together; fruits blue-black spherical berries, red when ripe.

Habitate: In the Himalayas, from 1,200 to 4,200 m.

Propagation: By Rhizomes.

Parts Used: Root stock.

Chemical Consistuents: N.A.

Uses: The root stock is sweet, cooling, emollient, aphrodisiac, galactagogue, depurative, vulnerary, febrifuge, expectorant and tonic. It is useful in burning sensation, agalactia, skin diseases, wounds, ulcers, tuberculosis, fever, vitiated conditions of *pitta*, cough, bronchitis and general debility.

1008. *Polygonatum kingianum* Coll. Et Hemsl. *(Liliaceae)*

Description: Perennial herbaceous plant 1-1.2m. high Rootstock horizontal, stout, whitish, strangled at the nodes. Leaves stalkless narrow 5-10 verticillate with a long, sharp and curling tip. Flowers red, in pairs, drooping in the axils. Berry oval, violet-blue when ripe.

Habitate: Found wild in the highlands above 1200m.

Propagation: By vegetative method.

Part Used: Rhizomes.

Chemical Constituents: The rhizomes contain mucilage, starch and sugars.

Uses: The rhizome is considered as a tonic and has a beneficial effect in the treatment of pulmonary diseases, dry cough and heamoptysis. It relieves general debility, lumbago and rheumatic pains. It is available in the form of a powder, decoction or alcoholic maceration.

1009. *Polygonatum multiflorum* *(Liliaceae)*

Vernacular Name: *Eng:* Solomon's seal.

Description: Perennial growing to about 50cm. Has arching stems, alternate elliptical leaves, delicate, greenish-white, bell-shaped flowers and blue-black fruit.

Habitate: Native to Europe and to temperate regions of Asia and North America.

Propagation: By seeds and vegetative method.

Parts Used: Rhizomes.

Chemical Constituents: Solomon's seal contains saponins, flavonoids and vitamin A.

Uses: Like arnica Solomon's seal is stimulate tissue repair. Used mainly in the form of a poultice, the rhizome has astringent and demulcent actions that undoubtedly contribute to its ability to accelerate healing Solomon's seal has also be recommended for tuberculosis, as a remedy for menstrual problems, and as a tonic. In Chinese herbal medicine, it is considered a *yin* tonic, and it thought to be particularly applicable to respiratory system problems-sore throats dry and irritable coughs, bronchial catarrh and chest pain.

1010. *Polygonatum odoratum* var. pluriflorum Ohwi *(Liliaceae)*

Vernacular Name: *Eng*: Solomon's seal, King-Solomon's-seal.

Description: Rhizoatous, perennial herb. Rhizome horizontal much jointed, with many scars. Stems to 30-50 cm or more, angled, arkching. Leaves alternate, sessile, elliptic-oblong to ovate, to 10 cm long, glabrous. Flowers greenish-white, axillary, to 2 cm long, fragrant, on 2-flowered peduncles; perianth cylindrical, 6-lobed; stamens 6, on perianth tube, filaments glabrous. Fruit a blue-black berry with several seeds.

Habitate: Meadows and sparse woods in lowlands and foothills.

Propagation: By vegetative method.

Parts Used Rhizome.

Chemical Constituents: Polysaccharide; odoratan. Flavonoids; cosmosiin, saponarin, vitexin, vitexin-2"-glucoside, polygonatiin. Saponins.

Uses: Used in convelescence, weakness and febrile diseases. Cardiotonic.

1011. *Polygonatum verticillatum* (L.) All. *(Liliaceae)*

Vernacular Name: *Eng*: Mahameda; *Hin*: Mahameda; *Kan*: Mahamedha; *Mal*: Mahameda; *San*: Mahameda; *Tam*: Mahameda; *Tel:* Mahameda.

Description: An erect glabrous herb upto 120 cm in height with thick root stock; upper part of the stem leafy, zig-zag and grooved; leaves whorled, sessile, linear or lanceolate; flowers 2-3 together, white, pinkish white or pale green in whorled racemes; fruits berries, red when ripe.

Habitate: In the Himalayas, at a height of 1,800 to 3,900 m.

Propagation: By vegetative method.

Parts Used: Root stock.

Chemical Consistuents: N.A.

Uses: The root stock is sweet, cooling, emollient, diuretic, aphrodisiac, galactagogue, appetising and tonic. It is useful in vitiated conditions of *pitta* and *vata*, burning sensation, fever, strangury, seminal weakness, anorexia and general debility.

1012. *Polygonum aviculare* *(Polygonaceae)*

Vernacular Name: *Eng:* Knotgrass, Bian xu; *Hin*: Machoti, ban-natia, banalia; *Beng*: Machutie.

Description: A highly variable annual herb, with prostrate stems and branches, up to 0 cm high; leaves elliptic or lanceolate; flowers small, green, tipped with red or white, in axillary clusters; nuts ovoid, minutely wrinkled.

Habitate: Knotgrass is found in temperate regions throughout the world. It thrives on wasteground and along shorelines.

Propagation: By Rhizomes.

Parts Used: Aerial parts.

Chemical Constituents: Knotgrass contains tannins, flavonoids, polyphenols, silicic acid and mucilage.

Uses: A herb with astringent and diuretic properties, knotgrass is used in European herbal medicine to treat diarrhoea and haemorrhoids, to expel worms, to staunch bleeding wounds, to reduce heavy menstrual flow and to stop nosebleeds. Knotgrass is also taken for pulmonary complaints, since its silicic acid content strengthens connective tissue within the lungs. In Chinese medicine, it is given to expel tapeworm and hookworm to treat diarrhoea and dysentery, and as a diuretic, particularly when urination is painful.

1013. *Polygonum bistorta* L. *(Polygonaceae)*

Synonyms: *Polygonum paleaceum* Wall.

Vernacular Name: *Eng:* Bistort; adderwort; dragonwort, snake root.

Description: A perennial herb, 50-80 cm high. Rootstock crooked, robust, woody, purplish-brown or black, as thick as the thumb or less. Stem erect, simpe, slender, glabrous. Basal leaves long-petiolate, oblong-lanceolate, 10-18 cm long by 2.5-5 cm side; apex acute; base obtuse-rounded or truncate, sometimes cordate, coriaceous; sheath of stipules tube-like, membranous. Cauline leaf linear or lanceolate, sessile or amplexicaul. Inflorescence a compact terminal spike, 3-10 cm long. Flowers reddish or white. Petals 5, elliptic. Stamens 8. Stigmas 3 nut very small, trigonous, glossy reddish-brown.

Habitate: On slopes, in grassland and under trees in China, Japan and India.

Propagation: By seeds and vegetative method.

Part Used: Rhizomes.

Chemical Constituents: Rhizomes and leaves contain tannin.

Uses: Diarrhoea, enteritis, bleeding haemorrhoids, skin inflammatin, stomatitis, gingivitis. Used in soups and stews; also recommended for silage. Root-stocks eaten. Rhizomes constitute the Anjubar of Arabs. They are used as a febrifuge, diuretic, expectorant, hemostatic. Preparations of this herb are used as a substitute for Peruvian Rhatany. Rhizomes and leaves contain tannin.

1014. *Polygonum chinense* L. *(Polygonaceae)*

Vernacular Name: *Eng:* Chinese knotweed; *Kan:* Bilichini, ganiglu.

Description: Undershrub aboug 1m. high. Stems cylindrical, glabrous, much branched. Leaves alternate, ovoid, entire with a tubular ocrea and sometimes a black marking like a

"V" on the upper face. Inflorescence in terminal panicled cyme; flowers small, white or pink, Nutlet trigonous, pulpy, dull-black when ripe.

Habitate: Grows wild every where.

Propagation: By seeds and vegetative method.

Part Used: Leaves.

Chemical Constituents: The whole plant contains rubin, rheum-emodin, oxy-methyl-anthraquinone, anthraquijnone, flucosides, myrcyl alcohol.

Uses: The leaves have antivacterial properties and are effective in the treatment of furunculosis, impetigo, ulceration of the helix, scalp scabs, cold sore, eczema, and streptococcal skin infections. Poultices made of pounded fresh leaves their juice or their concentrated extract are topically applied. A decoction of dried leaves is indicated for boils and dysentery. Snake-bite is treated by oral administration of juice of fresh leaves, the residue being applied to the bite as a plaster.

1015. *Polygonum dichrotomum* Blume. *(Polygonaceae)*

Description: Perennial sprawling herb with rooting lower nodes and ascending branches to 1 m tall. Leaves alternate, petiolate, blades lanceolate to lanceolate-ovate, up to 20 cm long and 5 cm wide, with a thin membranous sheath surrounding each node where the petiole attaches. Flowers white to pink, borne in terminal spike-like clusters. Fruit small, brown, 3-angled.

Habitate: Common in swamps, shallow water of lakes and ponds, and moist open areas from sea-level to mountain lake shores above 800 m elevation.

Propagation: By seeds and vegetative method.

Part Used: Whole plant.

Chemical Constituents: N.A.

Uses: Used in remedies for neuralgia, and to treat urinary tract infections. It is also used to treat gonorrhea.

1016. *Polygonum multiflorum* Thumb. *(Polygonaceae)*

Vernacular Name: *Eng:* Many-flowered knotweed.

Description: Perennial climber, Stems twining, branchlets and petioles violet-purple, Roots tuberous, brownish-red. Leaves alternate, ovate-cordate; apex pointed; ocrea thin, membranous. Inflorescence in axillary pancle; flowers small, white. Nutlet 3-angled, winged.

Habitate: Grows wild in the highlands; occasionally cultivated.

Propagation: By seeds and vegetative method.

Part Used: Tuberous roots.

Chemical Constituents: The tuberous roots contain rhponticin (rhapontin, ponticin), chrysophanic acid, emodin, physcion, rhein and polygonic acid.

Uses: The roots is a blood tonic and anti-inflammatory. It is effective in the therapy of renal and hepatic hypofunction, neurasthenia, dyspepsia, insomnia, hypogalactia, rheumatism, lumbago, spermatorrhoea, leucorrhoea, haematuria, bloody stools, prurigo and anaemia. Long-term administration has a rejuvenating effect and makes white hair grow black again.

1017. *Polygonum tinctorium* Lour. *(Polygonaceae)*

Vernacular Name: *Eng*: Polygonum.

Description: Annual herb, to 50-60 cm tall, cutivated as a source of dye. Stems appearing to be jointed. Leaves alternate, simple, ovate, 8 cm long, entire, stipular sheaths well developed; stipules tinged red. Flowers small, whitish pink, in terminal or axillary compact spikes; sepals 5; stamens 6-8. Fruit a small achene, 3-angular, 2 mm long, wholly enclosed by sepals. Leaves used for dark-blue dye.

Habitate: Open wet grassy areas.

Propagation: By seeds and vegetative method.

Parts Used: Leaf, fruit.

Chemical Constituents: Glucosides: indican. Tryptanthrin. N-Phenyl-2-naphthylamine.

Uses: Augmented leukocyte phagocytosis, anti-inflammatory, antipyretic activities, antifunal. Used as liver protection.

1018. *Polymnia uvedalia* *(Asteraceae)*

Vernacular Name: *Eng:* Bearsfoot.

Description: Perennial herb growing to 2m with large 3-lobed leaves and yellow flowers.

Habitate: Bearsfoot is native to the eastern US. It grows from New York southwards, preferring rich soil.

Propagation: By seeds and vegetative method.

Parts Used: Root.

Chemical Constituents: N.A.

Uses: Bearsfoot is perhaps best known for its use as a hair tonic, having traditionally been a popular ingredient in hair lotions. It is still used in this way, but today the root is more often taken internally as a treatment for non-malignant swollen glands and especially for mastitis. The root is thought to have a beneficial effect on the stomach, liver and spleen, and may be taken to relieve indigestion and counteract liver malfunction. The herb has laxative properties and it may also act to relieve pain.

1019. *Polyscias fruticosa* (L.) Harms *(Araliaceae)*

Synonyms: *Notho panax frutica* Sum.

Description: Shrub to small tree up to 4 m tall. Leaves alternate, petiolate, irregularly pinnately compound, the leaflets with conspicuous toothed margins, blades often yellowish in colour and fragrant if curshed. Flowers relatively small, yellowish-green, borne in umbels. Fruit is a small dry drupe with single seed.

Habitate: Commonly cultivated in gardens and possibly naturalized in some areas from sea-level to 500 m elevation.

Propagation: By seeds and vegetative method.

Part Used: Root, bark and leaves.

Chemical Constituents: Alpha-Bergamotene, gamma-trans-bisabolene,beta-elemene, flacarinol, germacrene D, polyacetylenes, and oleanolic acid.

Uses: The root is used as a diuretic. The juice from the bark is taken for thrush and an ulcerated tongue or throat. A poultice made from the bark is used on syphiltic sores. Liquid from the stem bark is given to aid in the exulsion of the afterbirth. A decoction of the leaves is used to treat sinusitis, headache and haemorrhoids. A decoction of the leaves, together with the decoctions of the leaves of some other species, is used to treatments for tonsillitis and migraine. High blood pressure is also treated with this plant.

1020. *Poncirus trifoliate* Raf. *(Rutaceae)*

Vernacular Name: *Eng*: Trifoliate orange, bitter orange.

Description: Deciduous shrub, to 3 m tall, with tangled rigid, green branches and stout green spines 3-5 cm long. Leaves alternate, trifoliate; leaflets 3-6 cm long, obovate or elliptic, cuneate at base, crenate; petioles slightly winged, 25 mm long. Flowers solitary, terminal or axillary, 1-2,3 cm across, white, scented, sepals and petals 5; stamens many. Fruit globose, 3-5 cm in diameter, fragrant when ripe, inedible.

Habitate: Woods in mountains and hills commonly planted as a fence Korea and China.

Propagation: By seeds and vegetative method.

Parts Used: Fruit.

Chemical Constituents: Flavonoids. Coumarins. Monoterpenes. Alkaloids: 5-hydroxy-noracronycine.

Uses: Sedative, angiotonic. Used in gastritis, hernia, sputum remedy and sinusitis.

1021. *Pongamia pinnata* (L.) Pierre *(Fabaceae)*

Synonyms: *Pongamia glabra* Vent.

Vernacular Name: *Eng*: Indian beech, Pongam oil tree, Karanj, *Hin*: Karanj, Karanja, *Kan*: Hongemara, *Mal*: Unnu, Ponnu, *San*: Karanjah, *Tam*: Ponka, Punkumaram, *Tel: Kan*ugacettu.

Description: A medium-sized semi-evergreen glabrous tree with a short bole and spreading crown upto 18 m or more in height, bark greyish green or brown, very often mottled with bark brown dots, specks, lines or streaks; leaves compound, leaflets 5-7, ovate acuminate or elliptic; flowrs lilac or pinkish white, fragrant in axillary racemes; fruits thick woody, smooth, compressed, with a short curved beak, seeds 1 or 2 per pod, reniform to nearly round, smooth or wrinkled.

Habitate: Throughout India, in tidal and beach forests; cultivated often as avenue trees.

Propagation: By seeds and vegetative method.

Parts Used: Root, bark, leaves, flowers, seeds oil.

Chemical Consistuents: Pongaglabrone, diketonepongamol, glabrin, karanjin, pongapin, kanjone.

Uses: The roots are good for cleaning foul ulcers, cleaning teeth, strengthening gums and gonorrhoea. A root paste is sued for to local application in scrofulous enlargements. The fresh bark is sweet and mucilaginous to taste, soon becoming bitter and acrid. It is anthelmintic and alexeteric and is useful in haemorrhoids, berieri, ophthalmopathy, dermatopathy, vaginopathy and ulcers. Leaves are digestive laxative and anthelmintic, and are good for flatulence, dyspepsia, diarrhoea, leprosy, gonorrhoea, and cough. A hot infusion of the leaves is good for rheumatalgia and for cleaning ulcers and wounds. Flowers are useful to quench dipsia in diabetes and for alleviating *vata* and *kapha*. The seeds are anthelmintic, haematinic, bitter, acrid and carminative. They are useful in inflammations, otalgia, lumbago, pectoral diseases, chronic fevers, hydrocele, haemorrhoids and anaemia. The oil is anthelmintic, stypic and depurative and is recommended for scabies, opthlamia, leprosy, haemorrhoids, ulcers, herpes and lumbago.

1022. *Popetia pinnata* J.R.&G.Forster *(Sapindaceae)*

Description: Tree upto 20 m high with buttressed trunk. Leaves alternate, pinnately compound, 18-30 cm long, leaflets 6-8, opposite, elliptical and unequal, bright red when young. Flowers minute, regular, 5-parted, whitish except for red stamens. Fruit a red juicy, globose drupe to 4 cm broad containing whitish pulp with one large seed.

Habitate: Common in lowland forest, forest edges, open woodlands, lava flows, and often cultivated in villages.

Propagation: By seeds and vegetative method.

Part Used: Leaves and bark.

Chemical Constituents: Anthocyanidins, lignin, oleanolic acid glycoside, tannins.

Uses: To treat deep pains in the bones, migraine headache, to aid expulsion of placenta after childbirth, to relieve rheumatic aching of muscles and joints, to relieve fever, as a remedy for flue and cold to cure diarrhoea, stomach trouble, cough, fever constipation, and diaper rash. An infusion of the bark is used as an emetic for mouth infections, colds and mucous congestion, and to treat abdominal pains. An infusion of the leaves is rubbed onto the heads of infants or is given internally to treat unclosed fontanelles.

1023. *Populus candicans* *(Salicaceae)*

Vernacular Name: *Eng:* Balm of Gilead.

Description: Deciduous tree growing to 25m. Has heart-shaped leaves, buds producing a sticky resin and female catkins.

Habitate: Naturalized in northern temperate region, balm of Gilead is also cultivated as an ornamental tree.

Propagation: By Cutting.

Parts Used: Buds, stem bark.

Chemical Constituents: Balm of Gilead buds contain flavonoids, phenolic glycosides and fatty acids. Salicin's analgesic, anti-inflammatory and fever-reducing actions rescrmble those of aspirin.

Uses: Balm of Gilead is a common ingredient of cough mixtures. Its expectorant, antiseptic and analgesic properties make it an excellent remedy for sore throats, dry irritable coughs, bronchitis and other respiratory ailments. In France and Germany, balm of Gilead is applied as a salve to grazes, small wounds, chapped and itchy skin, sunburn, chilblains and haemorrhoids. A preparation of balm of Gilead, applied externally, may also help relieve the pain of rheumatic joints and strained muscles. As culpeper noted, the plant is also thought to reduce breast milk production.

1024. *Populus tremuloides* *(Salicaceae)*

Vernacular Name: *Eng:* Quaking aspen.

Description: Deciduous, spreading tree growing to 20m. Has oval, slightly sticky buds and round, finely toothed leaves that quiver in the wind.

Habitate: Native to North America, quaking aspen prefers damp and moist areas, and grows alongside rivers.

Propagation: By vegetative method.

Parts Used: Bark.

Chemical Constituents: The bark contains phenolic glycosides and tannins. salicin and populin are salicylates, substances that have fever-reducing, pain-relieving and anti-inflammatory properties that are similar to those of aspirin.

Uses: Like willow bark, quaking aspen bark has widely recognized anti-inflammatory and pain relieving properties. The bark's significant astringent and antiseptic qualities make it useful for treating diarrhoea and the symptoms of irritable bowel syndrome. It is also used to treat urinary tract infections.

1025. *Portulaca oleracea* L. *(Portulacaceae)*

Vernacular Name: *San:* Brihalloni, lonika, lonamla; *Eng:* Garden purslane, common npurslane, purple flowered purslane, kitchen-garden purslane; *Hin:* khursa, baralaniya, kulfa; *Bang*: Baraloniya; *Tel:* Peddapayilijura, ganga-pavilikura; *Tam:* Karikeerai, paruppukiray, pullikirai; *Kan:* Dooddagooni soppu and *Mal:* Kariecheera.

Description: Prostrate annual herb. Stems succulent, green or reddish. Leaves altenate, fleshy, shining glabrous; base attenuate, apex truncatel nerves inconspicuous. Flowers bright yellow in terminal cluster, without stalks. Capsule globose or ovoid, opening transversely; seeds numerous, shining black.

Habitate: Commonly found wild in wet places.

Propagation: By seeds and vegetative method.

Part Used: Whole plant.

Chemical Constituents: The whole plant contains carotene, vitamins C, B_1, B_2, PP, Ca, Mg, Na, K salts; organic acids, nicotinic and oxalic, noradrenalin, and the biflavonoid liquiritin.

Uses: Except for the roots, the entire plant is used as an antibacterial, anti-inflammatory and anthelminthic. It is used in treating bacillary dysentery and dysuria. A combination with equal parts of Euphorbia thymifolia is also used. The juice extracted from 100g of pounded fresh plant and diluted with water serves as an anthelminthic against oxyuriasis and ascariasis. It is administered in the morning, for 3-5 days. Poultices of fresh leaves are used to treat mastitis, boils and impetigo.

1026. *Potentilla anserina* *(Rosaceae)*

Vernacular Name: *Eng:* Silverweed.

Description: A slender, perennial herb, up to 30 cm high; Root stocks very short, slender; levaes pinnate; stolons up to 30 cm. long arise from the leaf axils; leaf lets 12-24, linear-oblong to narrowly lanceolate; flowers large, solitary, golden yellow, achenes numerous, smooth.

Habitate: Silverweed is found in Europe, Asia and North America. In India it is distributed in W. Himalayas upto 2100-4800 m.

Propagation: By seeds and vegetative method.

Parts Used: Root.

Chemical Constituents: Silverweed contains 2-10% ellagitannins, flavonoids, choline and bitters.

Uses: Contemporary medical herbalists believe that silverweed's main medicinal value lies in its astringency. Silverweed makes an effected gargle for sore throats, and is a helpful remedy for diarrhoea. It is less astringent than its close relative tormentil, but it also has a gentler action within the gastro-intestinal tract. It is used externally as a lotion or ointment6 of bleeding haemorrhoids.

1027. *Potentilla chinensis* Ser. *(Rosaceae)*

Vernacular Name: *Eng*: Chinese cinquefoil.

Description: Pubescent perennial herb with stout rhizome, to 30-60 cm tall. Leaves pinnately compond, alternate, obovate to linear-lanceolate; leaflets 15-29, the lower smaller, the upper oblanceolate to narrowly oblong, 2-5 cm long, 8-15 mm wide, glabrous above, densely white-woolly tomentose beneath. Flowers many, 1-2 cm across, yellow; calyx segments ovate, acute; bracts lanceolate; receptacle hairy. Achenes broadly ovoid, longitudinally rugose, 1.3 mm long.

Habitate: Open sunny places lowlands Korea, Japan and China.

Propagation: By seeds and vegetative method.

Parts Used Whole plant.

Chemical Constituents: Gallic, catecholic tannins.

Uses: Antitumour, antipyretic, haemostatic and women's tonic.

1028. *Potentilla erecta* *(Rosaceae)*

Synonyms: *Potentilla tormentilla.*

Vernacular Name: *Eng:* Tormentil.

Description: Downy creeping perennial growing to 10cm. Has leaves bearing 5 leaflets, and many 4-petalled yellow flowers.

Habitate: Native to temperate regions of Asia and Europe.

Propagation: By seeds and vegetative method.

Parts Used: Root.

Chemical Constituents: Tormentil contains 15-20% tannins, catechins, ellagitannins and a phlobaphene.

Uses: Containing even more tannins than oak bark, all parts of tormentil are strongly astringent, finding use wherever this action is required. The plant makes a beneficial gargle for throat infections, and an effective mouthwash for treating mouth ulcers and infected gums. Tormentil may be taken for conditions that give rise to diarrhoea, such as irritable bowel syndrome, colitis, ulcerative colitis and dysentery, and for rectal bleeding. Applied externally as a lotion or ointment, tormential helps relieve heamorrhoids. In the form of a lotion, tormentil is used to help staunch wounds and protect areas of damaged or burned skin.

1029. *Premna obtusifolia* R. Br. *(Verbenaceae)*

Synonyms: *Premna corymbosa* Rottl., *Premna serratifolia* Linn., *P. integrifolia.*

Vernacular Name: *San:* Agnimanthah; *Eng:* Headache tree; *Hin:* Agetha, arani, ustabunda; *Beng*: Bhut-bhiravi, ganiari; *Tel:* Pomanti, pedda narva, gaebbu nelli; *Tam:* Munnay, muney kiray; *Kan:* Eegigida, agnimanda, takkite, bachanige mara; *Mal:* munna.

Description: A large shrub or a small tree upto 9 m in height with yellowish lenticellate bark, spinous large branches and yellowish brown woody aromatic root; leaves simple, opposite, sometimes, whorled, elliptic-ovate, membranous when young, coriaceous when mature, entire or irregularly toothed, primary lateral nerves 4-6 pairs; flowers small, greenish yellow or greenish white with a strong disagreeable odour in corymbiform cymost panicles; fruits globose drupes, black when ripe with the persistent saucer-shaped calyx surrounding its base.

Habitate: Throughout India in the plains.

Propagation: By stem cutting.

Parts Used: Roots, leaves.

Chemical Consisuents: The chief active principles are the three alkaloids, premnine, ganiarine and ganikarine.

Uses: The roots are astringent, bitter acrid, sweet, thermogenic, anodyne, anti-inflammatory, alexeteric, cardiotonic, alterant expectorant, depurative, digestive, carminative, stomachic, laxative, febrifuge, antibacterial and tonic. They are useful in vitiated conditions of *vata* and *kapha*, neuralgia, inflammations, cardiac disorders, hepatopathy, cough, asthma, bronchitis leprosy, skin diseases, dyspepsia, flatulence, colic, anorexia, constipation, haemorrhoids, fever diabetes and general debility. The leaves are stomachic, carminative and galactagogue, and are useful in dyspepsia, flatulence, colic, agalactia, cough and catarrh, fever, rheumatalgia, neuralgia, haemorrhoids and tumours.

1030. *Primula veris* *(Primulaceae)*

Vernacular Name: *Eng:* Cowslip.

Description: Hairy perennial growing to 10 cm. Has a basal rosette of slightly rough oblong leaves. Stems bear clusters of bright yellow, bell-shaped flowers.

Habitate: Cowslip grows in Europe and western Asia, preferring fields and pastures with chalky soils.

Propagation: By seeds and vegetative method.

Parts Used: Flowers, leaves, root.

Chemical Constituents: Cowslip contains triterpenoid saponins, flavonoids, phenols, tannins and a trace of volatile oil. The flavonoids, mainly in the flowers, are antioxidant, anti-inflammatory and antipsamodic. The triterpenoid saponins, which are concentrated in the root are strongly expectorant.

Uses: Cowslip is an under-used but valuable plant. The root is strongly expectorant, stimulating a more liquid mucus and so easing the clearance of phlegm. It is given for chronic coughs, especially those associated with chronic bronchitis and catarrhal congestion. The root is also thought to be mildly diuretic and antirheumatic and to slow blood clotting. The leaves have similar properties to the root, but are weaker in action. The flowers are believed to be sedative and are recommended for overactivity and sleeplessness, particularly in children. Cowslip flowers' antispasmodic and anti-inflammatory properties make them potentially useful in the treatment of asthma and other allergic conditions.

1031. *Prunella vulgaris* L. *(Lamiaceae)*

Synonyms: *Brunella Vulgaris* Linn.

Vernacular Name: *Eng:* Selfheal, heal-all, sicklewort.

Description: A low sprawling perennial herb, 45 cm high, faintly pubescent. Leaves petiolate, opposite, ovate or oblong, 2.5-5 cm long by 1 cm wide, entire or dentate, base rounded or wedge-shaped, faintly nervate. Flowers 1.3-2 cm long violet purple, in whorls of 6 crowded in erect, terminal spikes 2.5-5 cm long and bearing a pair of sessile leaves at the base; floral leaves bract-like, hairy, purple-margined, broadly ovate, acute, overlapping. Calyx tinged with purple, bell-shaped, 2-lipped; upperlip broad; 3-toothed; lower deeply 2-loved; mouth closed after flowering time. Corolla tube broad, slightly longer than the calyx; limb 2-lipped, upper lip erect, hood-like, notched; lower spreading, 3-lobed; middle lobe largest, minutely toothed, stamesn 4, in unequal pairs, ascending under the upper lip; filaments bearing a small tooth below the anthers. Fruit a collection of ovoid nutlets, smooth, 2-celled when young, splitting into 4 parts when mature, each part containing 1 seed.

Habitate: By roadsides and on forest edges.

Propagation: By seeds and vegetative method.

Part Used: Whole plant.

Chemical Constituents: N.A.

Uses: Dizziness due to hypertension; headache; tinnitus; conjunctivitis, dry cough, skin inflammation and boils. Expectorant and antispasmodic.

1032. *Prunus amygdalus* Batsch *(Rosaceae)*

Synonyms: *Prunus communis* Fritsch., *Amygdalus communis* Linn., *Prunus dulcis* (Miller) D. A. Webb.

Vernacular Name: *Eng*: Almond; *Hin*: Badam; *Kan*: Badamu; *Mal*: Badam Badamkotta; *San*: Vatadah, Vatamah; *Tam*: Vatamkottai; *Tel:* Badamvittulu.

Description: A middle sized tree upto 8 m in height; leaves simple, alternate grayish when fully grown, oblong-lanceolate minutely serrate; flowers white tinged with red, showy, appearing before the leaves or wit the early foliage from scaly buds; fruits velvety drupes about 3-6 cm long, separating into 2 valves on maturity exposing the compressed stones having minute holes, the stones enclose the valuable kernel.

Habitate: Cultivated in Kashmir and Punjab at an altitude of 760-2,400 m.

Propagation: By seeds and vegetative method.

Parts Used: Kernel, oil.

Chemical Consistuents: The chief protein of almond is a globulin, amandin an albumin is also reported. The essential amino acid make-up of amandin is; arginine, histidine, lysine, phenylalanine, leucine and valine. Tryptophan methionine and cystine are also present.

Uses: The kernel is sweet, thermogenic, emollient, aphrodisiac, laxative, diuretic, lithontriptic, nutritious, demulcent and nervine tonic. It is useful in cephalalgia, vitiated conditions of *pitta*, burning sensation, neuralgia, dysopia, cough, obstruction of the liver and spleen, amenorrhoea, otalgia, pharyngodynia, skin disease, pruritus, inflammation, ascites, colic, peptic ulcer, strangury, renal and vesical calculi and general debility. The oil is sweet, cooling antispasmodic, sedative, laxative, vulnerary and rejuvenating It is useful in hepatopathy, vitiated conditions of *pitta* and *vata*, delirium, cough, pharyngodynia, colic, wounds, ulcers, nephralgia,hepatodynia, splenalgia, gleet, otalgia, burning sensation, cracked skinand amentia.

1033. *Prunus armeniaca* L. *(Rosaceae)*

Vernacular Name: *Eng:* Apricot; common apricot; *Hin:* Azrdalu, khubani, chuari, kushmiaru.

Description: A medium-sized deciduous tree. Twiss glabrous. Leaves convoluted inbud, blade broadly ovate, 5-7 cm long by 3.805 cm wide, acuminate, crenate-glandular, hairy on the nerves beneath when young, sometimes sparsely hispid above; when mature glabrous except for the axils of the nerves beneath; petiole about 2.5 cm long, glanular; stipules lanceolate, glandular on the margins. Flowers in spring, pinkish at first then white, appearing before the leaves, solitary or fascicled, pedicle very short. Calyx-tube campanulate, puberulous. 5 mm long; loves rounded, pubescent, half the length of the tube. Petals sub-orbicular, 7.5-13 mm long. Stamens inserted at the mouth of the calyx-tube. Ovary and base of the style hairy. Drupe downy or glabrous, yellow tinged with red, stone smooth with a thickened sulcate margin.

The seed, used as a drug, is 1-1.9 cm long by 0.8-1.5 cm wide and 0.5-0.8 cm thick, and is flattened-cordate in shape; the taste is thin, brown and scurfy; one edge of the seed is more acute, the other more rounded, cotyledons 2, white, oily, odour none taste bitter.

Habitate: In mountains; commonly cultivated in China, India, Japan and Korea.

Propagation: By seeds and grafting.

Part Used: Seeds.

Chemical Constituents: The chief protein of almond is a globulin, amandin an albumin is also reported. The essential amino acid make-up of amandin is; arginine, histidine, lysine, phenylalanine, leucine and valine. Tryptophan methionine and cystine are also present.

Uses: Fruits edible. Kernels extracted during preparation of dry apricots are used for extraction of a fatty oil used for cooking, in pharmaceutical and cosmetic industry and for burning. Kernels of some varieties are sweet and eaten like almonds. Cake left after extraction of oil is used as manure or fuel; also yields an essential oil identical with Bitter Almond Oil, obtained from bitter almond cake. Apricot cake contains amygdalin and is unfit for use as cattle feed. French Almond Oil of commerce is practically pure apricot oil or its mixture with Peach Kernel Oil.

1034. *Prunus avium* *(Rosaceae)*

Vernacular Name: *Eng:* Sweet cherry.

Description: A tree up to 24 m. high, erect or pyramidal in habit; leaves oblong-ovate, acutely serrate, flowers in fascicles, white, long stalked, appearing with the leaves; fruits round, smooth, yellow, red or nearly black.

Habitate: Native to south-western Asia, sweet cherry is naturalized in Europe and cultivated in temperate regions around the world.

Propagation: By seeds and vegetative method.

Parts Used: Stems and fruit.

Chemical Constituents: The stems of sweet cherry contain phenols, including salicylic acid, and tannins. Cherry fruit contains small quantities of salicylates and cyanogenic glycosides, and vitamins A, B and C. The seeds also contain amygdalin, a cyanogenic glycoside.

Uses: In European herbal medicine, cherry stems have long been used for their diuretic and astringent properties. They have been prescribed for cystitis, nephritis, urinary retention and for arthritic problems, notably gout. Cherries can be a helpful part of an overall regime treating arthritic problems. Their high sugar content makes them mildly laxative.

1035. *Prunus cerasoides* D. Don *(Rosaceae)*

Synonyms: *Prunus puddum* (Wall.) Roxb. Ex Brandis.

Vernacular Name: *Eng*: Himalayan wild cherry, Bird cherry; *Hin*: Patmakath, Patmakh, Paddam; *Kan*: Padmaka; *Mal*: Patumukam, Patimukam, Patimukham; *San*: Padmakah, Padmagandhi; *Tam*: Patumugam; *Tel:* Padmakla.

Description: A medium sized or large tree with pale red wood and smooth brown bark peeling off in horizontal strips exposing a shining copper-coloured surface; leaves simple, alternate, glossy, ovate, long, acuminate, doubly-serrate, one or more conspicuous glands on the petiole; flowers white, pink or crimson in fascicles or umbels; fruits ovoid or globose drupes, yellow or red, stone ovoid, rugose and furrowed.

Habitate: In the Himalayas, at an attitude of 900 to 2,300 m.

Propagation: By seeds and vegetative method.

Parts Used: Heartwood.

Chemical Consisituents: N.A.

Uses: The heartwood is astringent, bitter, acrid anodyne, refrigerant, vulnerary, demulcent, digestive, constipating, diuretic, emmenagogue, depurative, antipyretic, and tonic. It is useful in vitiated conditions of *pitta*, burning sensation, sprains, neuralgia, wounds, ulcers, leprosy, skin decolourations, pruritus, dyspepsia, diarrhoea, strangury, amenorrhoea, dysmenorrhoea, erysipelas, hiccough, asthma, vomiting, ophthalmopathy, cephalalgia, cardiac debility, hallucinations and intermittent fevers.

1036. *Prunus domestica* L. *(Rosaceae)*

Synonyms: *Prunus communis* Huds.

Vernacular Name: *Eng*: Common plum, *Hin*: Alubukhara, *Kan*: Albokhala, *Mal*: Arukam, Plums, *San*: Arukam,Plums, *Tam*: Aluppukkarappalam, *Tel:* Alpagodapandu.

Description: An unarmed small tree upto 12 m in height with glabrous branches; leaves simple, large, alternate, dull green, coarsely serrate, wrinkled, ovate to obovate, obtuse; flowers white or cream-coloured, single, in pairs or in clusters on spurs along the branches; fruits drupes, varying in colours from green and golden yellow to red and dark purple; shape varying to a great extent, stones large, rough or pitted.

Habitate: Cultivated at high altitudes in Nilgiris and Himachal Pradesh.

Propagation: By seeds and vegetative method.

Parts Used: Fruits.

Chemical Consisituents: D-galactose, D-mannose, L-arabinose, D-xylose, L-rhamnose, glucuronic acid and probably traces of 4-O-methyl-glucuronic acid. The heartwood contains the flavonoid, kaempferol, dihydrokaempferol, kaempferide, dihydrokaempferide, and prudomestin, besides a leucoanthocyanidin.

Uses: The fruits are sweet, laxative, refrigerant, appestising, stomachic, digestive and tonic. They are useful in vitiated conditions of *pitta* dipsia, nausea, flatulence, colic, dyspepsia, and debility.

1037. *Prunus japonica* var. nakaii (Lev.) Rehder *(Rosaceae)*

Vernacular Name: *Eng*: Japanese bush berry, Japanese plum.

Description: Deciduous small shrub, to 1 m tall. Branches fine, elongate, often puberulent while young, glabrous. Leaves alternate, petiolate, ovate to ovate-oblong, sharply serrate, 2-7 cm long, long-pointed, glabrous above, pubescent beneath on the veins. Flowers before or with leaves, 2-4, in umbels, pale pink, to 2 cm in diameter; pedicels 1.7-2.2 mm long, with hairs or glabrous. Fruit glabose, red, glabrous; the stone globose, pointed at the ends, 12 mm long.

Habitate: Woods in mountains and hills.

Propagation: By seeds and vegetative method.

Parts Used: Seeds.

Chemical Constituents: Amygdalins. Saponins. Flavonoids; prunuside.

Uses: Used in constipation, laryngitis and acute gastritis. Purgative, deuretic.

1038. *Prunus mume* Siebold et Zucc. *(Rosaceae)*

Vernacular Name: *Eng*: Japanese apricot, Japanese flowering apricot.

Description: Round-crowned tree, up to 10 m tall. Twigs thin, green. Leaves alternate, ovate to elliptic, long-pointed, 3-10 cm long, sharply serrulate, pubescent beneath, at least on veins. Flowers 1-2, white to dark red, to 3 cm across; sepals and petals 5; stamens many, inserted with the petals on the calyx tube; pistil 1, with 2 ovules. Fruit roundd, 3 cm in diameter, yellow to greenish, slightly pubescent, sour and bitter; the stone furrowed.

Habitate: Mostly cultivated and naturalized, mountain woods.

Propagation: By seeds and vegetative method.

Parts Used: Fruit.

Chemical Constituents: Various organic esters, alcohols and acids. Amygdalin.

Uses: Broad spectrum antibacterial activity, antifungal, antiallergy, antioxidant. Used in bronchitis and cough.

1039. *Prunus persica* (L.) Batsch. *(Rosaceae)*

Synonyms: *Perscia vulgaris* Mill; *Prunus devidiana* (Carr.) Franch.

Vernacular Name: *Eng:* Peach, Nectarine and *Hin:* Aru, Shaftalu.

Description: A large deciduous shrub or small tree up to 8 m high. Stem erect, branched twigs glabrous; special dwarf shoots bear flowers or else the flowers arise from long branches. Leaves exstipulate, subsessile with many pairs of glands at the base of each leaf-blade; alternate, simple, elliptic-lanceolate, 8-15 cm long; apex acute; margin serrulate, glabrous. Flower, cup-shapoed, appearing before or with the leaves. Calyx a campanulate tube, 5-lobed; petals, pink, stamens many, as long as the petals. Carpel one. Fruit a flrshy and downy drupe enclosing a hard furrowed one-seeded stone.

Habitate: Commonly cultivated in China, India and Japan.

Propagation: By seeds and vegetative method.

Part Used: Seeds.

Chemical Constituents: Sugars, thiamine, ascorbic acid, vitamin A.

Uses: Peaches are favourite table fruits. Freestone peaches are soft and juicy when ripe and used as dessert; clingstone peaches are hard-fleshed and inedible, but are delicious on cooking in syrup, mostly used for canning. Peaches are used in beverages and for peach brandy and are a fair source of sugar, thiamine, and ascorbic acid; some types contain appreciable quantities of vitamin A. kernels yield a fatty oil, called Leaves yield a volatile oil. Infusion of leaves or bark given for whooping cough. Flowers anthelmintic. Root-bark yields a dye. Used in dysmenorrhoea; amenorrhoea, contusions and strains, constipation.

1040. *Prunus serotina* *(Rosaceae)*

Vernacular Name: *Eng:* Wild Cherry.

Description: Deciduous tree growing to 30m. Has elliptical to oblong leaves, white flowers and purple-black fruit.

Habitate: Native to North America, wild cherry grows throughout much of the US.

Propagation: By seeds and vegetative method.

Parts Used: Inner bark.

Chemical Constituents: Whild cherry contains prunasin, benzaldehyde, eudesmic acid, coumarins and tannins. Prunasin reduces the cough reflex.

Uses: Figuring in official pharmacopoeias and much used in the Anglo-American tradition, wild cherry bark is an effective remedy for chronic dry and irritable coughs. it combines well with coltsfoot as a treatment for asthma and whooping cough. The astringent bark also helps treat indigestion and the symptoms of irritable bowel syndrome, especially when these conditions are of nervous origin.

1041. *Pseudarthria viscida* (L.) Wight & Arn. *(Fabaceae)*

Vernacular Name: *Hin*: Chapakno; *Mal*: Muvvila; *San*: *San*aparni; *Tam*: Nirmalli, Muvilai; *Tel:* Muyyakuponna.

Description: A perennial viscid pubescent semi-erect diffuse undershrub, 60-120 cm long with slender branches, more or less clothed with whitish hairs; leaves 3-foliate, terminal leaflet rhomboid-ovate, the lateral ones obliquely ovate-oblong or subrhomboid, all more or less hairy above and densely grey-silky beneath; flowers purplish or pink, small, numerous, in distant fasciles along the rachis of terminal and axillary racemes or panicles; fruits pods, linear-oblong, flattened, covered with sticky hairs, seeds 4-6, compressed, brownish black.

Habitate: Throughout south India, upto 900 m in the hills, also in Gujarat.

Propagation: By seeds and vegetative method.

Parts Used: Roots.

Chemical Consistuents: N.A.

Uses: The roots are astringent, sweet, bitter, thermogenic, emollient, digestive constipating anthelmintic, nervine, tonic, anti-inflammatory, diuretic, cardiotonic, aphrodisiac, febrifuge, rejuvenating and tonic. They are useful in vitiated conditions of *pitta* and *vata*, cough, bronchitis, asthma, tuberculosis, helminthiasis, dyspepsia, diarrhoea, neurasthenia, inflammations, strangury, cardiopathy, fever, emaciation, haemorrhoids, gout, diabetes,hyperthemia, and general debility.

1042. *Psidium guajava* L. *(Myrtaceae)*

Vernacular Name: *San:* Mansala; *Eng:* Guava; *Hin:* Amrud, safed safari; *Beng*: Goaachhi, peyara, piyara; *Tel:* Ettajama, goyya, tellajama; *Tam:* Koyya; *Kan:* Sebe hannu, jam phala; *Mal:* Pera koyya.

Description: Shrub or small tree upto 10 m high with thin, smooth, patchy, peeling bark. Leaves opposite, short-petiolate, the blade oval with prominent pinnate veins, 5-15 cm long. Flowers somewhat showy, 4-5 merous, petals whitish and up to 2 cm long, stamens numerous Fruit a fleshy yellow globose to ovoid berry about 5 cm in diameter with an edible pink mesocarp containing numerous small hard white seeds.

Habitate: Common in disturbed places often forming thickets in pastures, plantations and other similar habitats.

Propagation: By seeds and vegetative method.

Part Used: Leaves, fruits and root.

Chemical Constituents: Tannins, vitamins B and C, 18 sesquiterpenes, 11 monoterpense, eugenol, quercetin, quaverin, gallic acid, lipids (seeds), Asiatic acid, brahmic acid, lupeol, maslinic acids, oleanolic acid, ellagic acid, derivatives, eugenol, catechin, amritoside, amyrins, arjunolic acid, trans-cinnamic acid, benzaldehyde, butyl acetate, daucosterol, acetyl furan, furfural derivatives, leucocyanidin, procyanidins, paramethylstyrene, ursolica acid derivatives, valeraldehyde, and alkaloids zeatin and zeatin nucleotide.

Uses: Juice from the leaves is used for treating diarrhoea, coughs, stomachache and dysentery. The leaves are pounded, squeezed in salt water and the solution is used to treat toothaches. An infusion of the leaves and roots is used to treat indigestion. The fruit is eaten to cure constipation. Tahitians use the plant in a treatment for skin tonic, as well as for painful menstruation, miscarriages, uterine bleeding and premature labour in women.

1043. *Psoralea corylifolia* L. *(Fabaceae)*

Vernacular Name: *San:* Bakuchi, kushthanashini, sugandhakantak; *Eng:* Malay tea scur pea; bawchee seed plant; *Hin:* Babchi, bavanchi, bukchi; *Beng*: Bavachi, kakuch, latakasturi; *Tel:* Baavanchalu, bapunga, bawuchee; *Tam:* Kaarboka arisi, karporgam; *Kan:* Bavanchigida, karbekhiga; *Mal:* Karpokkari, kaurkoalari.

Description: An erect annual herb, up to 90 cm high, wide blackish glands, leaves distinctly petioled, roundish-oval, 6-9 cm long by 5-7 cm wide; apex slightly acute; base truncate or slightly cordate, dentate at margin, both faces conspicuously dotted with black dots, nearly glabrescent. Flowers 10-30 in abundant dense long-peduncled heads. Calyx cupuliform, teeth 5, lanceolate, the lowest longest. Corolla yellow, little exserted. Stamens 10, ovary sessile. Fruit an oval pod, short, dry, indehiscent, black, glabrous, surrounded by the persistent calyx.

Habitate: On plains, in tussocks along streams but mostly cultivated in China. Found on waste places in many parts of India.

Propagation: By seeds and vegetative method.

Part Used: Seeds and fruits.

Chemical Constituents: Seeds yield raffinose, psoralen, isopsoralen, corylifolean, corylifolin, corylifolinin, psoralidin, isopsoralidin, bakuchiol, bavachin, isobavachin, 7-O-methylbavachin, bavachinin, 4-O-methylbavachalcone, isobavachalcone, neobavaisoflavone, bavachromene, traincontane, β-sitosterol-D-glucoside, corylidin, bavachalcone, isobavachalcone, neobavachalcone, bakuchalcone, isoneobavachalcone, psoralidin-2, 3-oxide diacetate and stigmasterol. limonene, αelemene, β-caryophylenoxide, 4-terpineol, linalool, geranylacetate, angelicin, psoralene, and bakuchiol are reported from the seed oil.

Uses: Diarrhoea due to poor health, enuresis in old men, frequent micturition, seminal emissions; impotence, lumbago and weakness in the legs, cough due to cold, vitiligo, psoriasis, tinea capitis, corns. Fruits commonly called seeds, are laxative, diuretic, diaphoretic, and aphrodisiac, specially recommended for leucoderma, leprosy, psoriasis, and inflammatory diseases of skin; used both internally and externally.

1044. *Psychotria insularum* A. Gray. *(Rubiaceae)*

Description: Small tree up to 4 m high. Leaves opposite, elliptical and 10-20 cm long. Flowers borne on narrow pedicels in branching axillary or terminal, cymose clusters. The corolla is tubular (4-8 mm long), 5-lobed, with 5 epipetalous stamens. Fruit a red oval beery up to 1 cm long with two longitudinally ribbed seeds.

Habitate: Occurs in coastal to lowland forest but is also found in cloud forests up to 1000 m.

Propagation: By seeds and vegetative method.

Part Used: Leaves.

Chemical Constituents: N.A.

Uses: It is used as remedies for piles inside the stomach or for stomach cancer, for appendicitis, heart attack, infertility, high blood pressure, shortness of breath in the lower chest and back pain. The plant is used to cure toothache and pig bites. The leaf infusion is also used for some types of swellings and inflammations which are though to have a supernatural origin.

1045. *Pterocarpus marsupium* Roxb. *(Fabaceae)*

Vernacular Name: *Eng*: Indian kino tree Malabar kino tree; *Hin*: Bijasal, Vijayasar, Bija; *Kan*: Hannemara; *Mal*: Venna; *San*: Asanah, Bijakah; *Tam*: Vengai; *Tel:* Beddagi, Asana.

Description: A medium sized to large tree, 15-30 m in height with dark brown of grey bark having shallow cracks, exfoliating in thin flakes and exuding a red gummy substance (Gum kino) on injury; leaves compound, imparipinnate, leaflets 5-7 coriaceous, oblong, obtuse, emarginated or even bilobed at apex, glabrous on both surfaces mina nervesnumerous, prominent; flowers yellow in terminal panicles, corolla with crisped margins; fruits nearly circular, glabrous, flat winged pods, convexly curved between stipe and style, wings veined, seeds, 1-2, convex bony.

Habitate: Throughout India, in deciduous and evergreen forests.

Propagation: By seeds and vegetative method.

Parts Used: Heartwood, leaves, flowers, gum.

Chemical Consistuents: *l*-epicatechin. The heartwood yields liquiritigenin, *iso*liquiritigenin, a neutral unidentified component, alkaloid an dresin. The wood also contains a yellow colouring matter and an essential oil and a semi-drying fixed oil. Kino contains a non-glucosidal tannin kinotannic acid, kinoin, and kino-red in addition to small quantities of catechol protocatechuic acid resin, pectin and gallic acid.

Uses: The heartwood is astringent, bitter, acrid, cooling, anti-inflammatory, union-promoter, depurative, urinary astringent, haemostatic,revulsive, anthelmintic, constipating, anodyne, alterant and elephantiasis, inflammations, fractures, bruises, leprosy, skin diseases, leucoderma, erysipelas, urethrorrhea, diabetes, rectalgia, rectitis, ophthalmopathy, haemorrhages, verminosis, diarrhoea, dysentery, odontalgia, gout, rheumatoid arthritis, cough, asthma, bronchitis and greyness of hairs. The leaves are useful in boils, sores and skin diseases. The flowers are bitter, sweet, cooling, appetizing and febrifuge, and are useful in vitiated conditions of *pitta,* anorexia and fevers. The gum is biter, styptic, vulnerary, antipyretic, anthelmintic and liver tonic. It is useful in spasmodic gastralgia, vitiated conditions of *pitta,* boils, gleet, urethrorrhea, odontalgia, diarrhoea, psoriasis, wounds and ulcers, helminthiasis, intermittent fevers, hepatopathy and ophthalmia.

1046. *Pterocarpus Santalinus* L.f. *(Fabaceae)*

Vernacular Name: *Eng:* Red Sandal wood; *Hin:* Lal chandan, Rakta-chandan; *Kan:* Agaru, Honne; *Mal:* Patrangam, Tilaparnni; *Mar:* Tambada chandana; *San*: Rakta chandana; *Tam:* Ratha Sandanam, Chenkunkumam, Sivappu chandanam, Sandana vengai; *Tel:* Agaru gandhamu, Yerra chandanamu, Rakta chandanam.

Description: Trees about 12 m height. *Bark* blackish brown, 1-1.5 cm thick, deeply cleft into rectangular plates by deep vertical and horizontal cracks. *Blaze* pale yellow with numerous pink streaks exuding copious red sticky thick gum. Branchlets drooping, hairless. Leaves 3-foliolate, 10-18 cm long; rachis swollen at base; *leaflets* usually 3, rarely 4 or 5, broadly egg-shaped or orbicular, 7-12 x 4-8 cm, base round or slightly heart-shaped, apex rounded or deeply notched, margin entire, leathery, shiny, hairless, distinctly stalked. *Flowers* bisexual, stalked, in axillary simple or sparingly branched racemes, yellow, about 2 cm long, fragrant. *Pods* unequally orbicular, flat, about 5 x 4.5 cm including the wing, gradually narrowed in to a short tip which is about1 cm long. *Seeds* 1 rarely 2, more or less kidney-shaped, 1-1.5 cm long, smooth, reddish brown.

Habitate: The drier, hilly zones of dry deciduous forests.

Propagation: By seeds and vegetative method.

Parts Used: Heart-wood.

Chemical Constituents: *San*talin quinonoid structure. The wood contains desoxy*San*talin supposed to be a naphthaquinonoid derivative, the yellow isoflavone *San*tal, and two unidentified pigments A and B, beside three colourless substances, viz., pterostilbene, ptterocarpin and homopterocarpin.

Uses: One of the ingredients of *Triphaladya ghrta*, used to cure chronic fever. The heartwood is rubbed with water, honey, ghee and oil, applied as collyrium to alleviate defects of vision. Also used for treating skin diseases, bone fracture, leprosy, spider poisoning, scorpion sting, hiccough, ulcers, general debility and mental aberrations. Wood paste applied on boils and other skin eruptions, infections, inflammation and on forehead to relieve headache. Decoction of fruits is used to cure chronic dysentery; also used by *Kani* tribes to check dermatological conditions including psoriasis. Wood and bark brew taken orally relieves chronic dysentery, worms, blood vomiting, weak vision and hallucination. Wood powder is used to control haemorrhage, bleeding piles and inflammation.

1047. *Pueraria lobata* (Willd.) Ohwi. *(Fabaceae)*

Synonyms: *Purerarla thunbergiana* (Sieb. & Zucc.); *Purerarla hirsuts* (Thunb.) Schneid.

Vernacular Name: *Eng:* Lobed kudzuvine; kudzu hemp.

Description: A hairy, twining perennial vine up to 8 m long. The root is cylindrical and sometimes reaches a length of 2 m. the stem bristles with rough brown hair. Leaves pinnate-trifoliate; leaflets entire or slightly lobate, the central leaflet 5.5-19 cm long by 4.5-18 cm wide, the lateral leaflets smaller, pubescent; petiole 10-20 cm long. Inflorescence an axillary or terminal raceme, dense, erect, nearly 25 cm long. Flower purplish-red, 1.5 cm long; July-September, calyx 5-toothed. Petals 5, nearly regular, stamens 10, monadelphous. Fruit a linear pod, straight, compressed, 5-12 cm long by 6-15 mm wide, hirsute, yellowish-brown.

Habitate: China, Japan.

Propagation: By roots.

Part Used: Roots.

Chemical Constituents: Protein, carbohydrate glucoside, daidzin.

Uses: Common cold with fever, thirst, acute gastro-enteritis; diarrhoea, palpitation. Tuberous roots may attain a weight up to 35kg or even more and are eaten as a vegetable after boiling. Dried roots are a source of starch which resembles cassava starch and may be used as food or in medicine (digestibility 21.9%. In China and Japan a kind of flour called Ko-fen is made from the roots; it is sweet and odourless used in soups. Decoction of root given in colds and dysentery and as a febrifuge. Shoots used as a lactagogue.

1048. *Pueraria tuberosa* (Roxb. ex Willd.) DC. *(Fabaceae)*

Vernacular Name: *Eng*: Indian kudzu, *Hin:* Viddarikand, Tirra, Sural, bilaikand, *Kan*: Gumadi gida, *Mal*: Palmutukku, *Mar*: Badra, *San*: Vidari, Vidarika, *Tam:* Darigummadi, Niala-gumodi, *Tel:* Dari, Gumidi.

Description: A large woody deciduous climbing shrub with huge tuberous root. *Tubers* globose or pot-like, about 25 cm across, white inside, starchy and mildly sweet. Branchlets with dense appressed velvety hairs. Leaves alternate, 3-foliolate; *leaflets* egg-shaped, about 18 x 16 cm, base rounded and unequal sided, apex acuminate, margin with fringed hairs, hairless above, densely pubescent below; leaf stalks up to 18 cm long; lateral nerves 7-8 pairs. *Flowers* bisexual, about 1.5 cm across, bluish purple to pale violet, shortly stalked, densely arranged in 15-25 cm long axillary panicles. *Pods* linear, 2-5 cm long, distinctly constricted between the seeds covered with dense bristly reddish brown hairs. *Seeds* 3-6.

Habitate: Dry deciduous to moist deciduous forests.

Propagation: By tubers, seeds, divisions and layers.

Parts Used: Tubers.

Chemical Constituents: Dry matter total carbohydrates, crude fibre, crude protein, ether extr, β-Sitosterol, sucrose, glucose and fructose have been identified.

Uses: Tubers used for treatment of dysuria, cough, rheumatism, erysipelas and malarial fever. The roots are said to be used in medicine as a demulcent and refrigerant in fevers as cataplasam for swellings of joints and as lactagogue.

1049. *Pulmonaria officinalis* *(Boraginaceae)*

Vernacular Name: *Eng:* Lungwort.

Description: Perennial growing to 30 cm. Has broad oval basal leaves, smaller upper leaves mottled with white spots, and clusters of pink-purple flowers.

Habitate: Lungwrot is native to Europe and the Caucasus.

Propagation: By seeds and vegetative method.

Parts Used: Leaves.

Chemical Constituents: Lungwort contains allantoin, flavonoids, tannins, mucilage, saponin and vitamin C. Unlike many of its relatives in the borage family, it does not contain.

Uses: Given its high mucilage content, lungwort is indeed a useful remedy for chest conditions, and it is particularly beneficial in cases of chronic bronchitis. It combines well with herbs such as coltsfoot as a treatment for chronic coughs and it can be taken for asthma. Lungwrot can also be used as a treatment for sore throats and catarrh. In the past, lungwort was given for the coughing up of blood arising from tubercular infection. Lungwort leaves are astringent, and have been applied externally to stop bleeding.

1050. *Pulsatilla chinesis* (Bunge) Regel . *(Ranunculaceae)*

Vernacular Name: *Eng:* Chinese pulsatilla.

Description: A perennial herb. Basal leaves 4-5, oval 4.5-14 cm long by 8.5-16 cm wide, divided feather-faschionl petiole 5-10 cm, densely covered with white long hairs; lateral leaflets 2, opposite, incised-lobate, coarsely dentate, sessile the terminal leaflet tripartite, petioluate, pubescent underneath. April-May. Scapes 1-2, 15-35 cm high. Flowers large, solitary, 2.5-5.0 cm in diameter; sepals 6; outside covered with white silky hairs; inside purple; no petals; stamens very numerous; styles accrete, plumose, after flowering the styles elongate and become covered with silvery hairs, cluster to form a glove and scatter a maturity.

Habitate: On grassy slopes in low hills, in thickets.

Propagation: By seeds and vegetative method.

Part Used: Roots.

Chemical Constituents: N.A.

Uses: Amoebic dysentery, leucorrhoes. Pharmacological studies show that Chinese pulsatilla decoction inhibits the growth of amoeba.

1051. *Pulsatilla koreana* Nakai *(Ranunculaceae)*

Vernacular Name: *Eng*: Korean pasque flower.

Description: Hairy, tufted, perennial herb. Leaves long-stalked in a basal rosette, pinnately compound; leaflets 5, white-wooly pubescent beneath, 3-4 cm long, 2-3 lobed. Flowers solitary, terminal on peduncle 30-40 cm long, scapose, pendent; perianth campanulate, 35 mm long, 12 mm across, red-purple, segments 6, petal-like, exterior selky; stamens in a central boss surrounded by a ring of staminoids. Fruit heads with long feather styles.

Habitate: Open wastelands and grassy places.

Propagation: By seeds and vegetative method.

Parts Used: Root.

Chemical Constituents: Protoanemonin, anemonin, saponins, hederagenin monodesmoside, hederagenin bisdesmoside.

Uses: Used in leucorrhoea, dysentery, scrofula, antiparasitic. Anemonin is a cardiotoxin and cardiotonic. Antiamoebal, antitrichomonas, antibacterial.

1052. *Punica granatum* L. *(Puniacaceae)*

Vernacular Name: *San:* Dadima; *Eng:* Pomegranate; *Hin:* Anar; *Beng*: Dalim; *Kan:* Dalimba; *Tel:* Danimma; *Tam:* Madulai; *Mal:* Matalam.

Description: Shrub to small tree up to 6 m high. Leaves mostly opposite, short-petiolate, blades oblong-elliptical up to 8 cm long. Flowers showy and up to 6 cm broad, bisexual, 5-8 petals, reddish and up to 2.5 cm long, numerous stamens surrounding a conspicuous hypanthial tube, the flowers usually occurring terminally or in axils. Fruit a red spherical berry. Flowers available during the summer.

Habitate: Commonly cultivated as an ornamental and fruit tree; possible naturalized in some areas.

Propagation: By seeds and vegetative method.

Part Used: Seeds and flowers.

Chemical Constituents: Apigenin glucoside, betulinic acid, callistephin, tannins, chrysanthemin, coniine, coumestrol, cyaniding and its diglucoside, cyanin, diadzein, diadzin, delphin,m delphinidin and its glucosides, ellagic acid and its deriative, estrone, freidelin, gallic acid, genistein, genistin, lipids, hygrine and norhygrine, luteolin glycosides, mannitol, pelargonin, pelletierine and its derivative, piperidine derivatives, polyphenols, sedridine, xanthoxylin, estradiol.

Uses: A decoction of the seed is used to treat syphilis. Juice of the fruit is used to treat jaundice and diarrhoes. The rind of the fruit is ground in water and drunk every morning by diabetics. The fruit together with the juice of *Cynodon dactylon* leaves is used for runny noses and olds. The juice of the flowers is used to treat nose bleeds. The fruit pulp and the seed are a stomachic. The root and the stem bark have astringent and anthelmintic properties.

1053. *Pygeum africanum* *(Boraginacae)*

Vernacular Name: *Eng:* Pygeum.

Description: Evergreen tree growing to 35m. Has oblong leaves, white flowers and red berries.

Habitate: Pygeum is native to Africa.

Propagation: By seeds and vegetative method.

Parts Used: Bark.

Chemical Constituents: Pygeum contains phytosterols, triterpenes, long chain alcohols and tannins.

Uses: In conventional medicine in France, the fat-soluble extract of pygeum bark has become the primary treatment for an enlarged prostate gland. In combination with other plants, pygeum may be valuable in the treatment of prostatic cancer.

1054. *Pyrrosia lingua* (Thunb.) Farw. *(Polypodiaceae)*

Vernacular Name: *Eng*: Tongue fern, Japanese felt fern.

Description: Scandent, epiphytic fern. Rhizomes wide-creeping, 3 mm in diameter, covered with stalked scales. Stipes 5-25 cm long, straw coloured, densely brown stellate hairy while young. Blades leathery, simple, lanceolate or ovate-lanceolate, covered with stellate hairs beneath; the sterile ones 10-25 cm long, 2-7 cm wide; the fertile ones 10-20 cm long, 1.5-3 cm wide. Costa raides beneath, the veins and veinlets concealed. Sori covering lower surface of leaves, indusia lacking.

Habitate: Rocks and old tree trunks in mountains China, Japan, and Indo-China.

Propagation: By Roots suckers.

Parts Used: Aerial part.

Chemical Constituents: Diplotene, chlorogenic acid, isomangiferin, mangiferin.

Uses: Antibacterial, antitussive, expectorant, antiasthmatic, hypolipidaemic (chlorogenic acid). Used in bloody urine and haemostasis.

1055. *Quercus robur* *(Fagaceae)*

Vernacular Name: *Eng:* Common oak.

Description: Slow-growing, long-lived deciduous tree reaching 45m. Hs deeply lobed leaves, long catkins and green to brown fruit.

Habitate: Common oak grows throughout the northern hemisphere, in woods, forests and long hedgerows.

Propagation: By seeds and vegetative method.

Parts Used: Bark, galls.

Chemical Constituents: Common oak bark contains 15-20% tannins. Oak galls contain about 50% tannins.

Uses: Common oak bark, prepared as a decoction, is used as a gargle to treat sore throats and tonsillitis. It may also be applied as a wash, lotion or ointment to treat haemorrhoids, annual fissures, small burns and other skin problems less commonly, a decoction of the bark is taken in small doses to treat diarrhoea, dysentery and rectal bleeding. Powdered oak bark may be sniffed to treat nasal polyps, or sprinkled on eczema to dry the affected area. Oak galls are very astringent. They are used, in small quantities, in place of bark.

1056. *Quillaja saponaria* *(Rosaceae)*

Vernacular Name: *Eng:* Soap bark.

Description: Evergreen tree growing to 20 m. Has glossy oval leaves, white flowers and star-shaped fruit.

Habitate: Soap bark is native to Chile and Peru, and is now cultivated in California and India for medicinal and industrial use.

Propagation: By seeds and vegetative method.

Parts Used: Inner bark.

Chemical Constituents: Soap bark contains up to 10% triterpenoid saponins, calcium oxalate and tannins. the saponins are strongly expectorant and can cause inflammation of the digestive tract.

Uses: Soap bark has a long tradition of use as a treatment for chest problems. Its strong expectorant effect is beneficial in the treatment of bronchitis, especially in the early stages of the illness. Like other medicinal plants that contain saponins, soap bark stimulates the production of a more fluid mucus in the airways, facilitating the clearing of phlegm through coughing. Soap bark is useful for treating any condition featuring congested catarrh within the chest, but it should not be used for dry irritable coughs. Soap bark is also used externally, appearing in the formulations of dandruff shampoos.

1057. *Quisqualis indica* L. *(Combretaceae)*

Synonyms: *Quisqualis densiflora* Wall. ex. Miq.

Vernacular Name: *Eng:* Rangoon creeper; *Hin:* Rangoon-ki-bel; *Tel:* Ettaguttilativva, rangonimalle, tige-ganneru and *Tam:* Irangunmalli, ilengaramalligai.

Description: A woody vine, 2-7 m long. Leaves opposite, petiolate oval or elliptic, 5-15 cm long by 2.6 cm wide; apex briefly acuminate; base broad-cuneate, rounded or nearly cordate, glabrous above, hairy beneath; nerves 6-8 pairs, membranous; petioles 7.5 mm long. Inflorescence a compact terminal spike 4-10 cm long; pubescent. Summer. Calyx a 5-lobed tube, green, pubescent. Petals 5, lanceolate, acute, white changing to pink. Stamens 10. Ovary cylindrical-fusiform, 5-angled, villous, glandular. Fruit a dry capsule, 5-sided, chestnut-brown, leathery, monospermous, tardily dehiscent.

Habitate: In forests and mountains in China, India, Laos, Malaysia, Philippines and Viet Nam.

Propagation: By seeds and vegetative method.

Part Used: Seeds.

Chemical Constituents: The kernels contain a fatty oil consisting of myristic, palmitic, stearic, oleic and linoleic acids; potassium salt of quisqualic acid; trigonelline, and phytosterols. The flowers yield cyaniding monoglucoside.

Uses: Ascariasis, ringworm disease, infant, malnutrition. Fruits and seeds anthelmintic; seeds soporific also. Ripe seeds roasted and given in diarrhoea and fever, also used in rickets. Macerated in oil, seeds used for application in parasitic skin troubles. Seeds yield a fatty oil with purgative action. Young shoots eaten raw or steamed. Long flexible stems used for basketry, flsh-weirs, and fish-traps. A native of tropical Africa and Indo-Malaysian region, grown in gardens throughout India.

1058. *Randia dumetorum* Lam. *(Rubiaceae)*

Synonyms: *Xeromphis spinosa* (Thunb.).

Vernacular Name: *San:* Madanab; *Eng:* Emetic nut tree, Common emetic nut; *Hin*: Mainphal, Madan; *Kan:* Banegaru, Kare, Mangarike, Mangri; *Mal:* Malankara, Karacculli; *Tam:* Madkarai, Marukkalankay; *Tel:* Manga, Marrga, Manda.

Description: A large deciduous armed shrub upto 9.0m in height with strong straight spines, horizontal rigid branches and dark brown or grey rough scaly bark; leaves simple, usually fascicled on the suppressed branches, obovate, obtuse, wrinkled, shining or more or less pubescent above and on nerves beneath, main nerves 6-10 pairs; flowers at first white, later turning yellow, fragrant, solitary or 2-3 together at the ends of short leaf-bearing branchless; fruits globose or broadly ovoid, smooth or obscurely longitudinally ribbed berries, yellow when ripe, crowned with the large calyx limb; seeds many, angular, embedded in the pulp.

Habitate: Throughout India in deciduous forests and exposed areas upto an elevation of 1.350m.

Propagation: By seeds and vegetative method.

Parts Used: Bark, fruits.

Chemical Constituents: Saponin, valerianic acids, vax, resin, colouring matter, d-mannitol and essential oil. A new glycoside and lupeol have been isolated from the ripe fruit. Bark gave randialic acid-A and randialic acid-B; whereas root contains scopolatin and d-mannitol. Pulp contains citric and tartaric acid, tannins, pectin, mucilage, saponins, dumetaronins and free sugars.

Uses: The bark is astringent, emetic, abortifacient, anodyne, constipating and antiseptic, and is useful in ostalgia during fever, diarrhoea, dysentery, bruises, cuts and vitiated conditions of *vata*. The fruits are bitter, astringent, acrid, sweet, thermogenic, emetic, anodyne, anti-inflammatory, carminative, anthelmintic, depurative, vulnerary, emmenagogue, expectorant, febrifuge, sudorific, abortifacient and antispasmodic, and are useful in vitiated conditions of *pitta* and *kapha*, pains and sprains, inflammations, gout, helminthiasis, leprosy, skin diseases, wounds, ulcers, tumours, amenorrhoea, dysmenorrhoea, cough, asthma, bronchitis, flatulence, colic, constipation and fever.

1059. *Ranunculus ficaria* *(Ranunculaceae)*

Vernacular Name: *Eng:* Lesser celandine, Pilewort.

Description: Mat-forming perennial growing to 15 cm. Has small tubers, fleshy heart-shaped leaves and shiny-petalled, brilliant yellow flowers.

Habitate: Lesser celandine in native to western Asia, North Africa and Europe.

Propagation: By cutting.

Parts Used: Aerial parts.

Chemical Constituents: Lesser celandine contains saponins, protoanemonin and anemonin, tannins and vitamin C. Protoanemonin is antibacterial and irritant; it is absent from the dried herb.

Uses: Lesser celandine makes a useful ointment or suppository for treating haemorrhoids.

1060. *Ranunculus sceleratus* L. *(Ranunculaceae)*

Synonyms: *Ranunculus umbellatus* Roxb ex. willd., *Ranunculus digitatus* Gilib., *Ranunculus carnosus* Wall.

Vernacular Name: *Eng:* Blister butter cup., Celery-leaved butter cup.

Description: An erect glabrous, much branched annual, up to 70 cm. in height. Leaves alternate, petionlate, upper ones simple, crenate, or of 3 linear-oblong segments; lower ones usually 3-partite, segments cuneate and again variously lobed or notched; cauline leaves sessile. Stem hollow, furrowed and glabrous. Flowers bracteate, bisexual, numerous, in cymose inflorescence with sepals 5, petaloid; petals 5, obovate; nectary present at the base of each petal; stamens many polyandrous; receptacle hairy.

Habitate: Wet patches in India, Asia, Europe and United States.

Propagation: By seeds and vegetative method.

Parts Used: Whole plant.

Chemical Constituents: Anemonin, Protoanemonin.

Uses: For complaints of boring and gnawing pain at one sport on left of vertex. Skin vesicular eruptions, with tendency to form large blisters, with acrid exudations, which makes surrounding part sore. Boring pain in extremities. Sudden burning sticking in right toes. Corns with burning and soreness. Bruised pain in chest with sore burning behind xiphoid cartilage. Sensation of a plug behind umblicus, with sensitiveness & pain over live region.

1061. *Raphanus sativus* L. *(Cruciferae)*

Vernacular Name: *San*: Moolaka; *Hin:* Muli; *Guj*: Moli, Mula, mura; *Tel:* Mullangi; *Tam*: Mullangi; *Kan*: Mullangi; *Mal*: Mullangi.

Description: Small root annual, growing rapidly. *Stem* 0.2-0.6 cm high, flexuose, fistular, branched in the upper part, glabrous or hispid. Lower *leaves* on hairy petioles 3 cm long. Lyrate-pinnatifid 3-4 rarely 5 jugate, terminal lobe, suborbicular or shortly ovate, rounded at the apex, with the margin crenate, and more or less confluent ith lateral lobes. All leaves roughly pilose, bright green. *Flowers* scented–sepals 6.5–10 mm long oblong, sometimes brown red; petals 1.5-2.2 cm long, blade obovate subemarginate at the apex white or lilac with yellow or pulple veins. *Roots* white cylindrical and fleshy with tiny rootlets from the surface.

Habitate: Cultivated all over India upto 5000 m and in many other temperate and warm countries.

Propagation: By seeds and vegetative method.

Parts Used: Leaves roots, seeds.

Chemical Constituents: Seeds contain an active antibacterial principle-Raphanin, stable between pH 3 and 8, giving reactions similar to coumarin. Other components are glycosinolates, enzymes, trace elements, acids, aldehydes, anthocyanin, pectin and arabinogalactan proteins. In the leaves Vitamin C has also been found.

Uses: Indigestion. Oedema. Skin infections. In Ayurveda it is used as a diuretic, carminative and a digestive. The flowers are cholagogue. The juice of fresh leaves is also used as a diuretic, a laxative and in flatulence.

1062. *Rauvolfia cambodiananpierre* ex pitard *(Apocynaceae)*

Vernacular Name: *Eng:* Cambodian rauvolfia.

Description: Erect evergreen undershrub 0.5-1.5m high. Stems erect, lenticellate. Leaves in whorl of three, attenuate at both ends; dark green above, pale below; margins entire. Inflorescence in axillary or terminal cyme with long stalk; flowers white, poinkish outside. Drupe obliquely ovoid, blackish-violet when ripe. All parts of the plant yield a milky juice.

Habitate: Grows wild; endemic in the mountains of the southern region.

Propagation: By seeds and vegetative method.

Part Used: Root-bark.

Chemical Constituents: The root-bark contains 2.64% alkaloids, mostly reserpine and ajmaline. In addition serpentine, reserpinine, ajmalicine and rauvomitine are found in R. vomitoria and canescine in R. canescens.

Uses: The root-bark, which possesses hypotensive and sedative properties, is widely used for the treatment of hypertension and pshychoses.

1063. *Rauvolfia serpentina* (L.) Benth. ex Kurz *(Apocynaceae)*

Vernacular Name: *Eng:* Serpentine root, *Hin:* Chota chand, Sarpagandha, *Kan:* Sarpagandha, *Mal:* Sarpaganthi, Amalpori, *Mar:* Harki, *San*: Sarpagandha, *Tam:* Sarpaganthi, Sivan amalpodi, *Tel:* Patalaganthi, Sarpaganthi.

Description: Herbs to undershrubs, 0.5-2 m tall. Stems woody at base. *Rootstock* thick and woody. *Bark* ashy white, thin. *Latex* water. Branchlets hairless. *Leaves* 3-4 in a whorl or sometimes opposite, elliptic or oblanceolate, 8-16 x 3-5 cm, base gradually tapering, apex acuminate, margin entire, papery, hairless, with distinct stalk; lateral nerves 8-15 pairs, faintly seen. *Flowers* bisexual, in terminal or axillary umbellate cymes, white with pale purple shade, about 2 x 1 cm. *Drupes* united in their lower half, stalkless, fleshy, ovoid, about 7 mm long, hairless, shiny, purplish black when ripe. *Seeds* 1, ovoid.

Habitate: Moist deciduous to evergreen forests.

Propagation: By seeds and vegetative method.

Parts Used: Roots.

Chemical Constituents: Canembine, Corynanthine, Seredine, Yohimbine, α-Yohimbine, β-Yohimbine, 3-Epi-α-Yohmbine, ψ-Yohimbine, Deserpidine, Isopseudoreserpine, Isoraunescine, Isoreserpine, Raugustine, Raunescine, Renoxidine, Rescidine, Rescinnamine, Reserpic Acid Methyl Etser, Reserpine, ψ-Reserpine, Deserpideine, Raujemedine, Ajmalicine, Aricine, Isoreserpiline, Isoreserpinine, Rauniticine, Raunitidine, Raumitorine, Rauvanine, Reserpiline, Reserpinine, Tetrahydro-Alstonine, Tetraphylline, Alstonine, Serpentine, Serpentinine, Neosarpagine, Sarpagine, Ajmalidine, Ajmaline Mauiensine Isoajmaline, Mitoridine, Picrinine, Purpeline, Rauvomitine, Rauwolfinine, *San*dwichine, Seredamine, Tetraphyllicine, Vincamajine, Vomalidine, Isoreserpiline-ψ-Indoxyl, Perakine, Vomilenine, Carapanaubine, Rauvoxine, Rauvoxinine, Ajmalinine, Alkaloid A, Alkaloid D, Alkaloid RPI, Alkaloid RP2, Alkaloid RP3, Amsoniaefoline, An Alkaloid, Chandrine, Neoreserpiline, Obscuridine, Obscurine, Pelirine, Raucaffricine, Raucaffridine, Raucaffriline, Raunamine, Rauwolfine, *San*dwicensine, Samatine, Semperflorine,.

Uses: The chief use of the drug is as a sedative and hypnotic and for reducing blood pressure. The drug is now largely used in insanity and high blood pressure. The alkaloids stimulate the central nervous system. It is more suitable for cases of mild anxiety or patients of chronic mental illness. The drug has tranquillising effect. Root is also considered as anthelmintic and an antidote to snake venom. Its decoction is given during labour pains to increase uterine contraction. Juice of the leaves is used for the cure of corneal opacity of the eyes.

1064. *Rehmannia glutinosa* (Gaertner) *(Scrophulariaceae)*

Vernacular Name: *Eng*: Glutinous rehmania.

Description: Perennial herb with tuberous roots, 20-30 cm. High, usually withered in the dry season. Leves oval base oblong, apex round, irregularly crenate-toothed, radiating in rosettel nerves reticulately veined. Flowers tubular, reddish-violet in long raceme. Capsule many-seeded. The whole plant is covered with soft hairs.

Habitate: An introduced species in many parts of the country.

Propagation: By seeds and vegetative method.

Part Used: Tubers and roots.

Chemical Constituents: The tuberous roots contain glucose, mannite, the glucoside rehmanin and carotene.

Uses: The tuberous root possesses reconstituent, antianaemic and diuretic properties. It is used in treating general debility, anaemia, epistaxis, polymenorrhoea, threatened abortion, internal haemorrhage, chronic nephritis, sore throat, erythema and dysentery. It is also prescribed as a depurative, cardiac tonic and soporific.

1065. *Rhamnus catharticus* L. *(Rhamnaceae)*

Synonyms: *Rhamnus xanthocarpa* Hort. ex. Koch., *Hramnus wicklia* Hort. ex. Koch.

Vernacular Name: *Eng:* Buckthorn.

Description: A deciduous thorny shrub or a small tree, up to 6 m. tall with some branches ending in short thorns. Leaves opposite, broadly elliptic, oblong, or elliptic obovate, minutely serrate, 3-6 cm. long, lateral veins commonly 3 on each side, strongly curved upward; petiolate, petioles a third to two third as long as the blade. Flower greenish-yellow, dioecious, in axillary clusters; sepals 4, 2mm. long, petals 4, erect, lanceolate, 1-1.3 mm. long in the staminate flowers, 0.6 mm. long in the pistillate; style 4-fid for about half its length. Drupe black 5-6 mm. in diameter, commonly with 4 stones.

Habitate: Throughout Europe, North Africa & U.S.A.

Propagation: By seeds and vegetative method.

Parts Used: Fruit.

Chemical Constituents: Rhamnin, Rhamnetin, Rhamnocathartin, Frangula-emodin, Chrysophanol, Rhamnosterin, Rhamnofluorin, Rhamnicoside.

Uses: Used for complaints specifically of copious watery diarrhoea with violent rumbling and griping especially cutting pain in ileo-caecal region. Vomiting. Fever with violent chill with skin sometime warm and sometime cold.

1066. *Rhamnus frangula* *(Rhamnaceae)*

Synonyms: *Frangula alnus.*

Vernacular Name: *Eng:* Alder buckthorn.

Description: Deciduous shrub or small tree growing to 5 m. Has smooth brown bark, oval to elliptical leaves, white flowers in late spring, and small round berries ripening from yellow to black.

Habitate: Alder buckthorn grows in Europe and in north-eastern parts of the US. It prefers marshy woodland. The bark of trees at least 3-4 years old is collected in late spring and early summer, and is dried and stored for at least 1 year before use.

Propagation: By seeds and vegetative method.

Parts Used: Bark.

Chemical Constituents: Alder buckthorn contains 3-7% anthraquinones, anthrones, anthranols, an alkaloid, tannins and flavonoids. The anthrones and anthranolds induce vomiting, but the severity of their effect lessens after long-term storage. The anthraquinones found in alder buckthorn and closely related species act on the wall of the colon, stimulating a bowel movement approximately 8-12 hours after ingestion.

Uses: Alder buckthorn is a laxative and a cathartic, and is most commonly taken as a treatment for chronic constipation. Once dried and stored, it is significantly milder than senna or common buckthorn the long-term to treat constipation and to encourage the return of regular bowel movements. Alder buckthorn is a particularly beneficial remedy if the muscles of the colon are weak, and if there is poor bile flow. The plant should not be used for constipation caused by excessive tension in the colon wall.

1067. *Rhaphidophora pertusa* (Roxb.) Schott *(Araceae)*

Synonyms: *Rhaphidophora laciniata* sensu Alston non (Burm.f.) Merr.

Vernacular Name: *San*: Sphotya bhujangam, *Kan*: Dodda thippali, *Mal*: Anai thippili, Gaja thippili, Elithadi, *Mar*: Ganeshkanda, *Tam*: Anai pirandai, Anai thippili, Ilatti mara vazhai, *Tel:* Enugan alleru.

Description: A lofty semi-epiphytic climbing shrub, with stout clinging roots. *Stems* cylindrical, dark green, sub-fleshy, about 10 cm girth, shiny, smooth, hairless, rooting at nodal regions. *Leaves* alternate, arranged in two rows, broadly elliptic to oblong, 18-45 x 12-26 cm, base rounded and unequal, apex shortly cuspidate, unlobed, or perforate or pinnately lobed, with many parallel nerves; leaf stalks 15-40 cm long, swollen and with a sheath at base, deeply grooved on the upper surface. *Flowers* bisexual, minute, greenish yellow, numerous, compactly packed in a special structure called 'spadix', which is cylindrical and about 8 x 2 cm. *Spadix* is partially covered by a hood-like structure known as 'spathe'. *Spathe* oblong, twisted, 7-14 x 4-6 cm, apex acuminate, greenish yellow. *Berries* numerous, small, many-seeded, red when ripe.

Habitate: Wet lowland forests from deciduous to evergreen.

Propagation: By stem cuttings, roots and air-layers.

Parts Used: Juice.

Chemical Constituents: N.A.

Uses: Used for treatment of snakebites and scorpion stings. Stems used for treating ulcers, pain in the colon, abdominal tumours and also in bronchiopathy. *Kani* tribes in Kerala orally administer the stem juice to cure ascites, inflammation of spleen and liver.

1068. *Rheum emodi* D. Don. *(Polygonaceae)*

Synonyms: *Rheum australe* Wall. ex.Meissn.

Vernacular Name: *San*: Gandhint, Pitamulika; *Tel:* Nattupasupu-chinngadda; *Hin*: Hindirevaandchini, doler; *Tam*: Nattu-ireval-chinni; *Beng*: Bengala revanchini; *Kan*: Nat-reva-chinni; *Guj*: Gamni-revanchini.

Description: A robust perennial herb with thick, long, roots; 1-15 m tall and grows on rocky lands. Roots are stout and the stem is hollow. Lower leaves are 20-50 cm in diameter, orbicular and are broadly ovate. Flowers are small and dark purple in colour. Fruits are purple and angled.

Habitate: The herb is distributed in the Himalayas from Kashmir to Sikkim at altitudes of 3300-5200 m. In Himchal Pradesh it is found growing in Chhota Bhangal & Bara Bhangal of Kangra; Pangi Bharmour of Chamba, Parvati valley of Kullu, Dodra kawar, Khashadhar and Rohru ranges of Shimla district, Kinnaur, Lahaul & Spiti districts.

Propagation: By seeds, rootstock and rootsuckers.

Part Used: Dried rhizomes and roots. Collection is done during September-November. The roots are cut into circular pieces dried and stored.

Chemical Constituents: Chrysophanic acid, emodin, starch, rhein, anthraquinone derivatives, essential oil, calcium oxalate and a resinous substance have been obtained from the roots. Leaves contain oxalic acid.

Uses: Rhizomes/ roots are purgative, astringent, tonic, stomachic and aperient. The petioles are pickled. Powdered roots are used for cleaning teeth and are sprinkled over ulcers for quick healing. In action, it is aperient, astringent, diuretic, emmenagogue, expectorant, purgative, stomachic and tonic. It is of special use for infant's stomach problems. The root is used along with madder and potash for dyeing fabrics. Red-leaf stalks are eaten either raw or boiled, sprinkled with salt and pepper. Root is regarded as a panacea in local home remedies and is used in stomach problems cuts, wound and muscular swellings, tonsillitis and mumps. It has been found as a potent anti-inflammatory drug.

1069. *Rheum moorcroftianum* Royle *(Polygonaceae)*

Vernacular Name: Archa, Chukri, Chuchi, Lechu, Usharerevand, Revandchini, Rhubarb.

Description: A stout, perennial herb, variable in size from 0.3-1.8 m high, stem lacking with radical leaves 10 to 60 cm in diameter, thick, coriaceous, margins undulate, usually cordate often puberulous beneath. Flowers are paleyellowish arising in stout, glabrous racemes from the middle of the large, stout radical leaves. Fruit is broadly oblong or orbicular in appearance and pink-purple in colour.

Habitate: *R. moorcroftianum* is found at altitudes of 3000 to 5200 m in the Himalayas, chiefly in Garhwal and Kumaon. In Himachal Pradesh, the plant is found chiefly in Lahaul-spiti, Kinnaur, Kangra and Bharmour areas in sub-alpine and alpine pastures.

Propagation: By seeds, cutting.

Part Used: Roots.

Chemical Constituents: Rhubarb contains as its chief constituents, certain anthraquinone derivatives, glucoside rhaponticin, chrysophanic acid, emodin, eugenol, a terpene alcohol and a product believed to be methyl heptyl ketone. Leaves contain oxalic acid.

Uses: The drug is used as purgative. Since it also contains tannins, after purgation it creates astringent effect as well. It is not suitable in cases of chronic constipation, but must be used in mild cases. Due to its astringent action, the drug is also given in certain types of diarrhoea. In villages, the lotion/paste made in water is used in cuts, wound swellings, rashes etc. It is similar in effect to that of iodine.

1070. *Rheum officinalis* Baillon. *(Polygonaceae)*

Synonyms: *Rheum paltatum* Linn.

Vernacular Name: *Eng:* Indian rhubarb, China rhubarb.

Description: Perennial herb, short with a thick vertical rhizome, bearing fleshy, spreading roots. Leaves numerous, long-petioled, arising from upper part of the vertical rhizome. Lamina cordate to somewhat orbicular, entire or coarsely dentate. Flowers greenish-white or white to red, on elongated leafy panicles. Fruit, an achene with three board thin wings and remains of the parianth at the base.

Habitate: India, China and Tibet.

Propagation: By seeds and Rhizomes.

Parts Used: Rhizome.

Chemical Constituents: Rutin. Anthraquinones of emodin, chrysophenol & physcion viz. Emodin, chrysophenol & physcion; Rhein; Erythroeretin; Sennosides A & B; Palmidin-A, B and C; Sennidin-C, Rheidin-B & Rheidin-C. Glucogallin. Tetrarin.

Uses: For complaints of children, especially during dentition, with difficult dentition and whole body smelling sour even after a bath. Stool sour smelling, pasty with shivering and tenesmus and burning in anus. Colicky pain about navel, worse by uncovering an arm or leg. Desires various kinds of food but cannot eat them. Constant sweat of scalp, whether asleep or awake. Cold sweat about mouth & nose. Mentally impatient, cries, desire many things but dislikes when offered.

1071. *Rheum palmatum* *(Polygonaceae)*

Vernacular Name: *Eng:* Chinese Rhubarb, Da huang.

Description: A thick-rhizomed perennial growing to 3m, with large palm-shaped leaves and small flowers.

Habitate: Native to China and Tibet, where the best-quality herb is still found.

Propagation: By seeds and vegetative method.

Parts Used: Rhizomes.

Chemical Constituents: Anthraquinones, rhein, aloe-emodin, emodin, Flavonoids, Phenolic acid, Tannins, Calcium oxalate.

Uses: Laxative, constipating, Astringent, Eases Stomach pain, Antibacterial.

1072. *Rheum undulatum* L. *(Polygonaceae)*

Vernacular Name: *Eng:* Rhubarb.

Description: Stout, perennial hert, to 1 m tall, with hollow stem. Leaves in basal clumps, with long petiole of purple tint, ovate, acute, cordate, margin undulate; leaves on flowering stems without petiole, wrapping stems, cordate. Flowers small, greenish, in panicled clusters on tall hollow stems, cordate. Flowers small, greenish, in rows; stamens 9, styles 3. Fruit a achene with wings.

Habitate: Wet places in grassy fields.

Propagation: By seeds and vegetative method.

Parts Used: Rhizomes.

Chemical Constituents: Anthraquinones; chrysophanol, emodin, aloe-emodin, rhein, physcion, citreorosin and their glucosides. Dianthraquinones; sennoside A, -F. Torachrysone-8-glucoside. Stibenes; rhaponticin, peceid, deoxyrhaponticin. 3,4′, 5-Trihydroxyustilbene-glucoside, gallic acid, glucogallin, catechol, 4-(ρ-hydroxyphenyl)-2-butanone glucoside, cinamic acid.

Uses: Purgative, bile and pancreatic secretory, antibacterial, astringent, anticarcinogenic, stomachic, ρ-glycosidase inhibitory activity (rhaponticin). Used in constipation and gastrointestinal disorders.

1073. *Rhododendron anthopogon* D. Don. *(Ericaceae)*

Vernacular Name: Dhoop, Nichni, Rattanbat, Nera, Kaizaban, Morua, Talisa, Talisri, Talsar, Talispatra.

Description: The plant is a small shrub or a scrub with an aromatic odour. Branchlets are scabrous and scaly. Leaves are 2.5-4 cm long, elliptic or broad-oblong, shining above and brown tomentose beneath having a short petiole. Flowers are yellow and in dense, terminal corymbs; calyx lobes are oblong, elliptic, membranous or ciliate; corolla is tubular with a dilated mouth. Tube is .2 cm long. Lobes are obovate, entire and spreading. Stamens are 6-8; ovary is scaly and the capsules are .5 cm long and ovoid. Seeds are oblong and sub-acute.

Habitate: The plant is found in the Himalaya from Kashmir to Bhutan at altitudes of 3000-5200 m. It Himachal Pradesh, the bush is found in Chansal peak rocks, Chansal-dhamkhari, Chounti slopes, Buraskandi, Mani-Mahesh, Rohtang peak, Thamsar and Dainasar areas between 3200-4500m elevation.

Propagation: By seed, stem cutting and rootsuckers.

Part Used: Leaves.

Chemical Constituents: Chemical screening needs to be done on this alpine shrub.

Uses: Leaves possess stimulant properties. These are aromatic and are administered as an errhine to produce sneezing.

1074. *Rhodomyrtus parviflora* Alston. *(Myrtaceae)*

Synonyms: *Rhodomyrtus tomentosa* (Ait.) Hassk.

Vernacular Name: *Eng:* Tomentose rose myrtle, downy rose myrtle, hill gooseberry, hill guava; *Tam:* Thaontay, koratta, thavattu; *Mal:* Thaontay, koratta, thavattu and *Kan:* Tavuti, guddade nelli.

Description: Small shrub, 1-3m. in height, much-branched. Young shoot angular, tomentose, Branches cylindrical, glabrous. Leaves opposite, oblong-ovate, thick, base 3-nerved, villous beneath. Flowers axillary, rose-pink, solitary or fascicled. Berry dark-violet when ripe, edible. Seeds numerous, small.

Habitate: Grows wild on the lower slopes of hills.

Propagation: By seeds and vegetative method.

Part Used: Young shoots, leaves, flower-buds, ripe fruit.

Chemical Constituents: The whole plant contains tannin. The fruit yields proteins, fatty substances, hydrocarbons, vitamin A, thiamine, riboflavin and nicotinic acid.

Uses: The buds and young leaves have a beneficial effect in colic, diarrhoea, dysentery, abscesses, furunculosis and haemorrhage. The concentrated decoction of leaves is used as an antiseptic wash for wounds, impetigo and abscesses. A combination of the ripe fruit and Caesalpinia sappan is also prescribed.

1075. *Rhus chinensis Mill.* *(Anacardiaceae)*

Synonyms: *Rhus javanica, Rhus semialata.*

Vernacular Name: *Eng:* Nutgall tree; *Hin*: Tatri.

Description: Deciduous, cough, abnormal sweating, haemorrhage. Leaves pinnately compound, 40 cm long; leaflets 7-13, ovate, 5-12 cm long, 2.5-6 cm wide, commonly toothed, brownish-pubescent beneath; rachis and often the petioles winged. Flowers creamy-white, in large terminal panicles, 15-30 cm long, with glandular hairs, 1-seeded, drupaceous.

Habitate: Thickers in foothills, lowlands and mountains in Korea, Japan, China and temperate Asia.

Propagation: By seeds and vegetative method.

Parts Used: Gallnut.

Chemical Constituents: Gallotannin, gallotannic acid, gallic acid, m-digallic acid.

Uses: Astringent, haemostatic, antibacterial, antifungal, antiviral. Used in diarrhoea, cough, abnormal sweating and haemorrhage.

1076. *Rhus glabra* *(Anacardiaceae)*

Vernacular Name: *Eng:* Smooth sumach.

Description: Deciduous shrub growing to a height of about 2m. Has straggling branches, compound leaves in pairs, large clusters of greenish-red flowers and downy deep red berries.

Habitate: Native to North America, smooth sumach is found on the borders of woods, along fences and hedgerows and in neglected sites.

Propagation: By seeds and vegetative method.

Parts Used: Root bark, berries.

Chemical Constituents: Smooth sumach contains tannins. its other constituents are unknown.

Uses: The astringent root bark of smooth sumach is often used as a decoction. It is taken to alleviate diarrhoea and dysentery, applied externally to treat excessive vaginal discharge and skin eruptions and used as a gargle for sore throats. The berries are diuretic, help reduce fever, and may be of used in late-onset diabetes. The berries are also astringent and can be used as a gargle for mouth and throat complaints.

1077. *Ribes nigrum* *(Saxifragaceae)*

Vernacular Name: *Eng:* blackcurrant.

Description: An erect shrub up to 2.0 m. high, leaves 3-5 lobed, serrate, 4-8 cm. long; flowers greenish purple in pendulous and acemes; berries globose, black, with a strong aromatic smell & taste.

Habitate: Blackcurrant is native to the temperate regions of Europe, western and central Asia and the Himalayas. It is cultivated for its sour-sweet fruit.

Propagation: By seeds and vegetative method.

Parts Used: Leaves, berries.

Chemical Constituents: Blackcurrant leaves contain a volatile oil, tannins and vitamin C; the berries contain anthocyanosides, flavonoids, pectin, tannins, vitamin C and potassium.

Uses: In Europe, blackcurrant leaves are used for their diuretic effect. By encouraging the elimination of fluid, the leaves help to reduce blood volume and thereby to lower blood pressure. The leaves are also used as a gargle for sore throats and mouth ulcers. Blackcurrant berries and their juice are high in vitamin C. they help improve resistance to infection and make a valuable remedy for treating colds and flu. The juice also helps to stem diarrhoea, and calms indigestion. Juice that is fresh or vacuum-sealed is more effective than concentrate.

1078. *Ricinus communis* L. *(Euphorbiaceae)*

Vernacular Name: *Eng:* castor Bean; *Hin:* Erandi; *Beng*: Bheranda; *Tam:* Amanakku kottai muthu; *Tel:* Amudamuchettu; *Kan:* Haralu and *Mal:* Avanakku.

Description: Shrub or small tree to about 4 m high with conspicuous ring-like scars on the hollow stem. Leaves alternate, long-petiolate, palmate with 7-11 lobes and serrated edges, 20-60 cm long and often tinged with red. The terminal inflorescence is a narrow panicle; there are separate unisexual flowers, Fruit a spiny subglobose schizocarp about 1.5 cm long, splitting into three sections when mature, each section containing one mottled smooth brown seed in each of three sections flowers and fruit available throughout the year.

Habitate: Common in disturbed areas and waste places from sea level to 500 m elevation.

Propagation: By seeds and vegetative method.

Part Used: Seeds.

Chemical Constituents: Beta-amyrin, ricins, 5-dehydro-avenasterol, beta carotene, tannins, brasicasterol, campesterol, beta-sistosterol, stigmasterol, lupeol, quercetin, casbene, chlorogenic acid, coumarin, ellagic acid, diethyleneglycol disulphide, hemaglutinin, quinic acid, indoleacetic acid, ricinine, N-demethylricinine, ricinus agglustinins, glycoproteins, vitamins B_6 and B_1. Seed saponins, Epicatechin hyperuside, kaempferol flycoside.

Uses: Seed oil is used as a purgative. An infusion of the bark is used to treat skin inflammations and rashes. A drink of the juice in water is taken to treat breast tumours and boils.

1079. *Rorippa sarmentosa* (DC) Macbr *(Cruciferae)*

Synonyms: *Nasturtium sarmentosum* Schinz & Gulliaumin.

Vernacular Name: *Eng:* Polynesian cress.

Description: Spreading herb to 60 cm high with short, solid stems, arising from a long, thick root. Leaves basal, pinnately compound, up to 15 cm long, the leaflets with settated margins, the largest leaflet being terminal. Flowers small and numerous, white or pale yellow. Borne in racemes up to 25 cm long, arising from the rosette. Fruit a siliqua up to 3 cm long. Seeds which are expelled when the mature pod bursts.

Habitate: Common in damp waste areas from near sea-level to more than 1000 m elevation.

Propagation: By seeds and vegetative method.

Part Used: Whole plant.

Chemical Constituents: Sinapin and cholyl sinapate.

Uses: The plant is used to induce miscarriages and to cure convulsions in children. It is used to cure swellings and itches.

1080. *Rosa canina* *(Rosaceae)*

Vernacular Name: *Eng:* Dog rose.

Description: Climbing perennial growing to 3m. Has curved thorns, leaves with 2-3 pairs of toothed leaflets, pink or white flowers and scarlet fruit.

Habitate: Native to Europe, temperate areas of Asia and North Africa.

Propagation: By Cutting.

Parts Used: Hips.

Chemical Constituents: Dog rose hips contain vitamins C, A, B^1, B^2, B^3 and K, flavonoids, tannins, invert sugar, pectin, plant acids, polyphenols, carotenoids, volatile oil and vanillin.

Uses: Dog rose hops have extremely high levels of vitamins. When consumed fresh, they provide vitamins and other nutrients in a form that is readily absorbed by the body. This makes rose hop syrup a nourishing drink for young children. The tannin content of rose hops makes them a gentle remedy for diarrhoea. The hips are mildly diuretic. Additionally, dog rose hips reduce thirst and alleviate gastric inflammation.

1081. *Rosa centifolia* L. *(Rosaceae)*

Vernacular Name: Eng.: Cabbage rose, Hundred-leaved rose, Pale rose; *Hin:* Gulab; *Kan:* Gulabi, Gulavihuvu; *Mal:* Paninir, Paninirppu, Rosappu; *San:* Satapatri, Saumyagandha; *Tam:* Eros, Paninirppu; *Tel:* Rojapuvvu, Gulavi.

Description: A small, erect, prickly shrub with unequal, large, hooked prickles and many bristles; leaves compound, alternate, leaflets usually five, rachis not prickly; flowers usually pink, very fragrant, very double on long slender pedicels, calyx tube globose, ovoid, the mouth contracted, lobes 4-5, imbricate, petals many, stamens many, inserted on the mouth of the calyx tube; carpels many in the bottom of the calyx tube, style subterminal, free, stigma thickened, ovules solitary, pendulous; fruit a fleshy hip enclosing bony achenes; seeds small, pendulous.

Habitate: Cultivated throughout India.

Propagation: By vegetative method.

Parts Used: Roots, leaves, flowers.

Chemical Constituents: Essential oil. Quercetin, kaempferol and cyaniding from whole plant; cyaniding 3,5-diglucoside from petals. Detection of citronell, nerol, geraniol and phenylethanol in essential oil. Flowers contain a bitter principle, tannin matter, fatty oil and organic acids. Hips contain the pigments lycopene, β-and y_carodtenes, rubixanthin, zeaxanthin, xanthophylls and taraxanthin.

Uses: The roots are astringent and vulnerary and are useful in intestinal ulcers, rickets, haemorrhages and diarrhoea. The leaves are useful in treating wounds, ophthalmia, hepatopathy and haemorrhoids. The flowers are bitter, astringent, sweet, cooling emollient aromatic, cardiotonic, anti-inflammatory, expectorant, digestive, carminative, aphrodisiac, depurative, febrifuge, intellect promoting styptic. Rejuvenating and tonic. They are useful in vitiated conditions of *vata* and *pitta*, inflammations, cough, asthma, bronchitis, wounds, ulcers, halitosis, amentia, dyspepsia, flatulence, colic, skin diseases, hyperhidrosis, cardiac debility, fever and general weakness. The rose water is cooling, fragrant, emollient and ophthalmic, and is good for hyperhidrosis, halitosis and ophthalmopathy. The 'rose Otto' is antibacterial and is useful in the treatment of biliary calculus.

1082. *Rosa gallica* *(Rosaceae)*

Vernacular Name: *Eng:* Rose.

Description: Deciduous shrub growing to about 1.5 m. Has a smooth stem, sharp thorns, serrated leaves with 2-3 pairs of leaflets, semi-double deep pink or red flowers and scarlet hips.

Habitate: Native to the Middle East, the rose is not now found in the wild except as a garden escape.

Propagation: By Cutting.

Parts Used: Flowers, essential oil.

Chemical Constituents: Rose contains a volatile oil consisting of geraniol, nerol, citronellol, geranic acid and other terpenes, and many other substances.

Uses: The rose is currently little used in herbal medicine, but it is probably time for a re-evaluation of its medicinal b benefits. The essential oil, call "attar of rose", is used in aromatherapy as a mildly sedative, antidepres*San*t and anti-inflammatory remedy. Rose petals and their preparations have a similar action. They also reduce high cholesterol leaves. Rosewater is mildly astringent and makes a valuable lotion of inflamed and sore eyes.

1083. *Rosa laevigata* Michaux *(Rosaceae)*

Vernacular Name: *Eng:* Cherokee rose.

Description: An evergreen, climbing shrub, 5 m tall. Stem with a few compressed, somewhat hooked prickles. Leaves alternate, pinnate; leaflets 3 rearely 5, oval-elliptical or oval lanceolate, 2-7 cm long by 1.5-4.5 cm wide, acute or acuminate, finely dentate, glossy, the terminal leaflet larger and long-petiolate. Flowers solitary, fragrant, white 6-8 cm in diameter. Calyx a cupuliform tube covered with hair; petals obcordate; stamens very numerous. Receptacles oblong, ovoid, or nearly globular, 1.5-3 cm long by 1-1.5 cm wide, reddish, covered with stiff hairs and crowned with the perstent calyx. The fruit tastes sour and astringent.

Habitate: On sunny slopes in China, Japan and Viet Nam.

Propagation: By stem cutting.

Part Used: Fruit.

Chemical Constituents: The fruit contains citric and malic acids, tannin, vitamin C, glucosides, saponins.

Uses: Malabsorption and diarrhoea, chronic cough, perspiration from no apparent cause; night sweats, enuresis; frequent micturition, leucorrhoes; massive uterine bleeding, seminal emissions.

1084. *Rosa laevigata* Michaux. *(Rosaceae)*

Vernacular Name: *Eng:* cherokee rose.

Description: Small vigorous shrub with thick hooked prickles. Leaves trifoliate, toothed; stipule at the base of petiole. Flowers large, white, solitary and terminal, odourless. Fruit ovoid, clothed with thin, sharp spines and crowned by the persistent calyx, brownish-yellow when ripe. Seeds numerous, compressed.

Habitate: Wild species, indigenous to Cao Bang and Lang son provinces; also cultivated as a hedge-plant.

Propagation: By seeds and vegetative method.

Part Used: Fruit.

Chemical Constituents: The fruit contains citric and malic acids, tannin, vitamin C, glucosides, saponins.

Uses: The fruit is regarded as a general tonic and is successfully employed in spermatorrhoea, leucorrhoea, enteritis, pollakiuria and neurasthenia. It is also used as haemostatic.

1085. *Rosa multiflora* Thunb. *(Rosaceae)*

Vernacular Name: *Eng:* Baby rose, Japanese rose.

Description: Prickly climbing shrub, to 2 m tall. Stems densely prickly. Leaves alternate, odd-pinnate; leaflets 5-1 1, obovate to lanceolate, to 3 cm long; stipules pectinate. Flowers white, many, in large clusters, 2 cm across; petals 5; stamens many; petals and stamens inserted on disc at the edge of the calyx tube; pistils many, borne on the inside of the deep hypanthium, styles glabrous. Fruit pea-size, red hip. May.

Habitate: In hills and mountains, often planted for ornamental purposes in Korea and Japan.

Propagation: By seeds and vegetative method.

Parts Used: Fruit.

Chemical Constituents: Flavonoid glycosides: multiflorin A, B, multinoside A, B, quercitrin, afzelin. Carotenoids: lycopin. Phenols methyl gallate. Steroids.

Uses: Purgative, antihyperglycaemic. Used in constipation and articularpain.

1086. *Rosa rugosa* Thunb. *(Rosaceae)*

Vernacular Name: *Eng:* Turkestan rose, Japanese rose.

Description: Prickly shrub, to 2 m tall. Stems densely prickly and bristly, tomentose. Leaves alternate, odd-pinnate, stipules adnate to petioles; leaflets 5-9, elliptic, 2-5 cm long dark green and furrowed above; pedicels bristly. Flowers rose, solitary, 6-9 cm in diameter; petals 5; stamens many; petals 5; stamens many; petals and stamens inserted on a disc at the edge of the calyx tube; pistils many, borne on the inside of the deep hypanthium. Fruit a fleshy hip containing the hairy achenes, 2-2.5 cm in diameter, red at ripening.

Habitate: Near seashores in Korea and Japan.

Propagation: By vegetative method.

Parts Used: Flower, fruit.

Chemical Constituents: Ruleixanthine, locopene, catechol tannin. Flavonol glycosides: quercetin, apigenin 7-O-glucoside. Anthocyanidin, anthocyanoside. Tannis: gallic acid glucoside gallate, etc. Essential oils: linalool, linaly; formate, citonellol, geraniol, etc. Sesquiterpenes.

Uses: Antihypercholesterolaemic. Used in vomiting, diarrhoea, diabetes.

1087. *Rosmarinus officinalis* *(Lameaceae)*

Vernacular Name: *Eng:* Rosemary.

Description: A exotic leafy evergreen shrub up to 2 m. high; leaves narrow, entire, with revoluts margins; flowers few, in axillary racemes; bluish or white or pale violet; nutlets smoth, ovoid sub-globose.

Habitate: Native to the Mediterranean, rosemary grows feely in much of southern Europe and is cultivated throughout the world.

Propagation: By seeds and vegetative method.

Parts Used: Leaves.

Chemical Constituents: Volatile oil, containing borneol, camphene, camphor, cineole., Flavonoids, Tannins, Rosmarininc acid, Diterpenes, Rosmaricine.

Uses: Tonic, Stimulant, Astringent, Nervine, anti-inflammatory, Carminative.

1088. *Rotula aquatica* Lour. *(Boraginaceae)*

Vernacular Name: *Kan:* Pasanabheda; *Mal:* Kallurvanci; *San:* Pasanabhedah; *Tam:* Seppunerinji; *Tel:* Pasanabheda.

Description: A small much branched shrub, 60-180 cm high with numerous short lateral arrested branchlets offten rooting; leaves simple, nearly sessile, spathulate, rouded at the apex, more or less hairy, crowded on the branches; flowers pink or reddish, shortly pedicellate, single or 2-3 together on short lateral branches, stamens exerted beyond the corolla tube; fruits subglobose, orange red drupes, tipped with the remains of the style.

Habitate: Throughout India in the sandy and rocky beds of streams.

Propagation: By seeds and vegetative method.

Parts Used: Roots.

Chemical Constituents: Allantoin, rhabdiol.

Uses: The roots are bitter, astringent, cooling, diuretic and laxative and are usefule in haemorrhoids, renaland vesical calculi, diabetes and venereal diseases.

1089. *Rhamnus frangula* L. *(Rhamnaceae)*

Synonyms: *Frangula alnus* Mill., *Rhamnus alnoides* Gray, S.F., *Rhamnus nemoralis* Salisb., *Rhamnus pentapetala* Gilib.

Vernacular Name: *Eng:* Alder Buckthorn.

Description: A thornless deciduous shrub, 4-5 m. tall. Branches subopposite, ascending at an acute angle to the main stem. Young twigs with thin, smooth glossy dark purple bark marked with transeversely elongated white lenticels and inner layers deep crimson coloured. Leaves 2-7 cm. long, petioled, obovate bluntly apiculate, entire with few marginal glands near the apex, undulate with caduceus brownish tomentum particularly beneath, shiny green but turning clear yellow and red in autumn; large lateral veins about 7 pairs. Flowers: 3 mm. in diameter, on rather stout pedicels in axillary fascicles, sessile umbels. Calyx lobes greenish, 5 ovate; petals 5, small. **Fruit:** 6-10 mm. in diameter changing from green to red and then violaet-black on ripening, 2-3 seeded.

Habitate: Europe, including Germany, United States.

Propagation: By seeds and vegetative method.

Parts Used: Bark of young branches.

Chemical Constituents: Emodine glycosides viz Trimethylanthraquinone, oxymethyl anther quinone Frangulosides including frangulin A and B Glucofrangulin A and B; Emodin dianthron, Palmidin, Emodine glycoside; Chrysophanol and physcione, Rhemmicoside absent.

Uses: Used for complaints of copious, dark-green thin, pasty diarrhoea with flatulent rumbling in the Ileo-caecal region, itching of anus along the transverse colon, with purging and weakness after stool and characteristic frequently sour vomiting. Urethritis with burning in urethra while urinating with frequent urging. Great sleepiness.

1090. *Rubia akane* Nakai *(Rubiaceae)*

Vernacular Name: *Eng:*-Asian madder.

Description: Twining perennial herb, to 1 m tall. Stems angled, short spines along the edges. Leaves whorled, ovate to ovate-cordate, with 5 nerves from the base, 4, two of them stipules, 2-4 cm long, 1-2 cm wide, short spines on the ribs of the back side and margins. Flowers in terminal cyme, pale yellow, small, 3.5 cm in diameter, 5-merous; corolla slightly campanulate. Fruit fleshy, black; seeds few.

Habitate: Thickets and edge of mountain woods in Korea, Japan and China.

Propagation: By seeds and vegetative method.

Parts Used: Root.

Chemical Constituents: Mecocyanin, pseudopurpurin, cyclic hexapeptides RA-III, -IV, -V, -VII, anthraquinones, triterpenes.

Uses: Antitumour, aldose reductase inhibition. Used in haemostatic, carbunde, leucorrhoea, dysmenorrhoea and emmenagogue.

1091. *Rubia cordifolia* L. *(Rubiaceae)*

Vernacular Name: Eng.: Indian madder; *Hin:* Mamjith, Majith; *Kan:* Manjusta, Citravalli, Somalate, Siragatti; *Mal:* Mancatti, Covvallikkoti, Sivoiikkoti; *San:* Manjistha, Yojanavalli; *Tam:* Sevfvelli, Manjitti; *Tel:* Tamravalli, Manjistatiga, Ciranji.

Description: A very variable prickly or scabrous climbing perennial herb with long cylindric, flexuose, smooth reddish, roots and 4-angled rough stems and branches; leaves very variable 2-8 in a whorl often only 4,cordate-ovate-lanceolate, 5-7, ribbed, scabrous above, base rounded or slightly cordate, petioles very long, provided with sharp recurved prickles on the edges, stipules absent; flowers white, greenish yellowish or reddish, sweet-scented, small, in terminal panicled glabrous cymes; fruits globose or slightly 2-lobed, fleshy, smooth, purplish black when ripe; seeds two, small.

Habitate: Throughout India in hilly districts upto 3,750m.

Propagation: By seeds and vegetative method.

Parts Used: Roots.

Chemical Constituents: Colouring metter in the roots is a mixture of purpurin and munjistin. Roots also contain small amounts of xnthopurpurin and pseudopurpurin. Munjistin, alizarin and its glucoside in plant.

Uses: The roots are sweet, bitter, astringent, thermogenic, anti-inflammatory, antiseptic, digestive, carminative, constipating, antidysenteric, anthelmintic, depurative, vulnerary, emmenagogue, diuretic, galacto-purifier, alterant, ophthalmic, febrifuge, rejuvenating and tonic. They are useful in vitiated conditions of *kapha* and *pitta*, rheumatoid arthritis, neuralgia, cephalalgia, dyspepsia, flatulence, colic, diarrhoea, dysentery, helminthiasis, leprosy, skin diseases, leucoderma, pruritus, wounds, ulcers, amenorrhoea, dysmenorrhoea, strangury, ophthallmoopathy, intermittent fevers, pharyngitis, cough, diabetes, discolouration of the skin, slow healing of broken bones, tubercular conditions of the skin and mucous tissue, otopathy, urethrorrhea, haemorrhoids, jaundice, hepaatopathy, spolenopathy, arthralgia, leucorrhoea, pectoral diseases and general debility.

1092. *Rubia tinctorum* *(Rubiaceae)*

Vernacular Name: *Eng:* Madder.

Description: A prickly or scabrid, dimbing herb with quadrangular stems; Root stock perennial, with fleshy roots; leaves 4-6 in whorls; usually elliptic, some times elliptic-lanceolate; flowers greenish yellow in terminal and axillary panicles of cymes; fruit globose, red to black.

Habitate: Madder is native to southern Europe, western Asia and North Africa. It flourishes on wasteground, in hedgerows and amid rubble. It is also found in Kashmir.

Propagation: By Seeds and cutting.

Parts Used: Root.

Chemical Constituents: Madder contain anthraquinone derivatives an iridoid, resin and calcium.

Uses: Madder fell largely out of use in the 19th century, and is now only rarely employed to treat kidney and bladder stones.

1093. *Rubus coreanus* Miq. *(Rosaceae)*

Vernacular Name: *Eng:*-Korean bramble.

Description: Deciduous, prickly shrub, to 3 m tall. Stems purplish red, covered with white powder, arching branches takes roots at the recurving tip on the ground. Leaves alternate, pinnately compound; leaflets 5-7, ovate or elliptic, acute, 3-7 cm long, irregularly serrate, pubescent, at least on vein; petioles with pricklets. Inflorescence corymbs at the terminals of branches. Flowers pink; sepals pubescent, ovate, lanceolate; petals shorter than sepals, obovate. Fruit an aggregate of small drupes, red at ripening, turned to black later.

Habitate: Thickets on mountain slopes of Korea.

Propagation: By seeds and vegetative method.

Parts Used: Fruit.

Chemical Constituents: Polysaccharides, vitamin A-like substances. Triterpenoids: naga-ichigoside F1, F2, suavissimoside R1, coreanoside F1, (+)-catechin, (-)-epicatechin, procyanidin B-4, sanguiin H-4.

Uses: Antibacterial, aldose reductase inhibition. Used in impotence, spermatorrhoea, back pain and as tonic.

1094. *Rubus fruticosus* *(Rosaceae)*

Vernacular Name: *Eng:* Blackberry.

Description: A large erect shrub with robust branches; stems arched with short stout prickles; leaves with white stellate tomentum beneath; flowers pink; fruits small, with many black, more or less hemispherical fleshy drupes.

Habitate: Native to temperate areas of Europe, blackberry is naturalized in the Americas and in Australia. It is commonly found on wasteground, in hedgerows and woodland. In India it is found in himalaya region.

Propagation: By vegetative method.

Parts Used: Leaves, berries.

Chemical Constituents: Blackberry leaves contain tannins, flavonoids, and gallic acid. The fruit contains anthocyanins, pectin, fruit acids and vitamin C.

Uses: Blackberry leaves are strongly astringent and may be used as a mouthwash to strengthen spongy gums and ease mouth ulcers, as a gargle for sore throats and as a decoction to relieve diarrhoea and haemorrhoids. The berries make a plea*San*t gargle for swallowing.,.

1095. *Rubus ideaus* *(Rosaceae)*

Vernacular Name: *Eng:* Raspberry.

Description: An upright and diffuse, glandless deciduous perennial, sucking by adventitious buds from the roots, armed with slender, straight subalate prickles, rarely un armed; leaves pinnate with 3-5 or 7 leaflets, flowers 1-10 in dense axillary or terminal cymes; fruit red, rarely pale yellow and cone shapea.

Habitate: Native to Europe and Asia, raspberry now grows wild and in cultivated in may temperate regions.

Propagation: By vegetative method.

Parts Used: Leaves, fruit.

Chemical Constituents: Raspberry leaves contain polypeptides, flavonoids and tannins. The fruit contains pectin, fruit sugars, fruit acids and vitamins A, B and C.

Uses: Raspberry leaves are still used to encourage easy labour. While the specific mode of action is unknown, the leaves are thought to strengthen the longitudinal muscles of the uterus, increasing the force of contraction and thereby hastening childbirth. The leaves also find use as an astringent external remedy-as an eyewash for conjunctivitis, a mouthwash for mouth problems, or a lotion for ulcers, wounds or excessive vaginal discharge. The fruit is nutritious and mildly astringent.

1096. *Rumex acetosella* *(Polygonaceae)*

Vernacular Name: *Eng:* Sheep's Sorrel.

Description: Slender low-growing perennial. Has arrow-shaped leaves and terminal spikes bearing small green flowers that turn red as their seeds ripen.

Habitate: Sheep's sorrel is found in most temperate regions of the world. It grows on wasteground and in meadows, and is gathered in early summer.

Propagation: By seeds and vegetative method.

Parts Used: Aerial parts.

Chemical Constituents: Sheep's sorrel contains oxalates and anthraquinones. In isolation, the anthraquinones are irritant and have a laxative effect.

Uses: Sheep's sorrel is a detoxifying herb, the fresh juice having a pronounced diuretic effect. Like other members of the dock family, it is mildly laxative, and holds out potential as a long-term treatment for chronic disease, in particular that of the gastro-intestinal tract.

1097. *Rumex chinesis* Campd. *(Polygonaceae)*

Vernacular Name: *Eng:* Chinese dock.

Description: Erect herb, 30-50cm. High, with brown tuberous roots. Stems deeply grooved. Leaves alternate, margins wavy, the lower broad and long-stalked, the upper narrow, subsessile. Inflorescence in terminal whorled cyme; flowers greenish-yellow. Small nut acutely trigonous, enclosed in persistent and thickened calyx.

Habitate: Grows wild in abandoned fiels and on river banks.

Propagation: By seeds and vegetative method.

Part Used: Roots and leaves.

Chemical Constituents: The roots and leaves contain anthraglucosides 3-3.4%, of which the free form 0.47%, the combined form 2.54%; tannin; resins.

Uses: The roots are prescrived as a laxative to cure constipation. Exernal application is effective for contusions, inflammation, acne, eczema, prurigo, scalp scabies and vulvitis: a maceration in vinegar or alcohol of fresh roots or leaves is prscribed for external use.

1098. *Rumex crispus* L. *(Polygonaceae)*

Synonyms: *Rumex elongatus* Guss., *Rumex japonicus* Meissn.

Vernacular Name: *Eng:* Curled dock.

Description: A smooth, perennial herb, with deep, spindle-shaped, yellow root. Stem, 90-120 cm. high, angular, furrowed, somewhat zigzag. Leaves lanceolate, petiolate, whorled, acute, wavy-curled, crisp margined, smooth and light green; the radical leaves long-petioled, truncate, or the radical leaves long-petioled, truncate, or scarcely heart-shaped at the base; the cauline, acute at both ends and nearly sessile. Flowers with 6 perianth sepaloid leaves, petals none, bisexual, green, small, numerous and on short rather stout pedicels, pedicels 5-10 mm., long visibly jointed at the base, forming crowded and dense whorled racemes. Inflorescence stalk jointed at the base. Inner fruiting perianth segments, green, cordate of truncate, entire each with 3 tubercles, unequal, the largest one ovoid, very turgid, tubercular, round at both ends. The nut, 2.5 mm. by 3.0 mm., ovoid, pointed and slimy brown.

Habitate: U.S.A., Mexico, New Zealand, India.

Propagation: By seeds and vegetative method.

Parts Used: Root.

Chemical Constituents: Anthraquinones viz. chrysophanol, Emodin, Nepodin, Physcion. Catechol; Brassidinic acid, Oxalic acid, chrysophanic acid. Rumicin.

Uses: For complaints predominantly of respiratory systems. Tubercular diathesis. Respiratory complaints from cold air, which aggravates such symptoms. Tickling in throat pit causing dry, teasing cough. Dry incessant, fatiguing cough, worse from cold air or lying down or touching/ pressing throat pit but with little or no expectoration. Sensation of lump in throat, descends on swallowing but returns immediately. Soreness of larynx & trachea, cannot eat meat because it ca**Uses** eructations & pruritus. Intense itching of skin, especially in lower extremities, worse by cold air.

1099. *Ruscus aculeatus* *(Liliaceae)*

Vernacular Name: *Eng:* Butcher's broom.

Description: Bushy evergreen perennial growing to 1 m. Has leaf like leathery branches with terminal spine, greenish-white flowers and shiny red berries.

Habitate: Butcher's broom is found throughout much of Europe, western Asia and North Africa. It is a protected species, growing wild in woodland and on uncultivated ground. Cultivated plants are gathered in autumn when in fruit.

Propagation: By seeds and vegetative method.

Parts Used: Aerial parts, rhizome.

Chemical Constituents: Butcher's broom contains saponin glycosides, including ruscogenin and neoruscogenin. These constituents have a structure similar to that of diosgenin, found in wild yam. They are anti-inflammatory and cause the contraction of blood vessels, especially veins.

Uses: Butcher's broom is not widely used today, bur, in view of its positive effect on varicose veins and haemorrhoids, it could be due for a revival. In the European tradition, both the a4erial parts and the rhizome are considered to be diuretic and mildly laxative.

1100. *Ruta chalepensis* L. *(Rutaceae)*

Vernacular Name: *Eng.*: Garden rue, Common rue; *Hin:* Pismaram, Sadab, Satari; *Kan:* Sadabu, Nagadali, soppu, Simesedanu; *Mal:* Aruta, Nagatali; *San:* Gucchapatra; *Tam:* Aruvadam, Arvada; *Tel:* Sadazpa, Aruda.

Description: An aromatic perennial herb upto 75cm high; leaves compound shortly petitolate, ultimate segments oblong or obovate-oblong; flowers yellow; fruits capsules, shortly pedicelled.

Habitate: Cultivated in Indian gardens.

Propagation: By seeds and vegetative method.

Parts Used: Whole plant, oil.

Chemical Constituents: Essential oil, rutin.

Uses: The plant is acrid, bitter, thermogenic, diuretic, laxative, aphrodisiac, febrifuge, abortifacient, digestive, carminative, emmenagogue and tonic. It is useful in vitiated conditions of *kapha* and *vata*, strangury, fever, flatulence, colic, amenorrhoea, epilepsy and hysteria. The oil acts as a stimulant for uterine and nervous systems. The fresh leaves are used for rheumatalgia. The juice obtained from the leaves is given to children for helminithic infections and is good for odontalgia and otalgia.

1101. *Ruta graveolens* *(Rutaceae)*

Vernacular Name: *Eng:* Rue.

Description: A strong-scented, erect, glabrous herb, 30-90 cm. high; leaves 2-3 pinnate, segments oblong to spathulate, covered with a bloom and strongly aromatic; flowers small, yellowish in corymbs; petals with dentate or wavy margin; capsules small with lobes some what rounded.

Habitate: Rue grows in the Mediterranean region, preferring open sunny sites. It is also cultivated in many parts of the world as both a garden ornamental and a medicinal plant.

Propagation: By seeds and vegetative method.

Parts Used: Aerial parts.

Chemical Constituents: Rue contains about 0.5% volatile oil, flavonoids, furanocoumarins, about 1.4% furoquinoline alkaloids. Rutin has the effect of supporting and strengthening the inner lining of blood vessels and reducing blood pressure.

Uses: Rue is chiefly used to encourage the onset of menstruation. It stimulates the muscles of the uterus and promotes menstrual blood flow. In European herbal medicine, rue has also been taken to treat conditions as varied as hysteria, epilepsy, vertigo, colic, intestinal worms, poisoning and eye problems. The latter use is well founded, as an infusion used as an eyewash brings quick relief to strained and tired eyes, and reputedly improves the eyesight. Rue has been used to treat many other conditions, including multiple sclerosis and Bell's palsy.

1102. *Sabal serrulata* *(Palmaceae)*

Synonyms: *Serenoa serrulata.*

Vernacular Name: *Eng:* Saw Palmetto.

Description: A small palm growing to 6m, with fans of yellow-green leaves and ivory flowers.

Habitate: Saw palmetto is indigenous to North America and can be found growing in *San*d dunes along the Atlantic and Caribbean coasts from South Carolina to Texas.

Propagation: By seeds and vegetative method.

Parts Used: Berries.

Chemical Constituents: Volatile oil, Fixed oil, Steroidal saponin, Polysaccharides, Tannins.

Uses: Tonic, Diuretic, Sedative, Anabolic, Oestrogenic.

1103. *Saccharum officinarum* L. *(Poaceae)*

Vernacular Name: *San:* Ikshu, khanda, sarkara; *Eng:* Sugar cane; *Hin:* Pundia, pounda; *Tel:* Cheruku; *Tam:* Poovan karumbu; *Kan:* Patta patti kabbu and *Mal*: Karimbu.

Description: Erect, perennial grass with stout culms and solid, sweet, juicy, green to purplish stems 3-4 cm in diameter and up to or exceeding 3 m in height. Leaves sheathing and overlapping, lance-shaped, upto to 2 m long and 6 cm broad. Mature plants bear erect, dense clusters of small wind-pollinated flowers. Flowers usually available throughout the years.

Habitate: Widely cultivated and also naturalized from sea-level to 1000 m or more in elevation.

Propagation: By vegetative method.

Part Used: Whole plant.

Chemical Constituents: Abscisic acid, apigenin and its glycoside, 5-o-methylapigenin, arabinose, arunodin, para-hydroxybenzoic acid, calcium, campesterol, coumarin, cylindrin, orientin and its derivatives, fructose, galactose, gibberellins, glucose, O-methyllupeol. Luteolin, phytosterol, potassium, saccharans, schaftoside and isoschaftoside, bets sitosterol, sucrose, invert sugar, swertiajaponin, swertisn, tarasxerol methyl ether, tricin and tricin glycosides, vicenin, xylose.

Uses: The leaf ash is use to treat sore eyes the stem juice is use to treat sore throats.

1104. *Saccharum spontaneum* L. *(Poaceae)*

Vernacular Name: *Eng*: Thatch Grass, Wild sugarcane; *Hin:* Kas Kus; *Mal:* Kusa, Nannana; *San:* Kasah; *Tam:* Pekkarimpu; *Tel:* Kaki ceruku, Kaki gaddi.

Description: A tall, erect, perennial grass upto 6 m in height with slender culms and aggressive rhizomes bearing extensive roots; leaves simple, sheathing, narrowly linear, finely acuminate, rigid, coriaceous, ligule ovate, membranous; spikelets in pairs, on kilky hairy panicles, pale or greyish white to purplish grey in colour; in each spikelet pair one is pedicelled and the other sessile, glumes 4, coriaceous and brown below, obscurely keeled, one-nerved; grains oblong to subglobose.

Habitate: Throughout India, upto 1,800 m.

Propagation: By seeds and roots.

Parts Used: Whole plant and Roots.

Chemical Constituents: N.A.

Uses: The roots are sweet, astringent, emollient, refrigerant, diuretic, lithotriptic, haemostatic, laxative, aphrodisiac and tonic. They are useful in vitiated conditions of *pitta* and *vata*, burning sensation, strangury, renal and vesical calculi, dyspepsia, haemorrhoids, menorrhagia, dysentery, agalactia, phthisis and general debility.

1105. *Salacia oblonga* Wall. ex Wight & Arn. *(Hippocrateaceae)*

Vernacular Name: *Mal*: Ponkoranti, *Tam*: Ponkoranti, Kadal azhinjil, *Beng:* Dimal, Modhuplal.

Description: A large woody climbing shrub; branchlets cylindrical, densely sprinkled with lenticels, hairless. *Leaves* opposite, oblong or elliptic-oblanceolate, 7-15 x 3-5 cm, base acute, apex acute or acuminate, margin toothed with rounded to saw-like teeth, hairless; lateral nerves 7-9 pairs, prominent beneath; leaf stalks 5-10 mm long. *Flowers* bisexual, about 5 mm across, greenish yellow, seen in shortly stalked axillary clusters, usually 3-6 together. *Drupes* sub-globose or pear-shaped, 5-6 cm across, orange-red when ripe. *Seeds* 1-6, angled, embedded in fleshy pulp.

Habitate: Moist deciduous to evergreen forests.

Propagation: By seeds and vegetative method.

Parts Used: Stem bark, rook bark.

Chemical Constituents: N.A.

Uses: The stem bark is considered useful in treating polyuria, diabetes, excessive thirst, discoloured spreading patches on the skin, diarrhoea and fever. Root bark is used for treatment of gonorrhea, rheumatism and skin diseases.

1106. *Salacia reticulata* wight *(Hippocrateaceae)*

Vernacular Name: *Kan:* Ekanayakam; *Mal:* Ekanayakam, Ponkoranti, Koranti; *San:* Vairi, Pitika; *Tam:* Ponkoranti; *Tel:* Anukudu cettu.

Description: A large woody climber with pale yellow bark; leaves simple, opposite, exstipulate, ovate or obovate-oblong, coriaceous, shortly acuminate very shallowly, crenate-serrate, blabrous and shining; flowers yellowish green, fasciled on woody axillary tubercles; fruits large, tuerculate, bright pinkish orange; seeds 1-4, immersed in pulp.

Habitate: Throughout India, in forests.

Propagation: By seeds and vegetative method.

Parts Used: Roots.

Chemical Constituents: N.A.

Uses: The roots are acrid, bitter, thermogenic, urinary astringent, anodyne, anti-inflammatory, depurative, emmenagogue, vulnerary, liver tonic and stomachic. They are useful in vitiated conditions of *vata*, diabetes, haemorrhoids, inflammations, leucorrhoea, leprosy, skin diseases, amenorrhoea, dysmenorrhoea, wounds, ulcers, hyperhidrosis, hepatopathy, dyspepsia, flatulence, colic and spematorrhoea.

1107. *Saliva miltiorrhiza* Bunge. *(Lameaceae)*

Vernacular Name: *Eng:* Dan-shen.

Description: A perennial herb, 30-100 cm tall, villous. The stem erect, tetragonal and often branched in upper parts. Leaves opposite, petiolate, compound-imparipinnate; leaflets usually 5, sometimes 3 or 7, ovate to oval, 2-7 cm long by 0.8-5 cm wide; tip acute or acuminate; base obliquely rounded; margin crenate; both surfaces densely covered with white pubescence. Inflorescence a verticillaster, with 3-10 flowers in each whorl, 4-5 whorls being grouped in each terminal or axillary spike. Calyx bilabiate, the superior lip entire, the inferior bidentate. Corolla bluish-purple, bilabiate; the superior lip falcate and longer than the tube, bifid, the inferior lip bifid. Stamens 3, longer than the corolla. Style bifid. Fruit a collection of oblong nutlets, obtuse, 3 mm long.

Habitate: On sunny slopes, by roadsides and on canal banks and edges of forests.

Propagation: By seeds.

Part Used: Roots.

Chemical Constituents: N.A.

Uses: Irregular menstruation; dysmenorrhoes; amenorrhoesm abdoimanial pain due to postpartum haematoma, irritability and insomnia; neurashthenia, palpitation, infection and ulcerous disease of the skin.

1108. *Salix alba* *(Salicaceae)*

Vernacular Name: *Eng:* White Willow.

Description: A deciduous tree growing to 25 m; leaves narrowly lanceolate, ash grey, silky; flowers in male and female catkins; capsule ovoid-conic; seeds small, ovoid, yellow, keeled.

Habitate: Native to much of Europe, also found in North Africa and Asia, thriving in damp areas, such as on river-banks.

Propagation: By cutting.

Parts Used: Bark.

Chemical Constituents: Phenolic glycosides-salicylic acid, Flavonoids, Tannins.

Uses: Anti-inflammatory, analgesic, Reduces fever, Antirheumatic, Astringent.

1109. *Salvadora persica* L. *(Salvadoraceae)*

Vernacular Name: *Eng*: Salt bush, Toothbrush; *Hin:* Pilu, Jhak; *Kan:* Goni mara, Kankhina; *Mal:* Uka; *San:* Piluh, Pilu; *Tam:* Kotumavali, Cittuva; *Tel:* Gogu, Varagogu, Gunia.

Description: A much branched evergreen shrub or small tree with short trunk and drooping branches; leaves somewhat fleshy, greyish green, ovate, oblong, often mucronate at the apex, main nerves 5-6 pairs; flowers small, greenish yellow in axillary and terminal compound lax panicles; fruits globose, smooth, red when ripe.

Habitate: On saline lands and black cotton soil of peninsular India and Sri Lanka.

Propagation: By seeds and vegetative method.

Parts Used: Bark, leaves, shoots, fruits.

Chemical Constituents: Alkaloid trimethylamine, β-sitosterol and elementaly-monoclinic sulphur from roots.

Uses: The roots bark is tonic, stimulant and emmenagogue and is said to relieve splenalgia. The stem bark is good for gastropathy. The leaves are antiscorbutic, deobstruant, diuretic, anthelmintic, astringent, expectorant and tonic. The are useful in asthma, bronchitis, cough, vitiated conditions of *vata*, strangury, painful tumours, scurvy, constipation, verminosis and haemorrhoids. Shoots and leaves are bitter and are useful in all types of poisons, cough and bronchitis. The fruits and sweet, acrid, bitter, thermogenic, aphrodisiac, emollient, alexeteric, stomachic, purgative and digestive. The are useful in gastropathy, constipation, seminal weakness and vitiated conditions of *kapha* and *vata*. Tender twigs are used as toothbrush.

1110. *Salvia moorcroftiana* Wall. ex Benth. *(Lameaceae)*

Description: It is a tall, robust, perennial 45-90 cm tall herb. Leaves are thick, long stalked, ovate or lblong, sinuately and irregularly lobed, hairy; lower surface white tomentose. Flowers are pale blue or licac or nearly white with rose coloured bracts arranged in distant whorls on a long spike. Nutlets are sub-globose, pale a green in colour and with dark reticulations.

Habitate: The plant is found in the temperate Himalayas from Kashmir to Kumaon. In Himachal Pradesh, it has chiefly been found growing in patched in Kullu-Bajaura, Kiarighat, Shoghi, Deothi-Sabathu and Military area Solan upto 1800 m elevation.

Propagation: By seeds.

Part Used: Roots, leaves and seeds.

Chemical Constituents: Essential oil and mucilage.

Uses: Roots are used in colds and coughs. Leaves are used for guinea-worm and are applied as poultice for boils, wounds and chronic affections of the skin. Seeds are emetic and are used in heamorrhoids, colic and dysentery. These are edible after peeling. Locally the root is used in stomach pains.

1111. *Salvia officinalis* *(Lameaceae)*

Vernacular Name: *Eng:* Sage.

Description: A hardy variable sub-shrub; stem shrubby, white woolly, 15-30 cm tall; flowering branches tomentose-pubescent; leaves aromatic, entire, petiolate, oblong, base narrowed or rotund; flowers blue, purple or white, in simple racemes.

Habitate: Native to the Mediterranean, sage is cultivated all round the world, thriving in sunny conditions. It is grown from seed in spring and the plants are replaced after 3-4 years. The leaves are picked in summer.

Propagation: By seeds.

Parts Used: Leaves.

Chemical Constituents: Volatile oil, Diterpene bitters, Flavonoids, Phenolic, acids, Tannins.

Uses: Astringent, antiseptic, aromatic, carminative, oestrogenic, reduces sweating, tonic.

1112. *Salvia sclarea* *(Lameaceae)*

Vernacular Name: *Eng:* Clary Sage.

Description: Square-stemmed biennial growing to 1 m. Has hairy wrinkled leaves and whorls of pale blue flowers.

Habitate: Native to southern Europe and the Middle East, clary sage is now cultivated in France and Russia for its essential oil.

Propagation: By Seeds.

Parts Used: Seeds, essential oil.

Chemical Constituents: Clary sage contains 0.1% volatile oil, diterpenes and tannins.

Uses: An antispasmodic and aromatic plant, clary sage is used today mainly to treat digestive problems such as wind and indigestion. It is also regarded as a tonic, claming herb that helps relieve period pain and premenstrual problems. Owing to its oestrogen-stimulating action, it is most effective when levels of this hormone are low. The plant can therefore be a valuable remedy for complaints associated with the menopause, particularly hot flushing.

1113. *Samadera indica* Gaertn. *(Simaroubaceae)*

Vernacular Name: *Eng*: Niepa bark tree; *Hin:* Lokhanti; *Kan:* Nipa, Samdera; *Mal:* Karinnotta, Karinnotta; *San:* Gucchakaranjah; *Tam:* Nibam, Karincottai; *Tel:* Lokanti.

Description: A small tree upto 11 m in height with stout branches and pale yellow bark; leave large, upto 25 cm long and 9 cm broad, elliptic-oblong or elliptic-lanceolate, shortly acuminate, entire, shining, base rounded; flowers pinkish yellow in few or many flowered axillary umbels, peduncles longer than the leaves, pedicels red; fruits large, flat, pear-shaped, much compressed, smooth reticulate, containing a large brown curved seed.

Habitate: Evergreen forests and along backwaters of south India.

Propagation: By seeds.

Parts Used: Bark, wood, seeds.

Chemical Constituents: N.A.

Uses: The bark and wood are stomachic, emmenagogue, febrifuge and tonic, and are useful in vitiated conditions of *vata*, dyspepsia, flatulence, colic, dysmenorrhoea and general debility. The leaves are useful in erysipelas and pruritus. The seed oil is astringent, acrid, thermogenic, depurative, emetic, purgative and febrifuge. It is useful in vitiated conditions of *vata* and *kapha*, leprosy, scabies, pruritus, skin diseases, constipation and bilious fever.

1114. *Sambucus nigra* *(Caprifoliaceae)*

Vernacular Name: *Eng:* Elder.

Description: A deciduous tree growing to 10m, with oval leaves, cream flowers and blue-black berries.

Habitate: Native to Europe, elder thrives in woods, hedges and on waste-ground. It is now found in most temperate regions, and is often cultivated.

Propagation: By cutting.

Parts Used: Flowers and Berries.

Chemical Constituents: Flowers: Flavonoids-rutin, Phenolic acids, Triterpenes, Sterols, Volatile oil, Mucilage, Tannins. ***Leaves:*** Cyanogenic glycosides. Berries: Flavonoids, Anthocyanins, Vitamins A and C.

Uses: Increases sweating, Diuretic, Anti-inflammatory.

1115. *Sanguinaria canadensis* *(Papaveraceae)*

Vernacular Name: *Eng:* Blood root.

Description: Perennial plant growing upto 15 cm. Has palm-shaped leaves and solitary flower stems bearing attractive white flowers with 8-12 petals.

Habitate: Native to north-eastern North America.

Propagation: By Seeds and root cutting.

Parts Used: Rhizome.

Chemical Constituents: Blood root contains isoquinoline alkaloids, notably *Sanguinarine*, and many others, including berberine. *Sanguinarine* is a strongly expectorant substance that also has strongly expectorant substance that also has antiseptic and local anaesthetic properties.

Uses: In contemporary herbal medicine, blood root is chiefly employed as an expectorant, promoting coughing and the clearing of mucus from the respiratory tract. The plant is prescribed for chronic bronchitis and–as is prescribed for chronic bronchitis and–as it also has an antispasmodic effect–for asthma and whooping cough. Blood root may also be used as a gargle for sore throats, and as a wash or ointment for fungal and viral skin conditions such as athlete's foot and warts. Conditions such as athete's foot and warts prepared as a powder, blood root may be prepared as a powder, blood root may be sniffed to treat nasal polyps.

1116. *Sanguisorba officinalis* L. *(Rosaceae)*

Synonyms: *Poterium officinale* (L.) A. Gray.

Vernacular Name: *Eng:* Great burnet; garden burnet.

Description: A perennial herb, 50-150 cm high. The whole plant is glabrous, leaves compound-imparipinnate, alternate; leaflets 7-19, oblong-elliptic, 2-7 cm long by 0.8-3 cm wide, apex obtuse, base subcordate or truncate, serrate. Inflorescence a compact terminal spike, ovoid or oblong. Flowers small, dark-purple.

Habitate: On slopes in China, Europe and Northern Asia.

Propagation: By seeds and vegetative method.

Part Used: Roots.

Chemical Constituents: N.A.

Uses: Haemoptysis; melaena; haematuria; haemorrhoids with bleeding, diarrhoea, chronic gastrio-enteritis, burns.

1117. *Sansevieria trifasciata* Hort. ex Prain *(Liliaceae)*

Vernacular Name: *Eng:* Browstring hemp, mother-in-law's tongue.

Description: Perennial stemless herb with erect leaves arising from an underground rhizome. Leaves thick and fibrous, up to 1 m long, with pointed apices, the blade splotched with bands of whitish and darker green. Flowers 6-parted, with green and white perianth parts, fragrant, borne on terminal racemes. Fruit a reddish berry with 1-3 seeds.

Habitate: A common ornamental garden plant and also naturalized in some areas from sea-level to 800 m elevation.

Propagation: By rhizome.

Part Used: Whole plant.

Chemical Constituents: Phthalate, N-butyl1-4-ol-N-propyl, glycosides, saponins.

Uses: The plant is used to treat ringworm and fungal diseases.

1118. *Santalum album* L. *(Santalaceae)*

Vernacular Name: *Eng*: Sandal tree, White-sandal tree; *Hin:* Safed candan, santal; *Kan:* Bavanna, Srigandadamara, Agarugandha; *Mal:* Candanam; *San:* Candanah, Srikhandam; *Tam:* Candanam; *Tel:* Candanamu, Gandhapucekka, Srigandapumanu, Tellagandhapucettu.

Description: A medium sized evergreen, semiparasitic, glabrous tree with slender drooping branches, reaching upto 18 cm m in height; bark dark grey or brownish black. rough with short vertical cracks; leaves simple, opposite, elliptic-lanceolate, glabrous, entire; flowers brownish purple, reddish purple or violet in terminal and axillary paniculate cymes; fruits globose drupes, purple black with ribbed endocarp; seeds hard, globose or obovoid. The heartwood is light yellowish brown when fresh, turning dark brown to dark reddish brown on exposure. The wood is highly scented.

Habitate: In the Southern regions of India, especially in Karnataka, Tamilnadu and Kerala, ascending upto 1,200 m.

Propagation: By seeds.

Parts Used: Heartwood.

Chemical Constituents: Leaves, fruits and seeds contain santalbic acid, palmitic acid, oleic acid, linoleic acid and sugar. Fruits yield betulic acid and B-sitosterol and a fatty oil. Betulinic acid, β-sitosterol, glucose, fructose and sucrose from leaves. Heartwood yields essential oil which contains α-, α-and β-santalenes, santenol, teresantanol.

Uses: The heartwood is bitter, sweet, acrid, aromatic, deodorant, disinfectant, refrigerant, depurative, intellect promoting, cardiotonic, diuretic, diaphoretic, expectorant, aphrodisiac, haemostatic, anodyne, antipyretic, restorative and tonic. It is useful in vitiated condition of *pitta*, burning sensation, dipsia, cephalalgia, foul odour due to hyperhidrosis, skin diseases, leprosy, forgetfulness, amentia, psychopathy, cardiac debility, haemoptysis, hyperacidity, jaundice, strangury, cough, bronchitis, inflammations, cystitis, dysentery, gastric irritability, menorrhagia, leucorrhoea, spermatorrhoea, intermittent fever and general debility.

1119. *Sapindus laurifolia* Vahl *(Sapindaceae)*

Synonyms: *Spindus mukorossi.*

Vernacular Name: Eng.: Soapnut tree; *Hin:* Ritta; *Kan:* Kugatemara, Kugatekaye, Antawala; *Mal:* Urunci, Uruvanci, Urulinci; *San:* Phenilah Aristakah; *Tam:* Puvankottai, Ponnankottai; *Tel:* Kunkutikaya, Kumkuticettu, Phenilamu, Kumkullu.

Description: A medium sized deciduous tree upto 20m in height with grey smooth bark, peeling off in scales; leaves pinnate, leaflets 2–3 pairs, terminal pair being the largest; flowers white, polygamous, male flowers many, bisexual flowers few, all in the same pubescent panicle; fruits fleshy drupes, the pulp becoming a saponaceous wrinkled rind on drying; seeds black.

Habitate: Throughout India, in forests at low elevations and also cultivated.

Propagation: By seeds.

Parts Used: Roots, bark, fruits.

Chemical Constituents: Saponins-sapindoside A and sapindoside B. Nuts contain kaempferol, quercetin and β-sitosterol. Saponin emarginatoside from fruits.

Uses: The roots and bark are expectorant and demulcent. The roots are good for hemicrania, hysteria and epilepsy. A decoction of the bark is good for cattle suffering from ulcers due to worm infestation after calving. The fruits are acrid, bitter, thermogenic, emetic, astringent, expctorant, anthelmintic, abortifacient and tonic. They are good for asthma, diarrhoea, cholera, lumbago, verminosis and gastralgia due to dyspepsia.

1120. *Saponaria officinalis* L. *(Caryophyllaceae)*

Synonyms: *Saponaria nervosa* Gilib., *Saponaria vulgaris* Pall.

Vernacular Name: *Eng:* Bouncing bet, soap root plant

Description: A perennial herb, up to 80 cm. high, with aerial erect stem arising from horizontal prostrate stolon, from the nodes of which arise underground roots. Stem coarse, simple often branched, leafy, clustered, glabrous. Leaves 7-10 cm. long, 2-4 cm. wide, elliptic to oblong-lanceolate, acute, glabrous, 3 nerved, rarely puberulent. Inflorescence compact, subcapitate to open corymbose, paniculate cyme up to 15 cm. long with primary bracts coriaceous, ultimate ones scarious. Roots blood-red externally, slender, branched. Flowers fragrant, frequently double. Calyx 1.5-2.5 cm. long, 20 nerved, glabrous, calyx tube toothed, teeth triangularly acuminate. Petals 5, white or pinkish, petal lobes oblong to oblong-ovate, 8-15 mm. long, entire, notched at the apex, auricles lacking, appendages conspicuous. Stamens 10, exserted. Ovary 1 celled. Fruit a capsule, elliptic-oblong.

Habitate: Europe, India.

Propagation: By seeds.

Parts Used: Root.

Chemical Constituents: Sponin, Sapotoxin, Saponarin and Saporubrinic acid.

Uses: Of great use in treatment of acute colds. Coryza, sore throat, will often break-up a cold. Other associated complaints for which it is used are depression; sleeplessness; headache with stitching supra-orbital pain worse on left side; throbbing over orbits; leftside weakness in gait; left sided trigeminal neuralgia. Violent eye pain with hot stitches deep in eyeball, ciliary neuralgia, worse left side. Photophobia. Exophthalmos.

1121. *Saposhnikovia divaricata* (Turcz.) Schischk. *(Apiaceae)*

Synonyms: *Siler divaricatum* (Turz.) Benth. Et Hook. f.

Vernacular Name: *Eng:* Divaricate laserwort.

Description: A perennial herb, 30-80 cm high. The whole plant is glabrous, stem erect, much branched. Leaves 2 or 3 times pinnatifid, the ultimate segment linear to narrowly obolanceolate, 2-3 lobes at the top, apex acute, petiole expanded, clasping the stem. Umbels compound, terminal rays 5-9. Flowers in autumn. No bracts, bracteoles 3-5, much shorter than the umbellules. Fruit oblong, laterally compressed; mericarp with 5 primary and 4 secondary ribs, all regular, warty when immature.

Habitate: In grassland or on slopes in China, Japan, Korea, Mongolia, Soviet Union.

Propagation: By seeds.

Part Used: Roots.

Chemical Constituents: N.A.

Uses: Common cold, headache; dizziness, migraine, reheumatic arthritis.

1122. *Saraca asoca* (Roxb.) de Wilde *(Caesalpiniaceae)*

Synonyms: *Saraca indica.*

Vernacular Name: Eng.: Ashoka; *Hin:* Asok, Asoka; *Kan:* Asokada Kengalimar, Aksunkara; *Mal:* Asokam; *San:* Asokah, Gatasokah; *Tam:* Asogam; *Tel:* Asokamu, Vanjalamu.

Description: A medium sized handsome evergreen tree upto 9 m in height with numerous spreading and drooping glabrous branches; leaves pinnate, 30-60 cm long having 2-3 pairs of lancelalate leaflets; flowers orange or orange-yellow in dense corymbs, very fragrant; fruits flat black pods, leathery, compressed; seeds 4-8 per pod, ellespsoid, oblong and compressed. The bark is dark brown to grey or black with a warty surface, fresh cut ends are pale yellowish red.

Habitate: Throughout India, in evergreen forests upto an elevation of about 750 m and cultivated.

Propagation: By seeds.

Parts Used: Bark, leaves, flowers, seeds.

Chemical Constituents: The bark contains tannin, catechol, sterol and organic calcium compounds. Its methanol fraction contains haematoxylene, tannin, and water-soluble glycoside. The latter has glucose, galactose and mannose as sugars.

Uses: The bark is bitter, astringent, sweet, refrigerant, anthelmintic, styptic, stomachic, constipating, febrifuge and demulcent. It is useful in dyspepsia, fever, dipsia, burning sensation, visceromegaly, colic, ulcers, menorrhagia, metropathy, leucorrhoea and pimples. The leaves are depurative and their juice mixed with cumin seeds is used for treating stomachalgia. The flowers are considered to be a uterine tonic and are used in vitiated conditions of *pitta*, syphilis, cervical adenitis, hyperdipsia, burning sensation, naemorrhoids, dysentery, scabiesin children and inflammation. The dried flowers are used in diabetes and haemorrhagic dysentery and seeds are used for treating bone fractures, strangury and vesical calculi.

1123. *Sarcostemma acidum* Voigt *(Asclepiadaceae)*

Synonyms: *Sarcostemma Brevistigma* Wight & Arn.

Vernacular Name: *San:* Soma, Somavalli; *Eng:* Moon Plant, Moon creeper; *Hin:* Somlata; *Kan:* Somalata, Hambukalli; *Mal:* Somalata; *Tam:* Somam, Kotikkalli; *Tel:* Kondapala, somalata, Palmakasturi.

Description: A perennial leafless, jointed shrub with green, cylindrical, fleshy glabrous, twining branches having milky white latex; leaves reduced to scales, opposite; flowers white or pale greenish white, fragrant, in umbels on branch extremities; fruits follicles, tapering at both ends; seeds flat, ovate, comose.

Habitate: Bihar, Bengal and south India in dry rocky places upto 1,350m.

Propagation: By seeds and vegetative method.

Parts Used: Whole plant.

Chemical Constituents: The plant contains malic acid, succinic acid, reducing sugar, sucrose, traces of tannin, an alkaloid, a phytosterol, α and β-amyrins, lupeol and lupeol acetate and β-sitosterol.

Uses: The plant is bitter, acrid, cooling, alternate, narcotic, emetic, antiviral and rejuvenating. It is useful in vitiated conditions of *pitta*, dipsia, viral infection, hydrophobia, psychopathy and general debility.

1124. *Sarothamnus scoparius* *(Leguminosae)*

Synonyms: *Cytisus scoparius.*

Vernacular Name: *Eng:* Broom.

Description: Tall deciduous shrub growing to 2 m. Has narrow ridged stems, small trefoil leaves and bright yellow flowers in leafy terminal spikes.

Habitate: Native to Europe, broom is commonly found on heaths, verges, and in open woodland.

Propagation: By Seeds.

Parts Used: Flowers.

Chemical Constituents: Broom contains quinolizidine alkaloids, phenethylamines, isoflavones, flavonids, a volatile oil, caffeic and p-coumaric acids, tannins and pigments. Sparteine reduces the heart rate and the isoflavones are oestrogenic.

Uses: Broom is used mainly as a remedy for an irregular, fast heart beat. The plant acts on the electrical conductivity of the heart, slowing and regulating the transmission of the impulses. Broom is also strongly diuretic, stimulating urine production and thus countering fluid retention. Since broom causes the muscles of the uterus to contract, it has been used to prevent blood loss after childbirth.

1125. *Satureja montana* *(Lameaceae)*

Vernacular Name: *Eng:* Winter savory.

Description: Semi-evergreen aromatic herb growing to 40 cm. Has lance-shaped leaves and white-pink flowers appearing in clusters.

Habitate: Native to southern Europe, winter savory thrives in sunny, well-drained sites. It is commonly sunny, well-drained sites.

Propagation: By Seeds and cutting.

Parts Used: Flowers, essential oil.

Chemical Constituents: Winter savory contains about 1.6% volatile oil, composed mainly of carvacrol, p-cymene, linalool and thymol.

Uses: Winter savory is most often used in cookery, but is also has marked medicinal benefits. It settles wind and stimulates the digestion, helping to alleviate flatulence and colic. It is warming and has been taken for chest infections and bronchitis. They essential oil is strongly antibacterial and may be used to treat candidiasis and other fungal conditions.

1126. *Sauropus androgynus* (L.) Merr. *(Euphorbiaceae)*

Synonyms: *Saurpous albicans* Blume.

Vernacular Name: *Tam:* Thavasai murungai.

Description: Evergreen plant, 0.8-1.5m. high, much-branched, Stems cylindrical, intirely glabrous. Leaves alternate, ovate, base round, apex pointed; petiole very short. Stipule small. Flowers greenish-yellow, male and female on the same plant. Capsule globos, white, dehiscent into 3 valves when ripe.

Habitate: Cultivated everywhere as a vegetable.

Propagation: By seeds and vegetative method.

Part Used: Leaves and roots.

Chemical Constituents: The leaves contain amino acids: lysine, methionine, tryptophane, phenylalanine, threonine, valine, leucine, isoleucine; nicotinic acid, vitamin C and carotene.

Uses: The fresh leaves or roots possess uterotonic activity and are used for the treatment of retained placenta. A mouth-wash made of the juice of fresh leaves and honey and applied to the tongue and gums cures thrush of the tongue in infants. The elaves are effective for erythema, measles and dysuria. The roots serve as a diuretic and relieve congestion.

1127. *Saussurea lappa* C.B. Clarke *(Asteraceae)*

Synonyms: *Saussurea costus* (Fale.) Lipsch.

Vernacular Name: *Eng:* Kuth, Costus; *Hin:* Kuth, Kur; *Kan:* Kostha; *Mal:* Kottam, Simakkottam; *San:* Kusttah; *Tam:* Kostam, Gostham; *Tel:* Kostamu, Cengala,.

Description: A robust, erect perennial with a stem upto 2 m in height; keaves nenbranous, basal ones very large, upper ones small, irregularly toothed, basal clasping the stems by twolobes; flowers bluish purple in axillary and terminal heads; fruits compressed, curved achenes. The roots are stout, upto 60 cm long having and a rough reticulated surface.

Habitate: At low elevations of the Western Ghats in Kerala and Himalayas.

Propagation: By seeds.

Parts Used: Roots.

Chemical Constituents: The roots contains 1.5-2.5 per cent of volatile oil, an alkaloid saussurine resin and tannins. Kushtin has also been isolated from the roots.

Uses: The roots are bitter, acrid, sweet, thermogenic, aromatic deodorant, aphrodisiac, anodyne, carmimative, digestive, stomachic, diaphoretic, stimulant, alternate, depurative, galactagogue, diuretic disinfectant, expectorant, febrifuge, rekivemating and tonic. They are useful in chronic and foul ulcers, cephalalgia, odontalgia, odontalgia, cough, asthma, bronchitis, dyspepsia, flatulence, colic, cholera, leprosy, erysipelas, leucodemma, pruritus, ringwoem, disrrhoea, dysentery fever, hiccough, hysteria, strangury, dysmenorrhoea, cardiopathy, gout, gemera; debility and vitiated conditions of *vata*.

1128. *Scaevola taccada* (Gaertner) Roxb. *(Goodeniaceae)*

Synonyms: *Scaevola sericea* (Forstl.f.) Vahl.

Description: Spreading freely branching shrub with thick stems, up to 3 m in height. Leaves opposite, short-petiolate (or wanting), fleshy, glossy, light-green, obovate, variable in size, but usually about 15 cm long and 5 cm wide. Flowers white, zygomorphic, moderate-sized, 5-lobed, borne on few-flowered axillary inflorescences. Fruit a white, juicy, globose drupe containing 1-2 seeds.

Habitate: Common along beaches and rocky shores often forming dense beach thickets.

Propagation: By seeds.

Part Used: Roots, bark and leaves.

Chemical Constituents: Scaevolin, chlorogenica acid, saponins, glycosides, lipids (seeds), alkaloids.

Uses: Liquid from the leaves is used to treat weakness after childbirth which leads to pneumonia. The roots are used to treat stomachache. A decoction of the bark and leaves is used to treat a relapse after an illness. The juice from the bark is used in treating ringworm. The roots are used to treat beriberi, syphilis and dysentery. Parts of the plant are used to treat coughs, tuberculosis and stings from the stingray.

1129. *Schefflera octophylla* (Lour.) Harms *(Araliaceae)*

Vernacular Name: *Eng:* Octophyllous aralia.

Description: Tree 10m. high. Leaves palmate with 6-8 leaflets, alternate, lower part of long petiole surrounding the stem. Trunk bark and leaves smell sweet when crushed. Inflorescence in axillary or terminal receme of umbels; flowers small, greenish or white. Berry globose, dark violet when ripe.

Habitate: Grows wild in secondary forest in mountainous regions.

Propagation: By seeds.

Part Used: Bark.

Chemical Constituents: The root-bark and stem-bark contain triterpenoid saponins that yield oleanolic acid on hydrolysis.

Uses: The root-bark and stem-bark possess tonic, anti-inflammatory and diuretic properties and are used in treating rheumatism, lumbago, ostedynia paresis, amnesia, vulval pruritis, impotence, dyspepsia, infantile rickets, oedema, dysuria and impetigo.

1130. *Schisandra chinensis* Baill. *(Schisandraceae)*

Vernacular Name: *Eng*: Chinese magnolia vine.

Description: Deciduous, dioecious, twining shrub. Leaves simple, alternate, congested on short shoots, broad-elliptic or ovate, to 10 cm long, 3-5 cm wide, glossy above, denticulate or serrate; petioles 1.5-3 cm long. Flowers axillary, clustered on pedicels to 4 cm long, creamy with reddish tint; perianth segments 6-9,5-10 mm long, ovate to long-elliptic; stamens 5; carpe many; receptacle to 5 cm long in fruit. Fruit berries 6-20, red, to 1.5 cm long.

Habitate: Thickets in mountains.

Propagation: By Seeds.

Parts Used: Fruit, barriers.

Chemical Constituents: Lignans: schizandrin, deoxyschizandrin, gomisins A-T and their angeloyl, tigloy1 and benzoy1 ester derivatives.

Uses: CNS depression, antitussive, antiallergic, kanti-inflammatory, antidepressant, antioxytocic. Used in cough and weakness.

1131. *Schizonepeta tenuifolia* Briq. *(Lamiaceae)*

Vernacular Name: *Eng:* Fineleaved schizonepeta.

Description: An aromatic annual herb, 60-80 cm high. Stem erect, quadrangular, upper part branching, lower part purplish, the whole plant covered with a shallow pubescence. Leaves opposite, subsessile, pinnately 3-5 parted. Segments linear or lanceolate, 1.5-2 cm long by 2-4 mm wide, entire, underside dotted with glands. Inflorescence a verticillaster, like a terminal spike consisting of many compact whorls of cymes; spike 3-8 cm long; leaf-like bracts linear, sessile. Flowers small. Fruit a collection of ovoid or elliptic nutlets, brown, glossy.

Habitate: On sunny mountain slopes, in gullies or in grass in China.

Propagation: By seeds.

Part Used: Whole plant.

Chemical Constituents: N.A.

Uses: Common cold, lack of perspiration, headache, fever, sore throat; scabies.

1132. *Schleichera oleosa* (Lour.) Oken *(Sapindaceae)*

Vernacular Name: *San*: Mukulakah, Raktamrah, Laksavrksah; *Eng*: Lac tree, Ceyolon oak, Macassar–oil tree; *Hin*: Kusum, Kausum; *Ken:* Sagade, Kendala, Jendalacekota; *Mal*: Puvam; *Tam*: Puvattipuvam, Pumarata; *Tel:* Posuku, Busi, Kodalipulusu, Madakapulusu, Botanga, Sagsdipusuku, Mavidavitiki.

Description: A medium sized to large tree 15-32 m in height with a dense spreading crown and smooth pale brown bark exfoliating in small irregular flakes: leaves paripinnate, ultimate, leaflets 2-4 pairs, elliptic or elliptic-oblong the lowest pairusually yellow, either male or bisdexual, fascicled in spike-like lateral racemes: fruits ovoid or globose, smooth or slightly prickly hand-skinned berrors, seeds 1-2 brown, oily, enclosed in succulent aril.

Habitate: Throughout India, in semi-evergreen and deciduous forests.

Propagation: By seeds.

Parts Used: Bark, oil.

Chemical Constituents: Seeds contains phenols and polyene pigments. Kusum oil contains cyanolipid. Leaves contain alcohols, alkanes, stigmasterol, β-sitosterol, campesterol, cholesterol, glucose, fructose, tartartaric acid and oxalic acid.

Uses: The bark is astromgemt and antipyretic, and is useful in pruritus, adenitis, ripening boils, notalgia, arthralgia, malaria, inflammations and ulcers. The seed oil is bitter, sour, sweet, stomachic, anthelmintic, purgative, trichogenous and tonic. It is useful in pruritus, burns, acne, dermatipathy, scald, trichopathy, ulcers, cephalalgia and vitiated conditions of *vata*.

1133. *Schrebera swietenioides* Roxb. *(Oleaceae)*

Vernacular Name: *Eng*: Weaver's Beam tree; *Hin:* Moka, Banpalas; *Kan:* Bula, Gante, Nagganti, Mogalingamara; *Mal:* Malamplasu, Muskkakavrksam, Maggamaram; *San:* Muskakah, Ksarasresthah; *Tam:* Kattupparutticceti, Mogalingam; *Tel:* Magalinga, Bullakaya, Tondamukkudi.

Description: A moderate sized deciduous tree upto 20 m in height with thick grey bark; leaves imparipinnate, leaflats opposite, 3-4 pairs, ovate, entire, unequal-sided, petioles thickened at the insertion of leaflets; flowers yellowish brown in terminal trichotomous, corymbose, compound cymes; fruits pendulous, pear-shaped, 2-valved capsules; seeds 8, ending in long wings.

Habitate: Throughout India, in deciduous forests upto an altitude of 1,200 m.

Propagation: By seeds and vegetative method.

Parts Used: Roots, bark, leaves fruits.

Chemical Constituents: Charcoal, acetic acid, formic acid, methyl alcohal.

Uses: The roots, bark and leaves are bitter, acrid, appetising, digestive, thermogenic, stomachic, depurative, constipating urinary astringent and anthelmintic. They are useful in vitiated conditions of *kapha*, dyspepsia, colic, flatulence, skin diseases, leprosy, diarrhoea, urethrorrhea, splenomegaly, anaemia, helminthiasis, boils, burns and rectal disorders. The fruits are reported to be useful in curing hydrocele. It is digestive, purgative and stomachic, and is useful in flatulence, anorexia, colic, anaemia, haemorrhoids, vesical calculi and diabetes.

1134. *Scindapsus officinalis* (Roxb.) Schott *(Araceae)*

Vernacular Name: *Hin:* Gajapipal, Pipalijhamgha, Baripippli; *Kan:* Dodda hippali, Gajahippali; *Mal:* Attittippali, Anattippali; *San:* Gajapippali; *Tam:* Attittippali, Yanaittippili; *Tel:* Enugutippali, Gajapippallu, pippalu.

Description: A large epiphytic climber with adventitious aerial roots growing on trees and rocks; leaves large, upto 25 cm long, leathery; flowers densely arranged in the spadix which is cylindric, spathe green outside and yellow within; fruit berries, confluent.

Habitate: In forests throughout India.

Propagation: By vegetative method.

Parts Used: Dried mature inflorescence.

Chemical Constituents: Glucosidic colouring compounds, scindapsin A and B which on hydrolysis yields the aglycones, scindapsinidine A and B respectively and glucose, 11-hydroxy-cis-5, 8-tetracosadienoic acid and cyclopropenoid fatty acids, free sugars, fructose, glucose, rhamnose, xylose together with some di-and trisaccharides isolated from the plant.

Uses: The dried inflorescence is acrid, sweet, thermogenic, stimulant, aphrodisiac, expectorant, diaphoretic, carminative and anthelmintic. It is useful in vitiated conditions of *vata* and *kapha*, diarrhoea, cough, bronchitis, pharyngopathy and helminthiasis.

1135. *Scoparia dulcis* L. *(Scrophulariaceae)*

Vernacular Name: *Eng:* sweet broom, toothbrush.

Description: Annual herbaceous plant, 40-70cm. High. Stems woody at th base, much-branched, quadrangular when young, leaves small 3-verticullate or opposite, coarsely toothed-serrate. Flowers white, crosded in the axil of the leaves. Capsule small, globose, many seeded.

Habitate: Common as a wild plant in abandoned fields, on roadsides and on river banks.

Propagation: By seeds and vegetative method.

Part Used: Whole plant.

Chemical Constituents: The roots contain alkaloids and a bitter substance, amellin.

Uses: The entire plant, including the roots, possesses anti-inflammatory, antifebrile and diuretic properties. It is used in treating coryza, hyperthermia, sore throat, cough, erythema, measles, boils, impetigo, manioc and other poisoning and menorrhagia. The fresh plant is especially active against dry cough.

1136. *Scopolia japonica* Maxim. *(Solanaceae)*

Vernacular Name: *Eng*: Japanese scopolia.

Description: Glabrous perennial herb with fleshy rhizome, 30-60 cm tall. Stems erect, sparsely branched in upper part. Leaves alternate, entire, narrowly oblong, 10-20 cm long, 3-7 cm wide, acute at both tips and base, petiolate. Flowers solitary in axil, pendent, 3-5 cm long, calyx unequally 5-lobed, accrescent; corolla companulate, 2 cm long, purplish yellow, limb 5-lobed; stamens 5. Fruit globose, 1 cm in diameter, enclosed in the accrescent calyx.

Habitate: Mountains woods of Japan and Korea.

Propagation: By Rhizomes.

Parts Used: Rhizome.

Chemical Constituents: Hyoscyamine, scopolamine, scopoletin.

Uses: Sedative, pleurisy.

1137. *Scorophularia ningpoensis* Hemsl. *(Scrophulariaceae)*

Vernacular Name: *Eng:* Ning-po figwort.

Description: Herbaceous plant, 1.5-2m. tall. Stems quadrangular, greenish, grooved. Leaves opposite, pointed at the apex; margins toothed. Inflorescence in short axillary and terminal raceme; flowers brownish-yellow. Fruit and seeds black.

Habitate: An introduced species, naturalized and widespread in the mountains, midlands and plains.

Propagation: By seeds.

Part Used: Roots.

Chemical Constituents: The roots contain scrophularin, asparagine, phytosterols, an essential oil, fatty acids and sugars.

Uses: The root possesses antifebril, antibacterial and anti-inflammatory properties. It is utilized in the treatment of evening feber, erythema, mouth dryness, constipation, prurigo, furunculosis, sore throat, ulcerous stomatitis and tonsilitis.

1138. *Scrophularia buergeriana* Miq. *(Scrophulariaceae)*

Vernacular Name: *Eng*: Buerger's figwort.

Description: Perennial herb of 4-angled stem, glabrous, to 80-150 cm tall. Leaves opposite, simple broad-ovate, acute, 5-10 cm long, 2.5-5 cm wide, serrate; petioles slightly winged or without wing. Flowers greenish-yellow, small in terminal cymes arranged in panicles, 1-2 cm long; calyx 5-lobed; corolla tube 6-7 mm long, urceolate, 2-celled. Fruit a round capsule.

Habitate: Grassy areas in lowlands.

Propagation: By seeds.

Parts Used: Root.

Chemical Constituents: Iridoids; harpagoside, 8-(o-methyl-R-coumaroyl)-harpagide. Oligosaccharides, R-methoxycinnamic acid.

Uses: Vasodilating, hypotensive, anti-inflammatory, hypoglycaemic, antipyretic. Used in phlegum, goitree, scrofula and erysipelas.

1139. *Scrophularia nodosa* *(Scrophulariaceae)*

Vernacular Name: *Eng:* Figwort.

Description: Upright perennial herb growing to 1 m. Has a square stem, oval leaves, small round brown flowers in clusters and green seeds capsules.

Habitate: Native to Europe, Central Asia and North America, figwort thrives in wet or damp places, in open woodland, on riverbanks and alongside ditches.

Propagation: By Seeds.

Parts Used: Aerial parts.

Chemical Constituents: Figwrot contains iridoids, flavonoids, cardioactive glycosides and phenolic acids. Harpagoside and harpagide are thought to account for its anti-arthritic activity.

Uses: Figwort is a herb that supports detoxification of the body and may be used as a treatment for various types of skin conditions. Taken internally as an infusion or applied externally, figwort is of value in treating chronic skin diseases such as eczema and psoriasis. Applied externally, it will also help speed the healing of burns, wounds, haemorrhoids and ulcers. The traditional use of figwort as a treatment for swellings and tumours continues in Europe to this dry. The herb is also mildly diuretic, and it is reputed to be effective when used to expel worms.

1140. *Scutellaria baicalensis* Georgi. *(Lamiaceae)*

Synonyms: *Scutellaria macrantha* Fisch.

Vernacular Name: *Eng:* Baikal skullcap.

Description: A spreading perennial herb 20-60 cm high, the stems erect, tetragonal, branching near the base, glabrous or pubescent at the corners. Leaves opposite, with short petioles; limb lanceolate, 1.5-4 cm long by 5 mm side; tip obtuse, entire. Flowers blue, in racemesl. Fruit a collection of small tuberculate nutlets, nearly globular, leathery.

Habitate: On exposed slopes or by roadsides in mountainous areas in China, Korea, Mongolia, Soviet Union.

Propagation: By seeds.

Part Used: Roots.

Chemical Constituents: N.A.

Uses: High temperature due to febrile disease; common cold, conjunctivitis, haemoptysis, epistaxis, general fatigue, jaundice, headache due to hypertension, enteritis; dysentery, fetal distress, skin inflammation, burns.

1141. *Scutellaria barbata* D. Don. *(Lamiaceae)*

Vernacular Name: *Eng:* Barbed skullcap.

Description: An annual or perennial herb, 15-40 cm high, glabrous, stem quardrangular and creeing below. Leaves opposite, the lower with short petioles, the upper sessile, blade ovate or lanceolate, obtuse, entire or crenate, 1-3 cm long by 0.5-1.5 cm wide. Flowers from April to October. Spikes 7-14 cm long, bracts quite entire, ovate or laneolate. Flowers axillary, subsessile or apicate. Nutlets very minute, smooth, granulate or hispidulous.

Habitate: On damp, shaded slopes in China, India and Japan.

Propagation: By seeds.

Part Used: Whole plant.

Chemical Constituents: N.A.

Uses: General fatigue, abdominal pain and ascites, pyodermas, snake bites, injuries.

1142. *Scutellaria lateriflora* *(Lameaceae)*

Vernacular Name: *Eng:* Skullcap, Virginian skullcap, Mad dog.

Description: A perennial growing to 60 cm, with an erect, many-branched stem and pink to blue flowers.

Habitate: A native of North America, skullcap still grows wild in much of the US and Canada.

Propagation: By seeds.

Parts Used: Seeds.

Chemical Constituents: Flavonoids, Bitter iridoids, volatile oil Tannins.

Uses: Sedative, Nervine tonic, antispasmodic, Mild bitter.

1143. *Securinega leucopyrus* (Willd.) Muell-Arg. *(Euphorbiaceae)*

Synonyms: *Fluggea leucpyrus* Willd.

Vernacular Name: *San:* Panduraphali Bhuriphali; *Eng:* Spinous fluggea; *Hin:* Hartto, Ainta; *Kan:* Bilculi, Gudahale, Huli; *Mal:* Ampuripaccila, Mulpulanni; *Tam:* Mulluppulatti, Vellaippulanci; *Tel:* Tellapulisara, Pulugudu, Puli, Callmunta.

Description: A large, rigid, thorny bush with somewhat straggling branches, usually ending in sharp thorns; leaves simple, alternate, obovate or obcordate or elliptic, reticulately veined beneath; flowers very small, male greenish yellow in clusters, female reddish, also in clusters; fruits globose, white fleshy berries.

Habitate: In dry localities throughout India.

Propagation: By seeds and vegetative method.

Parts Used: Whole plant.

Chemical Constituents: An unidentified alkaloid as wel as free triterpenes, diterpenes, steroids or related polycyclic substances are said to occur in the leaves. Stem bark contains tannins and friedelin.

Uses: The plant is sweet, cooling, diuretic, aphrodisiac and tonic, and is useful in vitiated conditions of *pitta*, burning sensation, strangury, seminal weakness and general debility.

The leaves act as a disinfectant and its paste is used by tribes to extract any extraneous materials from body tissues without surgery.

1144. *Selenicereus grandiflorus* *(Cactaceae)*

Vernacular Name: *Eng:* Night-blooming cereus.

Description: Climbing multi-branched perennial cactus with upright cylindrical stems and aerial roots. Produces large flowerbuds opening into night-blooming white flowers that grow to 20 cm across, and red oval fruit.

Habitate: Native to Mexico and Central America, night-blooming cereus is now rarely found in the wild.

Propagation: By Seeds and cutting.

Parts Used: Flowers, stems.

Chemical Constituents: Night-blooming cereus contains alkaloids, flavonoids and a pigment. Cactine's cardiotonic effect is considered similar to that of cardiac glycosides,.

Uses: As it is in short supply, night-blooming cereus in little used at present, but it is a valuable remedy for the heart. It stimulates the action of the heart, increasing the strength of contractions while slowing heart rate. It is prescribed as a treatment for various conditions, including angina and low blood pressure, and is often given as a tonic during recovery from a heart attack. In the Caribbean, the juice of the whole plant is used to expel worms, and the stems and flowers are used in the treatment of rheumatism.

1145. *Selinum vaginatum* C.B. Clarke. *(Apiaceae)*

Vernacular Name: Bhutheshi, Mathosla.

Description: A glabrous, stout herb, 1.0 to 1.5m tall with robust, aromatic rootstock beset with thick tuft of grey fibres, left over by the dying leaves. Roots, 12 to 18 cm long, abruptly tapering from the middle. Stem is hollow and finely grooved. Leaves, 1 to 2 pinnate; segments lanceolate, serrate, lobed or pinnatifid. Flowers-white, in long-stalked, compound umbels. Fruit-glabrous, flattened, ovate-oblong, 4 to 8 mm long with winged ridges.

Habitate: Distributed in Western Himalaya between 1800-3800 m. Found in temperate and alpine moist pastures in Chhota-Bara Bhangal area of Kangra, Holi Range of Chamba, Parvati Valley and Rohtang area in Kullu, Rampur and Rohru division of Shimla district.

Propagation: By seeds.

Part Used: Roots.

Chemical Constituents: Roots contain coumarins like selinidin, vaginidin, angelicin, oroselol and lomatin. A flavone derivative selinone has also been reported. Dried roots on steam distillation yield an aromatic oil containing 45.5% alphapinene, 25.3% limonene, 5.7% camphene, 5.2% beta-phellanetrine, 1.2% alphathujene, 3.2% fenchyl alcohol, 3.8% terpeneol and 2.6% an unidentified ketone.

Uses: The roots possess a sweet, musky odour with a bitter taste and are employed as incense. They are also used as nervine sedatives. The roots of S. vaginatum and S. wallichianum are often offered as a cheap substitute to jatamansi and also adulterated with the later. The oil obtained from the roots, has hypotensive, sedative and analgesic properties. Large scale collection from the area is possible and proper time is October.

1146. *Selinum wallichianum* (DC.) Raizada and Saxena ex. Raizada. *(Apiaceae)*

Synonyms: *Selinum tenuifolium* Wall.

Vernacular Name: Muramansi, Mathosal, Nesrawlo.

Description: An erect herb, 0.6 to 2.4 m tall with a perennial rootstock. Leaves-pinnately compound deeply cut into narrow, linear-lanceolate, acute segments. Flowers white in compound umbels. Fruits 0.5 cm, much dorsally compresded, lateral ridges are the broadest.

Habitate: Temperate Himalaya between 2000-4000m. In Himachal Pradesh, it is usually found in temperate pasture lands, forest shades and alpine pastures in Kangra, Kullu, Chamba, Kinnaur, Sirmour and Shimla district between 2400-4200m.

Propagation: By seeds.

Part Used: Rootstock.

Chemical Constituents: Three furanocoumarins-bergapten, heraclenin and heraclenol alongwith another coumarin ST-1 have been isolated from the roots. Angelicin and xanthotoxol are the two other coumarins and a mixture of long chain saturated fatty oils has also been detected. Seeds yield essential oil. The volatile oil from the roots contains an acetylenic compound-3, 5-nonadiyne.

Uses: Root is regarded as a nervine sedative and used as a substitute for Jatamansi. Frequently used as incense and in local brew, called as 'Dheli'. The oil from the root has hypotensive, sedative and analgesic properties. Leaves are regarded as a nutritious fodder for sheep and goats.

1147. *Semecarpus anacardium* L.f. *(Anacardiaceae)*

Vernacular Name: *San:* Bhallatakah, Arusharah; *Eng:* Marking nut tree, Oriental cashew; *Hin:* Bhela, Bhilava; *Kan:* Goddugeru, Karigeri, Bhallika; *Mal:* Ceru, Alakkuceru; *Tam:* Senkottai, Erimugi; *Tel:* Bhallatamu, Jidi.

Description: A medium sized to large tree, 15-25 m in height, with grey bark exfoliating in small irregular flakes; leaves simple, alternate, obovate-oblong, rounded at the apex, coriaceous, glabrous above and more or less pubescent beneath, main nerves 15-25 pairs; flowers greenishwhite, fascicled in pubescent panicles; fruits obliquely ovoid or obong drupes, 2.5 cm long, black when ripe, seated on a fleshy receptacle which is yellow when ripe.

Habitate: Throughout India, in semi-evergreen and moist deciduous forests.

Propagation: By seeds.

Parts Used: Fruits.

Chemical Constituents: Anacardic acid, cardol, catechol, anacardol and fixed oil; semicarpol, bhilawanol.

Uses: The fruits are acrid, bitter, astringent, weet, themogenic, emollient, digestive, carminative, anthelmintic, purgative, liver tonic, expectorant, alternate, aphrodisiac, antiarthritic, depurative, anticarcinomic, stimulant, urinary astringent, antiseptic, anti-inflammatory, cardiotonic, uterine stimulant, sudorific, febrifuge, rejuvenating and tonic. They are useful in beriberi, cancer, vitiated conditions of *kapha* and *vata*, sciatica, neuritis, cough, asthma, dyspepsia, constipation, flatulence, colic, haemorrhoids, helminthiasis especially hookworms, hepatophathy, splenopathy, leprosy, leucolderma, scaly skin eruptions, inflammations, cardiac disease, fever, diabetes, dysmenorrhoea, amenorrhoea, scrophulla, tumours, ulcers and general debility.

1148. *Semecarpus travancorica* Bedd. *(Anacardiaceae)*

Vernacular Name: *Kan*: Kadu gobbi, *Mal*: Avukkaram, *Tam*: Kattu chenkottai, Nattu chenkottai, Periya seran, *Tel:* attu sengote.

Description: Large evergreen trees, 10-30 m tall. *Bark* smooth; *Leaves* alternate, simple, crowded at the tip of branchlets, inverted egg-shaped-oblong to oblanceolate, 25-60 x 10-15 cm, base acute or rounded, apex round or retuse, margin entire, recurved, thick leathery, hairless, glossy, dark green turning yellow when old; *Male, female* and *bisexual flowers* are separately seen in the same plant, greenish yellow, distinctly stalked, arranged in axillary and terminal panicles, which are about 20 cm long. *Drupes* un equally oblong, about 3 cm long, ripening black, exude black acrid juice, seated on a cup-shaped, fleshy, about 1 cm across stalk called as 'hypocarp'.

Habitate: Evergreen forests.

Propagation: By seeds.

Parts Used: Bark, Gum, Oil.

Chemical Constituents: Phenolic and non-phenolic fractions catechol constituent laccol polymerizes on standing to a glossy, friable mass soluble in benzene acetone and chloroform.

Uses: Chopra *et al* in *"Glossary of Indian Medicinal Plants"* report that the medicinal properties of *S. anacardium* and *S. travancorica* are similar. Hence the latter could substitute the former, which has the following uses: Gum and bark is used for treating scrofulous, venereal and leprous infections and nervous debility. Nuts are used on bruises and applied to uteri to induce abortion; also given as a vermifuge. Oil from nuts is used externally to releave rheumatism and leprous nodules. Ashes of the plant in combination with other drugs are used for the treatment of snakebites and scorpion stings.

1149. *Sempervivum tectorum* *(Crassulaceae)*

Vernacular Name: *Eng:* Houseleek.

Description: Succulent perennial growing to 10 cm. Has round rosettes of leaves, and flowering stems bearing clusters of bell-shaped red flowers.

Habitate: Houseleek is native to central and southern Europe and now grows wild in northern Europe, North Africa and western Asia.

Propagation: By cutting.

Parts Used: Leaves, leaf juice.

Chemical Constituents: Houseleek contains tannin, mucilage, malic acid and formic acid.

Uses: Houseleek leaves and their juice are used for their cooling and astringent effect, being applied externally to soothe many skin conditions, including burns, wounds, boils and corns. As with many other remedies that are both astringent and soothing, houseleek simultaneously tightens and softens the skin. Traditionally, the leaves have been chewed to relieve toothache, and the juice has been sniffed to stop nosebleeds. Houseleek is still used externally, but internal use is not advised because in large does it induces vomiting.

1150. *Senecio aureus* *(Asteraceae)*

Vernacular Name: *Eng:* Life root, Squaw weed.

Description: Upright perennial growing to 1m. Has lance-shaped leaves and clusters of yellow daisy-type flowers.

Habitate: Native to eastern North America, life root is found in marshes, on damp ground and riverbanks.

Propagation: By Seeds.

Parts Used: Aerial parts.

Chemical Constituents: Life root contains a volatile oil, pyrrolizidine alkaloids, tannins and resin. In isolation, the pyrrolizidine alkaloids are highly toxic to the liver.

Uses: Until recently, life root was employed in Anglo-American herbalism much as it was in earlier times-as a means to induce menstrual periods and to bring relief to menopausal complaints. Today, the plant is recommended only for external use, as a douche for excessive vaginal discharge.

1151. *Senecio jacobeae* *(Asteraceae)*

Vernacular Name: *Eng:* Ragwort.

Description: Biennial or perennial plant growing to about 1 m. Has lobed compound leaves and dense clusters of bright yellow daisy-type flowers.

Habitate: Regwort is native to much of Asia, Europe and North Africa, and is naturalized in North America and Australia. It thrives in open grassland, meadows and verges.

Propagation: By Seeds.

Parts Used: Aerial part.

Chemical Constituents: Rragwort contains a volatile oil, pyrrolizidine alkaloids, tannins and resin. In isolation, pyrrolizidine alkaloids are highly toxic to the liver.

Uses: While no loner taken internally, ragwort still finds use as a poultice, ointment or lotion applied to relieve pain and inflammation. Conditions treated by ragwort include rheumatism and rheumatoid arthritis, and neuralgic conditions such as sciatica.

1152. *Sesamum indicum* L. *(Pedaliaceae)*

Vernacular Name: *San:* Tilah; *Eng:* Sesame, Gingelly; *Hin:* Til; *Kan:* Ellu; *Mal:* Ellu; *Tam:* Ellu, Eellu-cceti; *Tel:* Nuvvulu.

Description: An erect, pubescent annual upto 90 cm in height, branching from the base; leaves large, thin, the lower ones lobed, sparsely hairy, uppermost linear and intermediate usually ovate and toothed: flowers white, pink or purplish with yellow marks in racemes in the leaf axils; fruits quadrangular, oblong, compressed capsules, deeply 4-grooved, dehiscent from above to half way down; seeds many, black, brown or white.

Habitate: Cultivated throughout India in the plains and upto an altitude of 1200m.

Propagation: By seeds.

Parts Used: Roots, leaves, seeds, oil.

Chemical Constituents: Seeds are fairly rich in thiamine and niacin. The principal protein is a globulin. Seeds contain a fixed oil and leaves contain a gummy matter. A flavonoid glucoside pedalin isolated from leaves.

Uses: Roots and leaves are emollient and a decoction of them forms a good hair-wash which will promote hair growth and will blacken them. The leaves are useful in dysentery, cholera, vitiated conditions of *kapha*, nephropathy, uropathy, ophthalmopathy and dermatopaty. The seeds are sweet, astringent, bitter, acrid, emollient, themogenic, aphrodisiac, laxative, galactagogue, digestive, hair-restorer and tonic. They are useful in haemorrhoids, ulcers, burns, dysentery, vitiated conditions of *vata*, strangury, dermatopathy, migraine, alopecia, ophthalmopath and obesity. In medicated oils sesame oil forms a fat soluble medium. The oil is bitter, astringent, sweet, themogenic, digestive, anthelminitc, constipating and emollient, and is good for ophathalmopathy, burning sensation of the legs, gonorrhoea, otalgia, cephalalgia, obesity and emaciation. Externally it is used for dryness of the skin and leucoderma.

1153. *Sesbania grandiflora* (L.) Poir. *(Fabaceae)*

Vernacular Name: *San:* Agastyah; *Eng:* Swamp pea, Sesban; *Hin:* Hathya, Agast, Basna, Haddga; *Kan:* Agasi; *Mal:* Akatti, Agatti, Atti, Argatti; *Tam:* Attikkirai; *Tel:* Avesi, Avasinara.

Description: A short lived, quick growing, soft-wooded tree, 6-9 m high and 0.6 m in girth; leaves 15-30 cm long, abruptly pinnate; leaflets 41-61, linear-oblong, deciduous; flowers 6-10 cm long with showy, fleshy white, pink or red petals; pods 30 cm or more long, rather flat and somewhat 4-cornered, non-torulose, septate with swollen margins and 15-50 pale coloured seeds.

Habitate: Cultivated in gardens and betel-vine plantations.

Propagation: By seeds.

Parts Used: Root bark, leaves, flowers, fruits.

Chemical Constituents: Grandifloral, arginine, cystine, histidine, isolcucine, phenylalanine, tryptophan, valine, threonine, alanine, aspargine, aspartic acid and a saponin yielding oleanolic acid, galactose, rhamnose and glucuronic acid.

Uses: The root-bark of the red-flowered variety is useful in vitiated conditions of *vata* and arthralgia. The bark is astringent, cooling, bitter, tonic, anthelmintic and febrifuge. The pounded bark is externally applied to cure scabies. The juice of the bark is good for dyspepsia, diarrhoea and gastralgia. The leaves are acrid, bitter, sweet, cooling, aperient, tonic and diuretic, and contain a non-poisonous saponine-like substance. The leaf juice is used in nasal catarrh, nyctalopai and cephalalgia. Leaves are chewed to disinfect mouth and throat and are useful in stomatalgia. The flowers are cooling, bitter, astringent, acrid and antipyretic. The juice of the flowers is applied to the eyes for nyctalopia and is used for intermittent fevers. The fruits are sweet, bitter, laxative and alexiteric and are useful in flatulant-colic, anaemia, emaciation and vitiated conditions of tridosa.

1154. *Setaria italica* (L.) P. Beauv *(Poaceae)*

Vernacular Name: *San:* Kanguh, Kanguni; *Eng:* Indian millet, Fox-tail millet; *Hin:* Karmguni, Kamguni; *Kan:* Bilikorla-hullu; *Mal:* Tina, Tena, Tenayari; *Tam:* Tenai; *Tel:* Koralu, Nakka-korra.

Description: A herbaceous or robust annual with erect, tufted, fasciculated and prominently jointed culms, 0.6-1.5 m in height; leaves linear or lanceolate-linear, acuminate, sheath densely ciliate on margin and mouth; flowers in spikelets which are oval and borne on abbreviated branchlets of the panicle; grain oblong or ellipsoid and of various colours tightly enclosed in the hardended lemma and palea.

Habitate: Widely cultivated in India.

Propagation: By seeds.

Parts Used: Grains.

Chemical Constituents: Folic acid, nicotinic acid, riboflavin, thiamine, vitamin A; proteins: albumin, globulin, glutenin, prolamine, α-and β-setarins; alanine, arginine, lutamic acid, histidine, isoleucine, leucine, lysine, methionine, phenylalanine, proline, threonine, tryptophan, valine; α-D-glucan; phytic acid; arachidic, behenic, linoleic, linolenic, oleic, palmitic, stearic acids β-alanine, γ-aminobutyric acid; D-alanyl-Dalanine, betaine and betaine aldehyde dehydrogenase.

Uses: The grains are sweet, acrid, astringent, cooling, aphrodisiac, diuretic and laxative and are useful in rheumatism, burning sensation, fractures and for alleviating the pain of parturition.

1155. *Shorea robusta* Gaertn.f. *(Dipterocarpaceae)*

Vernacular Name: *Eng:* Sal; *Hin:* Sal, Sal; *Kan:* Kabba, Sala; *Mal:* Salavrksam, Mulappumarutu; *San:* Salah; *Tam:* Salam; *Tel:* Sarjakamu, Guggilamu.

Description: A large deciduous tree, 18-30 m in height with smooth or longitudinally fissured reddish brown or grey bark; leaves simple, ovate-oblong, acuminate, tough, coriaceous, glabrous, base cordate or rounded, lateral nerves 12-15 pairs; flowers yellowish, in lax axillary or terminal panicles, stamens upto 50, connectives with subulate bearded appendages, minutely 3-fid at the apex; fruits indehiscent, ovoid with 5 equal wings; seeds ovoid with fleshy unequal cotyledons.

Habitate: In North-East and Central India upto 1,700 m.

Propagation: By seeds.

Parts Used: Bark, leaves, fruits, resin.

Chemical Constituents: Presence of 2-(2-iminoacetic acid)–3-(2H)-benzo-furanone, glucoside of 4'hydroxychalcone, leuconathocyanidin, hopcaphenol, triterpenoids and a terpene alcohol, furfural, monomethylether and dimethyl ether of homocatechol, alkylbenzene derivatives, pentosans, lignan, tannin, amino-acids and fatty acids.

Uses: The bark and leaves are astringent, acrid, cooling, anthelmintic, alexeteric, anodyne, constipating, urnary astringent, union promoter, depurative and tonic. They are useful in vitiated conditions of *kapha* and *pitta*, ulcers, wounds otalga, bacterial affections, diarrhoea, dysentery, gonorrhoea, leucorrhoe, pruritus, leprosy, cough, hyperhidrosis, haemorrhoids and anaemia. The fruits are sweet, astringent, cooling, aphrodisia, cholagogue and tonic, and are useful in dipsia, burning sensation, tubercular ulcers, seminal weakness and dermatopathy. The resin is astringent, sweet, acrid, cooling, anodyne, vulnerary, antibacterial, deodorant, constipating, detergent, carminative, stomachic, aphrodisia, expectorant, ophathalmic and tonic. It is useful in hyperhidroses, vitiated conditions of *pitta*, wounds ulcers, neuralgia, burns, pruritus, fractures, fever, diarrhoea, dysentery, haemorrhoids, gonorrhoea, menorrhagia, splenomegaly, obesity, cephalalgia, odontalgia, burning of the eyes and ophthalmodynia.

1156. *Shorea tumbuggaia* Roxb. *(Dipterocarpaceae)*

Vernacular Name: *Hin*: Kala damar, *Mal*: *Tam*pakam, *Tam*: *Tam*bagam, Celai vakai, Karuppu dammar, *Kan*gu, *Tel:* Guggilamu, *Tam*ba jalory, Nalladam mara.

Description: Deciduous trees, growing up to 18 m tall. *Trunk* about 2 m girth. *Wood* hard and brown. *Bark* dark brown, thick, rough, longitudinally fissured; *Leaves* alternate, egg-shaped, 5-20 x 3-11 cm, base rounded to slightly heart-shaped, apex acuminate, margin entire, hairless on both surfaces; lateral nerves about 8 pairs, prominent at lower surface; leaf stalks 2-5 cm long, hairy. *Stipules* prominent. *Flowers* in axillary panicles, shortly stalked, 1.5 cm long, fragrant, white outside and yellow inside; flower buds densely hairy. *Fruit* is an indehiscent nut, oval-shaped, about 2 cm long, pubescent, with persistent 3 larger and 2 smaller sepal-like wings; larger wings, spoon-shaped, apex blunt, pubescent, about 4 x 1.5 cm, 8-10 nerved. *Seeds* solitary, egg-shaped.

Habitate: Dry deciduous forests.

Propagation: By seeds.

Parts Used: Gum.

Chemical Constituents: N.A.

Uses: The oleoresin is used as an external stimulant.

1157. *Sida cordata* (Burm.f.) Borssum *(Malvaceae)*

Synonyms: *Sida veronicaefolia* Lam.

Vernacular Name: *San:* Nagabala, Bhumibala; *Hin:* Bananiyar, Bhyunli; *Kan:* Bikkanatalegida; *Mal:* Vallikkuruntotti; *Tam:* Palampasi; *Tel:* Gayapuvaku, Gayapaku.

Description: A procumbent, diffuse, much branched hairy herb with a very short main stem and long selnder trainling branches that occasionally root at places of contact with the soil; leaves long-petioled, cordate to roundish with stellate hairs; flowers yellow, solitary or in pairs in the axils; fruits schizocarp located within the persistent calyx; seeds brownish, glabrous.

Habitate: Throughout India, as a weed on road sides and other waste place.

Propagation: By seeds.

Parts Used: Whole plant.

Chemical Constituents: It contains β-phenethylamines, quinazoline, carboxylated tryptamine, linoleic acid, malvalic acid, sterculic acid and gossypol.

Uses: The roots are sweet, sour, astringent, bitter, acrid, thermogenic and tonic, and are useful in fever, uropathy and arthritis. The bark of the root is used for leucorrhoea, gonorrhoea and hyperdiuresis. The leaves are good for diarrhoea. The flowers and ripe fruits are refrigerant and are useful in releiving burning sensation, hyperdiuresis, pectoral lesions and promoting strength.

1158. *Sida cordifolia* L. *(Malvaceae)*

Vernacular Name: *San*: Bala, *Hin*: Kungyi, *Beng*: Stetberela, Brela, Bala; *Guj*: Bala, Baldana; *Tel:* Tellaantisa, Tellagorra; *Tam*: Nilatutti, Paniartuthi; *Kan*: Hettuthi, Hettugigada, Kisangi; *Mal*: Kurunthatti, Velleoum.

Description: The plant is an undershrub, branched, softly hairy and with stellate hairs, nearly in all the parts of the plant. Leaves are 2.5-5 cm long, cordate, ovate-oblong, crenate, obtuse or subacute and not acuminate and the petioles are 1.2-3.8 cm long. Pedicels are solitary and few together, short, some upto 1.2-2 cm long bearing yellow flowers. Calyx is 6-8 mm long with ovate and acute lobes. Corolla exceed the calyx slightly. Fruit is 6-8 mm in diameter; strongly reticulated with two spiny projections on the top.

Habitate: The plant is a common weed distributed throughout tropical and sub-tropical India and Ceylon in waste places and scrub jungles upto an altitude of 1050 m.

Propagation: By seeds.

Part Used: Entire plant.

Chemical Constituents: Sida contains an alkaloid, a fatty oil, phytosterol mucin, resin, resin acids and potassium nitrate. The leaves, stem and root yield 0.085 per cent, and the seeds about 0.3 per cent alkaloid. The main portion of the alkaloid is ephedrine. Mehra, P.N. has reported 0.4 per cent rutin in the plant.

Uses: The plant is reputed for its tonic and aphrodisiac properties. The plant parts are used for the fever, fits, leucorrhoea, micturition, gonorrhoea, colic, nervous discorders, general debility and heart irregularity. The root juice is used for the healing of the wound and the juice of the whole plant is given for spermatorrhoea. The bark of the plant is effective in curing facial paralysis and sciatica and the leaves are used for curing the bloody flux. Useful in ophthalmia, rheumatism; shivering fits and improves sexual strength.

1159. *Sida rhombifolia* L. *(Malvaceae)*

Vernacular Name: *Hin:* Jamglimedhi; *Kan:* Ceruparuva, Malatanni; *Mal:* Kuruntotti; *San:* Bala; *Tam:* Kuruntotti; *Tel:* Cirubenda, Visaboddi, Cittimutti.

Description: An erect, minutely hairy, branched undershrub with a firm woody stem and intricate branches; leaves short-petioled, obovate, truncate of more often retuse and serrate; flowers yellow, solitary and axillary; cocci; seeds black, smooth.

Habitate: Throughout the warmer part of India, as a wed of waste places.

Propagation: By seeds.

Parts Used: Roots, leaves.

Chemical Constituents: Ephedrine, cellulose and lignin, quinazolines, β-phenethylamines, tryptamine derivative, sterculic, malvalic, linoleic acids.

Uses: The roots and leaves are bitter, sweet, emollient, cooling, aphrodisiac, unctuous, strengthening and prmote sexual vigour and vital factor. They are good for rheumatism, flatulence, colic, haemothermia, emaciation, vitiated conditions of tridosa, seminal weakness, arthritis and diarrhoea.

1160. *Sida spinosa* L. *(Malvaceae)*

Vernacular Name: *Eng:* Prickly sida; *Hin:* Bariyara, Gulsakari; *Kan:* Kadumentya; *Mal:* Anakkuruntotti; *San:* Mahabala; *Tam:* Mairmanikkam; *Tel:* Nagabala, Teranellabenda.

Description: A small, erect, grey, pubescent, branched undershrub with a slender erect stem, the young shoots being covered over with soft, grey stellate down; leaves with 2 or 3 small, stiff, minute spiny projections at the nodes adjacent to the place of insertion; flowers pale yellow to cream white, axillary and solitary on slender peduncles; fruits 5-6 or 3-chambered with one seed in each chamber; seeds brownish black, smooth.

Habitate: Throughout the hotter parts of India.

Propagation: By seeds.

Parts Used: Whole plant.

Chemical Constituents: Quinazoline, β-phenethylamines and tryptamine derivatives.

Uses: The roots are diaphoretic, antiperiodic, anphrodisiac and tonic. They are administered in debility, fever, malarial fever, vitiated conditions of *vata*, haemorrhoids, swellings and in irritability of the bladder. The leaves are emollient and refrigerant and are useful in gonorrhoea, gleet and scalding urine. The fruits are astringent and cooling.

1161. *Siegesbeckia orientalis* L. *(Asteraceae)*

Vernacular Name: *Eng:* Common St. Paul's wort.

Description: An annual herb about 50 cm tall. Stem stiff, erect with branches horizontal below and dichotomously branched above; stem and branches tinged with purple, terete, pubescent. Leaves opposite, 5-12.5 cm long by 3-7 cm wide, triangular-ovate, acute or acuminate, deeply and irregularl toothed, the uppermost leaves much smaller and nearly entire, all finely pubescent on both sides; base cuneate, running down wing-like into a somewhat obscure petiole. Flowers in October Heads small, peduncled, in leafly panicles, flowers yellow, those of the ray red underneath. Involucre bracts in 2 rows. Achenes each enclosed in a boat-shaped bract, glabrous, slightly rough, black. The leaves taste slightly bitter.

Habitate: On waste ground and at roadsides in Cambodia, China, India, Laos, Philippines, Sri Lanka, Viet Nam.

Propagation: By seeds.

Part Used: Whole plant.

Chemical Constituents: Essential oil, salicylic acid and bitter glucoside.

Uses: Rheumatic arthralgia, fatigue with fever, neurasthenia, ulcer; abscesses; boils.

1162. *Sinapis alba* L. *(Cruciferae)*

Vernacular Name: *Eng:* white mustard; salad mustard.

Description: An annual or biennial herb, up to 1 m high. Stem stout, the foliage villous-prickly. Leaves alternate, petiolate, lyrate-pinnatifid, with a large terminal lobe, the segments sinuatedentate. Inflorescence a terminal raceme, the pedicels erect, epanded, and as long as the valves, Flowers in summer, yellow. Fruit a cyluidrical embossed silique covered with white hairs, constricted between the seeds; valves with 3 prominent veins; beak compressed; tip attenuate, longer than the valves. Seeds 2-3 in each cell, yellowish-white, globular, 1.5-2 mm in diameter.

Habitate: Mostly cultivated in Asia, Europe, and North America.

Propagation: By seeds.

Part Used: Seeds.

Chemical Constituents: N.A.

Uses: Distension in the chest and hypochondrium, dyspnaea due to the accumulation of phlegm, joint pains, neuralgia; bruises; sprains; injuries.

1163. *Smilax china* L. *(Liliaceae)*

Vernacular Name: *San:* Dvipantaravaca, Madhusnuhi; *Eng:* China root; *Hin:* Cobcini; *Kan:* Cinipavu; *Mal:* Pavu, Cinappavu; *Tam:* Parankicekkai; *Tel:* Parangicekka.

Description: A hard tendril climber with sparsely prickled or unarmed stems and thick tuberous rhizomes; leaves simple, alternate, elliptic, rounded at the base, prominently nerved; flowers many, small, white in umbels; fruits red berries.

Habitate: In China and Japan.

Propagation: By seeds and rhizomes.

Parts Used: Rhizomes.

Chemical Constituents: Tannin, resin and cinchonin, along with smilacin, and a steroidal saponin, flavonoid glycosides, diosgenin, and rutin.

Uses: The rhizomes are bitter, acrid, thermogenic, anodyne, anti-inflammatory, digestive, laxative, depurative, aphrodisiac, diuretic, sudorific, febrifuge and tonic. They are useful in syphilis, leprosy, skin diseases, epilepsy, insanity, scrofula, vitiated conditions of *vata*, flatulence, dyspepsia, colic, neuralgia, constipation, helminthiasis, psoriasis, fever, strangury, seminal weakness and general debility.

1164. *Smilax zeylanica* L. *(Liliaceae)*

Vernacular Name: *Hin*: Jangli ashbha, Ramdatun, *Kan*: Kadu hambu thaavare, *Mal*: Kareelanchi, *Mar*: Goatvel, *San*: Vana madhusnahi, *Tam*: Kattu kodi, *Tel:* Sitapa, Kondaguruva tige.

Description: A prickly, tendril climber. *Tendril* usually two, arising on either side of the leaf stalk. *Prickles* short, bent, scattered on the stem. *Leaves* alternate, broadly egg-shaped to elliptic, 6-12 x 4-8 cm, base rounded to rarely slightly heart-shaped with a narrow leaf sheath, apex rounded to acute, sometimes notched, margin entire, hairless, leathery; nerves 3-7, arising from the base of the leaf; leaf stalks 1-3 cm long, twisted. *Male* and *female flowers* are separated, seen in the same plant, arranged in axillary 1-3 branched umbels, greenish white, about 6 mm long, 8 mm across, distinctly stalked. *Berries* globose, about 8 mm across, shiny, smooth, hairless, green turning red and becoming black when ripe. *Seeds* 3.

Habitate: Climbing on thickets and forest edges in deciduous to shola forests.

Propagation: By seeds.

Parts Used: Roots, Leaves.

Chemical Constituents: N.A.

Uses: Roots used for the treatment of venereal diseases, skin troubles, sores, swellings and abscess. Also applied for rheumatism and pains in the lower extremities.

1165. *Solanum indicum* auct.non Linn. (*Solanaceae*)

Synonyms: *Solanum anguivi* Lam.

Vernacular Name: *San:* Brhati, Simhi; *Eng:* Poison berry; *Hin:* Barhanta, Birhatta; *Kan:* Ramgulla, Vanvrntaki; *Mal:* Puttiriccunta, Cerucunta, Ceruvalutina; *Tam:* Karimulli, Puttiriccuntai; *Tel:* Cittimulage, Tellamulaka, Kakamunci.

Description: A much branched, common, very prickly undershrub 0.3-1.5 m in height; leaves simple, large, ovate, subentire, sinuate or lobed, sparsely prickly on both sides, base cordate, often unequal; flowers blue in extra-axillary cymes, penduncles stellately hairy and prickly; fruits globose berries, reddish or dark yellow; seeds smooth or minutely pitted.`.

Habitate: Throughout India, in the plains and at low elevations.

Propagation: By seeds.

Parts Used: Roots.

Chemical Constituents: Enzyme in fruits. Alkaloids solanine, solanidine in roots and leaves. Fruits contain 1.8% of alkaloids and can form a good source material for cortisone and sex hormone preparations.

Uses: The roots are bitter, acrid, astringent, thermogenic, anodyne, digestive, carminative, anthelmintic, stomachic, constipating, resolvent, demulcent, depurative, diuretic, expectorant, aphrodisiac, emmenagogue, febrifuge and cardiotonic. They are useful in vitiated conditions of *vata* and *kapha*, odontalgia, dyspesia, flatulence, colic, verminosis, diarrhoea, pruritus, leprosy, skin diseases, strangury, cough, asthma, bronchitis, amenorrhoea, dysmenorrhoea, fever, cardiac disorders and vomiting. The leaves and fruits are digestive, laxative and antibacterial, and are useful in odontalgia, pruritus and ringworm.

1166. *Solanum dulcamara* (*Solanaceae*)

Vernacular Name: *Eng:* Bittersweet.

Description: Slender-stemmed, woody climber growing to 4 m. Hs deeply lobed oval leaves, dark purple flowers with yellow anthers, and scarlet oval berries.

Habitate: Native to Europe, North Africa and northern Asia, bittersweet has been naturalized in North America.

Propagation: By Seeds.

Parts Used: Twigs, root bark.

Chemical Constituents: Bittersweet contains steroidal alkaloids, steroidal saponins and about 10% tannins.

Uses: Bittersweet has stimulant, expectorant, diuretic, detoxifying and antirheumatic properties. It appears to be most effective taken internally to treat skin problems such as eczema, itchiness, psoriasis and warts. Bittersweet may also be taken to relieve asthma, chronic bronchitis and rheumatic conditions, including gout.

1167. *Solanum erianthum* D. Don. *(Solanaceae)*

Synonyms: *Solanum verbascifolium* L.

Vernacular Name: *San:* Vidari; *Tel:* Rasagadimaanu; *Tam:* Chundai and *Mal:* Chundai.

Description: Small plant, 1-3m. high stems and twing covered with a dense yellowish tomentum. Leaves alternate, entire, velvety-pubescent on both sides. Inflorescence in axillary or terminal cyme; flowers white. Berry globose, many-seeded, yellow when ripe.

Habitate: Grows wild; common in the mountains and midlands.

Propagation: By seeds.

Part Used: Leaves.

Chemical Constituents: The leaves contain an essential oil, saponins and alkaloids: solanine, solasodine.

Uses: A locally applied poultice of pounded and heated fresh leaves is indicated for the relief of haemorrhoids and scrofula. It is better to apply poultices during the nigh. A plaster made of concentrated fresh leaf juice cures dermatomycosis and impetigo. An internally applied decoction of the elaves is used as a taeniafuge in buffaloes and oxen.

1168. *Solanum hainanense* Hance *(Solanaceae)*

Description: Procumbent prickly shrub. Leaves alternate, irregularly lobed, prickly on the upper face and covered with minute stellate hairs on the lower. Inflorescence in axillary cyme of 2-5 flowers, pale violet. Berry glovose, red when ripe; seeds numberous kidney-shaped, yellow.

Habitate: Grows wild, mainly on waste land.

Propagation: By seeds.

Part Used: Whole plant.

Chemical Constituents: The whole plant, especially the roots contain cholan saponins that on hydrolysis yield diosgenin, solasodinone, solasodine and flavonoids.

Uses: The entire plant, and especially the roots, possesses anti-inflammatory, antiallergic and and antiscelerotic properties. It is used in treating coryza, influenza, allertic diseases, lumbago, benign theumatoid polyarthritis, osteodynia and snake-bite. A liquid extract is used as gargle for gingivitis and parodontosis.

1169. *Solanum khasianum* C.B. Clarke. *(Solanaceae)*

Vernacular Name: Ban-bhindi, Kandiari, Kantkari, Bari kandiari.

Description: The plant is a stout, much-branched, under shrub, upto 1.5 m tall, with almost straight prickles. Leaves are ovate, lobed and the lobes are lanceolate or triangular, hirsute and prickly on both the surfaces. Flowers are white in colour and are in lateral, 1-4 flowered racemes. Berries are yellowish or greenish globose and 2.5 cm in diameter. Seeds are smooth, brown and compressed.

Habitate: Found in the Khasi, Jaintai and Naga hills of Assam and Manipur, Nefa, Sikkim, West Bengal, Orissa, the upper Gangetic plains upto an altitude of 1600m. Common in Hinachal Pradesh in the waste places, ravines and near habitations upto an elevation of 1500m.

Propagation: By seeds.

Part Used: Fruits.

Chemical Constituents: The berries contain solasodine, solakhasianin and diosgenin. Its berries are richest source of Solasodine.

Uses: Alcoholic extracts of the plant have been tested for the biological activity. They affect the contraction of the isolated ileum of guinea pig and also influence the central nervous system. It is much valued for its solasodine used in various formulation including it is used as a substitute for *Solanum indicum.*

1170. *Solanum melongena* L. *(Solanaceae)*

Vernacular Name: *San:* Varttaki; *Eng:* Brinjal, Egg plant; *Hin:* Bengan, Badanjan; *Kan:* Badanekaya, Doddabadane; *Mal:* Valutina; *Tam:* Kattirikkai; *Tel:* Vankaya, Niruvanga, Mettavanga.

Description: An erect or zsuffrustescent, herbaceous, armed or unarmed perennial; leaves simple, large, entire, lobed; flowers blue, in clusters of 2-5; fruits large, white, yellow or dark purple berries of different shapes capped with thick persistent calyx; seeds many, yellow or cream, discoid.

Habitate: Cultivated throughout India.

Propagation: By seeds.

Parts Used: Roots, leaves, unripe fruits.

Chemical Constituents: Solasodine from fruits. Arginine, aspartic acid.

Uses: The roots are laxative, analgesic and cardiotonic, and are useful in inflammations, neuralgia, cardiac debility and ulcers in the nose. The leaves are sialagogue, narcotic, and antiherpetic, and are useful in cholera, bronchitis, asthma, odontalgia and fever. The unripe fruits are bitter, acrid, sweet, aphrodisiac, cardiotonic and haematinic.

1171. *Solanum nigrum* L. *(Solanaceae)*

Synonyms: *Solanum rubrum* Mill.

Vernacular Name: *Eng:* Black night-shade; *Hin:* Makoy, Gurkkamai; *Kan:* Kakarundi; *Mal:* Manttakkali, Karintakali, Karimtakkali; *San:* Kakmaci; *Tam:* Manttakkali, Milagutakkali; *Tel:* Kamanci, Kacci, Kaccipandu, Gajjucettu.

Description: An erect, divaricately branched, unarmed, suffrutescent annual herb; leaves ovate or oblong, sinuate-toothed or lobed, glabrous; flowers 3-8 in extra-axillary drooping subumebellate cymes; fruits purplish black or reddish berries; seeds many, discoid, yellow, minutely pitted.

Habitate: As a weed, throughout dry parts of India.

Propagation: By seeds.

Parts Used: Whole plant.

Chemical Constituents: Leaf is a rich source of riboflavin, nicotinic acid and vitamin 'C'. besides these, β-carotene and citric acid are present. Fruits contain glucose and fructose, vitamin C and β-carotene. The immature green fruit of the plant contain four steroidal glyco-alkaloids viz. solamargine and α and β-solanigrine and all of them yield solasodine, as the aglycone. Diosgenin is also present in leaves, stem and fruits.

Uses: The plant is bitter, acrid, emollient, mildly thermogenic, antiseptic, anti-inflammatory, expectorant, anodyne, vulnerary, digestive laxative, diuretic, cardiotonic, depurative, diaphretic, febrifuge, hydragogues, rejuvenating, sedative, alterant and tonic. It is useful in vitiated conditions of tridosa, rheumatalgia, swellings, cough, asthma, bronchitis, wounds, ulcers, flaulence, dyspepsia, strangury, hepatomegaly, otalgia, hiccough, nasal catarrh, ophthalmopathy, vomiting, cardiopathy, leprosy, skin diseases, fever, splenomegaly, haemorrhoids, plant depresses the central nervous system and reflexes of the spinal cord and has influence on cardiac activity and in the regulation of blood pressure. The leaves are used as poultice for rheumatic and gouty joints and skin diseases. A decoction of the berries and flowers is useful in cough, erysipelas, rat bite, bronchitis, pulmonary tuberculosis, fever, diarrhoea, ophthalmopathy and hydrophobia. The seeds are useful in giddiness, dipsia, inflammatons and skin diseases. The root bark is useful in otopathy, ophthalmopathy, rhinopathy and hepatits. The leaves and berries are especially important as a cure for gastrohelcosis.

1172. *Solanum surattense* Burn.f. *(Solanaceae)*

Synonyms: *Solanum xanthocarpum* Schrad. & Wendl.

Vernacular Name: *Eng:* Yellow-berried nightshade; *Hin:* Remgani, Katali Kattay; *Kan:* Nelagulle; *Mal:* Kantakariccunta, Kantakarivalutana, Kantankattiri; *San:* Kantakari, Nidigdhika; *Tam:* Kantankattiri; *Tel:* Callamulaga, Pinnamulaka, Nelamulaka, Vakudu.

Description: A prickly, diffuse bright green suffrutescent, perennial undershrub, woody at the base, with zigzag branches that spread close to the ground covered over with strong, broad, sharp, compressed, straight, yellowish white prickles; leaves ovate or ovate oblong, stellately hairy on both sides, armed on the midrib and the nerves with long yellow sharp prickles; flowers blue or bluish-purple, in extra axillary cymes; fruits glabrous, globular drooping berry, yellow or white with green veins, surrounded by the calyx; seeds many, small, reniform, smooth and yellowish brown.

Habitate: Throughout India, in dry situation as a weed on roadsides and waste land.

Propagation: By seeds.

Parts Used: Whole plant.

Chemical Constituents: Fruits yield carpesteral and gluco-alkaloid, Solasodine, Solasonine and solanocarpine. Solanine-on hydrolysis yields alkaloid, Solanidine.

Uses: The plant is bitter, acrid, thermogenic, anthelmintic, antiinflammatory, anodyne, digestive carminative, appetiser, stomachnic, depurative, sudorific, febrifuge, expectorant, laxaative, stimulant, diuretic, rejuvenanting, emmenagogue and aphrodisiac. It is useful in vitiated conditions of *vata* and *kapha*, helminthiasis, dental caries, inflammation, arthralgia, flatulence, colic, constipation, dyspepsia, anorexia, leprosy, skin diseases, hypertension, rheumatoid fever, cough, asthma bronchitis, pharyngitis, hiccough, strangury, urolithiasis, amenorrhoea, dysmenorrhoea, lumbago, haemorrhoids, cardiac disorders, rhinopathy, epilepsy and catarrh.

1173. *Solanum tuberosum* L. *(Solanaceae)*

Vernacular Name: *Eng:* Potato; *Hin:* Alu; *Kan:* Batate, Alugadde; *Mal:* Urulakkilannu; *San:* Golakandah; *Tam:* Urulaikkilangu; *Tel:* Bangaldumpa, Urlagadda.

Description: A much branched spreading herb upto one meter in height with adventitious roots and swollen underground tubers; leaves pinnate with large terminal leaflets; flowers in cymose panicles, white pink or violet; fruits flobose berries; seeds many, flat, smooth. The underground tubers (potato) are the swollen tips of branches. They are yellowish brown in colour with several 'eyes' on the surface. In each eye there is a vegetative bud which can give rise to a new plant.

Habitate: Cultivated in higher elevations.

Propagation: By tuber.

Parts Used: Leaves, tubers.

Chemical Constituents: It content protein, amino acids, amides and nitrogenous bases. Principal protein is globulin. Potatoes are rich in a variety of enzymes.

Uses: The leaf extract is antispasmodic in chronic cough. The potato tuber is sweet, aphrodiasia, antiscorbutic, aperient, diuretic galactagogue and nervine sedative, rich in starch and vitamin C and is a tonic. It is good for strangury, constipation, hyperacidity, scabies and dermatopathy. A paste of it is used as a plaster for burns with much benefit. It is a tasty vegetable, which will cause flatulence if consumed in excess.

1174. *Solanum viride* Solander ex Forst F. *(Solanaceae)*

Synonyms: *Solanum upora* Dunal.

Description: Shrub to 2 m high Leaves alternate, petiolate, the blade ovate, 10-18 cm long, base unequal, with a tapering apex, Flowers whitish to yellowish, 5-parted with five spreading lobes, the flower about 3 cm broad and borne in small terminal or axillary clusters. Fruit a red berry.

Habitate: Occurring naturally or cultivated, especially on limestone soils at low elevations along coastlines, edges of forests, and open areas.

Propagation: By seeds.

Part Used: Leaves.

Chemical Constituents: Solasodine, Steroidal alkaloids.

Uses: Pressed fluid of the leaves is given to facilitate childbirth, especially the first birth. The leaves are cut in pieces and mixed with coconut oil to prepare a salve used to remedy body swellings. The plant is used as a sedative, diuretic, to treat infection of the eye (conjunctivitis) and to treat pus-filled infections. The swellings resulting from the parastic disease, filariasis, is remedied with a tea made from the leaves, Crushed leaves are applied to boils, fungal infections and tumours of the breast. The leaves are used to treat wounds.

1175. *Solena amplexicaulis* (Lam.) Ghandhi *(Cucurbitaceae)*

Synonyms: *Solena heterophylla* Lour.

Vernacular Name: *Hin:* Tarali, Amantamul; *Kan:* Bimpuli; *Mal:* Nerinnampuli; *San:* Amlavetasah; *Tam:* Pulivanci; *Tel:* Tiddanda, Tiyyadonda.

Description: A scandent dioecious perennial with several tuberous roots and with slender branched furrowed stems bearing simple tendrils; leaves polymorphous, ovate, suborbicular, oblong or narrowly lanceolate, 3-5 angled or lobed, usually cordate at base, reticulately veinved beneath, margins remotely denticulate; flowers small, yellow, males in subumbellate or umbellate racemes or fascicled, females solitary; fruits oblong ovoid, cylindric, brown ribbed, bright red when ripe; seeds many, white, subspherical, smooth.

Habitate: Throughout India upto 2100 m in the hills.

Propagation: By seeds.

Parts Used: Tuberous roots, leaves, seeds.

Chemical Constituents: N.A.

Uses: The tuberous roots are sour, astringent thermogenic, appetiser, carminative, digestive, purgative, stimulant, cardiotonic, diuretic, expectorant and invigorating. They are useful in vitiated conditions of *kapha* and *vata*, anorexia, dyspepsia, flatulence, colic, cardiac disorders, hiccough, asthma, bronchitis, vomiting, strangury, renal and vesical calculi, haemorrhoids, constipation, hepatosplenomegaly, gonorrhoea and spermatorrhoea. The leaves are useful in allergic inflammations and the seeds are used for their purgative action.

1176. *Solidago virgaurea* *(Asteraceae)*

Vernacular Name: *Eng:* Goldenrod.

Description: Perennial plant growing to 70 cm. Has toothed leaves and branched spikes of golden yellow flowers; fruit achene.

Habitate: Native to Europe and Asia and naturalized in North America, goldenrod prefers open areas, wasterground and hillsides. If is gathered in summer while in flower.

Propagation: By Seeds.

Parts Used: Aerial parts.

Chemical Constituents: Goldenrod contains saponins, diterpenes, phenolic glucosides, acetylenes, cinnamates, flavonoids, tannins, hydroxybenzoates, and inulin. The saponins are antifungal.

Uses: Antioxidant, diuretic and astringent, goldenrod is a valuable remedy for urinary tract disorders. It is used both for serious ailments such as nephritis, and for more common problems like cystits. The herb also has a reputation for helping to flush out kidney and bladder stones. Goldenrod's saponins act specifically against the *Candida* fungus, the cause of vaginal and oral thrush. The herb can also be taken for conditions such as sore throats, chronic nasal catarrh and diarrhoea. Due to its mild action, goldenrod is used to treat gastroenteritis in children. Externally, it may be used as a mouthwash or douche for thrush.

1177. *Sophora flavescens* Aiton. *(Fabaceae)*

Vernacular Name: *Eng:* Light-yellow sophora.

Description: A shrub, 1.3-3 m high. Stem erect, much branched. Young branches covered with sparse hairs. Leaves alternate, odd-pinnate; leaflets 11-29, oval-elliptic or lanceolate, 3-4 cm long by 1.2-2 cm wide; apex slightly acute or obtuse; base cuneate, entire; the top surface glabrous, the underside tomentose, glaucous. Inflorescence and axillary or terminal cluster, racemed. Flowers in May-July. Fruit a sliquaceous pod.

Habitate: On slopes and in grassland in China.

Propagation: By seeds.

Part Used: Roots.

Uses: Diarrhoea, abdominal pain, trichomonas, vatinitis; pruritis vulvae; burns.

1178. *Sophora japonica* L. *(Fabaceae)*

Vernacular Name: *Eng:* Japanese pagoda-tree; Chinese scholar tree.

Description: A deciduous, spreading, round-headed tree, 7-15 m high. Leaves alternate, compound-imparipinnate, leafles 7-13, ovate, 2.5-7.5 cm long by 1.5-3 cm wide; tip acute; base rounded, often oblique; margin entire, glaucous and puberulent on the underside. Inflorescence a loose, terminal panicle, 15-30 cm long. Flowers white, papilionaceous, 1.0-1.5 cm long, June-July. Fruit a cylindrical pod, 5-8 cm long, glabrous, fleshy, containing 1-6 seeds, contracted in the shape of a rosary.

Habitate: Often planted in streets as a shade tree in China, Japan, Korea and Viet Nam.

Propagation: By seeds.

Part Used: Floral buds, flowers.

Chemical Constituents: N.A.

Uses: Melaena, Haemorrhoids with bleeding, diarrhoea, metrorrhagia.

1179. *Sorbus aucuparia* *(Rosaceae)*

Vernacular Name: *Eng:* Rowan.

Description: Deciduous tree growing to 12 m. Has reddish bark, compound leaves, clusters of small white flowers and clusters of round red-orange fruit.

Habitate: Rowan grows throughout the Northern hemisphere, where it is found in woodland. It is also cultivated as an ornamental tree.

Propagation: By Seeds.

Parts Used: Fruit.

Chemical Constituents: The fruit contains tannins sorbitol, malic and sorbic acids, sugars and vitamin C. the seeds contain cyanogenic glycosides, which, in a reaction upon contact with water, produce the extremely poisonous prussic acid.

Uses: The astringent rowan is most often taken as a jam or an infusion to treat diarrhoea and haemorrhoids. In addition, infusions may be used as a gargle for sore throats and as a wash to treat haemorrhoids and excessive vaginal discharge.

1180. *Spermacoce hispida* L. *(Rubiaceae)*

Synonyms: *Borreria hispida* (Linn.) K.Schum.

Vernacular Name: *Kan:* Madanbadu, Megidda; *Mal:* Tartaval, Nattaccuri, Kutalccurukki; *San:* Vasukah, Bukah; *Tam:* Nattaiccuri; *Tel:* Madana, Madanagranthi.

Description: A hispid procumbent with long branches and quadrangular stems; leaves simple, opposite, subsessile, oblong or elliptic, scabrid; flowers pale mauve usually long tubed 4-6 in a whorl within the stipular cup; fruits capsules, ellipsoid, rounded at both ends, 5mm long, rounded on the back with a deep groove on the flat face.

Habitate: Throughout India upto 900 m in the hills and on all dry lands as a weed.

Propagation: By seeds.

Parts Used: Whole plant.

Chemical Constituents: N.A.

Uses: The plant is acrid, sweet, astringent, mildly thermogenic, emollient and stomachic. It is useful in vitiated conditions of *pitta* and *vata*, dyspepsia, colic, flatulence and general debility.

1181. *Sphaeranthus indicus* L. *(Asteraceae)*

Synonyms: *Sphaeranthus hirtus* Willd.

Vernacular Name: *Eng:* East Indian globe-thistle; *Hin:* Mundi; *Kan:* Gorakundi; *Mal:* Atakkamaniyan; *San:* Mudi, Sravani; *Tam:* Visnukkarantai, Kottakkarantai; *Tel:* Bodasaramu, Boddatarapu.

Description: A spreading aromatic herb with glandular hairy stem and branches with purple or pink flowers; stems with toothed wings; leaves alternate, toothed; flowers in close terminal, globose or ovoid heads.

Habitate: Throughout India.

Propagation: By seeds.

Parts Used: Whole plant.

Chemical Constituents: Essential oil containg methyl chavicol, α-ionone, d-cadinene, p-methoxycinnamaldehyde as major constituents and a-terpinene, citral, geraniol, geranyl acetate, β-ionone, sphaerene, indicusene and sphaeranthol as minor constituents. Leaves contain alkaloids.

Uses: The juice expressed from the plant is used in vitiated conditions of *vata*, epilepsy, hemicrania, jaundice, hepatopathy and gastropathy. A paste of the herb mixed with oil is good for pruritus and painful swellings. The roots are bitter, acrid, sweet, thermogenic, diuretic, expectorant, febrifuge and stomachic. They are useful in strangury, diabetes, leprosy, fever, pectoralgia, cough, gastropathy, hernia, haemorrhoids, helminthiasis and dyspepsia. An oil prepared by using the root is useful in scrofula. The powdered leaf is good for skin diseases and is considered as a nervine tonic. The flowers are highly esteemed as an alternant, depurative, refrigerant and tonic.

1182. *Spigelia marilandica* *(Loganiaceae)*

Vernacular Name: *Eng:* Pink root.

Description: Perennial plant with oval to lance-shaped leaves, spikes of brilliant red-pink flowers and a double seed capsule.

Habitate: Native to the southern regions of the US.

Propagation: By Seeds.

Parts Used: Root.

Chemical Constituents: Pink root contains alkaloids a volatile oil, tannin and resin. Spigeleine is emetic and irritant to the stomach.

Uses: Pink root is used today solely to expel intestinal worms–particularly tapeworms and roundworms. It is prescribed with other herbs such as senna and fennel to ensure the elimination of both the worms and the root itself, which is potentially toxic if it is absorbed through the gut.

1183. *Spilanthes acmella* L. *(Asteraceae)*

Synonyms: *Spilanthes mauritiana.*

Vernacular Name: *San:* Akarkara, Pokarmul, Akalkada; *Tel:* Maratimogga, Maratittega; *Kan*: Vanamugali, Himmugulu; *Mal*: Kuppamanjel.

Description: An annual herb, more or less pubescent, sometimes hairy. Stem 30-60 cm, usually decumbent near the base. Leaves opposite, stalked, ovate-lanceolate, about 5 cm x 3.75 cm, toothed or entire. Flower heads discoid or rediate, conical, solitary on long stalks. Flowers are white or yellow in colour, mostly bisexual. Achenes flattened, each enclosed in a scale.

Habitate: Throughout India, ascending to 1700 m, often found occurring as a weed in rice fields.

Propagation: By seeds.

Part Used: Leaves, flower heads and roots.

Chemical Constituents: Main ingredient is spilanthol obtained from roots, leaves and flowering heads.

Uses: Leaves are chewed to relieve toothache and affections of throat and gums. Tincture made from flower heads is reported to be used as a substitute for tincture of Pyrethrum to treat inflammation of Jaw-bones and caries. Plant boiled in water is given in dysentery and an ether extract of fresh flower-tops is effective against anopheles mosquito larvae. It increases the flow of saliva and is useful in fever especially during summers.

1184. *Spondias dulcis* Sol. ex. Parkinson *(Anacardiaceae)*

Synonyms: *Spondias cytherea.*

Vernacular Name: *Eng:* Otheite apple, Polynesian plum, june plum.

Description: Tree upto 20 m high with whitish bark. Leaves alternate, pinnately compound with 5-15 leaflets, the entire leaf up to 40 cm long. Flowers yellow or white, relatively small and 4-5 parted. Fruit an edible yellow to orange ovoid drupe containing one large seed. Flowers and fruit usually available throughout the years.

Habitate: Commonly cultivated in villages, or occurring in dry or secondary forests from sea-level to 500 m.

Propagation: By seeds.

Part Used: Fruit and bark.

Chemical Constituents: Tannins, amino acids, minerals, vitamin C, proteins, fibre, polysccharides and carotenoids.

Uses: Fruit is edible. Pressed liquid of the stem is given after a false pregnancy, and for weakness following childbirth. The shoots liquid of the bark is taken to cleans the bowels. The bark filtrate is also employed as an abortificient to promote sterility and to treat fish poisoning. A few drops of the pressed bark fluid are applied to the eyes as a remedy for cataracts.

1185. *Spondias pinnata* (L.f.) Kurz *(Anacardiaceae)*

Synonyms: *Spondias mangifera* Willd., *Spondias acuminata.*

Vernacular Name: *Eng:* Wild mango, Hogplum; *Hin:* Amra, Jungli-am; *Kan:* Ambatemarra, Amtakayi Vrksamia; *Mal:* Ampalam, Ampalam, Mampuli; *San:* Amratakah; *Tam:* Mampulicci, Ampalam, Kattimagirankai; *Tel:* Adavimamidi, Kondamamidi, Amratakamu.

Description: A medium sized aromatic, deciduous tree, upto 27 m in height and 2.5 m in girth; leaves compound, crowded at the ends of branches, leaflets large having parallel nerves meeting in an intramarginal nerve; bark thick, surface light grey to greyish brown, shallowly furrowed or cracked longitudinally, brittle, their fracture splintery; flowers many, in terminal spreading panicles; fruits fleshy drupes with woody endocarp surrounded by longitudinal interwoven fibres, young fruits green in colour, turning light yellow or greenish yellow on ripening.

Habitate: Throughout India, wild as well as cultivated.

Propagation: By seeds.

Parts Used: Roots, bark, leaves, fruits.

Chemical Constituents: β-Amyrin and oeanolic acid from fruits. Glycine, cystine, serine, alanine and leucine in fruits. Lignoceric acid, β-sitosterol and its glucoside in aerial parts.

Uses: The roots are useful in regulating menstruation. The bark is aromatic, astringent and refrigerant, and is administered in dysentery, diarrhoea, vomiting and muscular rheumatism. The leaves are aromatic, acidic, astringent and are used in dysentery. The juice of the leaves is recommended for local application in otalgia. The unripe fruits are astringent, sour, thermogenic, appetiser and aphrodisiac. The ripe fruits are sweet, astringent, cooling, emollient, tonic, constipating and antiscorbutic. They are useful in bilious dyspepsia, diarrhoea, general debility and vitiated conditions of tridosa.

1186. *Stachys officinalis* *(Lameaceae)*

Synonyms: *Stachys betonica.*

Vernacular Name: *Eng:* Betony.

Description: Mat-forming perennial growing to a height of 60 cm. Has toothed elliptical leaves and spikes of pink or white flowers.

Habitate: Grows throughout most of Europe, and occurs in Asia as far east as the Caucasus. It prefers meadows, heathland and hilly areas.

Propagation: By Seeds.

Parts Used: Aerial part.

Chemical Constituents: Betony contains alkaloids as well as betaine, choline and tannins.

Uses: No longer regarded as a panacea, betony nevertheless has real value as a remedy for headaches and facial pain. The plant is also mildly sedative, relieving nervous stress and tension. In British herbal medicine, betony is thought to improve nervous function and to counter overactivity. It is taken to treat "frayed nerves", pre-menstrual complaints, poor memory and tension. The plant has astringent properties and in combination with other herbs, such as comfrey and lime flowers, it is effective against sinus headaches and congestion. Betony may be taken alone or with arrow to help staunch nosebleeds. Betony is also mildly bitter. It stimulates the digestive system and the liver, and has an overall tonic effect on the body.

1187. *Stellaria dichotoma* L. *(Caryophyllaceae)*

Vernacular Name: *Eng:* Lanceolate starwort.

Description: A perennial herb 20-40 cm high. Stem erect. Upper parts divaricate, densely covered with shallow pubescence or glandular hairs, nodes dilated. Leaves opposite, sessile, lanceolate, up to 3 cm long by 4 mm wide; apex acute, base rounded; margin entire; with spares short hairs or glabrous on top, pubescent underneath. Flowers solitary. Capsule subglobose, 1-celled. Seeds numerous.

Habitate: On dry grassland or in crevices in the mountains in China, Mongolia.

Propagation: By seeds.

Part Used: Roots.

Chemical Constituents: N.A.

Uses: Hectic fever, infant malnutrition with fever.

1188. *Stellaria media* *(Caryophyllaceae)*

Synonyms*:* *Alsine media* L.

Vernacular Name: *Eng:* Chickweed.

Description: Sprawling perennial growing to about 15 cm. Has hairy stems, oval leaves and star like white flowers in cymes; capsules ovoid; seeds brown, acutely tuberted.

Habitate: Native to Europe and Asia, chickweed is now found in most regions of the world. It grows easily in wasteground, and is generally regarded as a troublesome weed. The plant is harvested in summer.

Propagation: By Seeds and root.

Parts Used: Aerial parts.

Chemical Constituents: Chickweed contains triterpenoid saponins, coumarins, flavonoids, carboxylic acids and vitamin C. the saponins may account for the herb's ability to help reduce itchiness.

Uses: Chickweed is chiefly used to treat irritated skin, being applied as juice, poultice, ointment or cream. In certain cases, chickweed may soothe severe itchiness where all other remedies have failed. It is often used to relieve eczema, varicose ulcers and nettle rash. An infusion of the fresh or dried plant may be added to a bath, where the herb's emollient properties will help to reduce inflammation–in rheumatic joints, for example–and encourage tissue repair. Chickweed may also be taken internally to treat chest ailments. In small quantities, this herb also aids digestion.

1189. *Stemona tuberosa* Lour. *(Stemonaceae)*

Synonyms: *Stemona minor* Hook.

Vernacular Name: *Tel:* Kaniputeega, ijedigadda.

Description: Perennial climbing shrub, reaching a length of 5-6m. with buberous roogs, fascicled. Leaves opposite or alternate, oblong heart-shaped; main nerves curved, secondary nerves very close. Flwoers in the axil of leaves, greenish-yellow externally, reddish-purple within fetid. Capsule ovoid-oblong, many-seeded.

Habitate: Grows wild in the hills and mountains.

Propagation: By seeds.

Part Used: Tuberous roots.

Chemical Constituents: The tuberous roots contain alkaloids, stemonine, tuberostemonine, isotuberostemonine, stemonidine, sinostemonine; glucides 2.3%, lipids 0.83%, proteins 9%, organic acids (citric, formic, malic, succinic).

Uses: The tuberous roots are well known for their antibacterial, antiparastic and expectorant properties. They are prescribed in the therapy of cough, ascariasis and oxyuriasis The decoction or extract is applied externally against impetigo and scabies. Can also be used as an insecticide against mosquito larvae, fleas and bugs.

1190. *Sterculia foetida* L. *(Sterculiaceae)*

Vernacular Name: *San:* Putidaru, Vatkhadirah; *Eng:* Pinari; *Hin:* Jamglibadam; *Kan:* Penari, Bhatala; *Mal:* Pinari, Pottakkavalam, Putiyanartti, Putimanatti; *Tam:* Pinari, Kutiraippitukku; *Tel:* Manjiponku, Gurapa, Guttapubadamu.

Description: A medium sized to large tree about 18m in height with reddish brown heartwood, whitish bark and whorled horizontal branches; leaves digitate, crowded at the ends of branches, leaflets 7-9, susessile, oblong lanceolate, acute or acuminate, pubescent when young, glabrous when mature, stipules caduous; flowers dull orange, fetid smelling in erect racemose panicles, unisexual, male flowers with curved long staminal column, female flowers with stout gynophore and deflexed style; fruits 1-5 oblong, boat-shaped, bright red follicles; seeds 10-15 ovoid-oblong black.

Habitate: Throughout India, in deciduous forests.

Propagation: By seeds.

Parts Used: Heartwood.

Chemical Constituents: Thiamine, riboflavin, nicotinic acid, vitamin C.

Uses: The heartwood is foetid, mildly thermogenic, depurative, febrifuge and vulnerarry. It is useful in convulsion, neuropathy, helminthiasis, leprosy, erysipelas, skin diseases, fever, ulcers and cephalalgia.

1191. *Stereospermum colais* (Buch.-Ham.ex Dillw.) Mabberley *(Bignoniaceae)*

Synonyms: *Stereospermum personatum* (Hassk.) Chatterjee.

Vernacular Name: *Eng:* Trumpet flower tree, Yellow snake tree; *Hin:* Paral, Patar, Padri; *Kan:* Hude, Kalludi, kala-adri; *Mal:* Puppatiri, Patiri; *San:* patala; *Tam:* Padiri, Pumpadiri; *Tel:* Kokkesa, Pagada, Pisulu, Kalagora, Arajavepa.

Description: A large deciduous tree 18-30 m in height with a straight trunk and fairly smooth yellowish brown bark; leaves imparipinnate, large, clustered towards the end of the branchlets, leaflets 3-6 pairs, short-stalked, often unequal-sided at the base, main nerves 8-10 pairs; flowers yellow, tinged with red, fragrant, in lax drooping terminal cymose panicles; fruits capsules, cylindric, slender, curved, some what rough with elevated white specks; seeds winged at each end, wings membranous.

Habitate: Throughout India, in deciduous forests upto 1200 m.

Propagation: By seeds.

Parts Used: Roots, leaves, flowers, fruits, seeds.

Chemical Constituents: N.A.

Uses: The roots are bitter, astringent, acrid, anodyne, appetiser, constipating, diuretic, lithontriptic, expectorant, cardiotonic, aphrodisiac, anti-inflammatory, antibacterial, febrifuge and tonic. They are useful in vitiated conditions of *vata*, dyspepsia, diarrhoea, strangury, renal and versical calculi, cough, asthma, hiccough, hyperdipsia, haemorrhoids, hyperacidity, vomiting, dropsy, fever and general debility. The leaves are useful in otalgia, odontalgia, rheumatalgia, malarial fever and wounds. The flowers are astringent, sweet, cooling, aphrodisiac, cardiotonic and tonic. They are useful in burning sensation, vitiated conditions of *pitta* and *vata*, cardiopathy, hiccough and general debility. The fruits are astringent, sweet and cooling, and are useful in vitiated conditions of *vata* and *pitta*. The seeds are useful for external application in hemicrania.

1192. *Stillingia sylviatica* *(Euphorbiaceae)*

Vernacular Name: *Eng:* Queen's Delight.

Description: Perennial growing to 4 ft. Has leathery leaves, yellow flowers without petals and 3-lobed fruit.

Habitate: It is native to the south-eastern US, where it prefers *San*dy soils.

Propagation: By Seeds and cutting.

Parts Used: Root.

Chemical Constituents: It contains alkaloids, diterpene esters, fixed oil, volatile oil, resin and tannins. The fresh root is considered most active.

Uses: It appears to promote general detoxification. It is taken internally to help clear constipation, boils, weeping eczema and scrofula. The root is also taken to treat bronchitis and throat infection. Externally, it is applied as a lotion to haemorrhoids, eczema and psoriasis.

1193. *Streblus asper* Lour. *(Moraceae)*

Vernacular Name: *Eng:* Siamese rough-bush; *Hin:* Sihora, Daheya; *Kan:* Mitlimara, Punji, Penalige; *Mal:* Paruv, Sakhotavrksam, parakam; *San:* Sakhotah, patrollekhataruh; *Tam:* Pirayamaram; *Tel:* Barinikacettu, Barinki, Pakki.

Description: A small, rigid evergreen tree, upto 15m in height with hairy scabrid twigs, milky white latex and light grey or greenish rough bark; leaves simple, alternate, rhomboid-elliptic, acute or acuminate, more or less crenate, scabrid on both surfaces, lateral nerves 4-6 pairs, prominent beneath; connected by intramarginal loops; flowers unisexual, dioecious, male heads globose, minute, yellowish green, female flowers solitary or 2-4 together, very small, fruits one-seeded succulent berries, yellow when ripe; seeds smooth, round, greenish white.

Habitate: Throughout India, in dry areas upto 600 m.

Propagation: By seeds.

Parts Used: Roots, bark, leaves, latex.

Chemical Constituents: It content cardenolides, cardenolide glycosides, kamaloside, asperoside, pyranoside, streboloside, indroside, lucknoside, cannodimethoside, strophalloside, strophanolloside, glucokamaloside, sarmethoside and α, β-unsaturated lactone.

Uses: The roots are astringent, bitter, acrid, thermogenic, vulnerary, anti-inflammatory, haemostatic, anticonvulsant, constipating, febifuge and antiseptic. They are useful in vitiated conditions of khapha, ulcers, sinusitis, inflammations, elephantiasis, boils, haemorrhages, haemoptysis, cough, bronchitis, convulsions, diarrhoea, dysentery, fever, syphilis and haemorrhoids. The bark is vulnerary, anti-inflammatory and constipating, and is useful in foul ulcers, diarrhoea, dysentery, inflammations and fever. The leaves are useful in sore heels, chapped hands, adenitis neuralgia and haemorrhages.

1194. *Streptocaulon juventas* (Lour.) Merr, *(Asclepiadaceae)*

Description: Branching perennial twiner, with long, fleshy roots. Stems twining, brown, leaves opposite, obovate, rounded or cordate at the base. Inflorescence in axillary cyme; flowers small, brownish-yellow. Double follicle, divergent. Seeds with a tuft of hairs at one end. All parts of the plant have a milky latex and a silky tomentum.

Habitate: Grows wild in the mountains and midlands.

Propagation: By seeds.

Part Used: Tuberous roots.

Chemical Constituents: The roots contain starch and alkaloids.

Uses: The roots are reconstituent and effective for anaemia, renal and hepatic hypofunction, dyspepsia, insomnia, neurasthenia, hypogalactia, chronic malaria, rheumatism, ostealgia, menstrual disorders, leucorrhoea, bloddy stools, prurigo and snakeObite. Long-term administration has a rejuvenating effect and white hair grows black again. For snake-bite, the root juice is swallowed and the residue used as a poultice.

1195. *Strobilanthes ciliatus* Nees *(Acanthaceae)*

Synonyms: *Nilgirianthus ciliatus* (Nees) Bremek.

Vernacular Name: *San*: Sahacarah, Sairyakah, *Hin*: Karvi, Kara, *Mal*: Karimkurunni, Kurunni, Vellakkurunni, *Tam*: Kurunji, Sinnakkurunji.

Description: A slender shrub with subquadrangular white dotted dark green, or purple stems and branches; leaves dark green, elliptic, acuminate at both ends serrate, glabrous, main nerves 6-7 pairs, raised above; flowers white to lilac in axillary slender glabrous spikes; fruits very rarely formed.

Adventitious roots arise from a few basal nodes also. The main roots as well as these nodal roots are used as raw material.

Habitate: Throughout the evergreen, forests of Western Ghats upto 1,200 m.

Propagation: By seeds.

Parts Used: Roots, leaves, bark.

Chemical Consistuents: Aromatic oil.

Uses: The roots are bitter, sweet, thermogenic, emollient, diuretic, febrifuge, diaphoretic, depurative, anti-inflammatory, expectorant and tonic. They are useful in rheumatalgia, lumbago, sciatica, limping, chest congestion, strangury, fever, leucoderma, skin diseases, inflammations, cough, bronchitis odontalgia and general debility. The leaves and bark are diaphoretic, expectorant, depurative and febrifuge, and are useful in whooping cough, fever, bronchitis, dropsy, leucoderma, leprosy, pruritus, inflammations, scrofula and fever.

1196. *Strobilanthes cusia* (Nees) Imlay *(Acanthaceae)*

Synonyms: *Strobilanthes flaccidifolius* Nees.

Vernacular Name: *Eng:* Assam indigo and *Assam*: Rum, rampat.

Description: Shrubby herbaceous plant, 50-70cm. High. Stems glbrous, swollen at the nodes. Leaves opposite, oblong-oval,with margins serrate. Inflorescence in axillary interrupted spike; flowers violet-blue or pink, corolla slightly curved. Capsule glabrous, narrow and long.

Habitate: Grows wild and is cultivated in damp valleys in the highlands.

Propagation: By seeds.

Part Used: Leaves.

Chemical Constituents: The leaves contain the glucoside indican, which yields glucose and indoxyl on hydrolysis. Indoxyl yields indigotin upon oxidation.

Uses: The leaves possess antivacterial, antifebrile, antioestrogenic, antiprogestogenic and uterostimulant properties. They are used in treating menorrhagia, metrorrhagia, sore throat, gingivitis and fever. A plaster of condensed extract helps to cure eczema and impetigo.

1197. *Strophanthus divaricatus* (Lour.). Hook. Et. Arn. *(Apocynaceae)*

Description: Shrub with milky juice. Stems and twings spreading, 3-4m. long, marked with lenticles. Leaves opposite, oblong; apex pointed, short-petioled. Inflorescence in terminal cyme; flowers yellow; petals prolonged into long narrow filaments veined with redish-brown, Fruit of 2 follicles, seeds numerous, brown crowned with a tuft of long hairs at one end.

Habitate: Grows wild on the lower hills and in coastal shrubland.

Propagation: By seeds.

Part Used: Seeds.

Chemical Constituents: The seeds yield the glucoside, divaricoside, which yield sarmentogenin and L-oleandrose on hydrolysis as well as divostroside, caudoside and sinoside.

Uses: D-strophantin is the purified glucosidal mixture extracted from the seeds. The drug enjoys a good reputatyion in the treatment of acute and chronic heart failure it is also destined fro patients who are intolerant of digitalis preparations.

1198. *Strophanthus kombe* *(Apocynaceae)*

Vernacular Name: *Eng:* Strophanthus.

Description: Woody vine climbing upto 10m. Has elliptical leaves, large yellow to white bell-shaped flowers and long slender seedpods.

Habitate: Strophanthus is native to eastern Africa. It grows wild in rainforests and is commercially cultivated.

Propagation: By Seeds.

Parts Used: Seeds.

Chemical Constituents: Strophanthus contains up to 10% cardiac glycosides. These slow the heart rate and improve the heart's efficiency. See foxglove.

Uses: Strophanthus may be prescribed like foxglove in the treatment of heart disease, but strophanthus's active constituents are less well absorbed. One authority recommended it as a gentle heart tonic, of particular benefit when combined with valerian and deadly nightshade. Like most herbs containing cardiac glycosides, strophanthus is strongly diuretic.

1199. *Strychnos nux-vomica* L. *(Loganiaceae)*

Vernacular Name: *Eng:* Strychnine tree, Snake-wood, Nux-vomica, Poison nut, Quaker button; *Hin:* Kucchla, Kajra; *Kan:* Kanjira, Hemmusti, Itti, Ittinji; *Mal:* Kanniram; *San:* Karaskarah; *Tam:* Etti, Kancirai; *Tel:* Musti, Mucidi.

Description: A medium sized deciduous tree, 15-20 m in height and upto 70 cm diameter with a fairly straight and cylindrical bole having dark grey or yellowish greey back and minute tubercles; leaves broadly elliptic, coriaceous, glabrous; flowers numerous, greenish white in terminal cymes; fruits globose, orange-red when ripe containing many discoid, compressed coin-like seeds in fleshy pulp; seeds concave on one side and convex on the other covered with fine grey silky hairs.

Habitate: Throughout India, in deciduous forests upto 1,200 m.

Propagation: By seeds.

Parts Used: Bark, leaves seeds.

Chemical Constituents: It content Strychnine, brucine, vomicine, α-colubrine, β-colubrine, pseudostrychnine, glycoside loganin, pseudobrucine etc.

Uses: The root bark is bitter and is useful in cholera. The leaves are applied as poultice in the treatment of chronic wounds and ulcers and the leaf decoction is useful in paralytic complaints. The pulp of the ripe fruit is used in treating paralytic affections of paws and foot. The seeds are bitter, acrid, alexeteric, aphrodisiac, appetiser, antiperiodic, anthelmintic, digestive, febrifuge, emmenagogue, purgative, stimulant and stomachic. They are useful in ananemia, asthma, bronchitis, constipation, diabetes, intermittent and malarial fevers, insomnia, cardiopalmus, skin diseases, paralysis and weakness of limbs.

1200. *Strychnos potatorum* L.f. *(Loganiaceae)*

Vernacular Name: *Eng:* Clearing nut tree, Clearing nut; *Hin:* Nirmali, Nelmal; *Kan:* Cilu, Cilledabija; *Mal:* Tettamaram, Tettamparal; *San:* Katakah, Ambuprasadah, Katakatphalam; *Tam:* Tettamaram, Tettankottai; *Tel:* Katakamu, Indupacettu, Cillacettu.

Description: A medium sized deciduous, glabrous tree about 12 m in height with cracked and scaly black bark and irregularly fluted trunk; leaves simple, opposite, ellipic, acute, chartaceous, upto 15 cm long and 6.25 cm broad, transverse nerves about 4 pairs joining the second pair of ribs to the mid rib, glabrous, shining; flowers white, fragrant, axillary cymes; fruits ovoid or globose, glabrous berries, black when ripe; seeds one or two, yellow, circular, not much compressed, 8 mm in diameter, shining with short appressed silky hairs.

Habitate: Deciduous forests of West Bengal, central and south India upto 1,200 m.

Propagation: By seeds.

Parts Used: Seeds.

Chemical Constituents: It content alkaloids, sucrose, loganin etc.

Uses: The seeds are sweet, bitter, astringent, refrigerant, demulcent, emetic, diuretic, digestive, anthelmintic, aphrodisiac, opthalmic, appetiser, alexiteric, tonic and water purifier. They are useful in vitiated conditions of *kapha* and *vata*, hepatopathy, nephropathy gonorrhoea, leucorrhoea, gastropathy, bronchitis, chronic diarrhoea and dysentery, strangury, renal and vesical calculi, diabetes, burning sensation, dipsia, conjunctivitis, scleritis, ulcers and other eye diseases. The leaves are used as a poultice for maggot-infested ulcers. Powdered bark is useful in cholera. The roots are useful in leprosy.

1201. *Strychnos wallichiana* Steud. Ex. Ed. *(Longaniaceae)*

Description: Woody climber with hooked tendrils, circinate, thickned upwards. Leaves opposite, strontly 3-nerved, inflorescence in terminal cormbiferous panicle; flowers pale yellow. Berry globose, 4-7cm. In diameter; seeds discoid, very compressed, covered on both sides with yellow silky haris.

Habitate: Grows wild in mountainous regions.

Propagation: By seeds.

Part Used: Bark.

Chemical Constituents: The stem-bark contains alkaloids 5.23% strychnine 2.37-243% brucine 2.8%.

Uses: The stem-bark and branch-bark are effective in treating rheumatism, ostealgia, paralytic cramp of the extremities, lumbago, sciatica, colic and diarrhoea, they are also used as an aphrodisiac. Caution must be exercised because of the preparation's high toxicity.

1202. *Styrax benzoin* *(Styraceae)*

Vernacular Name: *Eng:* Benzoin gum.

Description: Shrubby deciduous tree growing to 9 m. Has pointed oval leaves and clusters of white, fragrant, bell-shaped flowers.

Habitate: Native to South-East Asia, benzoin grows in tropical rainforests.

Propagation: By seeds.

Parts Used: Gum.

Chemical Constituents: Benzoin gum contains variable quantities of cinnamic, benzoic and sumaresinolic acid esters, free acids, benzaldehyde and vanillin.

Uses: Benzoin gum is strongly antiseptic and astringent. It may be used externally on wounds and ulcers to tighten and disinfect the affected tissue. When taken internally, benzoin gum acts to settle griping pain, to stimulate coughing, and to disinfect the urinary tract. Benxoin gum is an ingredient of Friar's Balsam, an antiseptic and expectorant steam inhalation for sore throats, head and chest colds, asthma and bronchitis.

1203. *Swertia chirayita* (Roxb. ex Flem.) Karsten *(Gentianaceae)*

Synonyms: *Swertia chirata* (Wall.) C.B. Clarke.

Vernacular Name: *Eng:* Clearing nut tree, Clearing nut; *Hin:* Nirmali, Nelmal; *Kan:* Cilu, Cilledabija; *Mal:* Tettamaram, Tettamparal; *San:* Katakah, Ambuprasadah, Katakatphalam; *Tam:* Tettamaram, Tettankottai; *Tel:* Katakamu, Indupacettu, Cillacettu.

Description: A medium sized deciduous, glabrous tree about 12 m in height with cracked and scaly black bark and irregularly fluted trunk; leaves simple, opposite, elliptic, acute, chartaceous, upto 15 cm long and 6.25 cm broad, transverse nerves about 4 pairs joining the second pair of ribs to the mid rib, glabrous, shining; flowers white, fragrant, axillary cymes; fruits ovoid or globose, glabrous berries, black when ripe; seeds one or two, yellow, circular, not much compressed, 8 mm in diameter, shining with short appressed silky hairs.

Habitate: Deciduous forests of West Bengal, central and south India upto 1,200 m.

Propagation: By seeds.

Parts Used: Seeds.

Chemical Constituents: Bitter principles, Ophelic acid, chiratin. Swertinin, swertianin, swerchirin, decussating, isobellidifolin, friedelin, and β-sitosterol.

Uses: The seeds are sweet, bitter, astringent, refrigerant, demulcent, emetic, diuretic, digestive, anthelmintic, aphrodisiac, opthalmic, appetiser, alexiteric, tonic and water purifier. They are useful in vitiated conditions of *kapha* and *vata*, hepatopathy, nephropathy gonorrhoea, leucorrhoea, gastropathy, bronchitis, chronic diarrhoea and dysentery, strangury, renal and vesical calculi, diabetes, burning sensation, dipsia, conjunctivitis, scleritis, ulcers and other eye diseases. The leaves are used as a poultice for maggot-infested ulcers. Powdered bark is useful in cholera. The roots are useful in leprosy.

1204. *Swertia corymbosa* (Griseb.) Wight ex C.B. Clarke *(Gentianaceae)*

Synonyms: *Swertia lawii* (Wight ex C.B. Clarke) Burkill.

Description: An erect branched herb, 30-75 cm tall. *Stems* 4-angled. *Leaves* opposite, egg-shaped-lanceolate to elliptic-oblanceolate, stalkless or minutely stalked, 2-4 x 1-2 cm, base rounded or truncate, apex bluntly apiculate, papery, hairless, with prominent 3-5 nerves arising from the base. *Flowers* in terminal branched 10-20 cm long corymbose cymes, about 1 cm across, densely arranged, white or pale blue with purplish veins, distinctly stalked. *Capsules* oblong, 5-6 mm long, dehiscing by 2-valves. *Seeds* many, minute.

Habitate: Grasslands of higher altitudes.

Propagation: By seeds.

Parts Used: Whole plant.

Chemical Constituents: N.A.

Uses: Several species of *Swertia*, including *S. corymbosa,* are accepted as substitutes for *S. chirayita,* the well known source of indigenous drug 'Chirayita'. Used for the treatment of fever, oedema, eruptie boils, haemorrhage and vomiting.

1205. *Symphytum officinale* L. *(Boraginaceae)*

Synonyms: *Symphytum album* Hort ex. Steud., *Symphytum patens* Sibth.

Vernacular Name: *Eng:* Common non-prickly comfrey.

Description: A perennial herb, with tuberous, thick dark blackish brown roots. Dried roots exhibit glistening crystals on the external surface and deep longitudinal wrinkles. Stem erect, branched, up to 1 m. high, sparsely to densely hirsute. Leaves decurrent, lanceolate obovate lanceolate, acute or acuminate, the lower up to 20 cm. long, narrowed at the base to a winged petiole; the upper progressively smaller on short petiole or sessile. Flowers white, yellowish, purple or rose coloured, in dense scorpioid cymes; sepals 5, petals 5, stamens 5. Nutlets 4, obliquely ovoid, brown, shining, rugose. Stomata on leaf anomocytic. Stomatal index for upper epidermis 14.00-15.50 and lower epidermis 15.50-20.00 root tastes mucilaginous.

Habitate: Great Britain, United States and Japan.

Propagation: By stem cutting.

Parts Used: Root.

Chemical Constituents: Symphytine, Symlandine, Echimidine, myoscorpine, Lycopsamine, intermidine, Lasiocarpine, Acetyllycopsamine, Acetylintermidine, Heliosupine, Lasiocarpine, Viridiflorine, Echiumine; Sitosterol, Stigmasterol, Isobauerenol; Arabinose, Glucuronic acid, Mannose, Mucilage; Allantoin, Chlorogenic acid, Choline, Rosmarinic acid, Silicic acid.

Uses: Used for gastric & duodenal ulcers. Gastralgia. Pruritus ani. Injuries to sinews, tendons and periosterum. Quickens formation of callus between broken surfaces of fractured bones. Of great use in wound penetrating to perineum & bones and in non-union of fractures. Irritable stumps after amputation. Irritability at the surface of fractured bones. Psoas abscess. Pricking pain & soreness of periosteum. Pain in eyes after a blow of an obtuse body. Traumatic injuries of eyes specially cured by this drug. Traditionally, it is used for colitis, gastric and duodenal ulcers, hemoptysis and haemotemesis.

1206. *Symplocarpus foetidus* *(Araceae)*

Vernacular Name: *Eng:* Skunk cabbage.

Description: Unplea*San*t-smelling perennial plant growing to 75 cm. Has a thick tuberous rootstock, cabbage-like leaves and numerous small purple flowers on a hooded spike.

Habitate: Native to northern North America, skunk cabbage thrives in meadows, swamps and marshes. The root and rhizome are collected in autumn or early spring.

Propagation: By Seeds.

Parts Used: Root and Rhizome.

Chemical Constituents: Skunk cabbage contains a volatile oil, serotonin and resins.

Uses: Skunk cabbage continues to be used primarily as an expectorant, treating cases of asthma, bronchitis and whooping cough. It is also taken for upper respiratory problems such as nasal catarrh and hay fever. Less commonly, skunk cabbage is used as a treatment for epilepsy, headaches, vertigo, and rheumatic problems and as a means to stop bleeding.

1207. *Symplocos cochinchinensis* (Lour.) Moore *(Symplocaceae)*

Synonyms: *Symplocos laurina* (Retz.)Wall. ex G. Don.

Vernacular Name: *Eng:* Chunga; *Hin:* Bholiya, Sodh; *Kan:* Lodha; *Mal:* Paccotti; *San:* Lodhrah; *Tam:* Kambli-vetti; *Tel:* Lodduga.

Description: A small evergreen tree upto 7 m in height with thin, smooth, light grey bark and white wood; leaves simple, alternate, very thick, lanceolate, elliptic or oblong, shortly acuminate at the apex, irregularly crenate or serrate; flowers yellowish white, fragrant, in close clusters, in axillary spikes; fruits globose, purplse, ribbed drupes; seeds 1-3, testa thin. The bark is greyish green to slight grey with patches of crustose lichens. The outer bark is thin and the inner greenish or light brown, the cut surface of the thick bark of a mature tree is reddish brown on drying; when broken, short thin fibre tips are seen.

Habitate: Throughout India, in evergreen forests, ravines and the Sholas upto 900 m.

Propagation: By seeds.

Parts Used: Bark.

Chemical Constituents: Bark contains two alkaloids, loturine and colloturine which are chemically related to harmine. Two new monomethyl pelargonidin glucosides and pelarggonidhin-3-O-glucoside isolated from trunk bank.

Uses: The bark is astringent, acrid, refrigerant, alternate, opthalmic, expectorant, anti-inflammatory, depurative, febrifuge, haemostatic, stomachic, constipating and suppurative. It is useful in vitiated conditions of *pitta* and *kapha*, opthalmopathy, asthma, bronchitis, dropsy, arthritis, ulcers, tumours, leprosy, skin diseases, fever, ulemorrhagia, haemorrhages, haemoptysis, dyspepsia, flatulence, leucorrhoea, diarrhoea, dysentery and gonorrhoea.

1208. *Symplocos paniculata* Wall. *(Symplocaceae (Styraceae))*

Synonyms: *Symplocos crataegoides* Buch-Ham.ex. D.Don.

Vernacular Name: Lodh, Lodar, Lodhra, Lojh.

Description: A deciduous shrub or a tree, upto 12 m in height. The bark is soft, friable, of light brown colour. The external surface is corky or much fissured transversely; while the internal part is of a lighter colour and of fibrous texture. Teaste is faintly balsamic and astringent. The leaves are obovate, serrate, 6.25 cm x 2.5-terminal panicles. Fruit is drupaceous, blue on maturity, l-seeded.

Habitate: The tree is common in the Himalayas from Himachal Pradesh to Assam and in the Kahsi hills, occurring at altitudes between 600 to 2400 m. In Himachal Pradesh, it is moderate to sporadic between 1600-2600 m in forests at Kharapathar, Kashdhar and Rohru Ranges; Parvativalley in Kullu; churdhar forest in Sirmour, Bilang; Barot in Mandi distt., Chhajpur, and Dalhousi-Kalatop forst. Its population is decreasing because the branches are frequently lopped for goat fodder.

Propagation: By seeds.

Part Used: Bark.

Chemical Constituents: The bark contains 2 alkaloids; loturine and colloturine and also a red colouring matter. The alkaloids are chemically related to harmine found in Peganum harmala. Seeds contain a fatty oil.

Uses: A water soluble fraction from the bark has been reported to exhibit anti-oxytoxic activity. Ethanolic extracts of the leaves shows activity against Entamoeba histolytica strain STA Ascaridia galli and Ranikhet-disease virus. It is also known to affect blood pressure in dogs and cats and has the effects on the ileum of guineapigs. Extract of the stem affects the blood pressure. The bark is also used in treatment of ophthalmia and a tonic to prevent abortion. It is also reported to be alterative, anti-leprotic, antidropsical, astringent, blood purifier, dentrifice, expectorant, febrifuge, haemostatic, stomachic, styptic and suppurative. It is useful in asthma, bleeding of spongy gums; bowel complaints, leucorrhoea, ulcers, tumors, uterine haemorrhages and in the diseases of eye, ear and liver. The bark powder alongwith coriander and calamus is used as a facial cosmetic.

1209. *Symplocos racemosa* Roxb. *(Symplocaceae)*

Synonyms: *Symplocos beddomei* C.B. Clarke, *Symplocos candolleana* Brand.

Vernacular Name: *San*: Rodhra, *Hin:* Lodh, *Kan:* Bala doddli, Lodhra, *Mal:* Pachotti, Mar: Lodhra, *Tam:* Vellilathi, *Tel:* Lodduga.

Description: Medium sized trees, 10-15 m tall, about 1 m girth. Branchlets hairless. *Leaves* alternate, elliptic-oblong, 8-15 x 3-6 cm, base wedge-shaped to rounded, apex acute to acuminate, margin toothed with rounded to saw-like teeth, obscurely recurved, papery, hairless, distinctly stalked; lateral nerves 8-11 pairs. *Flowers* bisexual, shortly stalked, in 6-17 cm long axillary racemes, about 1 cm across, white with pink tinge, fragrant. *Drupes* ellipsoid to ovoid, about 1.5 x 0.6 cm, hairless, ripening dark blue, turning yellow when dry. *Seeds* 1-2, oblong.

Habitate: North and East India, Himalayas upto 1400 m.

Propagation: By seeds and stem cuttings.

Parts Used: Bark.

Chemical Constituents: Loturine, loturidine, colloturine, sugars, oxalic acid, phytosterol, 3-monoglucofuranoside of 7-*O*-methyl leucopelargonidin.

Uses: Stem bark is used to treat haemorrhage, acne and pimples, leucorrhea, wounds, skin disorders, plant poisons, ascites, hoarseness of voice, fever, menstrual disorders, liver diseases, menorrhagia, bowel complaints, ulcers and to give firmness to spongy and bleeding gums.

1210. *Syzygium aromaticum* (L.) Merrill & Perry *(Myrtaceae)*

Synonyms: *Caryophyllus aromaticus, Eugenia caryophyllata, Eugenia aromatica.*

Vernacular Name: *Eng:* Clove tree, Cloves; *Hin:* Lavamg, Laumg; *Kan:* Lavanga; *Mal:* Karampu, Karayampu, Grampu; *San:* Lavangam, Devakusumam; *Tam:* Kirampu; *Tel:* Lavangamu, Devakusumamu.

Description: A pyramidal or conical evergreen tree usually upto 12 m in height with a single main stem bearing obliquely oriented branches; leaves simple, lanceolate, gland-dotted, fragrant; flower buds greenish to pink, clustered at the ends of the branches, highly aromatic; fruits fleshy, dark pink drupes; seeds oblong, grooved on one side.

Habitate: Cultivated in south India.

Propagation: By seeds.

Parts Used: Dried flower buds (cloves), oil.

Chemical Constituents: It content protein, carbohydrates, tannin, oleanolic acid, eugenol acetate, caryophyllene and eugenol.

Uses: The cloves are acrid, bitter, aromatic, refrigerant, ophthalmic, digestive, carminative, stomachic, stimulant, antispasmodic, antibacterial, rubefacient, aphrodisiac, appetiser, expectorant, emollient, anthelmintic, sialogogue, rejuvenating, galacto-purifier, diuretic, febrifuge and tonic. They are useful in halitosis, odontalgia, opthalmopathy, flatulence, colic, gastropathy, anorexia, cough, asthma, vitiated conditions of *kapha* and *pitta*, burning sensation, skin diseases, helminthiasis, agalactia, impurity of breast milk, strangury, fever, cephalalgia, neuralgia, lumbago, notalgia, dental caries, hyperacidity, vomiting, dipsia, hepatopathy, general debility and tuberculosis. The oil is useful in catarrh, cough, bronchitis, vitiated conditions of *vata*, gastrohelcosis, flatulence, colic, skin diseases, dyspepsia, vomiting, odontalgia, dental caries and cephalalgia. Extrenally the oil is used as a rubefacient and counterirritant.

1211. *Syzygium cornocarpum* (A. Gray) C. Muell. *(Myrtaceae)*

Description: Spreading cauliflorous tree upto 15 m tall. Leaves opposite, short-petiolate, the blade glossy, lanceolate or oblanceolate, up to 15 cm long. Flowers pinkish, borne in many-flowered, branching panicles which arise from branches or the trunk. Fruit a fragrant, red or purple elongated cylindrical berry 2-3 cm long containing 1-3 moderate-sized, hard seeds. Flowers available between July and January and fruit available between November and July.

Habitate: Common in dense wet forest from sea-level to 1000 m elevation.

Propagation: By seeds.

Part Used: Leaves and bark.

Uses: Used to treat severe boils or tumours of the breast. An infusion of the leaves is drunk to cure swelling of the breasts. Generally used as a tonic. An infusion of the bark or leaves is given to babies with teething problems. In Samoa, an infusion of the leaves is used in treating inflammations, skin sores and urinary tract problems.

1212. *Syzygium cumini* (L.) Skeel *(Myrtaceae)*

Synonyms: *Eugenia jambolana* Lam.

Vernacular Name: *Eng:* Jaman, Jambolan, Black plum; *Hin:* Jamun, Jambhal, Jaman; *Kan:* Nerale, Jambuva; *Mal:* Naval; *San:* Jambuh; *Tam:* Naval, Kottainaval; *Tel:* Neredu.

Description: A medium sized to large tree, 15-30 m in height with smooth light grey bark having dark patches; leaves simple, opposite, variable in shape, about 2.5 cm broad and 7.5-15 cm long, acuminate, nerves joining in a distinct intramagrinal nerve, gland-dotted, smooth and shiny; flowers greenish-white in trichotomous panicls; fruits oblong or ovoid-oblong, dark purple with pinkish juicy pulp; one-seeded.

Habitate: Throughout India, in forests upto 1,800 m usually along river banks and also cultivated.

Propagation: By seeds.

Parts Used: Bark, leaves, fruits.

Chemical Constituents: Seeds contain glycoside jambolin, ellagic acid, tannin, gallic acid, chlorophyll, fatty oil, starch, resin, sugar and traces of oil. Flowers give acetyl oleanolic acid two other triterpenoids, ellagic acid, isoquercitrin, quercetin, kaempferol and myricetin.

Uses: The bark is astringent, sweet, sour, acrid, refrigerant, carminative, diuretic, digestive, anthelmintic, febrifuge, constipating, stomachalgia, fever, gastropathy, strangury and dermatopathy. The leaves are antibacterial and are used for strengthening the teeth and gums. The tender leaves are used for vomiting. The fruits and seeds are sweet, acrid, sour, tonic and cooling, and are used in diabetes, diarrhoea, pharyngitis, splenopathy, urethrorrhea and ringworm.

1213. *Syzygium jambos* (L.) Alston *(Myrtaceae)*

Synonyms: *Eugenia jambos* Linn.

Vernacular Name: *Eng:* Rose-apple; *Hin:* Gulab-jamun; *Kan:* Pannerale; *Mal:* Campa, Malaykkacampa; *San:* Campeyah; *Tam:* Campai; *Tel:* Jambuneredu.

Description: A large shrub or small tree with spreading branches; leaves simple, opposite, lanceolate, narrowed into short petioles, secondary nerves joined by a prominent looping intramarginal vein; flowers greenish white in short terminal racemose cymes, stamens many, yellowish white; fruits pale yellow to pinkish white, blobose; seeds 1-2, grey in large cavity of the succulent pericarp.

Habitate: Cultivated throughout India upto 1,350 m.

Propagation: By seeds and vegetative method.

Parts Used: Bark, fruits.

Chemical Constituents: It content vitamin A, thiamine, riboflavin, nicotine acid, vitamin C, folic acid, alanine, aspartic acid, cystine, cysteine, glutamine, threonine and tyrosine.

Uses: The bark is astringent, bitter, sweet, haemostatic, depurative, vulnerary, antidiarrhoeal and anthelmintic. It is useful in gout, haemorrhages, syphilis, leprosy, dermatopathy, diarrhoea, colic helminthiasis, wounds, ulcers, stomatitis and vitiated conditions of *pitta*. The fruits are sweet and aromatic and are edible.

1214. *Syzygium malaccense* (L.) Merr. & Perry *(Myrtaceae)*

Synonyms: *Eugenia malaccensis* Linn.

Vernacular Name: *Eng:* Malay apple, mountain apple.

Description: Tree up to 20 m tall. Leaves opposite, petiolate, the blade oblong to ovate, up to 30 cm long, shiney green flowers 4-5 parted, pink, red, or rarely white, with numerous conspicuous excerted stamens. Fruit a fleshy drupe, obovoid, up to 7 cm. Long, often deep pink or pure whitish, fragrant and delicately flavoured.

Habitate: Common in villages, lowland secondary forests, and cultivated valleys from near sea-level up to 1000 m elevation.

Propagation: By seeds.

Part Used: Bark and leaves.

Chemical Constituents: Proteins, fibre, hemicellulose, cellulose, lignin, and silica; fruits contain vitamin C, fructose and glucose.

Uses: To treat cough, yellow urine and bad appetite; as a remedy for deep bone pains, diabetes, gonorrhea, swollen stomach after childbirth, sore throat, thrush, bronchitis and to relieve constipation. The bark is used to cure mouth sores in children. An infusion of the bark is used to treat stomachache and abdominal ailments. An infusion of the bark or leaves is used to treating mouth infections. The bark/leaf is used to treat mouth sores. A bark infusion is used to treat tuberculosis and digestive tract problems. It is used to treat venereal diseases. The leaves are used to treat red eyes.

1215. *Syzygium travancoricum* Gamble *(Myrtaceae)*

Description: Medium sized trees, 7-12 m tall. *Bark greyish* brown. Branchlets distinctly 4-angled, hairless. *Leaves* simple, opposite, egg-shaped to elliptic, 10-17 x 5-10 cm, base narrowed and decurrent, apex bluntly acuminate, papery, hairless, shiny; lateral nerves 10-15 pairs, distantly arranged, joining near margin; leaf stalks about 2 cm long. *Flowers* bisexual, about 3 mm across, white, mildly fragrant, arranged in 5-8 cm long axillary corymbose cymes. *Drupes* oblong-ellipsoid, smooth, hairless, about 1 cm long, purplish when ripe. *Seeds* single, white.

Habitate: Swampy areas along the Malabar Coast and in evergreen forests.

Propagation: By seeds and stem cuttings.

Parts Used: Bark.

Chemical Constituents: N.A.

Uses: The bark used in local medicine. Its relative *S. cumini* is used in treating diarrhoea, diabetes, intrinsic haemorrhage, vomiting, slugging digestion, maggots in ear and to heal wounds.

1216. *Tabebuia* Sp. *(Bignoniaceae)*

Vernacular Name: *Eng:* Lapacho, Pau D'arco.

Description: An evergreen tree reaching 30m, with pink flowers.

Habitate: An indigenous South American tree, lapacho grows well in mountainous terrains. In peru and Argentina it is found growing high up in the Andes. Lapacho is also found in low-lying areas, where it is thought to have originated.

Propagation: By seed.

Parts Used: Bark.

Chemical Constituents: Quinines, Bioflavonoids, Lapachenole, Carnosol, Indoles, Coenzyme Q, Alkaloids, Steroidal.

Uses: Antibiotic, antifungal, Immune-stimulant, anti-kinflammatory, Cleansing, Tonic, Anti-tumour.

1217. *Tabernaemontana divaricata* (L.) *(Apocynaceae)*

Synonyms: *Ervatamia coronaria* (Jacq.) Stapf; *Ervatamia divaricata* (Linn.) Burkill; *Tabernaemontana coronaria* (Jacq.) Willd.

Vernacular Name: *Eng:* East Indian rosebay; *Hin:* Candni; *Kan:* Kottubale, Nandibatlu; *Mal:* Nantyarvattam, Nantyavarttam; *San:* Nandivrkshah; *Tam:* Nantiyavattam, Atukunantiyarvattai; *Tel:* Gandhitagarapu, Nandivardhanamu.

Description: A blabrous, evergreen shrub 1.8-2.4 m in height with silvery grey bark and milky latex; leaves simple, opposite, elliptic or elliptic-lanceolate, smooth, glossy green, acuminate, margins wavy; flowers white, sweetly fragrant in 1-8 flowered cymes at the bifurcations of the branches, lobes of corolla overlapping to right in the bud; fruits follicles, 2.5-7.5 cm long, ribbed and curved, orange or bright red within, irregular, enclosed in a red puply aril.

Habitate: Throughout India, also cultivated as an ornamental plant.

Propagation: By seeds and vegetative method.

Parts Used: Roots, flowers, latex.

Chemical Constituents: It content coronaridine, voacristine, tabernaemontanine and dregamine. Bark of stem and root contains a crystaling substance and alkaloids tabernaemontanine and coronarine.

Uses: The roots are acrid, bitter, thermogenic, anodyne, astringent, vermifuge and tonic. They are useful in odonatalgia, opacity of the cornea, paralysis, strangury, vitiated conditions of *vata*, arthralgia burning sensation, ophthalmitis and dermatopathy. The latex is cooling and has an anti-inflammatory effect on wounds.

1218. *Tacca chantrieri* Andre *(Taccaeceae)*

Vernacular Name: *Eng:* Devil flower.

Description: Perennial herb. Root-stock many-noded, horizontally creeping, leaves radical, long-petioled, entire; margins wavy. Flowers dark-violet in umbel on an erect or curved scapel involucre of 4 bracts, 2 small and 2 larger; bracteoles filiform, concolorous. Capsule long. Seeds 3-angled, violet-purple.

Habitate: Grows wild in damp forests.

Propagation: By seeds and rhizome.

Part Used: Rhizomes.

Chemical Constituents: The rhizomes contain cholan saponins that yield diosgenin on hydrolysis, taccaoside and B-istosterol.

Uses: An alcholic maceration of the rhizome is used externally as a liniment in rheumatism,. Oral administration is prohibited. The rhizome is also used as raw material for the extration of diosgenin.

1219. *Tacca leontopetaloides* (L.) Kuntze *(Taccaceae)*

Synonyms: *Tacca pinnatifida* Forst. & Forst. f.

Vernacular Name: *San:* Surna; *Eng:* Polynesian arrowroot; *Tel:* Peddakandagadda, kanda, kaduchurngaed and *Mal:* Kattuchena-kizhangu.

Description: Coarse, stemless, perennial, tuberous herb upto 1 m high. Leaves large, petiolate, the petioles transversely striated, arising from a tuber up to 8 cm in diameter. Flowers small, bell-shaped, greenish, 6-parted, borne in a many-flowered umbel surrounded by leafy bracts and numerous long filaments, supported by an erect, hollow, transversely striated 1 m long stem arising from the tuber. Fruit a yellow, ribbed, globose berry up to 2.5 cm in diameter containing numerous longitudinally ridged seeds.

Habitate: Common on beaches and beach thickets and coastal woods with sandy soils to 250 m elevation.

Propagation: By seeds.

Part Used: Leaves and tubers.

Chemical Constituents: Alkaloids (unidentified), beta-sitosterol, ceryl alcohol, taccalin.

Uses: The inside of the root is squeezed in water and applied as rinse to injured eyes. The starch from the tubers of the plant was used as a remedy for diarrhoea and dysentery. Crushed leaf stalks of the plant are rubbed onto bee and wasp stings.

1220. *Tacca plantaginea* (Hance) Drenth *(Taccaeceae)*

Description: Stemless herb, 20-30cm. High. Root-stock round curved upwards. Leaves radical, entire, attenuate at the base; apex pointedl margins wavy, infloerescence in umbel of 6-10 flowers on a curved scape, bracts dark-violet; flowers violet, fruit capsular.

Habitate: Grows wild in wet places in mountainsous regions.

Propagation: By seeds.

Part Used: Tuberous roots.

Chemical Constituents: The tuberous roots contain cholan saponins that yield diosgenin on hydrolysis.

Uses: The roots are utilized for the relief of dyspepsia, colic, diarrhoea, jaundice folliwing viral hepatitis, menstrual disorders, hypertension, neurasthenia, sciatica, rheumatism and infantile polyyelitis.

1221. *Tagetes minuta* L. *(Asteraceae)*

Synonyms: *Tagetes glandulifera* Schrank.

Vernacular Name: Gaindri, Jangli-gainda, Gandloghas Tagetes.

Description: The plant is a highly aromatic annual, 1-2 m tall. Leaves are 7-15 cm long pinnatisect and the segments are 11-19; 4 cm or more long, linear or lanceolate. Flower-heads are pale-yellow, narrow, tubular, in corymbose clusters and the achenes are black.

Habitate: The plant, native to South America, is naturalized near waste places and on dry embankments in the north-west Himalayas, between altitudes of 1250 and 2500 m. In Himachal Pradesh, the plant has been found almost all over the state as a weed of waste places. Robust plant growth has been observed at Rohru, Samoli, Chirgaon-Tikkari, Dodra kawar, Shimla.

Propagation: By seeds.

Part Used: Entire herb/Foliage especially flowering tops.

Chemical Constituents: Aromadendrenem tagetone, phenylethyl alcohol, ocimens, salicylaldehyde, phenylacetaldehyde, eudesmol, linalylacetate, limonene, linalool and an un-identified carbonyl compound have been isolated from the plant.

Uses: The oil obtained from the herb, has synergistic activity and shows positive juvenile hormone activity. The ethanolic extracts of the entire herb show anti-viral activity against Ranikhet-disease virus. The roots show nematocidal activity and hence, the plant is grown in the tobacco fields. The plant has strong larvicidal effect and is also a slow repellent. It is suspected of poisoning cows and taints milk and butter. The juice of the herb ca**Uses** irritation of the eyes and skin. The flowers are used as a stomachic, aperient, diuretic and diaphoretic. They contain a volatile oil which exhibits tranquilizing, hypotensive, spasmolytic, bronchodilatory and anti-inflammatory properties.

1222. *Talinum patens* (L.) Willd. *(Portulacaceae)*

Description: Succulent perennial herb, 30-50cm. High. Stems greenish, occasionally purplish. Leaves ovoid, thick, entire; the lower alternate, the upper nearly opposite; nerves inconspicuous. Inflorescence in terminal compound raceme; flowers small, pink. Capsule brownish-purple;seeds comprssed, shining black.

Habitate: Grows wild in the mountains; is also cultivated fro ornamental and medicinal purposes.

Propagation: By seeds.

Part Used: Roots.

Chemical Constituents: N.A.

Uses: The roots possess tonic properties and are used in treating neurasthenia, cough, gastralgia an dpulmonary tuberculosis. They are also used ot treat dehydrating diarrhoea. A buillon made from the fresh laves is used as a stomachic.

1223. *Tamarindus indica* L. *(Caesalpiniacae)*

Vernacular Name: *Eng:* Tamarind tree; *Hin:* Imli, Amli, Ampli; *Kan:* Huli, Amli; *Mal:* Puli, Kolpuli, Valanpuli; *San:* Cinca, Tintrini; *Tam:* Puli Amilam; *Tel:* Cintapandu, Amlaki, Cintacettu.

Description: A large to very large evergreen tree upto 30 m in height with dark grey bark having longitudinal fissures and deep cracks; leaves paripinnate upto 15 cm long, rachis slender, channelled, leaflets 10-20 pairs, subsessile, oblong; flowers yellow, striped with red in laxz, few flowered racemes at the ends of the branchlets; fruits pods, brownish ash coloured, slightly curved, subcompressed, with a shallow oblong pit on each side of the flat faces; seeds enveloped by a toughy leathery membrane (the endocarp) and pulpy mesocarp, tests shining, hard.

Habitate: Throughout India, particularly in the South India, often cultivated.

Propagation: By seeds.

Parts Used: Roots, fruits, seeds.

Chemical Constituents: Fruit contains tartaric acid, citric maleic acid and potassium bitartarate and traces of oxalic acid. Kernel, polysaccharides. Leaves contain flavonoid glycosides saponaretin, vitexin, orientin and homoorientin. Hordenine isolated from leaves, bark and flowers.

Uses: The root bark is astringent constipating, emmenagogue and tonic, and is useful in diarrhoea, asthma, amenorrhoea, singivitis and ulcers. The leaves are sour, astringent, thermogenic, anthelmintic, anodyne, anti-inflammatory, antifungal, diuretic, febrifuge, aperient and opthalmic. They are useful in vitiated conditions of *vata*, swellings, fever, scalding of urine, gastropathy, helminthiasis, wounds, ulcers, jaundice, scabies, tumours, ringworm, boils, smallpox, otalgia and conjunctivitis. The fruits are sour, sweet, refrigerant, digestive, carminative, laxative, antiscorbutic, antiseptic, ophthalmic and febrifuge. They are useful in gastropathy, bilious vomiting, Datura poisoning, alcoholic intoxication dipsia, scabies, pharyngitis, pharyngodynia, stomatitis, constipation, haemorrhoids and ophthalmopathy. The seeds are astrigent, cooling, aphrodisiac, stomachic, constipating and tonic. They are useful in stomachalgia, diarrohea, dysentery, dipsia, burning sensation, haematuria, giddiness, vertigo, hepatopathy, inflammations, chronic ulcers, abscess, haemorrhoids, vaginopathy, metroptosis, diabetes and general debility.

1224. *Tanacetum parthenium* *(Asteraceae)*

Vernacular Name: *Eng:* Feverfew.

Description: A herbaceous perennial growing to 60cm, with numerous daisy-like flowerheads.

Habitate: Originally from South-eastern Europe, feverfew is now common throughout Europe, Australia and North America.

Propagation: By Seed.

Parts Used: Aerial parts.

Chemical Constituents: Volatile oil, Sesquiterpene lactones, Sesquiterpenes.

Uses: Analgesic, Reduces Fever, Antirheumatic, Promotes menstrual flow, Bitter.

1225. *Tanacetum vulgare* *(Asteraceae)*

Synonyms*:* *Chrysanthemum vulgare.*

Vernacular Name: *Eng:* Tansy.

Description: Strongly aromatic perennial growing to 1 m. Has an erect stem, feathery compound leaves and clusters of yellow disc-shaped flower in heads.

Habitate: Found throughout temperate zones in the northern hemisphere, tansy grows on wasteground, alongside roads and close to water.

Propagation: By Seeds.

Parts Used: Flowers.

Chemical Constituents: Tansy contains a volatile oil, which includes significant levels of thujone and camphor, sesquiterpene lactones, flavonoids and resin. The volatile oil strongly includes menstruation.

Uses: Tansy is little used today because of its potential toxicity. When the plant is taken, it is chiefly in order to expel intestinal worms, and, to a lesser degree, to help stimulate menstrual kill scabies, fleas and lice, but even external application of tansy preparations carries the risk of toxicity.

1226. *Taraxacum mongolicum* Hand.-Mazz. *(Asteraceae)*

Vernacular Name: *Eng:* Mongolian dandelion.

Description: A perennial acaulous herb with latex. Leaves basal, in rosette, hairy, linear-lanceolate, oblanceolate or obovate; apex acute or obtuse; base attenuate, irregular runcinate-pinnatifid; the segments triangular or dentate. Flowers yellow homogamous, all completely ligulate, 1.5-1.8 cm long by 2-2.5 mm wide; apex cuneate, 5-toothed; the lower part tubular Achene oblanceolate, 4-5 mm long, light yellowish-brown, 10-ribbed; ribs often muricate or echinate; beak often slender at the apex, pappus white.

Habitate: On hillsides, in grasslands and by roadsides in China, Korea, Mongolia, Soviet Union.

Propagation: By seeds.

Part Used: Whole plant.

Chemical Constituents: N.A.

Uses: Upper respiratory tract infection; acute tonsillitis; pharyngitis, gastritis, enteriris, general fatigue, relief of cholecystitis, abdominal pain, pyodermas; snake bits.

1227. *Taraxacum officinale* Weber *(Asteraceae)*

Vernacular Name: *Eng:* Common dandelion, Blow ball; *Hin:* Dudhal, Kanphul; *Kan:* Kadusevanti; *Mal:* Dugddhapheni; *San:* Dugdhapheni; *Tel:* Patri.

Description: A perennial herb with thick tap root and abundant milky juice in all parts; leaves radical, sessile, variable in shape, narrowly oblong, irregularly pinnatifid, lobes linear or triangular, toothed; flowers yellow in ligulate heads; fruits glabrous achenes, flattened, ribbed minutely, spiny on the upper half, crowned with white pappus hairs.

Habitate: Throughout India, in the hills from 300-5,400 m.

Propagation: By seeds and vegetative method.

Parts Used: Whole plant.

Chemical Constituents: The frug contains a bitter crystalline principle, taraxacin and a crystalline substance, taraxacerine; the phytosterols-taraxasterol and homotaraxasterol besides saponin. The milky sap contain cerylalcohol, lactuce-roltaraxacin, and choline. The root yields inulin, tannin and some ethereal oil; the leaves contain vitamin C and the flowers xanthophylls. Also contain Potassium and Vitamin A.

Uses: The plant is bitter, acrid, thermogenic, vulnerary, digestive, stomachic, anthelmintic, aperient, liver tonic, sudorific, febrifuge, diuretic, antibacterial, depurative, anti-inflammatory, cholagogue, stimulant and tonic. It is useful in vitiated conditions of *kapha* and *vata*, chronic ulcers, tuberculosis, dyspepsia, colic, flatulence, verminosis, constipation, strangury, nephropathy, fever, skin diseases, leprosy, inflammations, gout stiff joints, insomnia, hypochondria, jaudice, biliary calculi and other hepatic diseases and debility. Root is diuretic, tonic laxative, cholagogue, anti-rheumatic and aperient. The tender leaves are used as 'Salad' when harvested in spring, the plant has a slight inulin content and is used as a bitter for loss of appetite and stomach upsets. The drug promotes the secretion of gall and is a useful remedy for chronic disorders of kidney and liver. It has been in use for gallstones, cholecystitis, jaundice, atonic dyspepsia with constipation, muscular rheumatism and oligurea.

1228. *Tarenna sambucina* (A. Gray) dur ex. Darake (*Rubiaceae*)

Description: Compact or spreading shrub or small tree to 10 m tall. Leaves opposite, petiolate, lanceolate upto 20 cm long. Flowers white fragrant, borne in dense, branching, terminal cymose clusters. Fruit dark green to black, globose, hard and indehiscent, about 5 mm in diameter, containing several hard angular seeds.

Habitate: Common in coastal and grassland thickets, disturbed, dry open or dense forest, and even mangrove margins from sea-level to abut 500 m elevation.

Propagation: By seeds.

Part Used: Stem, bark and fruits.

Chemical Constituents: N.A.

Uses: Fluid from the stem of the plant is used for rheumatic aches and swellings of the muscles and joints. An infusion of the grated bark is used to treat children's fever or inflammation and diarrhoea as well as internal infuries. The fruit of the plant is used to make a salve or linament in Niue. A drink made from the boiled bark is used as a remedy for costipation and as a general tonic A tea made from the grated bark to treat stomachache, infertility, secondary amenorrhoea and dysmenorrhoea.

1229. *Taxus baccata* L. (*Taxaceae*)

Synonyms: *Taxus erecta* Hort. ex. Carr., *Taxus stricta* Hort. ex. Gord.

Vernacular Name: *Eng:* Yew; *San*: Manduparli, *Hin*: Thuno, Thuner, Birmi, *Beng*: Burmie, Bhirmie, Ilchujhu.

Description: A evergreen tree upto 18m. in height, usually with a short trunk, upto 1 m. in diameter. Bark reddish, flaky, deeply longitudinally fissured in old trees. Branches spreading forming a broad, low head, branchlets somewhat pendulous. ***Leaves:*** 2-ranked, linear usually falcate, shortly acuminate with a prominent mid-rib, dark green above, pale beneath 2-3.2 cm. long or shorter in some varieties. Male flowers are borne in a small catkin with bracts, while the female flowers take the form of fleshy apical disc with a few scales a its base. The fruit is red, fleshy, cup-like encasing a single seed. Seed brown, 0.60 cm. long.

Habitate: In India in temperate Himalayas between 2000-3500 m. and Khasia Hills.

Propagation: By seeds.

Parts Used: Twigs and leaves.

Chemical Constituents: Alkaloids: Taxine, Taxinine, Ephedrine, β-Sitosterl, Glucoside: Taxicatin, Taxiphyllin, Ecdysterone; Hydrocyanic acid. Formic acid. Resins.

Uses: Hysteria, Epilepsy, Headache, Giddiness. Coldness of extremeties. Sever biliousness antispasmodic. Emmenogogue. It is used as a remedy for pustular diseases of skin and night sweats, gout and chroninc rheumatism. Complaints of supra-orbital and temporal pain of right side, with lachrymation & dilated pupil. Pain in pit of stomach and region of navel with feeling of pain and needles at the pit of stomach. Sensation of emptiness of stomach, which makes one to eat frequently. Skin with lager, flat, itching pustules. Erysipelas.

1230. *Tectona grandis* L.f. *(Verbenaceae)*

Vernacular Name: *Eng:* Teak; *Hin:* Sagaun, Sagvan; *Kan:* Tega, Jadi, Tyagadamara; *Mal:* Tekku; *San:* Sakkah, Bhumishah; *Tam:* Tekku, Tekkumaram; *Tel:* Peddateku, Adviteku.

Description: A large to very large deciduous tree, 20-35 m in height with light brown or grey bark having shallow longitudinal furrows, fluted and buttressed base and characteristically quadrangular channeled branchlets; leaves simple, opposite, broadly elliptical or obovate, acute or acuminate, coriaceous, rough above, stellately-grey tomentose beneath, possessing minute glandular dots, main nerves 8-10 pairs; flowers many, white, small, sweet scented, in large erect terminal branched tomentose cymose panicles; fruits hard, bony, irregularly globose drupes enveloped by light brown bladder-like calyx; seeds usually 1-3, ovate, marble white.

Habitate: Throughout India, in deciduous forests upto 1,000 m, also cultivated.

Propagation: By seeds.

Parts Used: Whole plant.

Chemical Constituents: Wood contains in its cavities white crystellinee deposits of calcium phosphate, silica and ammonium and magnesium phosphate, also a resin. Seed contains a bland fatty oil.

Uses: The roots are useful in anuria. The bark is astringent, acrid, sweet, cooling, constipathing, anthelmintic and depurative. It is useful in bronchitis, hyperacidity, vitiated conditions of *pitta*, dysentery, verminosis, burning sensation, diabetes, leprosy and skin diseases. The leaves are cooling, haemostatic, depurative, anti-inflammatory and vulnerary. They are useful in inflammation, leprosy, skin diseases, pruritus, stomatitis, indolent ulcers, haemorrhages, haemoptysis and vitiated conditions of *pitta*. The fruits are diuretic and demulcent and are useful in strangury, vesical calculi, pruritus and stomatitis. The flowers are acrid, bitter, refrierant, depurative, diuretic and anti-inflammatory, and are useful in vitiated conditions of *pitta* and *kapha*, burning sensation, dipsia, leprosy, skin diseases, strangury and diabetes. The seeds are astringent, emollient, diuretic and demulcent and are useful in vitiated conditions of *vata*, strangury, skin diseases and pruritus. The wood is astringent, acrid, cooling, anti-inflammatory, anodyne, vermifuge, ophthalmic, expectorant, depurative, laxative and uterine sedative. It is useful in vitiated conditions of *pitta* and *kapha*, neuraglia, arthritis, inflammatory sweelling of the eyelids, dyspepsia, flatulence, cough, skin diseases, leprosy, leucoderma, hyperacidity, menorrhagia, leucorrhoea, abortion, dipsia, burning sensation, haemorrhoids and dysentery. The oil obtained from seeds, flowers and wood is trichogenous and is useful in the treatment of eczema and ringworm.

1231. *Tephrosia purpurea* (L.) Pers. *(Fabaceae)*

Vernacular Name: *Eng:* Wild indigo, Purple tephrosia; *Hin:* Sarphomka; *Kan:* Phanike, Empali, Koggili, Vajaranili; *Mal:* Kolinnil, Kattamari, Koluva, Kotikkolinnil; *San:* Sarapunkhah, Banah, Banapunkhah; *Tam:* Kattukkolincai; *Tel:* Vempali, Bontavempali.

Description: A much branched suberect herbaceous perennial, 30-60 cm in height with spreading branches; leaves imparipinnate, leaflets 11-21, narrow, oblanceloate; flowers red or purple in extra axillaty racemes; fruits slightly curved pods, 3-4.5 cm, long; seeds 5-10 per pod, grey, smooth.

Habitate: Throughout India, on waster lands and along roadsides.

Propagation: By seeds.

Parts Used: Whole plant.

Chemical Constituents: β-Sitosterol, lupeol, retin, delphinidin chloride, cyaniding chloride, isolonchocarpin, lanceolatins A and B, pongamol, karangin, kangone, 5,7-dimethoxy-8, flavanone, 2-methoxy-3-9-dihydroxycoumestone, flevichapparins B and C, methyl karanjic acid and purpurin.

Uses: The plant is bitter, astringent, acrid, thermogenic, anthelmintic, digestive, laxative, diuretic, uterine tonic, anti-inflammatory depurative, styptic, debostruant, alexiteric, alterant and antipyretic. The roots are useful in inflammations, skin diseases, scrofula, elephantiasis, dyspepsia, stomachalgia, flatulence, haemorrhoids, asthma, bronchitis, anaemia, hepatosplenomegaly, verminosis, strangury, dysmenorrhoea, chronic fever, boils pimples, odontalgia and gingivitis. The leaves are useful in dyspepsia, pectrol diseases, haemorrhoids, syphilis, gonorrhoea and bruises. The seeds are useful in skin diseases and rat poisoning.

1232. *Terminalia arjuna* (Roxb. ex DC) Wight & Arn. *(Combretaceae)*

Vernacular Name: *Eng:* Arjun; *Hin:* Arjun, Kahu, Kahua; *Kan:* Maddi, Vaidairya; *Mal:* Nirmarutu, Venmarutu, Attumarutu, Marutu, Pulamatti; *San:* Arjunah, Kakubhah; *Tam:* Attumarutu, Nirmarutu, Vellaimarutu, Marutu; *Tel:* Erramaddi.

Description: A large evergreen tree with butterssed trunk and spreading crown with drooping branches, bark smooth, grey outside and flesh coloured inside, flaking off in large flat pieces; leaves simple, subopposite, oblong or elliptic, coriaceous, crenulate, pale dull green above, pale brown beneath, often unequal sided, nerves 10-15 pairs, reticulate; flowers white in panicles of spikes with linear bracteoles; fruits ovoid or oblong with 5-7 short, hard angles or wings, the lines on the wings oblique and curving upwards.

Habitate: Throughout India.

Propagation: By seeds.

Parts Used: Bark.

Chemical Constituents: Arjunolic acid, tomentosic acid, B-sitosterol, ellagic acid, saponin and leucodelphinidin. Bark contains a crystalline compound arjunine, a laactone, arjunetin, essential oil, tannin pyrocatachol, large quantities of calcium salts and traces of aluminium and magnesium salts, reducing sugars and colouring matter.

Uses: The bark is astringent, sweet, acrid, cooling, aphrodisiac, demulcent, cardiotonic, styptic, antidysenteric, urinary astringent, expectorant, alexiteric, lithontriptic and tonic. It is useful in fractures, ulcers, urethrorrhea, leucorrhoea, diabetes, vitiated conditions of *pitta*, anaemia, cardiopathy, hyperhidrosis, fatigue, asthma, bronchitis, tumours, otalgia, dysentery, inflammations, internal and external haemorrhages, cirrhosis of the liver and hypertension.

1233. *Terminalia bellirica* (Gaertn.) Roxb. *(Combretaceae)*

Vernacular Name: *Eng:* Belliric myrobalan; *Hin:* Bahenda, Bahaira; *Kan:* Behara, Tanrikayi, Santikayi; *Mal:* Tani, Tannikka; *San:* Vibhitakah, Aksah; *Tam:* Tanni, Banrikkai; *Tel:* Tandra, Tani.

Description: A large deciduous butterssed tree, 20-30 m in height with thick brownish grey back having shallow longitudinal fissures; leaves simple, alternate, long-petioled, crowded about the extremities of the branches, broady elliptic, margins entire, main nerves 6-8 pairs, midrib prominent on both surfaces; flowers pale greenish yellow with an offensive odour, in axillary spikes, longer than the petioles but shorter than the leaves; fruits ovoid grey drupes, obscurely 5 angled, narrowed into a very short stalk.

Habitate: Throughout India, in deciduous forests upto an elevation of 900 m.

Propagation: By seeds.

Parts Used: Bark, fruits.

Chemical Constituents: Fruits contain about 17% tannin and β-sitosterol, gallic acid, ellagic acid, ethyl galate, galloyl glucose and chebulagic acid. Heartwood and bark contain ellagic acid and the seed-coat of the fruit contains gallic acid. A new cardiac glycoside-bellericanin. Kernel oil had a purgative action, and fruit extract produced fall in blood pressure and significant increase of bile secretion in experimental animals.

Uses: The bark is mildly diuretic and iseful in anaemia and leucoderma. The fruits are astringent, acrid, sweet, thermogenic, anti-inflammatory, anodyne, styptic, narcotic, digestive, anthelmintic, aperient, experctorant, ophthalmic, antipyretic, antiemetic and rejuvenating. They are useful in vitiated conditions of *kapha* and *vata*, cough, bronchitis, pharyngitis, insomnia, dropsy, dyspepsia, flatulence, dipsia, vomiting, haemorrhages, ophthalmopathy, strangury, splenomegaly, cephalalgia, skin diseases, leprosy, fevers, ulcers and general debility. The mature and dry fruit is constipating and is useful in diarrhoea and dysentery. The oil obtained from the seeds is trichogenous and is useful in dyspepsia, skin diseases, leucoderma and greyness of hair.

1234. *Terminalia catappa* L. *(Combretaceae)*

Vernacular Name: *Hin*: Deshi-badam; *Beng*: Bangla-badam; *Tel:* Badamuchettu, Vedam; *Tam*: Natvadom, *Mal*: Adamarram.

Description: Large, spreading tree to 30 m tall with leaves mostly near ends of branches. Leaves alternate, short-petiolate, the blades obovate to 30 cm long, deciduous and turning orange to red before falling. Flowers small, white borne in densely packed spikes. Fruit a reddish flattened ovoid drupe up to 6 cm long, with fibrous outer layer with a single edible seed within. Flowers and fruit available throughout the year.

Habitate: Common along beaches, rocky coats, upper margins of mangrove swamps, low land clearings and secondary forests.

Propagation: By seeds.

Part Used: Bark and leaves.

Chemical Constituents: Ellagic acid, corilagin, tannins, tannic acids, organic acids: palmatic, oleic, linoleic and myristic acids. Essential oils, reducing sugars, flavonoids amino acids.

Uses: The fluid from the bark is used to treat diabetes and as a tonic. It is used to treat thrush. The juice of the leaves is ingested for coughs. An infusion of the leaves is used to treat jaundice. The leaves are used to treat indigestion. The bark is used to treat mouth sores and stomachache. It is also used as an emetic for infants. Sore throats are treated with an infusion of the old leaves. Sores, pimples and fungal skin diseases are treated with the bark. The leaves are used to treat wounds and burns. The juice of the leaves is ingested for colic. An infusion of the bark is used to treat internal ailments in children. The leaves are used to treat bronchitis and tuberculosis.

1235. *Terminalia chebula* Retz. *(Combretaceae)*

Vernacular Name: *Eng:* Chebulic myrobalan; *Hin:* Hara, Harara, Harad; *Kan:* Harra, Karakkayi, Alalekayi; *Mal:* Katukka; *San:* Haritaki, Pathya, Abhaya; *Tam:* Katukkay; *Tel:* Karakkaya, Karitaki.

Description: A moderate sized to large (large in good soil, and moderate in dry rocky places) deciduous tree with a cylindrical bole, rounded crown and spreading branches; leaves ovate, elliptic or obovate, glabrous to tawny-villous beneath with a pair of large glands at the top of the petiole; fruits glabrous, shining, ellipsoidal, obovoid or ovoid drupes, yellow to orange brown in colour, faintly angled, upto 3.75 cm long; seeds hard, pale yellow.

Habitate: Throughout India, in deciduous forests on dry slopes upto 900m, especially in Bengal, Tamilnadu, West Coast and Western Ghats.

Propagation: By seeds.

Parts Used: Mature and immature fruits.

Chemical Constituents: Chebulin from flowers. Palmitic, stearic, oleic, linoleic, arachidic and behenic acids from fruit kernels. Fruits contain about 30% of an astringent substance; astringency is due to the charecteristic principle chebulnic acid. Also contain tannic acid 20-40%, gallic acid, resin etc. and a purgative glycoside of anthraquinone derivative. Chebulin exhibited antispanmodic action on smooth muscle similar to papaverine.

Uses: The Fruits are astringent, sweet, acrid, bitter, sour, thermogenic, anodyne, anti-inflammatory, vulnerary, alterant, stomachic, laxative, purgative, carminative, digestive, anthelmintic, cardiotonic, aphrodisiac, antiseptic, diuretic, febrifuge, depurative and tonic. They are useful in vitiated conditions of tridosa, wounds ulcers, inflammations, gastropathy, anorexia, helminthiasis, flatulence, haemorrhoids, jaundice, hepatopathy, splenopathy, pharyngodynia, hiccough, cough, urophathy, versical and renal claculi, cephalalgia, epilepsy, ophthalmopathy, skin diseases, leprosy, intermittent fever, cardiac disorders, stomatitis, neuropathy and general debility.

1236. *Terminalia crenulata* Roth. *(Combretaceae)*

Vernacular Name: *Eng:* Black murdah; *Hin:* Asaina, Kauha; *Kan:* Sadala, Asana; *Mal:* Karimarutu, Tempavu; *San:* Chagakarnah; *Tam:* Karumarudu,Karuppumarudu; *Tel:* Nallamaddi, Tani.

Description: A medium sized to large tree, 15-30 m in height with clear bole and greyish black bark having longitudinal fissures and transverse cracks exfoliating flakes; leaves simple, leathery, undersurface villous, linear-oblong with two large glands on the midrib; flowers in willous panicles; fruits large, glabrous with 5 equal wings.

Habitate: Throughout India, in semi-evergreen and mixed deciduous forests.

Propagation: By seeds.

Parts Used: Bark.

Chemical Constituents: N.A.

Uses: The bark is bitter; astringent, cooling, cardiotonic, diuretic, styptic, constipating, vulnerary, expectorant, anthelmintic and uterine tonic. It is useful in vitiated conditions of *pitta*, cardiopathy, strangury, wounds ulcers, haemorrhages, haemoptysis, diarrhoea, dysentery, cough, bronchitis, verminosis, leucorrhoea, gonorrhoea and burning sensation.

1237. *Terminalia nigrovenulosa* Pierre ex Laness. *(Combretaceae)*

Description: Big tree, reaching 10-30m. in heigh. Young twigs downy. Leaves opposite, coriaceous witth small white spots above and a pair of glands at the top of the petiole. Inflorescence in terminal compound panicle; flowers white, without petals. Fruit samaroid, largely 3-winged, purple, one-seeded.

Habitate: Grows wild in deciduous forests. Endemic in the southern part of the country.

Propagation: By seeds.

Part Used: Stem-bark.

Chemical Constituents: The stem-bark contains tannin. The fruit yield 20-40% tannin consisting of ellagic, gallic and luteolic acids and fatty oil 36.7%.

Uses: The trunk-bark is used as an antidiarrhoeic. The fruit and bark are used in treating chronic dysentery, sore throat, laryngitis and haemorrhoids,.

1238. *Terminalia paniculata* Roth. *(Combretaceae)*

Vernacular Name: *Eng:* Flowering murdah; *Kan:* Hanalu; *Mal:* Vellamarutu, Pullamarutu, Pumarutu; *San:* Asvakarnah; *Tam:* Pumarutu, Venmarutu; *Tel:* Putanallamanu, Namiri.

Description: A large deciduous tree, 20-30 m in height with a clear bole of about 10 m and brown to dark brown rough bark peeling off in thin flakes; leaves simple, upper alternate, lower opposite, oblong or elliptic, acute or acuminate, pale brown with two glands near the base of the midrib below, main nerves 10-15 pairs; flowers reddish brown, sessile, in rusty pubescent spikes; fruits reddish brown-winged, one wing broad and the other two narrow.

Habitate: In the Western and Eastern Ghats, in the semi-evergreen and moist deciduous forests upto 1,200 m.

Propagation: By seeds.

Parts Used: Bark.

Chemical Constituents: β-sitosterol, triterpene carboxylic acid, a new glucoside, dlmethyl ellagic acid.

Uses: The bark is astringent, bitter, cooling, expectorant, diuretic, cardiotonic, vulnerary, depurative and tonic. It is useful in vitiated conditions of *kapha* and *pitta*, cough, bronchitis, strangury, cardiac debility, diabetes, wounds and ulcers, skin diseases, leprosy and anaemia.

1239. *Tetrapanax papyriferus* K.Koch *(Araliaceae)*

Synonyms: *Aralia papyrifera.*

Vernacular Name: *Eng:*-Rice-paper plant, Chinese rice-paper plant.

Description: Evergreen shrub, upto 3 m tall. Leaves clustered at terminals, orbicular, 25-30 cm across, long petioled, deeply cut into 5-7 toothed lobes, each lobe divided again, densely tomentose beneath. Flowers in small, globose umbels arranged in large, terminal panicles, panicles to 45 cm across, woolly; petals 4, valvate; stamens 4; ovary 2-celled; styles 2, separate. Fruit a drupe; pyrenes 2, black.

Habitate: Mostly cultivated in warm parts of Korea.

Propagation: By seeds.

Parts Used: Medulla.

Chemical Constituents: Chikusaikosides I, II, tetrapanax papyriferus saponins R-3, R-1-a, R-4b, chikuetsusaponins I-B,IV, papuriogenins A,C,D,E, 16-epi-saikogenin C.

Uses: Diuretic, lactogenic oedema, dysuria, urodynia, analactia, galactostatis.

1240. *Teucrium chamaedrys* *(Lameaceae)*

Vernacular Name: *Eng:* Wall germander.

Description: Perennial herb growing to 24 cm. Has a woody root, toothed dark-green, oval leaves, and spikes of pink tubular flowers.

Habitate: Native to Europe, North Africa and western Asia, wall germander is commonly found growing on dry stony ground.

Propagation: By Seeds.

Parts Used: Aerial parts.

Chemical Constituents: Wall germander contains iridoid glycosides, diterpenes, a volatile oil, tannins and polyphenols.

Uses: Infusions of wall germander have long been used to treat gout, rheumatism, stomach problems, fever and catarrh. The plant has also been taken to aid weight loss, and is a common ingredient in tonic wines. Wall germander has been used as a mouthwash for sore gums, and as a lotion to help heal wounds.

1241. *Thalictrum foliolosum* DC. *(Ranunculaceae)*

Vernacular Name: Mamira, Pilijari, Chaitra, Sarphar, Bishkaral.

Description: An erect, rigid, perennial herb upto 2.5 m tall. Rootstock is fibrous yellowish-brown, resem-bling liquorice, but is knotty and extremely bitter and yellow inside. Leaves are pinnately decompound; leaflets 4-6mm, sub-orbicular, slightly lobulate. Flowers are usually pale-green often dingy-purple, polygamous, arising in branched terminal panicles. Achenes are 3.75 cm long, sharply ribbed.

Habitate: Temperate Himalayas and West Tibet between 1800-3500 m. In Himachal Pradesh, it is found in Chamba, Kangra, Kinnaur, Kullu, Mandi, Lahaul-spiti, Solan, Shimla and Sirmor districts upto an elevation of 3000 m.

Propagation: By seeds and vegetative method.

Part Used: Rhizomes.

Chemical Constituents: The rhizomes contain large quantities of water soluble salts of berberine besides magnoflorine, palmitine and jatrorrhizine. Since the rhizome loses its activity on storage, it is advisable to use the material fresh.

Uses: The rhizomes and the roots are used in the form of a decoction, extract or powder and are valued for the treatment of pohthalmia. The root is used as an antiperiodic, diuretic, aperient, and purgative; as bitter tonic during convalescence. It is also given for a tonic dyspepsia. The paste of the plant is locally used in skin diseases and to suppress boils.

1242. *Theobroma cacao* *(Sterculiaceae)*

Vernacular Name: *Eng:* Cacao, Cocoa.

Description: Evergreen tree growing to 8m. Has pale brown bark, glossy oval leaves, clusters of small yellow flowers, and large, pear-shaped, red-yellow seedpods.

Habitate: Native to Mexico and Central America, cacao is now a major crop throughout the tropics.

Propagation: By Seeds.

Parts Used: Seeds.

Chemical Constituents: The seeds pulp contains xanthines, a fixed oil and many constituents responsible for its flavour. The seeds contain very small amounts of endorphins, which are powerful painkillers that occur naturally within the body.

Uses: Though cacao is most often used as a food, it also has therapeutic value as a nervous system stimulant. In Central America and the Caribbean, the seeds are taken as a heart and kidney tonic. The plant may be used to treat angina, and as a diuretic. Cacao butter makes a good lip salve and is often used as a base for suppositories and pessaries.

1243. *Thespesia populnea* (L.) Soland ex correa *(Malvaceae)*

Vernacular Name: *San:* Gardha-bhanda; *Eng:* thespesia; *Hin:* Parsipu, porush, paras-pipal, gagjdanda; *Beng*: Dumbla, parespipal, palaopipal, gajashuni; *Tel:* Gangaraavi, munigangaraavi, gangareenu; *Tam:* Poovarasam, kallal, cheelanthi; *Kan:* Hoovarase, kandarola, adavi-bendi, jogiyarale and *Mal:* Poovarasu.

Description: Small tree to 12 m high. Leaves, alternate petiolate, dark green, glossy, blades cordate, about 8-16 cm long on equally long petioles. Flowers showy, yellow with a maroon to purple center, borne singly in the leaf axils. Fruit a brown flattened-globose capsule enclosing a sticky yellow sap and about 10 hairy seeds.

Habitate: Common along beaches, lowland river banks, forests and the margins of mangroves.

Propagation: By seeds and vegetative method.

Part Used: Leaves, bark and stems.

Chemical Constituents: Thespesin, gossypol, DL-gossypol, populinin, populetin, populneol, herbacetin, populnetin, glycosides of quercetin, gossypetin, epoxyleic acid, isoquercitrin, rutin, kaempferol 3-flucoside, lupenone, mansonones, myricyl alchohol, lipids, beta-sitosterol, thespesone, thespone.

Uses: A decoction of the leaves is used in treating cough, influenza, headache and relapses in illnesses. A cold infusion of the bark is used in treating dysentery, diabetes, gonorrhoes, yellow urine and thrush. Indigestion, pelvic infection, appetite loss, ulcers and worms are treated with the bark. The stem is employed in treating breast cancer. A decoction of the bark and fruit is mixed with oil and used to treat scabies. An infusion of the bark is used to treat intenstioanl diseases. The bark is used to treat thrush, and a leaf and bark induction is used to treat eye injuries. The inner bark is used to treat constipation and typhoid. The crushed fruit is used in treatment of urinary tract problems and abdominal swellings.

1244. *Thevetia peruviana* (Pers.) K. Schum. *(Apocynaceae)*

Synonyms: *Thevetia neriifolia* Juss.ex.

Vernacular Name: *San:* Ashvaghna, divyapushpa, haripriya, ashvamaraka, ashvantaka, shatakunda; *Eng:* Yellow olender, bastard oleander, lucky nut-tree, exile tree, exile oil plant; *Hin:* Pile kaner, zard kunel, kulkephul; *Beng*: Koklaphul, haldi korubi, china karabt; *Tel:* Pachaganneru; *Tam:* Pachaiyalari, tiruvachippu, manjalaleri; *Kan*: Kadukasi, kanogalu and *Mal:* Manja areli, pachcha areli.

Description: Small evergreen plant 2-3m. in height with milky juice. Stems scaled with scars of fallen leaves. Leaves alternate, linear-oblong, entire, only main nerve conspicuous. Inflorescence in axillary cyme of 2-3 flowers, bright yellow.Drupe angular, smooth; seeds brown.

Habitate: Cuiltivated for its elegant foliage and handsome flowers.

Propagation: By seeds and vegetative method.

Part Used: Seed and root.

Chemical Constituents: The seed and root contain cardiotonic glucosides: thevetin (A,B), 2-Oacetyl ceberoside, neriifolin, cerberin, peruvoside, theveneriin, and peruvonsidic acid. Glucosides thevetin, thevetoxin, a phytosterolin, abouain, kokilphin are obtained from the kernel of the seed. Nuts yielded a new heteroside neriifolin. Seeds contain glucosides neriifolin, acetyleriifolin and thevetin.

Uses: The purified glucoside thevetin, extracted from the seed and root is prescrived as a cardiotonic drug. The crushed seeds can be used as an insecticide. Caution is needed because of their high toxicity. Kernel of seed used as acro-narcotic poison. Bark is a bitter tonic, cathartic, febrifuge and useful in different kinds of intermittent fevers. All parts of the plant including latex are poisonous. The cardiac glycosides obtained from the kernels, bark and flowers are useful for heart diseases.

1245. *Thuja occidentalis* *(Cupressaceae)*

Vernacular Name: *Eng:* Arbor-vitae.

Description: Evergreen tree growing to 10 m. Has scale-like leaves aromatic; male cones round, yellow; female cones ovoid, purplish; fruits radish brown; seed winged.

Habitate: Native to the north-eastern US, arbor-vitae flourishes in wet, marshy ground and along riverbanks. It has become a popular ornamental tree in Europe.

Propagation: By Seeds.

Parts Used: Leaves.

Chemical Constituents: Arbor-vitae contains a volatile oil, flavonoids, wax, mucilage and tannins.

Uses: Arbor-vitae has an established anti-viral activity. It is most often used to treat warts and polyps, being prescribed both internally and externally for these conditions. It is also used as part of a regime for treating cancer–especially cancer of the uterus. Arbor-vitae makes an effective expectorant and anti-catarrhal remedy, and may be used to treat acute bronchitis and other respiratory infections. It induces menstruation and can be taken to bring on delayed periods, though this use is inadvisable if menstrual pain is severe. Arbor-vitae is diuretic and is used to treat acute cystitis and bed-wetting in children. Extracts may be painted on painful joints or muscles as a counter-irritant, improving local blood supply and easing pain and stiffness.

1246. *Thuja orientallis* L. *(Cupressaceae)*

Vernacular Name: *Eng:*-Oriental arborvitae.

Description: Coniferous, evergreen, monoecious tree, upto 25 m tall, 1m in diameter, but often densely branched shrub. Branchlet 2-ranked, in a vertical plane. Leaves scalelike, less than 3 mm long, glandular, grooved. Male cones at the terminals of branches of the last year, 2-2.5 mm long, with 10 scales. Female cones larger, erect, the 3-9 pairs of scales fleshy when young, becoming woody, strongly hooked at apex, 15-20 mm long; seeds wingless. April.

Habitate: Mountain thickets India, China, Japan and Korea.

Propagation: By seeds.

Parts Used: Leaf, seed.

Chemical Constituents: Terpenoids: pinusolide, pinusolidic acid, cedrol, totarol. Essential oil. Flavonoids: quercetin, myricetin, hinokiflavone, amentoflavone. Thujic acid.

Uses: Antiplatelet aggregation, topical anti-inflammatory, antitussive, expectorant, antiasthmatic, antibacterial, antifungal (thujaplicins), haemostatic activities. Colony formation inhibition. ***Seeds:*** lever tonic, weak ness of body.

1247. *Thunbergia grandiflora* (Roxb ex Rottle) Roxb. *(Acanthaceae)*

Vernacular Name: *Hin:* Mulluta; *Beng*: Nul-lata; *Assam*: Kukualoti.

Description: Climbing plant, stems twining, pubescent. Leaves opposite, long-petioled; base cordate, irregularly loved, inflorescence in terminal drooping leafy receme, rarely axillary; flowers large gright blue or violet-blue, Capsule glabrous, apiculate.

Habitate: Grows wild in sunny places, but is also cultivated as an ornamental plant.

Propagation: By seeds and vegetative method.

Part Used: Leaves.

Chemical Constituents: The leaves are rich in potassium salts. The flowers contain amino acids: aspartic acid serine, flycine, alanine, valine; flavonoids: apigenin 7-glucoronide, luteoline, anthycyanin, malvidin; saccharose, glucose and fructose.

Uses: The leaves are commonly used against snake-bite. The petioles are removed and the juice of 30 to 50g of pounded fresh leaves is used to massage the site of the snakeObite, from the top downwards, the residue is applied topically. The leaves are used on their own or in combination with *Ablemoschus moschatus* leaves and clausena lanisum seeds. Poulticing with a moschatus leaves and clusena lansium seeds. Poulticing with a moistened fine powder of dried leaves is also prescribed.

1248. *Thymus serpyllum* L. *(Lameaceae)*

Vernacular Name: Banajwain, Lepto, Lepte, Masho, Hasha, Pangduma, Padumba, Wild thyme.

Description: The plant is a variable, aromatic, hairy, prostrate and evergreen perennial herb; 10-25 cm high and is one of the most effective ground covers, forming dense mats. Rootstock is woody and the leaves are small, elliptic or oblong-ovate or lanceolate, 6-15 mm long, subsessile and glandular. Flowers are polygamous pink, in globose, terminal whorls. The male flowers are larger in size. The plant is pungent in taste.

Habitate: The plant is found in the Himalayas from Kashmir to Nepal at altitudes of 1500-4500 m and is reported to be grown in the gardens of Western India.

Propagation: By rootsuckers.

Part Used: Whole plant.

Chemical Constituents: The leaves and floral tops yield a volatile oil known as oil of wild thyme 0.27 per cent from fresh and 0.60 per cent from dried plants. Three flavonoides, i.e. scutellarin heteroside, luteolin 7-glucoside, and apigenin, have been isolated from the plant. The floral tops and leaves are reported to yield 0.75 per cent of ursolic acid. Its nectar is rich in ascorbic acid. Oil contains chiefly thymol.

Uses: The herb possesses anti-spasmodic, anti-septic, expectorant, carminative, anthelmintic and stimulating properties. The leaves and floral shoots and employed for the treatment of whooping cough, epilepsy, suppression of urine and menstrual catarrh. An infusion of the leaves is used in the treatment of itch and skin eruptions. The leaves are used in biliousness and their juice is considered emetic. The leaf juice is applied over bald patches of alopecia. The seeds are considered antifebrile and anthelmintic. It is a popular remedy in the hills for stomach complaints, cough and colds. Infusion of leaves with 'gur' acts as a diuretic.

1249. *Thymus vulgaris* *(Lameaceae)*

Vernacular Name: *Eng:* Thyme, Garden thyme.

Description: An aromatic shrub growing to 40 cm, with woody stems, small leaves and pink flowers.

Habitate: Thyme is a cultivated variety of wild thyme, also known as mother of thyme, which is native to southern Europe.

Propagation: By seeds.

Parts Used: Leaves.

Chemical Constituents: Volatile oil with variable content, Flavonoids, Tannins.

Uses: Antiseptic, Tonic, Relievers muscle spasms, Expectorant, Expels worms.

1250. *Tieghemopanax fruticosus* Vig. *(Araliaceae)*

Description: Small plant, 0.5-1.5m. high with handsome foliage, leaves, alternate, tripinnate, the lower part surroujnding the stem; margins toothed, inflorescence in terminal raceme of umbels; flowers small, grayish-white. Fruit globose, flat all parts of the plant, especially the leaves, are sweetly scented.

Habitate: Cultivated as an ornamental plant.

Propagation: By seeds.

Part Used: Roots and leaves.

Chemical Constituents: The roots contain triterpenoid saponins.

Uses: The roots are well known for their reconstituent properties and are used for treating general debility, fatigue, dyspepsia, feber, headache, mastitis, hypogalactia, cough, haemoptysis, oliguria, rheumatism and lumbago. They improve the resistance of the body to various noxious agents. A gruel made with 50 to 100g of fresh leaves is galactagogic. A poultice of pounded fresh leaves is effective for wounds, furunculosis, phlegmon and mastitis.

1251. *Tilia vulgaris* Hayne. *(Tiliaceae)*

Synonyms: *Tilia intermedia* D.C., *Tilia europaea* Linn., *Tilia officinarum* Crantz.

Vernacular Name: *Eng:* Common large leaved Linden

Description: A deciduous tree up to 3-6 m. with young branchlets glabrous. Leaves broadly ovate, abruptly accuminae, oblique, cordate or truncate at the base, serrate with short pointed teeth covered with aphids secretions, dark green above light green beneath, glabrous except axillary tufts of hairs, 7-10 cm. long; petiole about half as long as the blade. Flowers 5-10, yellowish white, fragrant in peduncular cyme arising half way the leaf-like bracts. A flower consists of 5-ovate calyces, 5-claweed corolla and 35 stamens. Staminodes absent. Staminal stalks long and very much coiled.

Habitate: Found in North America.

Propagation: By seeds and stem cutting.

Parts Used: Blossom twigs.

Chemical Constituents: Linarin, Glycoside: Tiliacine; Phytosterol Tocopherol; Volatile oils viz. Citral, Citronellal, Citronellol, Eugonol, Limonen, α-pinene, Nerol, Terpineol, Farnesol; Mucilage polysacchrides. Galacturonic and Glucuronic acids. Flavonoids viz. Quercetin, myricetin & Kaempferol.

Uses: For complaints specifically of muscular weakness of eyes, Purrperal metritis, diseases of antrum. Sensation of a guage before eyes. Imperfect binocular vision. Head neuralagia, with veil before eyes, diminished vision. Much violent itch and burning like fire after scratching. Warm, profuse sweat while sleeping. Excruciating leucorrhoeai with intense soreness of the uterus.

1252. *Tinospora capillipes* Gagnep. *(Menispermaceae)*

Description: Slender evergreen pernnial climber. Young shoots slightly pubscent. Roots tuberous long, thickened, brownish-yellow outside, whitish inside, leaves alternate, long-oetioled; base sagittate; apex pointed, nerves plamate and downy, inflorescence in axillary raceme; flowers yellowish-green. Drupe oblong, Seeds round, compressed.

Habitate: Occurs in wet and shady places.

Propagation: By seeds and vegetative method.

Part Used: Roots.

Chemical Constituents: The roots contain columbin.

Uses: The roods have beneficial effect for the relief of sore throat, laryngitis, hoarseness, colic and diarrhoea. A poultice of pounded roots is effective in treating abscess and phlegmon.

1253. *Tinospora Cordifolia* (Willd.) Miers ex Hook.f. & Thoms. *(Menispermaceae)*

Vernacular Name: *Eng:* Gulancha tinospora, Tinospora; *Hin:* Gulanca, Giloy, Amrta; *Kan:* Amrtaballi, Yuganiballi, Madhuparni; *Mal:* Cittamrtu, Amrtu; *San:* Guduci, Amrta; *Tam:* Amurutavalli, Cintilikkoti; *Tel:* Tippatiga, Amrta.

Description: A large extensively spreading glabrous, perennial deciduous twiner with succulent stems and papery bark; leaves simple, alternate, cordate, entire, glabrous, 7-9 nerved; flowers yellow in lax racemes, flowers usually solitary; fruits drupes, red when ripe. The surface of the stems appears to be closely studded with warty tubercles and the surface skin is longitudinally fissured. On removal of the surface skin the dark greenish mucilaginous stem is seen.

Habitate: Throughout India.

Propagation: By seeds and vegetative method.

Parts Used: Stem.

Chemical Constituents: The plant contains tinosporin, columbin, chasmanthin, palmarin, berberine, tinosporon, tinosporic acid, tinosporol, giloin, giloinisin, substituted pyrrolidine, a diterpenoid furanolactone, 18-norclerodane diterpene-O-glucoside, an aryltetrahydrofuranolignan, octacosanol, nonacosan-15-one and β-sitosterol.

Uses: The stem is bitter, astringent, sweet, thermogenic, anodyne, anthelmintic, alterant, antiperiodic, antispasmodic, anti-inflammatory, antipyretic, antipyretic, antiemetic, digestive, carminative, appetise, stomachic, constipating, cardiotonic, depurative, haematinic, expectorant, aphrodisiac, rejuvenating, galacto-purifier and tonic. It is useful in vitiated conditions of *vata*, burning sensation, hyperdipsia, helminthiasis, dyspepsia, flatulence, stomachalgia, intermittent fevers, chronic fevers, inflammations, gout, vomiting, cardiac debility, skin diseases, leprosy, erysipelas, anaemia, cough, asthma, general debility, jaundice, seminal weakness, uropathy and splenopathy.

1254. *Tinospora sinensis* (Lour.) Merr. *(Menispermaceae)*

Synonyms: *Tinospora malabarica* (Lam.) Hook. f. & Thoms.

Vernacular Name: *San*: Vatsadani, Sudarsana, Amrta, *Hin:* Giloy, Gruch, *Kan:* Sudarsana balli, *Mal:* Pee-amerdu, Kattu amirthu, *Tel:* Thippa theega.

Description: Deciduous, climbing shrubs. *Stem* with prominent, scattered lenticels. *Bark* papery, greyish white. *Latex* watery. Tender branches with distinct white hairs. *Leaves* alternate, broadly egg-shaped, 7-17 x 4-13 cm, base heart-shaped, apex acuminate, margin entire, sparingly pubescent in upper surface and densely pubescent in lower surface, basal nerves 5-7; leaf stalk up to 10 cm long, hairy. Flowers are formed in racemes from the axils of fallen leaves and also on the old stem, greenish yellow, many, 5 mm across. *Male* and *female flowers* are seen separately in the same plant. *Drupes* 1-3 in cluster, spherical-shaped, about 1.5 cm across, turning orange-red when ripe.

Habitate: Along streams, rocky valleys and in disturbed forests from deciduous to semi-evergreen.

Propagation: By stem cuttings and seeds.

Parts Used: Stems.

Chemical Constituents: Almost as C. cordifloia.

Uses: Stems are used for treating piles, ulcerated wounds, liver complaints, chronic rheumatism and also as muscle relaxant.

1255. *Toddalia asiatica* (L.) Lam. *(Rutaceae)*

Synonyms: Toddalia *aculeata* Pers.

Vernacular Name: *Eng:* Forest pepper, Lopez-root tree, Wild orange tree; *Hin:* Jangli-Kalimirc, Kanc; *Kan:* Musimullu, Mullumasige, Kadumaraju; *Mal:* Mulakutanni, Mulakutali, Kara; *San:* Tiksnaksah, Kancanah; *Tam:* Milagaranai, Kattumilagu; *Tel:* Kondakasinda, Errakasinda, Mirapakanda.

Description: A variable prickly sarmentose rambler upto 15m in height, circular lenticels and hooked prickles; leaves digitately trifoliate, leaflets oblong, elliptic or obovate, crenulate, glabrous and gland-dotted; flowers white or greenish yellow in axillary and terminal pubescent panicles, polygamous, fruits subglobose, fleshy, orange coloured; seeds reniform, surrounded by colourless mucilage.

Habitate: Throughout India, upto 2,500 m, also in dry places in the plains.

Propagation: By seeds.

Parts Used: Roots, leaves, flowers, fruits.

Chemical Constituents: Essential oil. Alkaloid berberine. Roots contain a poisonous resin which product abortion in guinea pigs and in large doses paralysis and death. Leaves contain toddaline and toddalinine, toddalolactone, pimpinellin, isopimpinellin, resins and glycosides. Tow new coumarins-norbraylin, 5, 7, 8-trimethoxycoumarin isolated.

Uses: The roots are acrid, astringent, bitter, sweet, aromatic, diaphoretic, antiperiodic, antipyretic, digestive, arminative, constipating, expectorant, antibacterial, vulnerary and tonic. They are useful in vitiated conditions of *vata* and *kapha* odontalgia, paralysis, malarial and intermittent fevers, dyspepsia, colic, flatulence, diarrhoea, cough, bronchitis, nausea, wound, filthy ulcers, epilepsy, gonorrhoea, and general debility. The unripe fruits and leaves are good for vitiated condition of *vata*. Flowers useful as an external application in wasp-stings.

1256. *Toona ciliata* Roemm *(Meliaceae)*

Synonyms: *Cedrela toona* Roxb. ex Rottler.

Vernacular Name: *San:* Tunah; *Eng:* Toon, Red cedar; *Hin:* Tun, Mahanim, Tun-ka-ped; *Kan:* Mandurike; *Mal:* Vempu, Madagirivempu, Ikana, Patukarana; *Tam:* Cantanavempu, Tunamaram, Sevvagil; *Tel:* Nandicettu.

Description: A large tree, 20-30 m in height with a large crown; leaves abruptly pinnate, leaflets 4-5 pairs, base oblique; flowers white, fragrant in large terminal drooping panicles; fruits capsules, 2-2.5 cm long, seeds with membranous wings at each end.

Habitate: West Coast tropical evergreen and semi-evergreen forests.

Propagation: By seeds.

Parts Used: Bark, flowers.

Uses: The bark is bitter, acrid astringent, tonic aphrodiasiac, expectorant, anthelmintic, depurative and antiperiodic. It is useful in chronic infantile dysentery, cough, bronchitis, intermittent fevers, verminosis, leprosy, dermatopathy, and ulcers. The flowers are emmenagogue and are useful in menstrual disorders.

1257. *Torilis japonica* (Houtt.) DC. *(Umbelliferae)*

Vernacular Name: *Eng:* Japanese torilis.

Description: Biennial herb with short setose hairs throughout, to 30-70 cm tall. Leaves ternately 2-pinnate, 5-10 cm long, acuminate; leaflets ovate to lanceolate, sharply serrate; petioles becoming wide at base to wrap stems. Umbels few, pedunculate; the involucral bracts 4-8, linear, 1 long; the involucel bractlets linear, appressed to the pedicels, rather unequal. Fruit 4-10, ovate, 2.5-3 mm long, covered with dense, short, slightly uncinate prickles.

Habitate: Open grassy places in lowlands in Japan, China and Korea.

Propagation: By seeds.

Parts Used: Fruit.

Chemical Constituents: Essential oil: a-cadinene,torilin. Fatty oils: petroselin, linolein. Torilolide, oxytorilolide. (-)-Germacrene-D, germacra-4-trien IB-ol. Oppositane sesquiterpenes.

Uses: Antifungal, antiviral, anthlmintic, antitrichomonas, sex hormone-like activities. Used in Amnesia, pruritus, acidosis and scabies.

1258. *Torreya nucifera* Siebold et Zucc. *(Taxaceae)*

Vernacular Name: *Eng:*-Japanese torreya.

Description: Evergreen, dioecious tree with widespreading brownish branchlets, to 15 m tall, 2 m in diameter. Leaves appearing 2-ranked, linear, 15-25 mm long, 3 mm wide, rigid, glabrous, dark-green above, midrib and 2 impressed stomatal bands beneath, petiole 3 mm long. Stamens clustered in 4-8 whorls, subtended with about 10 scales; anther 4-locular; ovule single or 2-3 in cluster, subtended with 5-6 scales, 6 mm long, surrounded by a fleshy aril. Seed narrowly ellipsoidal, 2.5 cm long, greenish, tinged with purple.

Habitate: Mountains.

Propagation: By seeds.

Parts Used: Seed.

Chemical Constituents: Vitexin, kayaflavone, hinokiol, ferruginol, 18-hydroxyferruginol, 18-oxoferruginol, kayadiol.

Uses: Anthelmintic activity, aldose reductase inhibition. This parasites to tapeworm, pinworms, hookworms and round worms.

1259. *Trachelospermum jasminoides.* *(Apocynaceae)*

Vernacular Name: *Eng:* Chinese star jasmine; confederate jasmine.

Description: An evergreen high-climbing, woody vine. Stem terete, reddish-brown, many branched; nodes slightly dilated with aerial root. Leaves opposite, briefly petiolate, elliptical to ovate lanceolate, 5-10 cm long by 2-4.5 cm wide; tip acute or obtuse; margin entire; base cuneate, glabrous or pubescent beneath. Inflorescence a sparse, long-pedunculate cyme; Arial-May. Flowers white, 2 cm in diameter, very fragrant. Fruit consisting of 2 long, slender follicles.

Habitate: Climbing on stone walls and tree trunks in China, Viet Nam.

Propagation: By seeds and vegetative method.

Part Used: Stem with leaves.

Uses: Rheumatic pains, muscular spasm, soreness and pain in limbs and knees. Pharyngitis, skin inflammation, injuries.

1260. *Trachyspermum roxburghianum* (DC.) Craib *(Apiaceae)*

Synonyms: *Trachyspermum involucratum* Wolff. non Marie; *Carum roxburghianum* Benth. ex Kurz.

Vernacular Name: *Eng:* Ajowan; *Hin:* Ajmud, Randhuni; *Kan:* Ajamodhavoma; *Mal:* Ayamodakam; *San:* Ajaoda; *Tam:* Asamtavomam; *Tel:* Ajumoda, Vamu.

Description: An erect branched annual herb, stems striate; leaves 2-pinnate, ultimate segements all linear; flowers pure white in compound umbels; fruits ovoid, ultimately shining, yellow, aromatic cremocarps, mericarps with faint ridges, compressed.

Habitate: Cultivated throughout India.

Propagation: By seeds.

Parts Used: Fruits.

Chemical Constituents: d-limonene, α-terpinene, d-linalool, dl-terpineol, thymohydroquinone, thymol, dl-piperitone, cuminic acid, cumminaldehyde, unidentified esters d-limonene and dipentene mixture.

Uses: The fruits are acrid, bitter, thermogenic antispasmodic, stimulant, tonic, digestive, anthelmintic and carminative. They are useful in flatulence, dyspepsia, diarrhoea, pharyngitis, rheumatoid arthritis, bronchitis, cough, asthma and strangury. They have been shown to possess antibiotic and diuretic properties. They are used as an household remedy for dysperpsia. They are also very rich in calcium and iron.

1261. *Tragia bicolor* Miq. *(Euphorbiaceae)*

Vernacular Name: *San*: Duralabha, *Tam:* Malai chenthatti.

Description: A perennial twining or climbing shrubs, with stinging hairs throughout. The younger parts densely clothed by golden-brown hairs. *Leaves* alternate, unlobed, egg-shaped-oblong, 5-15 x 3-9 cm, base heart-shaped, apex acuminate, margin doubly toothed, papery, tomentose; leaf nerves 3-5 arising from the base of the leaves; leaf stalks 1-4 cm long, hairy. *Male* and *female flowers* are separately seen in the same flowering branch. Flowers are arranged in terminal or leaf-opposed spikes, minute, about 3 mm across, greenish yellow; male flowers placed in the upper portion of the spike, and the female below. *Capsules* 3-lobed, about 1 cm across, enveloped within the enlarged perianth lobes. *Seeds* 3, spherical.

Habitate: Evergreen forests.

Propagation: By seeds.

Parts Used: Roots.

Chemical Constituents: N.A.

Uses: Used in the Ayurvedic system of medicine. It possess the same medicinal properties as that of *T. involucrate* whose roots are used for the treatment of pruritic skin eruptions, venereal diseases, haemorrhoides, diabetes, vomiting, stomach troubles, guinea worms, to purify blood and in relieving giddiness, melalgia and brachialgia.

1262. *Tragia involucrata* L. *(Euphorbiaceae)*

Vernacular Name: *Eng:* Indian stinging-nettle; *Hin:* Barhanta; *Kan:* Turaci, Dulondi, Haligilu; *Mal:* Kotuttuvva, Kottittuvva, Coriyannam; *San:* Dusparsa, Duralabha; *Tam:* Kancori, Kandudi; *Tel:* Duradagantatiga, Cinugantatiga.

Description: A perennial evergreen, climbing hispid herb with scattered stinging haris; stems slender, elongate, twining leaves simple, alternate, stipulate, oblong-lanceolate to broadly ovate, serrate, base rounded of cordate; flowers shortly pedicellate, in terminal axillary and leaf-opposed racemens, male flowers many in the upper part, female flowers few in the lower part; ovary 3-lobed, styles 3; fruits capsules, 3-lobed; seeds globose, smooth.

Habitate: Throughout India, ascending upto 750 m.

Propagation: By seeds and vegetative method.

Parts Used: Roots, leaves.

Chemical Constituents: N.A.

Uses: The roots are bitter, acrid, sweet, cooling, diuretic, diaphoretic, antiperiodic, depurative and alternant. They are useful in pruritic skin eruptions, venereal diseases, haemorrhoids, diabetes, gastropathy, guinea worms, blood impurities, dipsia, vomting, giddiness, vitiated conditions of *pitta*, melalgia and brachilalgia. The leaves are good for cephalalgia.

1263. *Tragopogon pratensis* *(Asteraceae)*

Vernacular Name: *Eng:* Goat's Beard.

Description: Erect annual or perennial growing to 60 cm. Has narrow leaves and large solitary yellow flowers succeeded by handsome dandelion-like "clocks".

Habitate: Native to Europe, goat's beard is found in dry grassy sites. The root is unearthed in autumn.

Propagation: By Seeds.

Parts Used: Root.

Chemical Constituents: The root contains inulin, inositol, mannitol and plant sterols.

Uses: Like its cousin dandelion, goat's beard is considered a useful remedy for a detoxifying action, and may stimulate the appetite and digestion. Its high inulin content makes this herb a useful food for diabetics. Inulin is a nutrient made of fructose rather than glucose units, and therefore does not raise blood glucose levels.

1264. *Trapa natans* L. var. bispinosa (Roxb.) Makino. *(Trapaceae)*

Synonyms: *Trapa bispinosa* Roxb.

Vernacular Name: *Eng:* Water chestnut, Caltrops, Singhara nut; *Hin:* Simghara, Simghada; *Kan:* Singara; *Mal:* Karimpolam, Vankottakkaya; *San:* Smgtakah; *Tam:* Cimkhara; *Tel:* Kubjakamu.

Description: An aquatic floating herb with flexuose ascending stems and green photosynthetic submerged roots; leaves simple, alternate, croweded at the upper parts of stems in rosettes; rhomboidal, apex triangualr, irregularly inciso-serrate in the upper part, dark green above, reddish purple beneath, petioles dilated near the apex into a large spongy float; flowers white, opening above the surface of water in the afternoon, axillary and solitary; fruits obovoid, bony, angular with a short conical beak in the centre at the apex and a spreading, flattened, very sharp spinous horn on either side, indehiscent, one-seeded; seeds white, starchy.

Habitate: Throughout India, in ponds, lakes and tanks; also cultivated.

Propagation: By seeds.

Parts Used: Fruits.

Chemical Constituents: Thiamine, riboflavin, nicotinic acid, vitamin C, vitamin A, oxalates, β-amylase.

Uses: The fruits are sweet, astringent, coolin, constipating, haemostatic, diuretic, aphordisiac, antipyretic, appetiser and tonic. They are useful in vitiated conditions of *pitta*, burning sensation, dipsia, dyspepsia, haemorrhages, haemoptysis, diarrhoea, dysentery, strangury, intermittent fevers, loeprosy, fatigue, inflammation, urethrorrhea, fractures, erysipelas, lumbago, pharyngitis, bronchitis and general debility.

1265. *Tribulus terrestris* L. *(Zygophyllaceae)*

Vernacular Name: *Eng:* Land-caltrops, Puncture-vine; *Hin:* Gokharu; *Kan:* Negalu, Sennanegalu; *Mal:* Narinnil; *San:* Goksurah, Svadamstra; *Tam:* Nerinci; *Tel:* Palleru, Cinnapalleru.

Description: An annual or perennial, prostrate herb with many slender, spreading branches and silky-villous young parts; leaves abruptly simple, pinnate, opposite, leaflets almost sessile, rounded or oblique at the base, mucronate at the apex; flowers bright yellow, solitary, pseudo-axillary or leaf-opposed; fruits, a 5 angled or winged spinous tuberculate woody schizocarp, separating into five cocci, each coccus having two long, stiff, sharp divaricate spines towards the distal half and two shorter ones nearer the base; seeds one or more in each coccus.

Habitate: Throughout India, upto 5400m, as a weed along roadsides and waste places.

Propagation: By seeds.

Parts Used: Whole plant.

Chemical Constituents: The plant contains saponins, diosgenin, gitogenin, chlorogenin, ruscogenin, and 25 D-spirosta-3.5-diene. Kaemprerol, kaempferol-3-glucoside, kaemperol-3-rutinoisde and new flavonoid tribuloside.

Uses: The roots and fruits are sweet, cooling, diuretic, aphrodisiac, emollient, appetiser, digestive, anthelmintic, expectorant, anodyne, anti-inflammatory, alternate, laxative cardiotonic, styptic, lithontriptic and tonic. They are useful in strangury, dysuria, vitiated conditions of *vata* and *pitta*, renal and vesical calculi, anorexia, dyspepsia, helminthiasis, cough, asthma, consumption, inflammations, cardiopathy, haemoptysis, spermatorrhoea, anaemia, scabies, ophthalmia, ulocace and general weakness. The leaves are astringent, diuretic, aphrodisiac, depurative, anthelmintic and tonic. They are useful in gonorrhoea, gleet, ulitis, inflammation, menorrhagia, strangury, leprosy, skin diseases, verminosis and general weakness. The seeds are astringent, strengthening and are useful in epistaxis, haemorrhages and ulcerative stomatitis. The ash of the whole plant is good for external application in rheumarthritis.

1266. *Trichodesma indicum* (L.) R.Br. *(Boraginaceae)*

Vernacular Name: *Hin:* Andhahuli, Chotta-kulpha; *Kan:* Athomukhi, Kattetumbesoppu; *Mal:* Kilukkamtumpa; *San:* Adhahpuspi, Andhapuspi; *Tam:* Kiluttaitumpai, Kallutaitumpai; *Tel:* Guvvagutii.

Description: A hispid, much branches, erect annual herb, upto 45 cm in height; leaves simple, opposite, very variable in shape, sessile, ovate, oblong or lanceolate-oblong, obtuse or subacute, clothed with stiff hairs, arising from tubercles; flowers pale blue, changing to pink or white on drooping axillary stalks, sometimes in terminal few-flowered cymes; cone of anthers alrge and very pointed clothed on the back with dense white hairs; fruits pyramidal 4-ribbed nutlets, smooth on the outer, rugose, regularly pitted on the inner face.

Habitate: Throughout India, on roadsides and stony dry wastelands, upto 1500 m.

Propagation: By seeds.

Parts Used: Whole plant.

Chemical Constituents: N.A.

Uses: The plant is acrid, bitter, thermogenic, emollient, alexeteric, anodyne, anti-inflammatory, carminative, constipating, diuretic, depurative, ophthalmic, febrifuge and pectoral. It is useful in vitiated conditions of *vata* and *kapha*, arthralgai, inflammations, dyspepsia, diarrhoea, dysentery, strangury, leprosy, skin diseases, ophthalmopathy, expulstion of the foetus, dysmenorrhoea, sores and fevers.

1267. *TrichoSanthes dioica* Roxb. *(Cucurbitaceae)*

Vernacular Name: *San*: Patola, *Hin:* Palwal.

Description: The plant has harsh broad, sinate or cordate five-lobed and serrated *leaves* upper surface downy, tendrils bifid; *flowers* are white and fringed; *fruit* is oblong, narrow and pointed at both the ends, 4-8 cms long, glaucous, of a greenish white colour and marked with few irregulr, longitudinal strips; *stem* is rather quadrangular, twining and striated, sometimes woody and scabrous. *Seeds* are minute, compressed and corrugate on the margin.

Habitate: It is grown as a vegetable all over India-Northern India, Gujarat to Assam, Bengal and in Sri Lanka.

Propagation: By Seeds.

Parts Used: Fruit and Root.

Chemical Constituents: The root has bitter active principles which are strongly laxative, it is likely that cucurbitacins of steroidal structure are also present in this plant, as in other members of the same natural order.

Uses: Constipation. Fever. Skin infections/wounds. Alopecia areata. The unripe fruit and the tender shoots and capsules are laxative. The vegetable is given to improve appetite and digestion. The root is a s1trong purgative. Chakradatta recommends a decoction, patoladikwath in fever. The same author also recommends another compound decoction useful as a valuable alternative tonic and febrifuge given in boils and other skin diseases. After the use of this medicine, light food only, such as gruel should be taken. The leaf juice is applied to patches of alopecia areata.

1268. *Trichosanthes lobata* Roxb. *(Cucurbitaceae)*

Vernacular Name: *Eng:* Wild snake gourd, Bitter snake gourd; *Hin:* Jamgali cicinda, Tikta cicinda; *Kan:* Kiripodla, kadupodavalu; *Mal:* Patolam, Kaypanpatolam, Kattupatolam, Peppatolam; *San:* patola, Tiktapatola; *Tam:* Kattupeppudal, Peppudal; *Tel:* Cetipotla, Cedupotla, Kommupotia.

Description: A slender, annual, monoecious climber with furrowed stems and 2-3 fid tendrils; leaves simple, broader than long, orbicular-reniform or broadly ovate, more or less deeply 5 lobed, distantly denticulate, some what glabrous; flowers white, males in axillary recemes, females axillary, solitary; fruits ovoid, fusiform, indehiscent berries, tapering at both ends, striped with whte when immature, scarlet red when ripe; seeds semi-ellipsoid when ripe, compressed, surrounded with red pulp.

Habitate: Throughout India, in plains and in lower hills, also cultivated.

Propagation: By seeds.

Parts Used: Whole plant.

Chemical Constituents: N.A.

Uses: The plant is bitter, acrid, thermogenic, emollient, laxative, depurative, alexeteric, anthelmintic, appeatiser, carminative, digestive, cholagogue, stomachic, anodyne, expectorant, cardiotonic, suppurative, vulnerray, anti-inflmmatory, antipyretic and tonic. It is useful in vitiated conditions of tridosa, leprosy, leucoderma, pruritus, anorexia, dyspepsia, flatulence, colic, dipsia, hyperacidity, hepatopathy, jajundice, helminthisasis, haemorrhoids, cephalalgia, cough, asthma, bronchitis, cardiac debility, wounds ulcers, inflammtions, intermittent fever, alopecia, boils and general debility. In higher doses it is emetic and purgative.

1269. *Trichosanthes tricuspidata* Lour. *(Cucurbitaceae)*

Synonyms: *Trichosanthes bracteata* (Lam.) Voigt; *Trichosanthes palmata* Roxb.

Vernacular Name: *Hin:* Indrayan, nanakal; *Kan:* Avagudehannu; *Mal:* Kakkattonti; *San:* Kakansa, Dhvamksanasa; *Tam:* Korattai, Ankorattai; *Tel:* Avaduta.

Description: A large, branched woody tendril climber, older part of stem light grey and younger smooth green, tendrils 2, commonly cleft into 3; leaves palmately 3-5 lobed, dark green above, pale beneath with dark-coloured circular gland scattered along the lower side; flowers unisexual, males in axiallary racemes, bracts broadly ovate, many-nerved, fringed and gland dotted, female flowers solitary and axillry; fruits globose, red when ripe with 10 orange streaks; seeds numerous, smooth.

Habitate: Throughout India, upto an altitude of 2500 m.

Propagation: By seeds.

Parts Used: Roots and fruits.

Chemical Constituents: Punicic acid; cycloeucalenol, hexacosanoic acid, trichonin, santholin, β-sitosterol, α-spinosterol, cyclotrichosantol, bryonolic acid, cucurbitacins B and D, and trichotetrol.

Uses: The roots are bitter, astringent, acrid, thermogenic, carminative, emetic, abortifacient and purgative. They are good for hemicrania, carbuncles and gonorrhoea. The fruits are very valuable in curing otitis and rhinitis and are also recommended for hemicrania, inflammations, weakness of lymphs, vitiated conditions of *vata*, asthma, ophthalmia, epilepsy and leprosy.

1270. *Trifolium pratense* *(Fabaceae)*

Vernacular Name: *Eng:* Red clover.

Description: Perennial herb growing to 40 cm. Has a hairy upright stem, leaves with 3 oval leaflets with a white crescent marking, and pink to purple egg-shaped flowersheads.

Habitate: Native to Europe and Asia, and naturalized in North America and Australia.

Propagation: By Seeds.

Parts Used: Flowers.

Chemical Constituents: Red clover contains flavonoids, phenolic acids, volatile oil, sitosterol, starch and fatty acids. Flavonoids in the flowers and leaves are oestrogenic.

Uses: Red clover is used to treat skin conditions, normally in combination with other purifying herbs as burdock and yellow dock. It is also expectorant and may be used for spasmodic coughs. Red clover's oestrogenic effect may help menopausal complains.

1271. *Trigonella foenum-gracum* L. *(Fabaceae)*

Vernacular Name: *Eng:* Fenugreek, Greek hayes; *Hin:* Meti, Mutti; *Kan:* Mentya, Mentesoppu, Mente; *Mal:* Uluva; *San:* Methika, Methi, Kalanusari; *Tam:* Ventayan; *Tel:* Mentulu, Mentikura.

Description: An aromatic, erect annual, 30-60 cm in height; leaves pinnte, 3-foliate, leaflets toothed; flowers white or yellowish white, axillay; fruits pods, 5-7.5 cm long with long persistent beak; seeds 10-20 per pod, greenish brown along with a deep groove across one corner.

Habitate: Wild in Kashmir, Punjab and upper Gangetic plains, also cultivated in many other part of India as a pot-herb.

Propagation: By seeds.

Parts Used: Leaves and seeds.

Chemical Constituents: The endosperm of the seed is rich in galactomannan, young seeds mainly contain carbohydrates and sugar; mature seeds content amino acid, fatty acid, vitamins, saponins etc., it also content diosgenin, gitogenin, neogitogenin, homoorientin, saponaretin, neogigogenin and tigogenin.

Uses: The leaves are refrigerant and aperient and are given internally for vitiated conditions of *pitta*. A poultice of the leaves is applied for swellings and burns. Seeds are bitter, mucilaginous, aromatic, carminative, tonic, thermogenic, galactagogue, atringent, emollient and anphrodisiac. They are good for fever, vomiting, anorexia, cough, brounchitis, and colonitis. Extermally in the form of poultics they are used for boils, abscess and ulcers. An infusion of the seeds is good cool drink for smallpox patients. Powdered seeds find application in verinary medicine. An aqueous extract of the seeds possesses antibacterial property.

1272. *Trillidium govanianum* (D. Don.) Kunth. *(Liliaceae)*

Synonyms: *Trillium govanianum* Wall. ex. D. Don.

Description: A tuberous rooted herb often upto 30 cm tall, growing frequently in forest shades with three leaves in one whorl at the summit of the stem and a solitary, purple flower in the center. Leaves are broadly ovate, acute and conspicuously stalked, 3.5-10 cm long. Flowers brown purple with narrow, spreading petals; the outer 3 narrowly lanceolate, the inner 3, linear. Anthers large, yellow; styles 3; long and conspicuous. Fruit is a red, flobular berry, 1-2 cm in diameter.

Habitate: Pakistan to Bhutan between 2700-4000 m in forests. In Himachal Pradesh, it is found growing in patches in forest shade rich in humus at Panju in Chhajpur and Rahlarohtang slopes in Kullu.

Propagation: By seeds and tubers.

Part Used: Roots.

Chemical Constituents: Roots contain Trillarin, which on hydrolysis yields 2.5% diosgenin-a corticosteroid hormone.

Uses: The cortico-steroid hormone isolated from the plant is used in various preparations like sex hormones, cortisone and allied preparation used in rheumatism, birth control, regularization of menstrual flow and the like. It can form a commercial source of diosgenin.

1273. *Trillium erectum* *(Liliaceae)*

Vernacular Name: *Eng:* Beth root.

Description: Attractive perennial with an erect stem growing to 40 m. Has 3 wavy leaves and an unplea*Sa*nt-smelling, 3-petalled, red to yellow flower.

Habitate: Native to North America, beth root grows in shady positions in woodlands.

Propagation: By Rhizome.

Parts Used: Rhizome.

Chemical Constituents: Beth root contains saponins, tannin, resin, fixed oil, and a trace of volatile oil.

Uses: Beth root is a valuable remedy for heavy menstrual or intermenstrual bleeding, helping to reduce blood flow. It is also used to treat bleeding associated with uterine fibroids. Beth root may also be taken for bleeding within the urinary tubules and less commonly, for the coughing up of blood. It remains a valuable herb in facilitating childbirth. A douche of beth root is useful for excessive vaginal discharge and thrush.

1274. *Triticum aestivum* L. *(Poaceae)*

Synonyms: *Triticum sativum* Lam.

Vernacular Name: *Eng*: Common wheat, Bread wheat; *Hin:* Gehum; *Kan:* Godhi; *Mal:* Gotampu, Kotampu; *San:* Godhumah; *Tam:* Kodumai; *Tel:* Godumalu.

Description: A tufted annual grass, 60-150 cm in height, stems hollow, tufted, erect, semi-erect or prostrate, leaves very long and narrow with ligule and auricles; inflorescence a spike or 2-ranked compressed spikelets; grains oblong, more or less swollen with groove on one face, blunt at both ends.

Habitate: Widely cultivated in India.

Propagation: By seeds.

Parts Used: Grains.

Chemical Constituents: p-Aminobenzoic acid, biotin, carotene, choline, folic acid, inositol, nicotinic acid, pantothenic acid, riboflavin, thiamine, α-tocopherol, β-tocopherol, α-and β-tocotrienols etc.

Uses: The grains are sweet, refrigerant, emollient, laxative, rejuvenating, appetiser, vulnerary, demulcent, aphrodisiac and tonic. They are useful in vitiated conditions of *vata* and *pitta*, anorexia, flatulence, boils, pruritus, skin disease, ulcers, constipation, menorrhagia and general debility.

1275. *Tropaeolum majus* *(Tropaeolaceae)*

Vernacular Name: *Eng:* Common nasturtium.

Description: Climbing annual growing to 3m. Has straggling stems, rounded leaves and orange to yellow trumpet-shaped flowers with a long spur.

Habitate: Native to Peru, common nasturtium flourishes in sunny sites.

Propagation: By vegetative method.

Parts Used: Flowers, leaves, seeds.

Chemical Constituents: Common nasturtium contains glucocyanates, spilanthol, myrosin, oxalic acid and vitamin C.

Uses: All parts of common nasturtium appear to be antibiotic but the constituents responsible are unknown. An infusion of the leaves may be used to increase resistance to bacterial infections and to clear nasal and bronchial catarrh-apparently the remedy both reduces catarrh formation and stimulates the clearing and coughing up of phlegm. In addition, common nasturtium makes an effective antiseptic wash for external use. The juice of the plant has been taken internally for the treatment of scrofula. The piquant-tasting leaves and flowers of common nasturtium are high in vitamin C, and make a good salad vegetable, while the ground seeds have purgative properties.

1276. *Tsuga canadensis* *(Pinaceae)*

Vernacular Name: *Eng:* Canada spruce.

Description: Evergreen tree growing to 30 m. Has reddish-brown bark, short narrow needle laves and small male and female cones.

Habitate: Hemlock spruce is native to eastern parts of North America, growing in woodland and marshy sites.

Propagation: By Seeds.

Parts Used: Bark.

Chemical Constituents: Hemlock spruce contains volatile oil, 10-14% tannins and resin.

Uses: The bark of hemlock spruce is astringent and antiseptic. A decoction may be taken to treat diarrhoea, colitis, diverticulitis and cystitis. Externally, hemlock spruce can be employed as a douche to treat excessive vaginal discharge, thrush and a prolapsed uterus; as a mouthwash and gargle for gingivitis and sore throats; or as a wash to cleanse and tighten wounds.

1277. *Turnera diffusa* *(Turneraceae)*

Synonyms*: Turnera diffusa var. aphrodisiaca.*

Vernacular Name: *Eng:* Damiana.

Description: An aromatic shrub growing to 2m, with smooth, pale green leaves and small, single yellow flowers.

Habitate: Damiana is native to the Gulf of Mexico, southern California, the northern Caribbean Islands, and Namibia. It is also cultivated in these areas. Damiana is grown from seed in spring and prefers a hot, humid climate. The leaves are harvested when the herb is in flowers in summer.

Propagation: By seeds.

Parts Used: Leaves.

Chemical Constituents: Arbutin, Volatile oil, dalta-cadinene, thymol, Cyanogenic, glycoside, resin, gums.

Uses: Tonic, stimulant, Mild, laxative & diuretic, antidepres*San*t, testosterogenic, reputed aphrodisiac.

1278. *Tussilago farfara* L. *(Asteraceae)*

Synonyms: *Tussilago vulgaris* Lam., *Tussilago rupestris* Wall.

Vernacular Name: *Eng:* Celtsfoot

Description: A white-wooly scapiferous herb with leaves radical, slightly fragrant, long-petioled, broadly ovate-reniform cordate-orbicular, 7.5-25 cm. board, angularly lobed and toothed with red-brown teeth along the margins, palmately 5-9 nerved, appearing after flowering, white-tomentose beneath; heads bright yellow; 40 central staminate and tubular florets surrounded by about 300 pistillate florets with very narrow, bright yellow ligulate corolla having rounded apices without teeth; heterogamous with ray and disc-florets; achenes 5 to 10 ribbed; pappus soft, snow-white. Rhizomes spreading white horizontaql with many fibrous roots; flowering branches with alternate reddish bracts. Involucre also reddish, linear, cottony, each terminating in a small dark gland.

Habitate: Himalayas from Kashmir to Nepal at 1,500 to 3,500 m.

Propagation: By seeds.

Parts Used: Whole plant.

Chemical Constituents: Pyrrilozidine type alkaloids: Senkirkine, Senecionine, Tussilagine; Ferulic acid, Caffeic acid, Malic acid; Mucilage; Kaempferol, Quercetin; Choline, Phytosterols, Triterpene, Tussilagone.

Uses: Used as an intercurrent medicine in phthisis pulmonalis. Scrofulous affections. Gonorrhoea. Traditionally also used for asthma, bronchitis, laryngitis and pertussis. In house hold, it is used for chronic cough. Bronchial catarrh.

1279. *Tylophora indica* (Burm.f.) Merrill *(Asclepiadaceae)*

Synonyms: *Tylophora asthmatica* (Linn.f.) Wight & Arn.

Vernacular Name: *Eng*: Emetic swallow-wory, Indan or Country ipeacacuanha; *Hin:* Jamgli pikvam, Antamul; *Kan:* Nipaladaberu, Antamula; *Mal:* Vallippala; *San:* Lataksiri; *Tam:* Naippalai, Nancaruppan; *Tel:* Vettipala, Verripala, Tellayadala, Kakapala.

Description: A slender, much branched, tough laticiferous climber with long fleshy, knotty roots; leaves simple, opposite, somewhat fleshy, ovate to orbicular, cordate, often apiculate, glabrous, acute or acuminate, more or less pubescent beneath; flowers in umbels, greenish yellow outside, purplish within, pedicels filiform with a number of filiform hairy bracts at their base; fruits fusiform, divaricate, glabrous, follicles tapering to a fine point at the apex; seeds ovate with long coma.

Habitate: Throughout India, in hedges and open forests upto 900m.

Propagation: By seeds and vegetative method.

Parts Used: Roots, leaves.

Chemical Constituents: Contains three alkaloids A, B and C, Alkaloid B is desmethyl-tylophorine and alkaloid C is desmethyl tylophorinine. Alkaloid A is not identified. It also contains a substance with emetic properties and essential oil. Leaves yield α-amyrin, tylophorine, kaempterol and quercetin.

Uses: The roots and leaves are sweet, acrid, aromatic, emetic, pugative, expectorant, vulnerary, diaphoretic, stomachic and antiviral. They are useful in asthma, bronchitis, whooping cough, dysentery, diarrhoea, hydrophobia, wounds, ulcers, dyspepsia, flatulence, haemorrhoids, gout, vitiated conditions of *vata*, cancerous tumours and murine leukaemia.

1280. *Typha angustifolia* L. *(Typhaceae)*

Vernacular Name: *Eng:* Narrow-leaved cat's-tail; small reedmace, narrow-leaved reedmace.

Description: A perennial lake herb, with creeping rhizomes. Stem erect, cylindrical, reaching 3 cm in height. Leaves elongated-linear 4-8 mm wide, rather thick and spongy, Flowers in vary dense superposed cylindrical spikes, the male and female similar, the male above, 20-30 cm long; pollen simple; the female below, 9-28 cm long, reddish-brown; the two sexes remove from each other. Flowers June to September. The pollen, used as a drug, is a fine, golden dust.

Habitate: Grows at the side of pools.

Propagation: By seeds.

Part Used: Pollen.

Chemical Constituents: N.A.

Uses: Dysmenorrhoes, abdominal pain during the puerperium, stomach-ache, contusions and strains, haemoptysis, nosebleeds; haematuria; functional uterine haemorrhage, aphthae; skin inflammation.

1281. *Typha orientallis* J. Preslw *(Typhaceae)*

Vernacular Name: *Eng:* Cat tail.

Description: Monoecious perennial herb of wet places, with creeping rootstocks and tall, erect, unbranched stems, 1-1.5 m tall. Leaves long, linear, 0.5-1cm wide, flat, erect, parallel-veined. Flowers in a dense terminal spike, spike 3-5 cm long, male above, female below; male flowers with 2-5 united stamens; female flowers with ovary, superior, 1-celled, 1-ovuled, style and stigma 1. Fruit and achene, subtended by capillary bristles.

Habitate: Riverbanks and ponds in lowlands in Korea, Japan, China and Philippines.

Propagation: By Rhizomes.

Parts Used: Pollen.

Chemical Constituents: γ-Cadinene (1,2). Alkanes.

Uses: Hypercholesteraemia, angina, pectoris, haematemesis.

1282. *Typhonium trilobatum* schott *(Araceae)*

Vernacular Name: *Beng*: Gherkochoo; *Tel:* Durada-kandagadda; *Tam:* Karunai-kizhangu; *Kan:* Kandagadde; *Mal:* Karunakizhanga.

Description: Annual herb, 20-30 cm. High. Rootstock thick and round. Leaves trifoliate, base sagittate; pertiole long with lax sheath. Inflorescence in spadix enclosed by a spathe, greenish overlaid with purple, bearing male flowers above, female below, foul-smelling. Berriers numerous, red when ripe.

Habitate: Grows wild in wet soils.

Propagation: By seeds and vegetative method.

Part Used: Rhizomes.

Chemical Constituents: The rootstocks contain proteins and inorganic substances Ca, P, I, F, Fe, Na, K; thiamine, niacin, carotene, folic acid sterols and B-sitosterol.

Uses: The rhizome is used with effect for treating vomiting, couth asthma, excessive expectoration, pyogenic sore throat, headache, gastric ulcer, abscess and snake-bite. Must be used very cautiously in treating pregnant women.

1283. *Ulmus macrocarpa* Hance *(Ulmaceae)*

Vernacular Name: *Eng:* Elm.

Description: Deciduous small tree. Branches well corky, young branches pubescent. Leaves alternate, simple, toothed, obovate, acute, asymmetrical at base, 3.5-15.5 cm long, 2-9 cm wide, coarse on both sides; petioles, 2-3 cm long, pubescent. Flowers inconspicuous, appearing before leaves in spring in axils of leaves. Fruit a flat, 1-celled, 1-seeded samara with the wings surrounding the nutlet and notched at apex.

Habitate: Mountain woods in Korea and Japan.

Propagation: By seeds.

Parts Used: Bark.

Chemical Constituents: Tannic acid, sugars, Fatty acids.

Uses: Antimicrobial, nematocidal. Used in chronic diarrhoea, antiparasites.

1284. *Ulmus rubra* *(Ulmaceae)*

Vernacular Name: *Eng:* Slippery elm.

Description: A large tree growing to 18m, with a brown trunk and rough grey-white bark on the branches.

Habitate: Slippery elm is a native of the US and Canada, and is most commonly found growing in the Appalachian Mountains. The tree thrives on high ground and dry soil. The inner bark of the trunk and branches is collected in spring.

Propagation: By seeds.

Parts Used: Bark.

Chemical Constituents: Mucilage, Starch, Tannins.

Uses: Demulcent, Emollient, Nutritive, Laxative.

1285. *Uncaria rhynchophylla* (Miq.) Jacks. *(Rubiaceae)*

Vernacular Name: *Eng:* Sharpleaved gambir.

Description: An evergreen climbing shrub up to 10 m long, branches 4-angled, brownish, glabrous, occasionally bearing compressed, curved spines. Leaves opposite, with short petioles, elliptical or ovoid-lanceolate, 6-10 cm long by 3-6.5 cm wide; apex acuminate, base attenuate or rounded, entire, glossy on top, glaucous and puberulous underneath, stipules 2-partite, linear-subulate, inflorescence an axillary or terminal peduncled solitary head. Flowers yellow. Fruit a dry capsule.

Habitate: In woods or ravines, on stream banks in China, Japan.

Propagation: By seeds.

Part Used: Unciferous branches.

Chemical Constituents: N.A.

Uses: Infantile convulsions; high fever; night screming vision due to hypertension.

1286. *Uraria picta* Desv. *(Fabaceae)*

Vernacular Name: *Hin:* Dabra, Prisniparni, Prishtaparni, Chitraparni; *San*: Prasniparni; *Beng*: Sankarjata; *Guj*: Pilvan; *Tam*: Sittirappaladai.

Description: It is an erect, little-branched, perennial herb, 90-180 cm tall. Leaves are very variable, 1-3 foliolate, upto 30 cm long and blotched white. Leaflets are 4-6, rarely 9, linear, oblong or lanceolate, obtuse and mucronate with subulate stipules. The flowers are purple in colour and are in dense, long, cylindrical, terminal racemes. Pods are 3-6 jointed, polished and whitish in colour.

Habitate: The plant is found in the dry grasslands, waste places and open forest in the Sub-Himalayan tract from Kashmir to West Bengal and Assam, upto an altitude of 1800 m, and all over the plains of India. In Himachal Pradesh, it is found in the districts of Una, Hamirpur, Bilaspur, Sirmour.

Propagation: By seeds.

Part Used: Whole plant.

Chemical Constituents: N.A.

Uses: The plant is one of the components of 'Dashmoola' and is credited with fracture healing properties. Its total extract has been found to effect better and quicker healing of fractures in the experimental animals due to early accumulation of phosphorus and more deposition of calcium. In Ghana, the plant is used for treating the heart trouble. The root is credited with aphrodisiac properties and itd decoction is prescribed for coughs, chills and fevers. The leaves are considered to be antiseptic and are used in gonorrhoea. The roots and pods are employed in Bihar to treat prolapse of anus in infants and for the treatment of sore-mouth in children.

1287. *Urginea indica* (Roxb.) Kunth. *(Liliaceae)*

Synonyms: *Scilla indica* Roxb.

Vernacular Name: *Hin:* Jungli-piyaz, Ban-piyazi, Ban-palandu; *Eng:* Indian squill, White squill, Sea-onoin; *San*: Vanapalandu; *Kan*: Adairirulli; *Mal*: Kattulli; *Tel:* Nakkavulligadda; *Tam*: Narivangayan.

Description: A glabrous herb. Bulb dull white or pale, ovoid, 2.5-5 cm diameter or more. Leaves radicle, flat, narrow pointed. Flowers appearing before the leaves, drooping or spreading, distant in a terminal raceme, 15-50 cm long. Perianth 10.8 cm long, bell shaped. 6-parted; segments white, with 3 green ribs in the center, tapering downwards; ovules several valved; seeds many, flat, black.

Habitate: Western Himalaya below 1400m; Bihar, Konkan and Coromandal. In Himachal Pradesh, it is found growing in lower parts of Solan and Sirmour, Bilaspur, Mandi and Hamirpur. Planted in Herbal Garden at nauni-Solan.

Propagation: By bulbs and seeds.

Part Used: Bulbs.

Chemical Constituents: Fresh squills yield at least two glycosides, scillarin-A, which is crystalline and scillarin-B, which is amorphous.

Uses: The bulb in action is anthelmintic, cardiac, stimulant, deobstruent, digestive, diuretic, emmenagogue, and expectorant. Useful in asthma, ailments of hearts, calculous affections, ailments of hearts, calculous affections, cough and bronchitis, paralytic affection, promotes urination, in reheumatism and skin diseases. Bulbs are source of raticide, and is used as an expectorant, stimulant, and cardio-tonic in small doses. Squill is used chiefly in chronic bronchitis and asthma. Alcoholic extracts of the bulbs possess anticancer activity against human epidermoid carcinoma. Also employed in dropsy, reheumatism and skin troubles. Externally used for removing corns and warts.

1288. *Urginea maritima* *(Liliaceae)*

Synonyms: *Drimia maritima.*

Vernacular Name: *Eng:* Squill.

Description: Perennial growing to 1.5 m from a large white or red bulb. Has a single flowering stem, a rosette of large basal leaves and a dense spike of white flowers.

Habitate: Native to southern Spain, the Canary Islands and south Africa, squill is cultivated in the Mediterranean region. The bulb of the white variety is unearthed in late summer.

Propagation: By Bulbs.

Parts Used: Bulb.

Chemical Constituents: Squill contains cardiac glycosides, flavonoids, anthocyanidins and mucilage. The cardiac glycosides are strongly diuretic and relatively quick-acting. They do not have the same cumulative effect as those present in foxglove.

Uses: Squill is a diuretic, emetic, cardiotonic and expectorant plant that finds use in a wide range of conditions. It makes a good diuretic in cases of water retention. Since its active constituents do not accumulate to a great degree within the body, it is a potential substitute for foxglove in aiding a failing heart. At low dosage, squall is an effective expectorant. At higher doses, the herb acts as an emetic. Squill is also used in homeopathic.

1289. *Urtica dioica* L. *(Urticaceae)*

Vernacular Name: *Eng:* Nettle; *Hin*: Bichhu booti.

Description: A perennial growing to 1.5m, with lance-shaped leaves and green flowers with yellow stamens in axillary cymes.

Habitate: Nettle grows in temperate regions throughout the northern hemisphere, southern Africa, the Andes and Australia.

Propagation: By Seeds.

Parts Used: Root.

Chemical Constituents: Flavonoids, amines, Glucoquinone, Minerals, Plant sterols, Phenols.

Uses: Diuretic, Tonic, Astringent, Prevents hemorrhaging, anti-allergenic, Increases breast-milk, production, reduces prostate enlargement.

1290. *Uvaria narum* (Dunal) Wall. ex Wight *(Annonaceae)*

Vernacular Name: *Kan:* Kariballi; *Mal:* Narumpanal, Kuril; *San:* Nilavalli, Vallisakhotah; *Tam:* Puliccan.

Description: A large woody stellately pubescent straggling shrub with dark bluish green leaves; leaves oblong lanceolate, acute or acuminate, glabrous on both sides, petioles shorts, less than 6mm, bruised leaves smell like cinnamon; flowers reddish, solitary, terminal or leaf-opposed, 2.5 cm in diameter, stamens with anthers concealed by the overlapping connectives, carpels numberous, scarlet-red; seeds chestnut brown.

Habitate: In the forests of Western Ghats upto an altitude of 1200m.

Propagation: By seeds.

Parts Used: Roots, leaves.

Uses: The roots are astringent sweet, aromatic, emollient, fragrant, stomachic, depurative and febrifuge. They are useful in vitiated conditions of *vata* and *pitta*, gastropathy, eczema, pruritus, erysipelas, jaundice and eclampsia. The leaves are astringent, sour, sweet, cooling, anti-inflammatory and febrifuge. They are useful in vitiated conditions of *vata* and *pitta*, inflammations, jaundice and fever.

1291. *Vaccinium myrthillus* L. *(Vacciniaceae)*

Vernacular Name: *Eng:* Bilberry.

Description: Deciduous shrub growing to about 40 cm. Has erect multi-branched stems, pointed oval leaves, small white or pink flowers, and spherical berries that ripen to purple-black.

Habitate: Bilberry is native to Europe and north America. It thrives in heathland, on moors and in undergrowth.

Propagation: By seeds and vegetative method.

Parts Used: Fruit and leaves.

Chemical Constituents: The fruit contains about 0.5% anthocyanosides, vitamins B^1 and C, pro-vitamin A, 7% tannins, and plant acids. The anthocyanosides have a tonic effect on the blood vessels.

Uses: Ripe berries are mildly laxative due to their fruit sugar content. The dried fruit, however, is markedly binding and has an antibacterial action. A decoction of the dried fruit is useful for treating diarrhoea in children. Bilberry's high anthocyanin content makes it a potentially valuable treatment for varicose veins, haemorrhoids and capillary fragility. A decoction of the fruit is used as a mouthwash. The leaves may be helpful in pre-diabetic states, but are not an alternative to conventional treatment. They may be taken for urinary tract infection.

1292. *Valeriana fauriei* Briq. *(Valerianaceae)*

Vernacular Name: *Eng:*-Faurie's valerian.

Description: Perennial herb with strong-smelling taproots, to 40-80 cm tall. Leaves opposite, pinnatifid to pinnate; segments 5-7, oblong-lanceolate to oblanceolate, 2-5 cm long, 7-15 mm wide. Flowers small, pink, inclustered cymes, calyx inrolled at first, becoming pappuslike in fruit; corolla rotate, 5-7 mm long, with slender long tube; stamens 3, long-exerted; ovary inferior, 3-celled at base. Fruit and achene lanceolate 4 mm long, crowned by persistent calyx.

Habitate: Wet, shaded places in woods and thickets in Korea, Japan and China.

Propagation: By seeds.

Parts Used: Root.

Chemical Constituents: Essentail oils, sesquiterpenes, iridoid glycosides.

Uses: Atnidepressant (a-kessyl alcohol). Used as antispasmodic, sedative.

1293. *Valeriana hardwickii* Wall. *(Valerianaceae)*

Vernacular Name: *Hin:* Muskbala, Tagar, Nihani; *Beng:* Tagar.

Description: Erect, pubescent herbs, 20-60 cm tall. Redical leaves few, ovate-orbiculate, entire or crenulate, pilose, cauline leaves 3-7 pinnate, terminal lobe the largest. Lobes ovate-lanceolate, crenate, serrate. Flowers white in axillary or terminal paniculate cymes or corymbs. Achenes pubescent, longer than the upper bracts.

Habitate: Pakistan to South-west China, Burma, South-east Asia, frequent on moist slopes in the Himalayas and Khasi hills in shrubberies and open slopes between 1500-4000 m elevation. In Himachal Pradesh, it has been found in Bharmour division of Chamba, Kanda area of Karsog and Chansil of Rohru forest division.

Propagation: By seeds and rootstock.

Part Used: Roots.

Chemical Constituents: Contains a crystalline acid. A new oxide, hydrocarbons a polyoxygenated crystalline solid together with alpha-eudesmol, beta-eudesmol, edemol, angelicin, 4-hydroxy thymol dimethyl ether have been isolated.

Uses: The roots are used as insecticide. It is also used in the mental disorders. Also used for scenting hair. Locally much used as a hair tonic and in dhoop manufacturing. It is a substitute for the drug valerian obtained from *V. officinalis L.*

1294. *Valeriana jatamansi* Jones *(Valeriancaceae)*

Synonyms: *Valeriana wallichii.*

Vernacular Name: *Eng:* Indian valerian; *Hin:* Tagar; *Kan:* Tagara; *Mal:* Takaram; *San:* Tagarah, Hatah; *Tam:* Takaram; *Tel:* Tagara.

Description: A tufted, hairy, herbaceous perennial upto 45 cm in height with thick horizontal root-stock basal radical leaves long-stalked, deeply cordate-ovate, usually toothed or sinuate, cauline leaves only a few, much smaller, entire or sometimes pinnate; flowers white or tinged with pink in terminal corymbs, often unisexual, the male and female on different plants; fruits oblong, compressed, hairy or nearly hairless.

Habitate: In the Himalayas, upto 3000 m.

Propagation: By seeds and vegetative method.

Parts Used: Roots.

Chemical Constituents: Actinidine, carotene, calarene, calarenol, elemol, jatamols A and B, jatamansic acid, jatamansone, nardol, nardostachonol, norseychelanone, seychellane, seychellene, spirojatomol, valeranal, valeranone, virolin; angelicin, jatamansin, jatamansinol, oroselol.

Uses: The roots are bitter, acrid, astringent, thermogenic, alexteric, emollient, anodyne, vulenerary; hypontic, carminative, digestive, stomachic, laxative, hepato and cardiotonic, trichogenous, expectorant, diuretic, emmenagogue, aphrodisiac, febrifuge, ophthalmic and tonic. They are useful in vitiated conditions of *kapha* and *vata*, arthralgia, ulcers, wounds epilepsy, convulsions, dyspepsia, flatulence, colic, ascites, constipation, jaundice, cardiac debility, dry cough, asthma, strangury, amennorrhoea, dysmenorrhoea, seminal weakness, chronic and intermittent fevers, ophthalmopathy, skin diseases, falling or hair, splenopathy, nephropathy, gleet, pharyngitis, leprosy, erysipelas and general debility.

1295. *Valeriana officinalis* Linn. *(Valerianaceae)*

Synonyms: *Valeriana excelsa* Poir., *Valeriana repens* Host.

Vernacular Name: *Eng:* Heal-all valerian, Great wild Valerian.

Description: A deciduous herb, with a tuberous, short, rhizome, bearing numerous slender, fleshy tapering, pale-brown rootlets and one or more stolons. Leaves both radical and cauline, the radical being on long petioles whereas the cauline are opposite or alternate, exstipulate and pinnatisect with 11-22 segments with clasping petoles. Basal leaves also divided into numerous segments. Leaflets sessile, lanceolate, dentate. Flowers numerous, small, white or pink, in racemes of cymes. Calyx many-toothed. Corolla 5-lobed, pink. Fruit oblong-ovate 4-ridged, 1-seeded achenes with a feathery persistent calyx. Fruits ciliate.

Habitate: India and Europe including U.K.

Propagation: By Rhizomes and seeds.

Parts Used: Rhizome.

Chemical Constituents: Alkoloids viz. Actinidine, skyanthine, Chatinine, Valerianine, Valerine. Caffeic & chlorogenic acids. β-sitosterol, choline. Terpenes: α-& β-pinene, Camphene, Borneol, Eugenol, isoeugenol, β-bisabolene, caryophyllene, Valeranone, ledol, pacifigorgiol, Valerianol, Valerenol. Valerenal acid, Valerenic acid. Valtrates viz. Valtrate, Valtrate isovaleroxyhydrin, Acevaltrate, Valechlorine; Didrovaltrates viz. Didrovaltrate, Homodidro valtrate, Deoxydidro-valtrate, Homodeoxydidro-valtrate, isovaleroxy-hydroxydidro-valtrate; isovaltrates, Bornyl valerate. Bornyl formate.

Uses: For complaints specifically of hysteria, over sensitiveness, nervous affections. Hysterical spans with changeable disposition. Feeling of excessive lightness of the body and floating in the air. Over sensitiveness of all senses. Sensation of great coldness of head. Sensation a thread handing in throat. Earache from cold draught exposure.

1296. *Vanda roxburghii* R.Br. *(Orchidaceae)*

Synonyms: *Vanda tessellata.*

Vernacular Name: *San*: Rasna; *Hin:* Nai-Rasna, Banda, Rasna; *Tel:* Chittiveduri; *Kan*: Vandakigidda; *Beng*: Nai, Rasna.

Description: A small epiphytic herb. *Roots* white, shiny, silvery grey coloured. The plant develops two kinds of roots, the clinging roots and aerial roots. *Leaves* coriaceous in two rows oblique at apex; *flowers* axillary racemose or solitary.

Habitate: This is a common orchid epiphytic on mango and other trees. It grows all over India and in Sri Lanka.

Propagation: By seeds and vegetative method.

Parts Used: Whole plant.

Chemical Constituents: The plant contains alkaloids and glycoside. The plant also contains tannins, saponins, sterols, fatty oils, resins and colouring matter.

Uses: Rheumatic disorders. Local swellings. Indigestion. The root of the plant is useful in inflammations, rheumatic disorders, osteoarthritis and allied disorders. It has been used for indigestion. It is also used as a laxative and stimulant to liver. The medicated oil is used for external application in rheumatic pains.

1297. *Vateria indica* Linn. *(Dipterocarpaceae)*

Vernacular Name: *Eng:* Indian copal tree, Piney varnich-tree, White dammar; *Hin:* Saphed dammar, Kahruba; *Kan:* Rala, Hugadamara, Bilagaggala; *Mal:* Vellappayin, Velutta Kunturukkam; *San:* Ajakarnah, Sarjah; *Tam:* Vellaikuntirikkam, Vellaidamar, Painimaram, Dhup-maram; *Tel:* Telladamara, Dupadamaru.

Description: A large, evergreen tree 20-30 m in height with grey thick bark often blotched with green and white; leaves simple, alternate elliptic-oblong or ovate, rounded at the base, thick and coriaceous with 12-15 pairs of nerves; flowers white, fragrant, in large drooping panicles; fruits ovoid, rough, pale brown, 3-valved capsules, valves one-seeded; seeds reddish white or cream-coloured. The resin which exudes out through cuts becomes yellowish white or reddish white in colour on soliditying.

Habitate: In the Western Ghats, upto 1200 m along the streams.

Propagation: By seeds.

Parts Used: Bark, resin, oil.

Chemical Constituents: Damar resin, 1.06% essential oil in fruit. dl-Epicatechin, fistinidol and afzelechin from bark. Seeds yield a semi-solid fat, known as PINEY TALLOW or DHUPA FAT.

Uses: The bark is bitter, acrid, thermogenic, alexeteric, depurative, expectorant, vulnerary and tonic. It is useful in vitiated conditions of *vata* and *kapha*, cough, asthma, leprosy, skin eruptions, wounds, ulcers, otorrhoea, dysentery, urethrorrhea and anaemia. The resin is bitter, alexeteric, bechic, carminative, expectorant, detergent and tonic. It is useful in chronic bronchitis, tubercular glands, haemorrhoids, hemicrania, vitiated conditions of *vata*, amenorrhoea, dysmenorrhoea, diarrhoea and ringworm. The fatty oil obtained from the seeds is antibacterial and is useful in chronic rheumatism and neuralgia.

1298. *Vateria macrocarpa* B.L. Gupta *(Dipterocarpaceae)*

Vernacular Name: *Mal:* Vella payin.

Description: Trees, 10-20 m tall. *Trunk* about 1 m girth. *Bark* surface grey mottled with white and green, smooth, resinous. *Leaves* alternate, elliptic-oblong or oblong-lanceolate, 15-40 x 6-20 cm, base rounded or slightly heart-shaped, apex rounded or shortly acuminate, margin entire, leathery, hairless on both surfaces, rarely with a few minutely star-shaped hairs on the main nerve beneath; lateal nerves 15-20 pairs, prominently seen on lower surface; leaf stalks 2.5-6 cm, swollen at the tip, minutely pubescent. *Stipules* prominent. *Flowers* in axillary panicles, about 2.5 cm across, white. Panicles shorter than the leaves, drooping, robust. Stamens numerous. *Capsules* more or less cylindrical, narrowing towards apex, 10-15 cm long and 5-6 cm broad, splitting into 3 valves from the top towards the base when mature. *Seeds* solitary.

Habitate: Rocky slopes of evergreen forests.

Propagation: By seeds.

Parts Used: Resin.

Chemical Constituents: N.A.

Uses: Like the resin obtained from *Vateria indica*, the resin of *V. macrocarpa* could also be used for similar purpose as the former finds extensive use in indigenous medicine.

1299. *Ventilago madraspatana* Gaertn. *(Rhamnaceae)*

Vernacular Name: *Eng:* Red creeper; *Hin:* Pitti; *Kan:* Pappali, papudi; *Mal:* Vempata; *San:* Dinesavalli, Raktavalli; *Tam:* Vempatam, Surubattaikkoti; *Tel:* Errasurugudi, Suralatige.

Description: A large, much branched, woody climber with branches hanging down and dark grey bark having vertical cracks exposing the inner vermilion surface; leaves simple, alternate, oblong-lanceolate or elliptic-ovate, obtuse or acute, entire or crenate, base rounded or acute, main nerves-4-8 pairs; flowersgreenish with an offensive odour in drooping pubescent terminal panicles, petals much smaller than the sepals; fruits yellowish globular nuts, supported by the persistent calyx, wing linear-oblong. 1-nerved, rounded at the apex.

Habitate: Throughout India, in forests.

Propagation: By seeds.

Parts Used: Bark.

Chemical Constituents: Trihydroxy-methyl-anthranolmonomethyl ether; emodinmonomethyl ether in root bark. Lupeol, B-sitosterol and its glucosidee in fruits, leaves and stem. Friedelin in stem bark.

Uses: The bark is bitter, astringent, thermogenic, digestive, carminative, stomachic, alexeteric, vulnerary, depurative, stimulant and tonic. It is useful in vitiated conditions of *kapha*, dyspepsia, colic, flatulence, erysipelas, leprosy, scabies, prurits, and other skin disease, fever and general debility.

1300. *Veratrum maackii* var. japonicum T. Shimizu *(Liliaceae)*

Vernacular Name: *Eng:* Japanese hellebore.

Description: Erect perennial herb with thick rhizomes, to 40-100 cm tall. Stems stout, leafy. Leaves alternate, radical and lower cauline, glabrous, narrowly oblong to linear-lanceolate, 20-35 mm long, 3-5 cm wide, gradually tapered towards the base. Inflorescence 15-50 cm long, branched, slender, the bracts shorter than the branches. Flowers loosely arranged, brown-purple, 10 mm across; pedicels 4-7 mm long; sepals broadly lanceolate, subobtuse, twice as long as the stamens. Capsules elliptic, 12-15 mm long.

Habitate: Mountain woods in Korea and Japan.

Propagation: By Rhizomes and seeds.

Parts Used: Root.

Chemical Constituents: Jervine, germerine, verazine, 15-O-(2-methylbutanoyl) germine, verussurinine, germidine.

Uses: Antibacterial, teratogenic, hypotensive, insecticide against cockroaches. Used in mucosal, irritation, nausea, vomiting.

1301. *Verbascum thapsus* *(Scrophulariaceae)*

Vernacular Name: *Eng:* Mullein.

Description: Upright biennial growing to 2m. Has slightly hairy, grey-green, oval to lance-shaped leaves, and spikes of bright yellow flowers.

Habitate: Mullein is native to central and southern Europe and western Asia. It is now also naturalized in many other temperate regions.

Propagation: By Rhizome.

Parts Used: Leaves and flowers.

Chemical Constituents: Mullein contains mucilage, flavonoids, triterpenoid saponins, volatile oil and tannins.

Uses: Mullein is a valuable herb for coughs and catarrh, and is a specific treatment for tracheitis and bronchitis. The leaves and the flowers may be used as an infusion to reduce mucus formation and stimulate the coughing up of phlegm. Mullein combines well with other expectorants such as coltsfoot and thyme. Applied externally, mullein is emollient and makes a good wound healer. In Germany, the flowers are steeped in olive oil, and the resulting fixed oil is used as a remedy for ear infections and haemorrhoids.

1302. *Verbena officinalis* *(Verbenaceae)*

Vernacular Name: *Eng:* Vervain, Ma Bian Cao.

Description: A slender perennial growing to 1m, with stiff, thin stems and spikes of small lilac flowers.

Habitate: Vervain grows wild throughout much of Europe and North Africa as well as in Chin and Japan.

Propagation: By Seeds.

Parts Used: Aerial parts.

Chemical Constituents: Bitter iridoids, Volatile oil, Alkaloids, Mucilage, Tannins.

Uses: Nervine, Tonic, Mild sedative, Stimulates bile secretion, Mild bitter.

1303. *Vernonia anthelmintica* Willd. *(Asteraceae)*

Synonyms: *Centratherum anthelminticum.* O.Kize.

Vernacular Name: *Eng:* Purple fleebane; *Hin:* Kalijira, Baksi; *Kan:* Kadujirage; *Mal:* Krmisatru, Kattujirakam; *San:* Aranyajiraka, Brhatpali; *Tam:* Kattuccirakam, Cittilai; *Tel:* Adavijilakarra.

Description: A tall robust, stout, erect annual 60-90 cm in height with pubescent branches; leaves long, lanceolate or ovate-lanceolate, acute, coarsely serrate, membranous, more or less pubescent on both sides, base tapering into petiole; flowers purplish in subcorymbose head, outer involucral bracts linear and hairy, green with purplish obtuse tips, innermost bracts longest; fruits achenes, oblong, cylindric, 10-ribbed, pubescent, pappus reddish, inner pappus long, outer short.

Habitate: Throughout India, as a weed.

Propagation: By seeds.

Parts Used: Fruits.

Chemical Constituents: Amino acids, linoleic myristic, oleic, palmitic, stearic and vernoleic acids, brassicasterol, stigmasterol an elemanolide lactone, vernodalol from seeds.

Uses: The fruits are bitter, acrid, thermogenic, anthelminitic, astringent, anti-inflammaoty, anodyne, expectorant, depurative, demulcent, purgative, diuretic, stomachic, febrifuge, galactagogue and tonic. They are useful in inflammations, hiccough, cough asthma, leprosy, skin disease, pruritis, leucoderma, dyspepsia, colic, strangury, fever, ophthalmopathy, vitiated conditions of *vata,* and are very specific for roundworm and threadworm.

1304. *Vernonia cinerea* (L.) Less. *(Asteraceae)*

Synonyms: *Conyza cinerea* Linn.

Vernacular Name: *Eng:* Ash-coloured fleabane; *Hin:* Sahadeyi, Sadodi; *Kan:* Sahadevi, Sadodi; *Mal:* Puvvamkuruntila, Puvvamkurunnila; *San:* Sahadevi; *Tam:* Puvamkuruntal, Naycitti; *Tel:* gharitikamini, Garitikamma.

Description: An erect or somewhat decumbent annual herb, 12-75 cm in heights with cylindric, striate, more or less pubescent branched stem; leaves simple, alternate, variable in shape, ovate, or lanceolate, shortly mucronate, irregularly toothed or shallowly crenate-serrate; flowers many, pinkishvilet, in small heads, involucral bracts oblong, lanceolate, acuminate, awned, silky on the back; fruits oblong, lanceolate, acuminate, awned, silky on the back; fruits oblong achenes, slightly narrowed at the base; clothed with appressed white hairs.

Habitate: Throughout India, as a weed on roadsides and open places.

Propagation: By seeds.

Parts Used: Whole plant.

Chemical Constituents: Seeds yield 38 per cent fatty oil. Plant contains β-Amyrin acetate; β-amyrin benzoate; lupeol and its acetate; β-sitosterol, stigmasterol, a-spinasterol and KCL.

Uses: The plant are bitter, acrid, thermogenic, anthelminitic, depurative, diuretic, lithontriptic, anodyne, anti-inflammatory, sudorific, stomachic, alexeteric, antibacterial, antifungal, antivitral and antiperiodic. The roots are useful in diarrhoea, stomachalgia, cugh, inflammations, skin diseases, leprosy, strangury, renal and versical calculi, chronic and intermittent fevers and vitiated conditions of *vata*. The leaves are useful in humid herpes, eczema, ringworm, guineaworms and elecphantiasis. The flowers are useful in conjunctivitis, vitiated conditions of *vata* and fever. The seeds are useful in roundworms, threadworms, cough, flatulence, leucoderma, psoriasis, chronic, skin diseases, colic and dysiria. The plant possesses anticancerous activities and is good for canerous malformations.

1305. *Veronicastrum sibiricum* (L.) Pennell *(Scrophulariaceae)*

Vernacular Name: *Eng:* Blackroot.

Description: Tall perennial herb, to 50-90 cm tall. Stems simple or sparsely branched in upper part. Leaves whorled, 3-8, sessile, simple, long elliptic or elliptic, acute, 6-17 cm long, 2-4 cm wide, serrate. Inflorescence terminal; spikes erect, 20-30 cm long, densely flowered; calyx deeply 5-lobed; the lobes lanceolate, slightly unequal; corolla tube 7-8 mm long, shallowly 4-lobed, purple, pubescent inside; stamens 2, exerted; ovary 2-celled; style exerted, white, glabrous. Fruit ovate-conical capsule.

Habitate: Grassy areas in mountains and lowlands in Korea and Japan.

Propagation: By seeds.

Parts Used: Root.

Chemical Constituents: Mannital, luteolin-7-b-neohesperidoside, luteolin-7-b-glucoside. Iridoids; minecoside, 6-O-veratryl catalpol ester, catalpol, aucubin, 6-deoxy-8-isoferuloy1 herpagide. Phenyl propanoids.

Uses: Antimicrobial (minecoside). Used in common colds and liver tonic.

1306. *Vetiveria zizanioides* (L.) Nash *(Poaceae)*

Synonyms: *Andropogon muricatus* Retz.

Vernacular Name: *Eng:* Vetiver, Khas-khas, khus-khus; *Hin:* Khas, Khas-Khas; *Kan:* Vattiveru, Lamnci, Karidappasajjehallu; *Mal:* Ramaccam; *San:* Usirah, Sevyah, Sugandhimulah; *Tam:* Vettiver; *Tel:* Kuruveru, Vettiveru.

Description: A densely tufted perennial grass, with aromatic roots and rhizomes; leaves narrow, linear, erect, sheaths compressed, ligules reduced to a scrious rim, midrib slender, lateral nerves close, spikelets grey, green or purplish in apanicle of numberous selnder racemes, sesile spikelets linear-lanceolate, glabrous, pedicelled spikelets 2-flowered; fruits oblong, grains, slightly oblique at the apex.

Habitate: Throughout India, in the plains and lower hills upto 1200m.

Propagation: By seeds.

Parts Used: Roots.

Chemical Constituents: Essential oil containing β-vetivone. Isobisabolene, khusol and azulene from oil.

Uses: The roots are bitter, sweet, acrid, refrigerant, aromatic, diaphoretic, depurative, digestive, carminative, stomachic, antiemetic, constipating, haematinic, haemostatic, expectorant, diuretic, febrifuge, stimulant, anthelmintic, emmenagogue, alexeteric, soporific, antispasmodic and tonic. They are useful in vitiated conditions of *pitta,* and *vata,* hyperdipsia, burning sensation, ulcers, skin diseases, nausea, obstinate vomiting, dyspepsia, flatulence, colic, anaemia, haemorrhages, haemoptysis, cough, asthma, hiccough, strangury, bilious fever, gout, lumbago, sprains, halitosis, cephalalgia, spermatorrhea, hysteria, insomnia, diarrhoea, hyperhidrosis, amentia, cardiac debility, amenorrhoea, dysmenorrhoea, helminthiasis, spasmodic affections, erysipelas, emaciation and general debility.

1307. *Viburnum opulus* L. *(Caprifoliaceae)*

Synonyms: *Viburnum americanum* Mill., *Viburnum lobatum* Lam., *Viburnum glandulosum* Salisb.

Vernacular Name: *Eng:* True cramp bark, Cranberry tree bush, Wild Guelder Rose.

Description: A deciduous shrub, 4 m. high. Leaves opposite, petiolate, broadly ovate, palmately-veined, 3-lobed, with middle lobe elongated, margins irregularly toothed or entire, apex acuminate, petiole grooved on upper surface, with stalked or sessile glands towards apex and elongated slender, glandular stipules at base. Flowers both fertile and infertile, in broad and stalked compoined cyme; fertile flowers small and green; infertile large, greenish-white and marginal. Fruit scarlet, sub-globular drupe with succulent sarcocarp and flat stony endocarp, enclosing a seed.

Habitate: Southern Canada, Northern United States, Great Britain and Europe.

Propagation: By vegetative method and seeds.

Parts Used: Stem bark.

Chemical Constituents: A phenolic glucoside, Esculetin, Scopoletin.

Uses: For complaints specifically of uterine cramps, colicky pains in pelvic organs, spasmodic and congestive affections of ovarian and uterine origin. Menses too late, too scanty, offensive with crampy pains extending down thighs. Bearing down pains before menses. Aching in sacrum & pubes extending in thighs. Spasmodic dysmenorrhoea. Excrociating leucorrhoea. Smarting & itching of genitals. Frequent & early miscarriages. Pains extending from back to pubes, loins & then to thighs. Sudden cramps and colic pains in abdomen. Urination on coughing & walking.

1308. *Viburnum prunifolium* L. *(Caprifoliaceae)*

Synonyms: *Viburnum* lentago Duroi.

Vernacular Name: *Eng:* Black Haw, Plum-leave Viburnum.

Description: A tall shrub or small tree, with the stem and foliage glabrous or sparsely scurfy when young. Petiole slender, 5-12mm. long, wingless or very narrowly wing-margined. Leaf-blades oblong or elliptic to obovate, rounded to apiculate or acute at apex. Finely serrate, obtuse to rounded at the base, without any lobes, those sub-tending the cyme mostly 3-5 cm. long at anthesis, those of sterile stems eventually 6-8 cm. long. Cyme sessile, 3 rayed or usually 4 rayed, 5-10 cm. wide. Flowers 4-7 mm. wide. Drupe blue black, ellipsoid to subglobose. Stone flat, oval, scarcely grooved.

Habitate: Central and Eastern United States of America.

Propagation: By seeds.

Parts Used: Stem bark.

Chemical Constituents: Viburnin; Salicin; Esculetin; Scopoletin; Isovaleric acid; Salicylic alcohol.

Uses: For complaints specifically of habitual abortion and miscarriage, bearing down pains in uterus after menses, cancer of tongue, obstinate hiccough, menstrual irregularities of sterile females with uterine displacements. Acts as a uterine sedative.

1309. *Vigna marina* (Burm) Merr. *(Fabaceae)*

Synonyms: *Vigna retusa* Walp.

Vernacular Name: *Eng:* beach bean.

Description: Herbaceous creeping vine without tendrils. Leaves alternate, trifoliate, leaflets obovate, up to 10 cm long and somewhat fleshy. Flowers small, pea-like, yellows. Fruit a black pod (legume), 5-8 cm long with several to many pea-like seeds.

Habitate: Common on sandy seashores and among coastal vegetation and plantations.

Propagation: By seeds.

Part Used: Leaves.

Chemical Constituents: Alkaloids.

Uses: Healing of fractured bones; remedy for food poisoning; to treat weakness after childbirth and to treat headache; to cure stomachache. An infusion of the leaves is used as a potion, is applied as drops to the eyes, nose and mouth and is rubbed onto the body to treat disease though to be caused by spirits. Mouth infections are also treated with this plant. Leaf infusion to treat a certain type of fever in children. The plant is also used in remedies for carbuncles and abscesses. Also used to clean out the female reproductive system.

1310. Vigna mungo (L.) Hepper *(Fabaceae)*

Synonyms: *Phaseolus mungo* Linn.

Vernacular Name: *San:* Masah; *Eng:* Black gram; *Hin:* Urd; *Kan:* Uddu; *Mal:* Ulnnu; *Tam:* Ulunthu; *Tel:* Uddulu, Minumulu, Nallaminumulu.

Description: An erect hairy annual with long twining branches; leaves triloliate, leaflets ovate, entire; flowers small, yellow on elongating peduncles; fruits cylindrical pods, hairy with a short, hooked beak; seeds 1-4 per pod, generally black with a white hilum protruding from the seeds.

Habitate: Cultivated all over India.

Propagation: By seeds.

Parts Used: Roots, seeds.

Chemical Constituents: It contains genistein, kievitone, dalbergioidin, cyclokievitone, isoferreirin, eurenol, glycinol, demethylvesititol, kievitone hydrate, cyclokievitone hydrate, hemicellulose A, hemicellulose pectin, starch and hexosans.

Uses: The roots are narcotic and are used for ostalgia, abscess and inflammations. The seeds are sweet, emollient, thermogenic, diuretic, aphrodisiac, tonic, nutritious, galactagogue, appetise, laxative and nervine tonic. They are useful in dyspepsia, anorexia, strangury, constipation, vitiated conditions of *vata*, haemorrhoids, hepatopathy, neuropathy and agalactia. They are used in the form of decoction, powder, paste etc.

1311. *Vigna pilosa* Baker *(Fabaceae)*

Synonyms: *Dolichos pilosus* Roxb.

Vernacular Name: *Hin:* Banmumg, Mumgvan; *Kan:* Kaduhesaru; *Mal:* Kattupayar, Kattucerupayar; *San:* Mudgaparni; *Tam:* Kattuppayar; *Tel:* Adavipesalu, Pillipesaru.

Description: A slender extensively spreading hairy twiner with strong wiry branches and well developed root system bearing large sized root nodules of various shapes; leaves alternate, trifoliate, leaflets large, ovate, acute, the end one deltoid at base; flowers medium sized, under 2 cm, reddish or bluish on axillary racemose peduncles; fruits pendulous, linear, very long pointed velvety pods, seeds reniform with a dark drown shining seed coat.

Habitate: Throughout India, in forests at low altitudes.

Propagation: By seeds.

Parts Used: Roots and seeds.

Chemical Constituents: Friedelin, epifriedelin, stigmasterol and tannins.

Uses: The roots are bitter, sweet, aphrodisiac, germicidal and cooling. They are used for curing consumption, cough fever, diarrhoea, haemorrhoids, ophthalmopathy, burning sensation, dyspepsia and vitiated conditions of *vata*, *pitta* and *kapha*.

1312. Vigna radiata (Linn.) Wilczek *(Fabaceae)*

Synonyms: *Phaseolus sublobatus* Roxb.

Vernacular Name: *Eng:* Wild black gram; *Hin:* Banurd; *Kan:* Kadu-uddu; *Mal:* Kattulunnu; *San:* Masaparni; *Tam:* Kattu uluntu; *Tel:* Adavi-uddulu.

Description: A suberect or twining annual or perennial with short slender stem and several long branches clothed with spreading or deflexed reddish brown hairs; leaves 3-foliate, petioles fairly long, leafltes ovate or ovate-rhomboid, entire or often lobed, acute, silky hairy on both sides, prominently 3-nerved from the base; flowers yellow, papilionaceous in 6-12 flowered short axillary racemes; fruits nearly cylindric, greenish, rusty pubescent, beaked 2-valved pods; seeds 10-15 per pod, dark grey to dark brown, truncate at the ends.

Habitate: Throughout India, on plains and on hills upto 300 m.

Propagation: By seeds.

Parts Used: Roots.

Chemical Constituents: Thiamine, riboflavin, nicotinic acid, pyridoxine, inositol, vitamin B_{12}, ascorbic acid and vitamin K.

Uses: The roots are bitter, sweet, refrigerant, digestive, emollient, constipating, depurative, anti-inflammatory, aphrodisiac, haemostatic, galactagogue, roborant, febrifuge and tonic. They are useful in dyspepsia, pyresiza, diarrhoea, skin diseases, leprosy, inflammations, cough, haemoptysis, agalactia, emaciation, consumption, facial paralysis, hemiplegia, vitiated conditions of *vata* and *pitta*, fever and general debility.

1313. *Vigna unguiculata* (Linn.) Walp. *(Fabaceae)*

Synonyms: *Vigna sinensis* (Linn.) Hassk; *Vigna catjang* (Burm.f.) Walp.

Vernacular Name: *Eng:* Cow pea; *Hin:* Lobiya, Santa; *Kan:* Tadagunni, Alasandi; *Mal:* Payar, Vellappayar, kottappaya; *San:* Rajamasah, Mahamasah; *Tam:* Karamani; *Tel:* Boberlu, Duntapesalu, Alusendi.

Description: A suberect or twining bushy glabrous annual; leaves pinnately 3 foliate, leaflets 7.5-15cm long, broadly or narrowly ovate, often rhombiodal, retire or slightly lobed; flowers white, pale violet or purple with a yellow eye, in subcapitate racemes; fruits pods, upto 90 cm long, slightly depressed between the seeds, 10-20 seeded; seeds vary in size, shape and colour.

Habitate: Throughout India, cultivated.

Propagation: By seeds.

Parts Used: Seeds.

Chemical Constituents: Carotene, thiamine, riboflavin, niacin, vitamin C, carotene, thiamine, riboflavin, niacin folic acid.

Uses: The seeds are sweet, astringent, appetiser, laxative, anthelmintic, anaphrodisiac, diuretic, galactagogue and liver tonic. They are useful in vitiated conditions of *kapha* and *pitta*, anorexia, constipation, helminthiasis, strangury, agalactia, jaundice and general debility.

1314. *Vinca minor* *(Apocynaceae)*

Vernacular Name: *Eng:* Lesser periwinkle.

Description: A mainly ground-hugging evergreen shrub arching to 45 cm. Has rooting stems, shiny elliptical leaves and 5-petalled, violet-blue flowers.

Habitate: Native to Europe, lesser perivwinkle grows in hedgerows and along woodland borders. It is also cultivated as a garden plant.

Propagation: By seeds.

Parts Used: Leaves.

Chemical Constituents: Lesser periwinkle contains about 7% indole alkaloids, a bisindol alkaloid and tannins. vincamine increases blood flow and oxygen supply to the brain.

Uses: Lesser periwinkle is employed as an astringent and blood-staunching herb. Its astringency makes it a useful mouthwash for sore throats, gingivitis and mouth ulcers. Its staunching ability is effective against internal bleeding, heavy menstrual bleeding and nosebleeds. Since vincamine was discovered in the leaves, lesser periwinkle has been used to treat arteriosclerosis and for dementia due to insufficient blood flow to the brain.

1315. *Viola odorata* Linn. *(Violaceae)*

Vernacular Name: *San*: Banaphasha, *Hin:* Banaphasha; *Eng*: Sweet violet; *Beng*: Banafshah, *Kan*: Violethoo; *Tam*: Vialettu.

Description: The plant is a creeping herb, colour brownish, without any stem, consists of leaves and *flowers*-yellow, white, blue purplish or pink with long filiform stalks. *Roots* dry, thready, fibrous pale yellow knotty, slender as thick as a quill. *Leaves* cordate at the base, heart shaped carpels three nerved and brown.

Habitate: A glabrous or pubescent herb found in Kashmir and the temperate western Himalayas above 1800 m, distributed to Northern and West Asia. North Africa and Europe.

Propagation: By seeds.

Parts Used: Flowers.

Chemical Constituents: Violate flower and root contain an emetic principle named 'voiline'. It forms salts with acids. It is volatile oil. Roots contain several coloruing matters-ionone and ionine. The plant also contains glucoside, methol salicylic ester and saponins.

Uses: Sore throat. Fevers. The root is laxtive, good febrifuge, tonic, expectorant, diuretic; it alleviates thirst, relieves inflammation. The medicated oil of *Viola odorata* is used for abdominal pain. It relieves cough and acts as a sedative. The root is an emetic. A syrup, made from the flower petals, is good medicine for cough, hoarseness of voice. The syrup, when mixed with almond oil, is a gentle laxative for children and also helps to soothe irritative cough and to relieve sore-throat. It is considered antipyretic and diaphoretic and very useful in relieving febrile symptoms.

1316. *Viola serpens* Wall. *(Violaceae)*

Synonyms: *Viola biflora, Viola caneseens, Viola patrinii.*

Vernacular Name: Banfshah, Banaksha, Gule-banaksha, Violet.

Description: A small perennial herb, with short tufted root-stocks. Stem short, but distinct, covered with withered scales, often producing runners. Leaves are ovate-cordate, crenate-serrate. Flowers lilac, blue or sometimes white. Capsule globose, only a few seeded.

Habitate: A hirsute or glabrous herb, found throughout the temperate Himachal Pradesh, it is found in Chamba, Kangra, Kinnaur, Kullu, Mandi, Sirmour, Bilaspur, Shimla and Solan districts.

Propagation: By seeds and stem cutting.

Part Used: Whole plant.

Chemical Constituents: Roots contain glucoside methyle salicylate; yields an alkaloid, voiline; a glycoside, viola quercitrin, which is probably identical with rutin and a saponin. Roots contain saponin and an alkaloid. Roots, leaves and blossoms contain methyl-salicylate in the form of a glucoside.

Uses: In action, it is aperient, antipyretic, cooling, demulcent, diaphorectic, diuretic, emetic, emollient, expectorant, febrifuge and purgative. Useful in asthma, bleeding piles, cancer of the throat, constipation, cough, fever, headache and skin diseases. Made into a syrup, it is given in infantile disorders.

1317. *Viola tricolor* *(Violaceae)*

Vernacular Name: *Eng:* Heartsease.

Description: Annual, biennial or perennial plant growing to 38 cm. Has lobed, oval leaves and handsome violet, yellow and white pansy-type flowers.

Habitate: Heartsease is native to Europe, North Africa and temperate regions of Asia, and has become naturalized in the Americas. It thrives in many habitats. From grassy mountainous areas to coastal sites, and is also cultivated as a garden plant. The aerial parts are gathered in summer.

Propagation: By Seeds.

Parts Used: Aerial parts.

Chemical Constituents: Heartsease contains flavonoids, methyl salicylate, mucilage, gums, resin and a saponin.

Uses: In western herbal medicine, heartsease is used as a purifying herb, and is taken for skin conditions such as eczema. An infusion also makes a useful wash for itchiness. Being expectorant, heartsease is used to treat bronchitis and whooping cough. The plant's diuretic action makes it useful for treating rheumatism, cystitis and difficulty in passing urine.

1318. *Viola yedoensis* Makino. *(Violaceae)*

Vernacular Name: *Eng:* Tokyo violet.

Description: An annual herb. The whole plant has white hairs; main root thick, white. Leaves basal, upper part of stalk usually winged; the petiole is often shorter than the blae; limb narrowly laneolate or ovate-lanceolate; after flowering the limb grows larger and often triangular-lanceolate. Flowers in spring, usually purple, the pedicels shorter than the leaves. Fruit an oblong capsule, 3-celled. Seeds numerous.

Habitate: On hills, roadsides, lawns in China, Japan.

Propagation: By seeds.

Part Used: Whole plant.

Chemical Constituents: N.A.

Uses: Skin inflammation, boils, snake-bite, jaundice, genital discharge.

1319. *Viscum album* L. *(Loranthaceae)*

Synonyms: *Viscum costatum* Gamble.

Vernacular Name: Bhulu-ka-banda, Ujjral, Banda, Kahbung, Mistletoe.

Description: A large, epiphytic, profusely branching shrubby perennial, forming rounded clumps over the host trees. It is green all over; branches dichotomous or whorled. Leaves about 5 by 10 cm, sessile, cuneate-oblong, or oblanceolate, with 3-5 longitudinal, basal nerves. Flowes are dioecious, sessile; in clusters of 3-5, supported by cocave bracts. Perianth-segments 3-4, triangular, deciduous. Fruit small, ellipsoid, white, smooth, almost transparent, mucilaginous.

Habitate: Jaunsar and Tehri-Garhwal upto 2000m. In Himachal Pradesh, it is parasitising chiefly or Rosaceous trees and shrubs, on elm, walnut and willows between 1200-2600 m.

Propagation: By seeds.

Part Used: Whole plant.

Chemical Constituents: Main constituents are fatty acids, nicotine alkaloids, amines. Other constituents include flavonoids, chaleone derivatives and flavonone derivatives; terpenoids-beta-amyrin, betalinic acid, lupeol and ester combinations; oleanoilic acid resin acid, ursolic acid, betasitosterol, sterol A, phytosterol glucoside, viscotoxin; mucilage, polyoles; sugars, starch, syringin and tannin, also contains a sticky greenish resin, "Viscin", fatty oil, lutein, alpha and beta carotene and vitamin C.

Uses: The extract and powder of the leaves were official in the French Pharmacopoiea stabilizers. In Europe, the leaves, stems and berries constitute a drug used for hypertension, arteriosclerosis, tumors and arthrosis. Also used for hysteria, epilepsy and ear diseases. The drug is reputed as a cardiotonic, antiseptic, antispasmodic, diuretic, purgative and emetic with narocotic action. It is employed as a decoction or tincture in intermitted fevers. Also considered useful in splenic and hepatic enlargements; in lumbago and piles. Locally used as a fodder for milch cattle. It is believed that the large quantity of mucilage in the fruits increases milk yield.

1320. *Vitex agnus-castus* L. *(Verbenaceae)*

Synonyms: *Vitex verticillata* Lam.

Vernacular Name: *Eng:* Chaste tree.

Description: A deciduous shrub or a tree of about 3-4 m. height. Leaves opposite, petiolate and digitate, 3-5 palmately partite, dark green on upper surface, grey on under surface with margins entire or undulated, the smallest leaflets are usually sessile. Flowers white, in panicles, terminal or axillary or supra-axillary, forming a pyramidal inflorescence, composed of numerous paired, many-flowered, sessile or subsessile cymules. Calyx densely white-puberulent, each 5-toothed. Corolla also densely white puberulent. Fruit a drupe, grayish hard.

Habitate: Southern Europe, shores of Mediterranean, France and Greece. Also cultivated in Indian gardens.

Propagation: By seeds.

Parts Used: Berries.

Chemical Constituents: Viticin, Casticin, Penduletin, Chrysophanol-D, Aucubin, Agnuside, Cineol, Pinene and Castine.

Uses: Eye diseases. Stomac-ache. Complaints of excessive sexual desire in both sexes and therefore acts as antiaphrodisiac. Premature old age due to abuse of sexual power. Complete impotence, relaxation, flaccidity, coldness of genitalia. No sexual power. Gleet with absence of sexual desire or erections. In females for abhorrence of sexual intercourse, relaxation of genitals with transparent yellow leucorrhoea. Traditionally for menstrual problems resulting from corpus luteum deficiency including spasmodic dysmenorrhoea, menstrual neurosis.

1321. *Vitex negundo* L. *(Verbenaceae)*

Vernacular Name: *Eng:* Five-leaved chaste tree; *Hin:* Samhalu, Saubhalu, Nirgandi; *Kan:* Niragundi, Lakkagida, Nekka, Nakkilu; *Mal:* Karunocci; *San:* Nirgundi; *Tam:* Nirkundi, Nallanocci; *Tel:* Nallavavili, Vavili, Tellavavili.

Description: An aromatic large shrub or small tree of about 3 m in height with quadrangular branches; leaves opposite, exstipulate, long petioled and digitately 3-5 foliolate, all leaflets with petiolules, the middle one longer, flowers bluish purple in panicles upto 30 cm long; fruits globose or ovoid or obovoid, four-seeded drupe, black when ripe.

Habitate: Throughout India, on waste lands upto 1500m.

Propagation: By seeds and vegetative method.

Parts Used: Whole plant.

Chemical Constituents: Leaves contain two alkaloid nishindine and hydrocotylene. Fresh leaves yield a pale greenish yellow oil.

Uses: The plant is bitter, acrid, thermogenic, anthelmintic, expectorant, carminative, digestive, stomachic, anodyne, anti-inflammatory, antiseptic, cephalic, alternate, antipyretic, diuretic, emmenagogue, depurative, rejuvenating, ophthalmic, vulnerary and tonic. The roots are useful in vitiated conditions of *vata*, cephalalgia, otalgia, arthritis, inflammations, dyspepsia, colic, verminosis, flatulence, dysentery, uropathy, wounds ulcers, bronchitis, cough, malarial fever, haemorrhoids, dysmenorrhoea, leprosy, dematopathy, ophthalmopathy and general debility. The leaves are useful in vitiated conditions of *vata*, *kapha*jajvara, cephalalgia, sprains, orchitis, gout, splenohepatomegaly, otorrhoea, inflammations and ulcers. The bark is useful in vitiated conditions of vat, odontalgia, verminosis and ophthalmopathy. The flowers are useful in diarrhoea, cholera, fever, haemorrhages, hepatopathy and cardiac disorders.

1322. *Vitex rotundifolia* L.f. *(Verbenaceae)*

Vernacular Name: *Eng:* Round-leaf vitex.

Description: Evergreen, procumbent or ascending shrub densely covered with short hairs throughout. Stems slightly 4-angled. Leaves opposite, simple, ovate to broad-elliptic, 2-5 cm long, 1.5-3 cm wide, rounded or abruptly acute at base, thinly puberulent above, densely grayish puberulent beneath. Inflorescence panicles at terminal, densely flowered, 4-7 cm long, short-pediceled; corolla purple, subbilabiate, 13 mm across; stamens 4, exerted, didymous; styles bifid, 1.5 cm long. Fruit globose, 5-7 mm in diameter.

Habitate: *San*dy areas by the sea in Asia, China, Korea and Japan.

Propagation: By seeds and stem cutting.

Parts Used: Fruit.

Chemical Constituents: Camphene, pinene. Diterpenes: rotundifuran, prerotundifurn, vitexilactone, previtexilactone. Flavones: vitexicarpin, luteolin, artemetin. R-Hydroxybenzoic acid, vanillin, vitricine (alkaoid). Glycosides: agnuside, eurostoside.

Uses: Antibacterial, antioxidant, antianaphylactic, aldose reductase inhibition. Used in common colds, headache, migraine, sore eyes.

1323. *Vitex trifolia* L.f. *(Verbenaceae)*

Synonyms: *Cayratia carnosa* (Wall.) Gangep. *Vitis carnosa* Wall.

Vernacular Name: *San:* Aranyavasini, atyamlaparni; *Eng:* Indian wild pepper; *Hin:* Amal-bel, ramchana; *Beng*: Amal-lata, bundal; *Tel:* Kurudinne, kamputige; *Tam:* Tumans; *Kan:* Heggoli and *Mal:* Sorivalli.

Description: Small tree, bark smooth pale grey. Young twigs quadrangular, pubscent. Leaves opposite, trifoliate or simple variable, leaflets mostly sessile, elliptic, ovate or ovovate-oblong, with a dense white tomentum beneath and a strong smell when crushed. Inflorescence in terminal cyme; flowers pale violet. Drupe globose, embraced by the persistent calyx.

Habitate: Grows well on the sea-coast.

Propagation: By seeds and vegetative method.

Part Used: Fruits.

Chemical Constituents: The fruit contains the alkaloid vitricine. The leaves yield an essential oil consisting of L-a-pinene, camphene, terpinyl acetate, diterpene alcohol; flavonoids; aucubin, agnusid, casticin, orientin, isoorientin, luteolin 7-glucoside.

Uses: The fruid is used in treating coryza, fever, headache, photopsia, vertigo, opthalmalgia, glaucoma, rheumatism and neuralgia.

1324. *Vitis vinifera* L. *(Vitaceae)*

Vernacular Name: *Eng:* Common grape-vine, Wine grape, European grape; *Hin:* Dakh, Drakh; *Kan:* Draksa; *Mal:* Muntiri; *San:* Draksa, Mrdvika; *Tam:* Kotumuntiri, Tiratcai; *Tel:* Draksa.

Description: A large, deciduous tendril climber, tendrils leaf-opposed, often bifid; leaves simple, more or less deeply 3-5 lobed, orbicular-cordate, irregularly toothed, glabrescent above, grey tomentose beneath, thin, membranous; flowers small green in leaf-opposed, panicled cymes; fruits bluish black, purplish or greenish berries, ovoid to globose; seeds 2-4 with a discoidal tubercle on the back.

Habitate: Cultivated throughout India.

Propagation: By seeds and vegetative method.

Parts Used: Ripe fruits (dried), leaves, stems, flowers.

Chemical Constituents: The leaves contain thiamine, niacin, biotin, tocopherol, Hulme, hexokinase, catalase, ascorbic acid oxidase, perosidase, polyphenol oxidase, ascorbic acid oxidase, peroxidase and polyphenol oxidase.

Uses: The fruits are sweet, refrigerant, laxative, emollient, intellect promoting, cardiotonic, haematinic, haemostatic, diuretic, aphrodisiac, rejuvenating, nervine tonic, febrifuge, depurative, antispasmodic, digestive, stomachic, suppurative, expectorant and tonic. They are useful in vitiated conditions of *pitta* and *kapha*, burning sensation, dipsia, contipation, amentia, cardiac debility, haemoptysis, haemorrhages, anaemia, strangury, emaciation, fever, leprosy, skin diseases, dyspepsia, colic, flatulence, cough, asthma, bronchitis. opthalmopathy, pharyngopathy, jaundice and general debility. The leaves are astringent, anodyne, diuretic and depurative, and are useful in cephalalgia, strangury, scabies, skin diseases, syphilis, haemorrhoids, splenomegaly, vomiting and stomatorrhagia. The ash of the stem is good for arthralgia, vesical calculi, haemorrhoids and orchitis. The flowers are expectorant, emmenagogue and haematinic, and are useful in bronchitis, hepatopathy, anaemia, amenorrhoea and dysmenorrhoea.

1325. *Wedelia calendulacea* Less. *(Asteraceae)*

Synonyms: *Wedelia chinensis* Merrill.

Vernacular Name: *San:* Bhringaraja, kesaraja, putabhringi; *Hin:* Bhanra, bhangra, pila-bhangra; *Beng*: Bhimra, kesraj; *Tam:* Postaley-kaiantageerai, potralai kaindha-keerai, manjal karisalan kanni; *Kan:* Kaesarji, gargari and *Mal:* Aswagandhi.

Description: Prostrate perennial herb with erect stems, 20–40 cm. High. Leaves opposite, subsessile, coarsely toothed, with coarse haris on both side. Infloreescence in axillary and terminal solitary head on long stalk; flowers yellow, the outer linear and the inner tubular. The fruit is an achene. All parts of the herb have an almond–oil odour when crushed.

Habitate: Grows wild in wet places and is cultivate.

Propagation: By seeds.

Part Used: Whole plant.

Chemical Constituents: The whole plant contains tannin, saponins, carotene, isoflavonoids and wedelolactone.

Uses: The whole plant, except for the roots, is well known for its antibacterial, demulcent and antiferbrile properties. It is indicated in the treatment of phelegmon, boils, impetigo, mastitis, abscesses, cystitis, cold and eruptive fever. A decoction of the fresh plant is used for bathing babies to prevent lichen tropicus.

1326. *Wedelia chinensis* (Osbeck) Merrill *(Asteraceae)*

Synonyms: *Wedelia calendulacea* Less.

Vernacular Name: *Hin:* Pilabhamgara; *Kan:* Kalsarji, Gargari; *Mal:* Mannakkannunni; *San:* Pitabhrngarajah, itabhrnga; *Tam:* Manjalkarilamkanni, Patalai, Kayyantakarai; *Tel:* Guntagalagara.

Description: A procumbent perennial herb upto 1 m in height with stems rooting at the lower nodes; leaves simple, opposite, subsessile, linear-oblong, oblanceolate, scabrous with short white hairs; flowers yellow in tetragonous rayed axillary or terminal heads;

fruits truncate, compressed or tubercled achenes without papus or with a ring of round scales.

Habitate: Throughout India, in wet places and coastal areas.

Propagation: By seeds.

Parts Used: Whole plant.

Chemical Constituents: Lactone, benzofuran-3-carboxylic acid, norwedelic acid, carotene; demethyl, wedelolactone, wedelolactone; stigmasterol and its glucoside, tannin from the herb.

Uses: The plant is astringent, bitter, acrid, thermogenic, anti-inflammatory, vulnerary, ophthalmic, cardiotonic, anthelmintic, diuretic, aphrodisiac, sudorific, febrifuge and trichogenous, and is useful in vitiated conditions of *kapha* and *vata*, inflammation, elephantiasis, otalgia, cephalalgia, wounds, ulcers, nyctalopia, dysopia, hepatosplenomegaly, colic, dyspepsia, helminthiasis, strangury, anaemia, seminal weakness, fever, baldness and greyness of hair. The plant is very specific for 'viral hepatitis'.

1327. *Wikstroemia indica* (L.) C.A. Mey. *(Thymelaeaceae)*

Synonyms: *Wikstroemia viridiflora* Meissn.

Vernacular Name: *Eng:* Small-leaf salago.

Description: Bushy shrub. Stems and branches at first downy, then glabrous, bearing scars of fallen leaves. Leaves subsessile, alternate or opposite, coriaceous, glabrous, dark green above, pale beneath. Inflorescence in terminal fascicle; flowers greenish-yellwo. Drupe ovoid, scarlet when ripe.

Habitate: Grows wild in mountainous regions.

Propagation: By seeds.

Part Used: Leaves and bark.

Uses: The leaves are particularly suitable for external use in poultices against furunculosis and phlegmon. They are crushed and mixed with poeanut oil to alleviate their irritant action. They can be also used as an insecticide in agriculture. Bark vesicant, purgative, and piscicidal, used for schistosomiasis. Fibre used for ropes. Bark used for the manufacture of high grade paper.

1328. *Withania somnifera* (L.) Dunal *(Solanaceae)*

Vernacular Name: *Eng:* Winter cherry; *Hin:* Asgandh, Punir; *Kan:* Viremaddinagaddi, Kiremallinagida; *Mal:* Amukkuram; *San:* Asvagandha, Varahakarni; *Tam:* Amukkira, Amukkirakkilangu; *Tel:* Vajigandha, Pannirugadda, Pulivendramu.

Description: An erect branching undershurb reaching about 150 cm in height usually clothed with minutely stellate tomentum; leaves ovate upto 10cm long; flowers greenish or lurid yellow in axillary fascicles; fruits globose berries which are orange coloured when mature enclosed in a persistent calyx. The fleshy roots when dry are cylindrical, gradually tapering down with a brownish white surface and pure white inside when broken.

Habitate: Throughout the drier parts of India, in waste places also cultivated.

Propagation: By seeds.

Parts Used: Roots, leaves.

Chemical Constituents: Roots contain several pyrazole alkaloids. Withasomnine and steroldal lactones, withaferin A and withanolides. They also contain starch, reducing sugars, hentriacontane, glycosides, dulcitol, withaniol, an acid and a neutral compound. Withaferin is a bacteriostatic and antitumerous agent.

Uses: The tuberous roots are astringent, bitter, acrid, somniferous, thermogenic, stimulant, aphrodisiac, diuretic and tonic. They are useful in vitiated conditions of *vata*, leucoderma, constipation, insomnia, tissue-building and nervous breakwdown. The leaves are bitter and are recommended in fever, painful swellings and ophthalmitis. A paste of the roots and bruised leaves are applied to carbuncles, ulcers and painful swellings.

1329. *Wollastonia biflora* (L.) DC. *(Asteraceae)*

Synonyms: *Wedelia biflora* (L.) DC.

Vernacular Name: Beach sunflower, wedelia.

Description: Coarse, branching, trailing to erect herbaceous subshrub up to 3 m high. Leaves opposite, blade ovate, more or less palmately veined and 8-20 cm in length on a petiole half as long. Flowers borne in dense sunflower-like heads in terminal clusters; the yellow florets are numerous, fruiting heads are subglobose, brown and 8-15 mm wide containing many dry, single seeded, wedge-shaped, black fruits (achenes), each about 2 mm long. Flowers and fruit available throughout the year.

Habitate: Common in littoral and coastal areas, forest margins, margins of mangroves, roadsides, waste places from sea-level to 500 m elevation.

Propagation: By seeds.

Part Used: Leaves and stems.

Chemical Constituents: Esential oil, kaurene diterpenoids.

Uses: The leaves from which they squeeze out the juice and apply to cuts and wounds to prevent tetanus. An infusion of the stem bark or leaves is ingested to treat gonorrhoea and urinary tract infections.

1330. *Woodfordia fruticosa* (L.) Kurz *(Lythraceae)*

Synonyms: *Woodfordia floribunda* Salisb.

Vernacular Name: *San:* Dhataki, Madaniyahetu; *Eng:* Fire-flame bush, Shiranjitea, Woodfordia; *Hin:* Davi, Tavi, Dhay; *Kan:* Bela, Tamrapuspi; *Mal:* Tatiri, Tatirippu; *Tam:* Dhattari, Jargi, Velakkai; *Tel:* Dhataki, Jargi, Serinji.

Description: A much branched, beautiful deciduous shrub, attaining a height of about 3-7 m with many long arching branches and reddish brown bark; leaves simple, opposite, entire, ovate-lanceolate, acute, subcoriaceous, with black glandular dots on the undersurface; flowers numberous, brilliant red in dense, axillary paniculate-cymoseclusters; fruits ellipsoid, irregularly dehiscent capsules about 1 cm long; seeds obovoid, smooth, brown.

Habitate: Throughout India, but more abundant in north India upto 1600m.

Propagation: By seeds and vegetative method.

Parts Used: Flowers.

Chemical Constituents: Extract of flowers possessed significant abortifiacient activity in mice. Flowers contain ellagic acid, β-sitosterol polystachoside, octacosanol, myricetin-3-galactoside, cyaniding-3, 5-diglucoside, pelargonidin-3,5-diglucoside, chrysophanol–8-O-B-D-glucopyranoside.

Uses: The flowers are astringent, acrid, refrigerant, stimulant, depurative, styptic, uterine sedative, anthelmintic, constipating, antibacterial, vulnerary, corrective of urinary pigments, alexeteric and febrifuge. They are useful in vitiated conditions of *kapha* and *pitta*, leprosy, skin diseases, burning sensation, haemorrhages, menorrhagia, leucorrhoea, haemoptysis, erysipelas, diarrhoea, dysentery, foul ulcers, diabetes, bilious fever, hepatopathy and verminosis.They are an important ingredient in Aristam and Asavam as they aid in fermentation; they are also highly valued as a stimulant in pregnancy.

1331. *Wrightia tinctoria* (Roxb.) R.Br. *(Apcynaceae)*

Vernacular Name: *Eng:* Pala indigo plant; *Hin:* Mitaindrajau, Dudhi; *Kan:* Kirikodasige, Bepalli, Kodamurki; *Mal:* Dantappala, Ayyappala, Tinnampala; *San:* Svetakutajah; *Tam:* Tontampalai, Veppalai; *Tel:* Jeddapala, Tedlapala.

Description: A small deciduous tree, upto 10m in height with pale grey, smooth, thin bark abounding in yellow milky juice with opposite divaricate branches; leaves simple, opposite, elliptic-ovate or obovate oblong, acuminate, glabrous, main nerves 6-12 pairs; flowers white, frangrant, in lax teminal cymes; fruits follicles in pairs, pendulous, cylindrical, tips adhering at first; seeds linear, pointed at the apex with a deciduous coma.

Habitate: Throughout India, upto 1200m.

Propagation: By seeds.

Parts Used: Leaves, bark, seeds.

Chemical Constituents: Indican. Seeds yield 30-49 % fixed oil. β-Sitosterol, β-amyrin and its acentate and lupeol benzoate from the bark.

Uses: The leaves are acrid, thermogenic, anodyne and hypotensive, and are useful in odontalgia, vitiated conditions of *vata* and hypertension. The bark and seeds are bitter, astringent, acrid, thermogenic, carminative, digestive, stomachic, constipating, depurative, anthelmintic, aphrodisiac and febrifuge. They are useful in vitiated conditions of *pitta* and *kapha*, dyspepsia, flatulence, colic, diarrhoea, leprosy, psoriasis, haemorrhoids, dipsia, helminthiasis, fever, burning sensation and dropsy. The latex of the bark and unripe fruits are used by hill tribes for coagulating and solidifying milk.

1332. *Xanthium strumarium* L. *(Asteraceae (Asteraceae))*

Vernacular Name: *San:* Arishta; *Eng:* Ditch bur, louse-bur, broad cocklebur; *Hin:* Banokra, gokhru, chota-gokhru, chota-dhatura, adhasisi; *Beng*: Banokra, chota-dhatura; *Tel:* Marulamathangi; *Tam:* Maruloomatham and *Kan:* Maruluummatti.

Description: An erect, tall, coarse, unarmed weed with triangular, cordate or sub-orbicular, often three-lobed, irregulary toothed, scabrid or hispid leaves. Flowers numerous, white or green in terminal and axillary racemes with both male and female flowers on the same plant; male heads upper most, globose, about 0.75 cm in diameter. Female heads ovoid, 1.25 cm long with hooked bristles. Achenes obovoid, thick, enclosed in the hardened, involucral bracts and clothed with strong hooked spines.

Habitate: Distributed throughout India. Widely distributed throughout the world in tropical and temperate region. Found as a weed in Himachal Pradesh in all part upto 2500 m elevation.

Propagation: By seeds.

Part Used: Roots, leaves and fruits, seed oil.

Chemical Constituents: The aerial parts of the plant contain a mixture of alkaloids which are said to be toxic i.e. the sesquiterpene lactones-xanthinin. The sterioisomers-xanthinim and xanthatin. The seeds on solvent extraction yield 30-35% of semidrying oil, resembling sunflower oil. It has the same taste as other vegetable oils.

Uses: The herb is reputed as a medicine in Europe, China, Indo-Chine, Malaysia and America. The drug is credited with powerful diaphoretic properties. The does of half to one ounce is recommended in chronic malaria, leucorrhoea and urinary diseases. It is also useful as a styptic and is considered a prophylactic against hydrophobia. In clinical experiments, its pollens have been found to cause asthma and rhinitis; also produce dermatitis in senstitive/susceptible persons especially during autumn when the plant is in pre-fruiting stage. The leaves are given internally in scrofula and herpes in powder form. The root is bitter tonic, useful in cancer and scrofula. Its extract is used locally over ulcers, boils and abscesses. The fruits are used as tonic, diuretic, diaphoretic, sedative, cooling and demulcent and are also given in small-pox. The seeds are used for resolving inflammatory swellings. The herb is reported to be used in snake bite also.

1333. *Xylocarpus granatum* Koenig. *(Meliaceae)*

Synonyms: *Carapa granatum* (Koening) Alston.

Vernacular Name: *Eng:* Puzzlenut tree; *Hin:* Pussur; *Beng*: Pussur; *Tam:* Kandalangay.

Description: Spreading tree upto 15 m high. Leaves alternate, pinnately compound with usually 4 oblong leaflets 6-14 cm long. Flowers greenish-white, the flowers borne in axillary or cauliflorus panicles. Fruit a large, green to light brownish, pendulous, subglobose capsule with several irregularly shaped seeds.

Habitate: Common in littoral forest, inner margins of mangrove swamps, lowland river banks, coastal thickets and rocky coasts.

Propagation: By seeds.

Part Used: Bark.

Chemical Constituents: Acetonyl-dihydrochelerythrine, xylomollin,N-methylfindersin, fructose, gedunin, glucose, mexicanolide, 7-alphaacetoxy dihydronomilin, sucrose, tannins, limonoids (xyloccenisins) xylomollin (monoterpene).

Uses: Used as a remedy for blood in the urine, weakness after childbirth, relapsed weakness, fever and high fever accompanied by a "black furry tongue". Also used as an anti-diarrhetic. A decoction of the bark is taken for stomachache, coughs and internal injuries, which have filed to heal. Also use the plant to treat peptic ulcer.

1334. *Zanonia indica* (Linn.) *(Cucurbitaceae)*

Vernacular Name: *Hin:* Cirpoti; *Kan:* Kuntali; *Mal:* Pinarvalli; *San:* Cirpota, Parpoti; *Tam:* Pinarvalli; *Tel:* Dirga patramu.

Description: A stout climbing shrub, upto 15 m in height with cylindric woody stem and glabrous tendrils; leaves petiolate, ovate-oblong, coriaceous, entire, acute, bright green, glabrous, 3-nerved from a rounded or slightly cordate base; male flowers greenish yellow in racemes or panicles, female flowers in racemes; fruits cylindric obconic, pale yellowish or brown apsules, slightly tapering towards the base; seeds winged, much compressed pale yellow, smooth.

Habitate: Throughout India, in forests.

Propagation: By seeds.

Parts Used: Leaves, fruits.

Chemical Constituents: N.A.

Uses: The leaves are anti-inflammatory and antispasmodic, and are useful in nervous irritation due to boils, inflammations and spamodic affections. The fruits are cooling, purgative, expectorant and antiseptic. They are useful in vitiated conditions of *pitta*, constipation, cough, asthma, cuts, wounds and ulcers.

1335. *Zanthoxylum americanum* *(Rutaceae)*

Vernacular Name: *Eng:* Prickly Ash, Toothache tree.

Description: A deciduous shrub growing to 3m, with thorny grey branches and compound leaves.

Habitate: Prickly ash is native to southern Canada and northern, central and western parts of the US, preferring moist, shady sites such as woodlands.

Propagation: By seeds.

Parts Used: Bark and berries.

Chemical Constituents: Alkaloids, Herclavin, Lignans, Neolherculin, Tannins, Resins, Volatile oil.

Uses: Circulatory stimulant, increases sweating, Antirheumatic, Carminative.

1336. *Zanthoxylum armatum* DC. *(Rutaceae)*

Synonyms: *Zanthoxylum alatum* Roxb.

Vernacular Name: *Eng:* Toothache tree; *Hin:* Tumru, Tejphal; *Kan:* Tumburudu, Dhiva; *Mal:* Tumpunal, Tumpuni; *San:* Tumburuh; *Tam:* Tumpunalu; *Tel:* Gandhalu.

Description: An armed shrub or a small tree, upto 6 m in height with dense glabrous foliage and straight pickles on stmes, blaze yellowish brown rapidly darkening on exposure; leaves compound, imparipinnate, rachis winged, often bearing pink prickles, leaflets 5-11, lanceolate, more or less serrate, each serrature with a pellucid gland, glabous, dark glossy green above, pale beneath, the terminal larger than the laterals; flowers yellow or gree in dense terminal or axillary panicles, polygamous; fruits reddish subglobose glabrous follicles; seeds solitary, globose, shining, black.

Habitate: In the Himalayas upto 2100 m and in Andhra Pradesh upto 1350 m.

Propagation: By seeds.

Parts Used: Bark, fruits.

Chemical Constituents: It contains Pipevine, linalool, linalyl acetate, citral, cinnamatic, limonene, sabinene.

Uses: The bark and fruits are acrid, bitter, aromatic, deodorant, antiseptic, stimulant, digestive, carminative, stomachic, anthelmintic, liver tonic, diuretic, constipating, sudorific, febrifuge, depurative and tonic. They are useful in vitiated conditions of *kapha* and *vata*, tumours odontalagia, cephalalgia, otopathy, ophthalmopathy, dyspepsia, colic, flatulence, helminthiasis, diarrhoea, hepatopathy, splenopathy, strangury, fever, leucoderma leprosy, skin diseases, cough, asthma, paralysis, gout, convulsions, diabetes, wounds ulcers, stomatopathy, pharyngopathy, cardiac debility and general debility.

1337. *Zanthoxylum nitidum* (Roxb.) DC. *(Rutaceae)*

Synonyms: *Zanthoxylum hamiltonianum* Wall. ex. Hook.f.

Vernacular Name: *Assam*: Tezamul, tejmoi, baghanchora, tejmuri.

Description: Climbing shrub, prickly. Branches spreading, with pale brown bark and scattered lenticles. Leaves alternate, imparipinnate; leaflets 5, entire, prickly on main nerve and petiole, inflorescence in axillary raceme; flowers small, white, unisexual. Fruit of 1-5 carpels. Seeds shining black.

Habitate: Found wild in mountainous regions.

Propagation: By seeds and vegetative method.

Part Used: Root, bark and fruits.

Chemical Constituents: Nitidin, flavoneglycoside, linalool, methyl cinnamate.

Uses: The fruit is used for treating dyspesis, cough, colic vomiting, diarrhoea, toothache, paresis, rheumatism and ascariasis. The roots are used for treating fever, paresis and rheumatism. The fruit is also used as a spice. Topical application of an alcoholic maceration of the fruit is effective against toothache. A powder made from the fruit is used to tret snake-bite.

1338. *Zanthoxylum piperitum* DC. *(Rutaceae)*

Vernacular Name: *Eng:* Japan pepper.

Description: Deciduous, small, compact tree or shrub with aromatic bark, to 3 m tall. Branchlets with paired spines at base of leaves. Leaves alternate, odd-pinnate, to 15 cm long; leaflets 9-19, broad-lanceolate to ovate, 1-3.5 cm long, obtusely toothed, glandular-dotted. Inflorescence paniculate-cymose, terminal on short branchlets. Flowers greenish yellow, small, unisexual; calyx 5-lobed, small, imbricate, stamens 5; carpels free. Fruit a 2-valved follicle.

Habitate: Thickets and woods in hills and mountains in Korea Japan and China.

Propagation: By seeds.

Parts Used: Fruit.

Chemical Constituents: Essential oil: dipentene, citronellal, B-phellandrene, geraniol, citronellol, citral. Acid amides: a-sanshools, sanshoamide. Flavonoids: quercitrin, afzelin, hesperidin. Isoquinoline alkaloids.

Uses: Anthelmintic antifungal, CNS toxic (xanthotoxin). Prostaglandin synthesis inhibition, nematocidal, antibacterial.

1339. *Zea mays* L. *(Poaceae)*

Vernacular Name: *Eng:* Maixe, Indian corn; *Hin:* Makai, makka, bhutta, junri, kukri, bara-jowar; *Beng*: Janar, bhutta, jonar; *Tel:* Mokka-janna, makka jonnalu; *Tam:* Makka-cholam; *Kan:* Mekkejola, musukojola, goinjol; *Mal:* Cholam.

Description: Robust annual herbaceous plant, 1-2m. tall. Leaves strap-shaped, distichous. Margins ciliate, wavy. Flowers unisexual, both sexes on the same plant; the male in a terminal spike, the febale closely crowded in the axil of the leaves, enclosed in numerous large foliaceous bracts; style silky, elongate, the fruit is a caryopsis.

Habitate: Cultivated everywhere.

Propagation: By seeds.

Part Used: Styles with stigmas.

Chemical Constituents: The styles contain potassium salts. The grains contain starch, flucose, fructose, sucrose, raffinose, ftty compounds, vitamins E, C. K, B-carotene.

Uses: Maize silk (styles with stigmas), is used as a diuretic in the treatment of heart disease, hypertension, cystitis, urethritis, urinary lithiasis, cholecystitis, hepatitis, rheumatism and diabetes mellitus. It is also used in combination with vitamin K as a haemostatic.

1340. *Zehneria umbellate* Thw. *(Cucurbitaceae)*

Synonyms: *Solena amplexicaulis* (Lam.) Gandhi; *Solena heterophylla* (Lour.) Cogn.; *Melothria heterophylla* (Lour.) Cogn.

Vernacular Name: *Hin*: Tarali; *Tam:* Pulivanji; *Beng*: Kudri.

Description: Scandant climber. Leaf coriaceous, ovate, suborbicular, variously lobed. Tendrils simple. Male flowers various. Calyx tube campanulate. Corolla lobes spreading. Anthers suborbicular. Female flowers solitary or with axillary male flowers. Fruits oblong-ovoid, bright red and when ripe, pulpy. Seeds many, grey, subspherical, turgid, smooth.

Habitate: In thickets and hedges almost throughout India.

Propagation: By seeds.

Parts Used: Leaves and root.

Chemical Constituents: Linoleic, linolenic and oleic acids (seeds); columbin in the root.

Uses: Leaves soothing, the juice finds local application in skin inflammation caused by marking nut juice; ***root:*** invigorating, purgative, stimulant; useful in dysuria and spermatorrhoea.

1341. *Zingiber officinale* Rosc. *(Zingibeaceae)*

Vernacular Name: *Eng:* Ginger; *Hin:* Adarak; *Kan:* Haisunti, Ardraka; *Mal:* Inci, Erukkilannu; *San:* Ardrakam; *Tam:* Inci; *Tel:* Allamu, Ardrakamu.

Description: A slender, perennial rhizomatous herb; leaves linear, sessile, glabrous; flowers yellowish green in oblong, cylindric spikes, ensheathed in a few scarious, glabrous bracts; fruits oblong capsules. The rhizomes are white to yellowish brown in colour, irregularly branched, somewhat annualated and laterally flattened. The growing tips are covered over by a few scales. The surface of the rhizome is smooth and if broken a fewfibrous elements of the vascular bundles project out from the cut ends.

Habitate: Cultivated throughout India, run wild in some place in the Western ghats.

Propagation: By rhizomes.

Parts Used: Rhizomes (raw as well as dry).

Chemical Constituents: α-Curcumene, α-curcumene, β-D-curcumene; α-bergamotene, β-and camphene, γ-bisabolene, β-bourbornene, d-borneol and its acetate, calamene, d-camphene, car-3-ene, α-cedrol, citral, citronellol.

Uses: The raw ginger is acrid, thermogenic, carminative, laxative and digestive. It is useful in anorexia, vitiated conditions of *vata* and *kapha*, dyspepsia, pharyngopathy and inflammations. The dry ginger is acrid, thermogenic, emollient, appetiser, laxative, stomachic, stimulant, rubefacient, anodyne, aphrodisiac, expectorant, anthelmintic and carminative. It is useful in dropsy, otalgia, cephalalgia, asthma, cough, colic, diarrhoea, flatulence, anorexia, vitiated conditions of *vata* and *kapha*, dyspepsia, cardiopathy, pharyngopathy, cholera, nausea, vomiting, elephantiasis and inflammations. It is also much used in several domestic preparations.

1342. *Zingiber zerumbet* Rosc. ex. Sm. *(Zingiberaceae)*

Synonyms: *Amomum zerumbet* Linn.

Vernacular Name: *San:* Karpooraharidra; *Eng:* Wild ginger; *Hin:* Narkachur; *Beng*: Narkachur; *Tel:* Karrallamu and *Mal:* Kattinji.

Description: Erect herb to 2 m tall arising from thick yellowish aromatic underground rhizome. Leaves parallel-veined, ligulate, lanceolate, up to 30 cm long arising in 2 ranks from unbranched, fleshy aerial stems. Flowers white to yellowish, borne on a fleshy spike with each flower arising from under a green to reddish bract, the inflorescence many-flowered, but usually only 1-3 flowers open at once. Fruit small capsule with tiny seeds. Flowers December through April.

Habitate: Common in moist forests, beach thickets, mangrove margins from sea-level to over 500 m.

Propagation: By rhizome.

Part Used: Rhizome.

Chemical Constituents: Alkaloids; camphene, camphor and other monoterpenoids; gingerol, zingeberol, zingerone, sesqui-terpenoids including zerumbone and zerumbone epoxide, oxalic acid, kaempferol derivatives, and flabonoids such as afzelin, flavonoid glycosides, essential oils, chlorgenic acid, ferulic acid.

Uses: To treat fish poisoning. It is used as a cough remedy and to treat the bacterial disease, thrush, and diabetes. The rhizome is used as stimulant, antihypertensive, carminative and flavouring agent; to treat dyspepsia wounds, haemorrhoids and flatulent colic for the cure of stomach trubles and fever. Used in peptic ulcers and related stomach problems as well as mouth infections.

1343. *Ziziphus jujuba* Mill. *(Rhamnaceae)*

Vernacular Name: *Eng:* common jujube; Chinese date.

Description: A spiny deciduous shrub or s small tree upto 10 m high. Leaves alternate, ovate to ovoid-lanceolate, 3-7 cm long by 2-3.5 cm wide; apex slightly obtuse; base oblique; margin closely serrulate, 3-veined, inflorescence an axillary cyme; April-May. Flowers perfect, 7-8 flowers in each cluster, greenish-yellow. Drupe 1.5-5 cm long, ovate to oblong, dark reddish-brown when ripe, containing a single stone surrounded by fleshy pulp; September-October.

Habitate: Commonly cultivated in India, Japan, China, Africa, Malaysia, Afghanistan and Australia.

Propagation: By seeds and vegetative method.

Part Used: Fruit.

Chemical Constituents: Carbohydrates, fat protein, amino acids, anthocyanins from fruit, seeds and leaves. Leucocyanidin from bark. Leucopelargonidin, betulinic and ceabothic acids from wood. Rutin from leaves. Mauritines A, B, C, D, E, and F, frangufoline and amphbines B, D and F.

Uses: Poor apetiate, general fatigue; loss bowels, palpitationl insomnia; night sweats, hysteria.

1344. *Ziziphus mauritiana* Lam. *(Rhamnaceae)*

Synonyms: *Ziziphus jujuba* (Linn.) Gaertn. non Mill.

Vernacular Name: *Eng:* Indian jujube, Common jujube, Chinese date; *Hin:* Ber, Beri; *Kan:* Bore, Yalaci, Elanji; *Mal:* llanta, Lantappalam, llantappalam, Peruntutali; *San:* Badarah, Kolah, Joli; *Tam:* llantai, llantappalam; *Tel:* Gangaregu, Regu.

Description: A low, much branched, thorny, dediduous tree with spreading crown, dark greyish black bark having irregular cracks and strong reddish hardwood; leaves oblong-elliptic, ovate or suborbicular, minutely serrulate or apex distinctly toothed, prominently 3-nerved; flowers greenish yellow in axillary dense fascicles or sessile or short peduncled cymes; fruits oblong, globose or ovoid drupes, turning from yellow to orange and finally red, the fleshy pulp enclosing a hard stone.

Habitate: Throughout India, in dry deciduous forests upto 1500m.

Propagation: By seeds.

Parts Used: Whole plant.

Chemical Constituents: Carbohydrates, fat protein, amino acids, anthocyanins from fruit, seeds and leaves. Leucocyanidin from bark. Leucopelargonidin, betulinic and ceabothic acids from wood. Rutin from leaves. Mauritines A, B, C, D, E, and F, frangufoline and amphbines B, D and F.

Uses: The roots are bitter, cooling anodyne and tonic and are useful in vitiated conditions of *pitta*, fever, wounds and ulcers and cephalalgia. The bark is astringent, constipating and tonic, and is useful in dysentery, diarrhoea, gingivitis and boils. The leaves are bitter, cooling, astringent, anthelmintic, diaphoretic antipyretic, and are useful in stomatitis, ulorrhea, wounds syphilitic ulcers, asthma, typhoid fever, diarrhoea and obesity. The fruits are sweet, cooling, anodyne purgative, mucilanginous, pectoral, styptic, aphrodisiac, invigorating, depurative, appetiser and tonic. They are useful in vitiated conditions of *pitta*, burning sensation, hyperdipsia, consumption, vomiting, constipation, flatulence, dyspepsia, nausea, leprosy, skin diseases, pruritus, wounds and ulcers, haemorrhages and general debility. The seeds are acrid, sweet, astringent, soporific and tonic. They are useful in encephalopathy, ophthalmopathy, dipsia, cough, asthma, wounds vitiated conditions of *pitta*, burning sensation, diarrhoea, vomiting, leucorrhoea, general debility and insomnia.

1345. *Ziziphus oenoplia* (L.) Mill. *(Rhamnaceae)*

Vernacular Name: *Eng:* Jackal jujube; *Hin:* Makkay; *Kan:* pargi, Barige, karisurimullu, Harasurali; *Mal:* Tutali, Ceriyalanta, Tutari; *San:* Karkandhauh; *Tam:* Suraimullu, Surai ilantai; *Tel:* paraki, Pragi, Paringi.

Description: A very thorny straggling shrub with rusty-tomentose young branches with paired prickles, one straight and the other recurved; leaves simple, alternate, distichous, ovate to ovate-lanceolate, often oblique, three prominent nerves with numberous transverse nervules; flowers green in subsessile pubescent axillary cymes; fruits globose or obovoid drupes, black, shining, pulp scnty; seeds woody or horny.

Habitate: Throughout India, in dry forests and open bushy places.

Propagation: By seeds.

Parts Used: Roots.

Chemical Constituents: The root bark contains two new cyclopeptide alkaloids, zizyphine-A and zizpyhine-B. betulinic acid, d-glucose, d-fructose, sucrose and unidentified polysaccharides. Betulinic acid.

Uses: The roots are astringent, bitter, anthelmintic, digestive and antiseptic. They are useful in hyperacidity, ascaris infection, stomachalgia and healing of wounds.

1346. *Ziziphus spinosa* Hu. *(Rhamnaceae)*

Vernacular Name: *Eng:* Spiny Chinese date.

Description: A spiny, deciduous shrub 1-3 m high, leaves alternate, elliptic or ovoid-lanceolate, 2-3.5 cm long by 0.6-1.2 cm wide. Apex obtuse; base rounded, slightly oblique; margin serrupate, 3-veined, inflorescence an axillary cyme;summer-autumn. Flowers perfect, 2-3 in each cluster. Drupe 1.0-1.5 cm long, oval, dark reddish-brown when mature. The fruit tastes sour. Seed compressed-rounded or compressed-elliptic, 5-9 cm long by 5-7 mm wide and 3 mm in thickness, purplish-red or purplish-brown, smooth and shiny.

Habitate: On dry slopes and hills and by roadsides in India, China, Korea, Mongolia.

Propagation: By seeds and vegetative method.

Part Used: Seeds.

Chemical Constituents: N.A.

Uses: Neurasthenia; insomnia; absentmindedness, palpitations, night sweats.

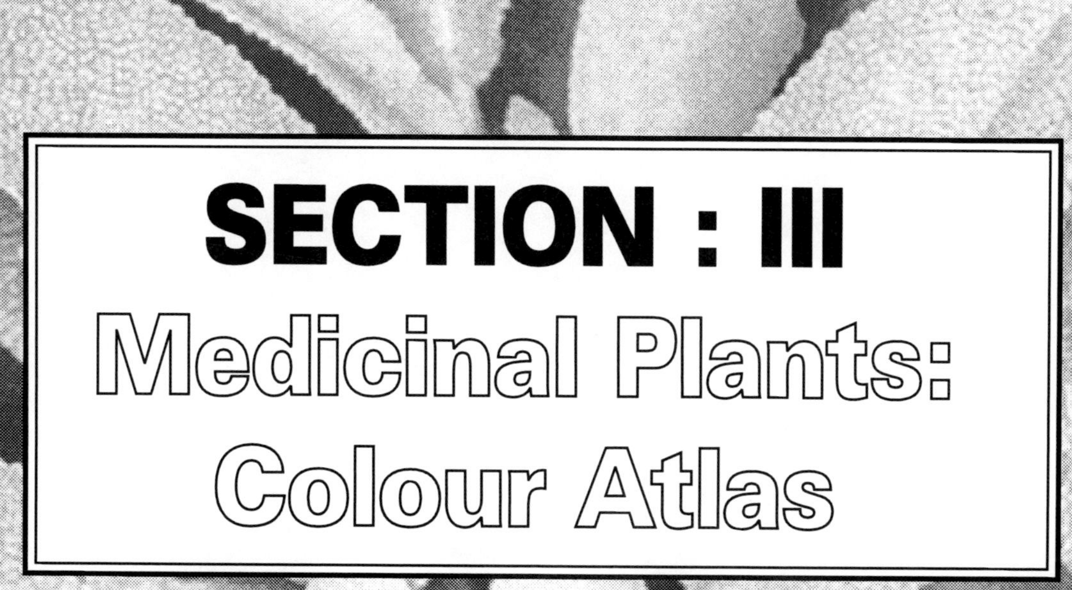

SECTION : III

Medicinal Plants: Colour Atlas

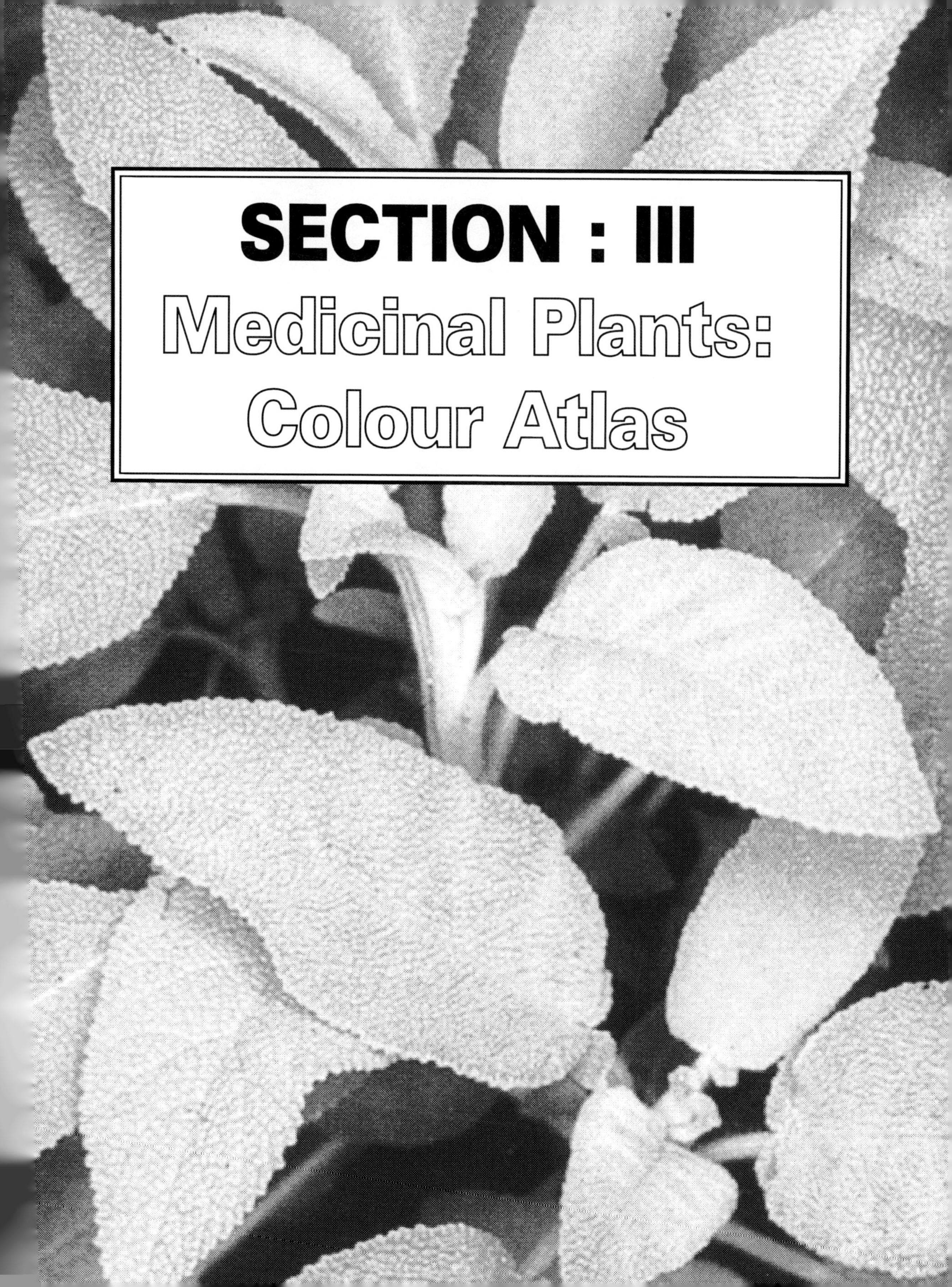

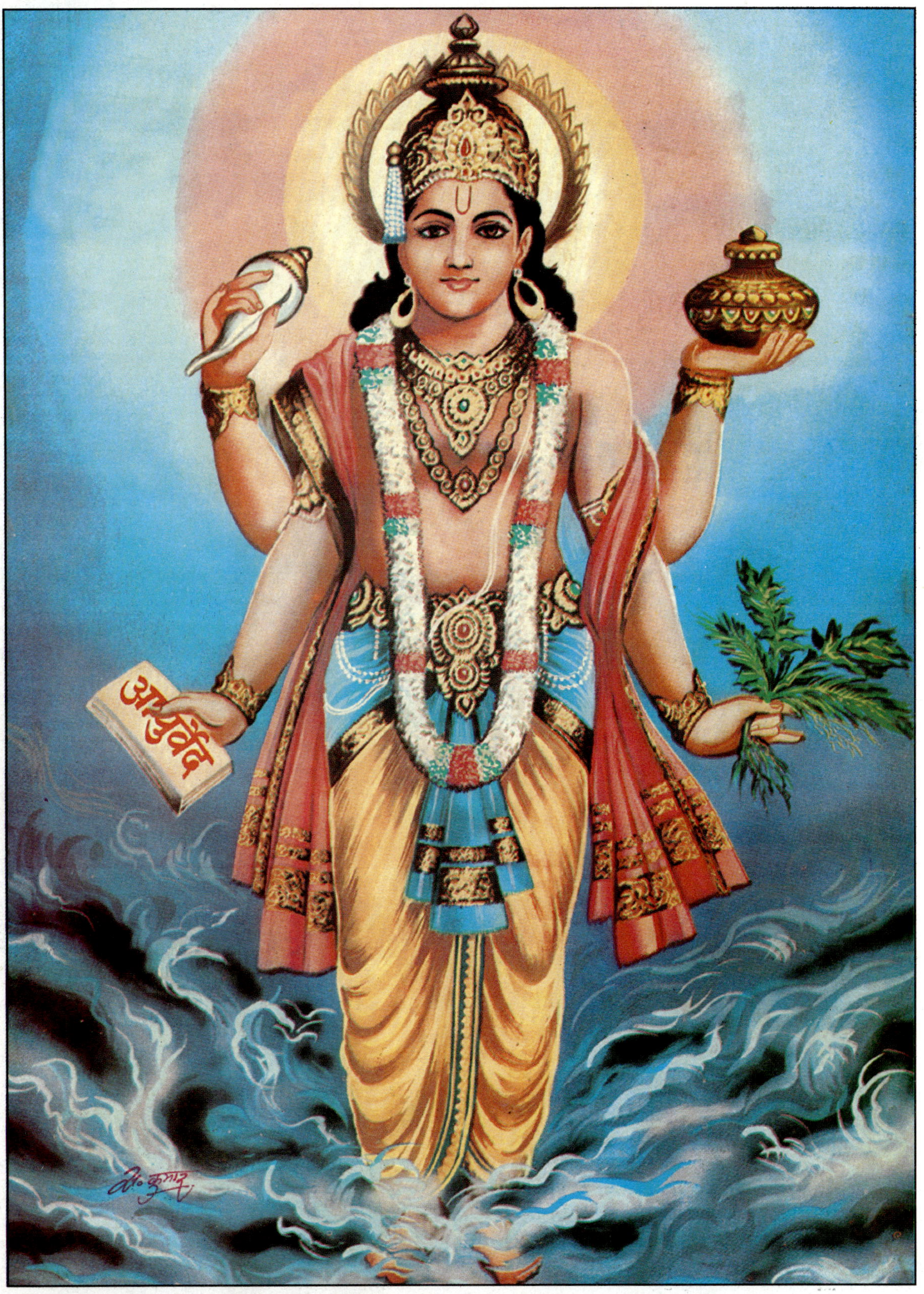
आयुर्वेद

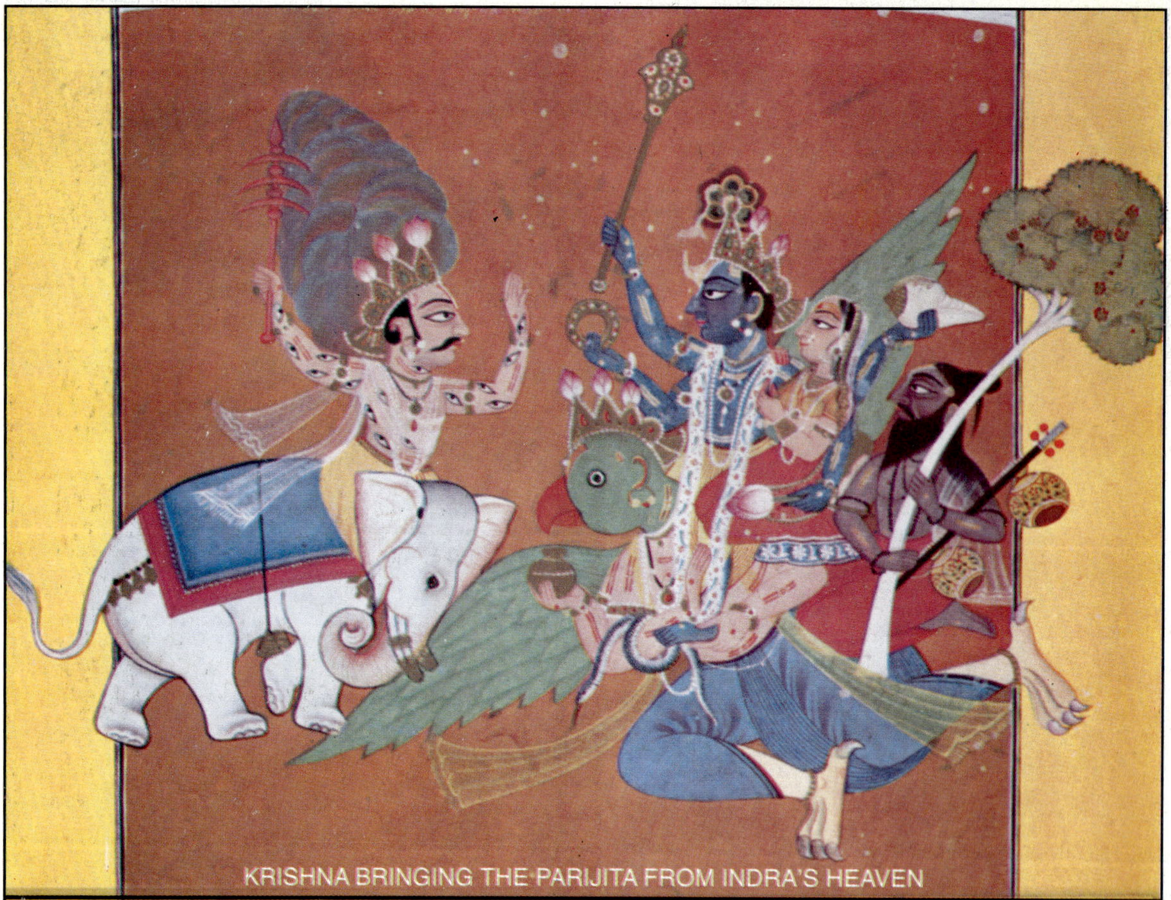

KRISHNA BRINGING THE PARIJITA FROM INDRA'S HEAVEN

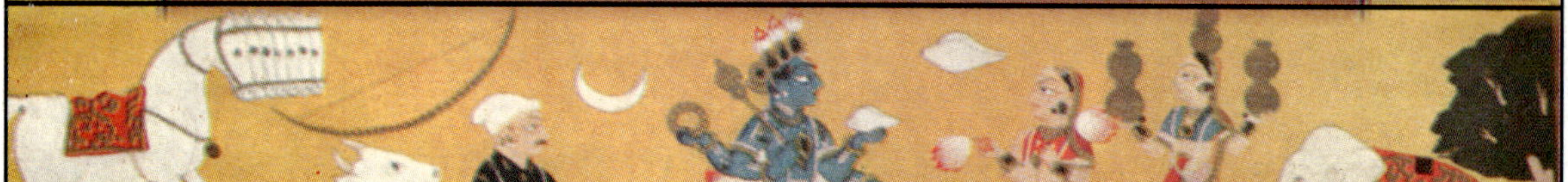

THE CHURNING OF THE OCEAN OF MILK

PLATE : 1

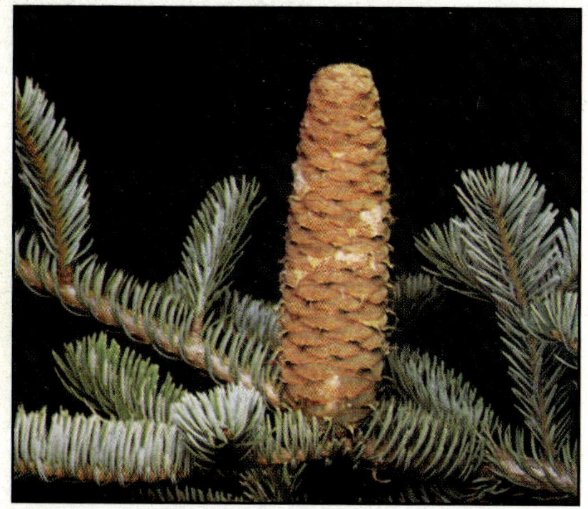

Abies alba

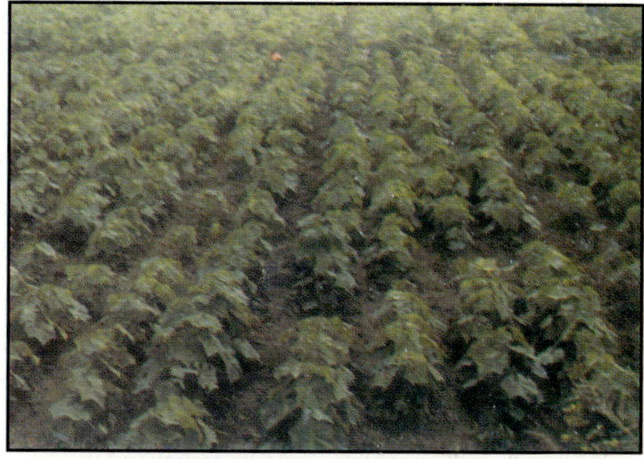

Abelmoschus moschatus

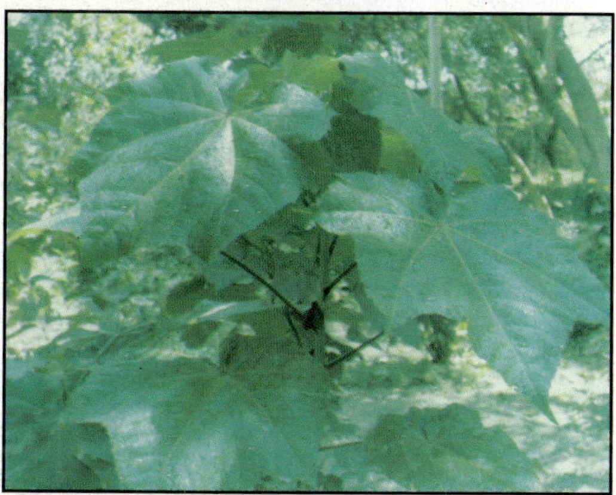

Abroama augusta

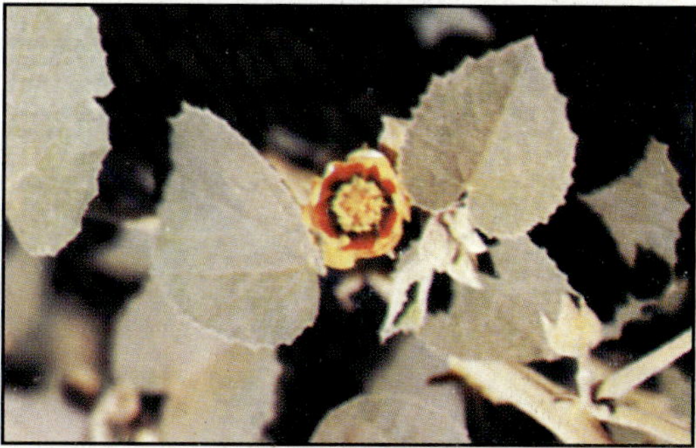

Abutilon figarianum

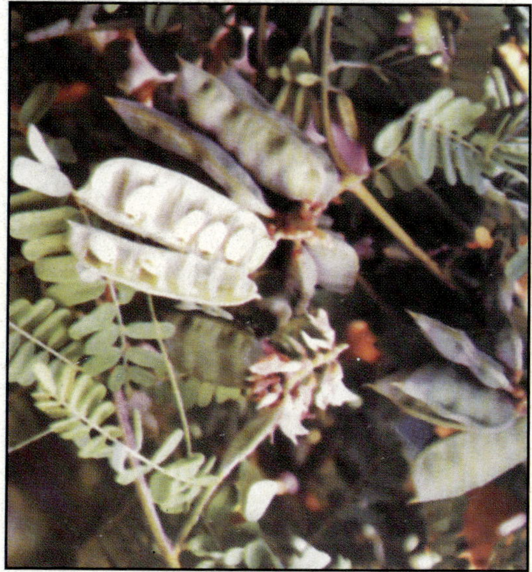

Abrus precatorius

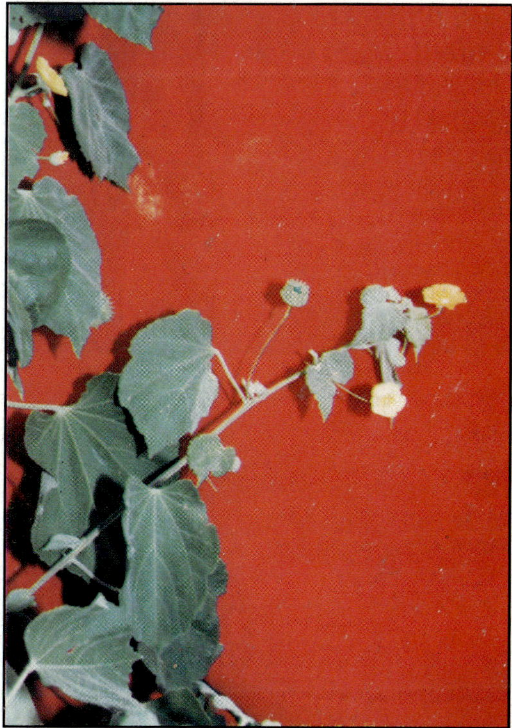

Abutilon indicum

PLATE : 2

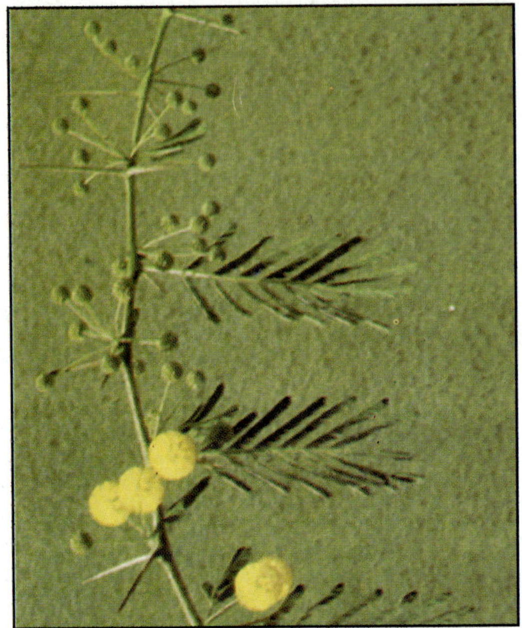

Acacia arabica

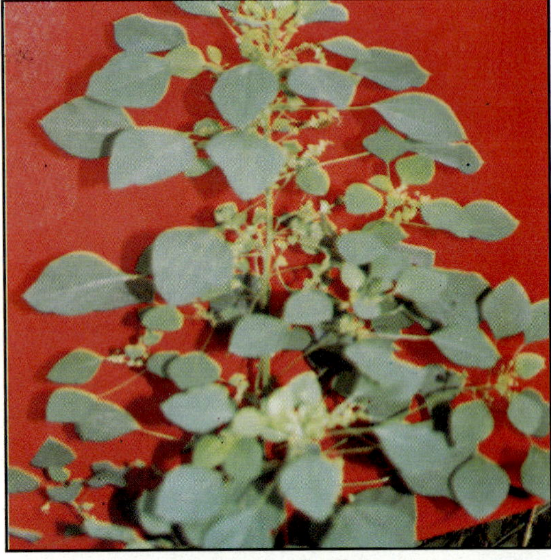

Acalypha indica

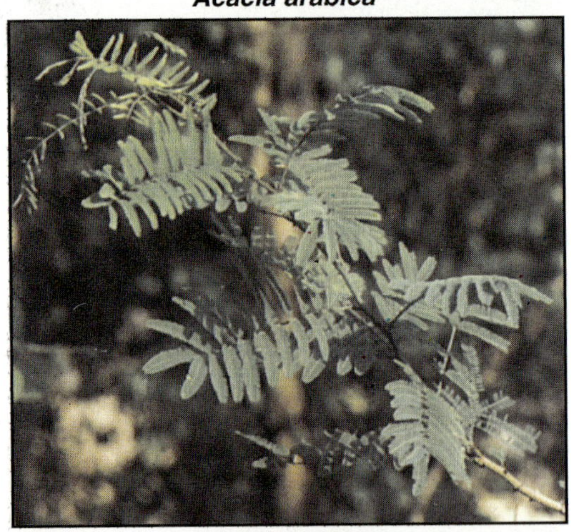

Acacia catechu

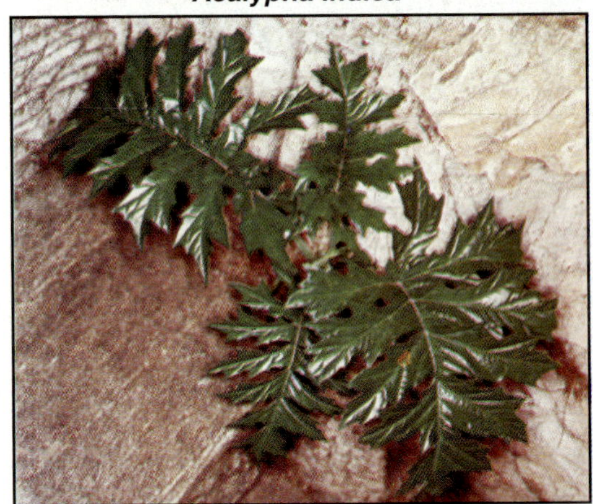

Acanthus mollis

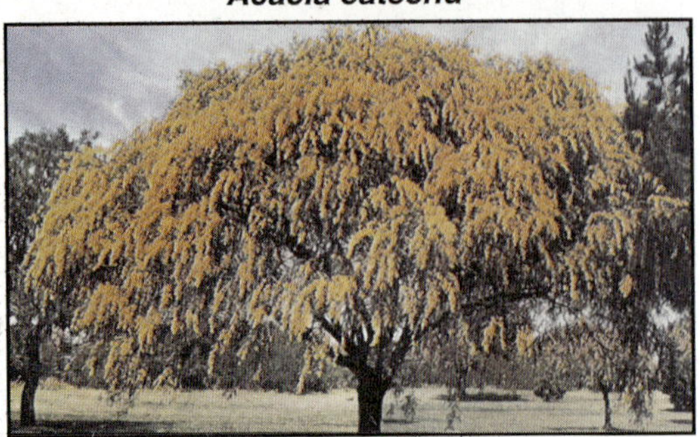

Acacia pycantha

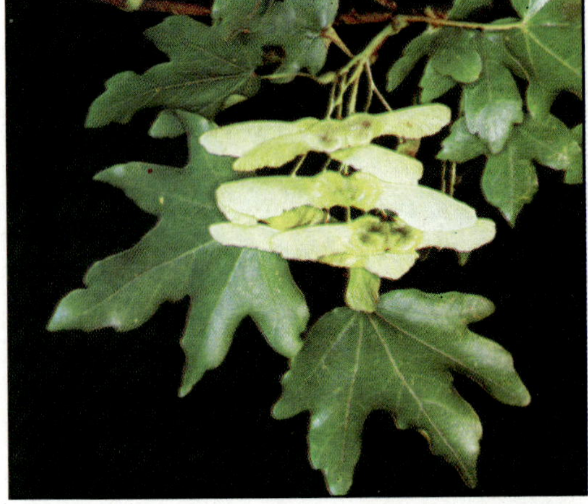

Acer campestris

PLATE : 3

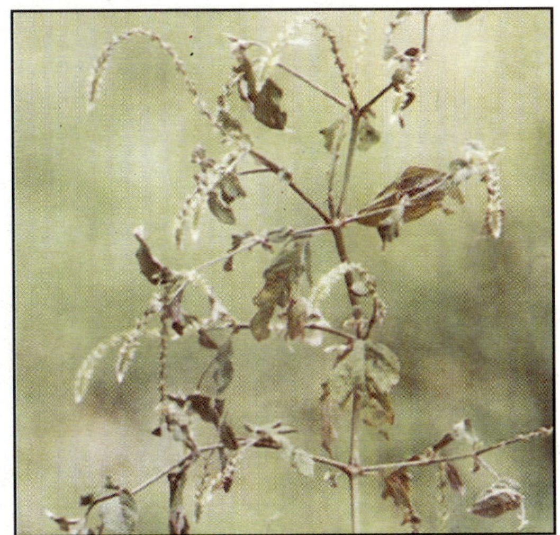

Achyranthes bidentata

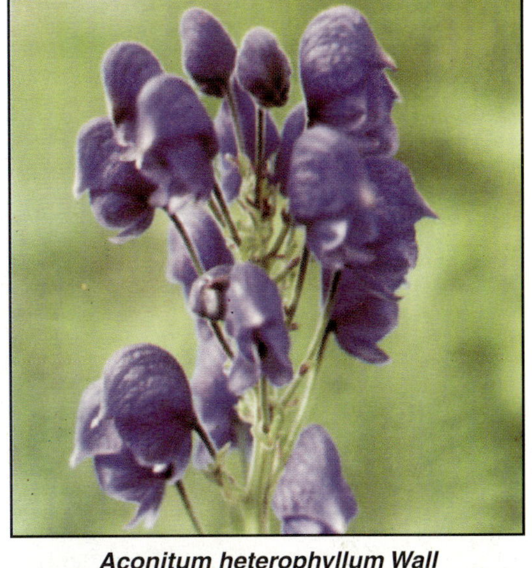

Aconitum heterophyllum Wall

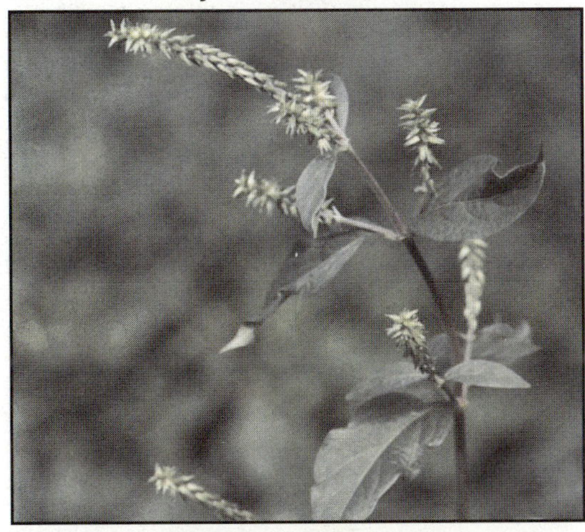

Achyranthes japonica

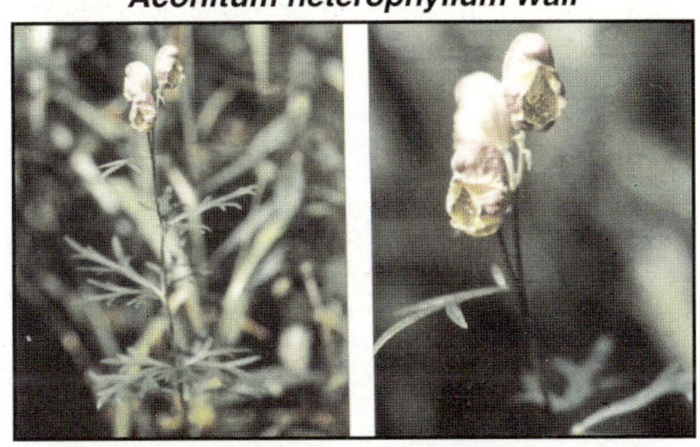

Aconitum koreanum

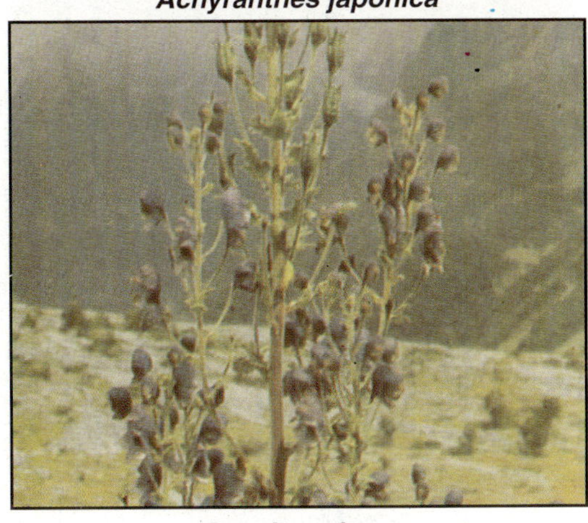

Aconitum ferox

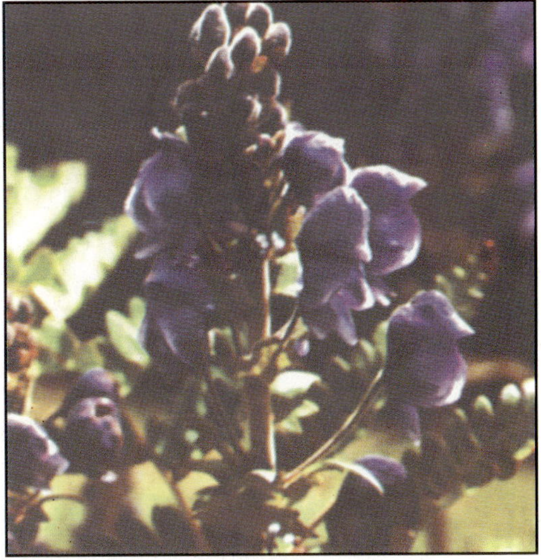

Acontium balfourii

PLATE : 4

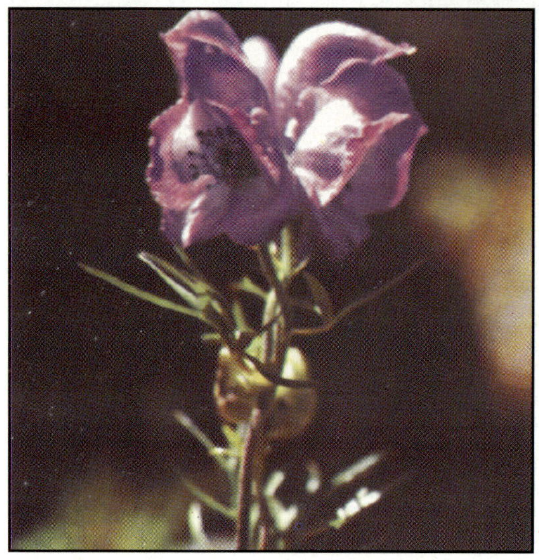

Acounitum violaceum

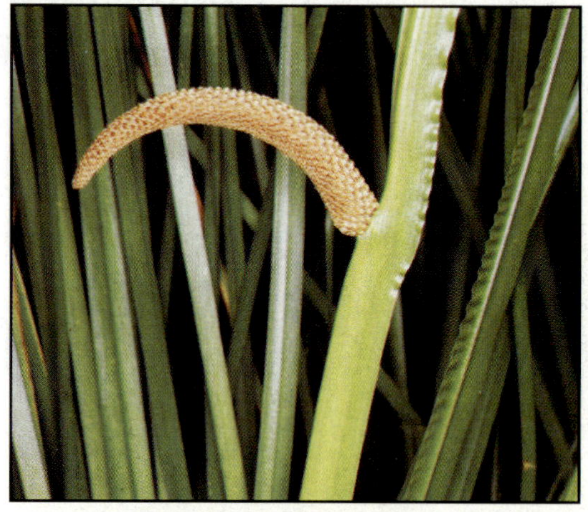

Acorus calamus

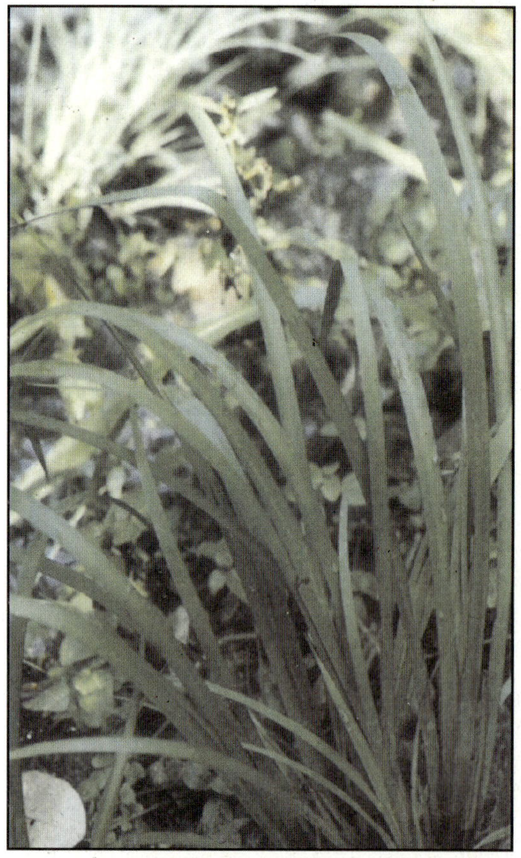

Acorus gramineus

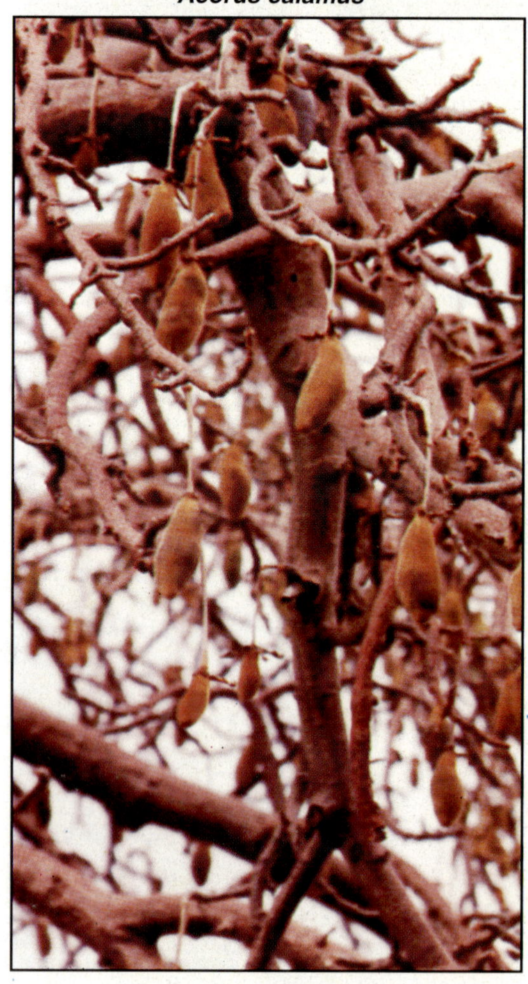

Adansonia digitata

PLATE : 5

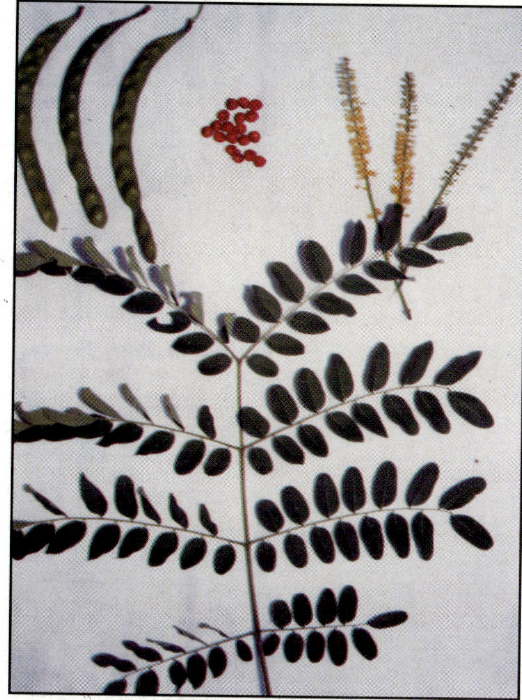

Adenanthera pavonia

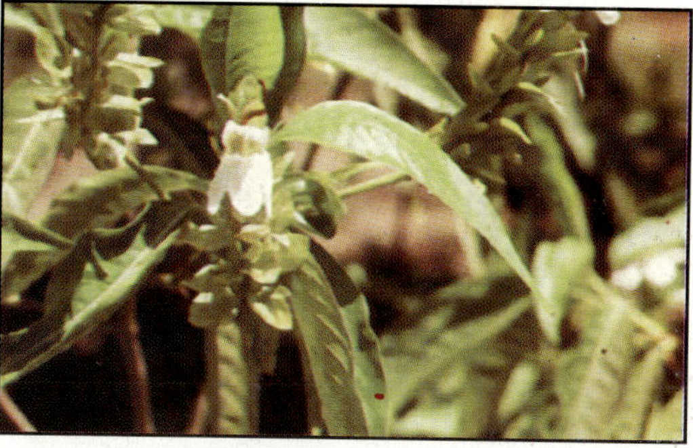

Adhatoda vasica

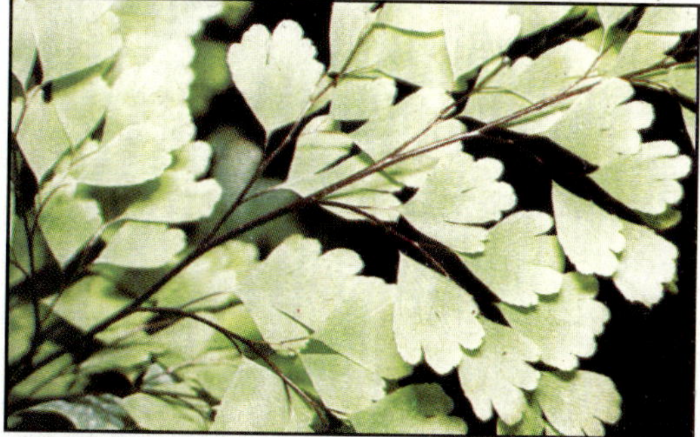

Adiantum capillus-veneris

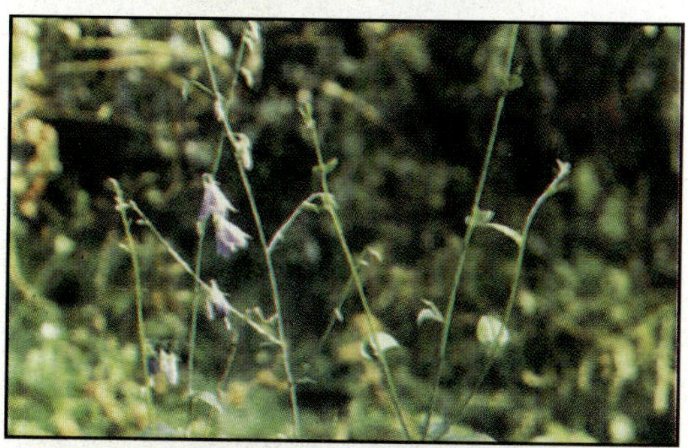

Adenophora stricta

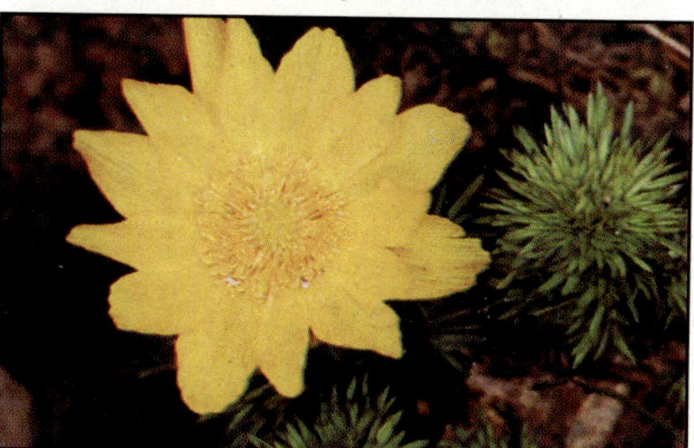

Adonis vernalis

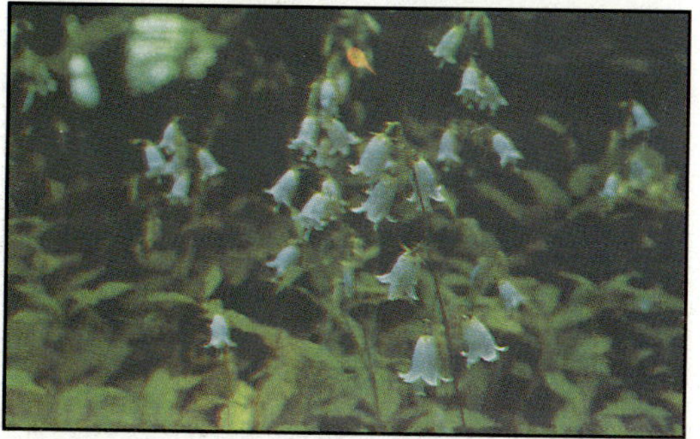

Adenophora triphylla

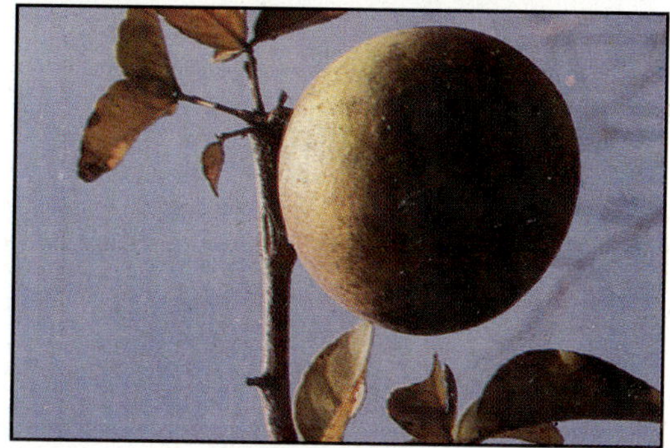

Aegle marmelos

PLATE : 6

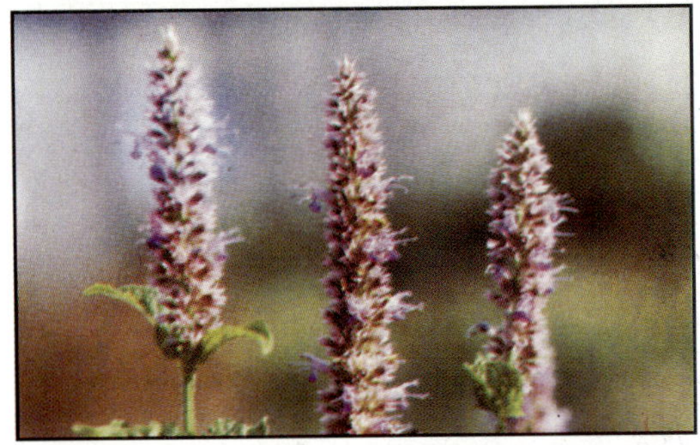

Agastache rugosa

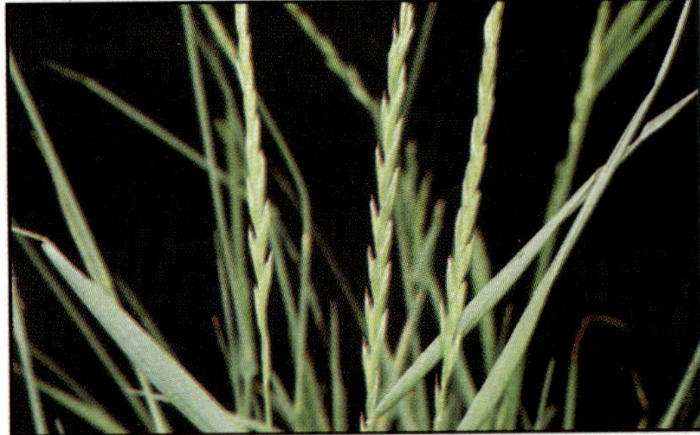

Agropyrun repens

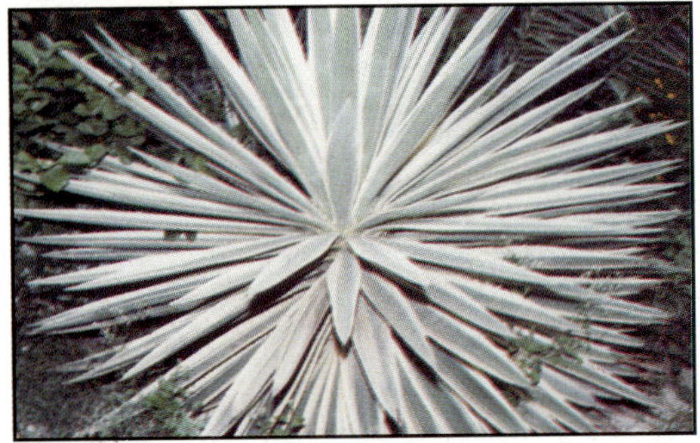

Agave americana

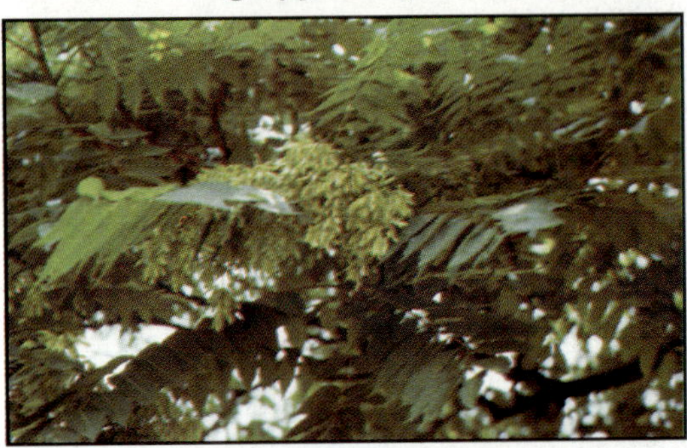

Ailanthus altissima

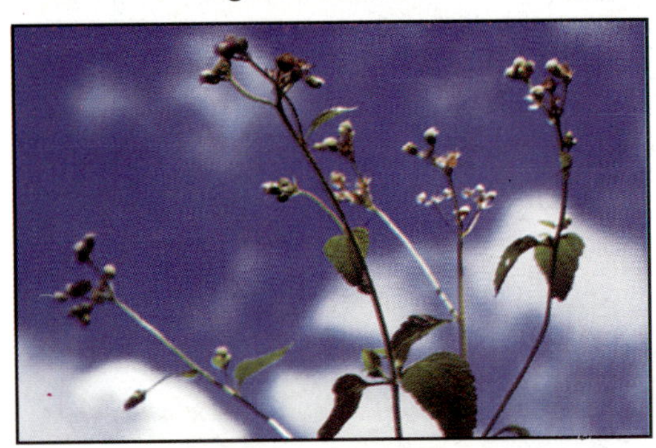

Ageratum conyzoides

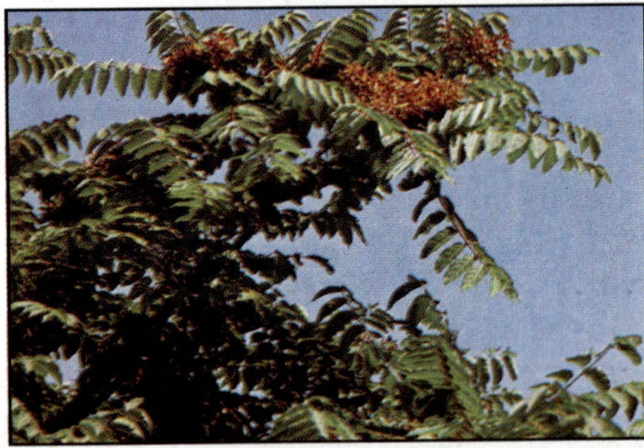

Ailanthus altissima

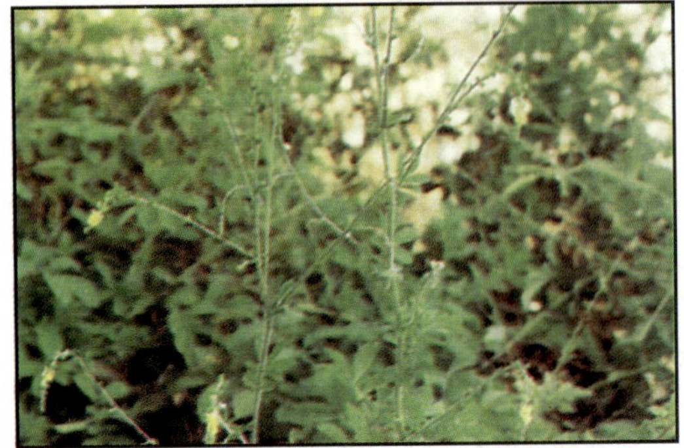

Agrimonia pilosa

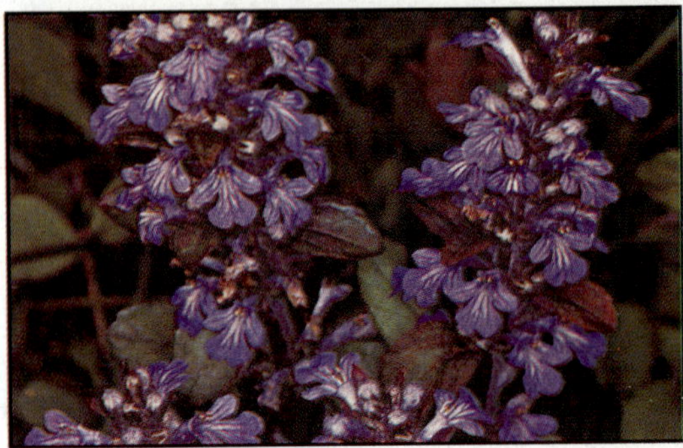

Ajuga reptans

PLATE : 7

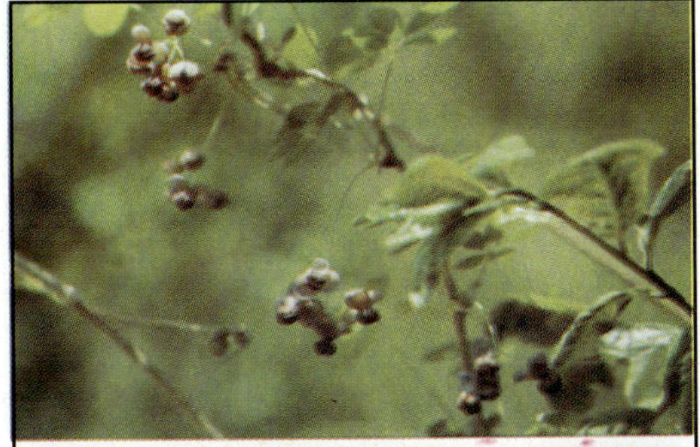

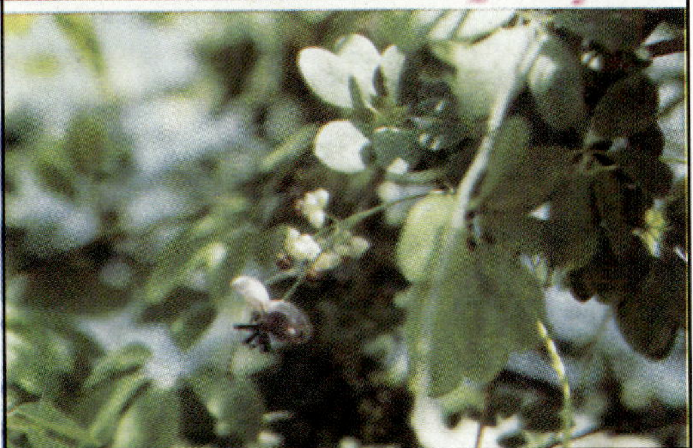

Akebia quinata

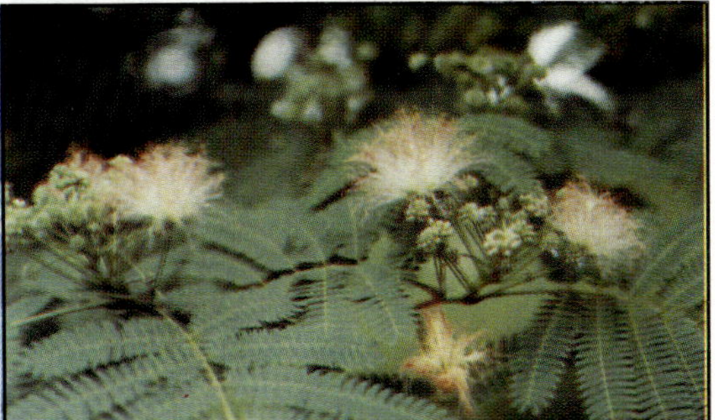

Albizia julibrissin

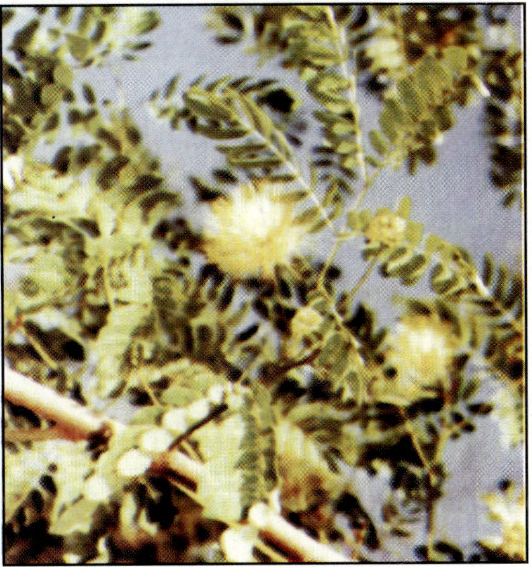

Albizia lebbeck

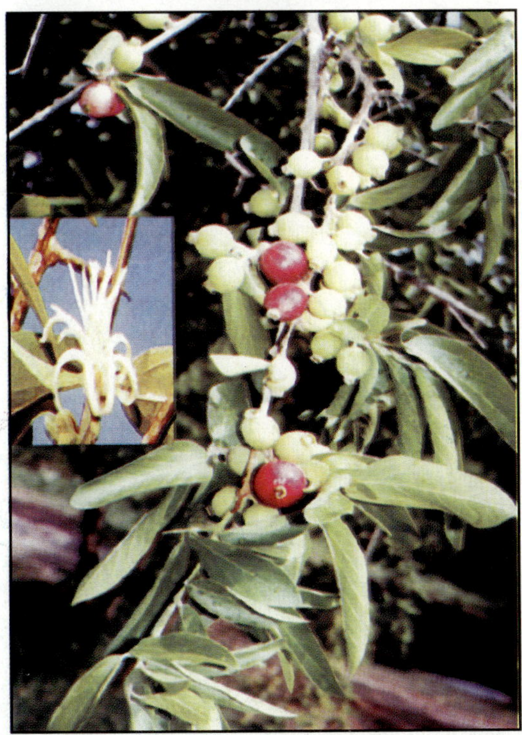

Alangium salviifolium

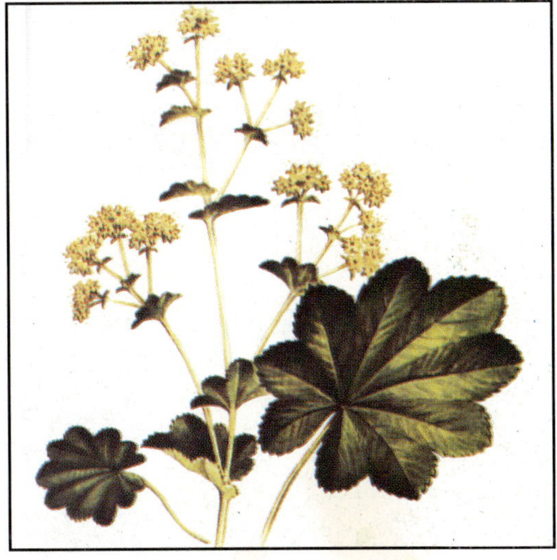

Alchemilla vulgaris

PLATE : 8

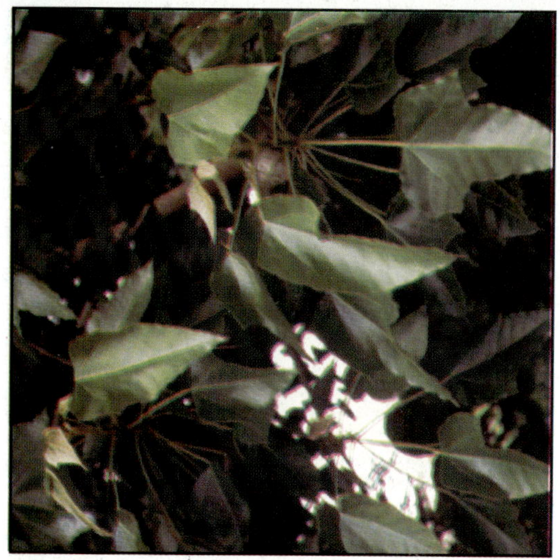

Aleurites moluccana

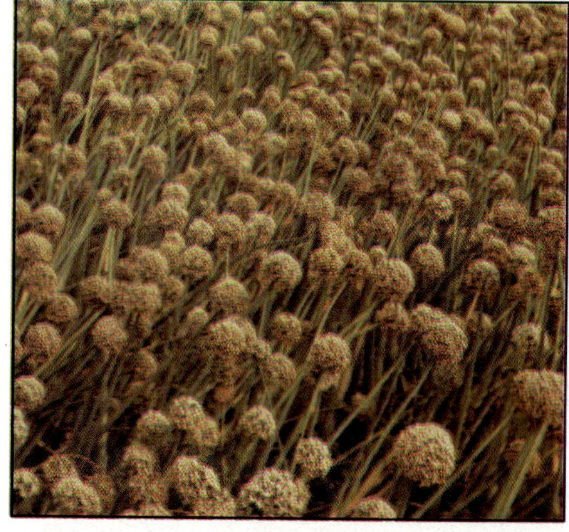

Allium cepa

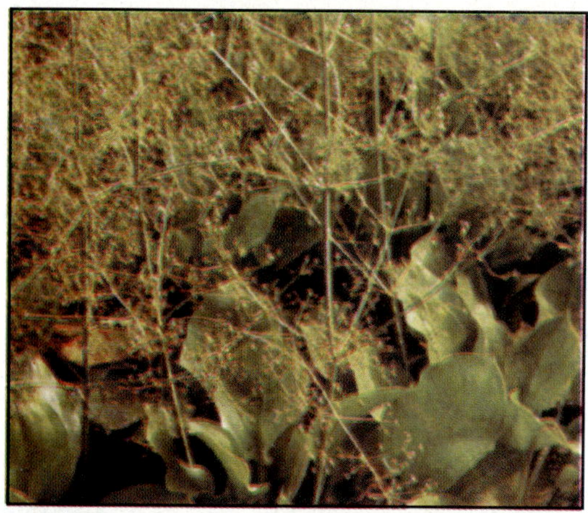

Alisma orientalis

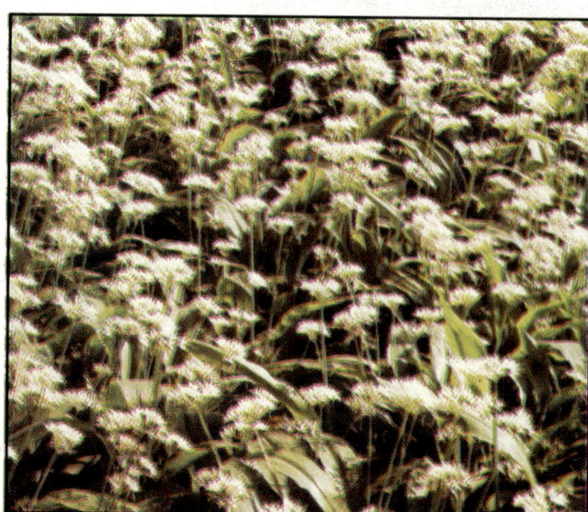

Allium ursinum

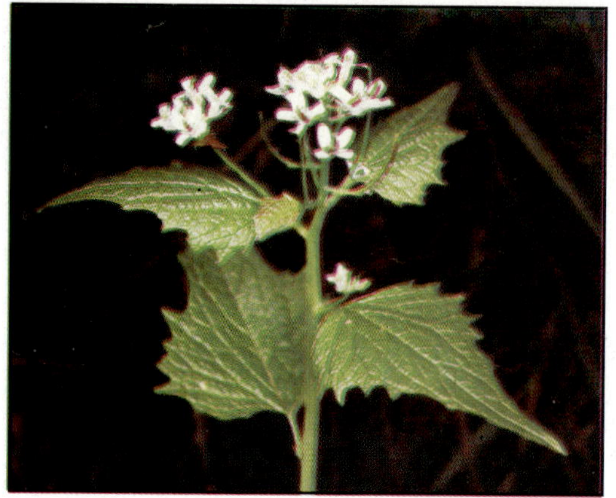

Alliaria petiolata

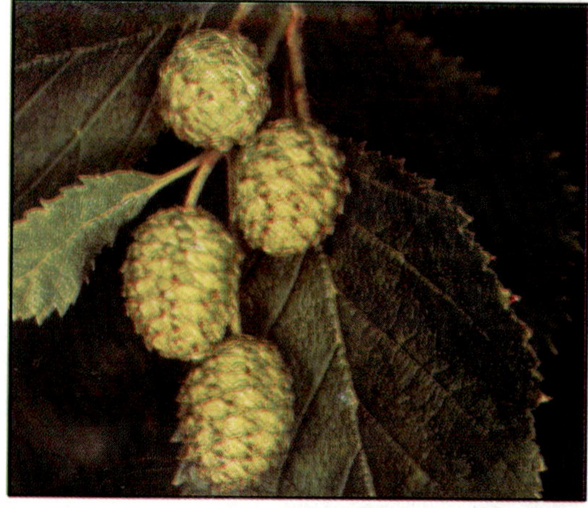

Alnus glutinosa

PLATE : 9

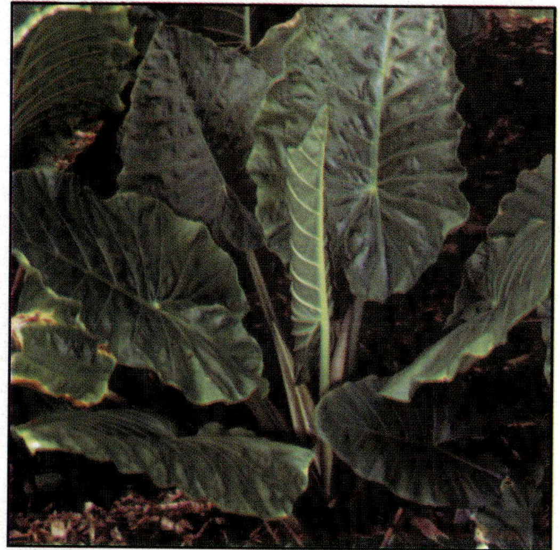

Alocassia macrorhiza

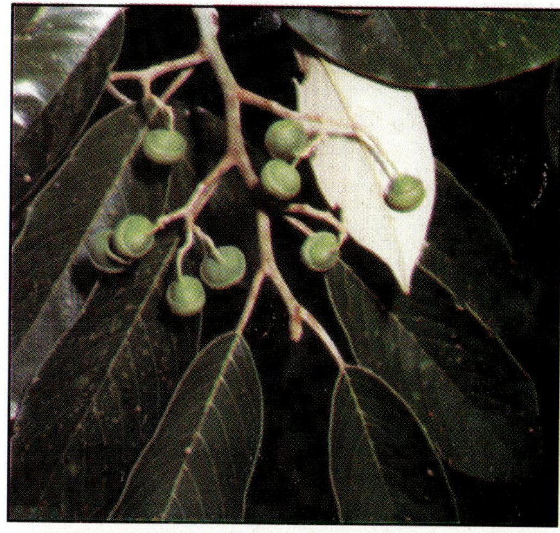

Alphitonia zizyphoides

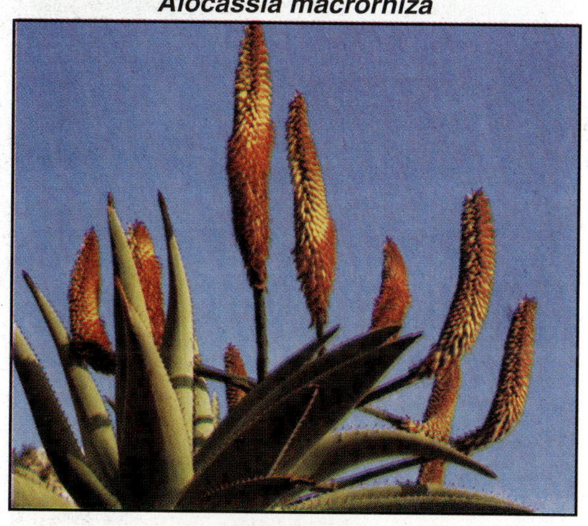

Aloe ferox

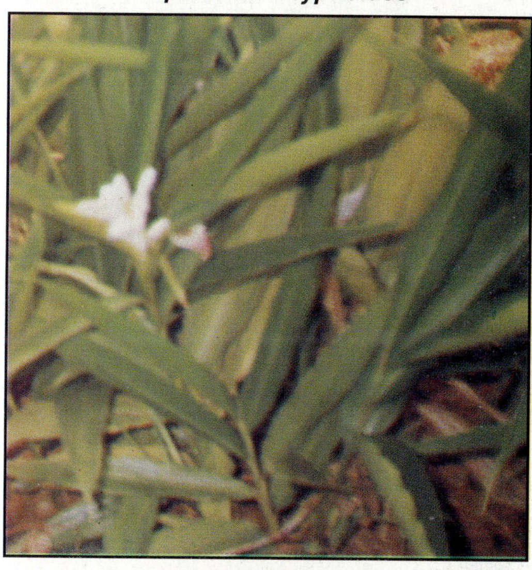

Alpinia calcarata

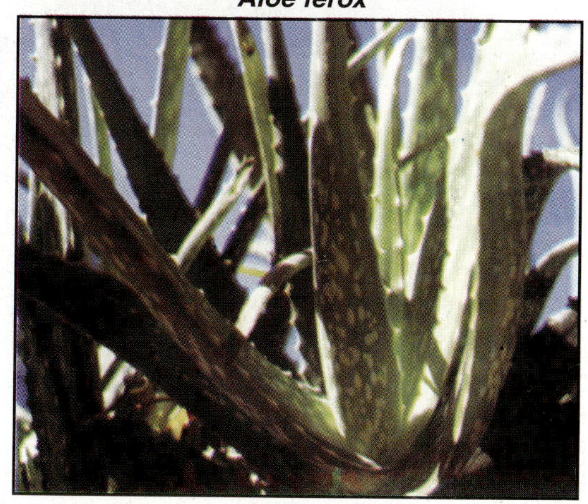

Aloe vera

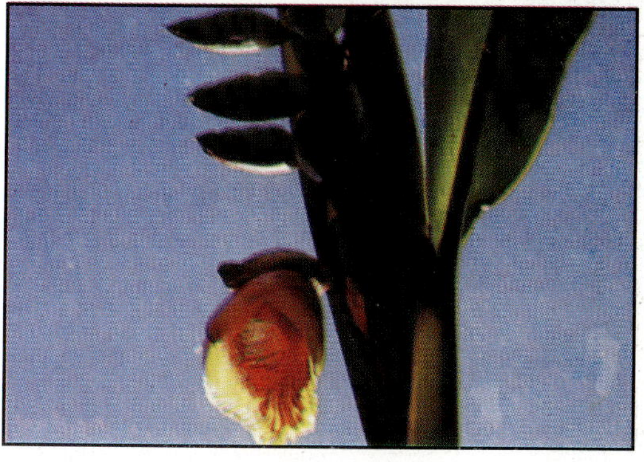

Alpinia galanga

PLATE : 10

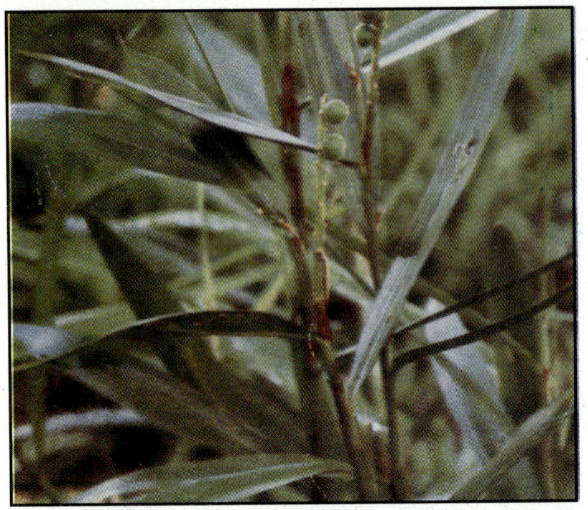

Alpinia officinarum

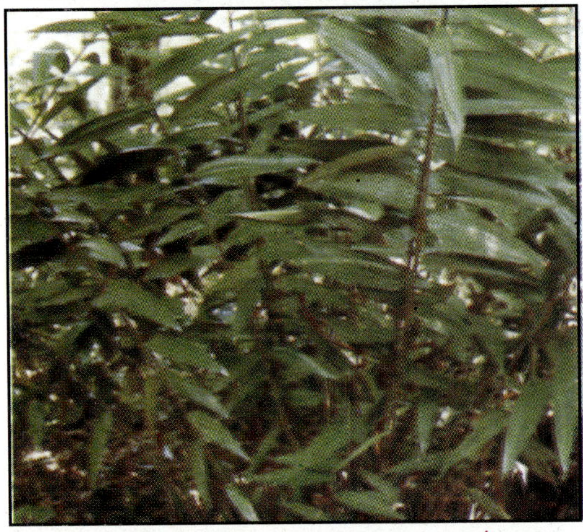

Alpinia oxyphylla

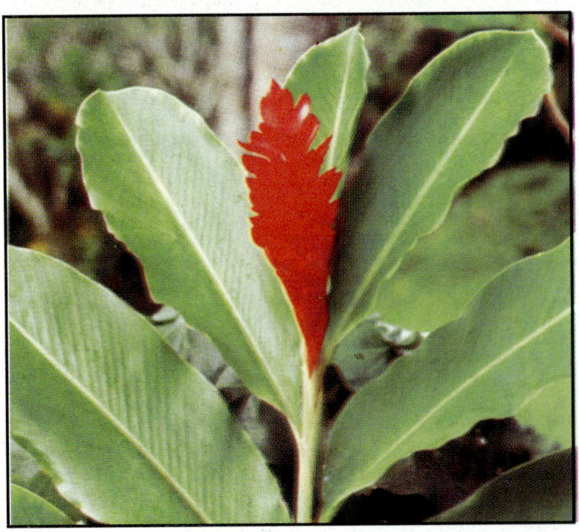

Alpinia purpurata

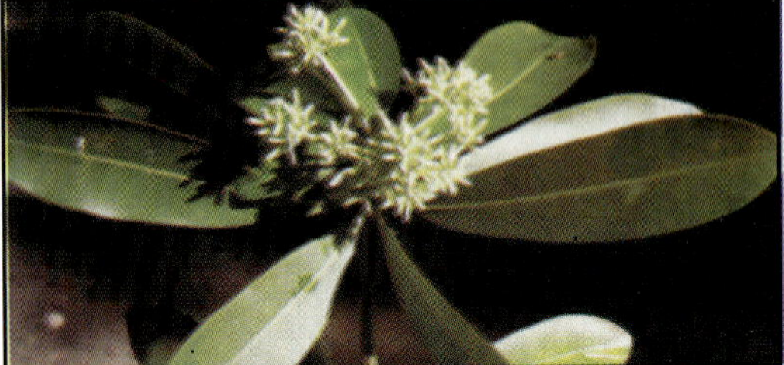

Alstonia scholaries

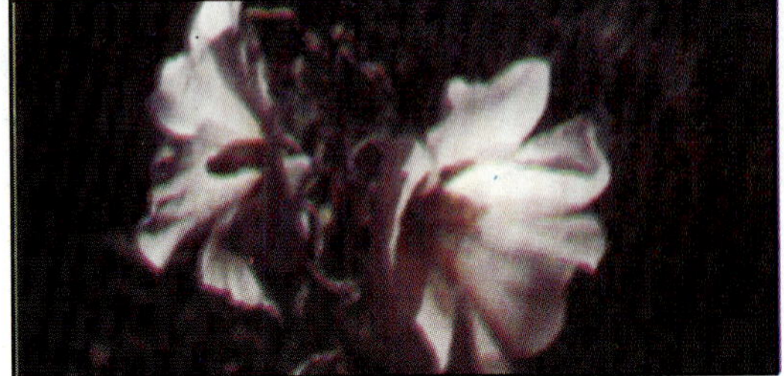

Althaea rosea

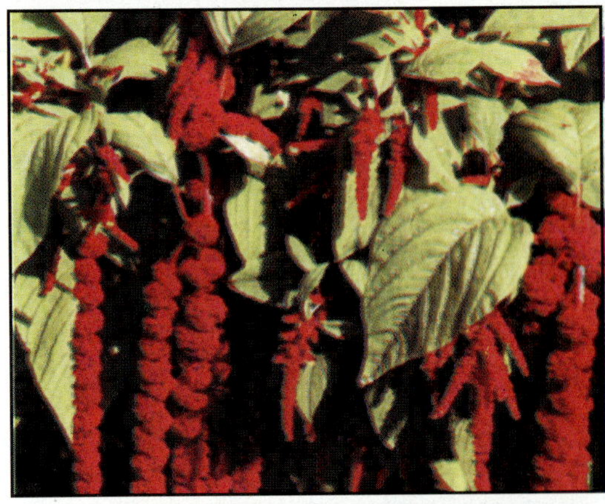

Amaranthus caudatus (red)

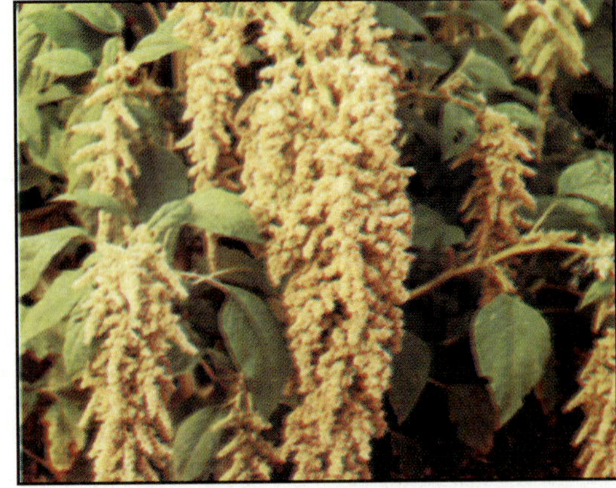

Amaranthus caudatus (yellow)

PLATE : 11

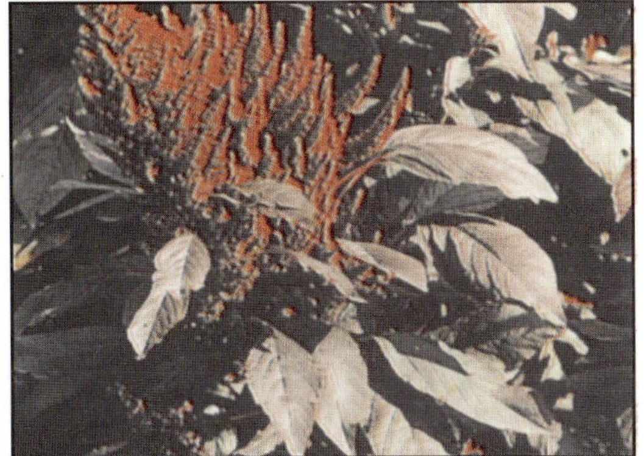

Amaranthus hypodriacus

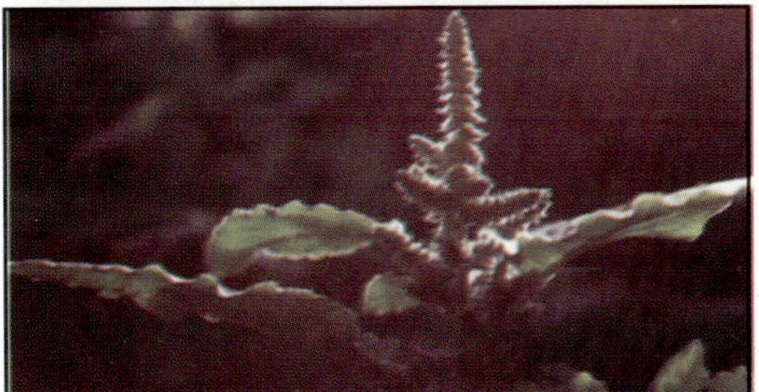

Amaranthus retroflaxus

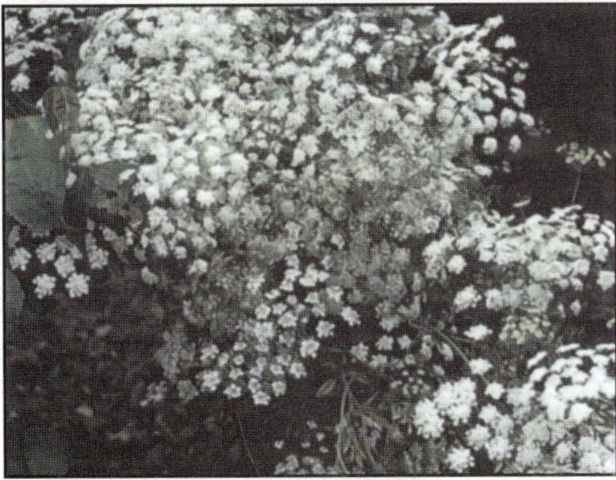

Ammi majus

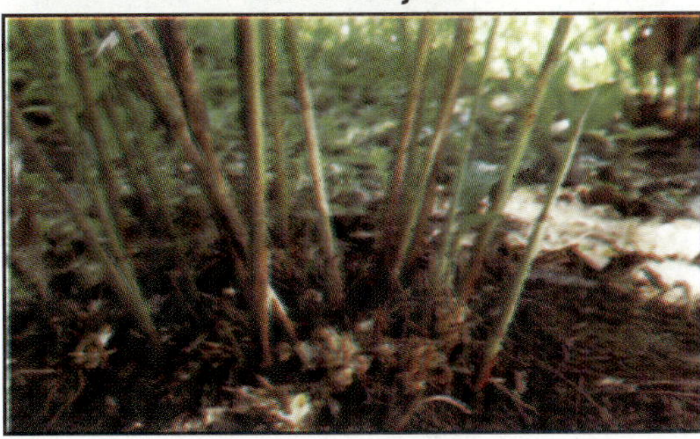

Amomum krervanh

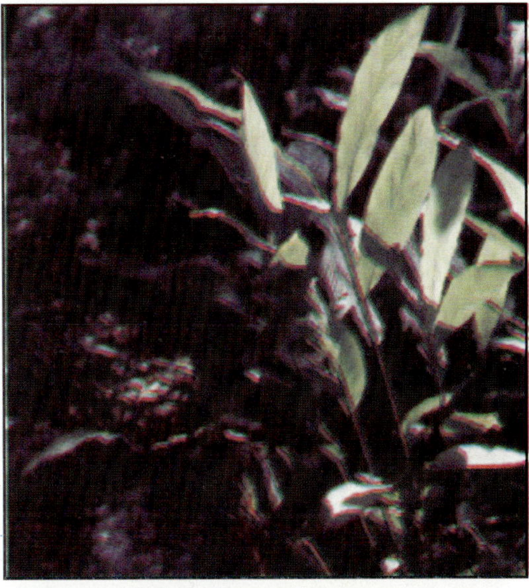

Amomum subulatum

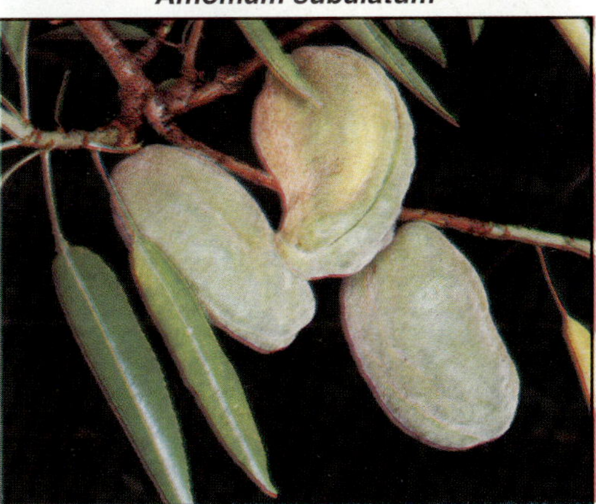

Amygdalus cammunis dulcis

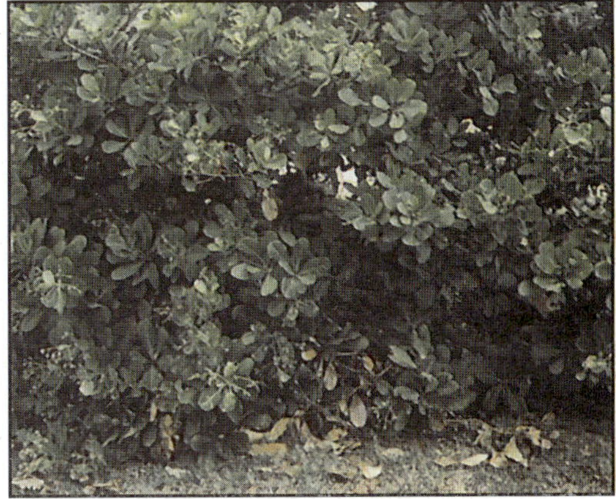

Anacardium occidentale

PLATE : 12

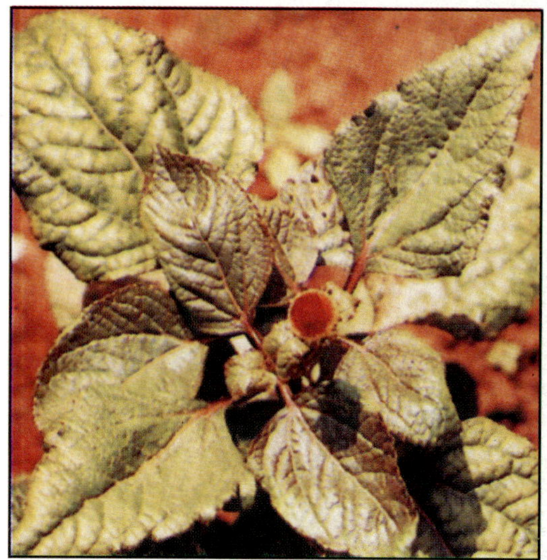

Anacyclus pyrethrum

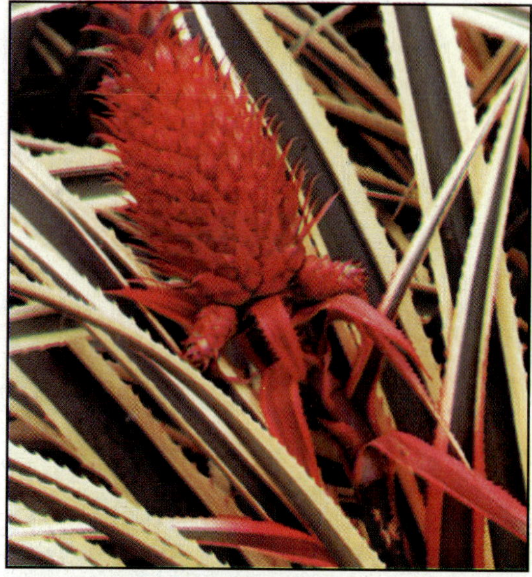

Ananas comosus

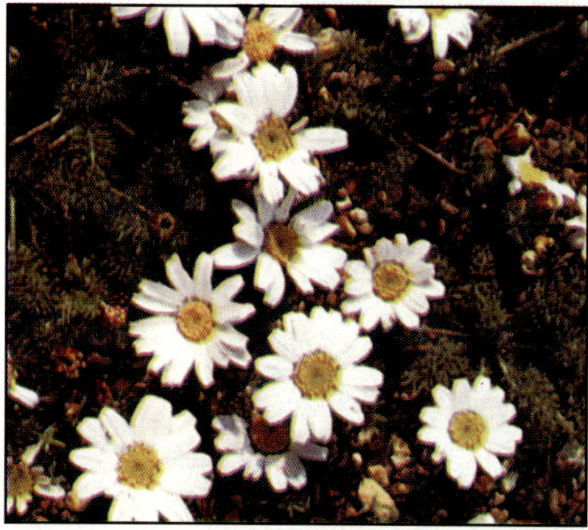

Anacylus pyrethrum

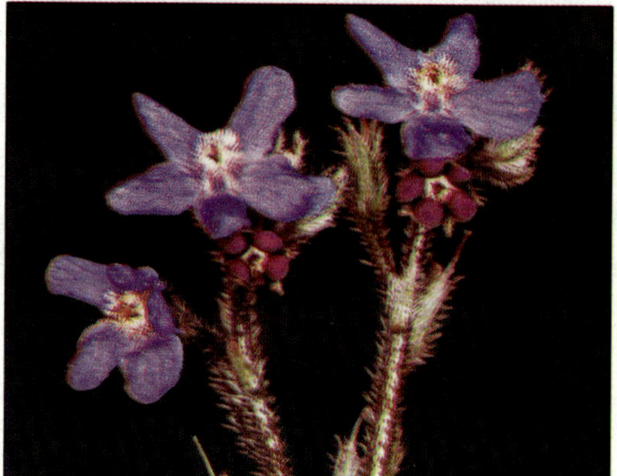

Anchusa azurea

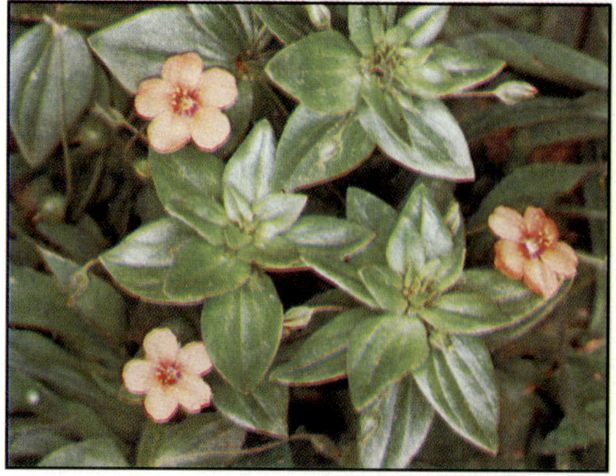

Anagallis arvensis

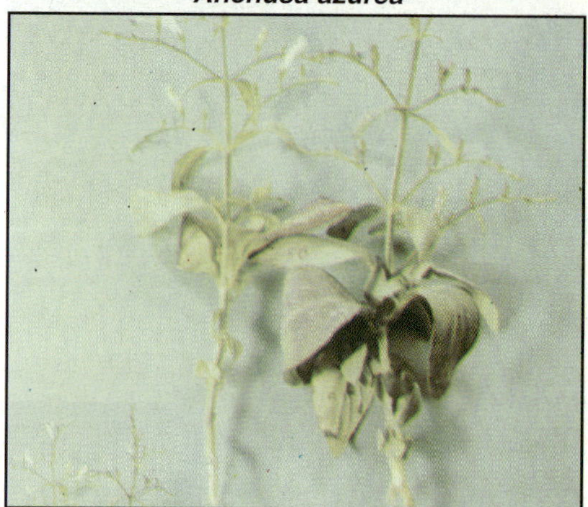

Andrographis paniculata

PLATE : 13

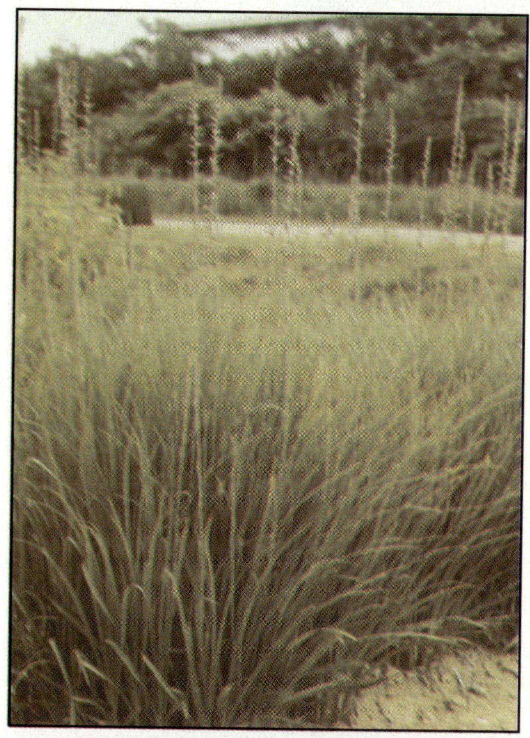

Anemarrhena asphodeloides

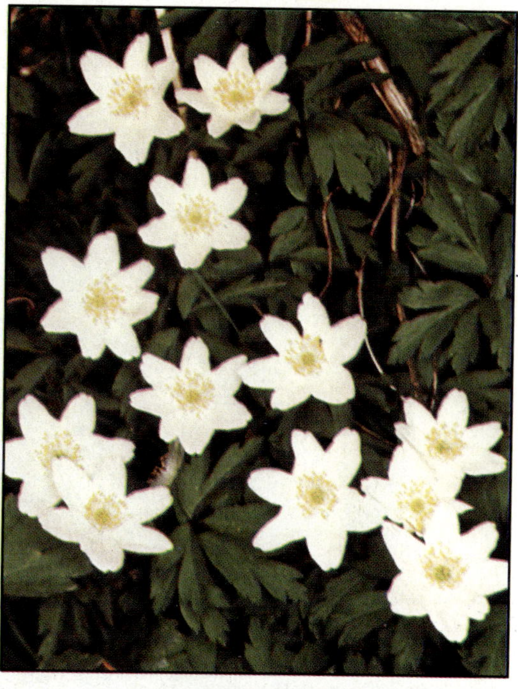

Anemone nemorosa

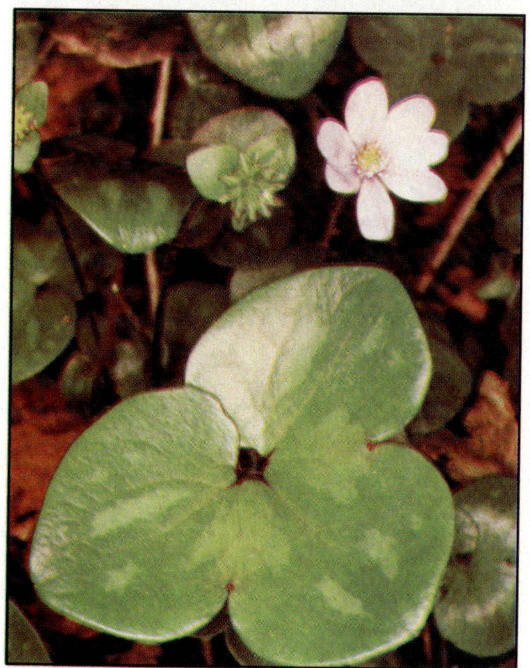

Anemone hepatica

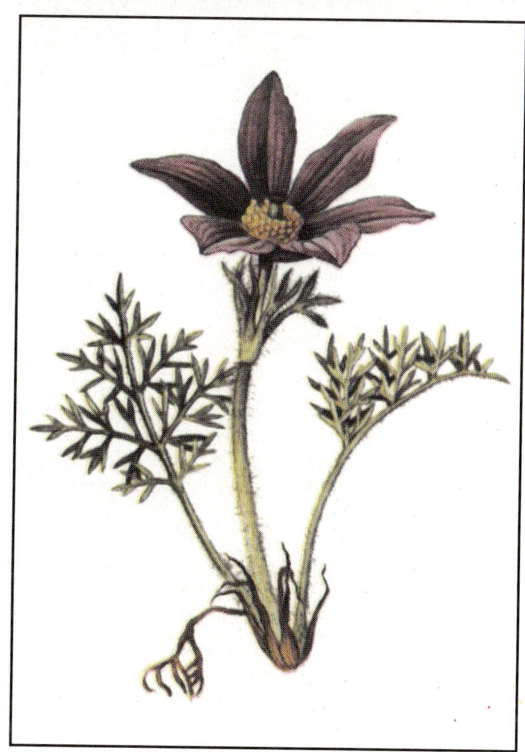

Anemone pulsatilla

PLATE : 14

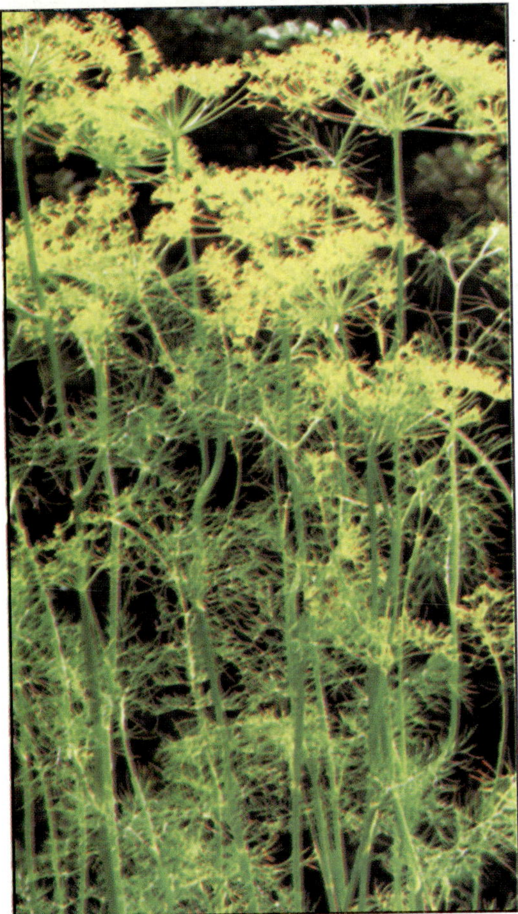

Anethum graveolens

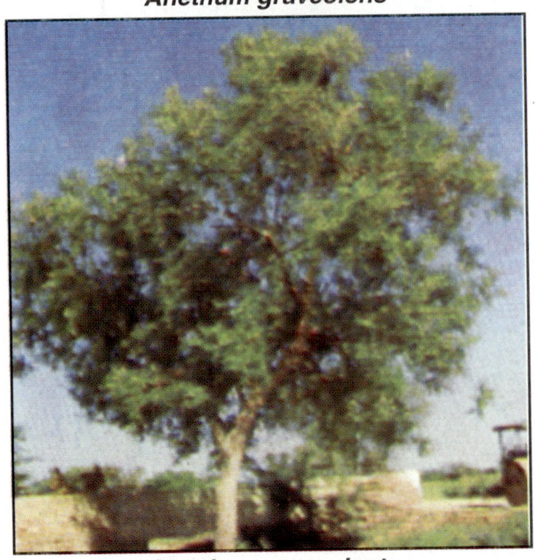

Angeissus acuminata

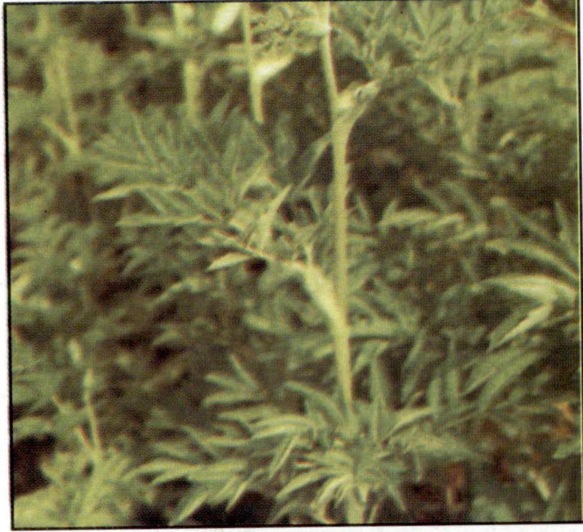

Angelica dahurica

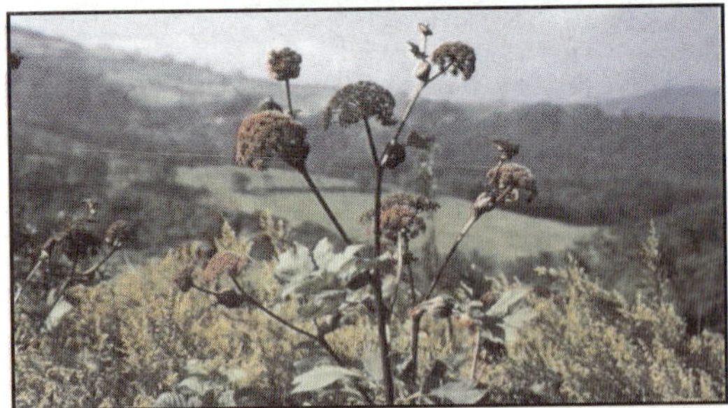

Angelica gigas

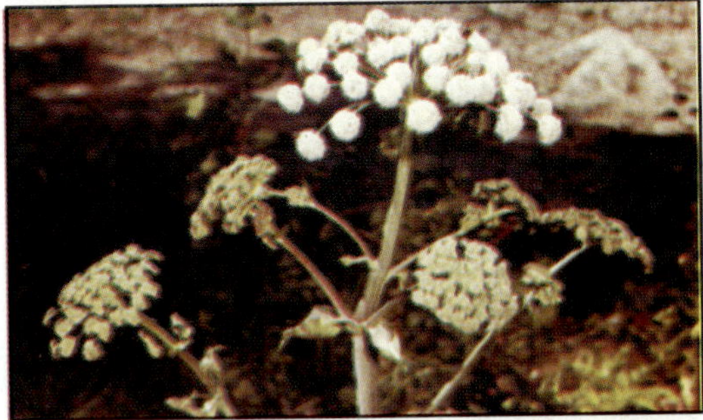

Angelica sylvestris

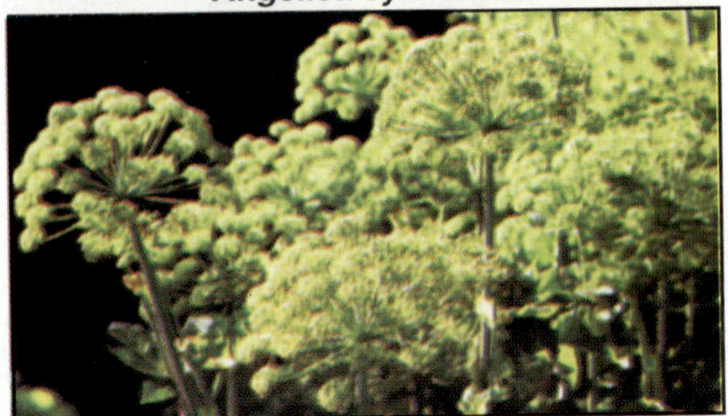

Angelica archangelica

PLATE : 15

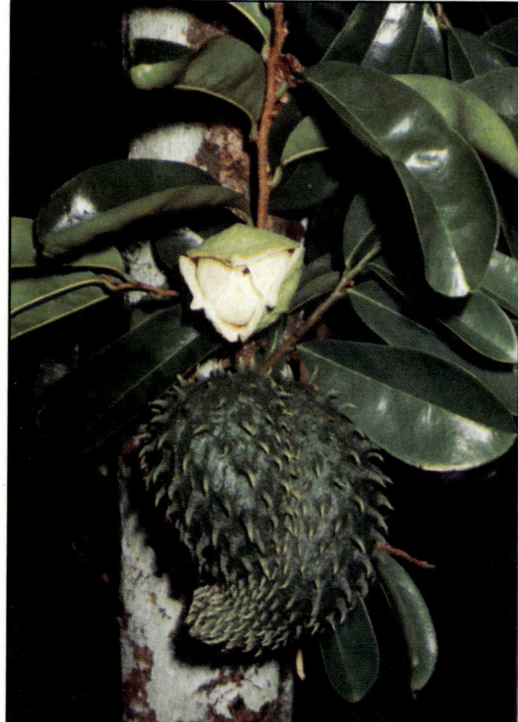

Annona muricata

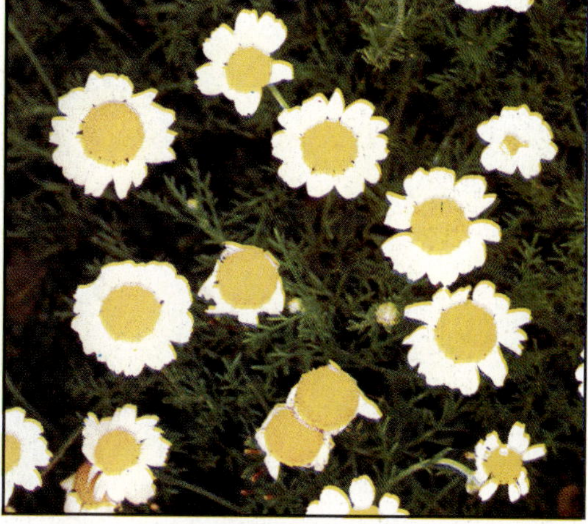

Anthemus nobilis

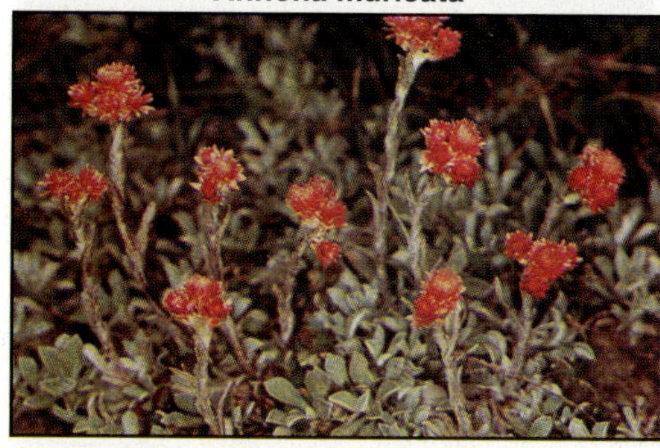

Antennaria dioica

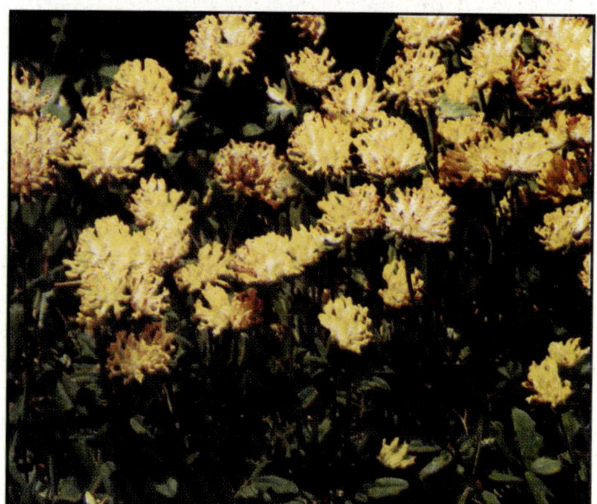

Anthyllis vulneraria

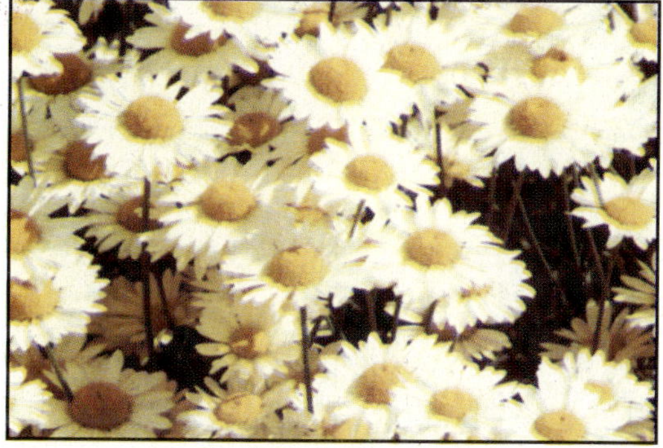

Anthemis tinctoria

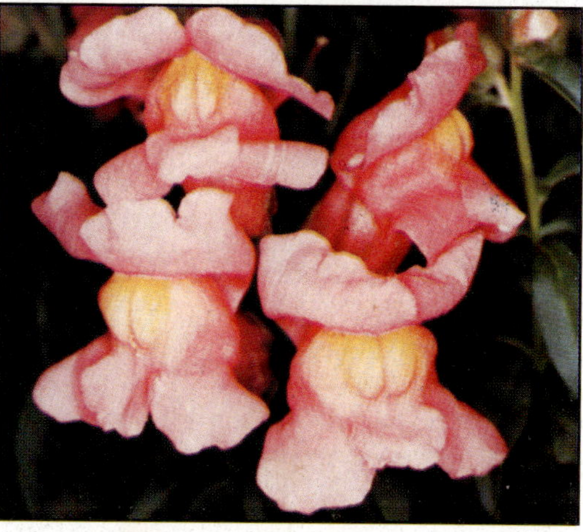

Antirrhinum majus

PLATE : 16

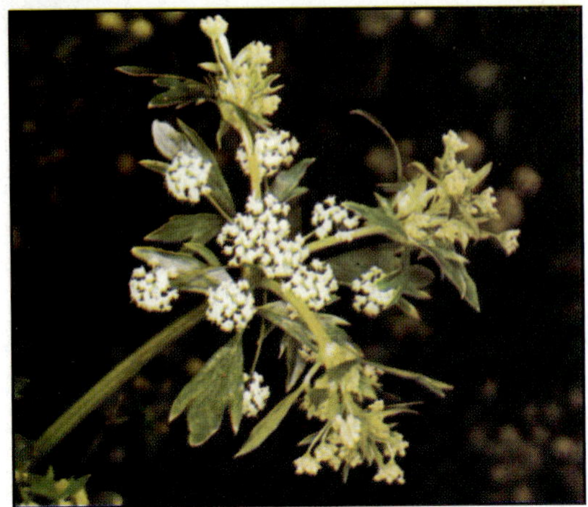

Apium graveolens

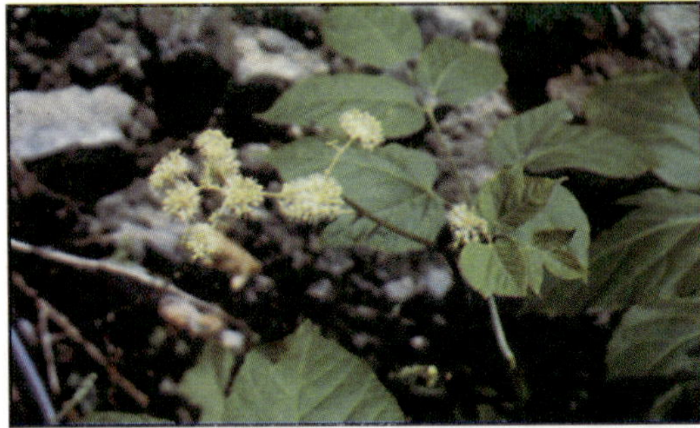

Aralia cordata

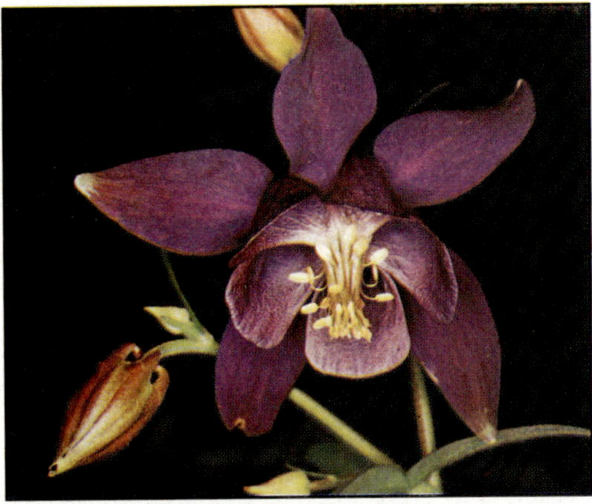

Aquilegia vulgaris

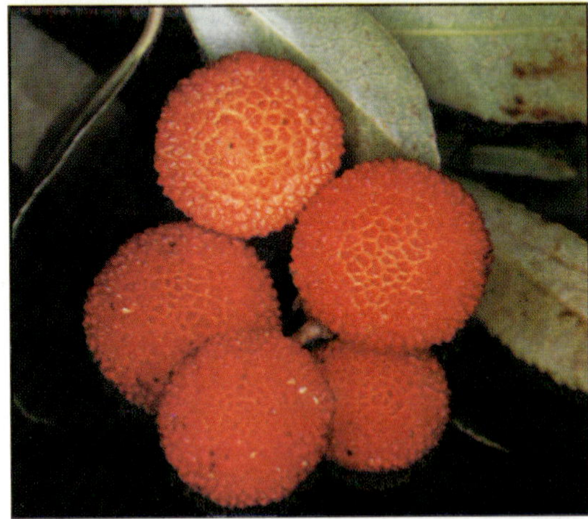

Arbutus unedo

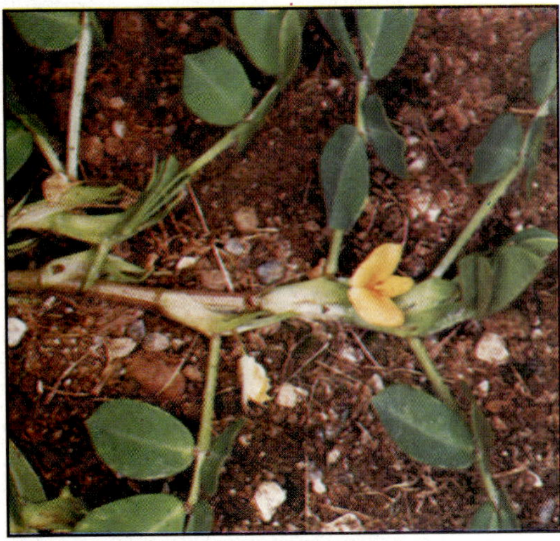

Arachis hypogaea

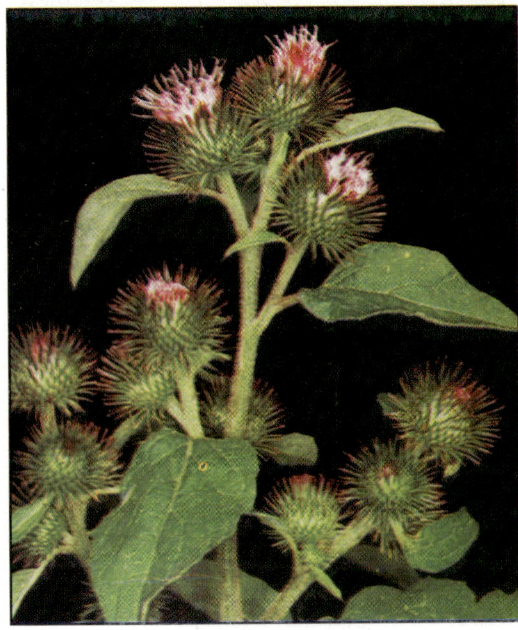

Arctium lappa

PLATE : 17

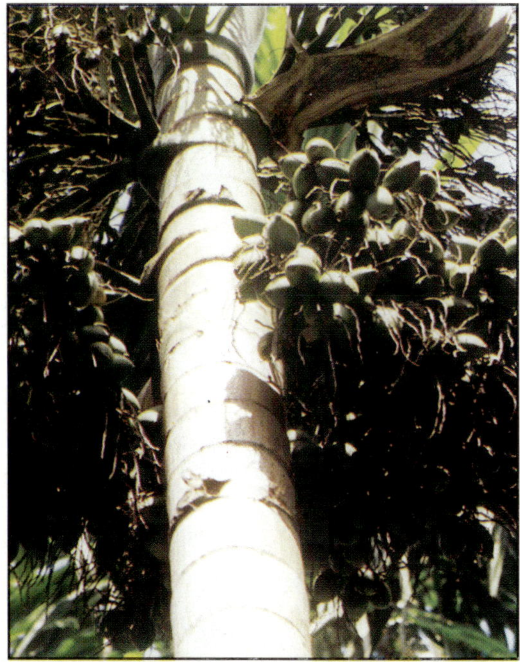

Areca catechu

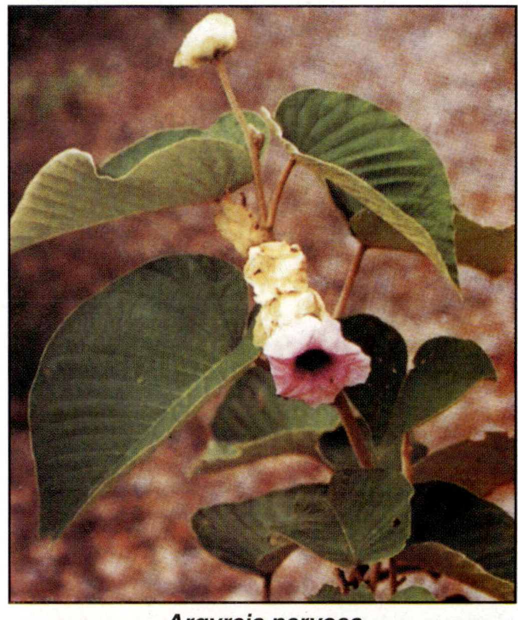

Argyreia nervosa

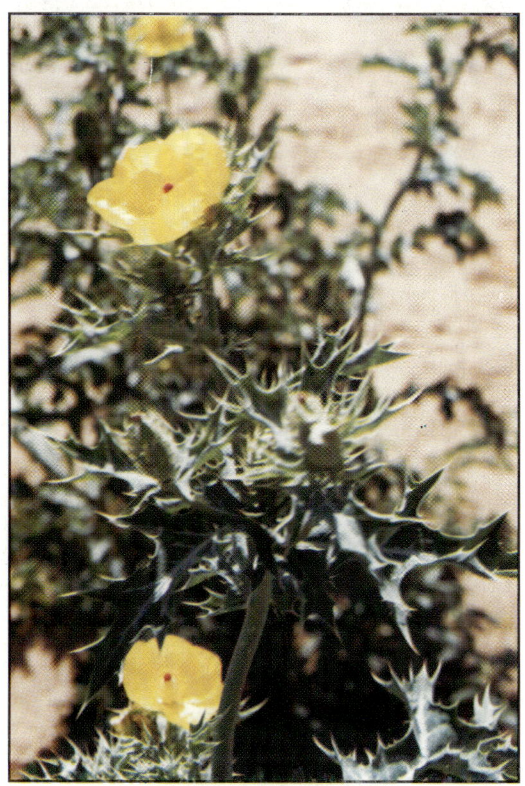

Argimone Maxcicana

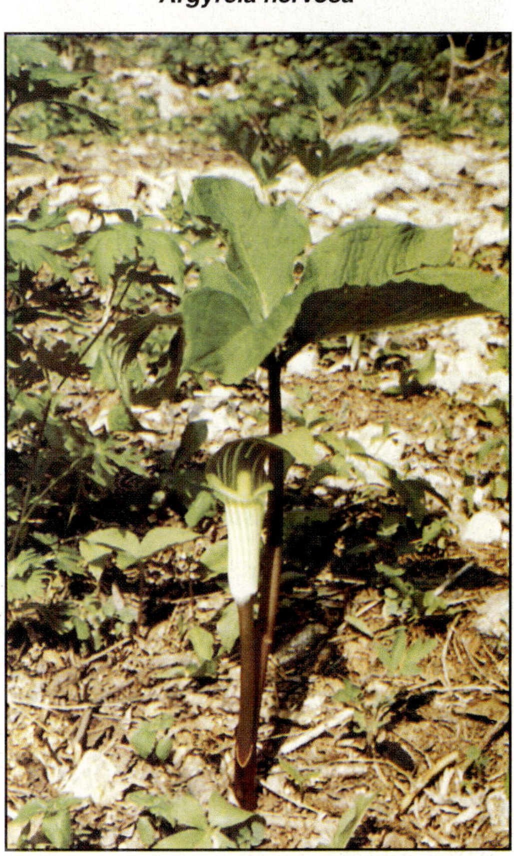

Arisaema amurense

PLATE : 18

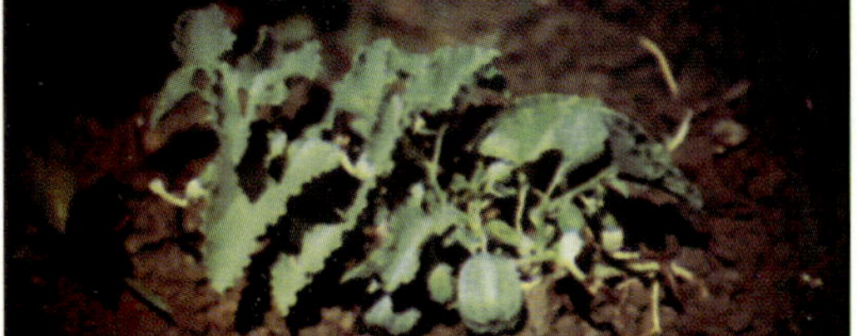

Aristolochia bracteolata

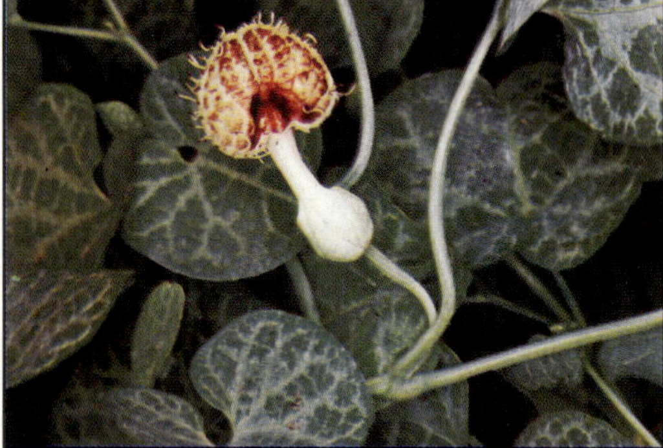

Aristolochia rotunda

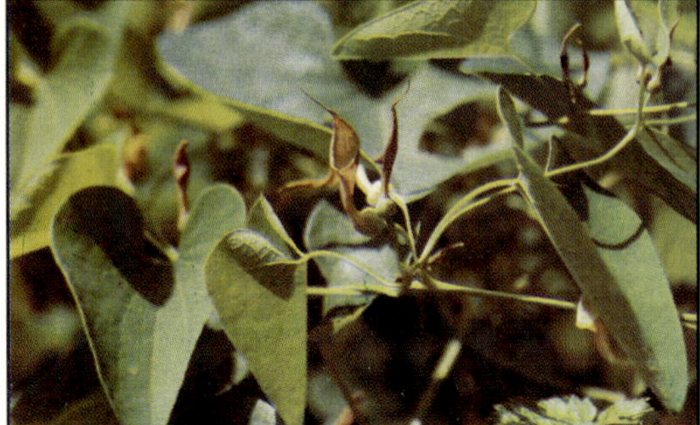

Aristolochia contorta

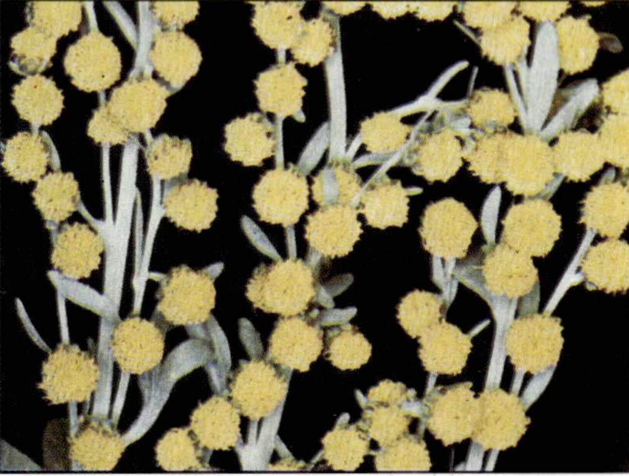

Artemisia absinthium

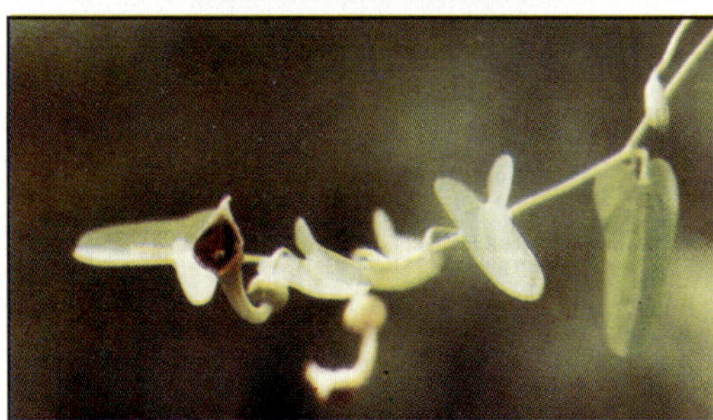

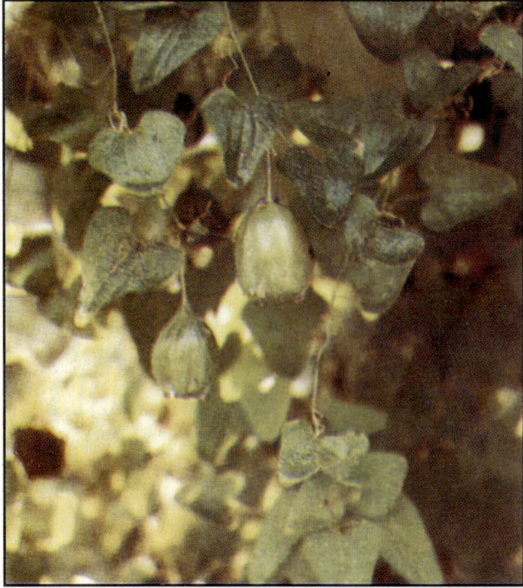

Aristolochia debilis

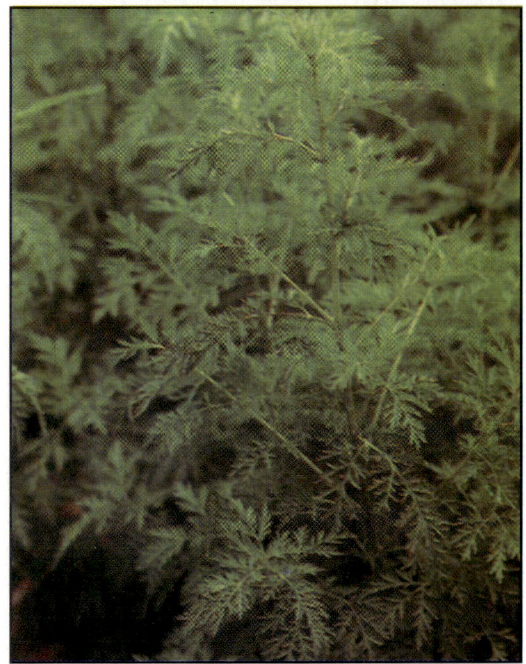

Artemisia annua

PLATE : 19

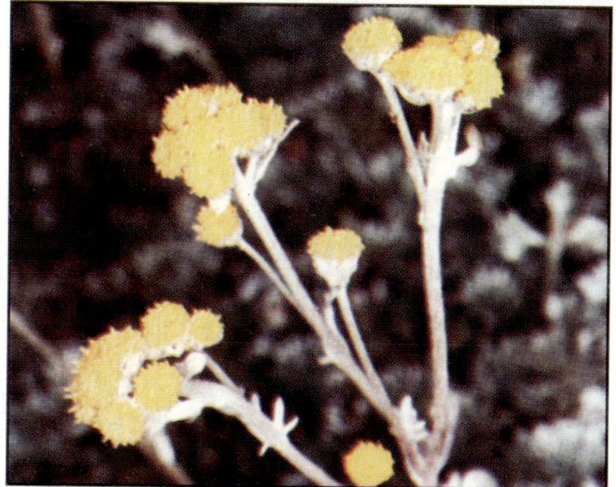

Artemisia glacialis

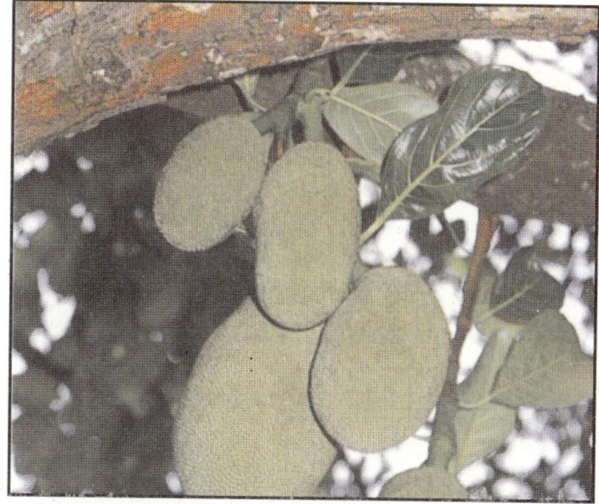

Artocarpus heterophyllus

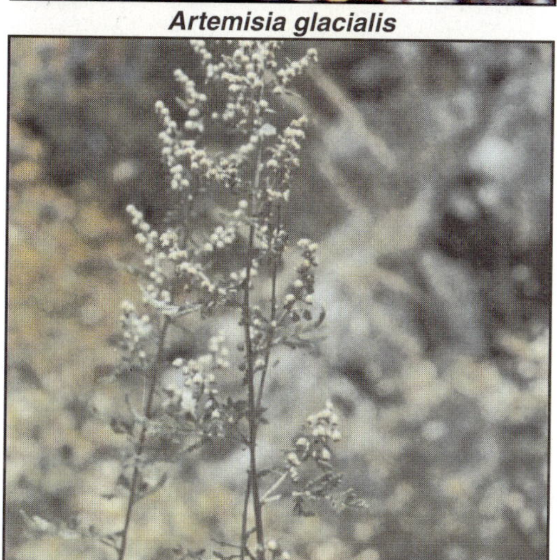

Artemisia gmelini

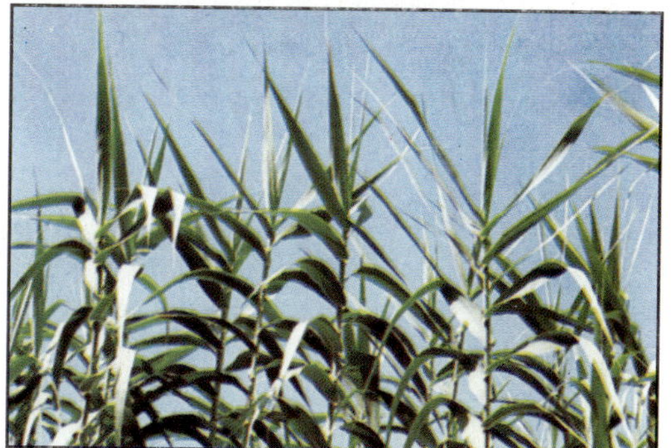

Arundo donax

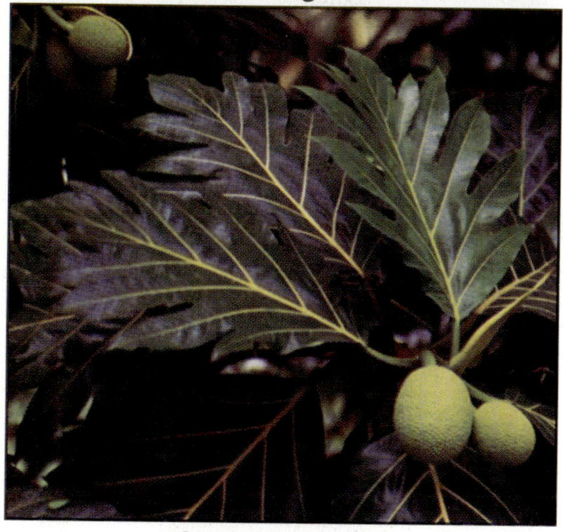

Artocarpus altilis

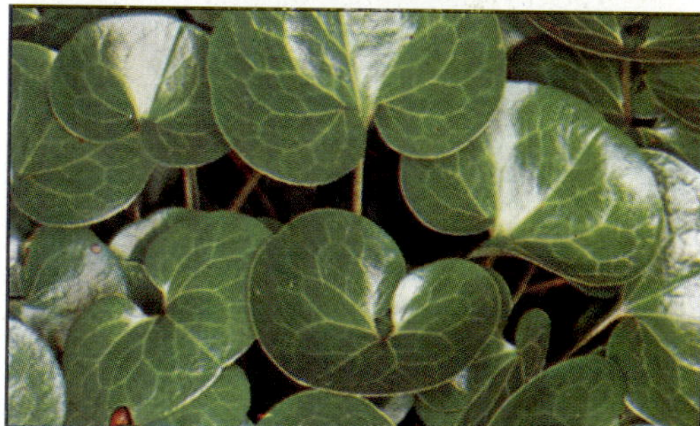

Asarum europaeum

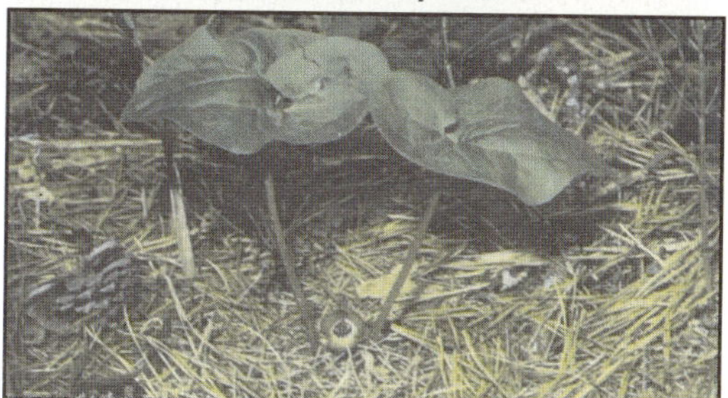

Asarum sieboldii

PLATE : 20

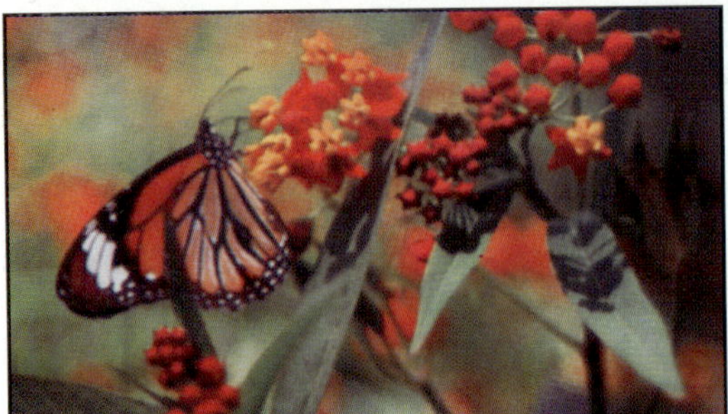

Asclepias curassavica

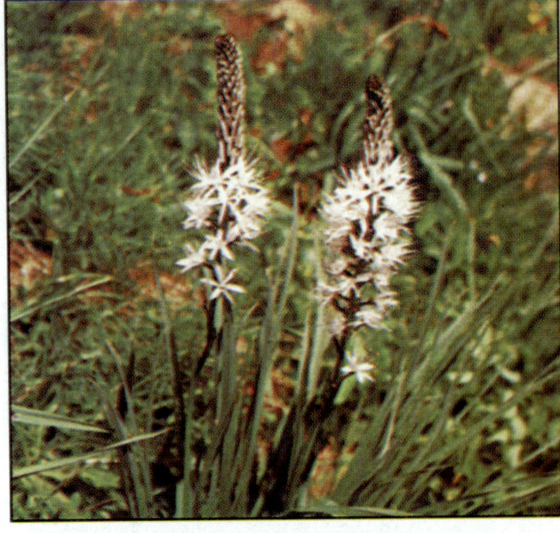

Asphodelus albus

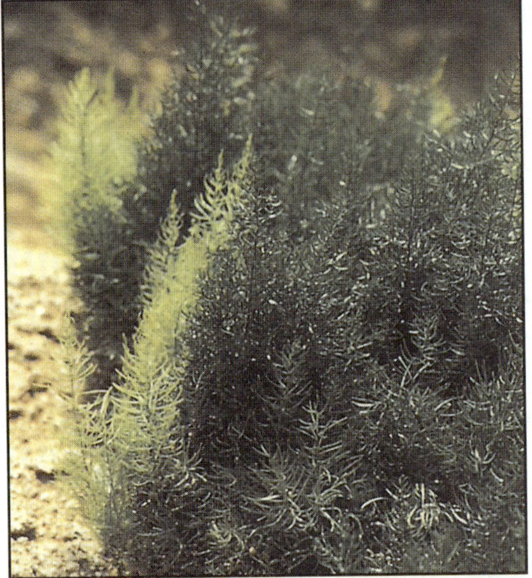

Asparagus cochinchinensis

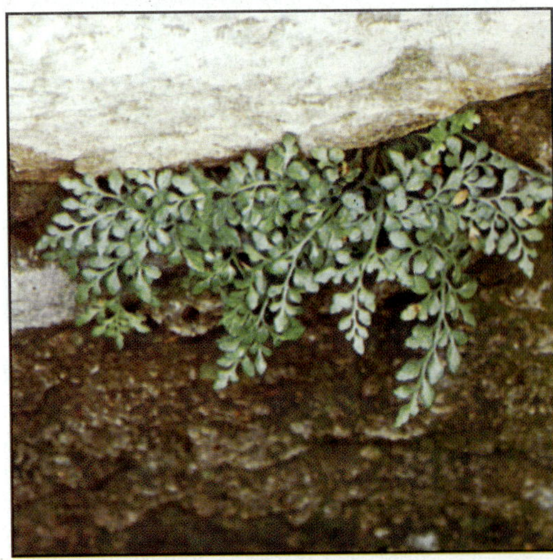

Asplenium ruta-muraria

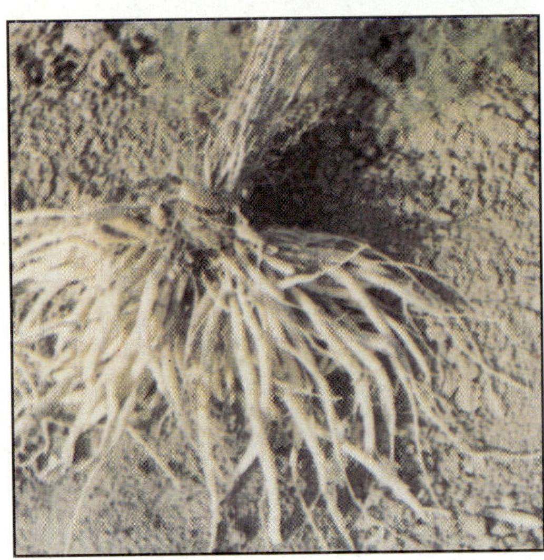

Asparagus racemosus

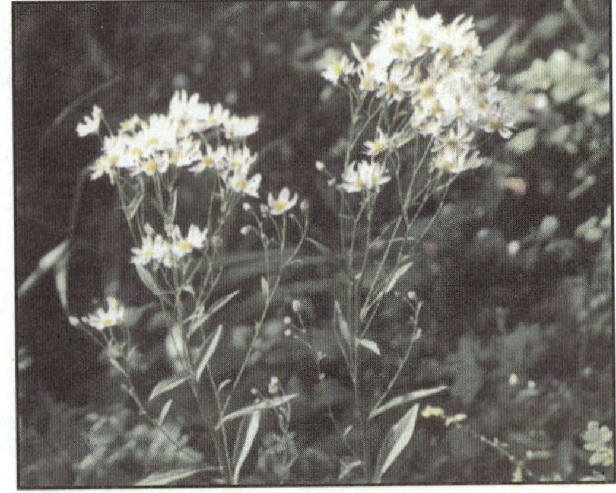

Aster tataricus

PLATE : 21

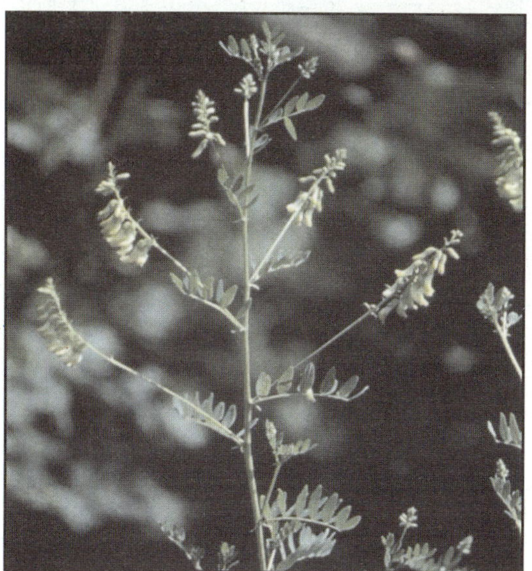

Astragalus membranaceus

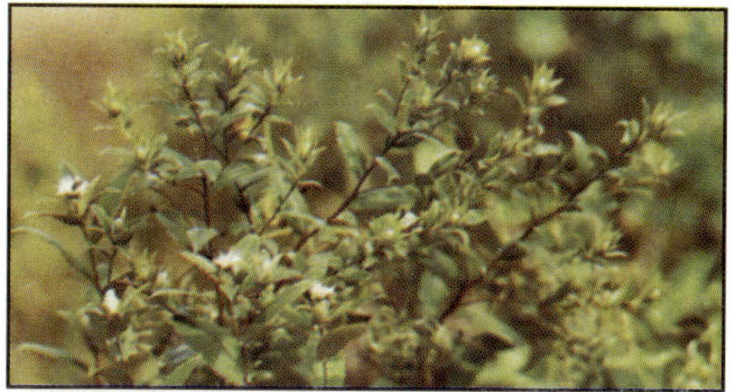

Atractylodes lancea

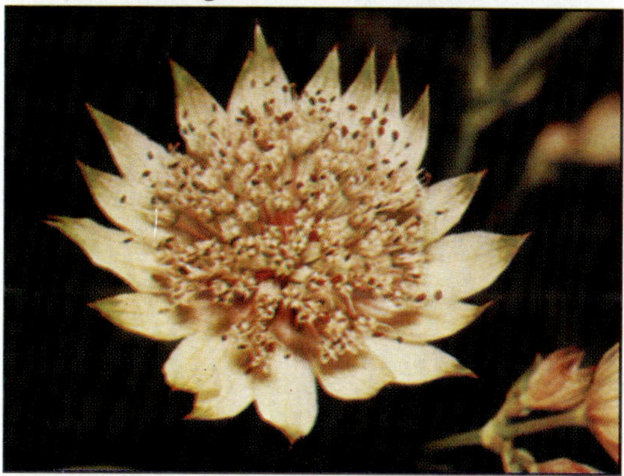

Astrantia major

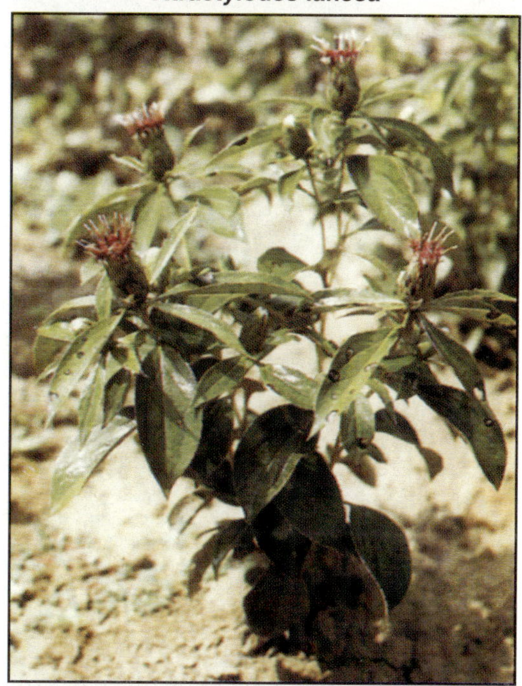

Atractylodes macrocephala

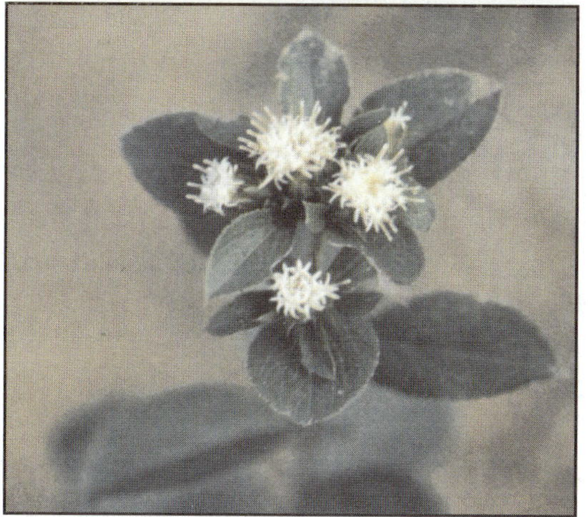

Atractylodes japonica

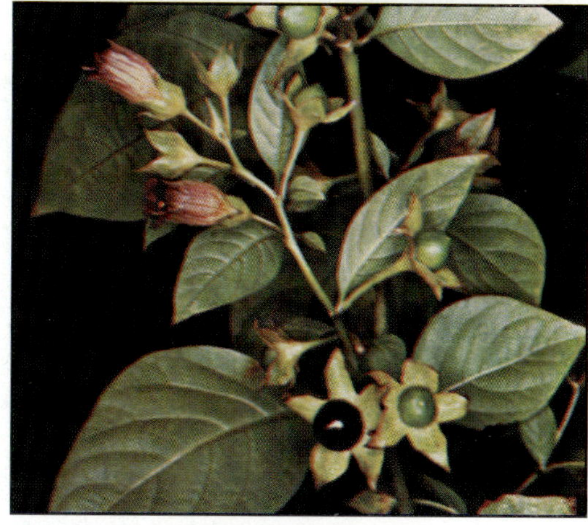

Atropa belladonna

PLATE : 22

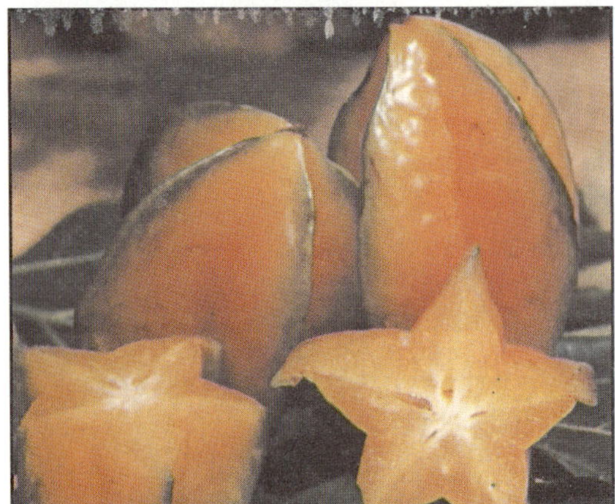

Averrhoa carambola

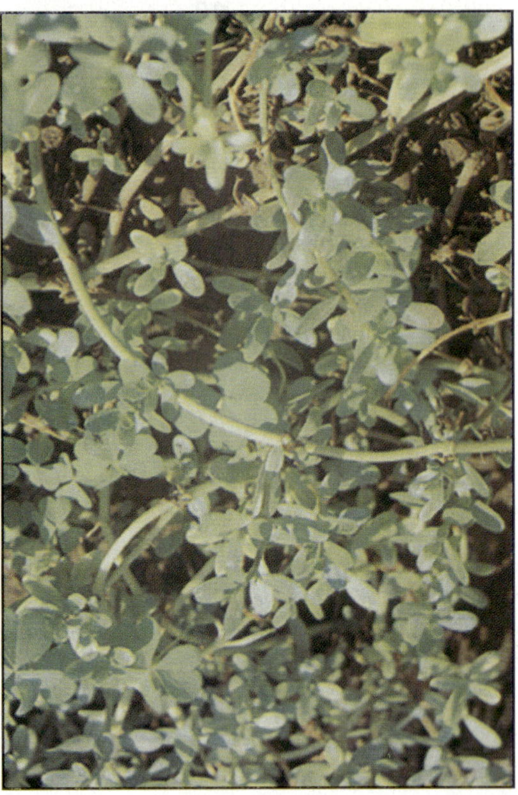

Bacopa monneiri

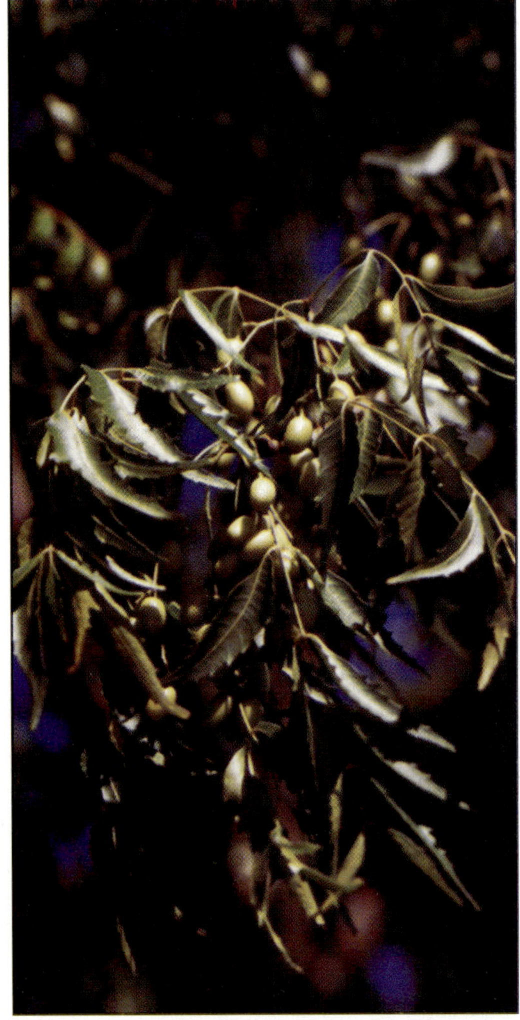

Azadirachta indica

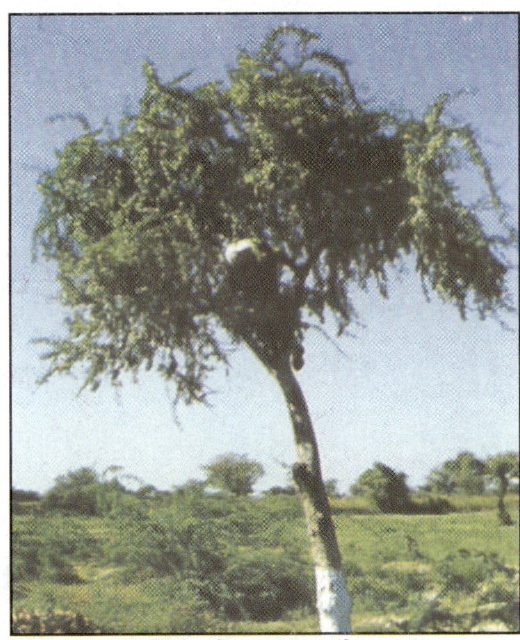

Balanites aegyptiaca

PLATE : 23

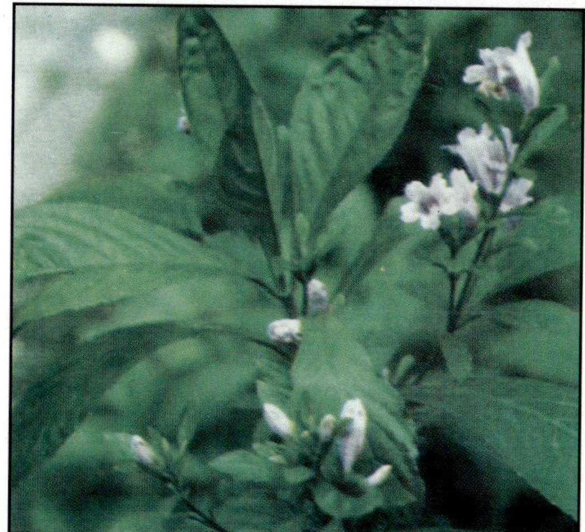

Baphicacanthus cusia

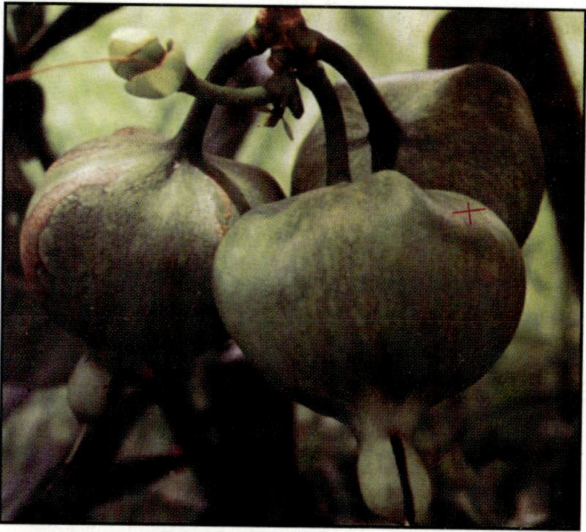

Barringtonia asiatica

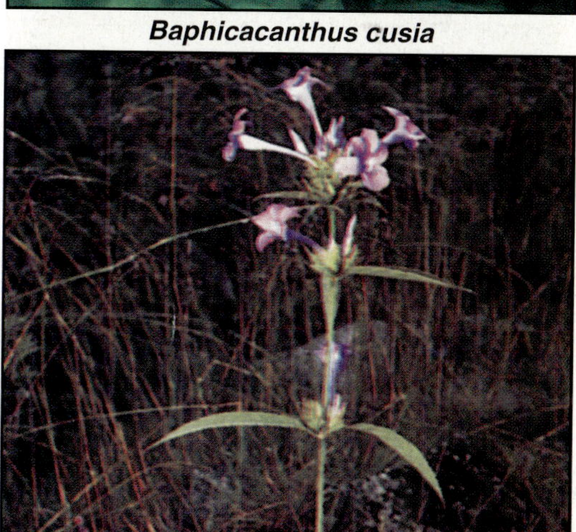

Barleria cristata

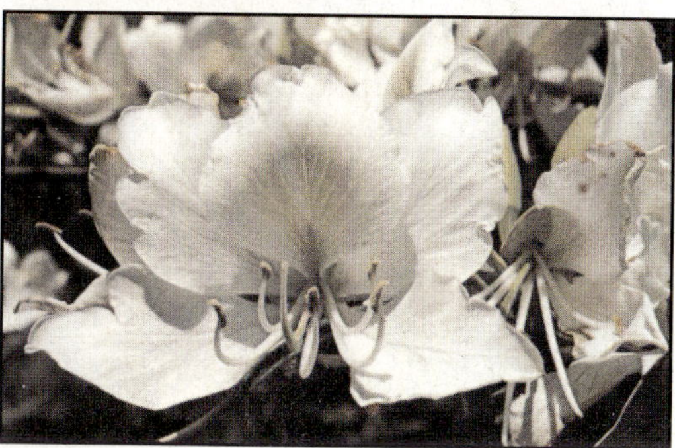

Bauhinia variegata

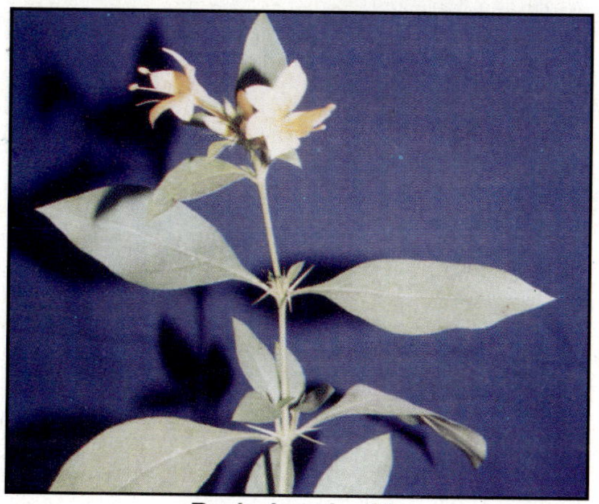

Barleria prionitis

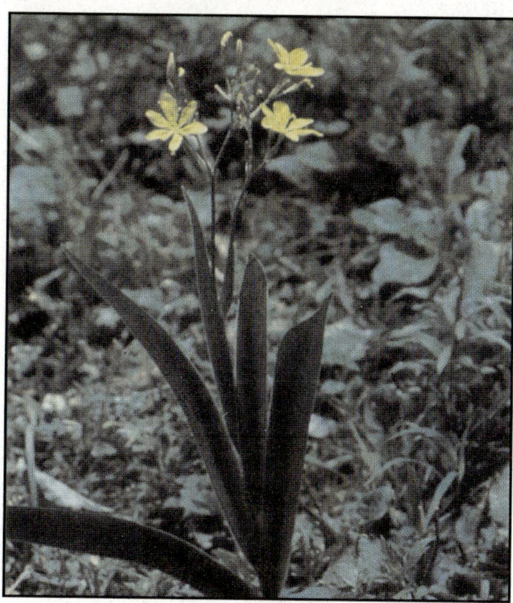

Belamcanda

PLATE : 24

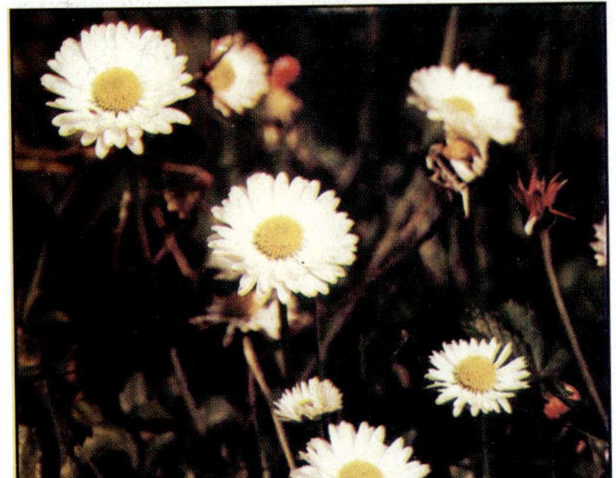

Bellis perennis

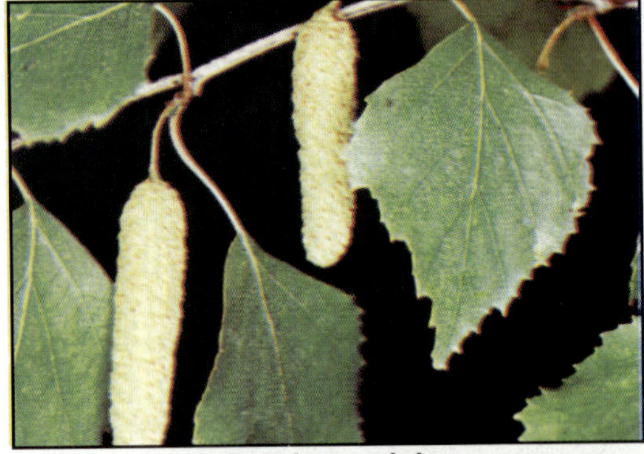

Betula pendula

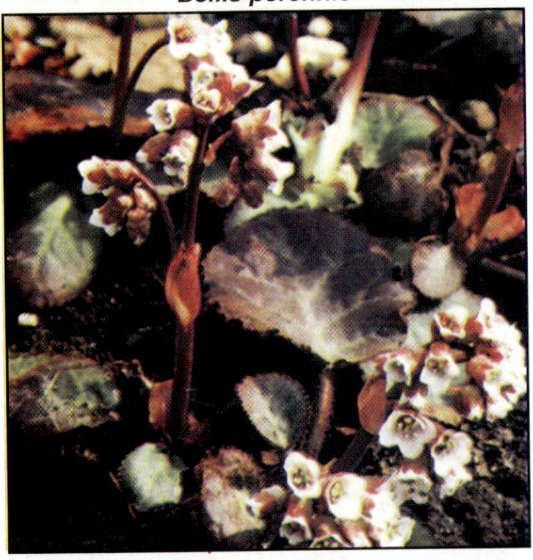

Bergenia ciliata

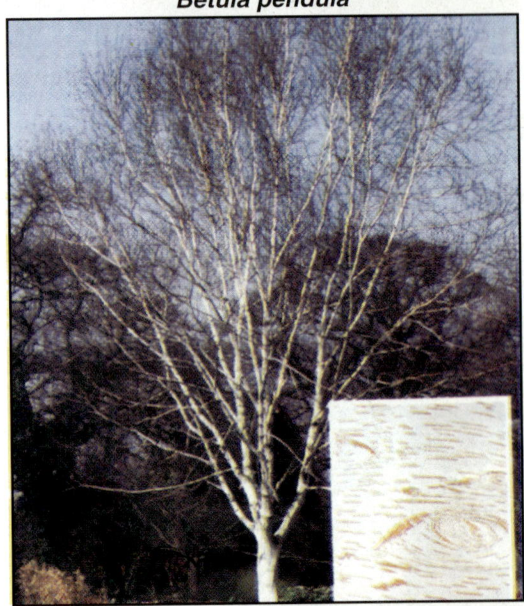

Betula utilis

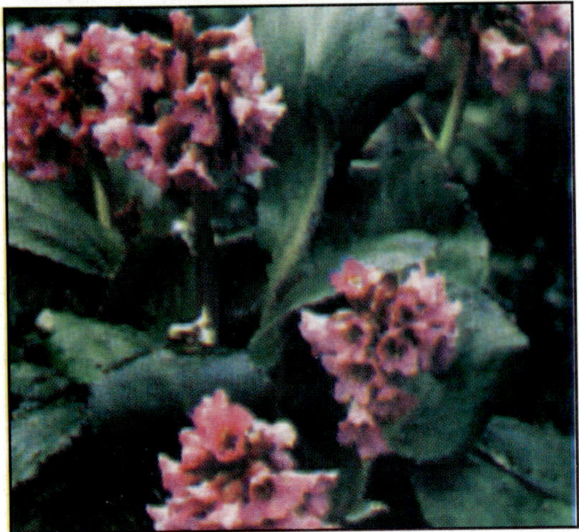

Bergenia stracheyi

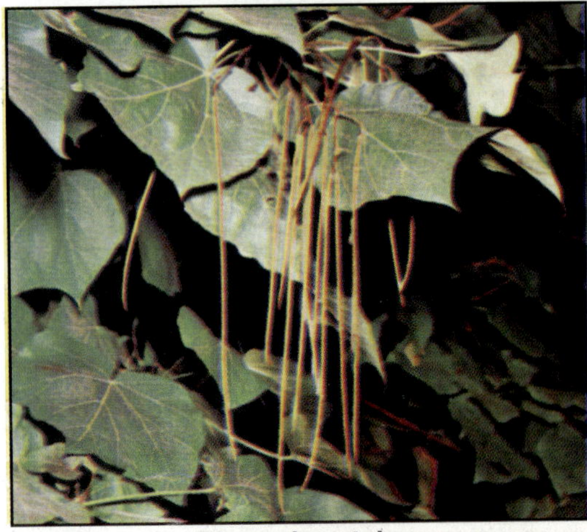

Bignonia catalpa

PLATE : 25

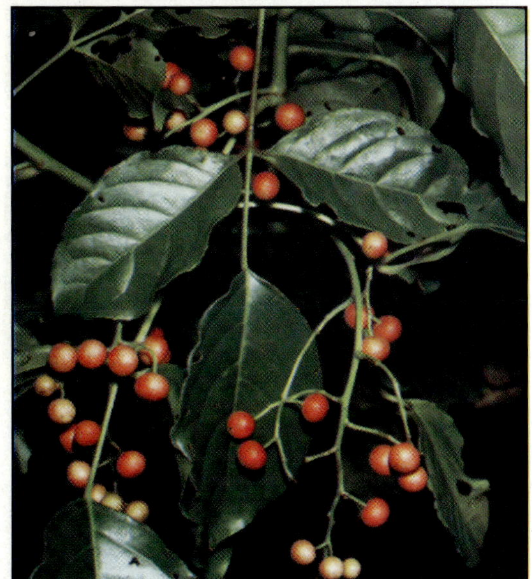

Bischofia javanica

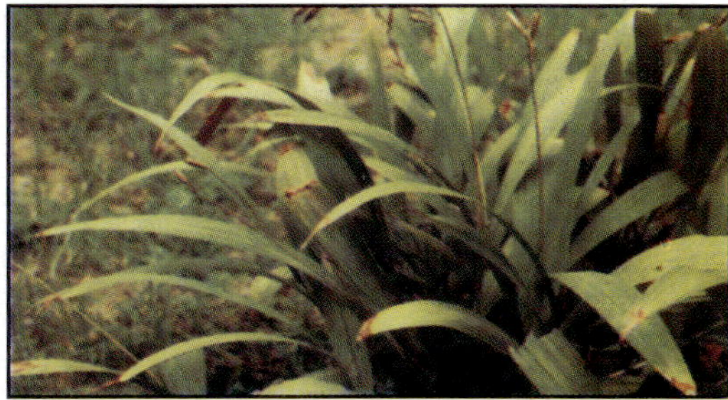

Bletilla striata

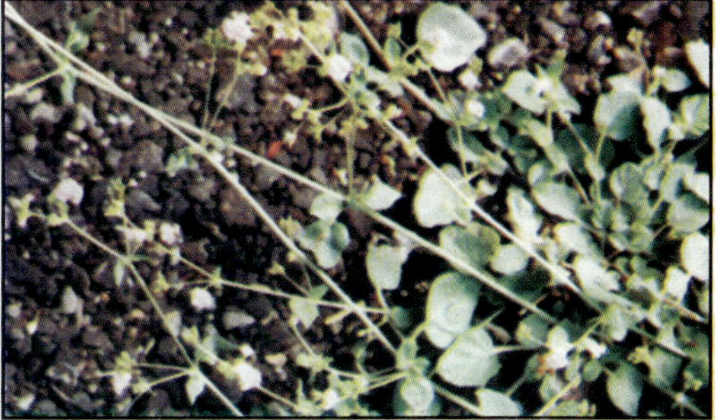

Boerhavia diffusa

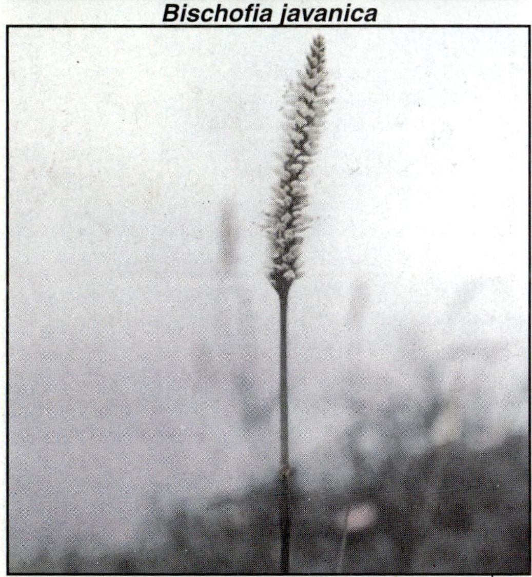

Bistorta manshuriensis

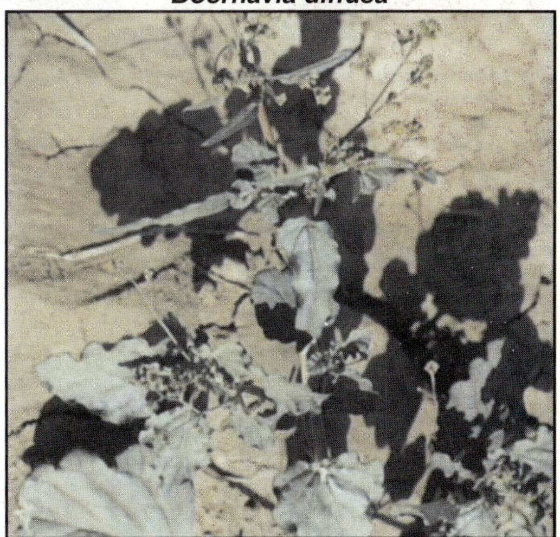

Boerhavia erecta

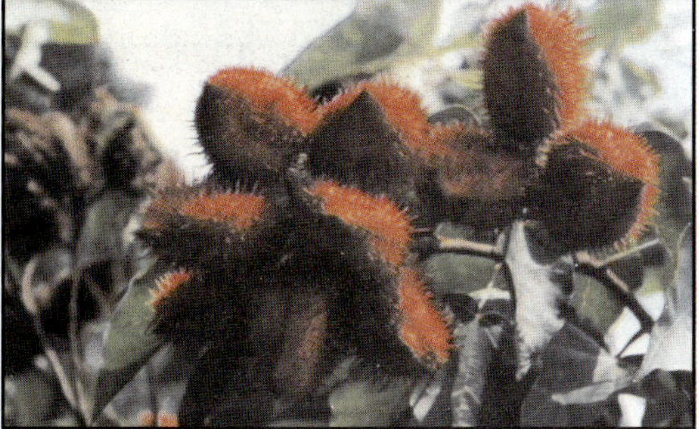

Bixa orellana

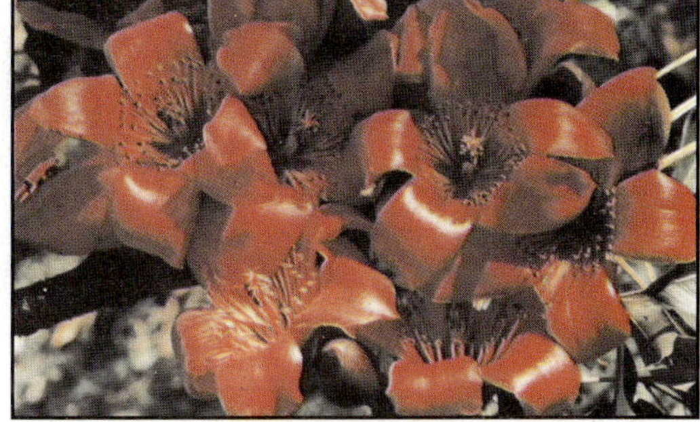

Bombax ceiba

PLATE : 26

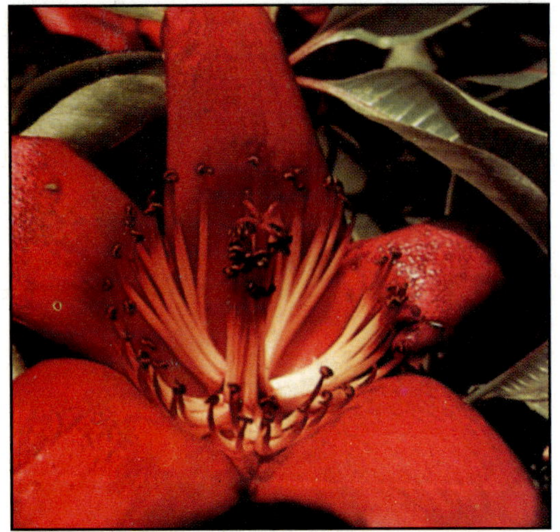

Bombax malabaricum

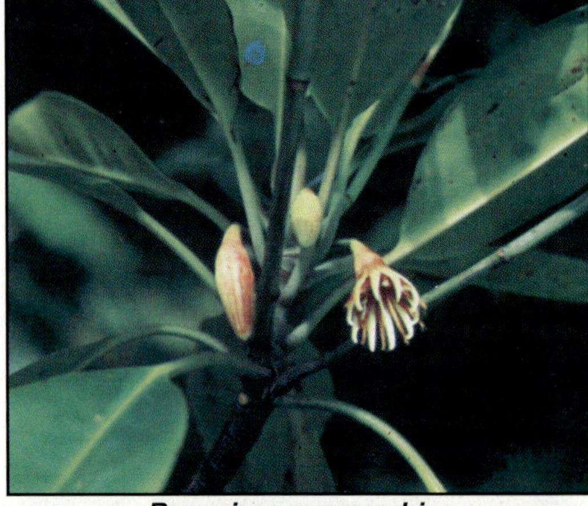

Bruguiera gymnorrhiza

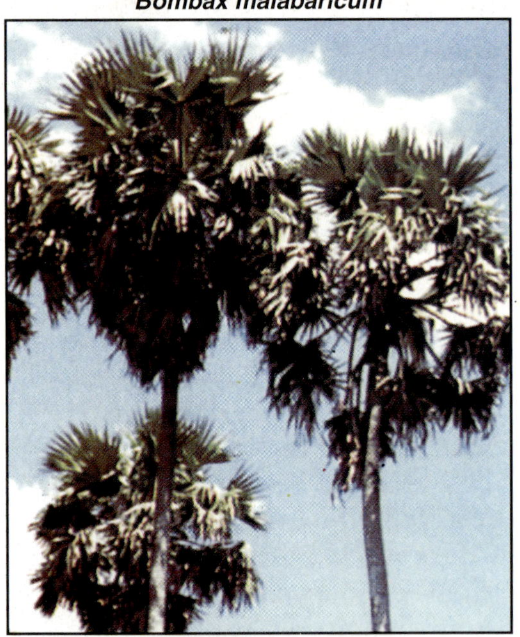

Borassus fladellifer

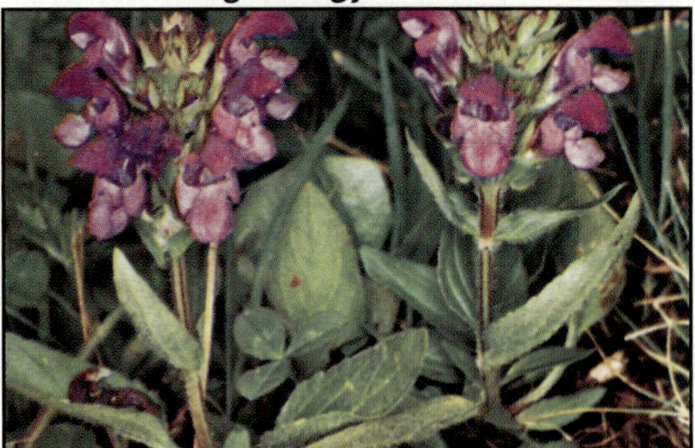

Brunella vulgaris

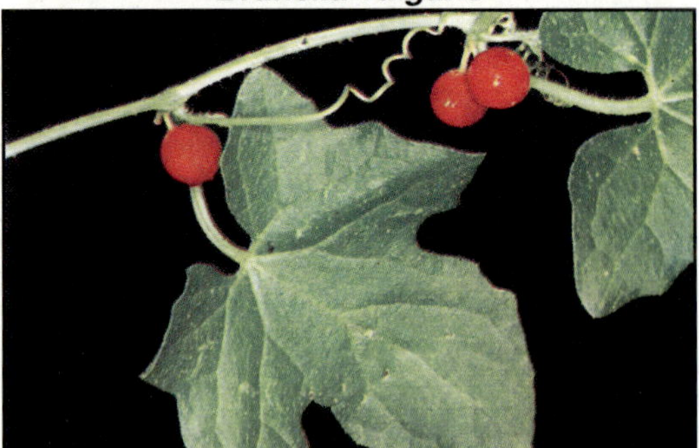

Bryonia cretica

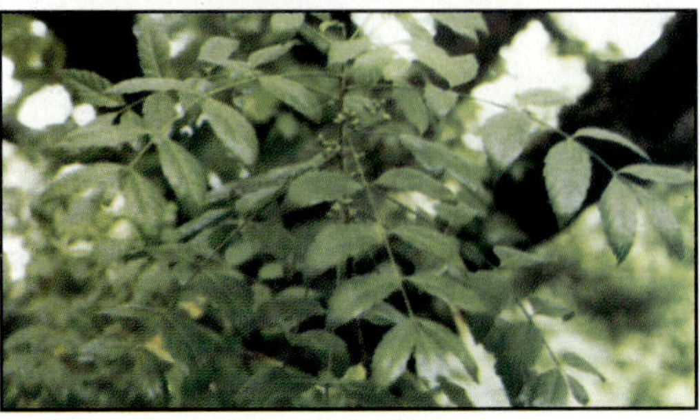

Brucea javanica

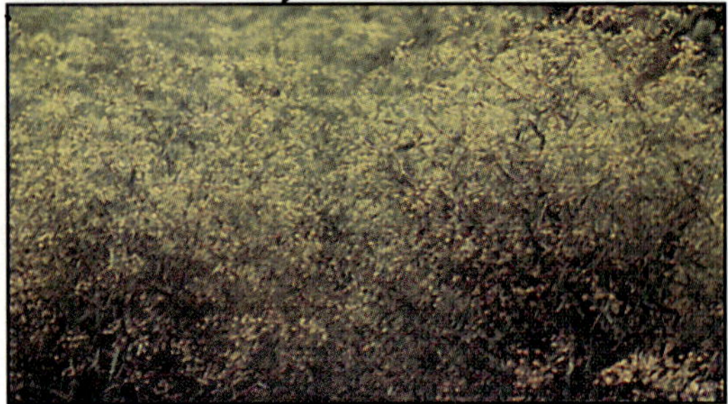

Bupleurum chinense

PLATE : 27

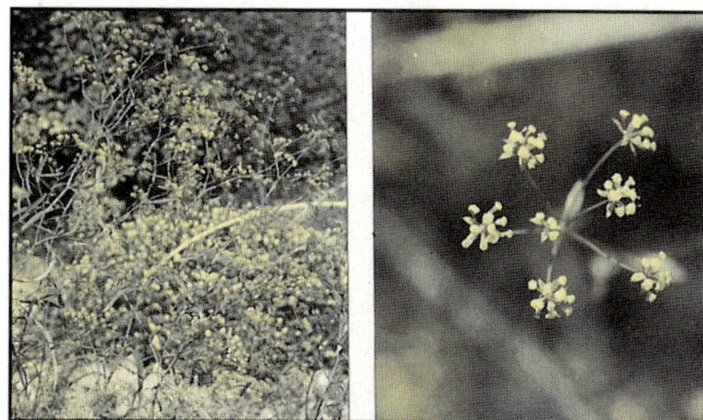

Bupleurum falcatum

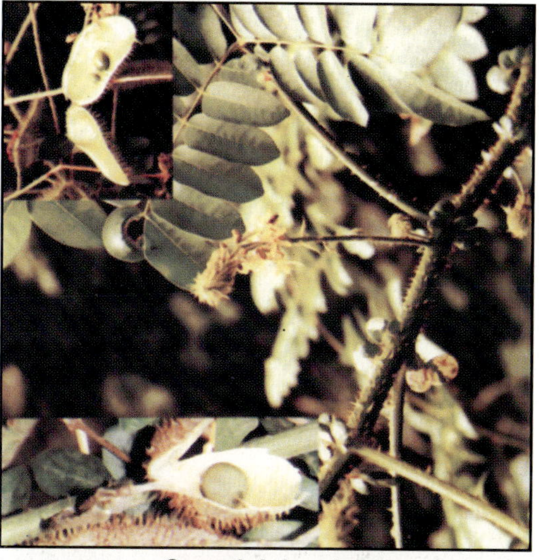

Caesalpinia crista

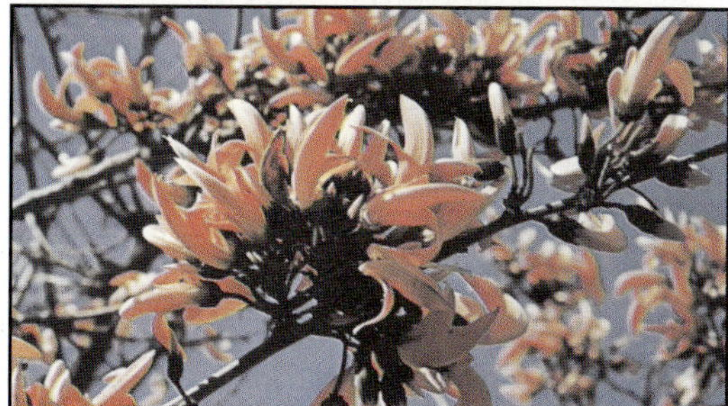

Butea frondosa

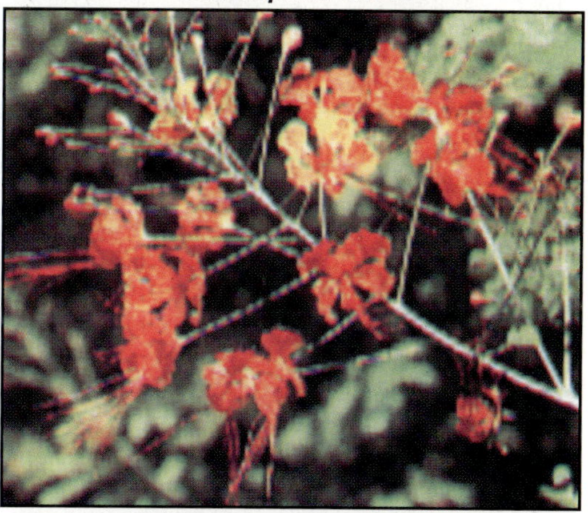

Caesalpinia pulcherrima

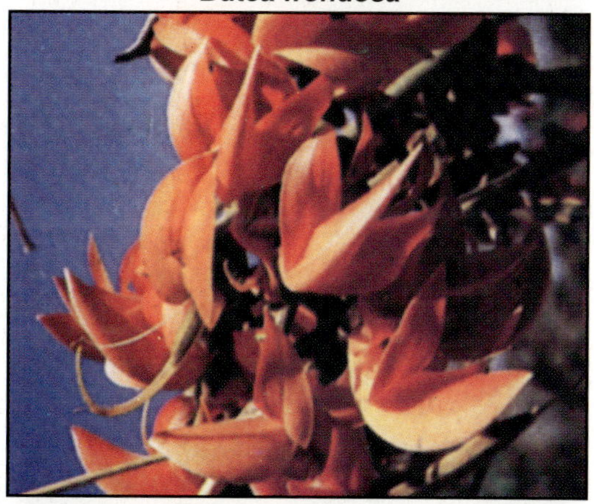

Butea monosperma

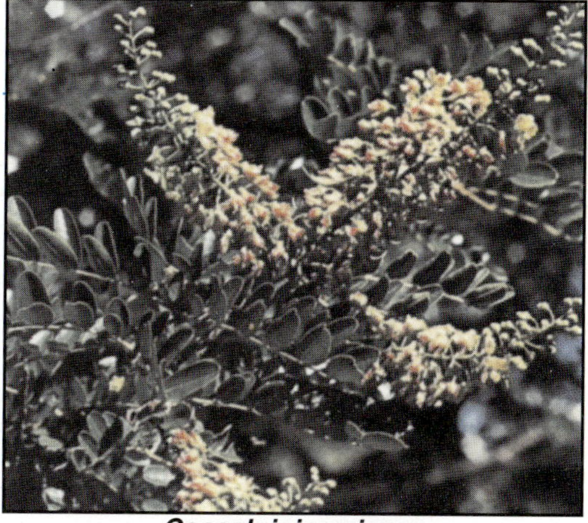

Caesalpinia spinosa

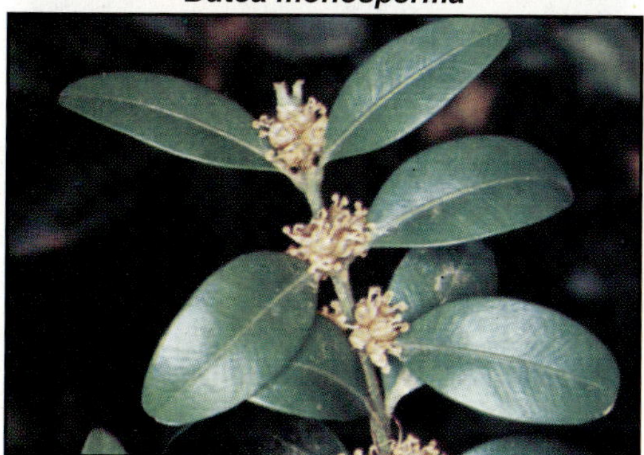

Buxus sempervirens

PLATE : 28

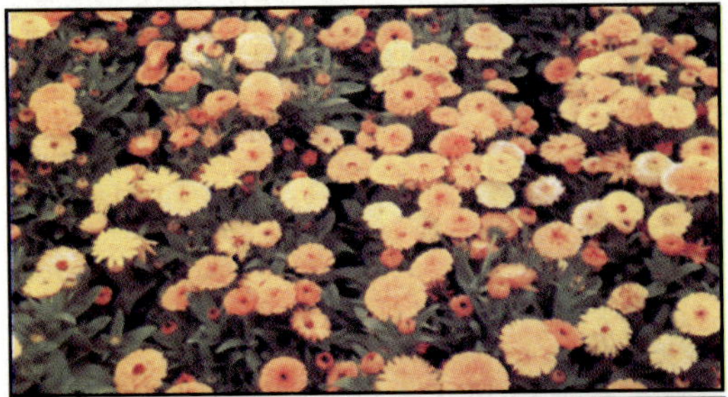

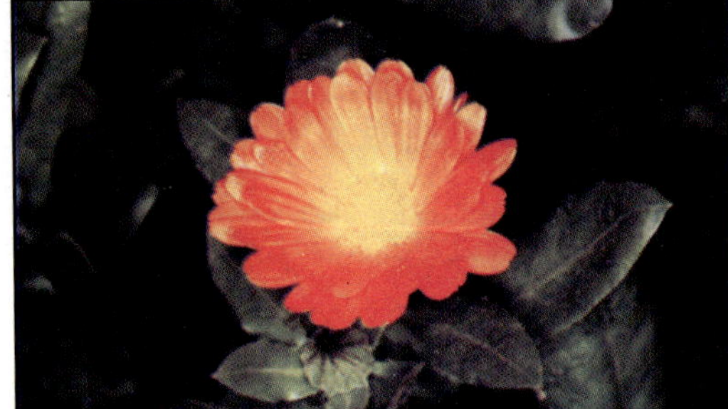

Calendula officinalis

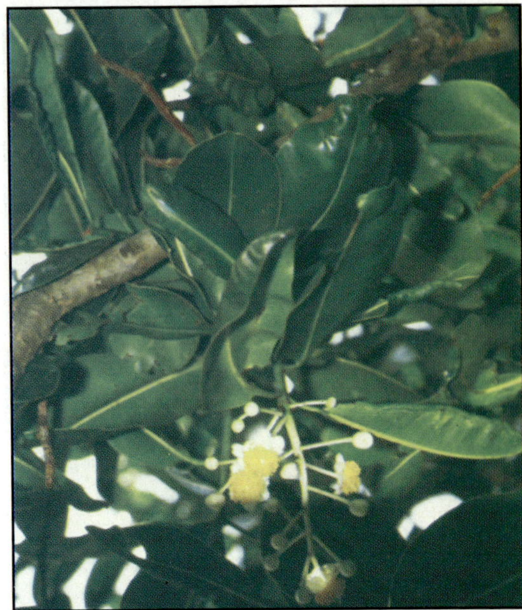

Calophyllum inophyllum

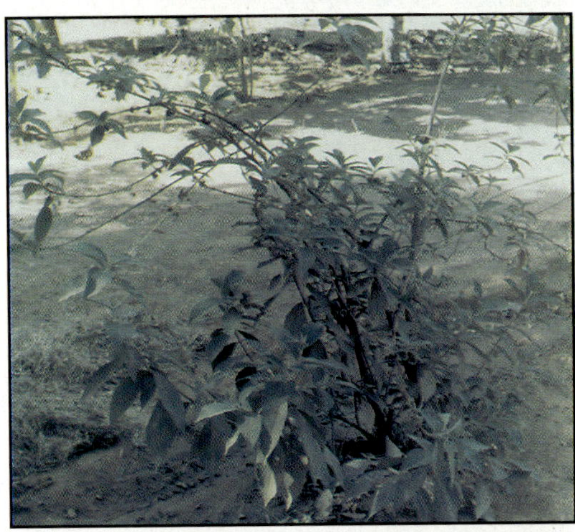

Callicarpa macrophylla

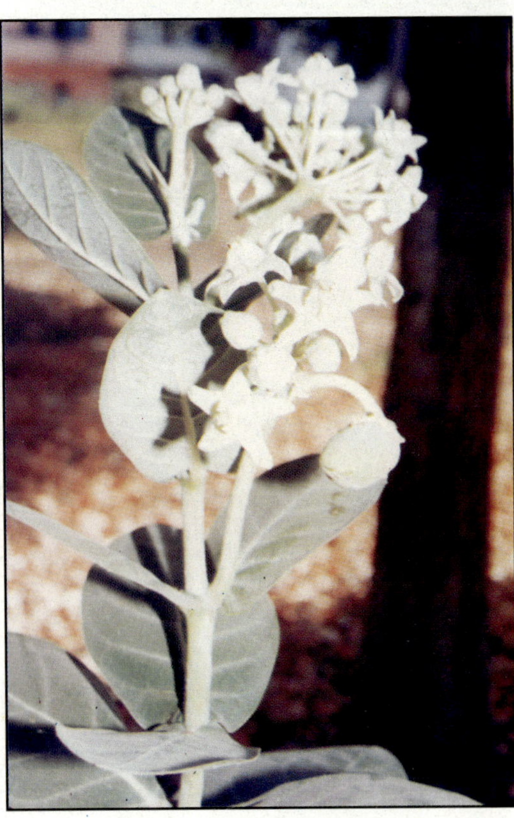

Calophyllum inophyllum

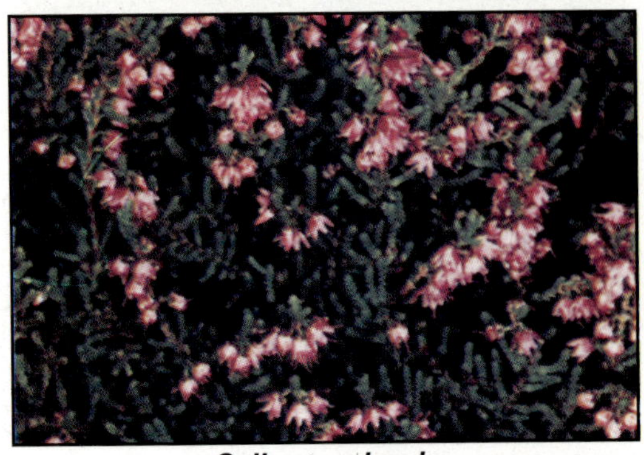

Calluna vulgaris

PLATE : 29

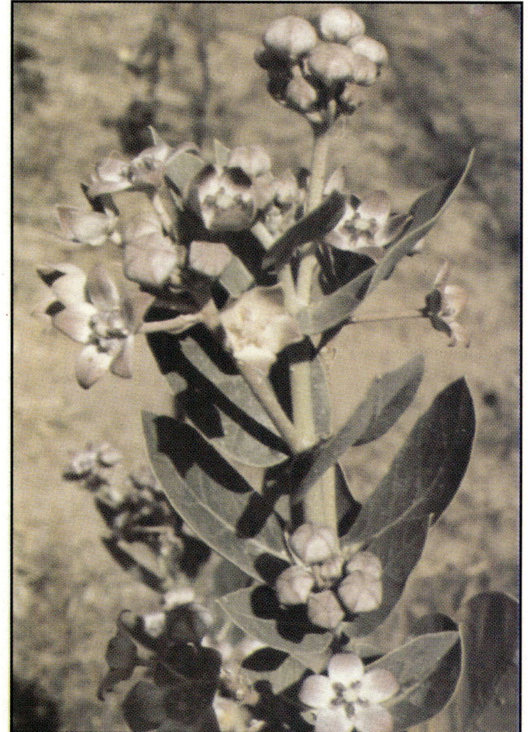

Calotropis procera

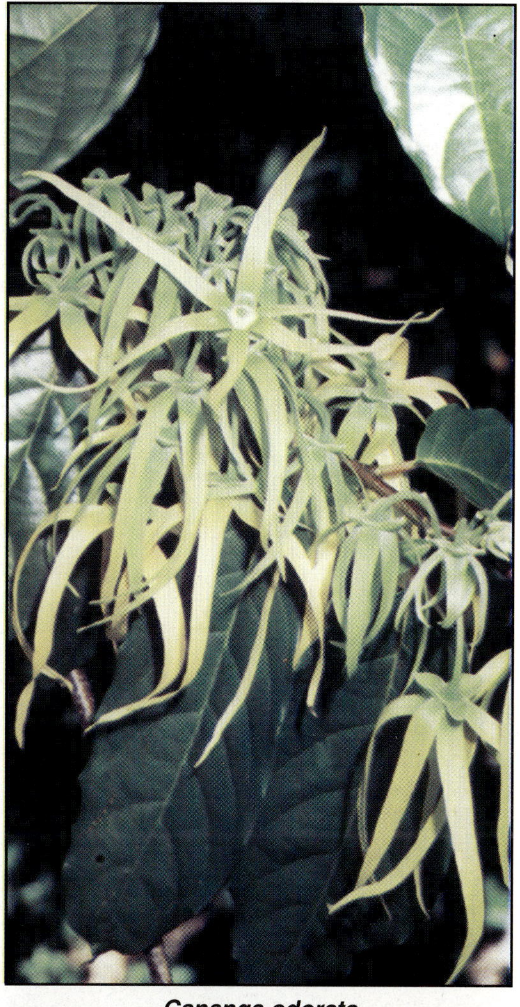

Cananga odorata

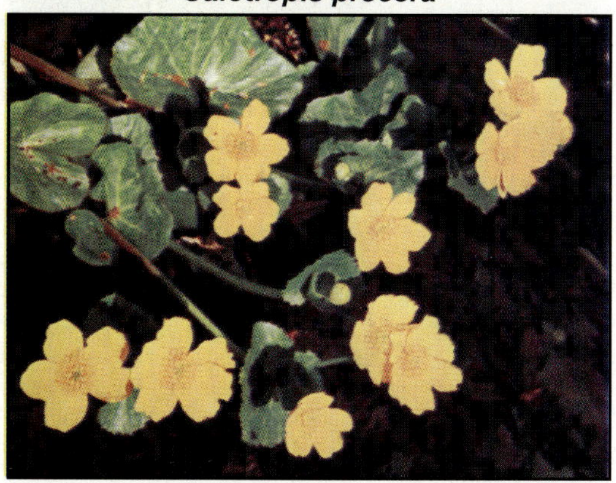

Caltha palustris

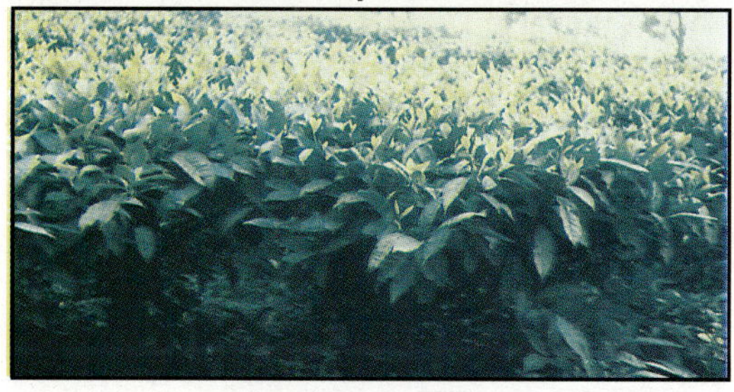

Camellia sinensis

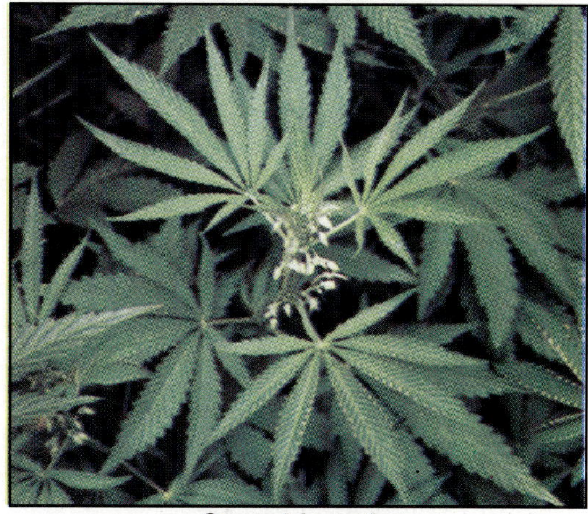

Cannabis sativa

PLATE : 30

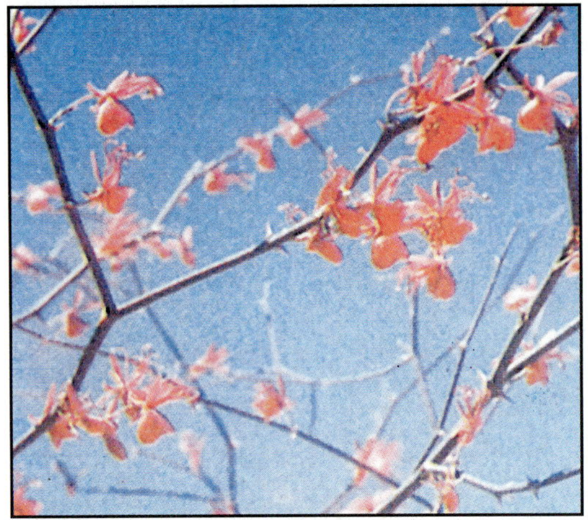

Capparis decidua

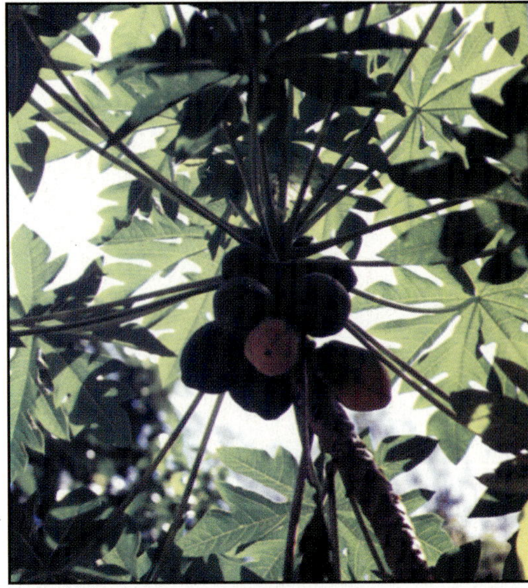

Carica papaya

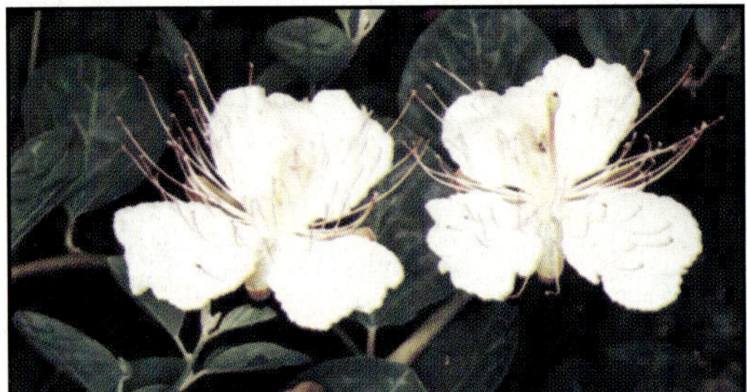

Capparis spinosa

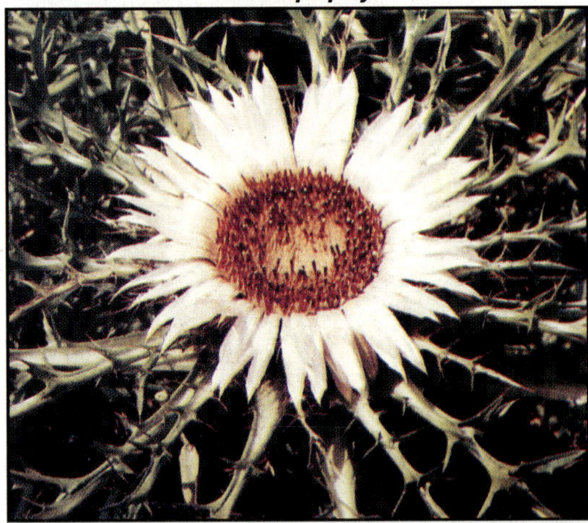

Carlina acaulis

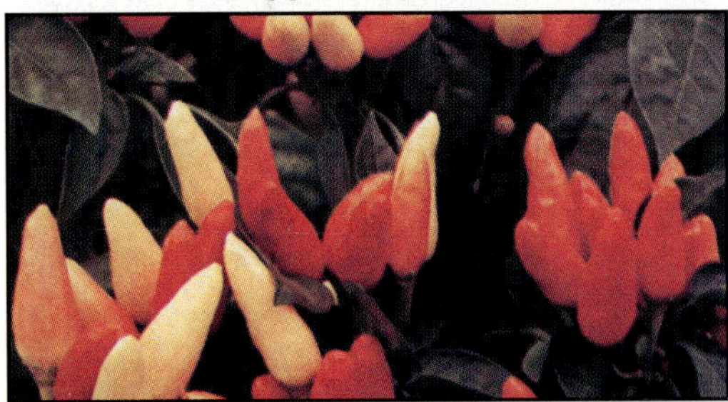

Capsicum annuum

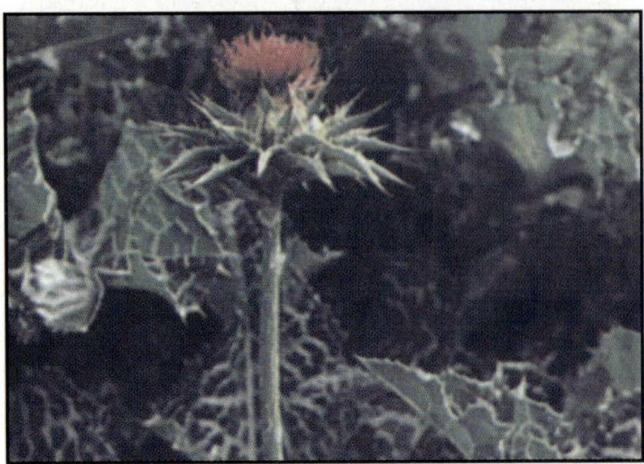

Carduus marianus

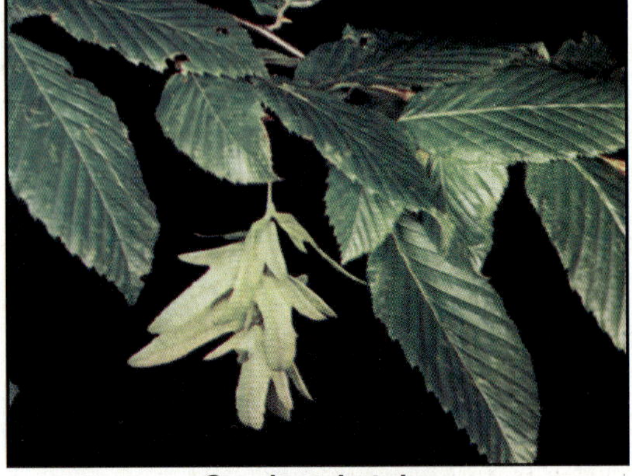

Carpinus betulus

PLATE : 31

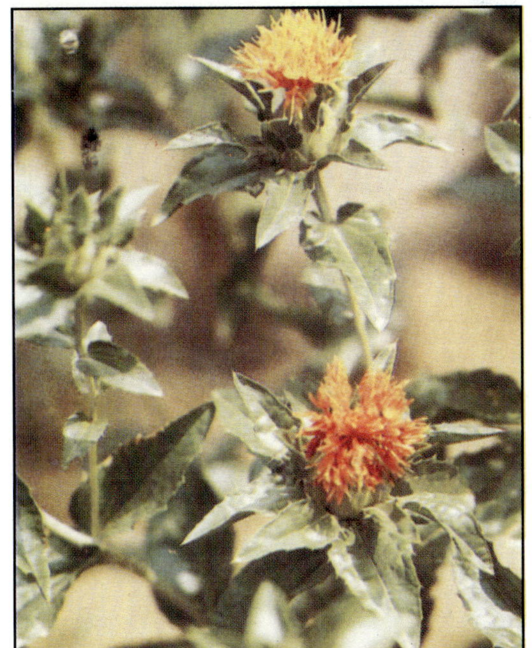

Carthamus tinctorius

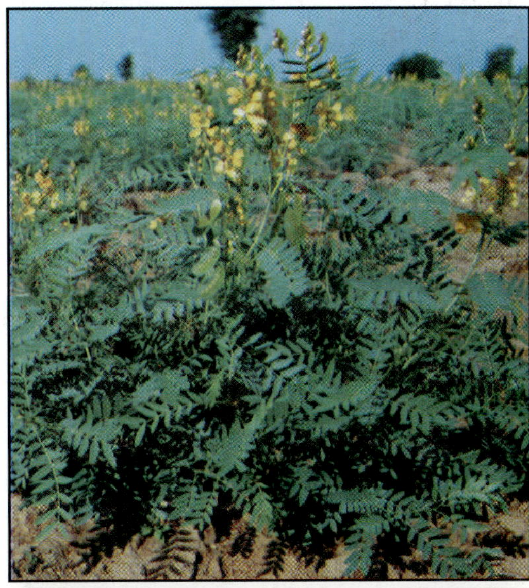

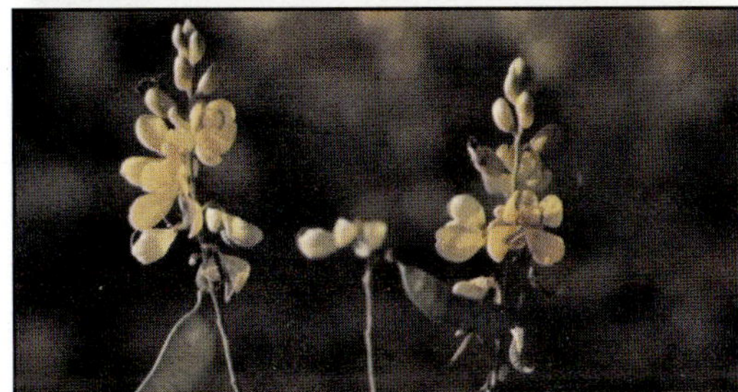

Cassia angustifolia

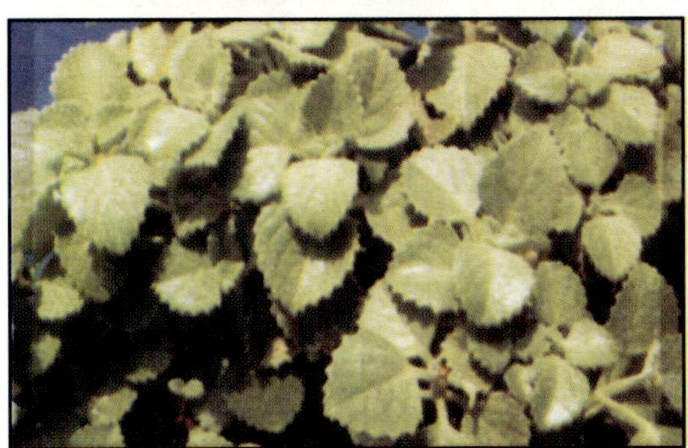

Carum copticum

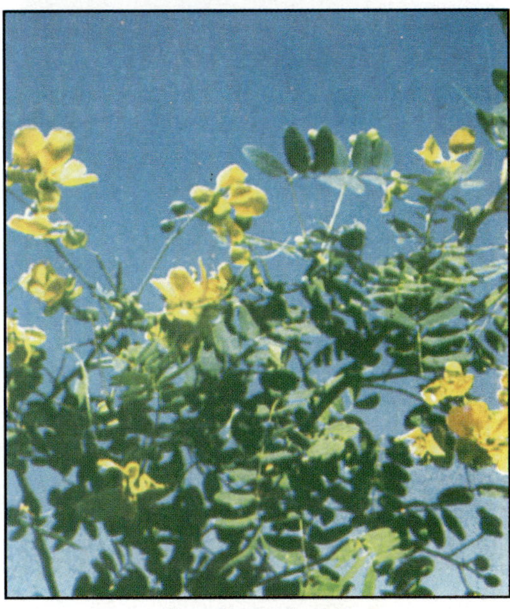

Cassia auriculata

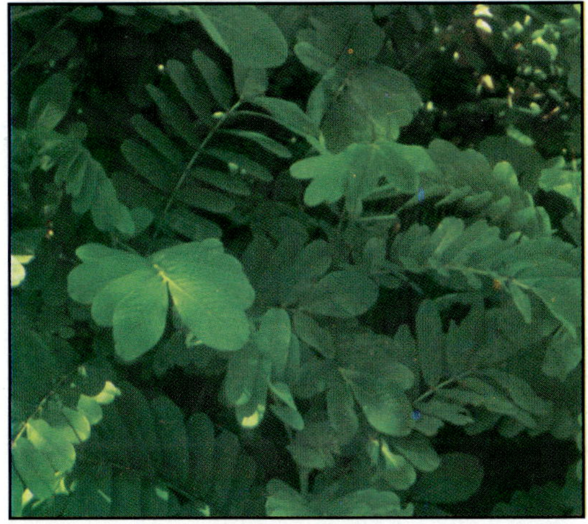

Cassia alata

PLATE : 32

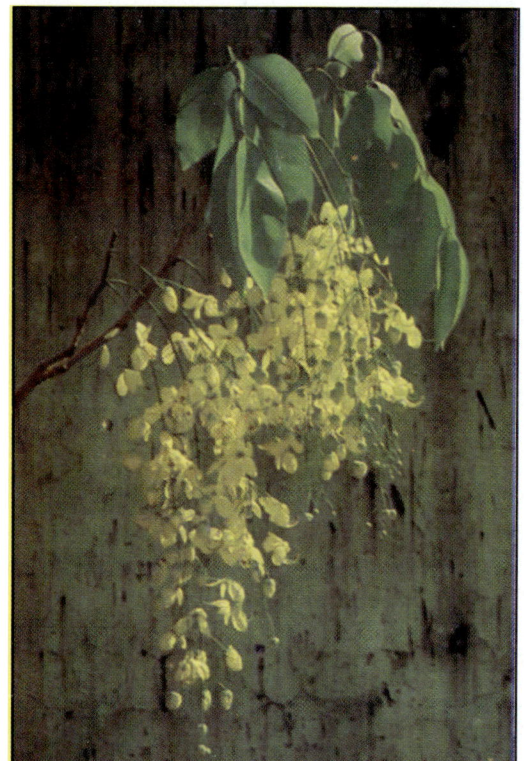

Cassia fistula

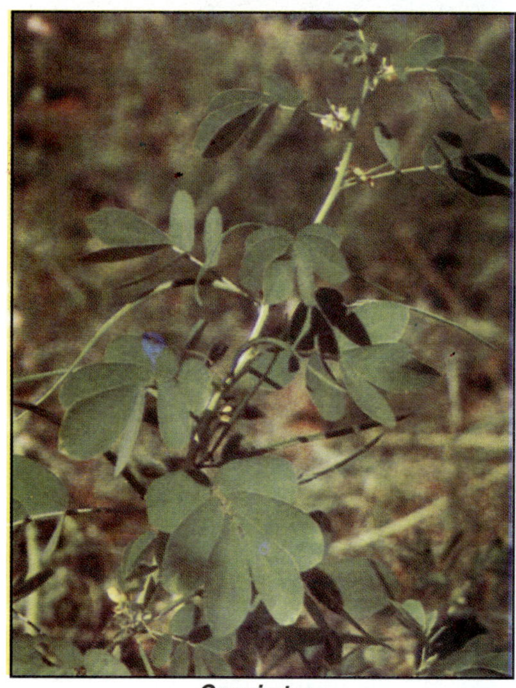

Cassia tora

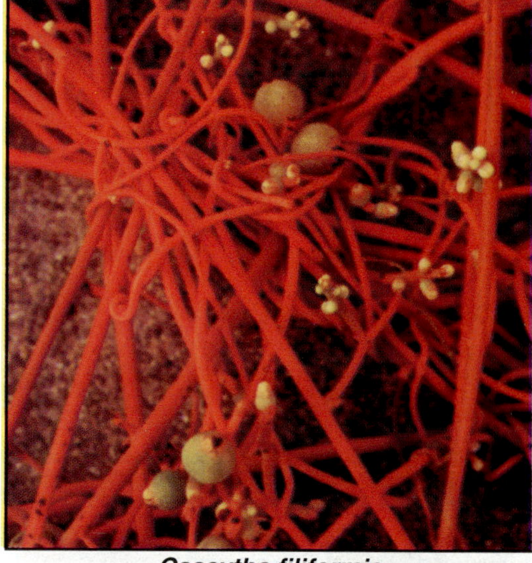

Cassytha filiformis

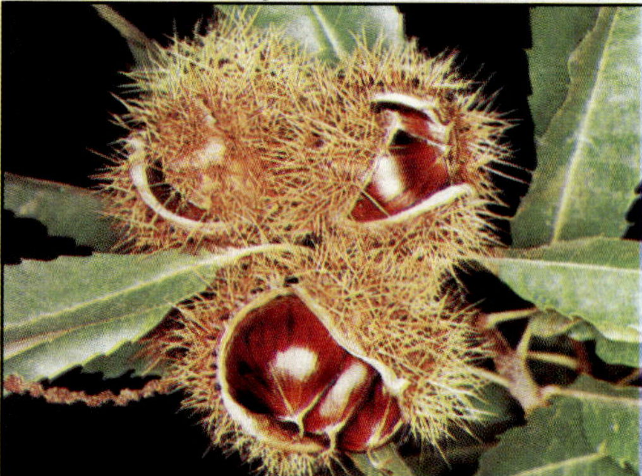

Castanea sativa

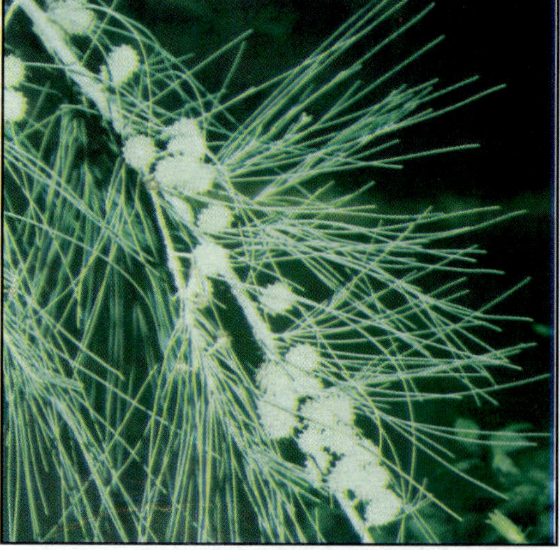

Casuarina equisetifolia

PLATE : 33

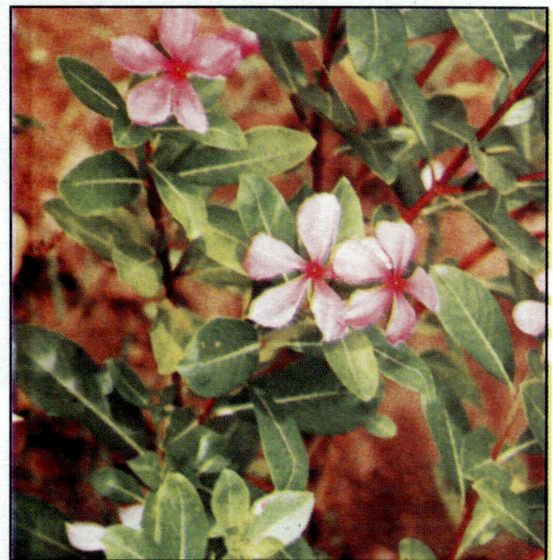

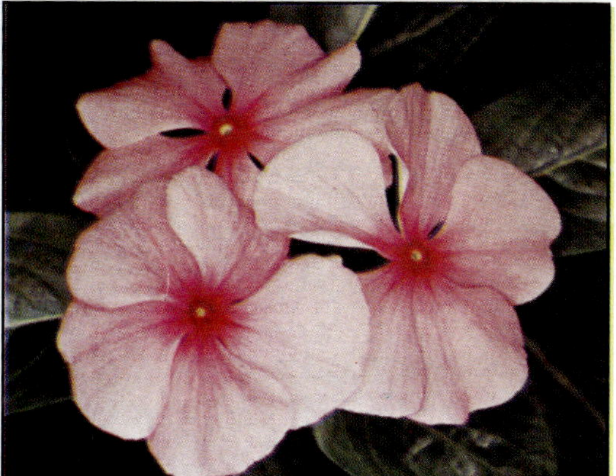

Catharanthus roseus

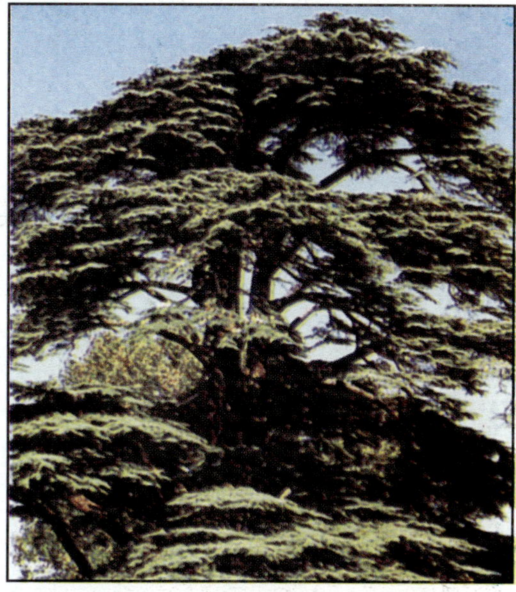

Cedrus libani

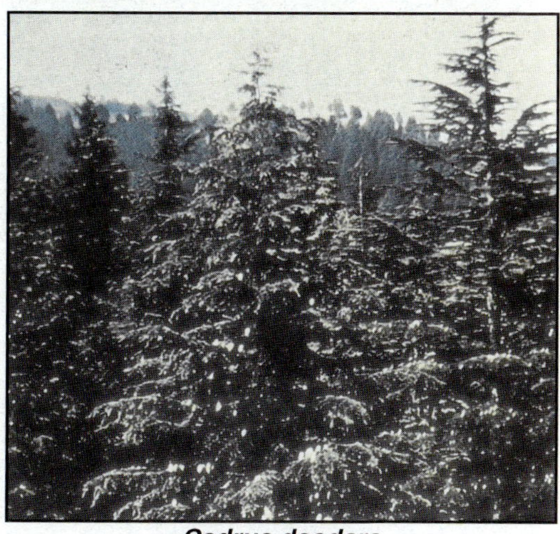

Cedrus deodara

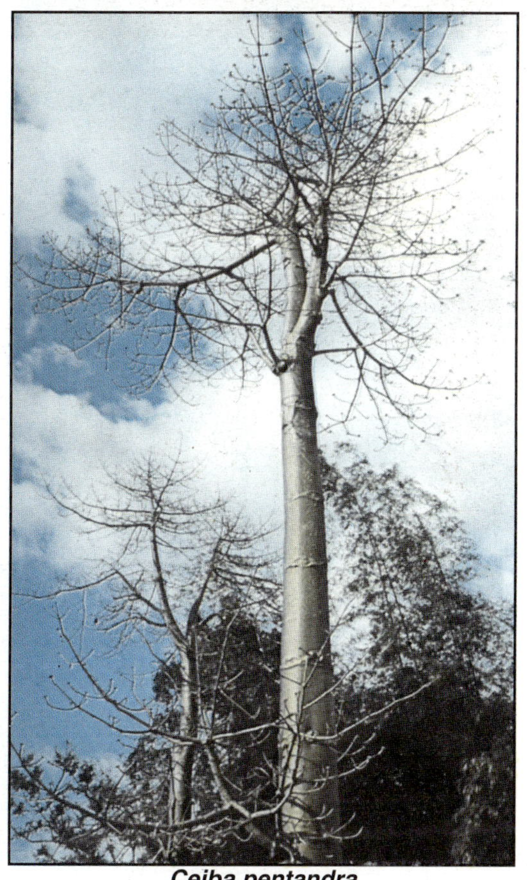

Ceiba pentandra

PLATE : 34

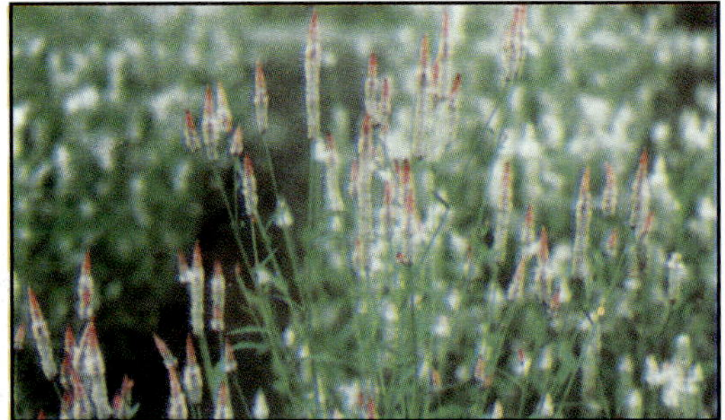

Celosia argentea

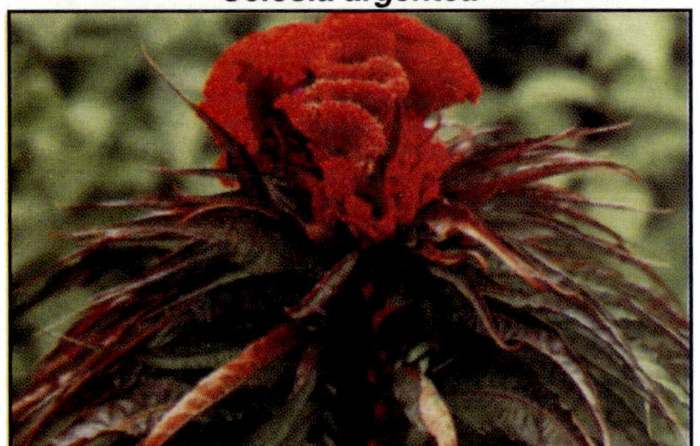

Celosia cristata

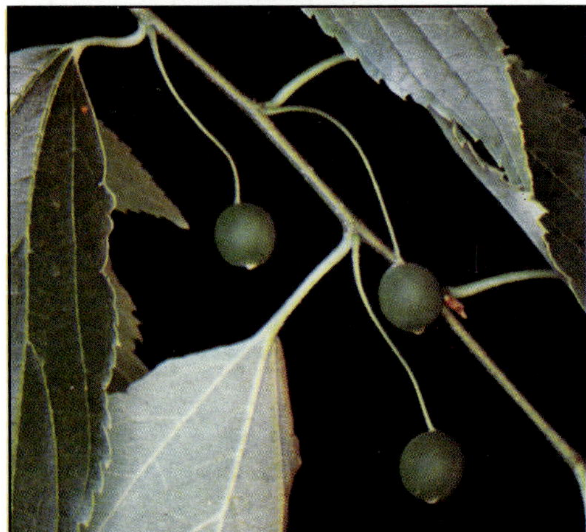

Celtis australis

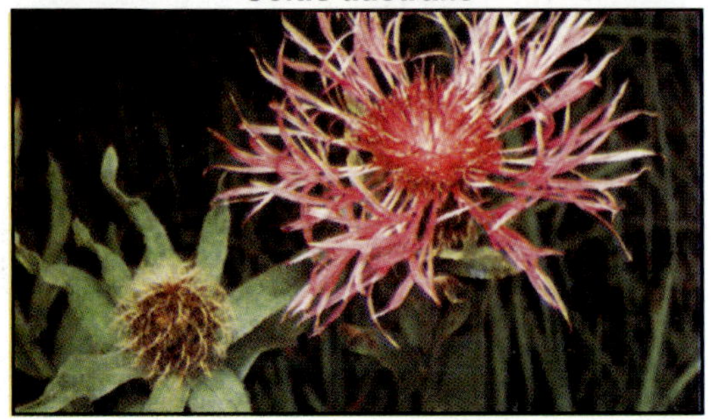

Centaurea centaurium

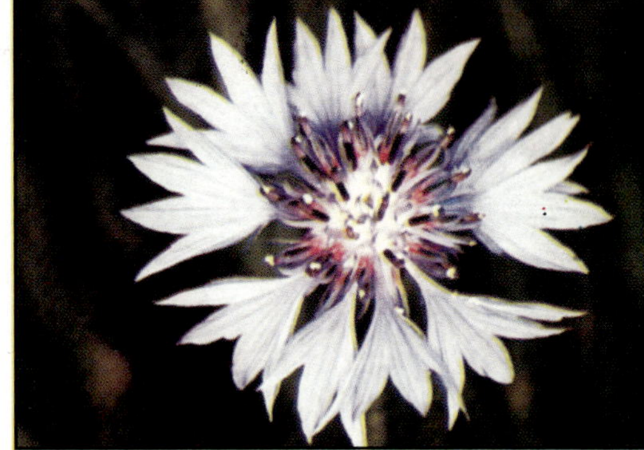

Centaurea cyanus

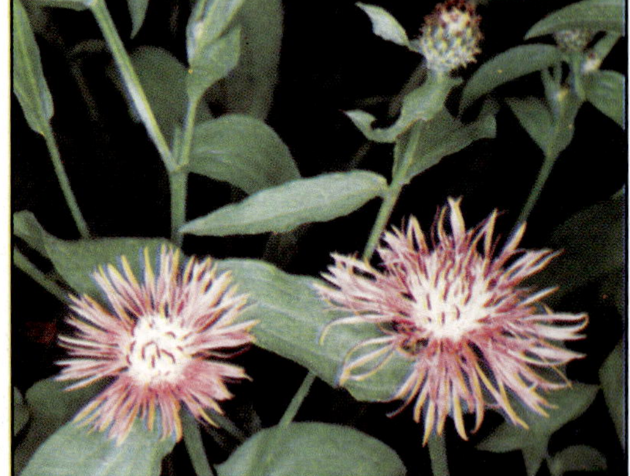

Centaurea jacea

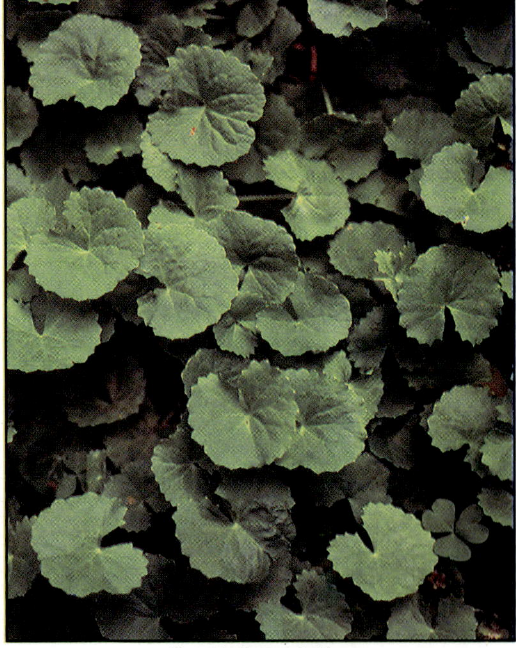

Centella asiatica

PLATE : 35

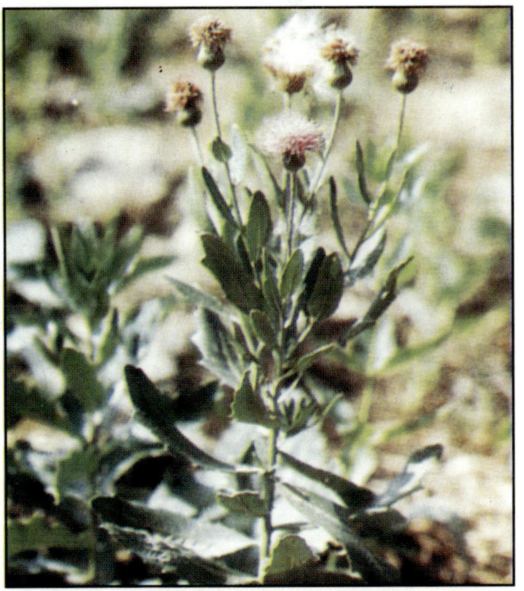

Cephalonploa segetum

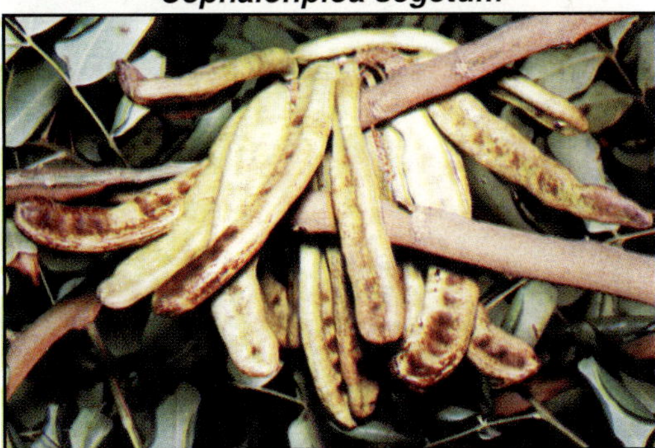

Ceratonia siliqua

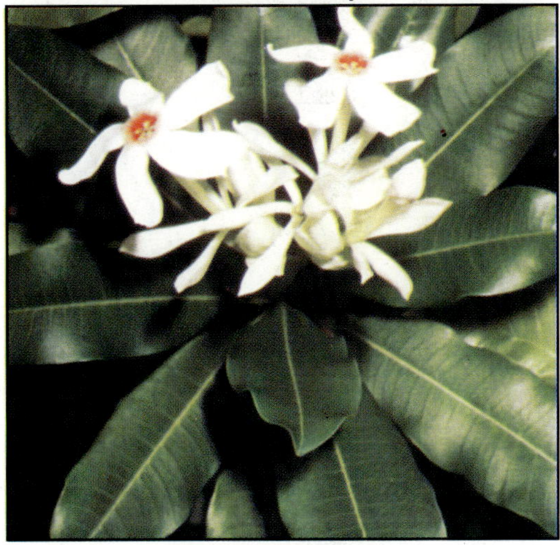

Cerbera manghas

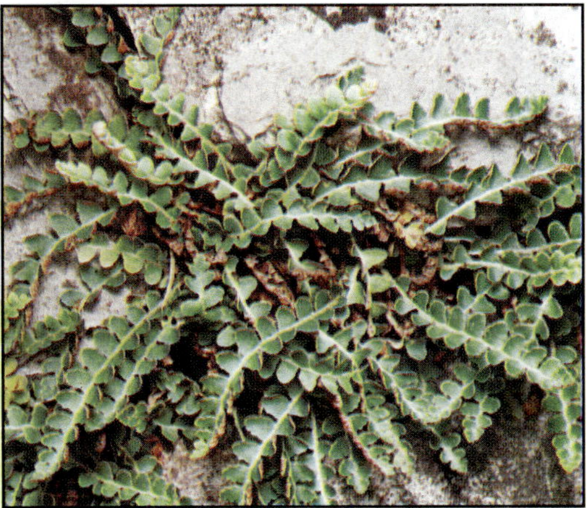

Ceterach officinarum

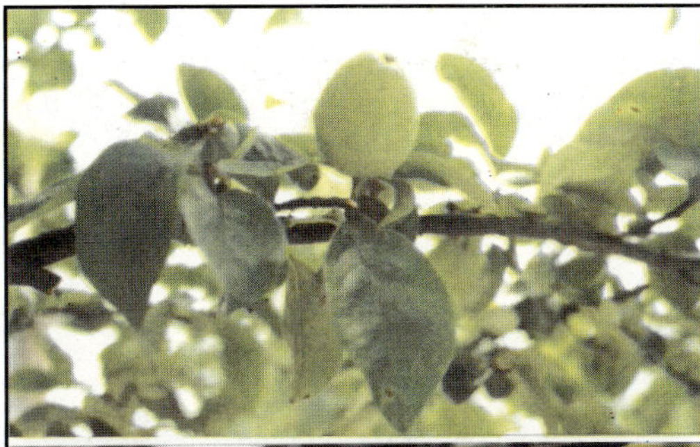

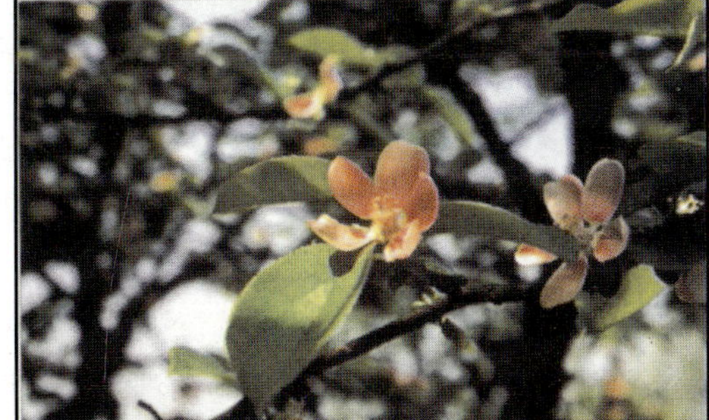

Chaenomeles sinensis

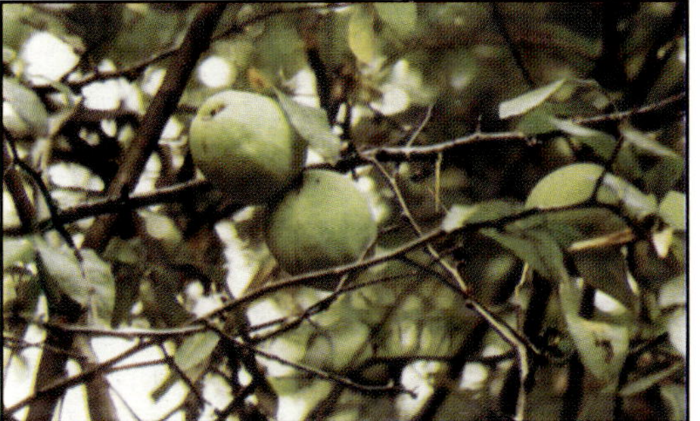

Chaenomeles speciosa

PLATE : 36

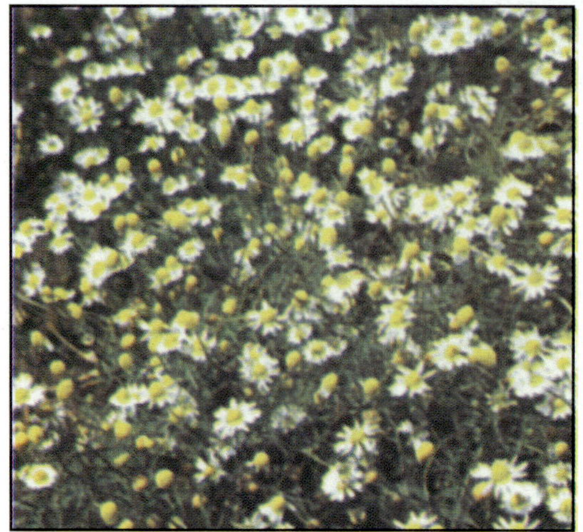

Chamomilla recutita

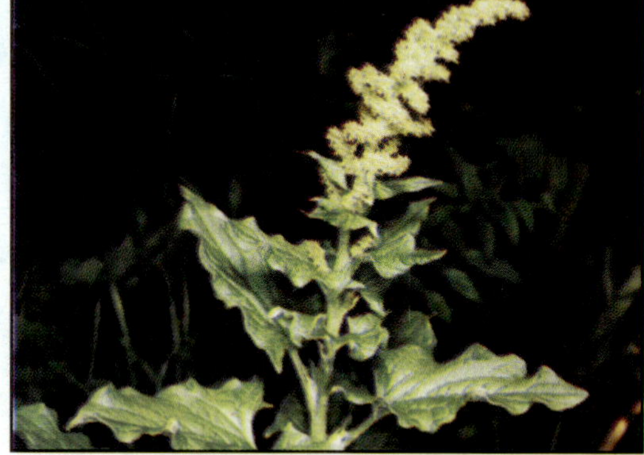

Chenopodium bonus-henricus

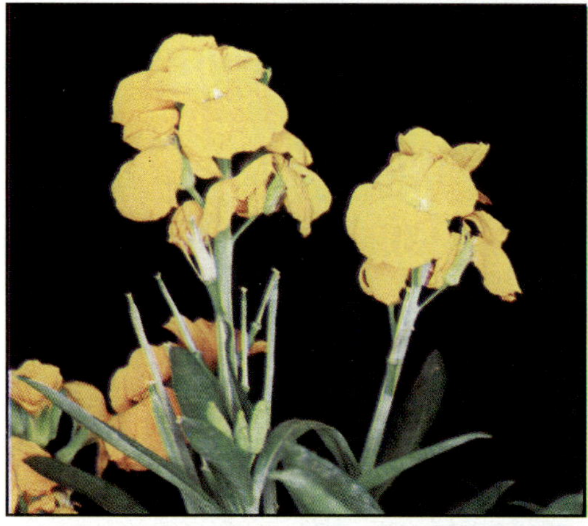

Cheiranthus cheiri

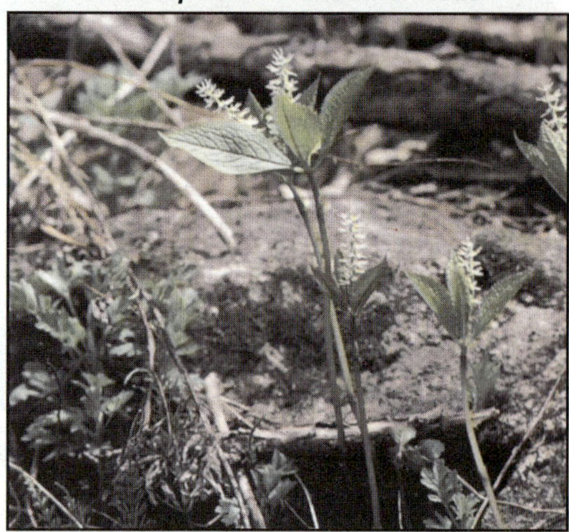

Chloranthus joponicus

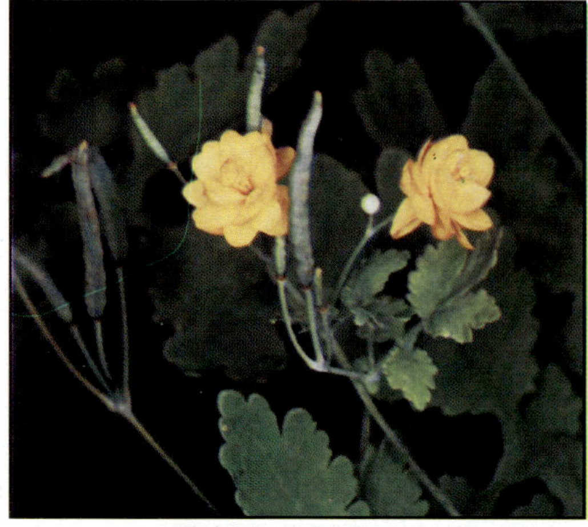

Chelidonium majus

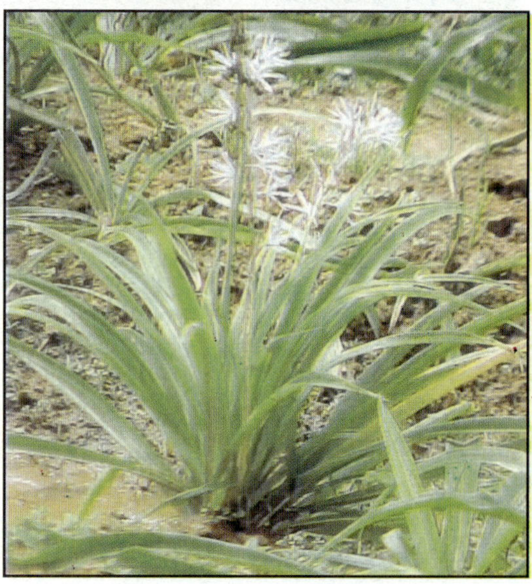

Chlorophytum borivilianum

PLATE : 37

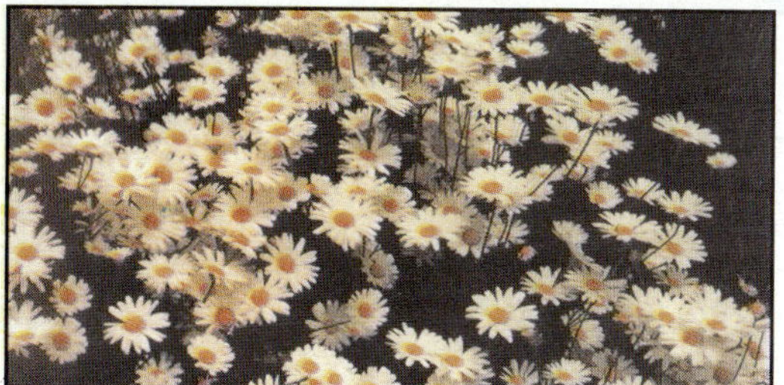

Chrysanthemum cinerariifolium

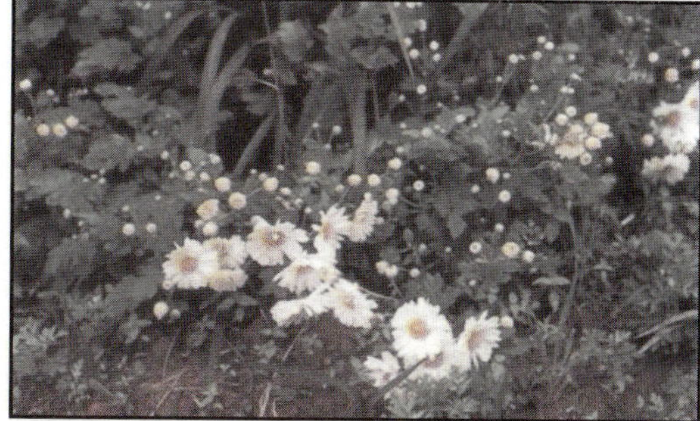

Chrysanthemum morifolium

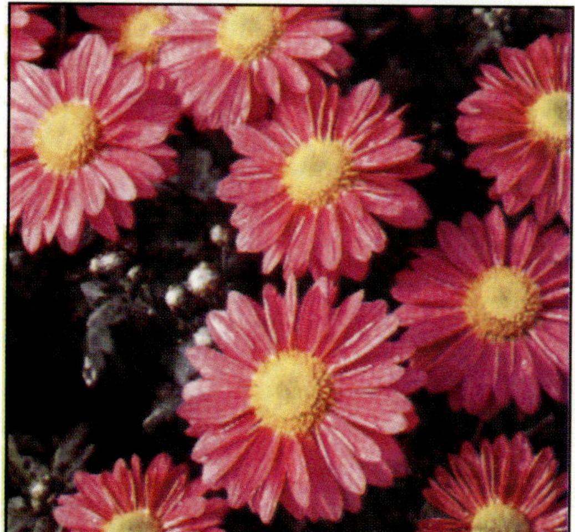

Chrysanthemum coronarium

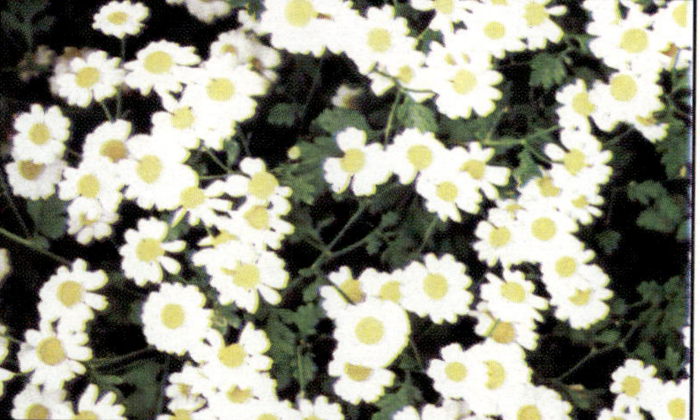

Chrysanthemum parthenium

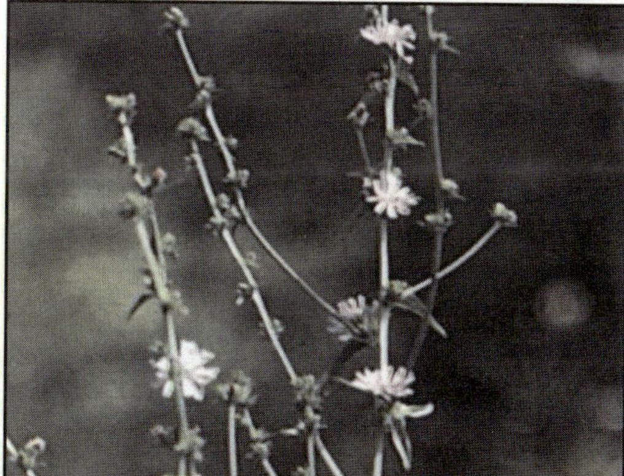

Cichorium intybus

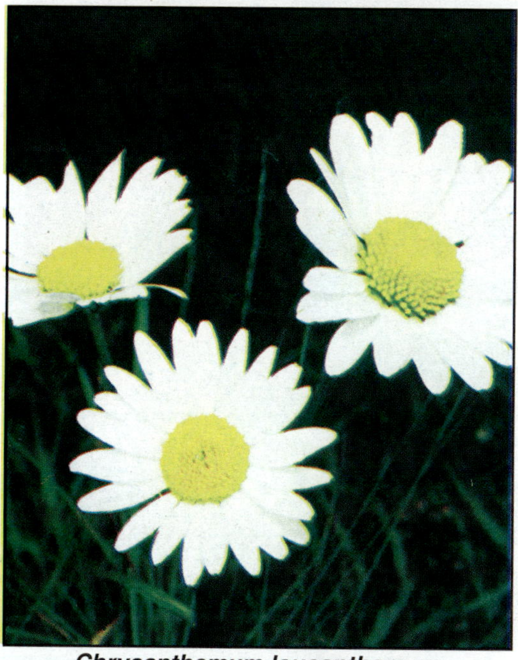

Chrysanthemum leucanthemum

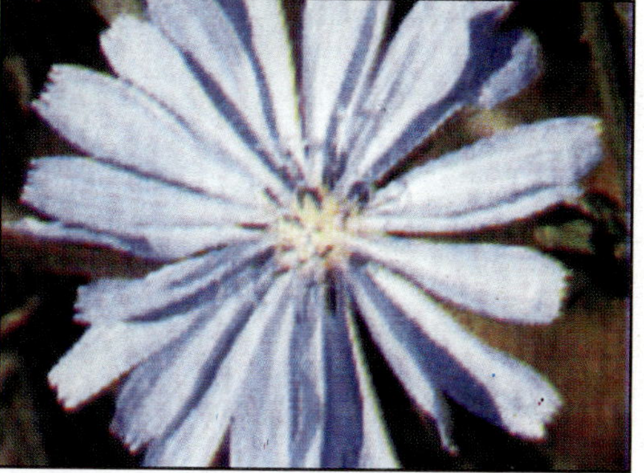

Cichoriun intybus

PLATE : 38

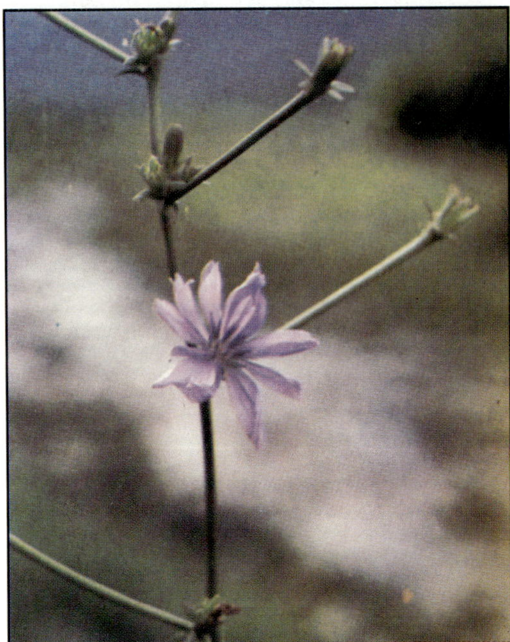
Cichorum endivia

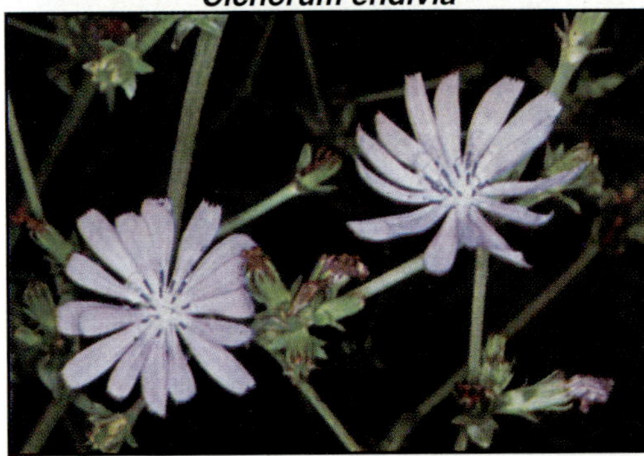
Cicjorium intybus

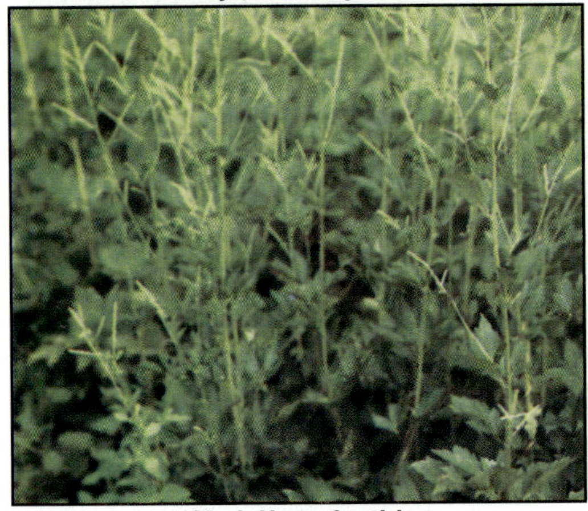
Cimicifuga foetida

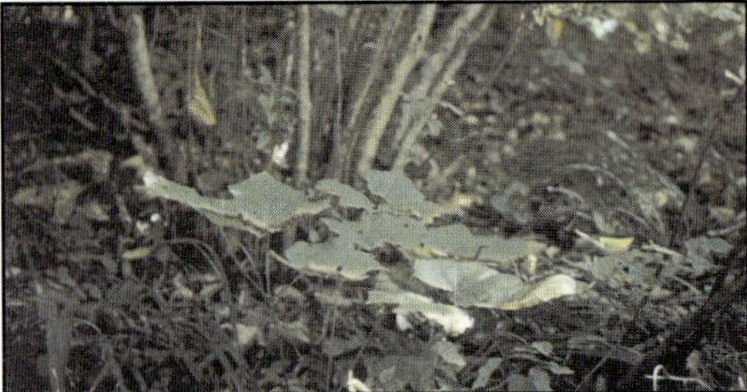
Cimicifuga heracleifolia

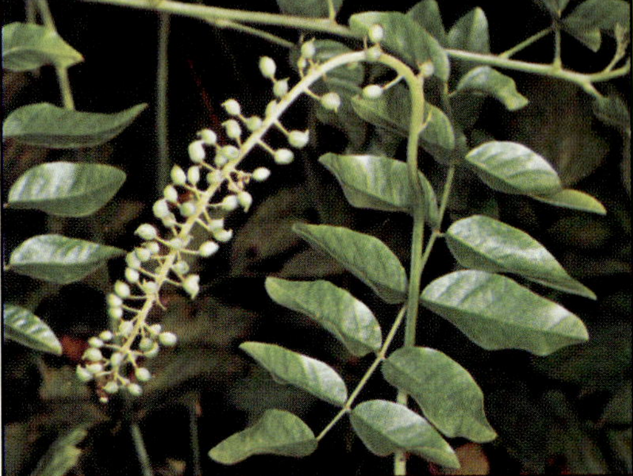
Cimicifuga racemosa

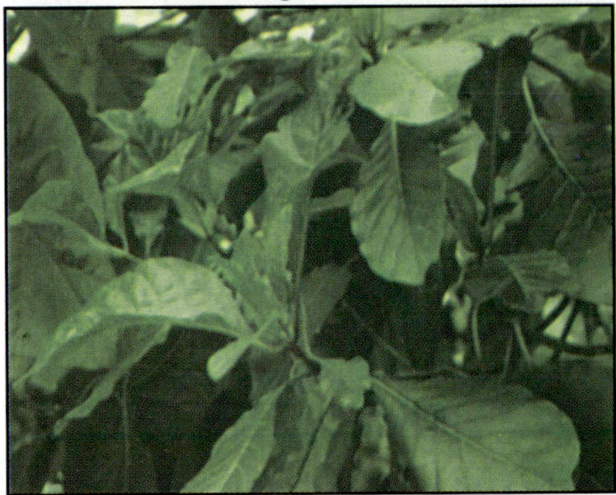
Cinchona officinalis

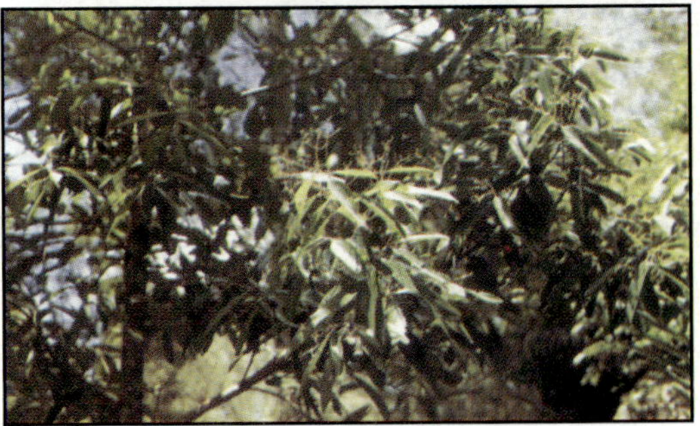
Cinnamomum cassia

PLATE : 39

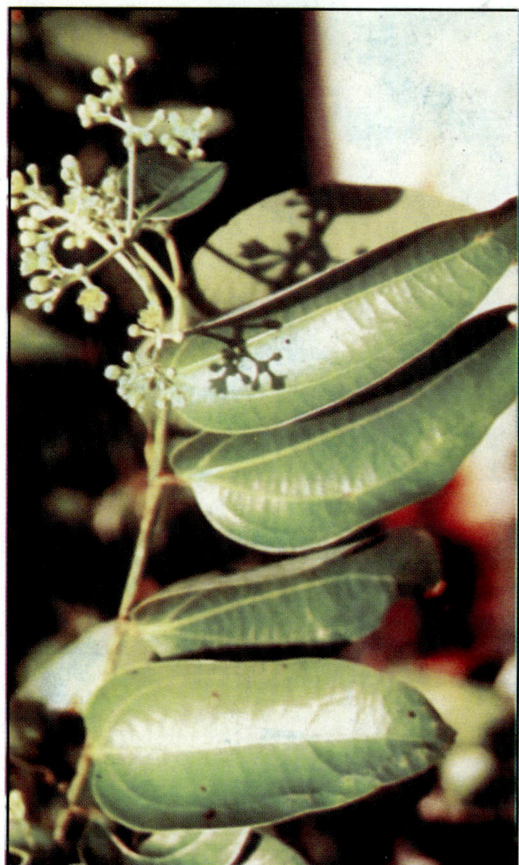

Cinnamomum tamala

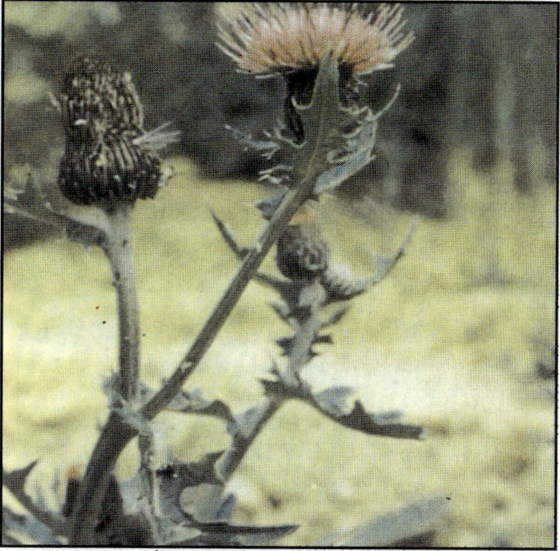

Cirsium japonicum

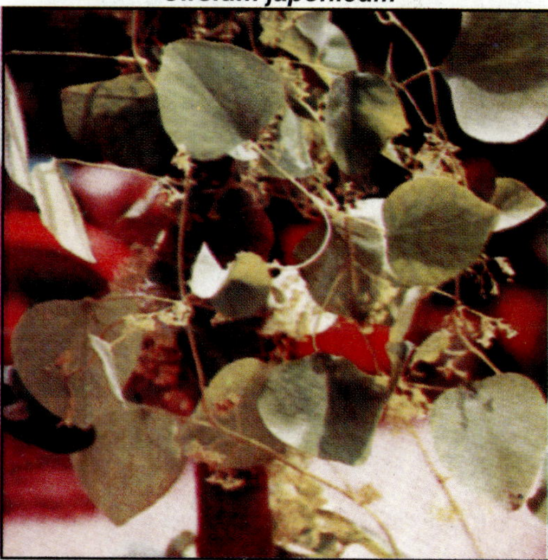

Cissampelos pareira

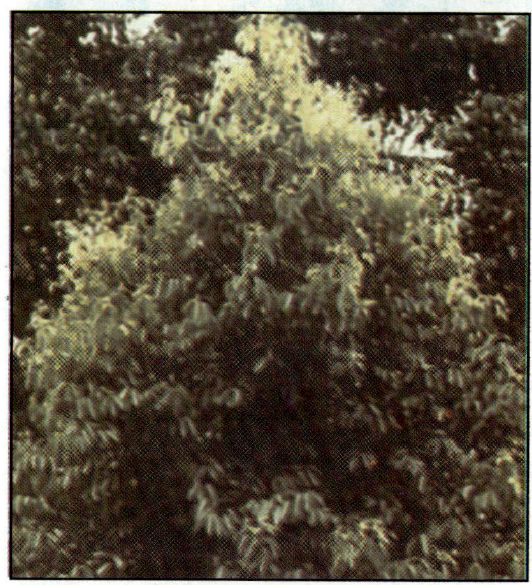

Cinnamomum verum

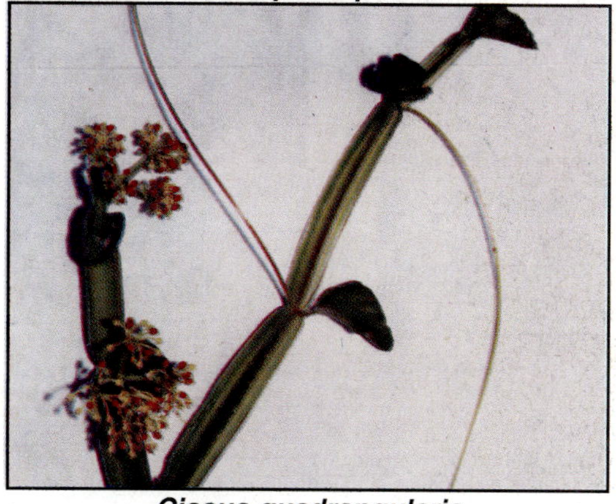

Cissus quadrangularis

PLATE : 40

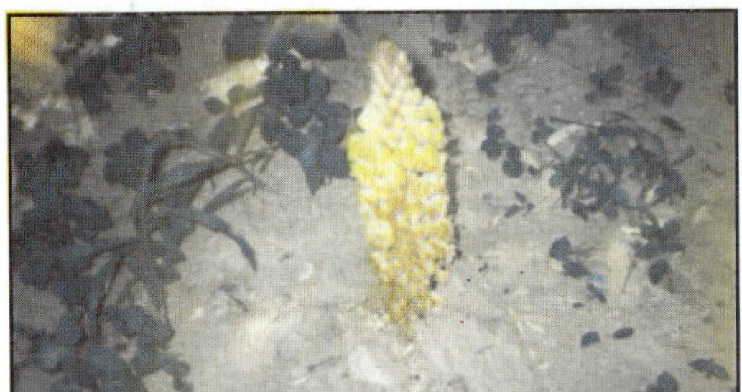

Cistanche tubulosa

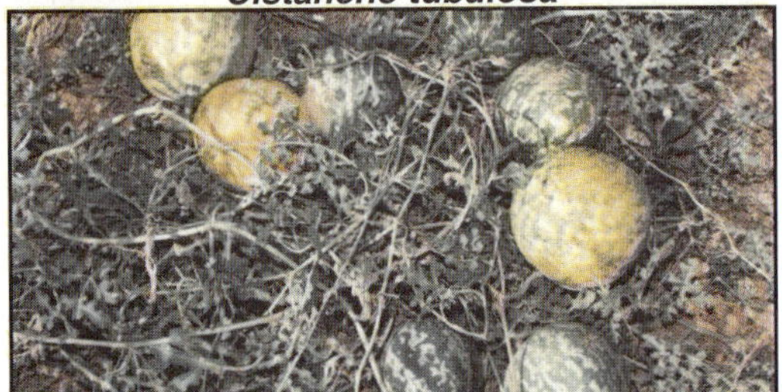

Citrullus colocynthis

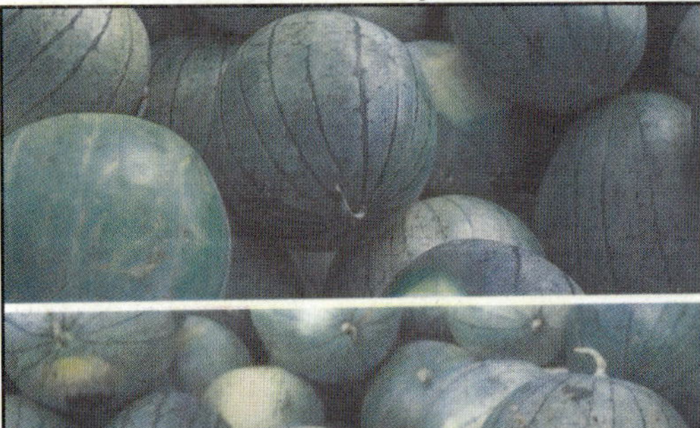

Citrullus lanatus

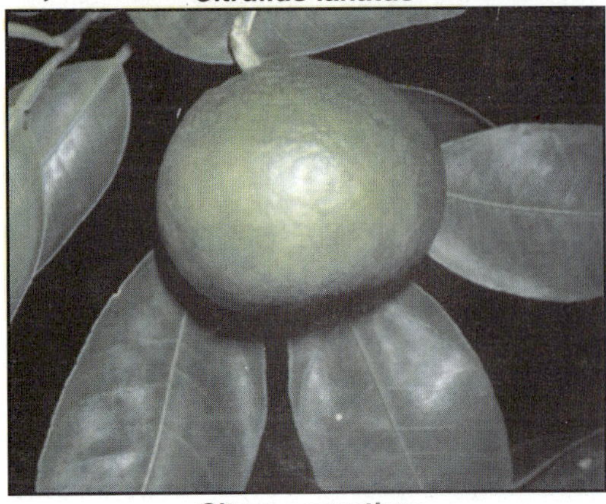

Citrus aurantium

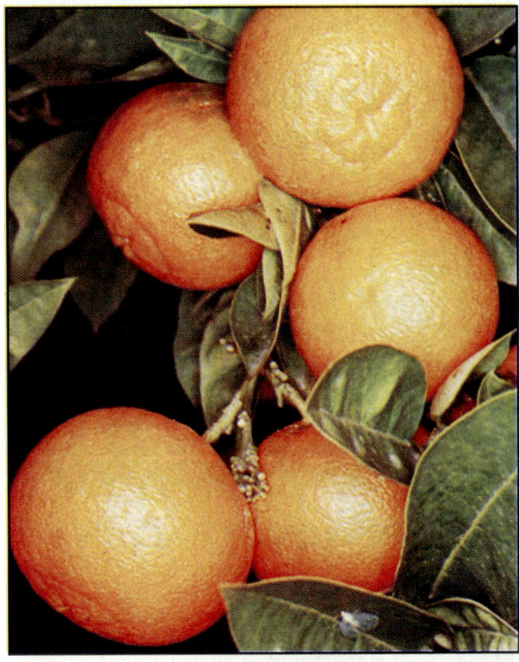

Citrus aurantium

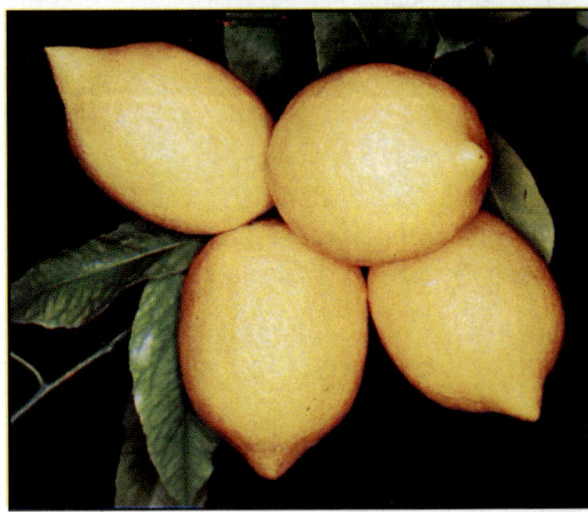

Citrus limon

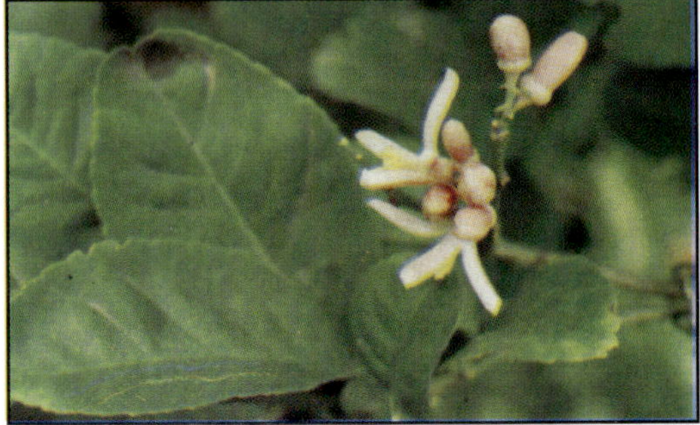

Citrus medica Linn

PLATE : 41

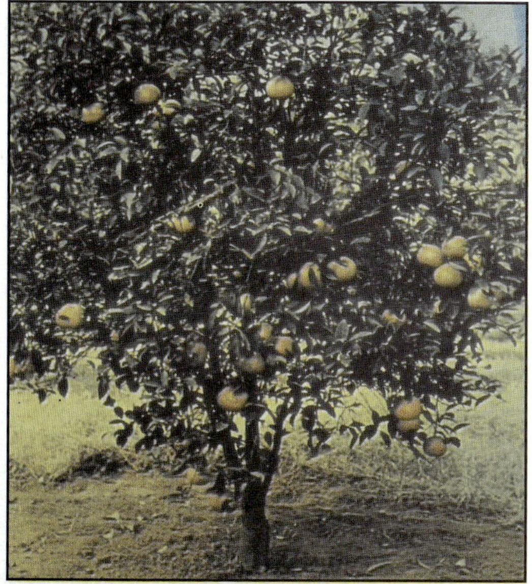
Citrus reticulata

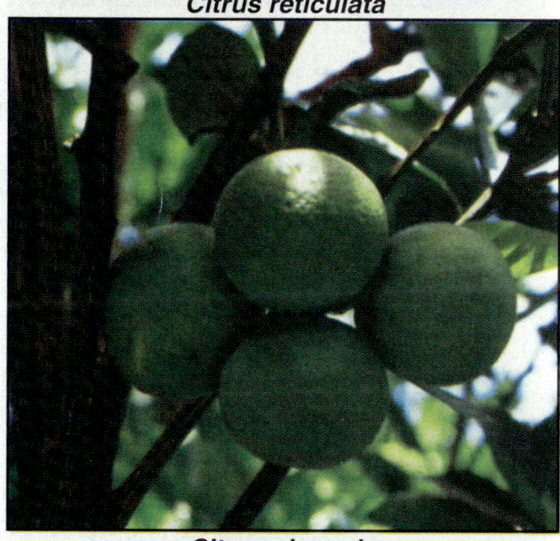
Citrus sinensis

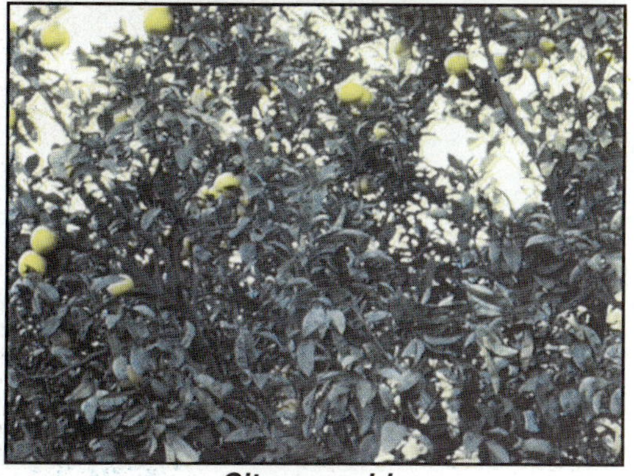
Citrus unshiu

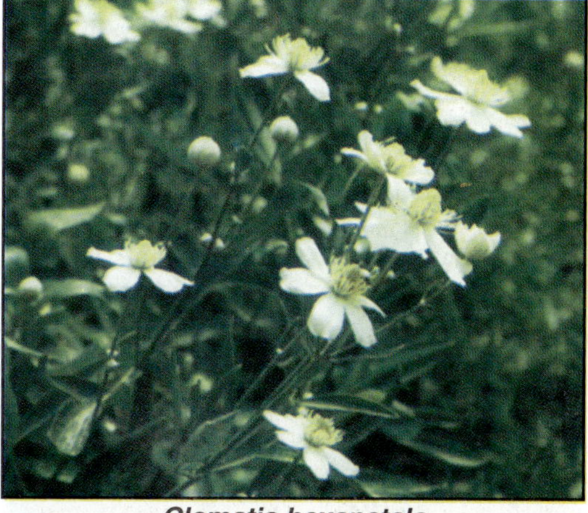
Clematis hexapetala

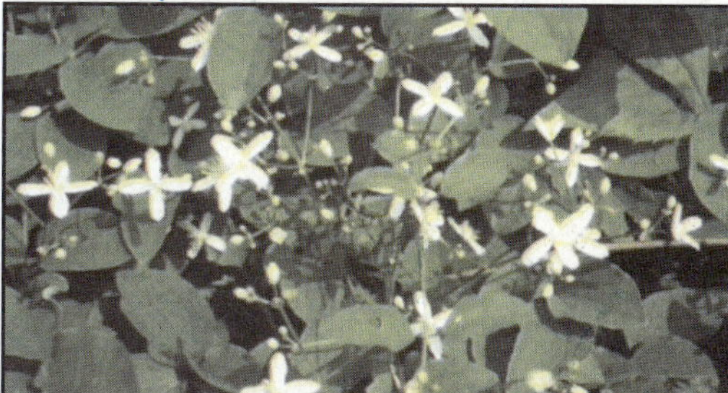
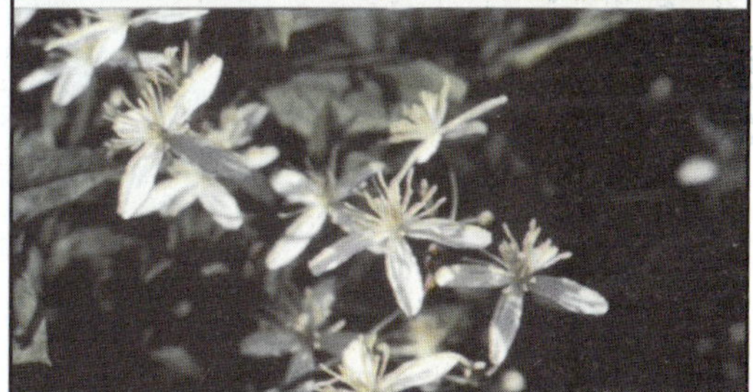
Clematis mandschurica

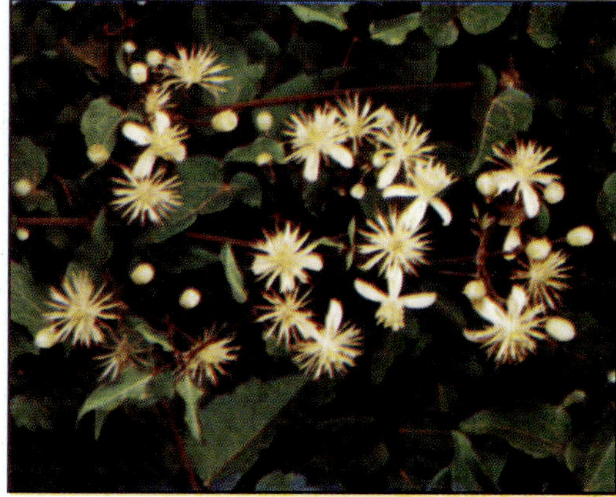
Clematis vitalba

PLATE : 42

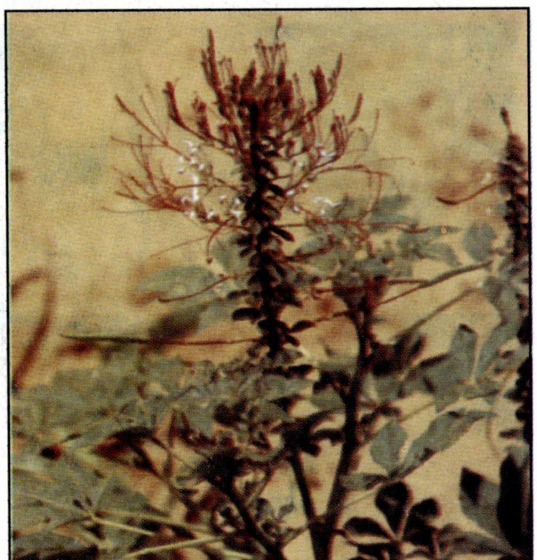

Cleome gynandra

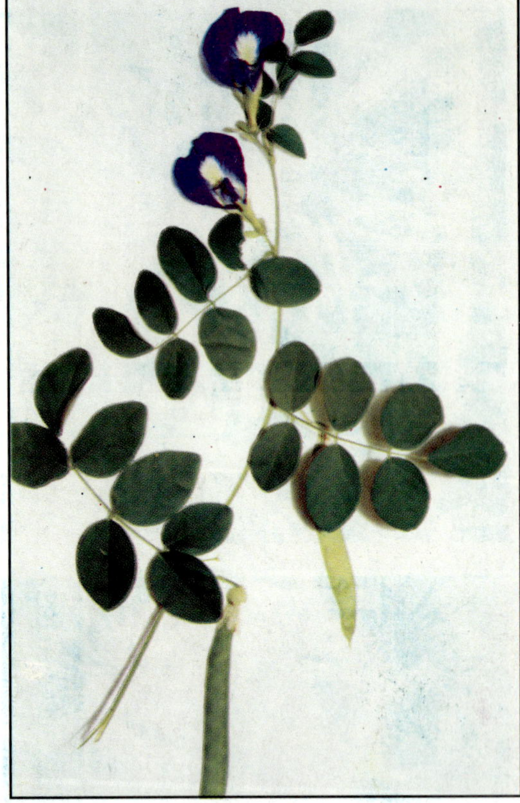

Clitoria ternatea

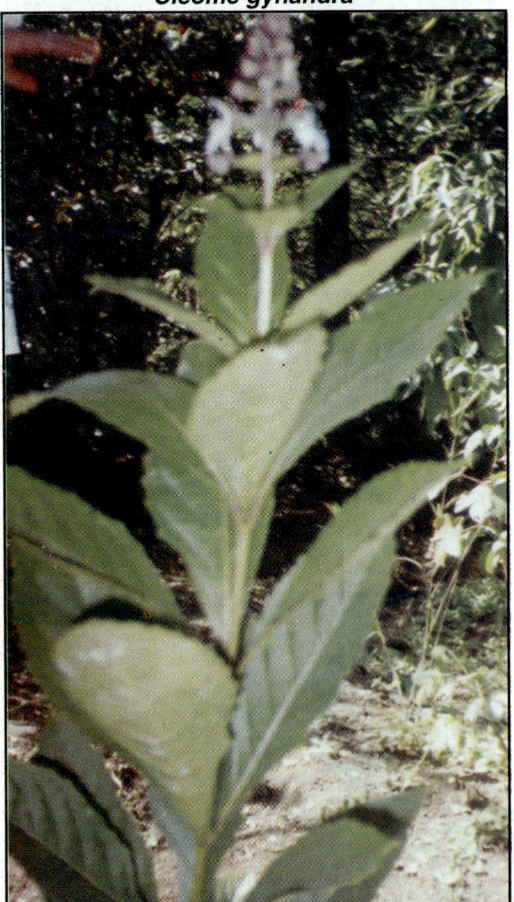

Clerodendrum serratum

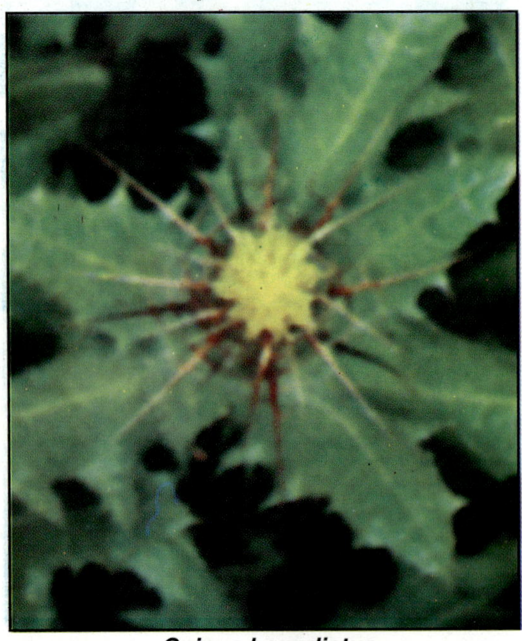

Cnicus benedictus

PLATE : 43

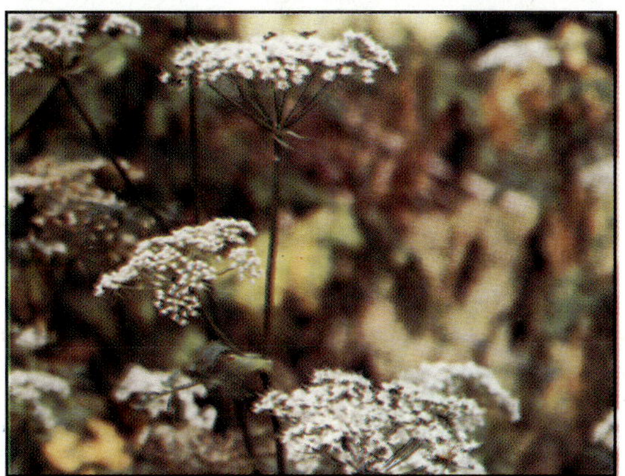

Cnidium officinale

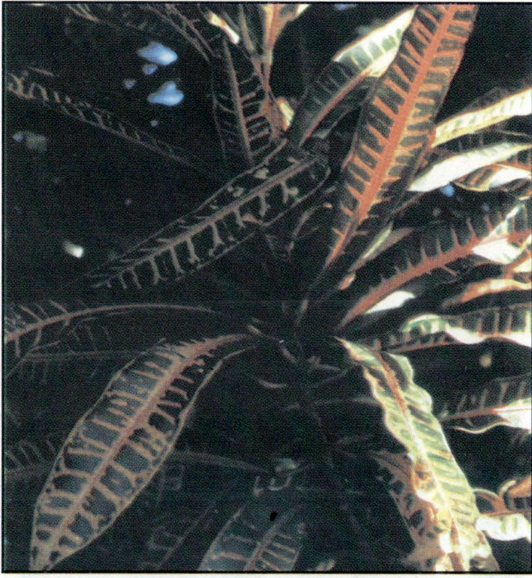

Codiaeum variegatum

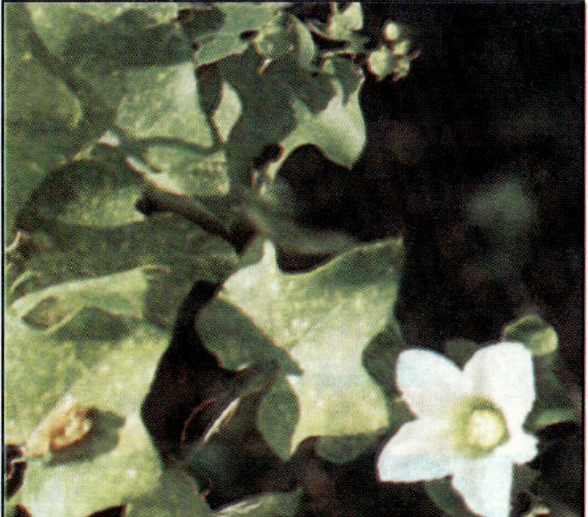

Coccinia grandis

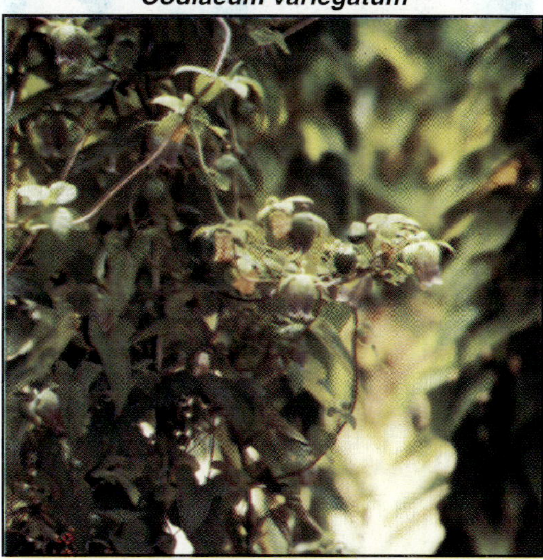

Codonopsis pilosula

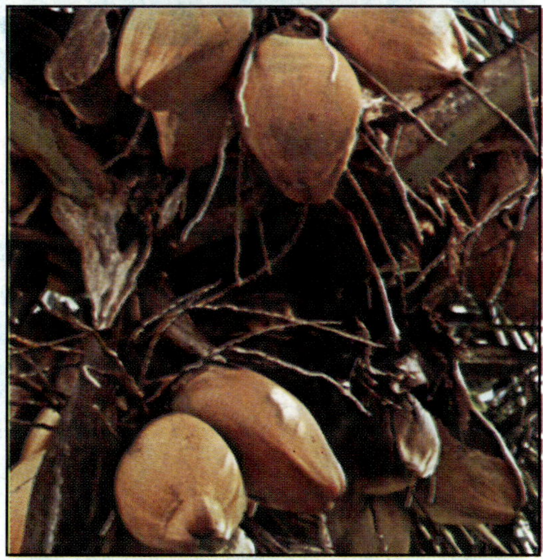

Cocos nucifera

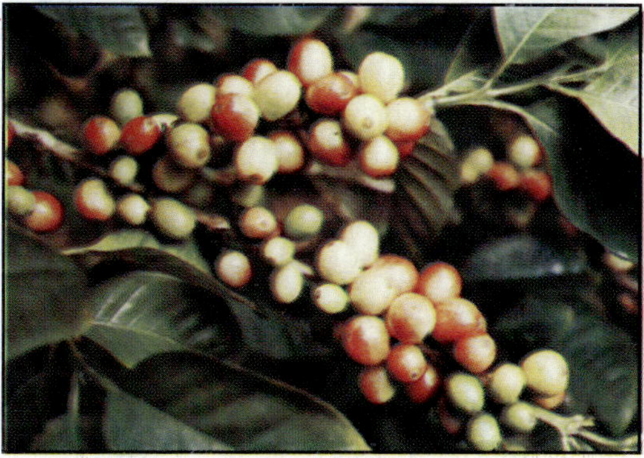

Coffea arabica

PLATE : 44

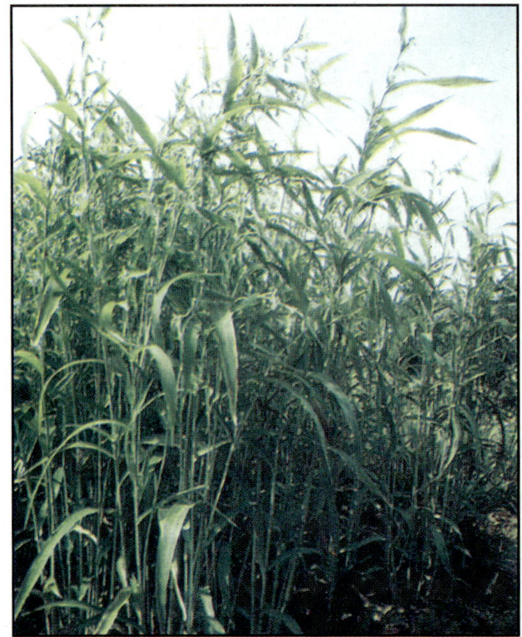

Coix lacryma-jobi

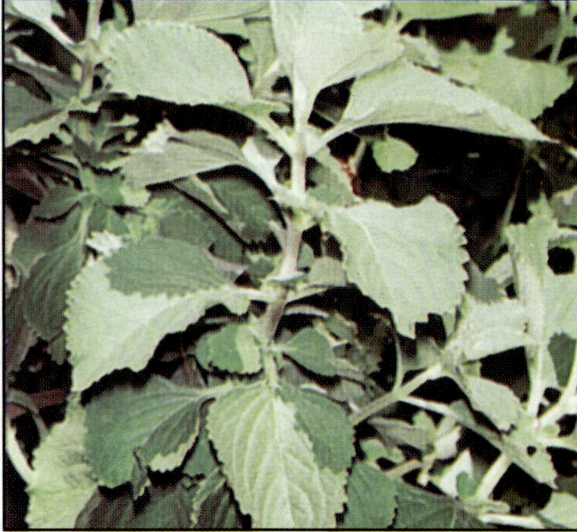

Coleus Forskohlii

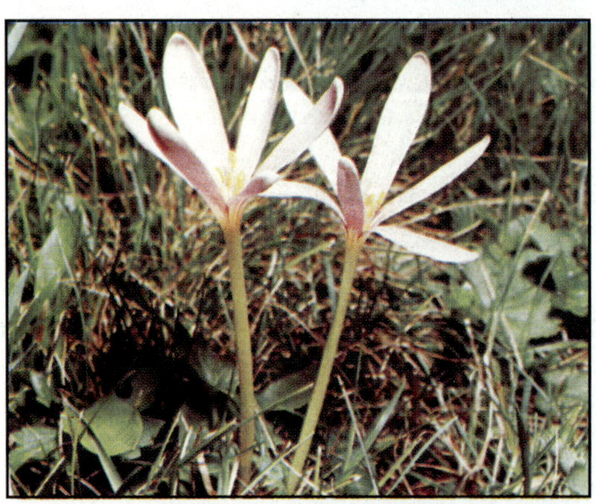

Colchicum autumnale

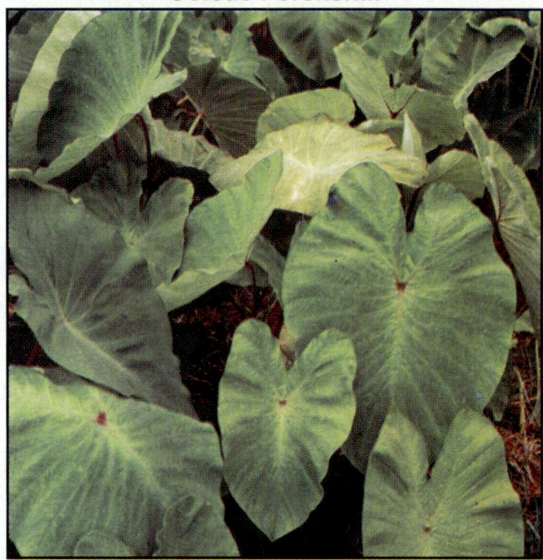

Colocasia esculenta

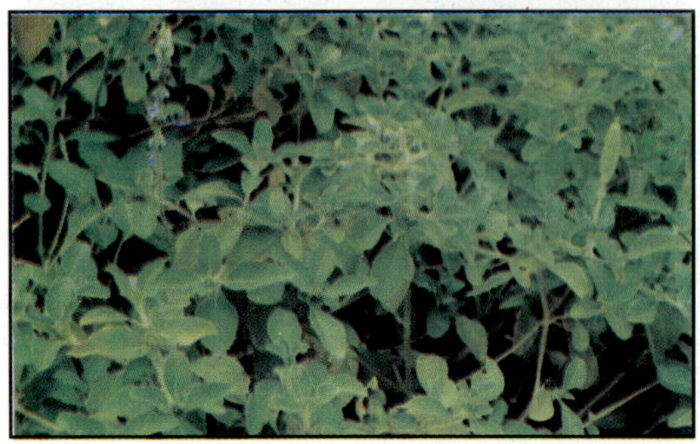

Coleus barbatus

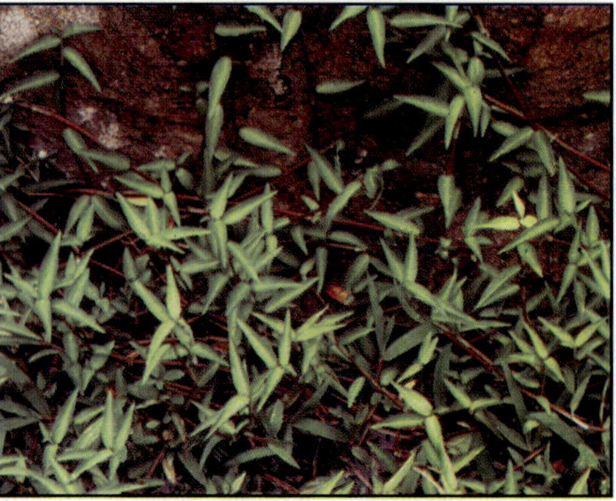

Commelina diffusa

PLATE : 45

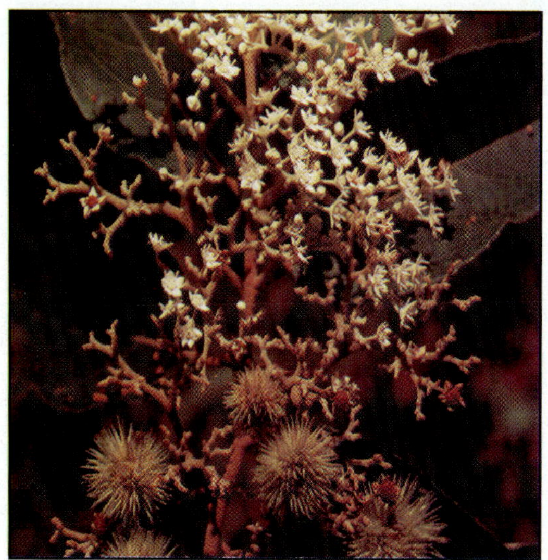
Commersonia bartramia

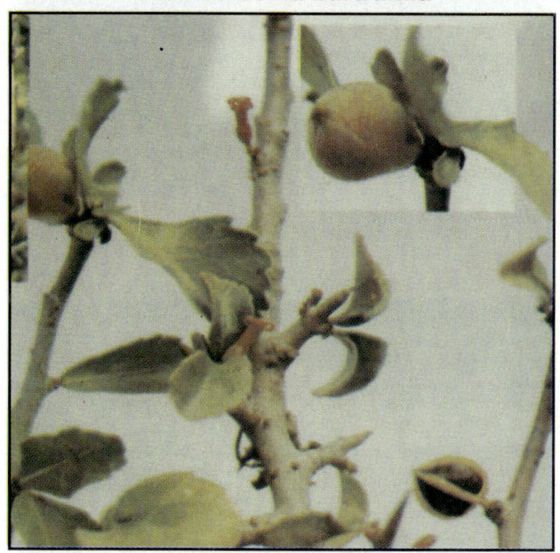
Commiphora wightii

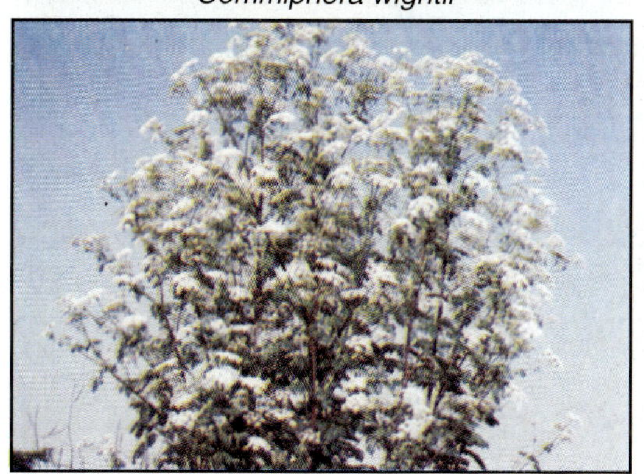
Conium maculatum

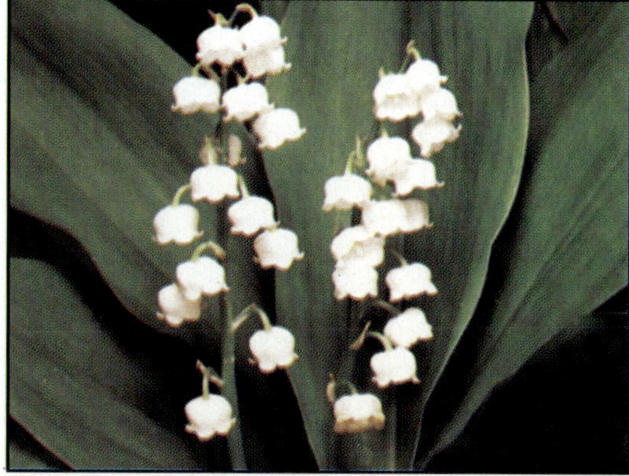
Convallaria majalis

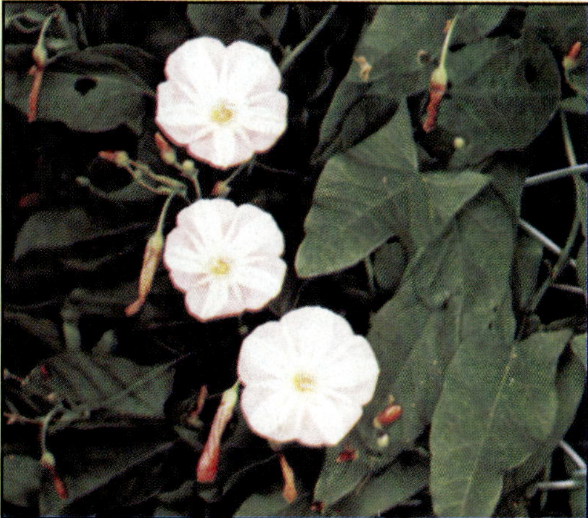
Convolvulus arvensis

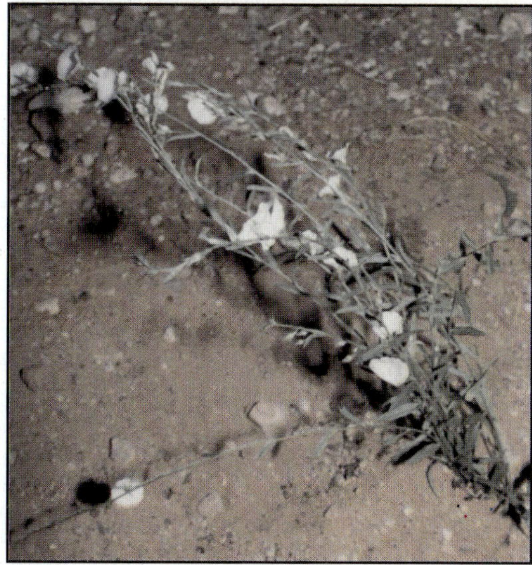
Convolvulus microphyllus

PLATE : 46

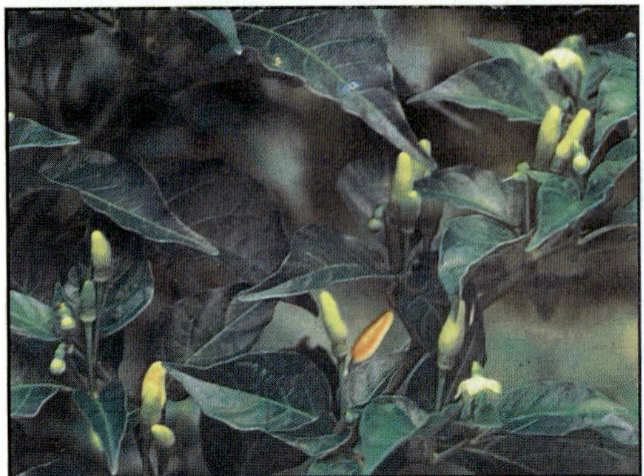
Copsicum frutescens

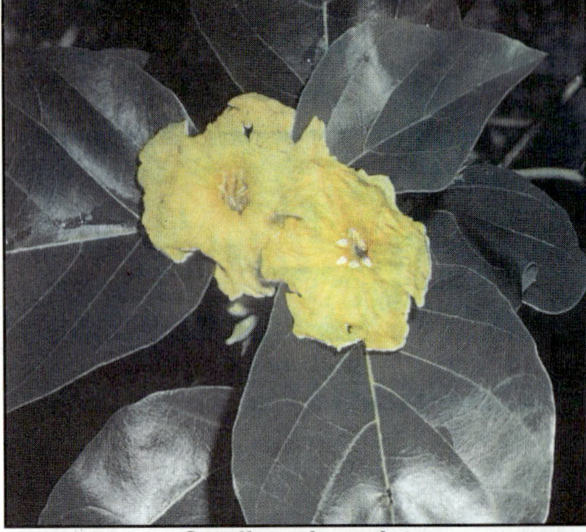
Cordia subcordata

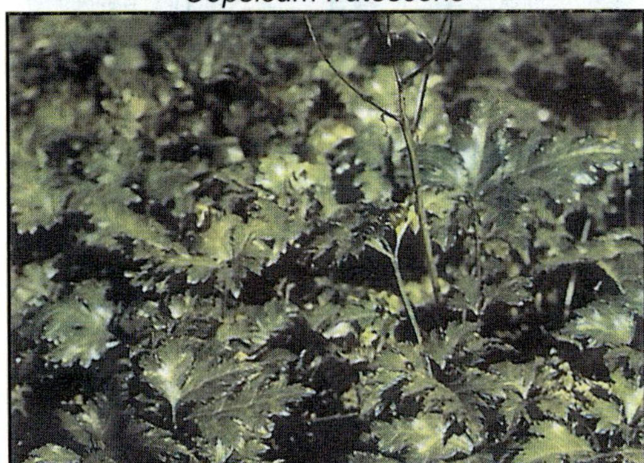
Coptis chinensis

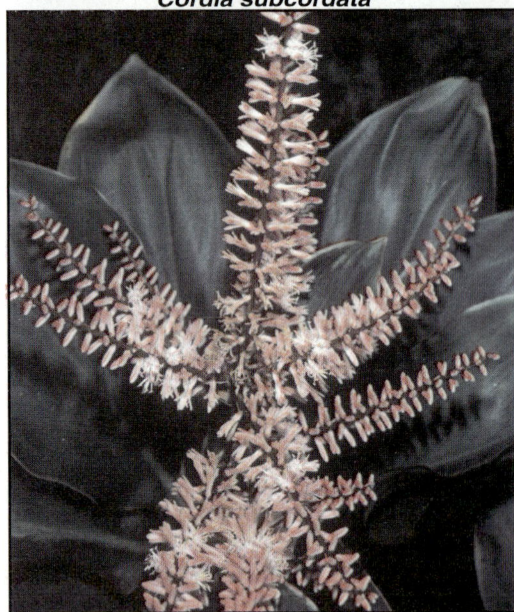
Cordyline fruticosa

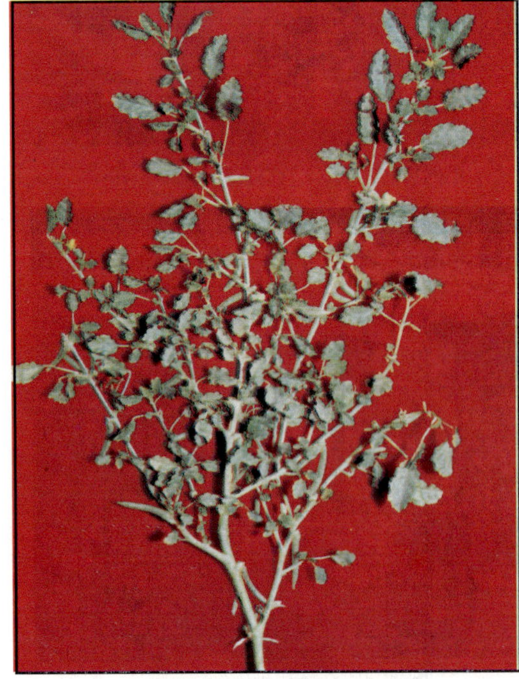
Corchonus dipresces

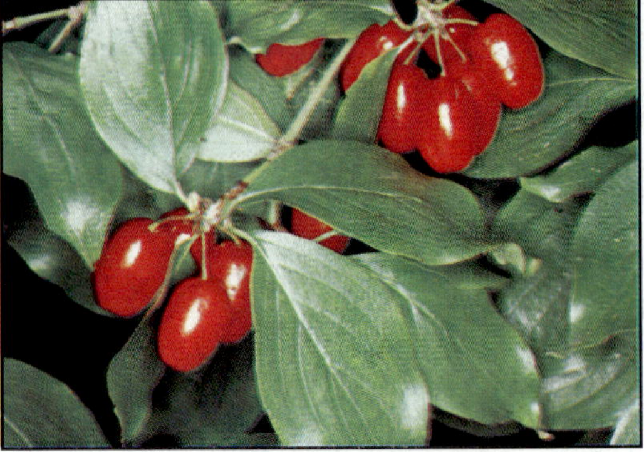
Cornus mas

PLATE : 47

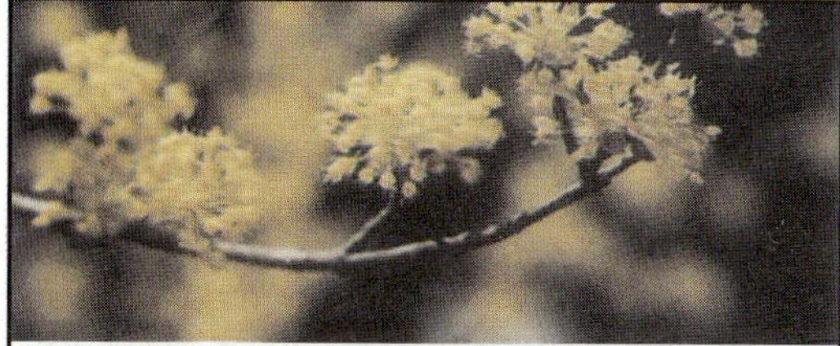

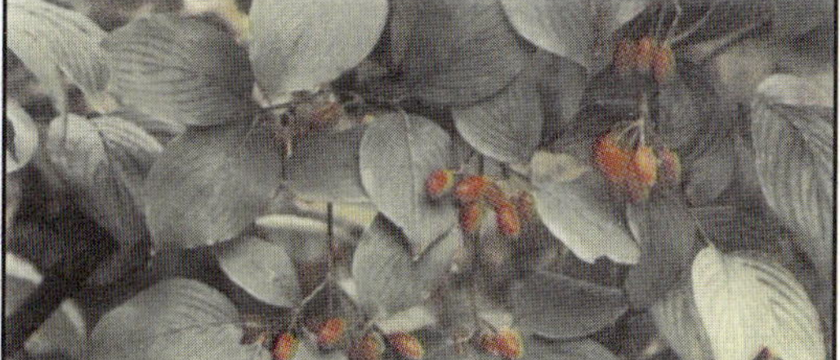

Cornus officinalis

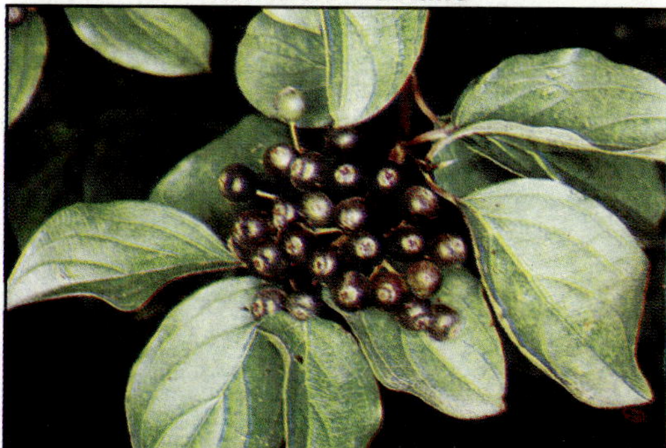

Cornus sanguinea

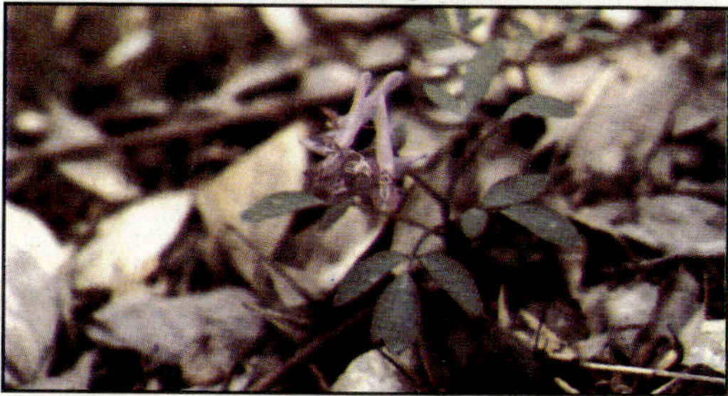

Corydalis ternata

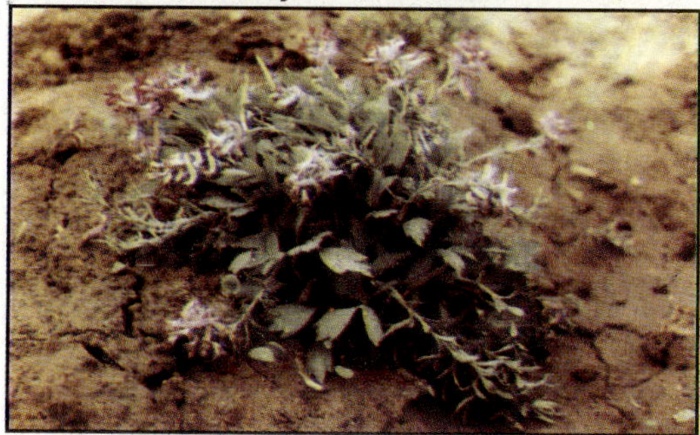

Corydalis yanhusuo

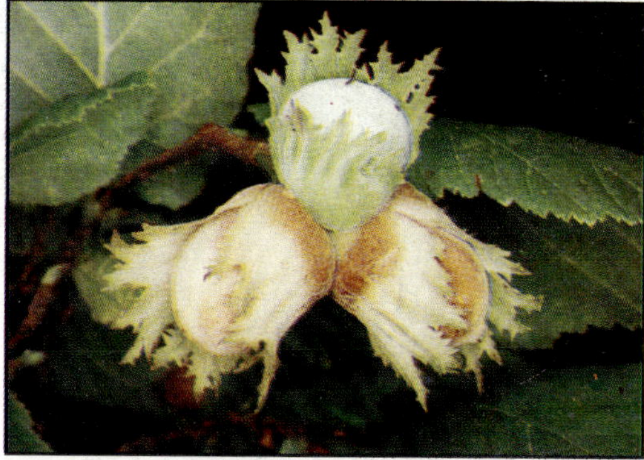

Corylus avellana

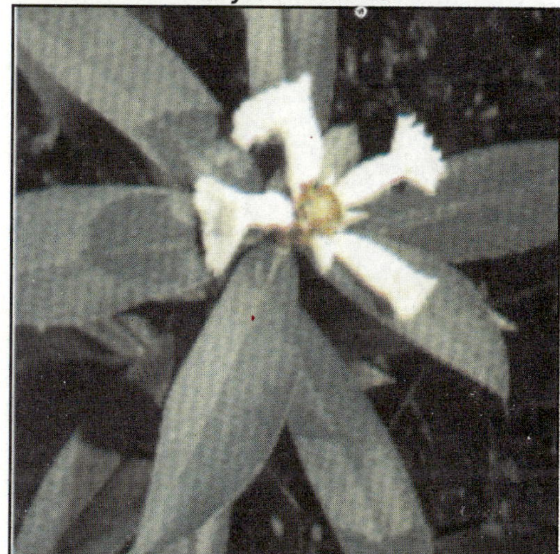

Costus speciosus

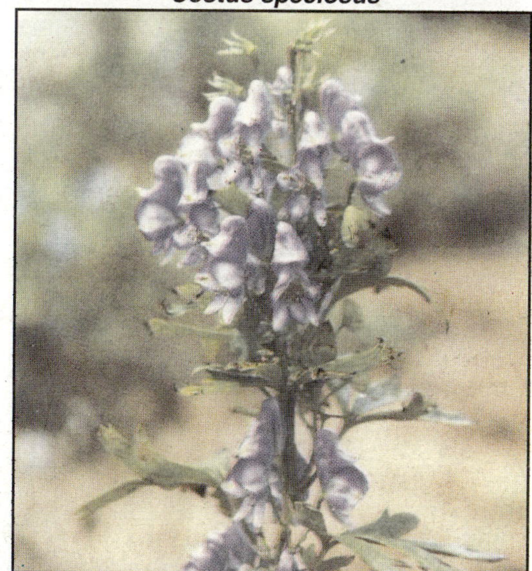

Countium kusnezoffii

PLATE : 48

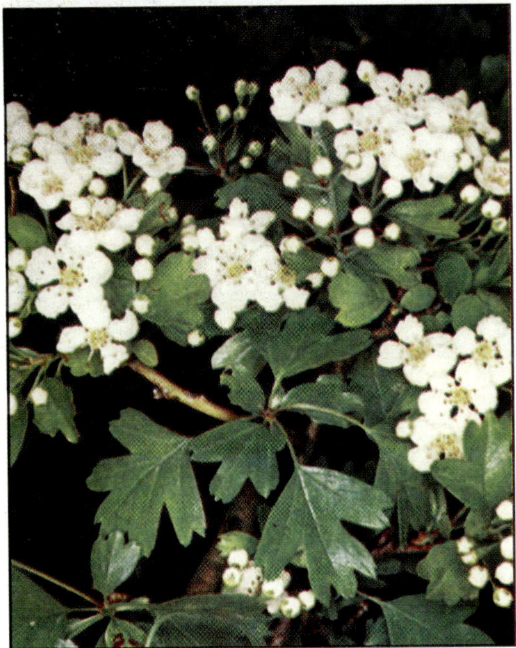

Crataegus monogyna

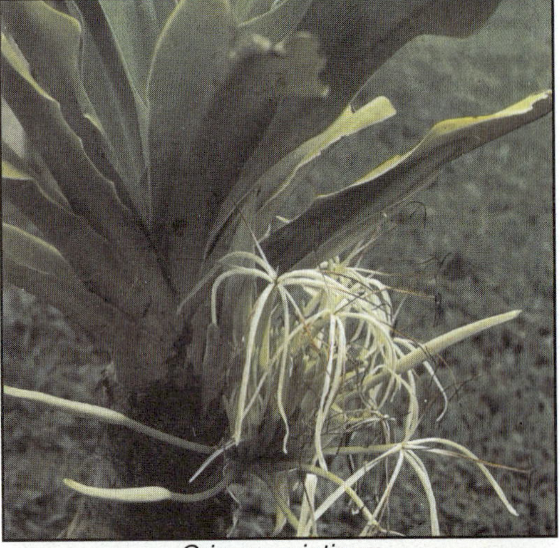

Crinum asiaticum

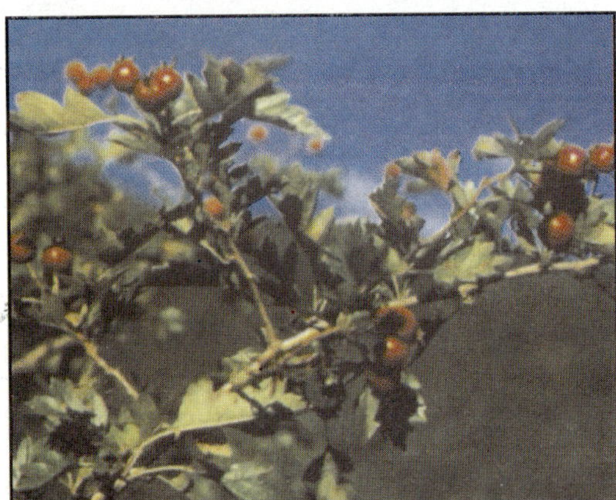

Crataegus pinnatifida

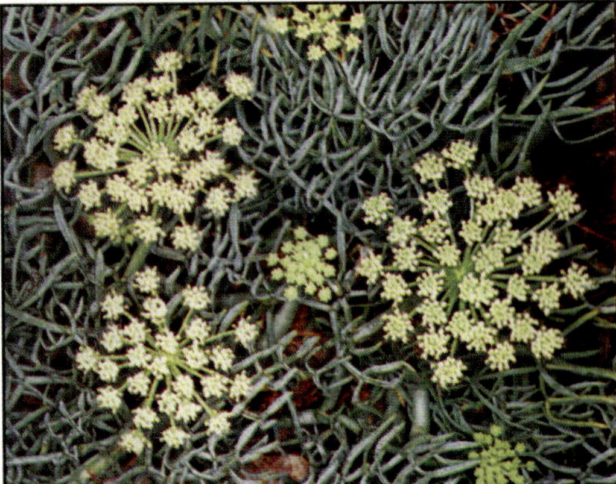

Crithmum maritimum

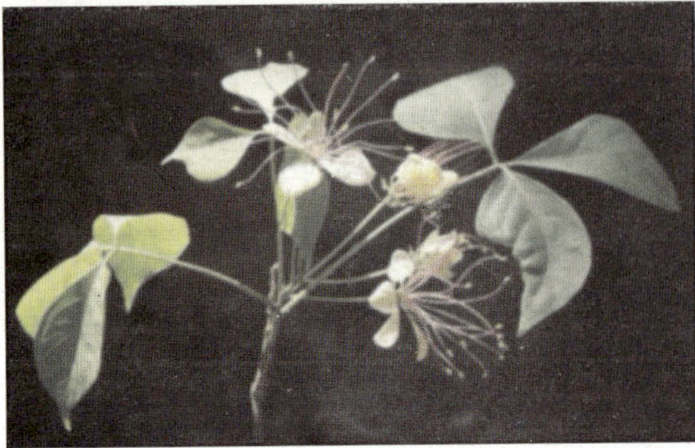

Crataeva nurvala

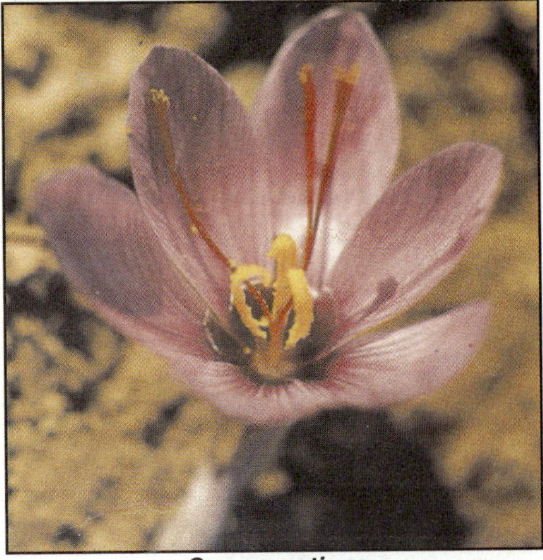

Crocus sativus

PLATE : 49

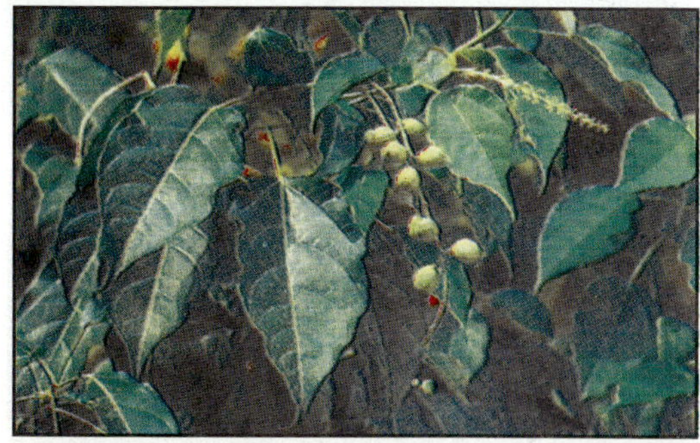

Croton tiglium

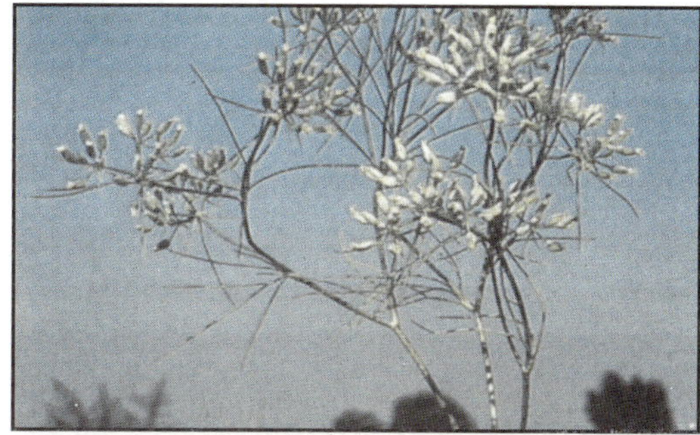

Cuminum cyminum

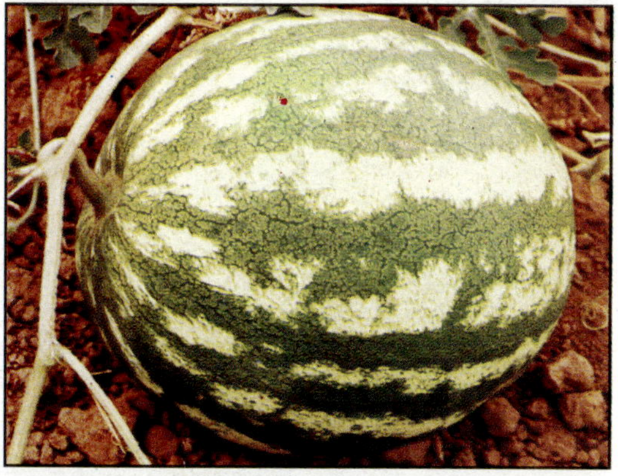

Cucumis citrullus

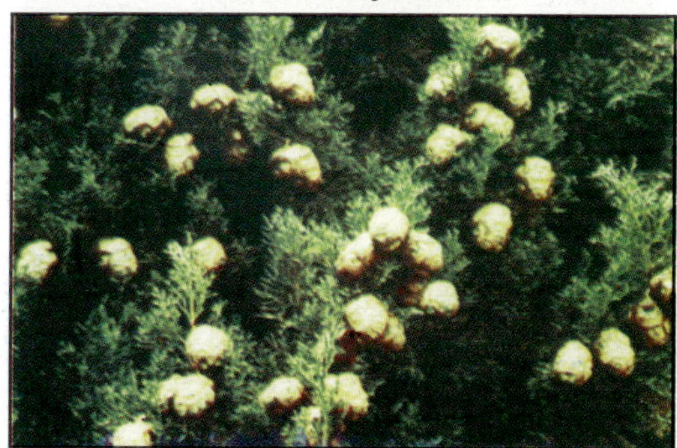

Cupressus sempervirens

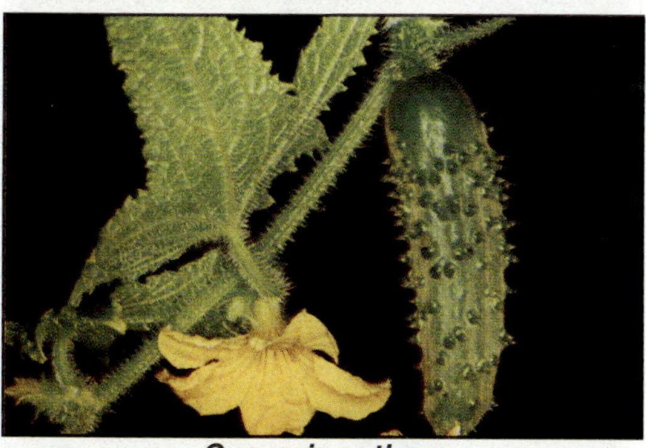

Cucumis sativus

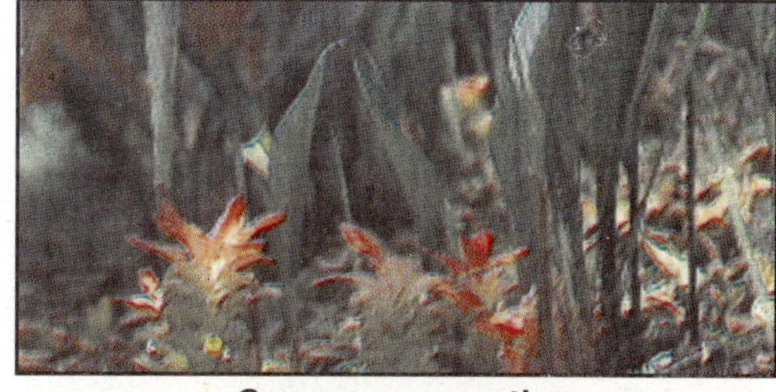

Curcuma aromatica

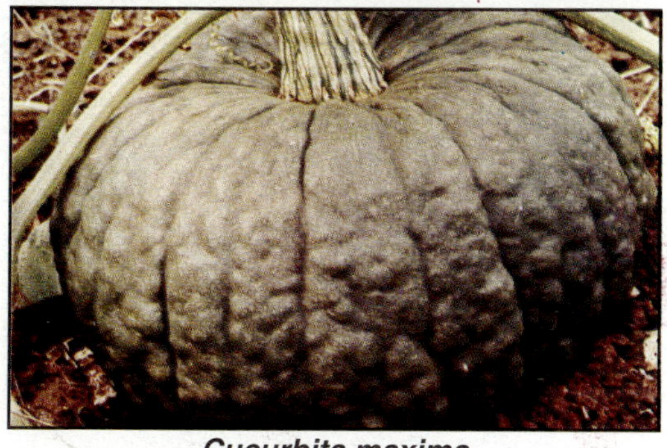

Cucurbita maxima

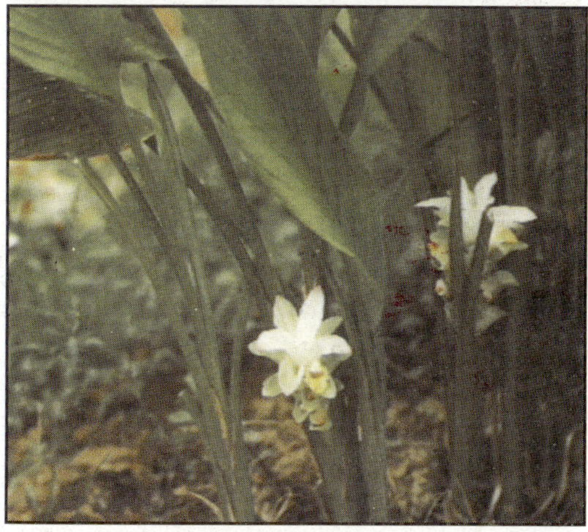

Curcuma longa

PLATE : 50

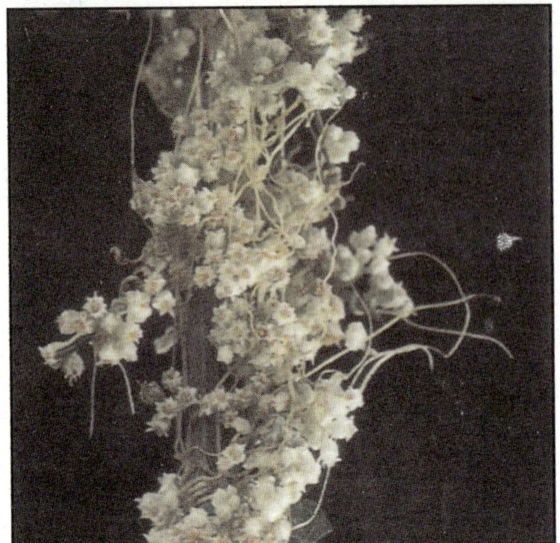

Cuscuta chinensis

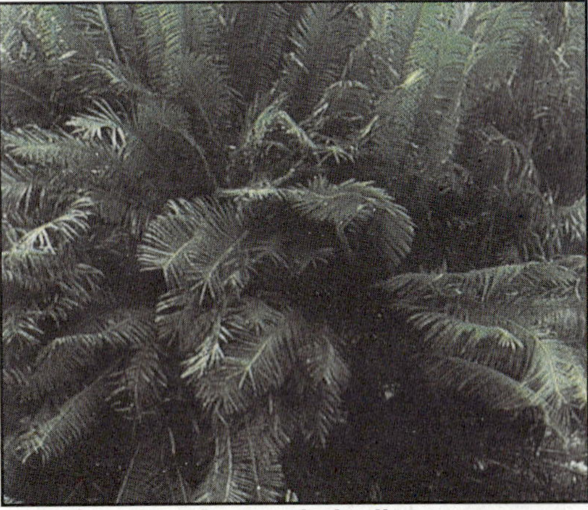

Cycas circinalis

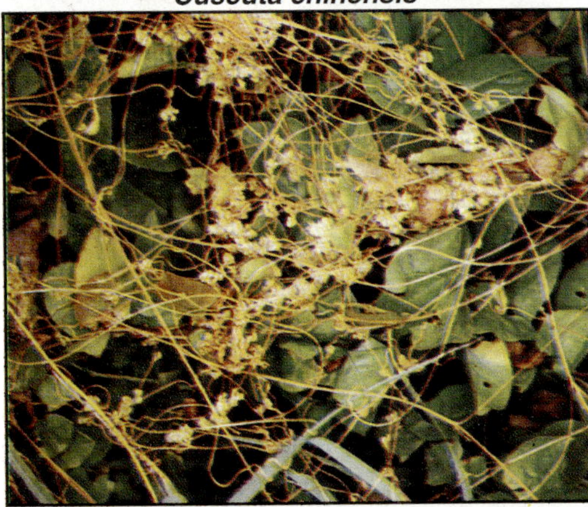

Cuscuta epithymum

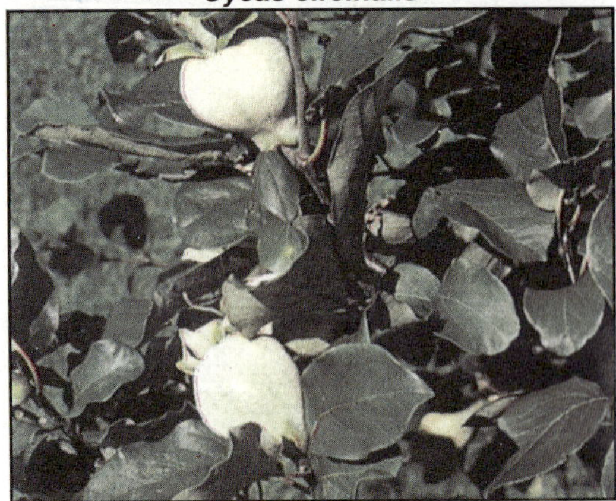

Cydonia oblonga

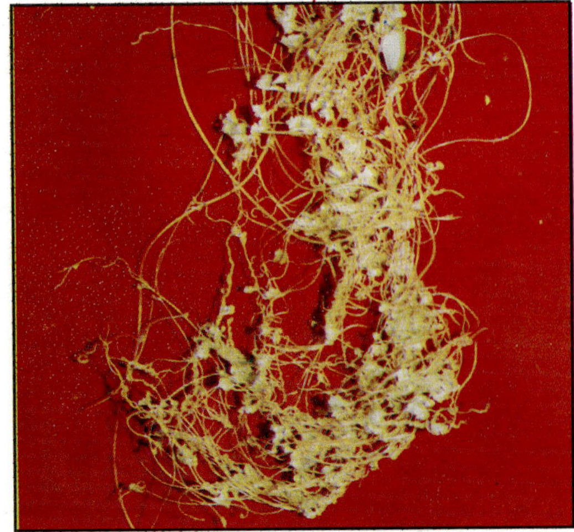

Cuscuta reflexa

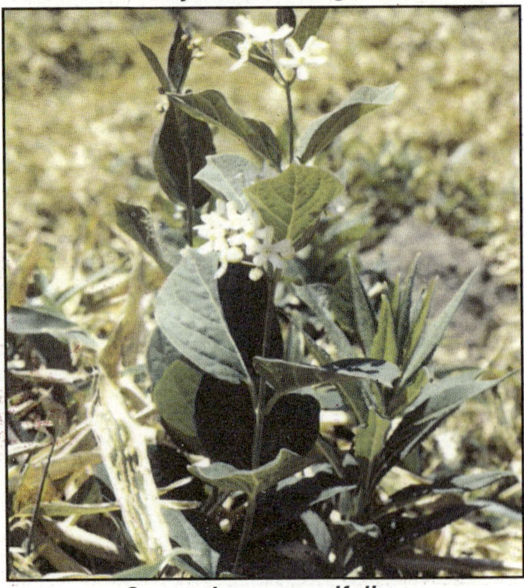

Cynanchum ascyrifolium

PLATE : 51

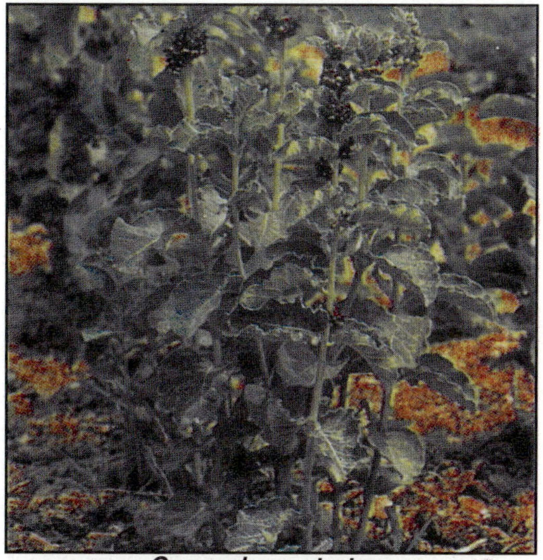
Cynanchum atratum

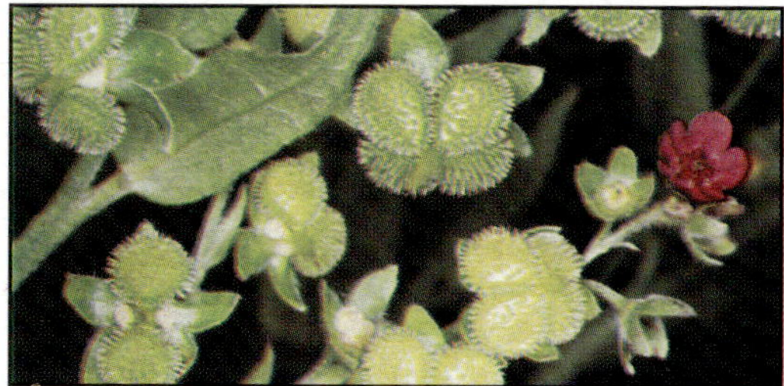
Cynoglossum officinale

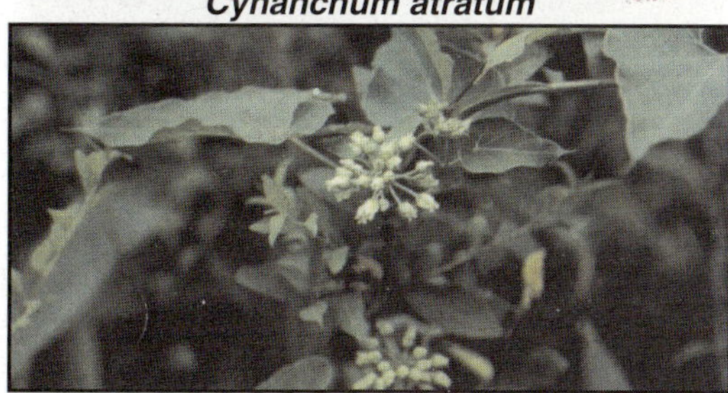
Cynanchum wilfordii

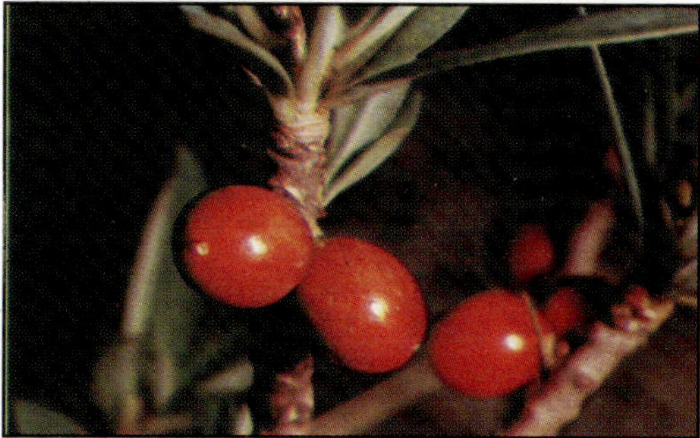
Daphne mezereum

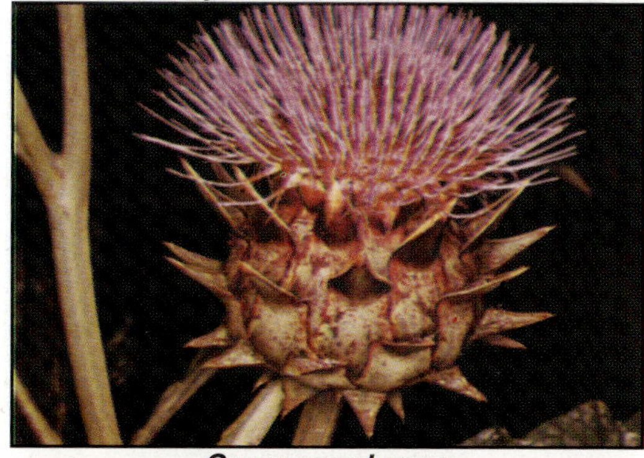
Cynara scolymus

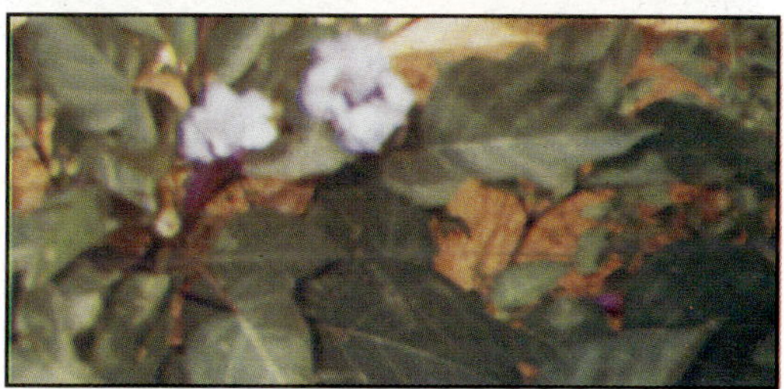
Datura innoxia

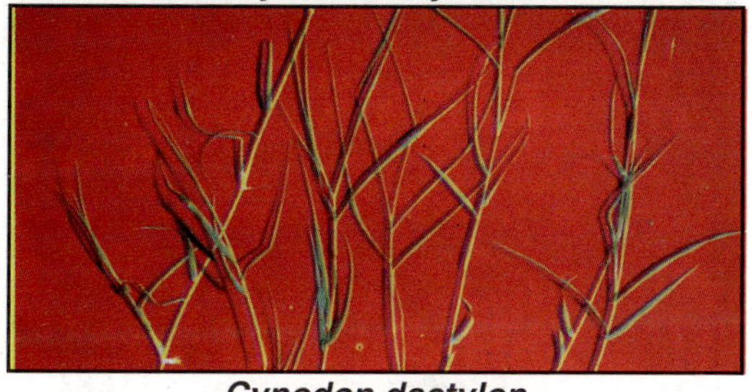
Cynodon dactylon

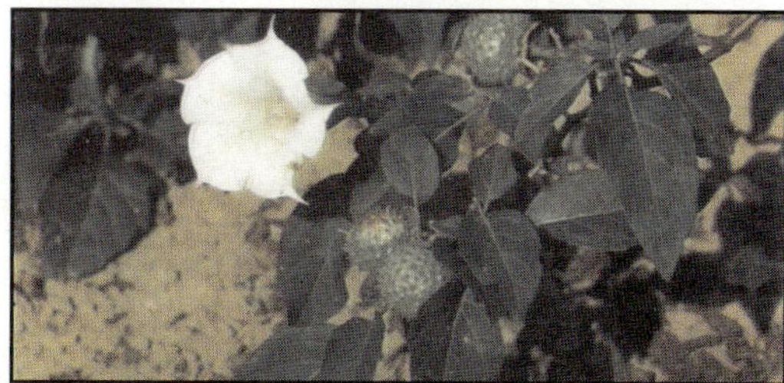
Datura Metal

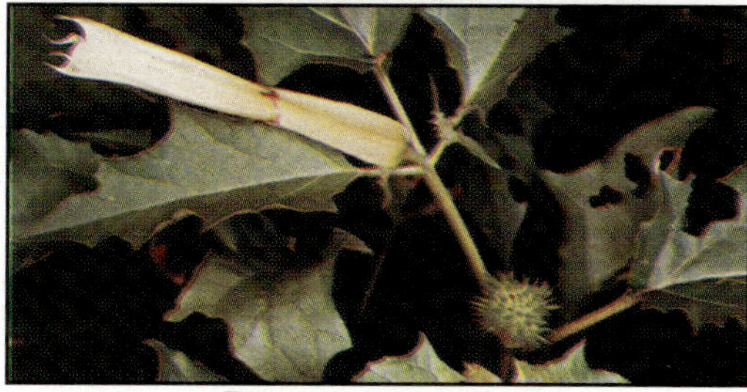
Datura stramonium

PLATE : 52

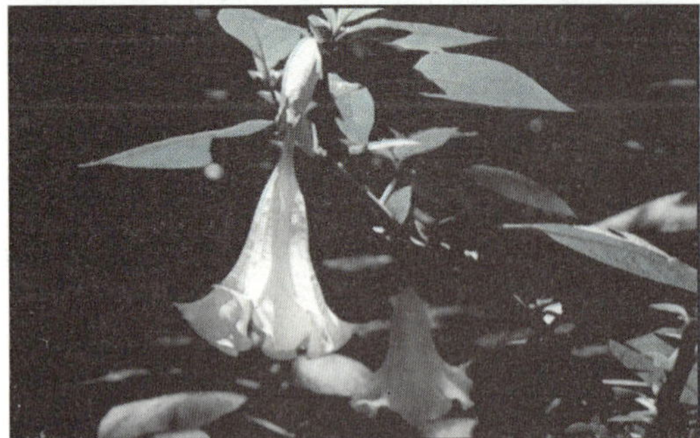
Datura suaveolens

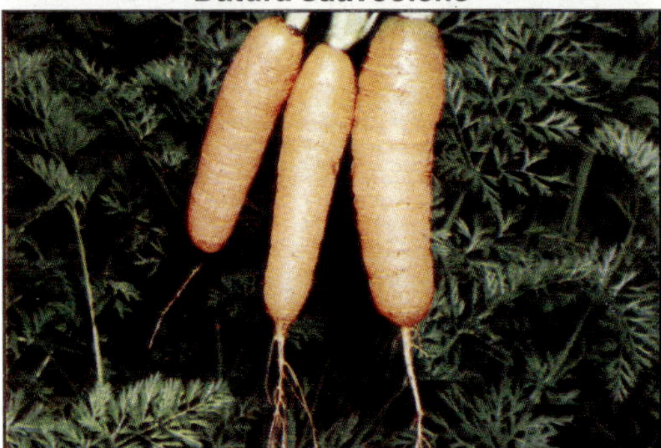
Daucus carota

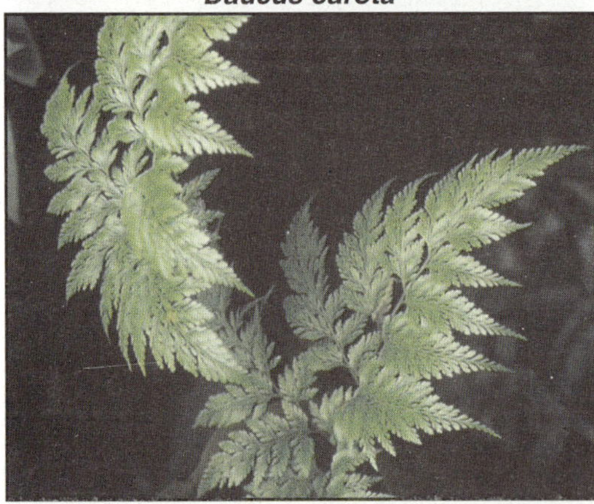
Davallia fijiensis

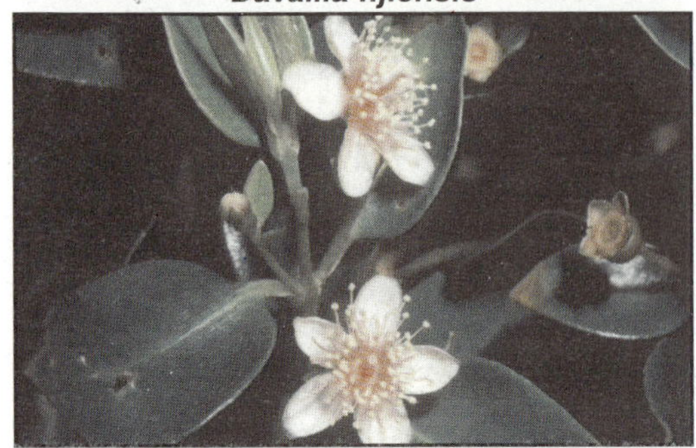
Decaspermum fructicosum

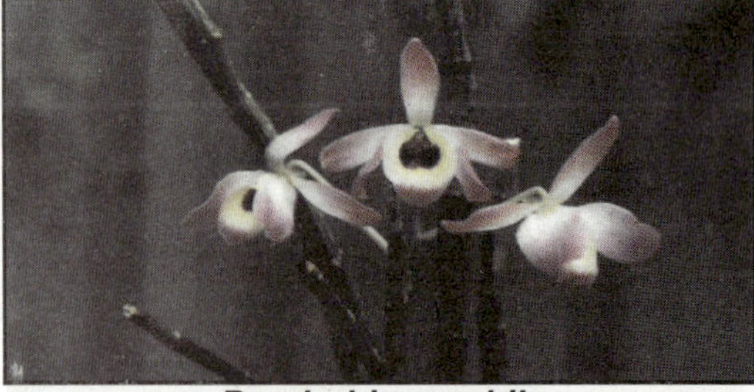
Dendrobium nobile

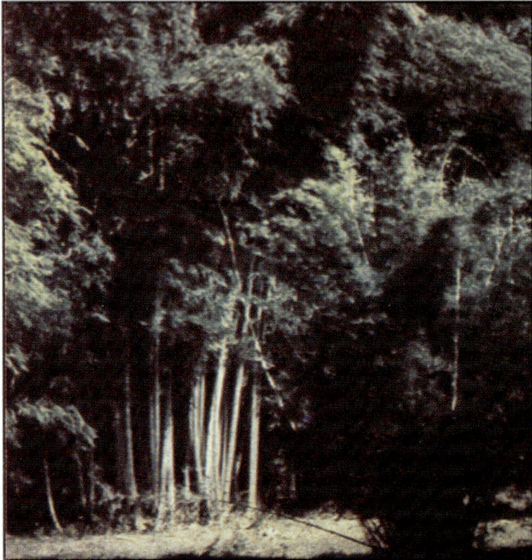
Dendrocalamus giganteus

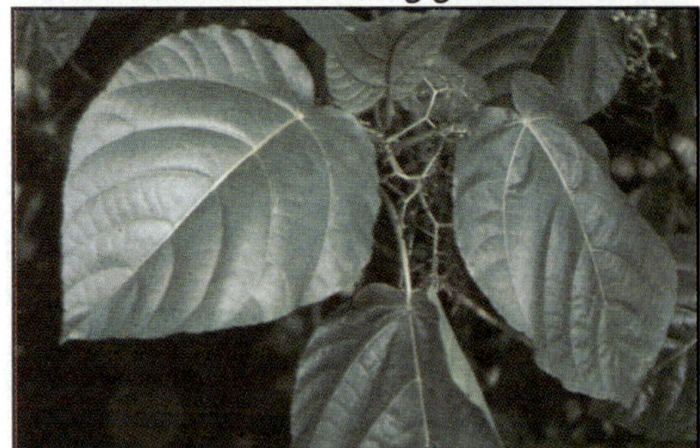
Dendrocnide harveyi

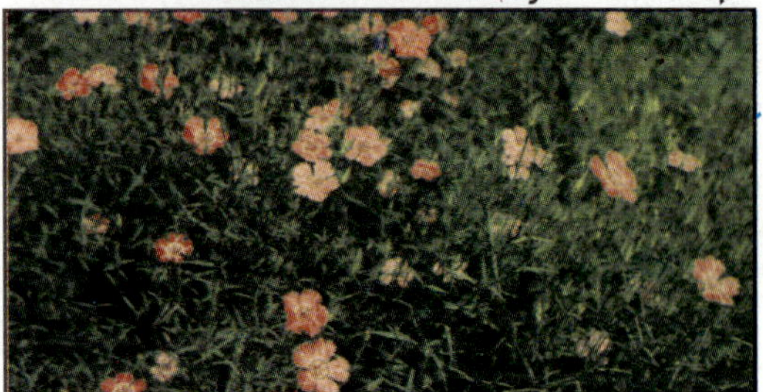
Dianthus chinensis

PLATE : 53

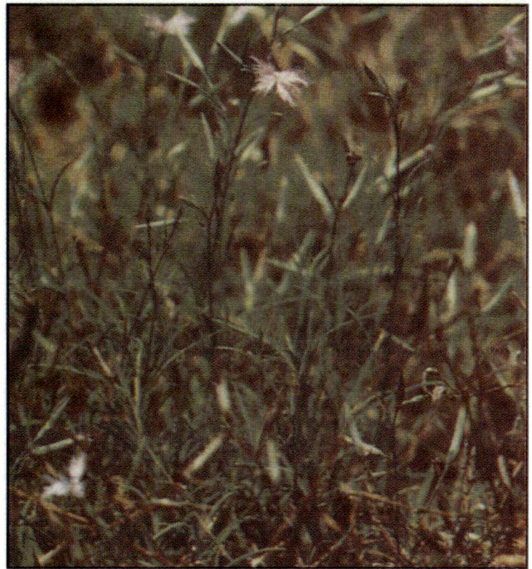
Dianthus superbus

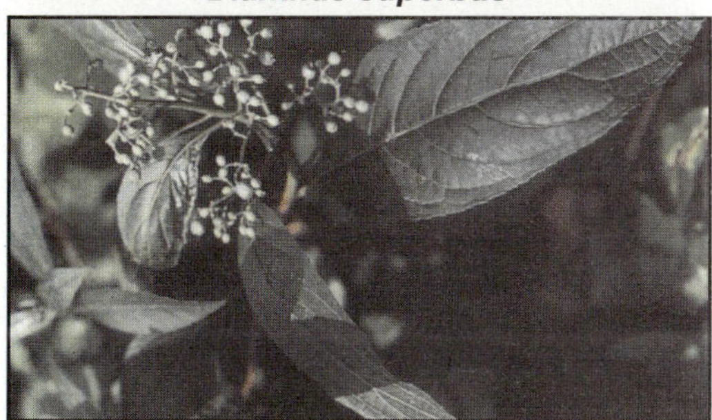
Dichroa febrifuga

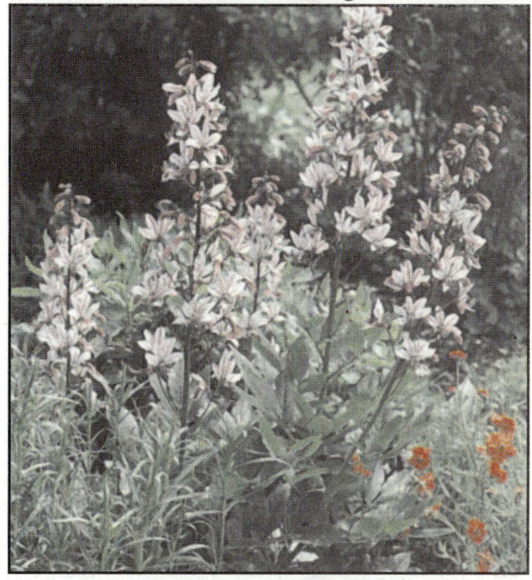
Dictamnus albus

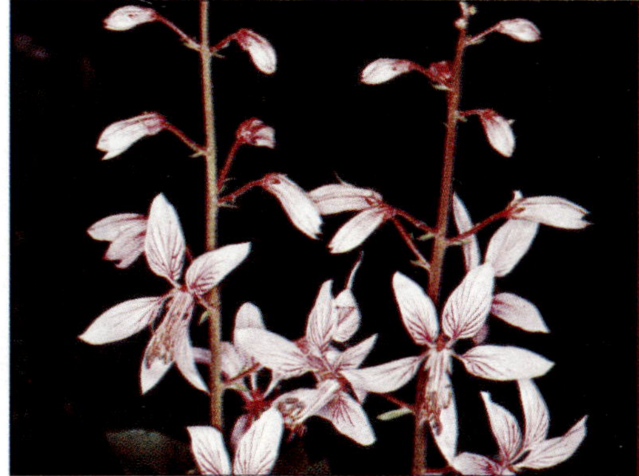
Dictamnus albus

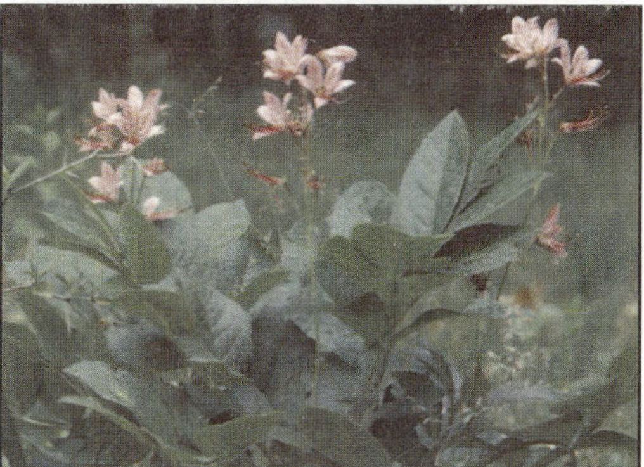
Dictamnus dasycarpus

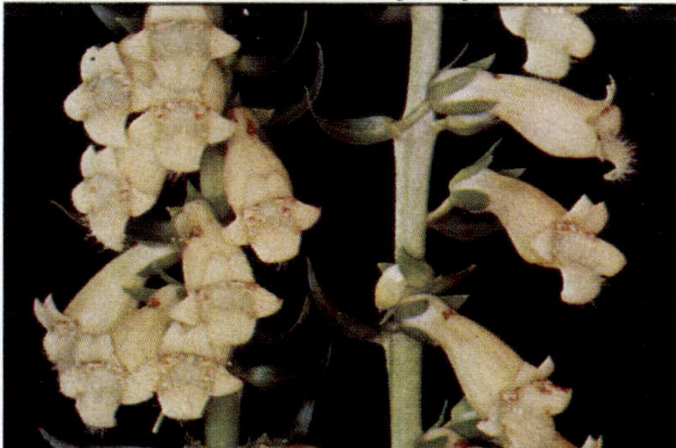
Digitalis lutea

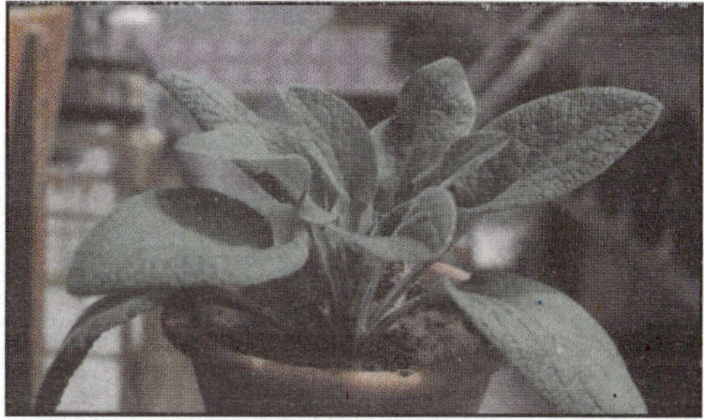
Digitalis purpurea

PLATE : 54

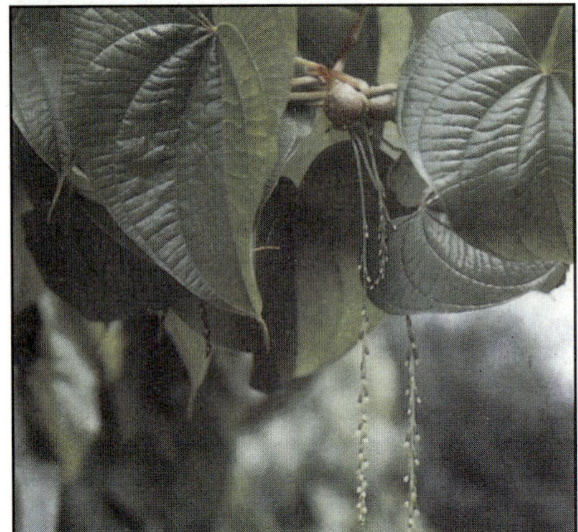

Dioscorea bulbifera

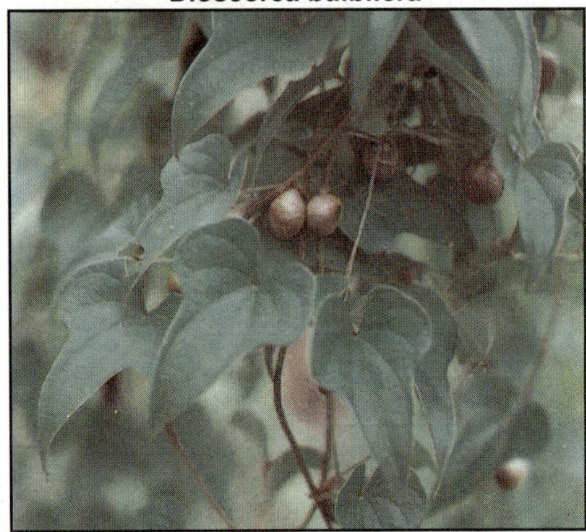

Dioscorea opposita

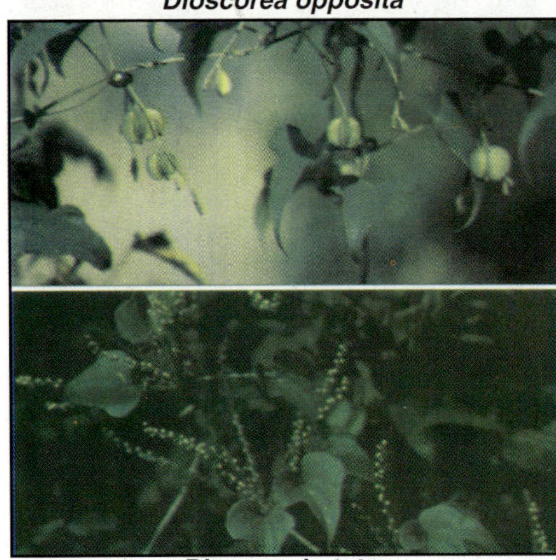

Diosorea batatas

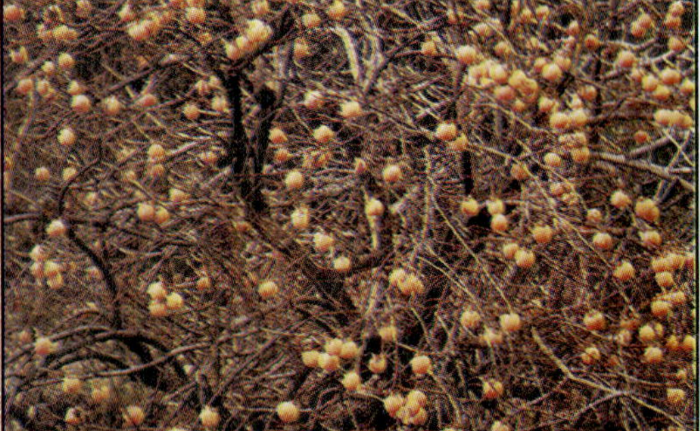

Diospyros kaki

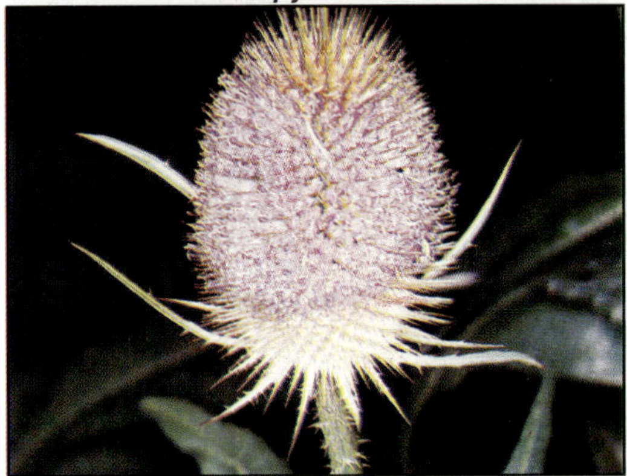

Dipsacus fullonum

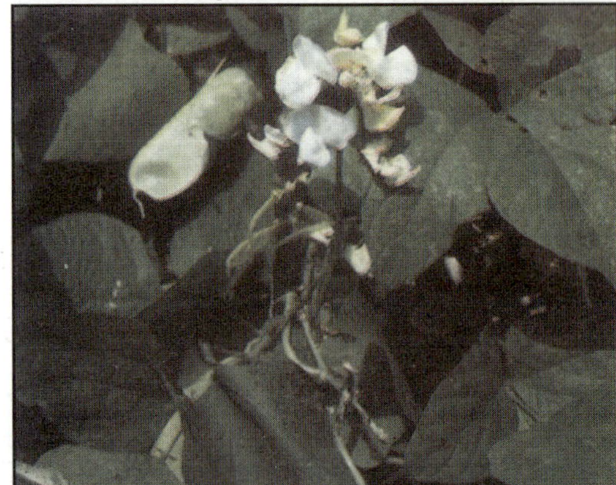

Dolichos lablab

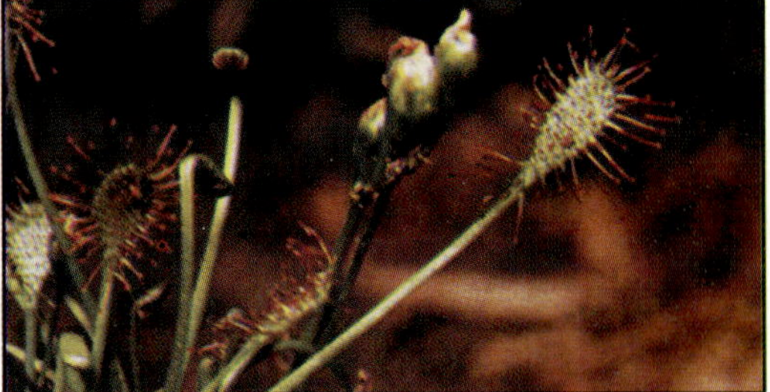

Drosera rotundifolia

PLATE : 55

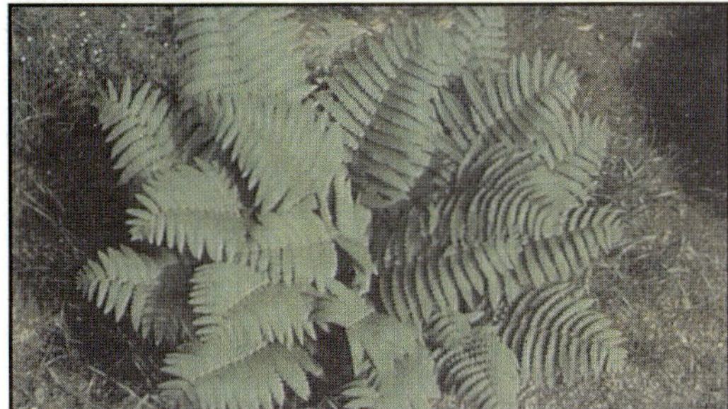

Dryopteris crassirhizoma

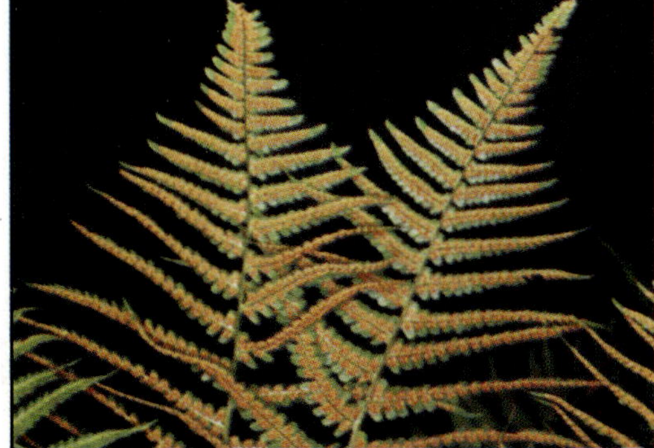

Dryopteris filix-mas

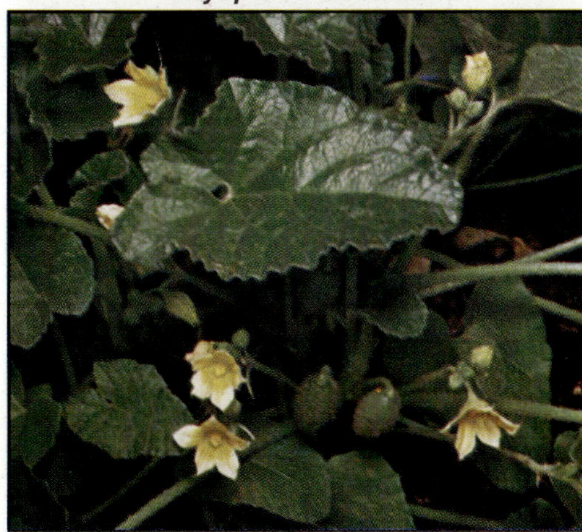

Ecballium elaterium

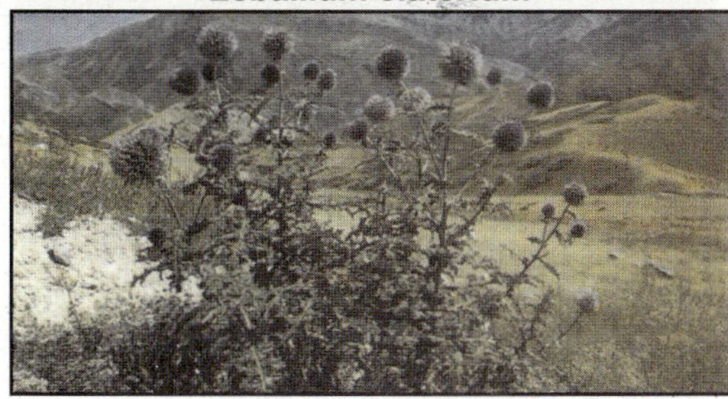

Echinops latifolius

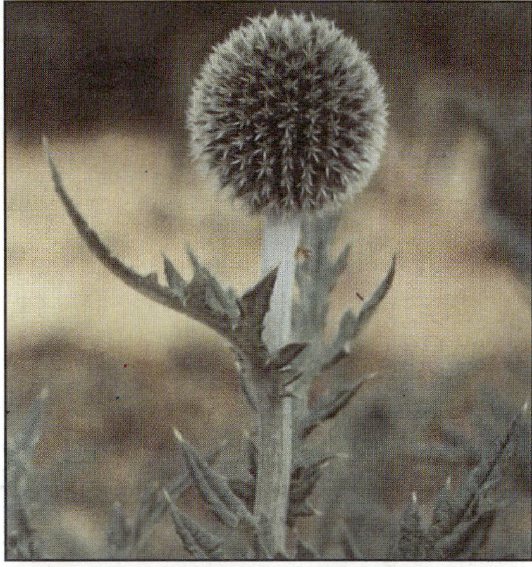

Echinops setifer

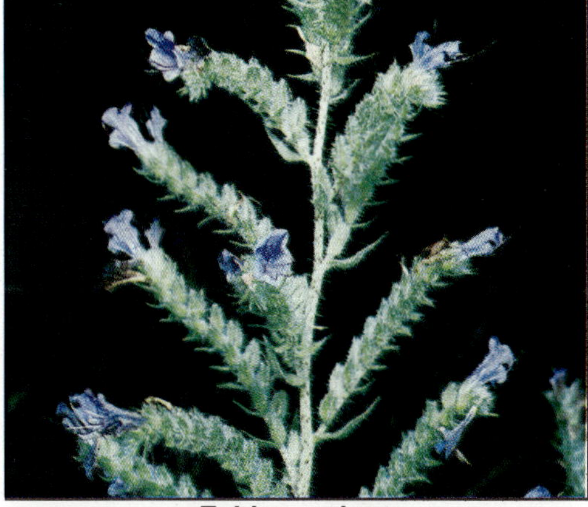

Echium vulgare

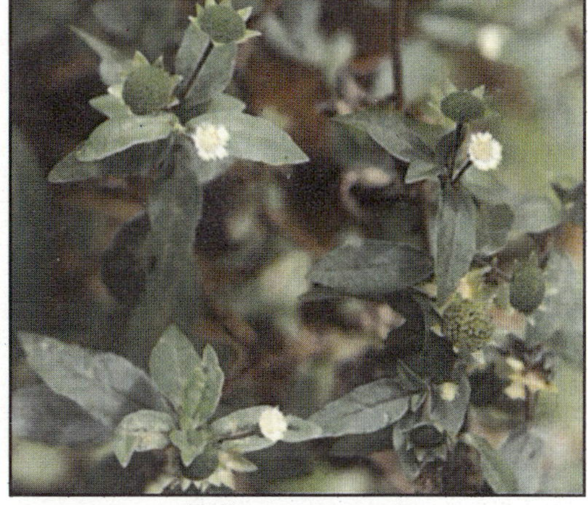

Eclipata prostrata

PLATE : 56

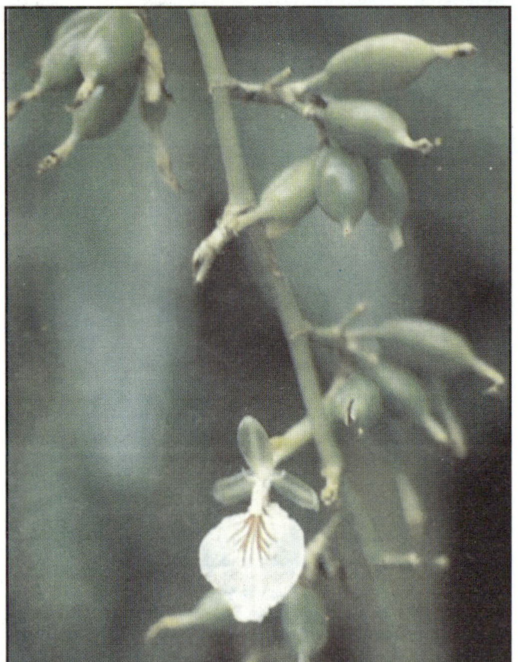

Elettaria cardamomum

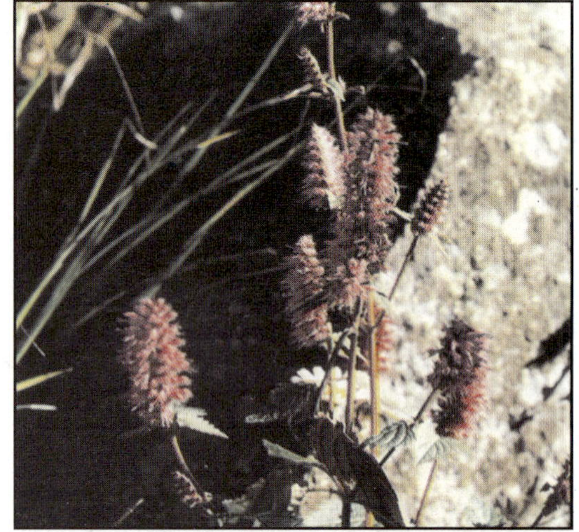

Elsholtzia splendens

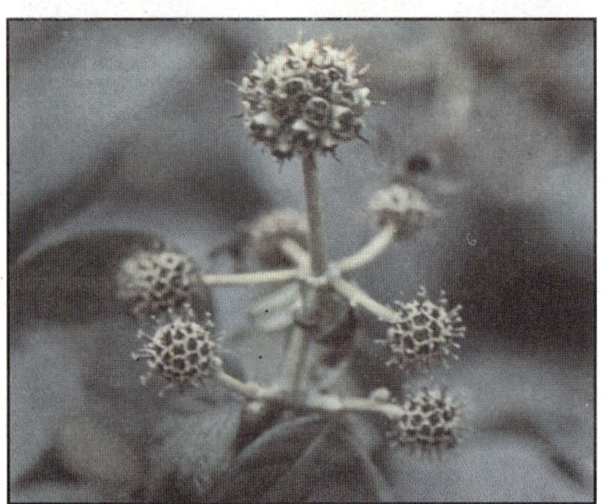

Eleutherococcus sessiliflorus

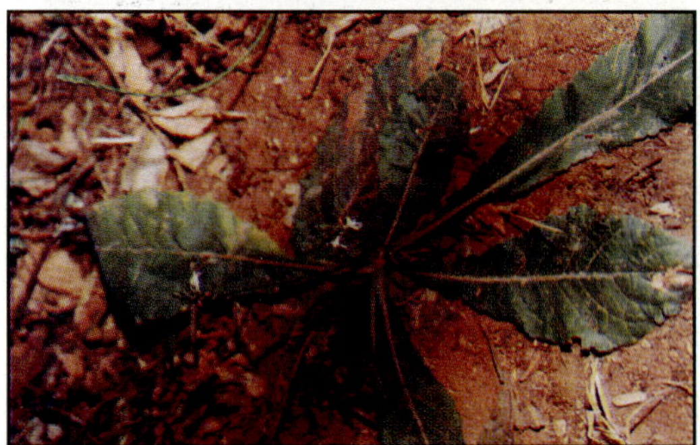

Elytraria acholis

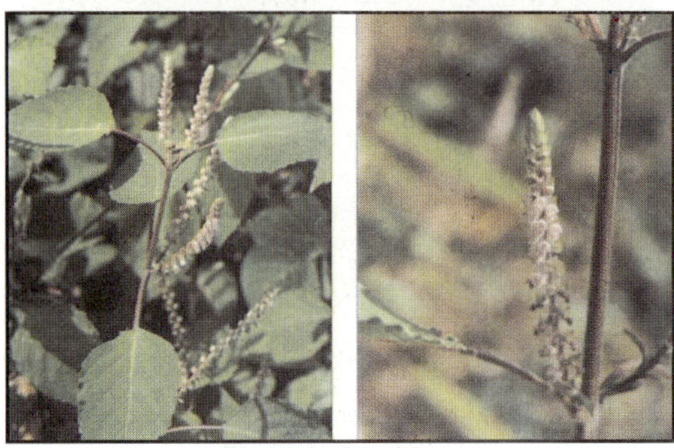

Elsholtzia ciliata

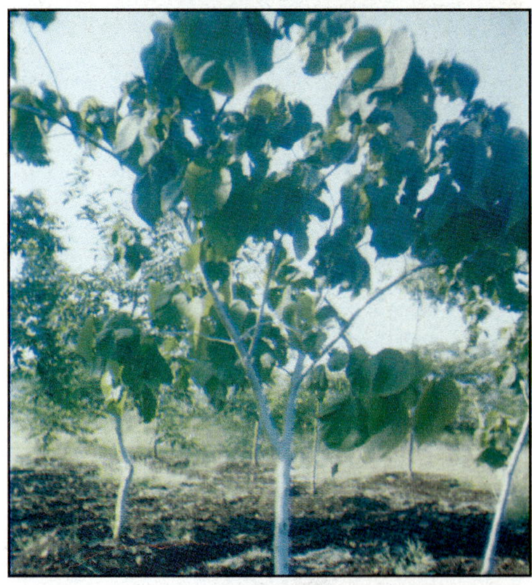

embelia ribes

PLATE : 57

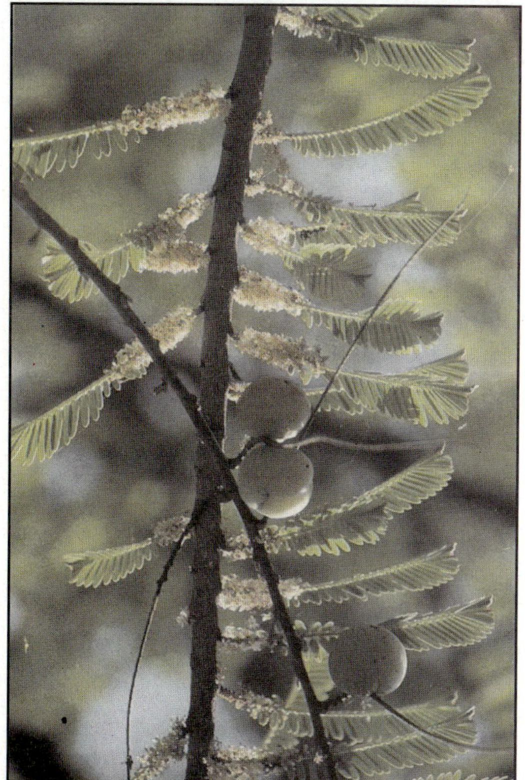

Emblica offcinalis

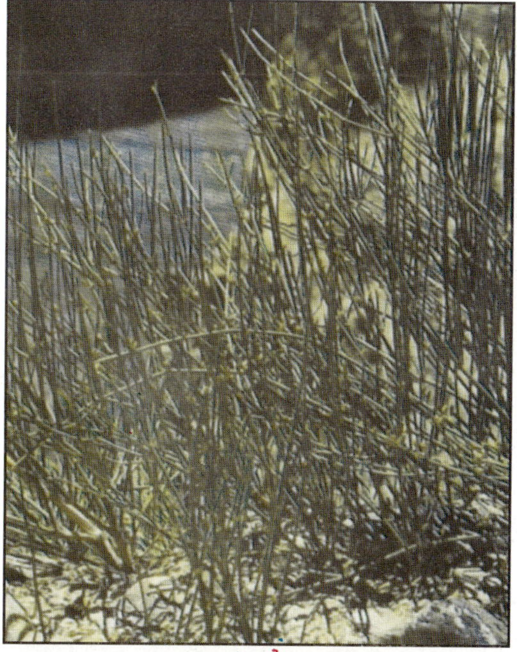

Ephedra gerardiana

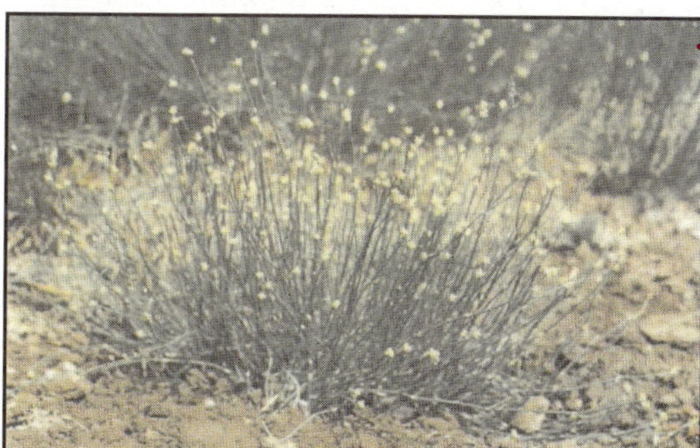

Ephedra sinica

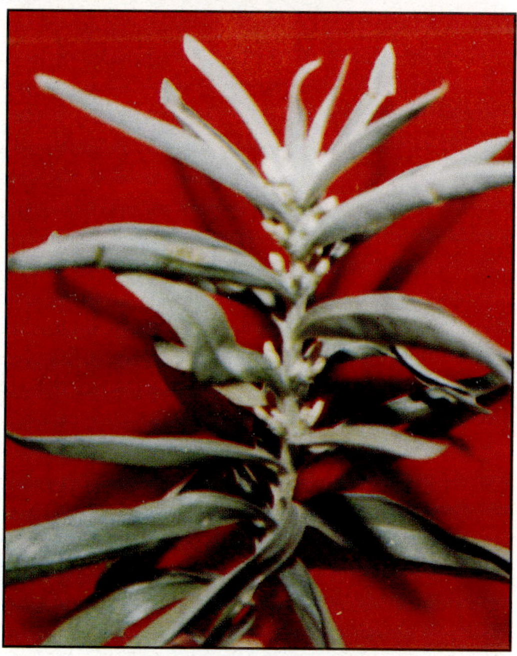

Enicostema hysopefolium

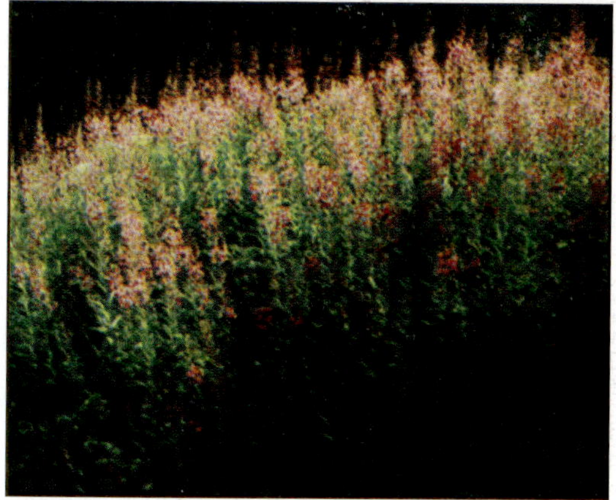

Epilobium angustifolium

PLATE : 58

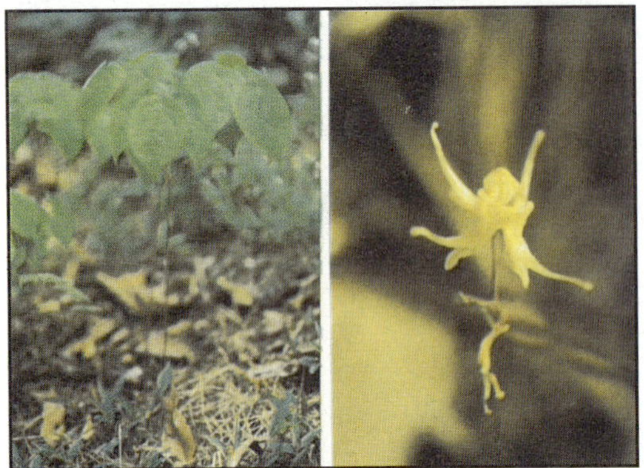

Epimedium koreanum

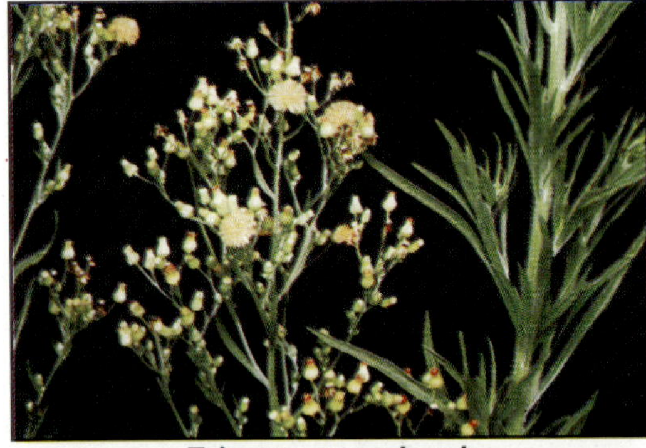

Erigeron canadensis

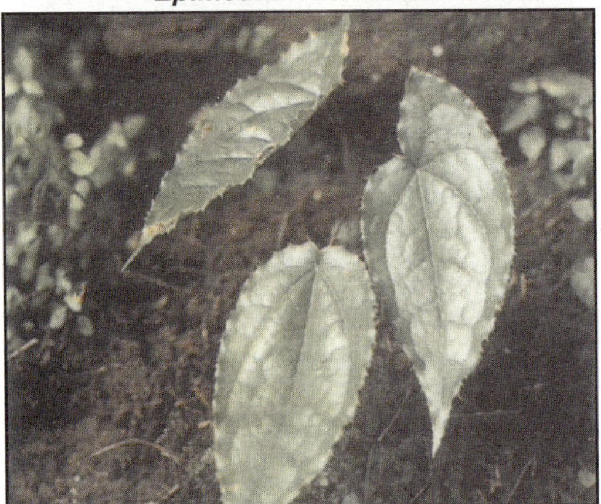

Epimedium sagittatum

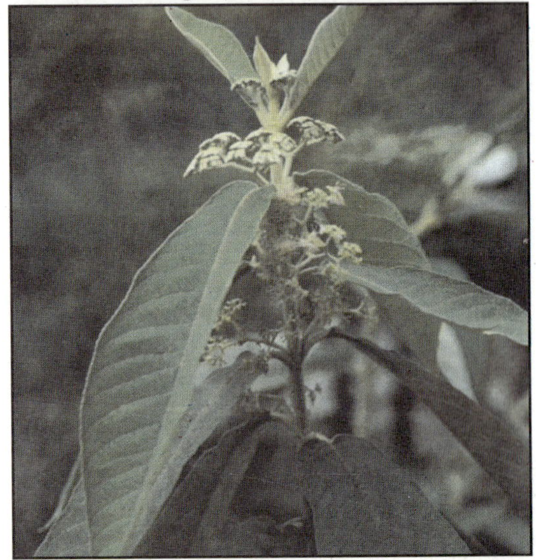

Eriobotrya japonica

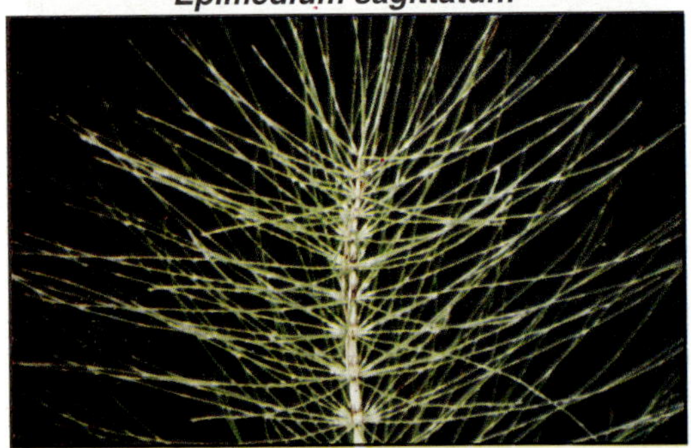

Equisetum arvense

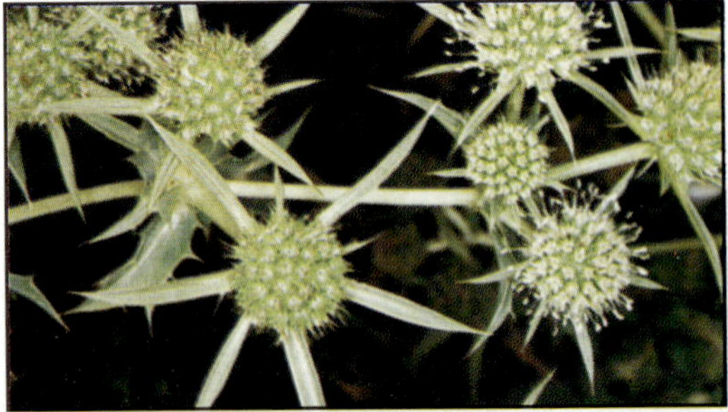

Eryngium campestre

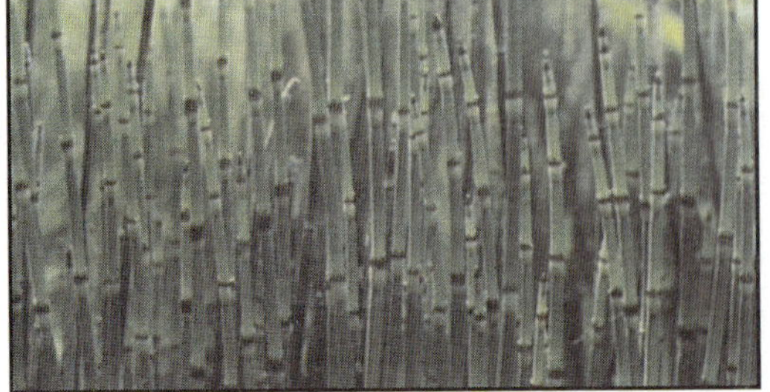

Equisetum hyemale

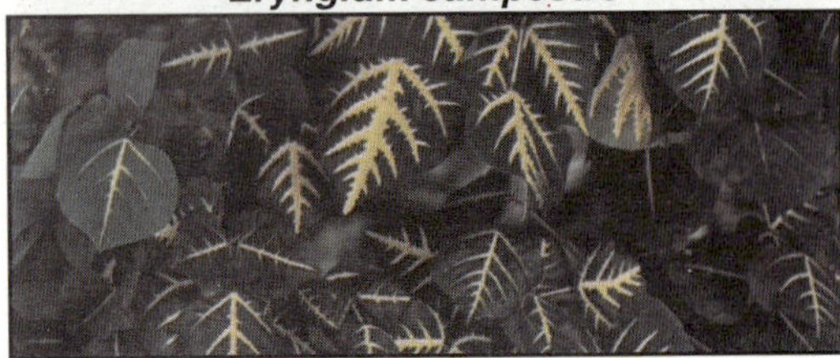

Erythrina variegata

PLATE : 59

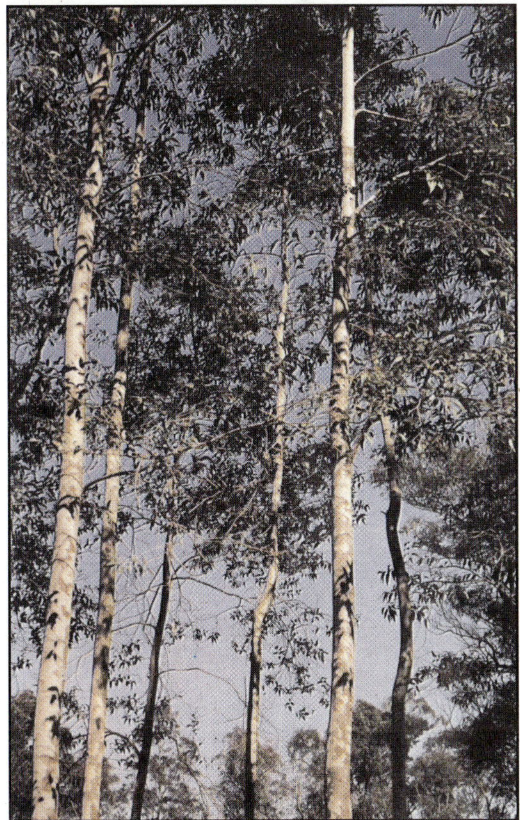

Eucalyptus citriodora

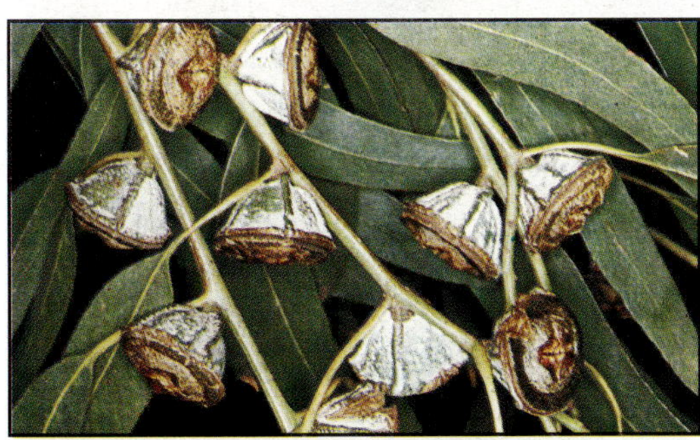

Eucalyptus globulus

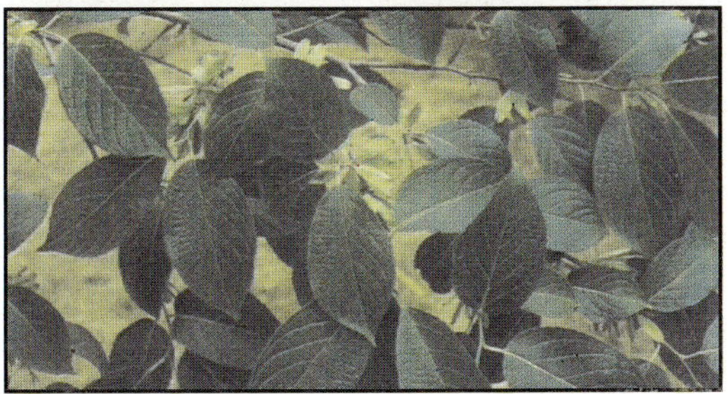

Eucommia ulmoides

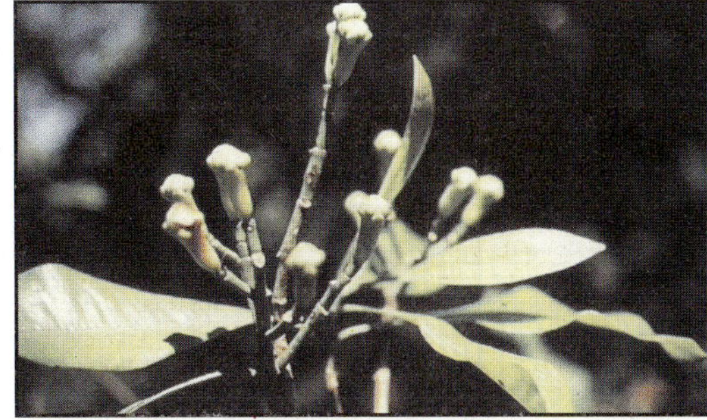

Eugenia aromatic

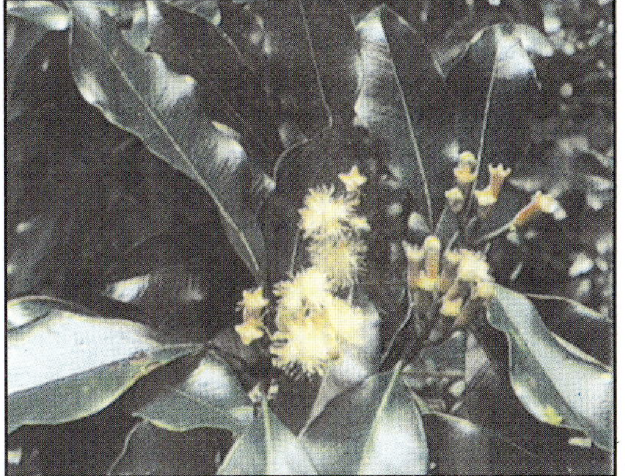

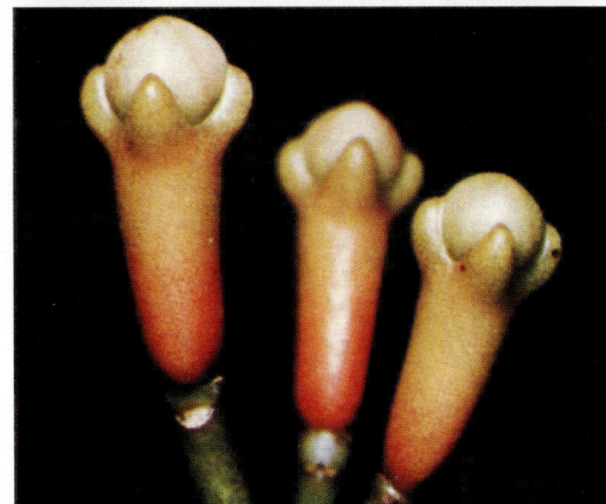

Eugenia caryophyllata

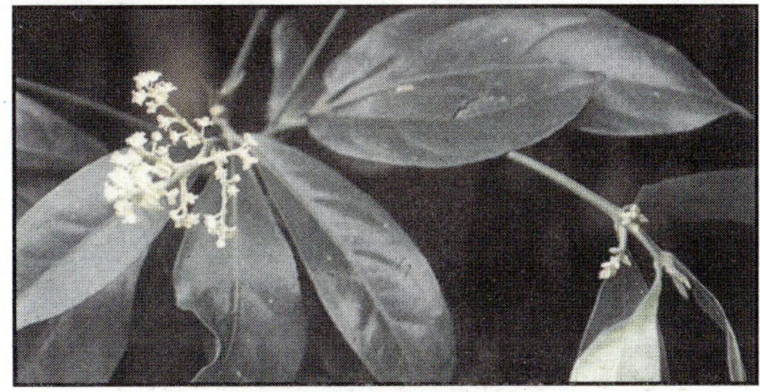

Euodia hortensis

PLATE : 60

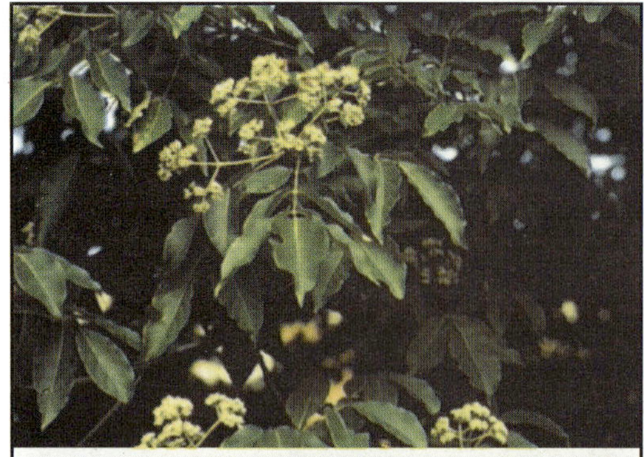

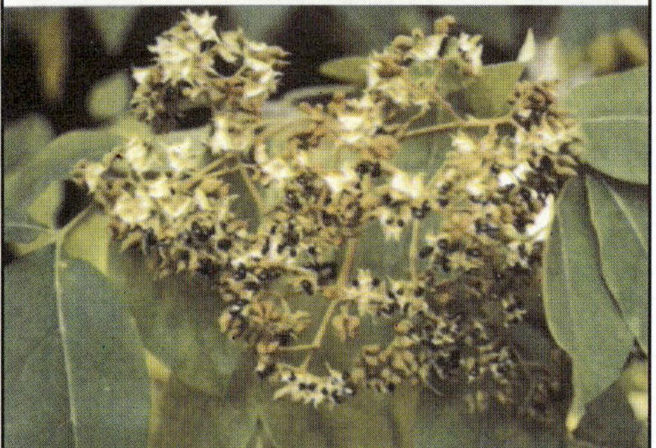

Euodia officinalis

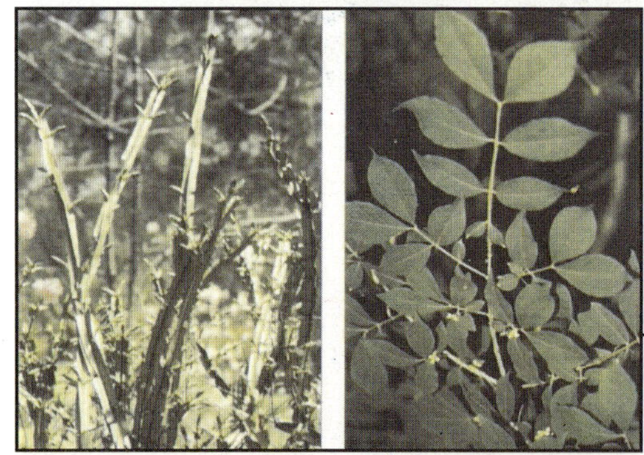

Euonymus alatus

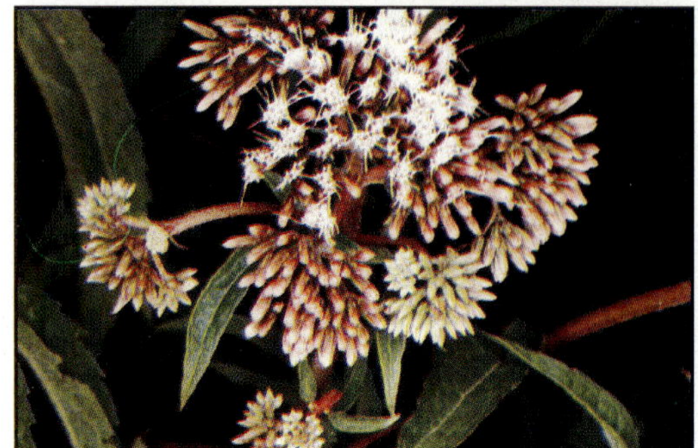

Eupatorium cannabinum

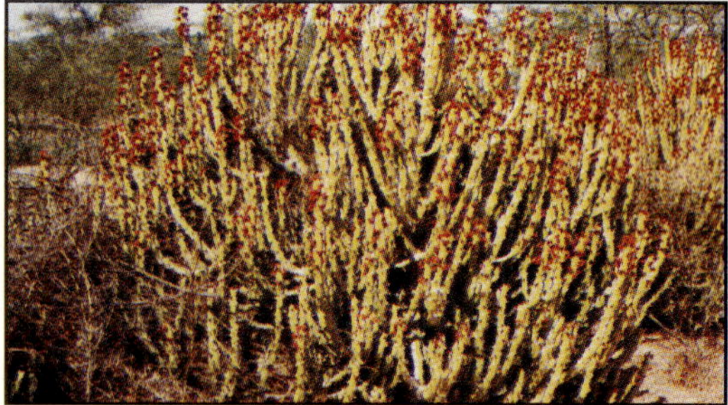

Euphorbia caducifolia

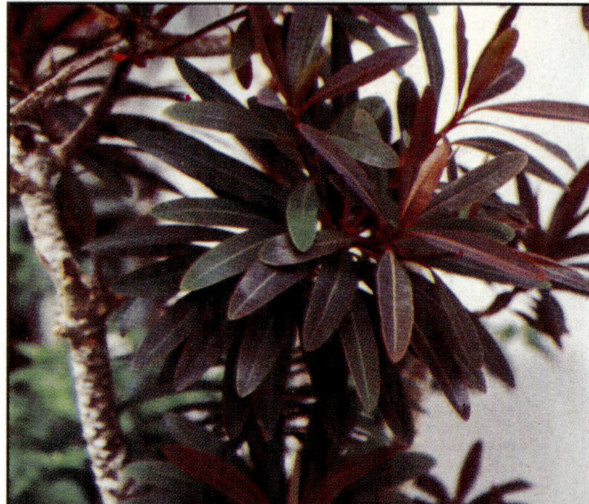

Euphorbia fidjiana

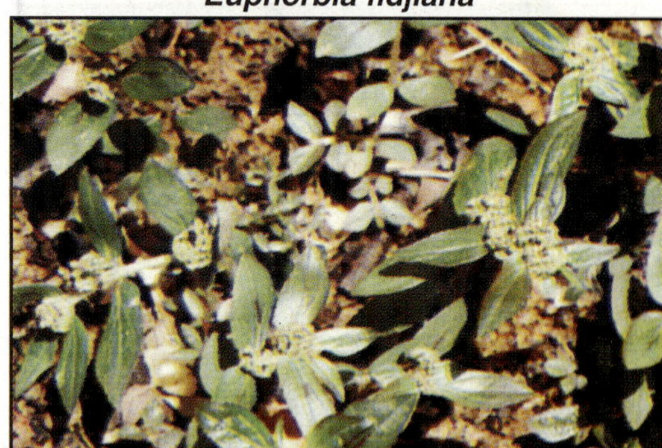

Euphorbia hirta

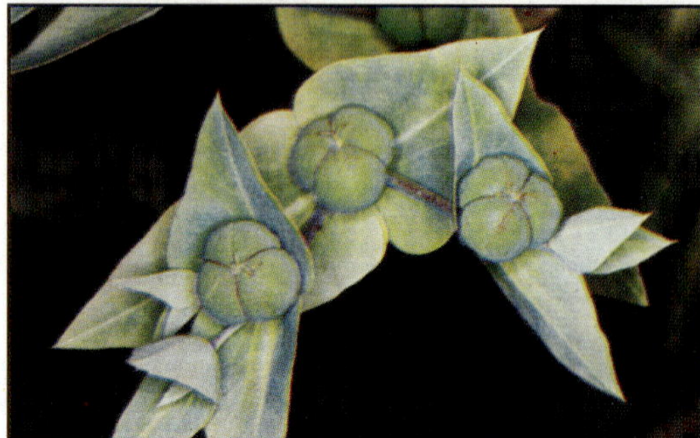

Euphorbia lathyrus

PLATE : 61

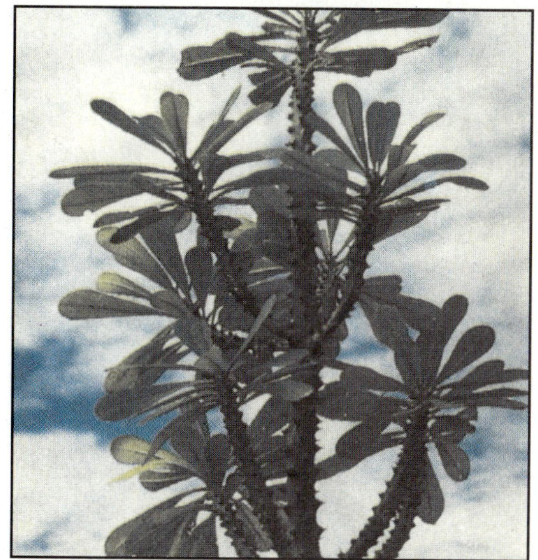
Euphorbia neriifolia

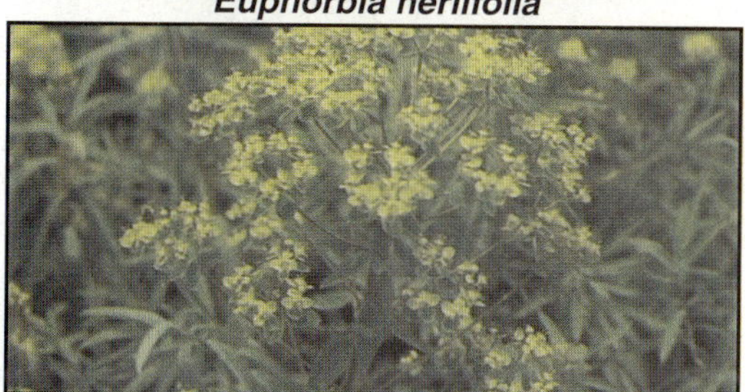
Euphorbia pekinensis

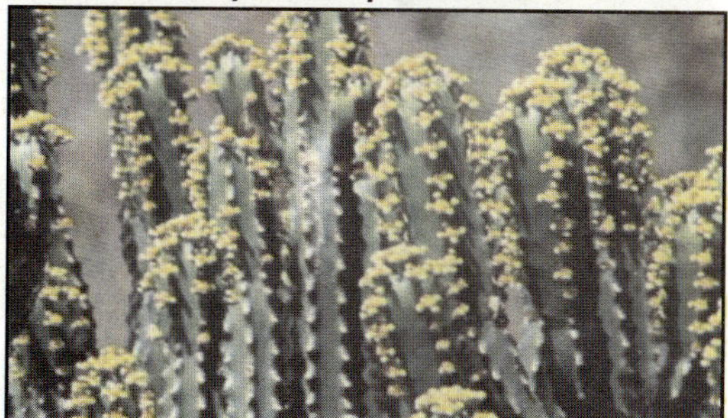
Euphorbia royleana

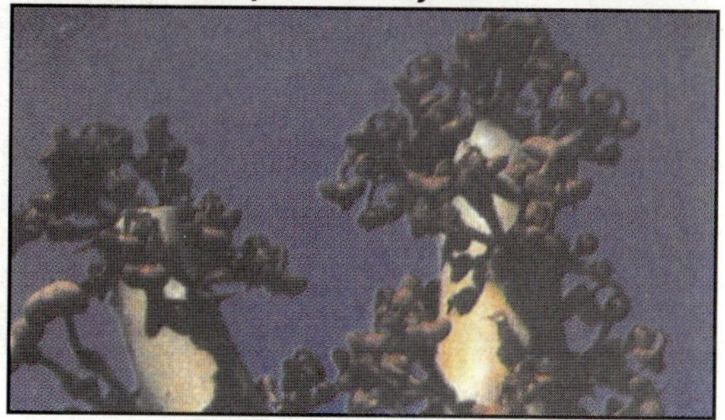
Euphorbia caducifolia

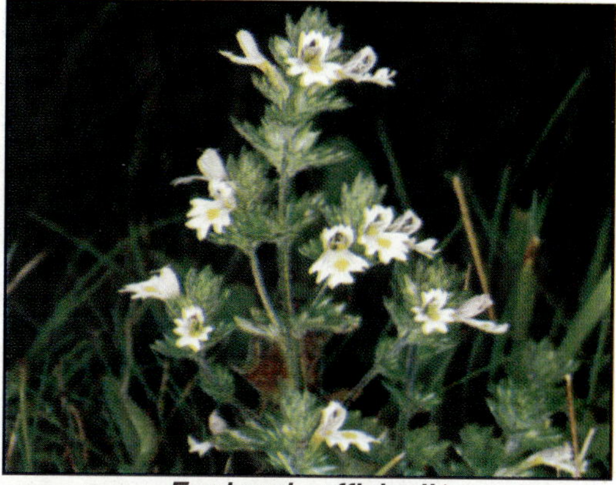
Euphrasia officinalis

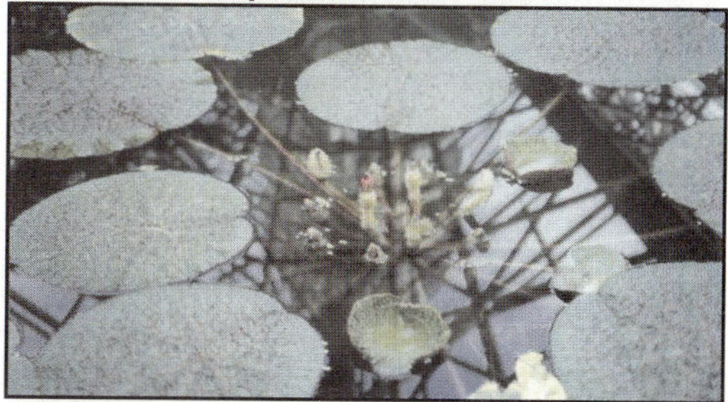
Euryale ferox

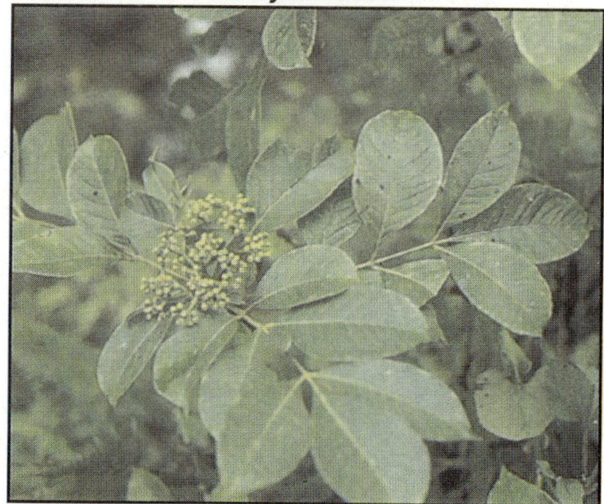
Evodia rutaecarpa

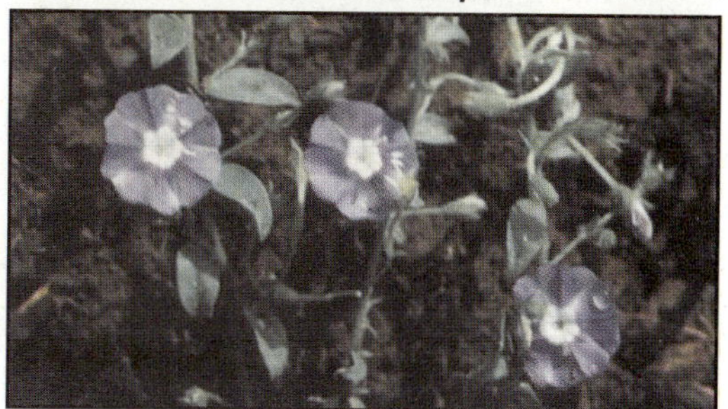
Evolvulus alsinoides

PLATE : 62

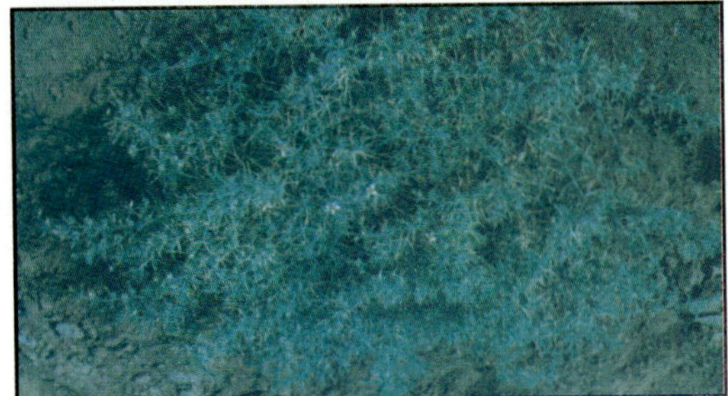

Fagonia cretica

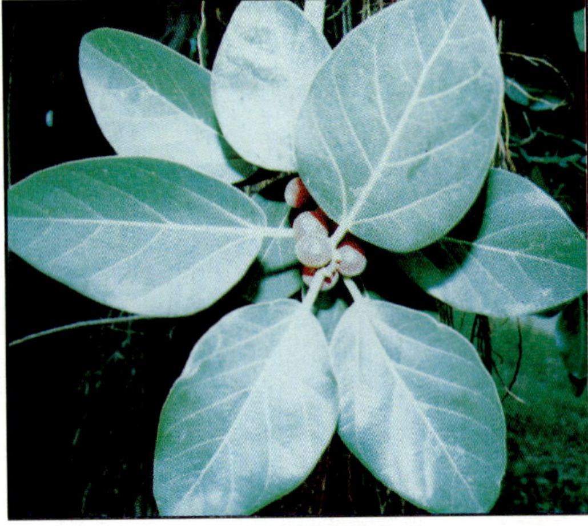

Ficus bengalensis

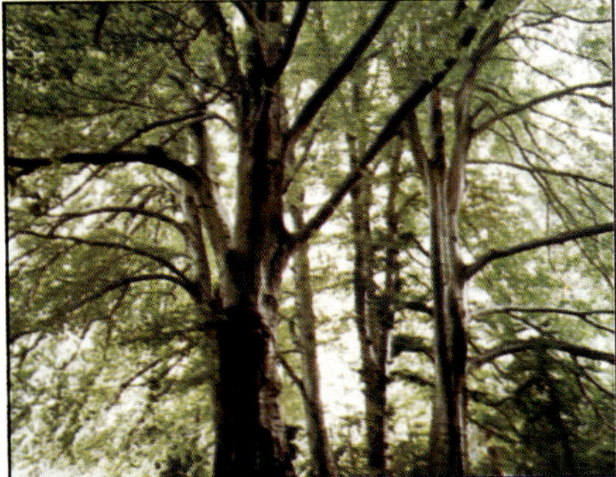

Fagus aylvatica

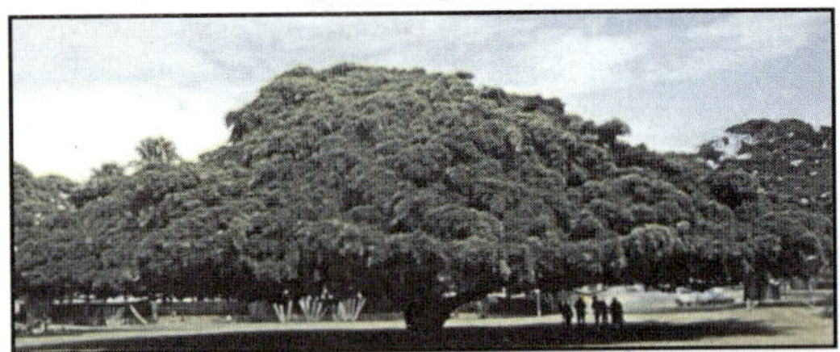

Ficus benjamina

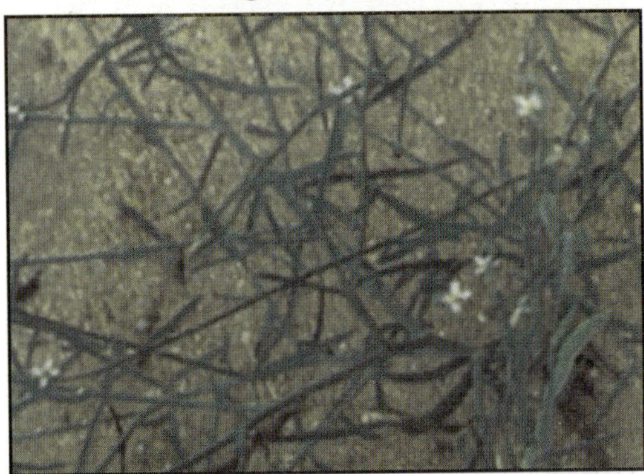

Farsetia hamiltonii

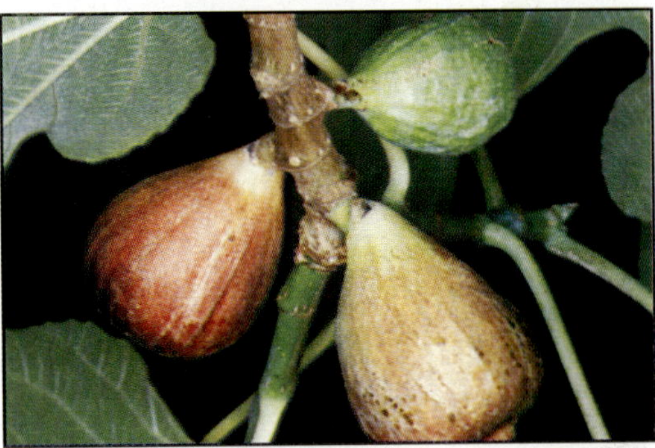

Ficus carica

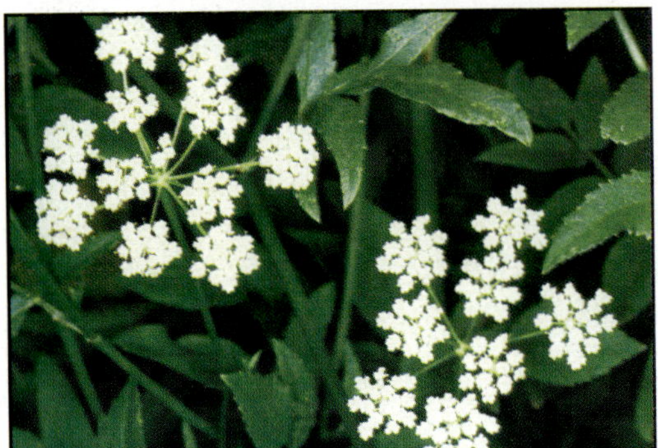

Ferula asafoetida

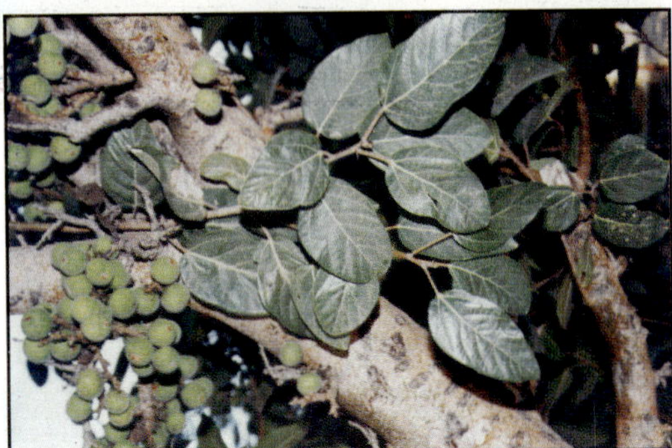

Ficus glomerata

PLATE : 63

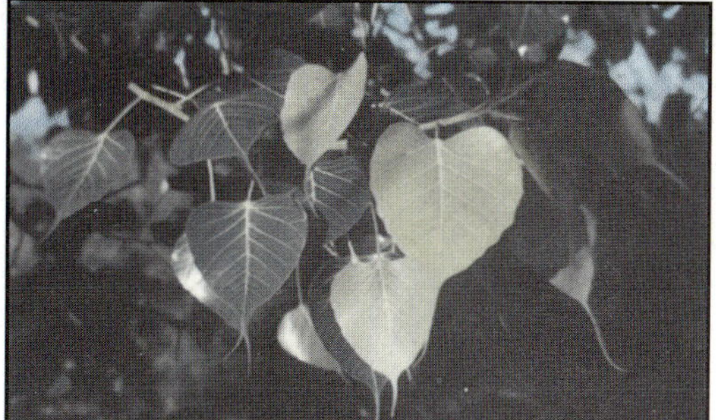

Ficus religiosa

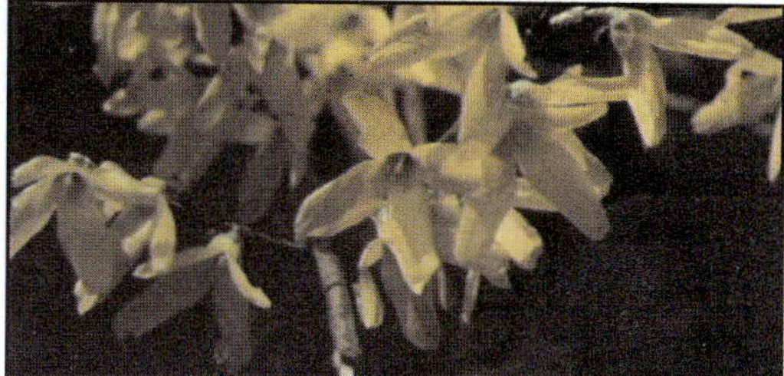

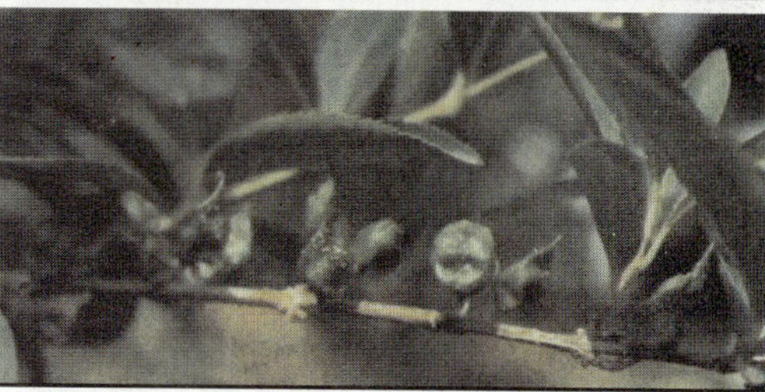

Forsythia viridissima

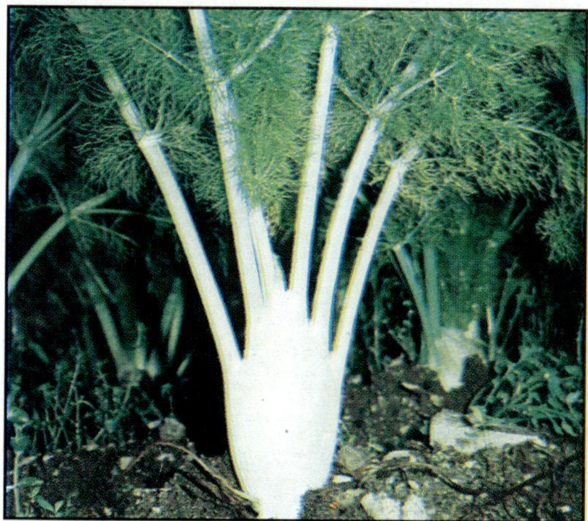

Foeniculum vulgare

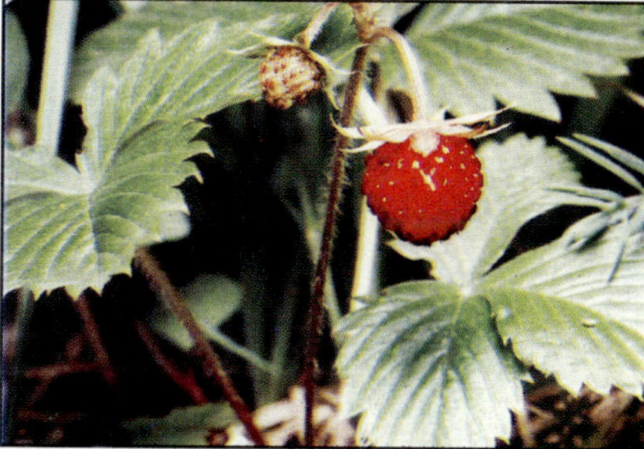

Fragaria vesca

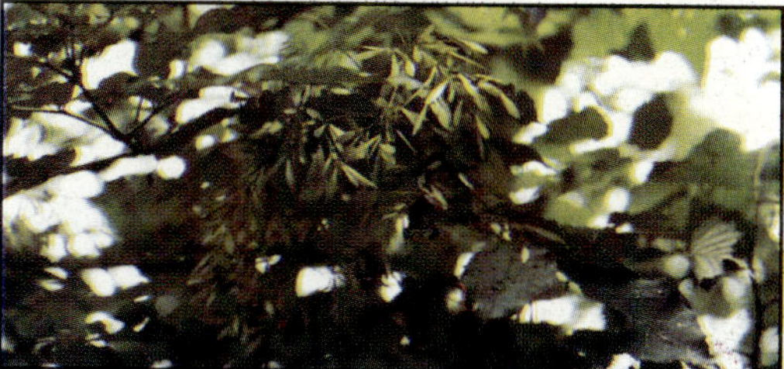

Frainus rhynchophylla

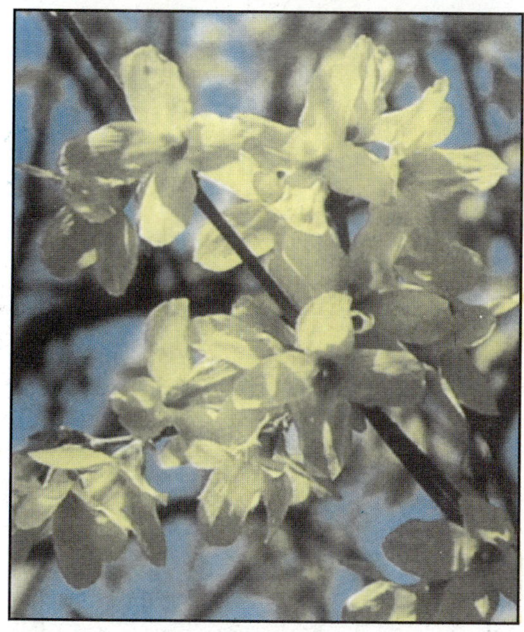

Forsythia suspensa

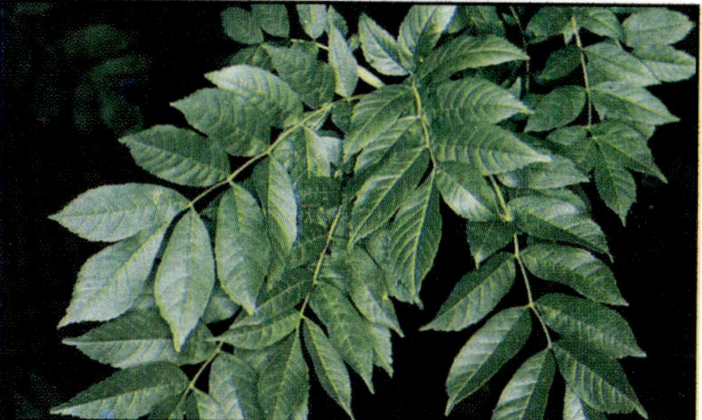

Fraxinus excelsior

PLATE : 64

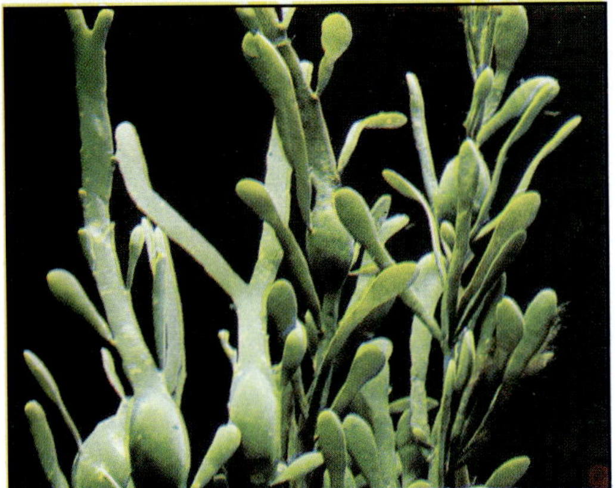

Fucus vesciculosus

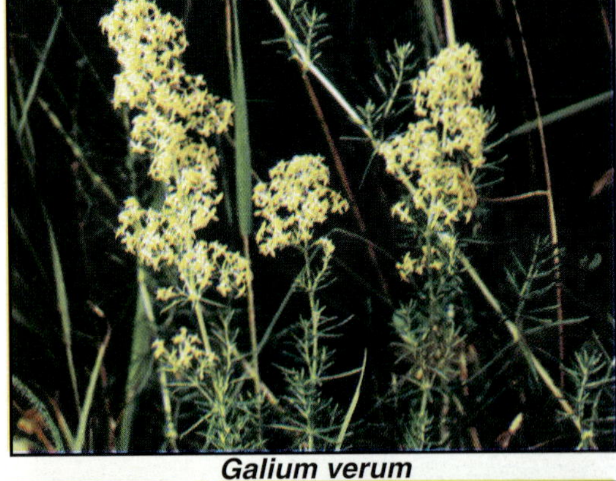

Galium verum

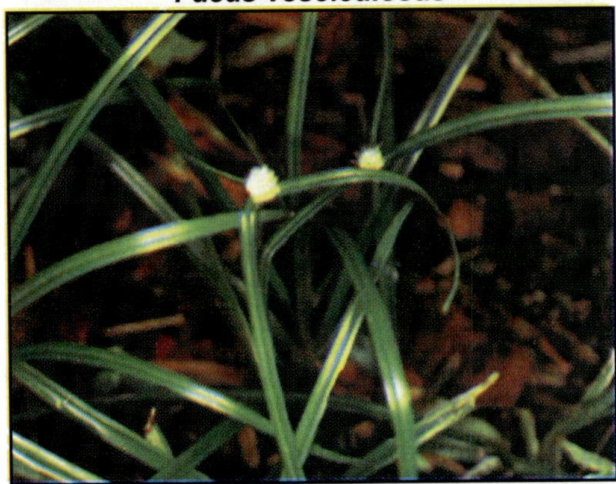

Fyllinga brevifolia

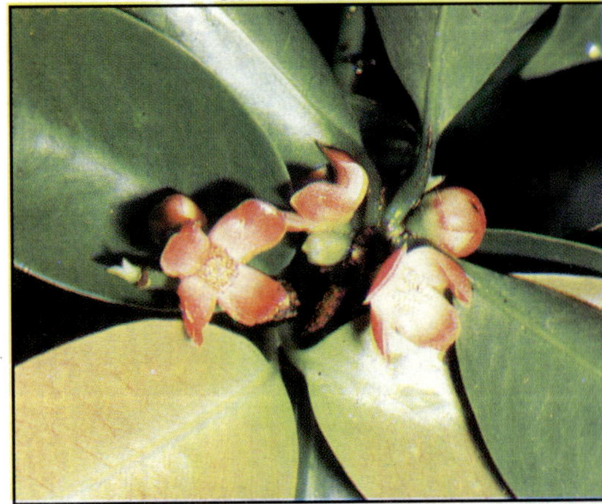

Garcinia sessilis

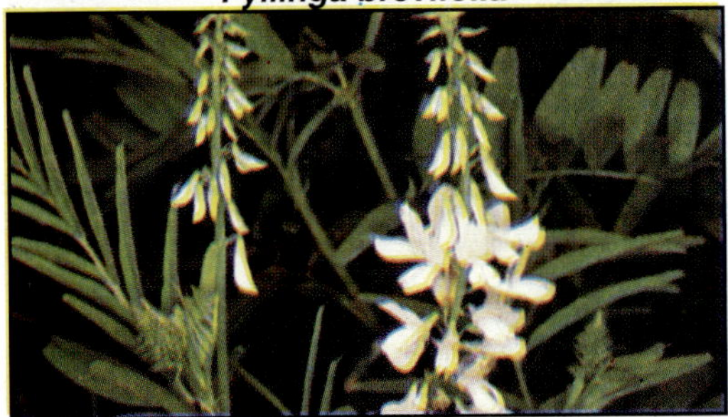

Galega officinalis

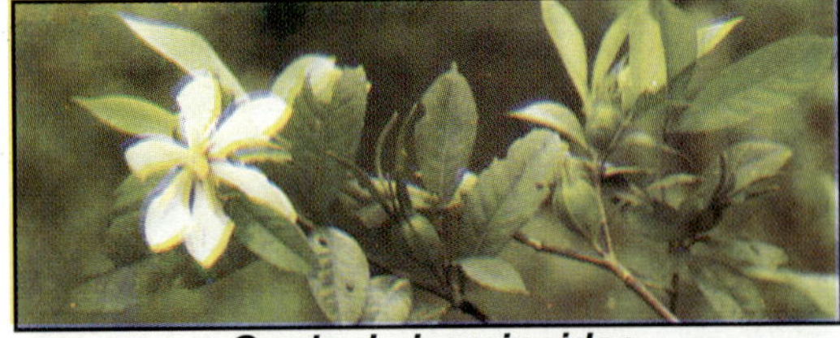

Gardenia jasminoides

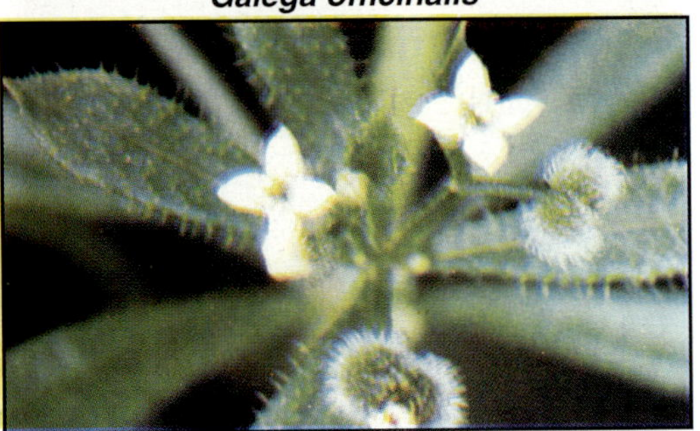

Galium aparine

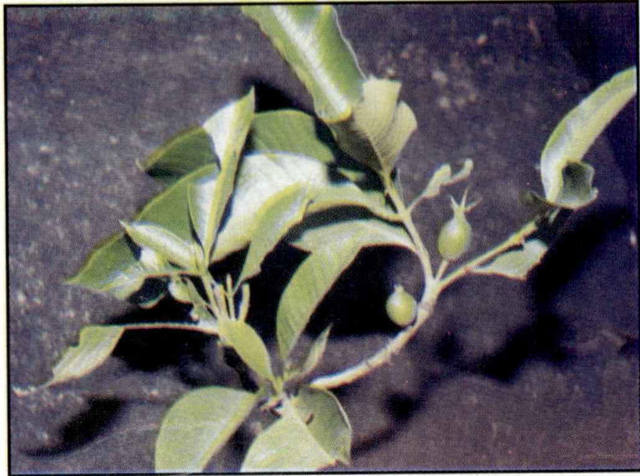

Gardinia gummifera

PLATE : 65

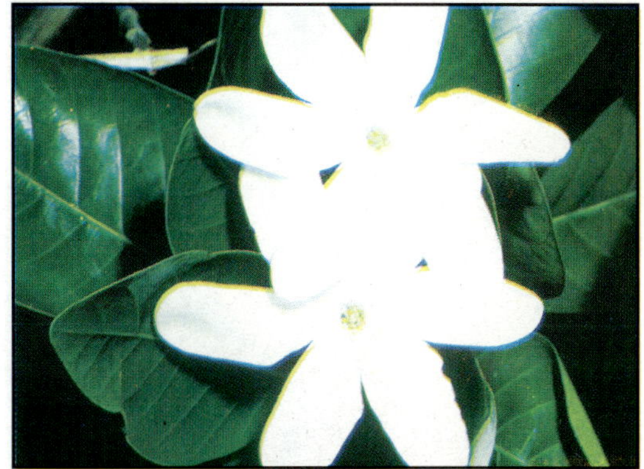

Gardenia taitensis

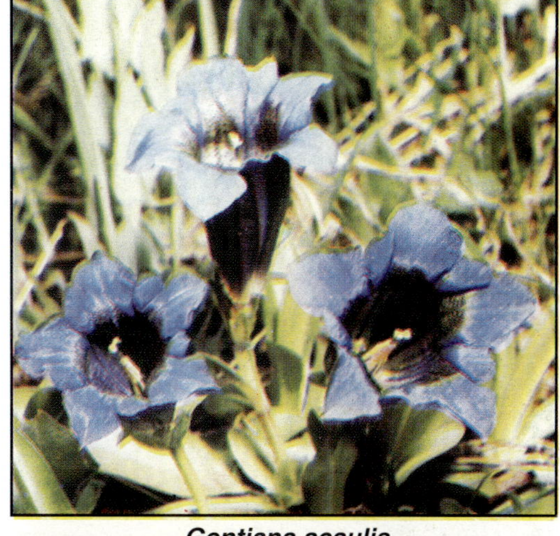

Gentiana acaulis

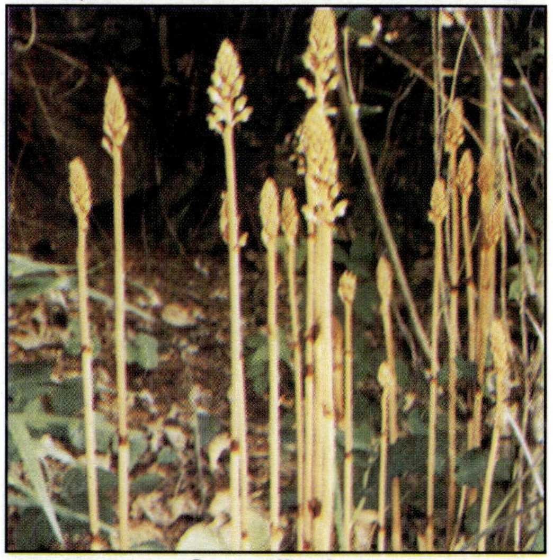

Gastrodia elata

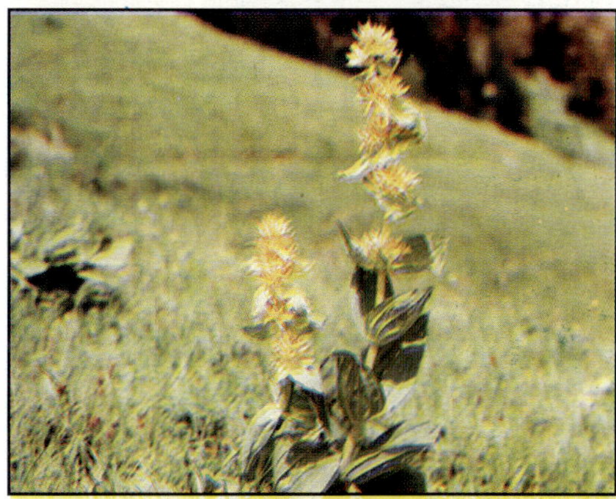

Gentiana litea

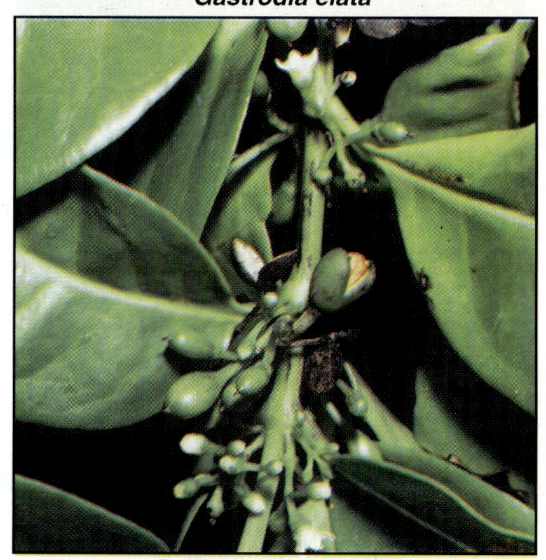

Geniostoma rupestre

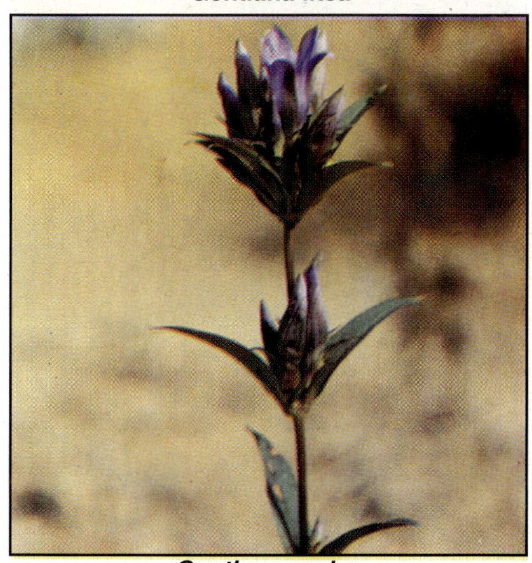

Gentiana scabra

PLATE : 66

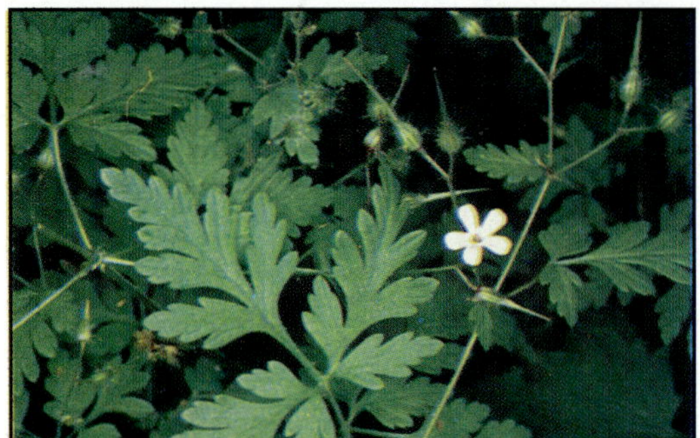

Geranium robertianum

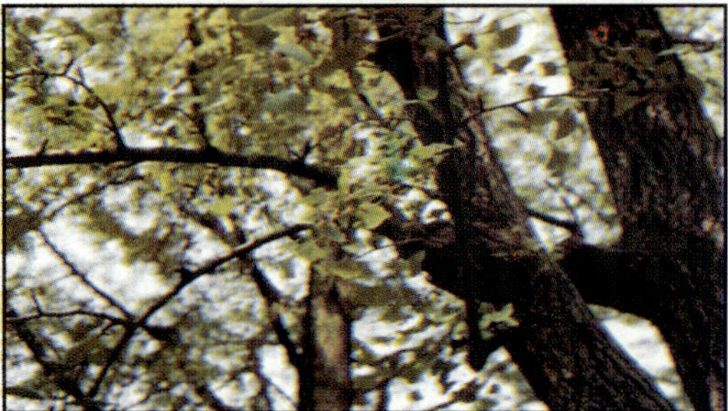

Ginkgo biloba

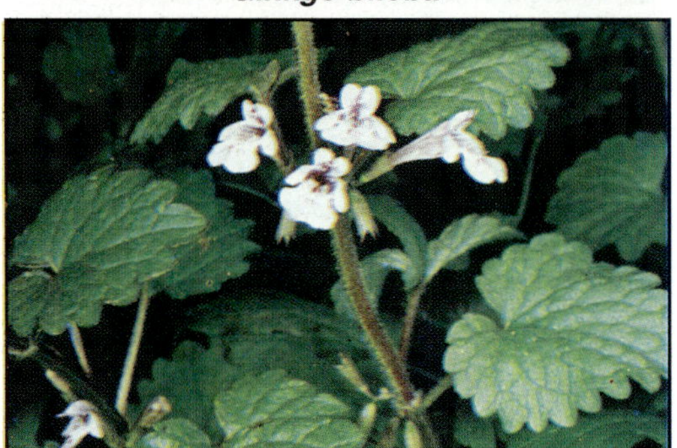

Glechoma hederacea

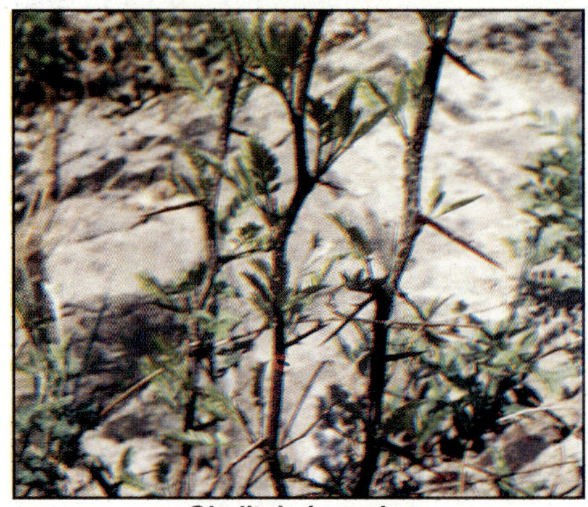

Gleditsia japonica

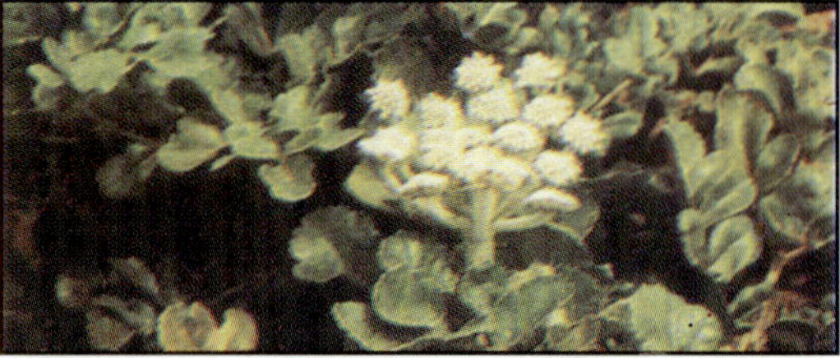

Globularia vulgaris

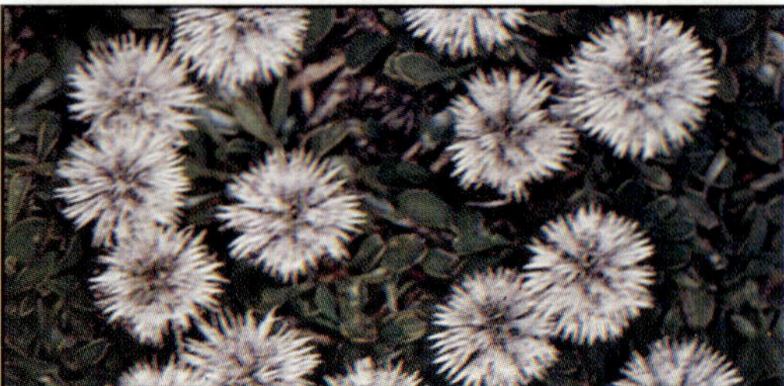

Glehnia littoralis

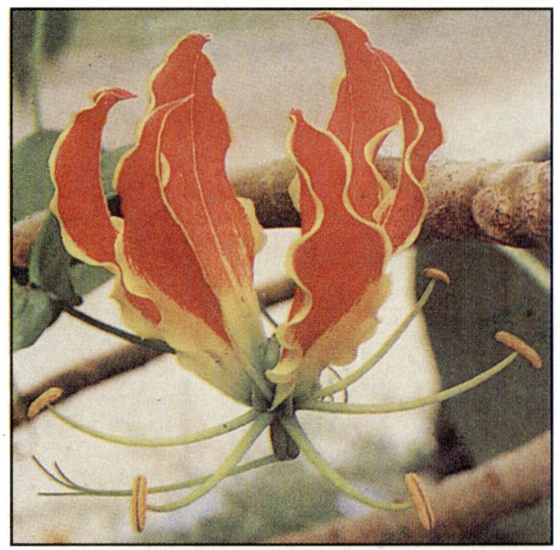

Gloriosa superba

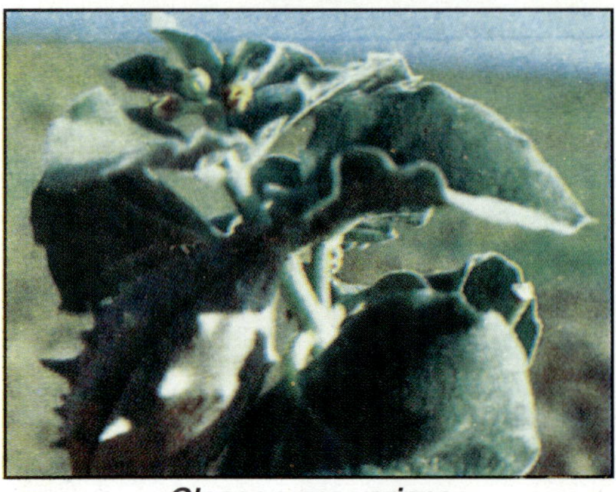

Glossonema varians

PLATE : 67

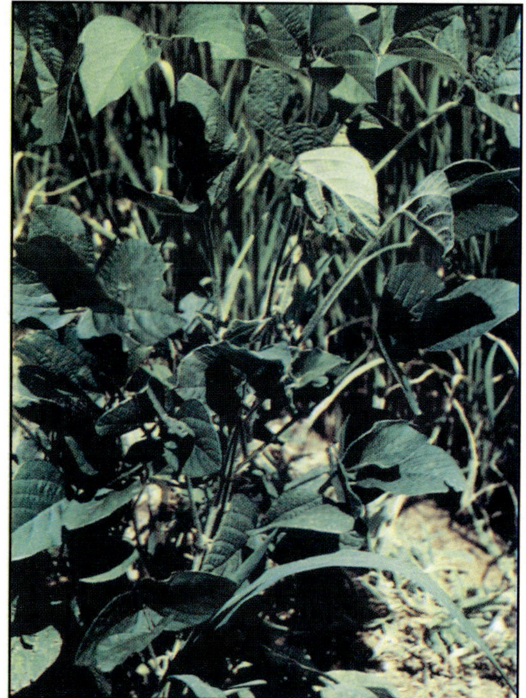

Glycine max

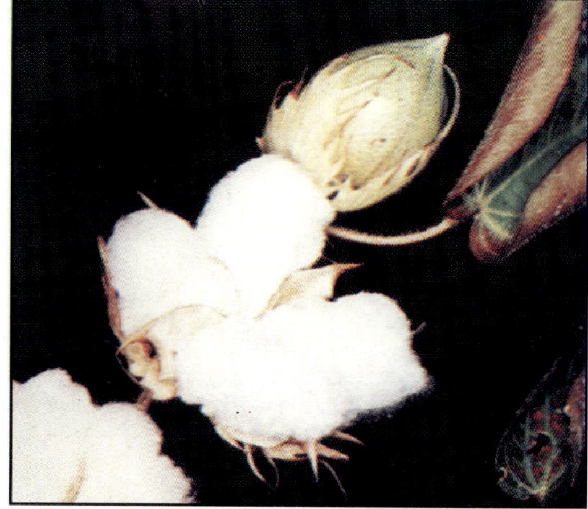

Gossypium herbaceum

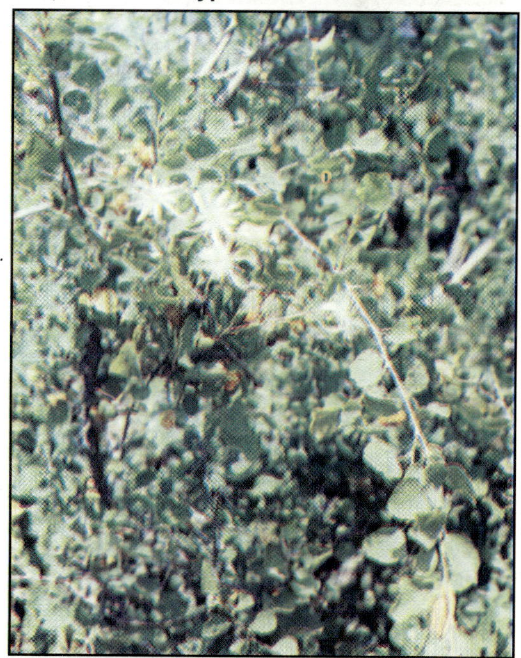

Grewia tenax

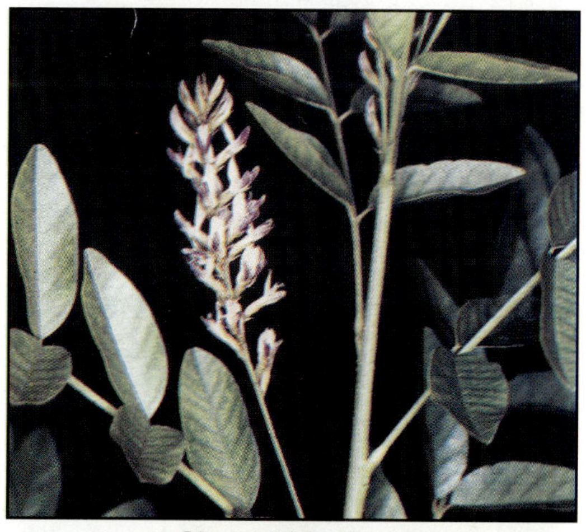

Glycyrrhiza glabra

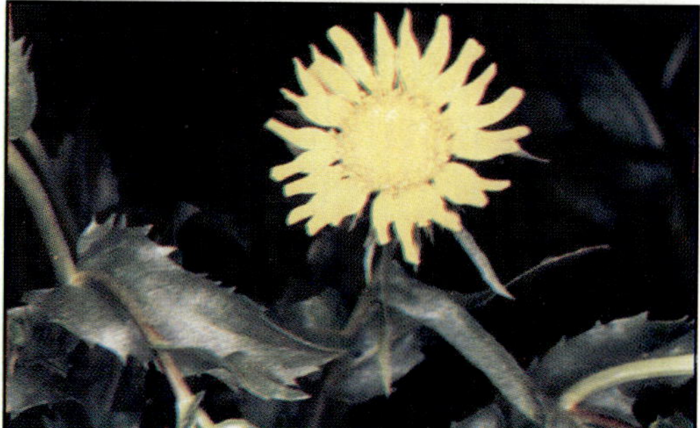

Grindelia robusta

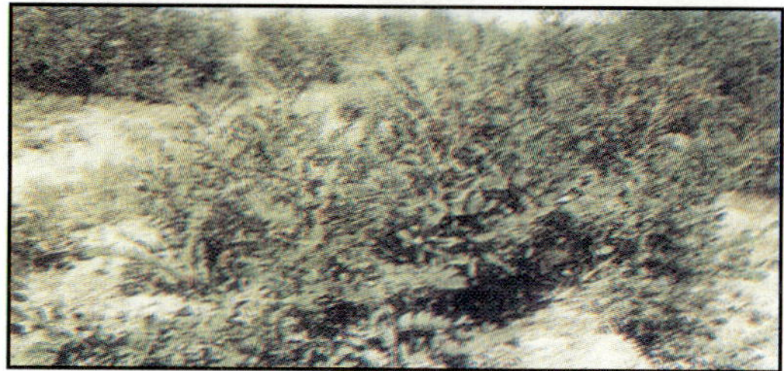

Glycyrrhiza uralensis

PLATE : 68

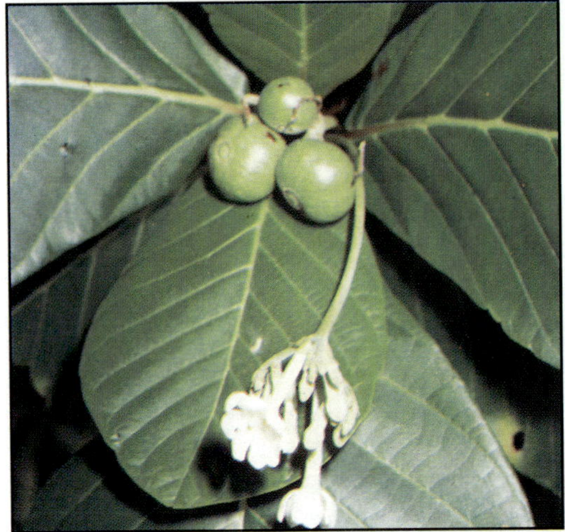

Guettarda speciosa

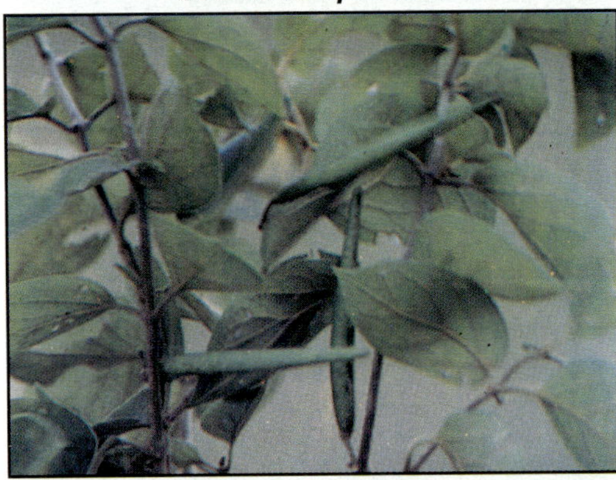

Gymnema sylvestre

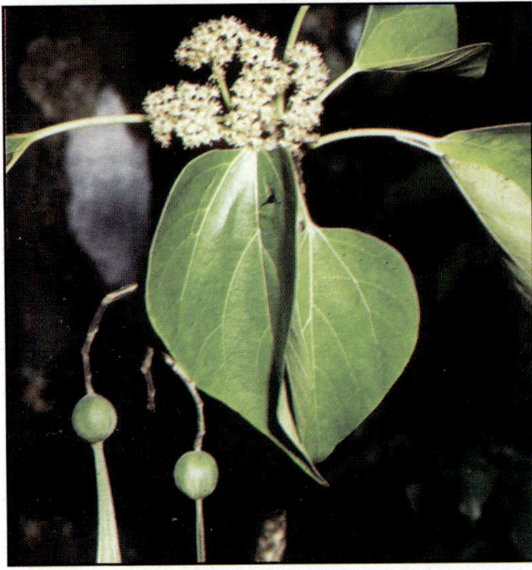

Gyrocarpus americanus

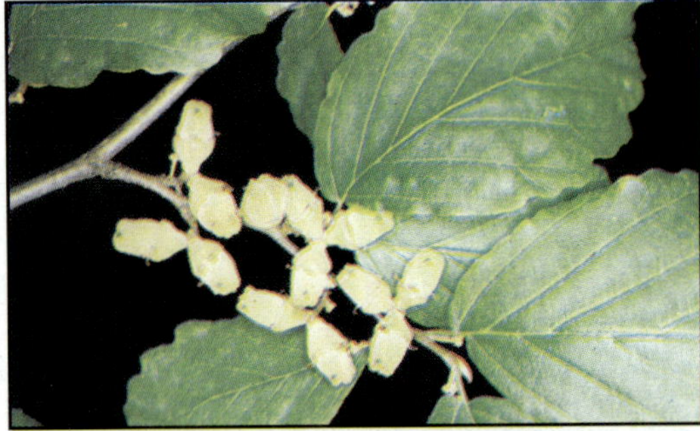

Hamamelis virginiana

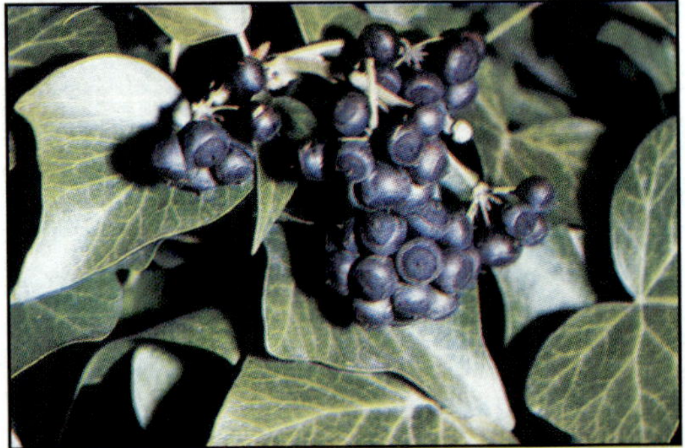

Hedera helix

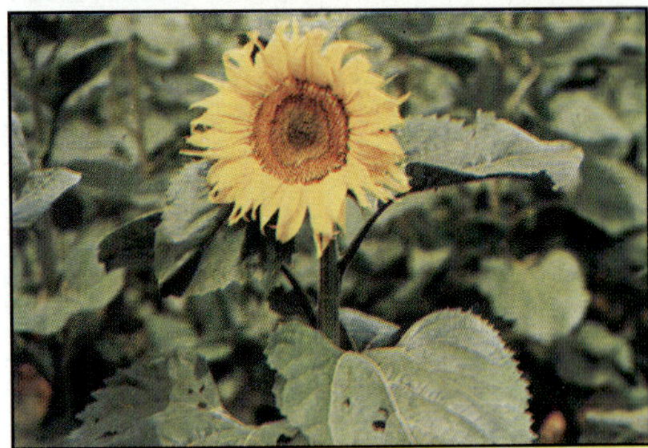

Helianthus annuus

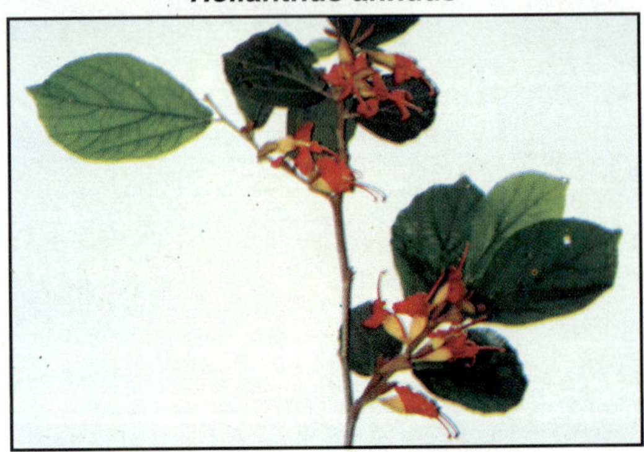

Helicteres isora

PLATE : 69

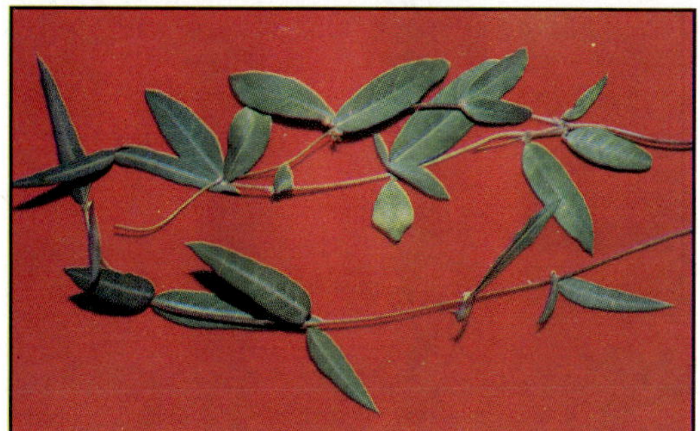

Hemidionius indicus

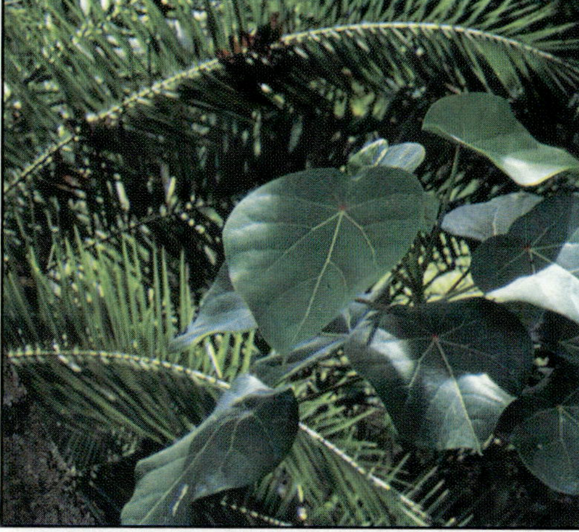

Hernandia nymphaeifolia

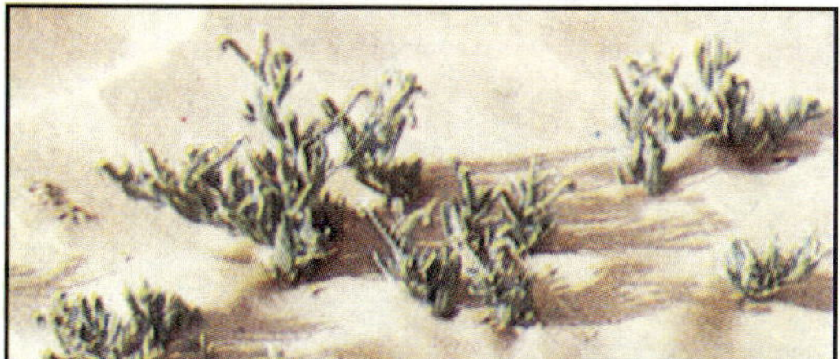

Heliotropium curasavicum

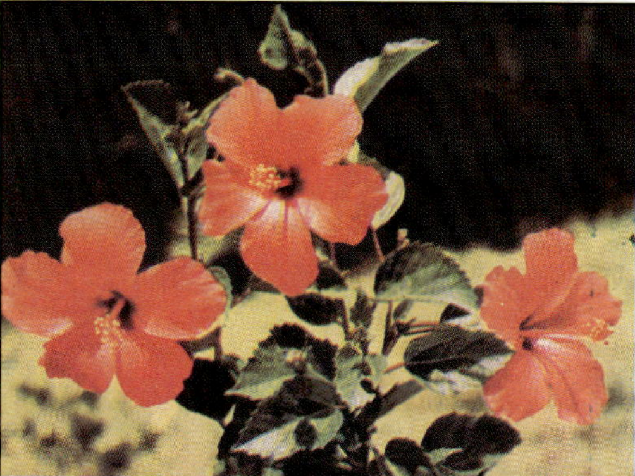

Hibiscus rosa-sinensis

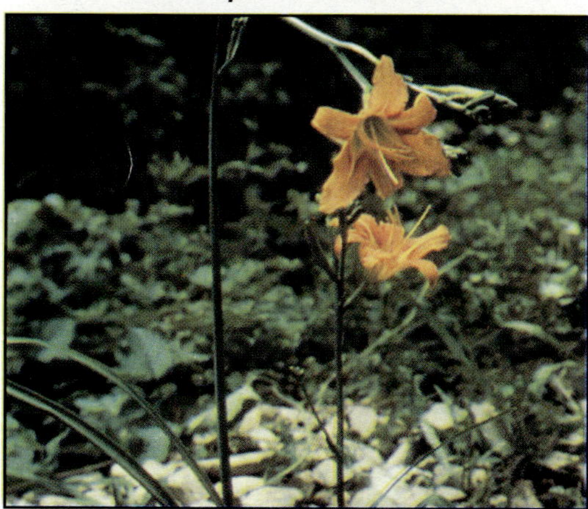

Hemerocallis fulva

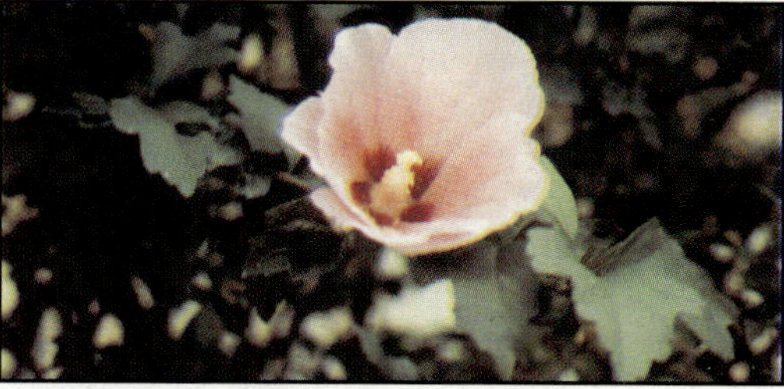

Hibiscus syriacus

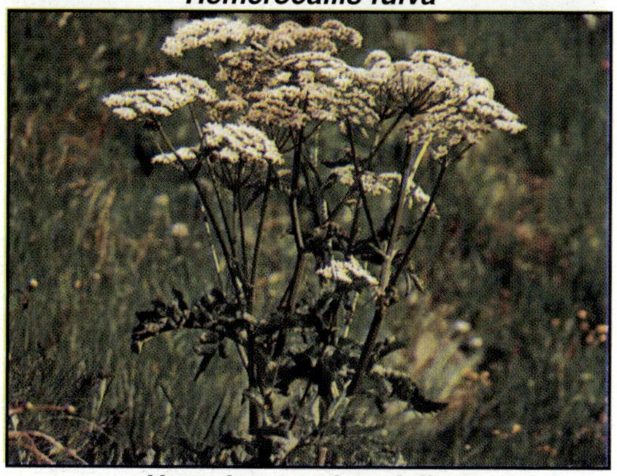

Heracleum sphondylium

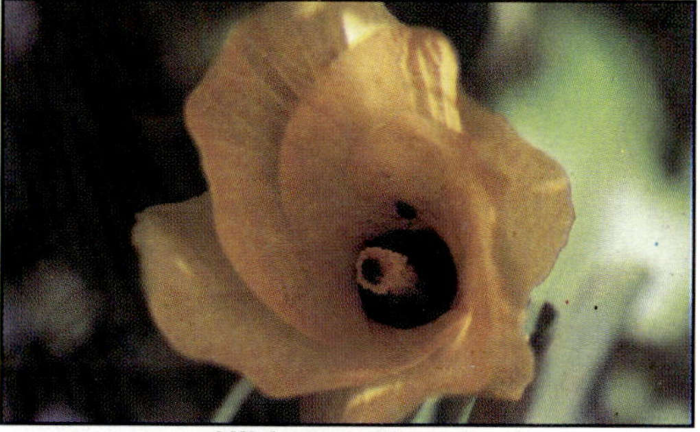

Hibiscus tiliaceus

PLATE : 70

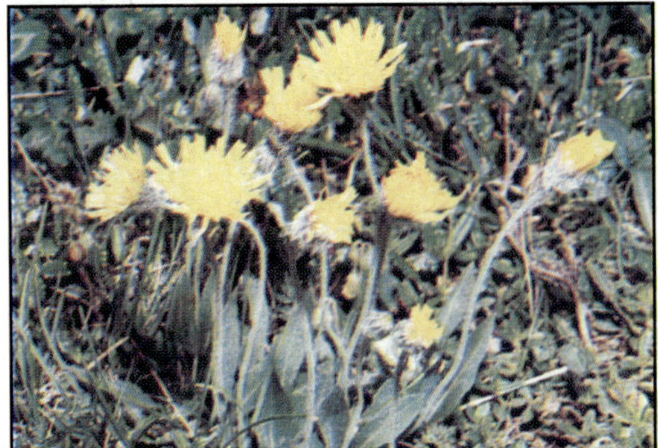
Hieracium pilosella

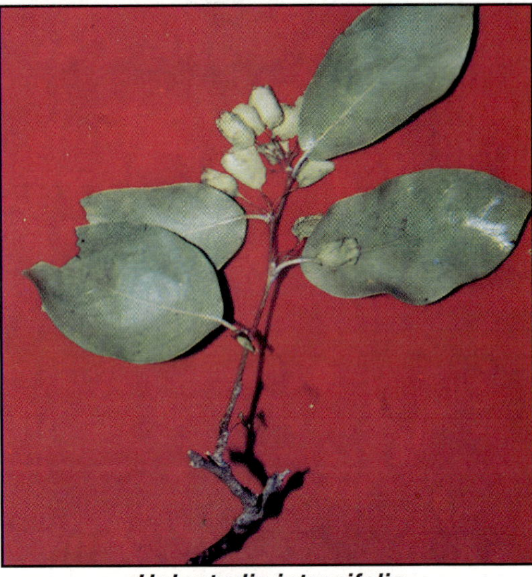
Holoptarlia intragifolia

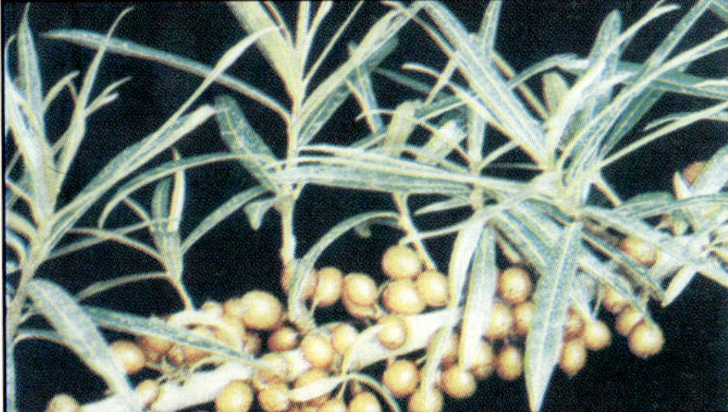
Hipophae rhamnoides

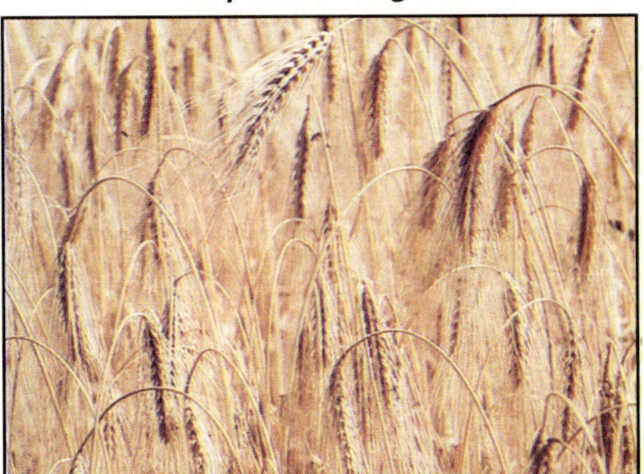
Hordeum vulgare

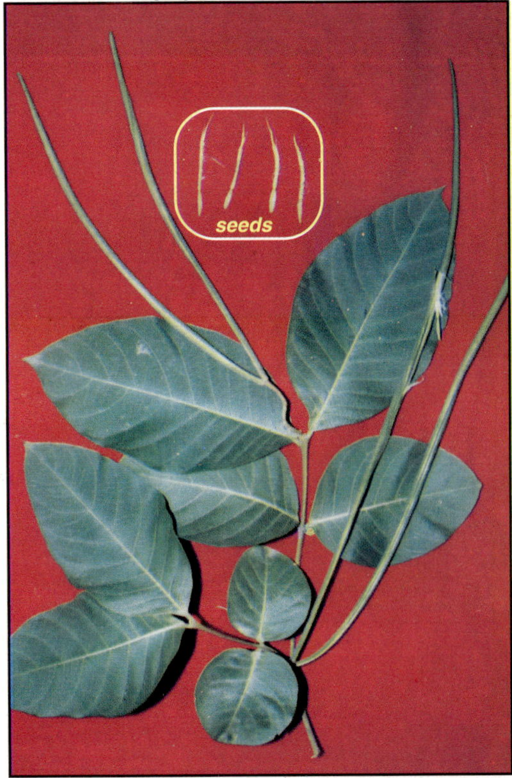

Holarrhena antldysenterica

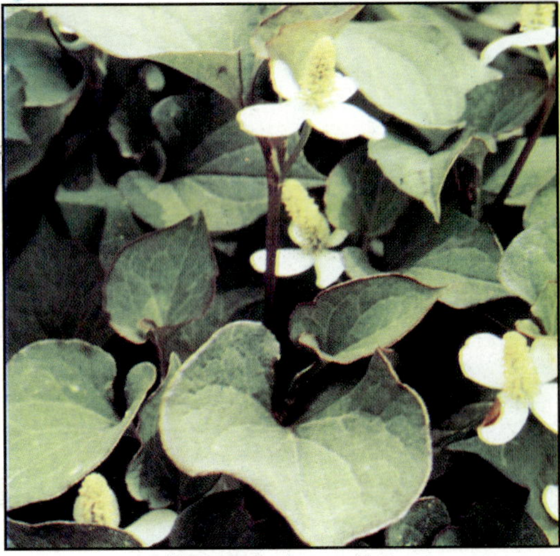
Houttuynia cordata

PLATE : 71

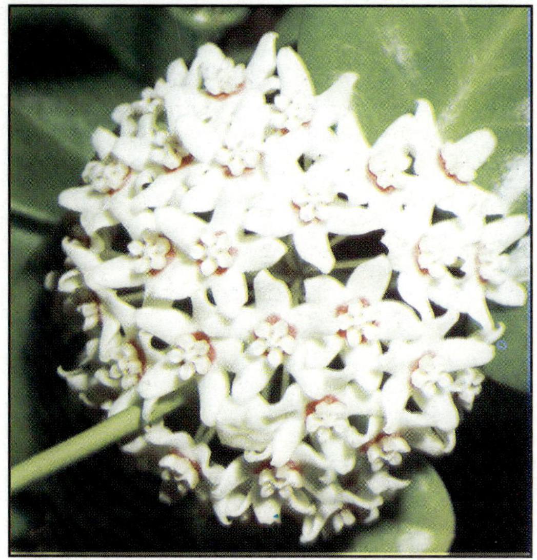

Hoya australis

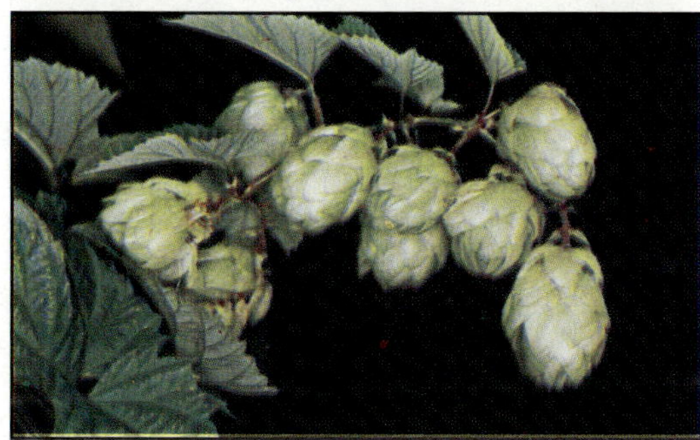

Humulus lupulus

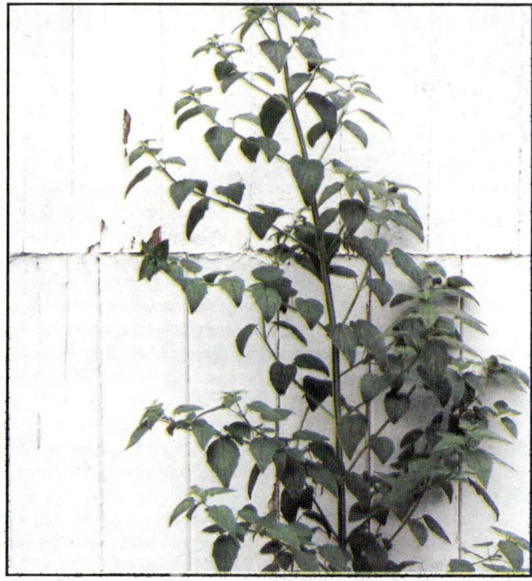

Hyatis pectinata

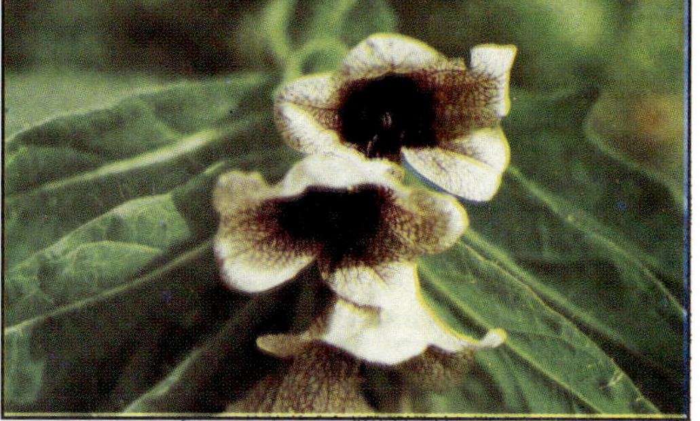

Hyoscyamus niger

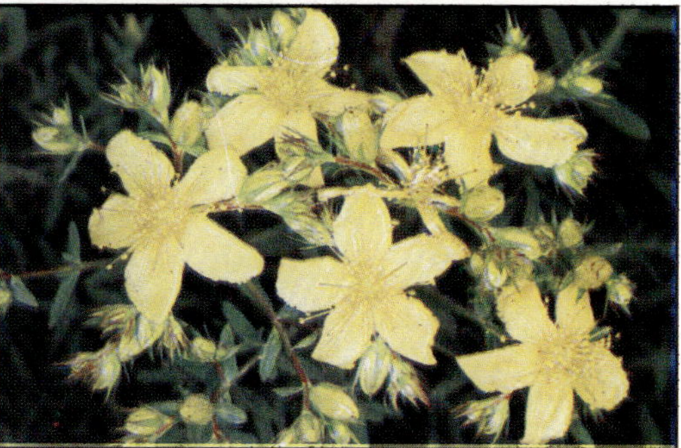

Hypericum perforatum

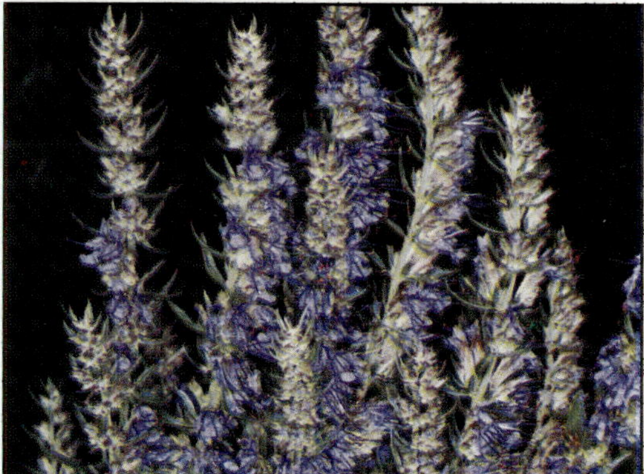

Hyssopus officinalis

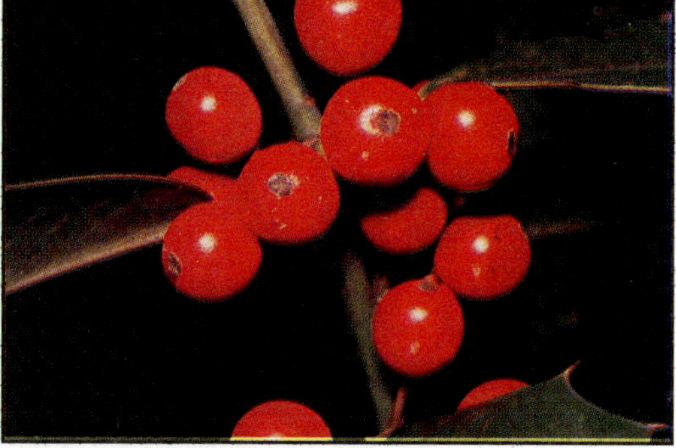

Ilex aquifolium

PLATE : 72

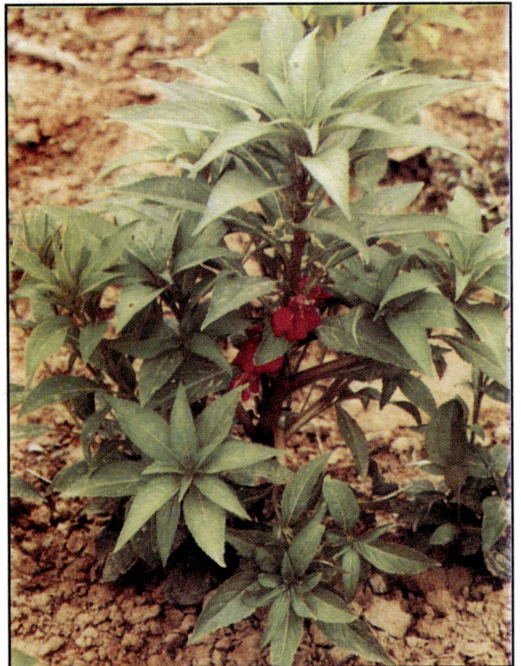

Impatiens balsamina

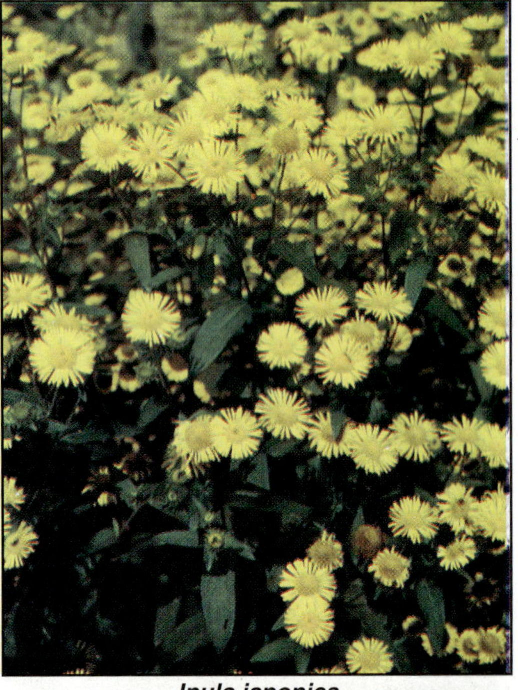

Inula japonica

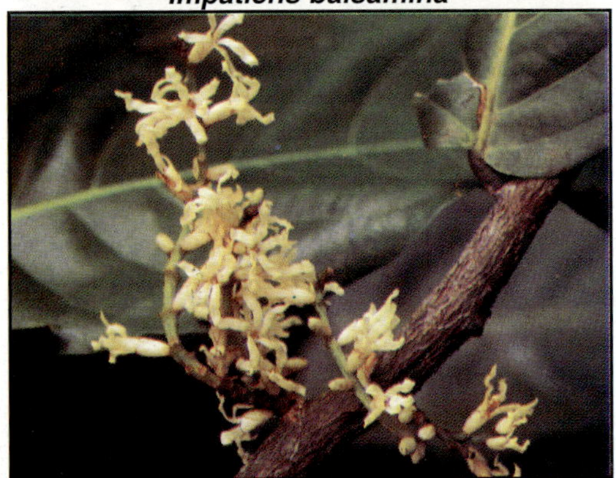

Inocarpus fagifer

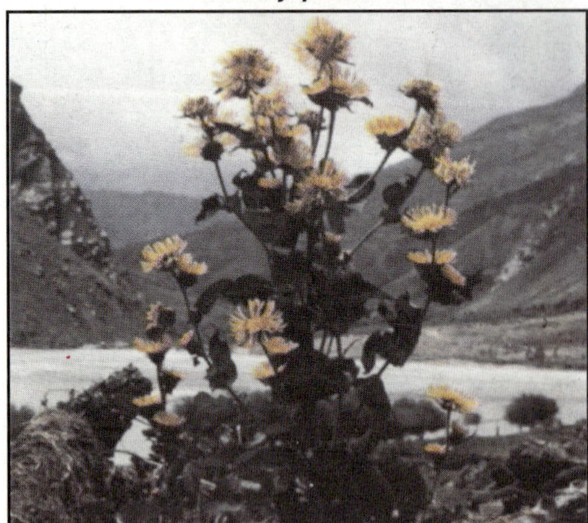

Inula racemosa

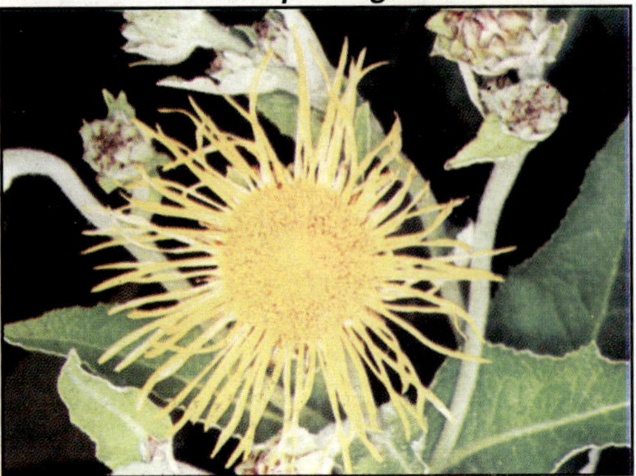

Inula helenium

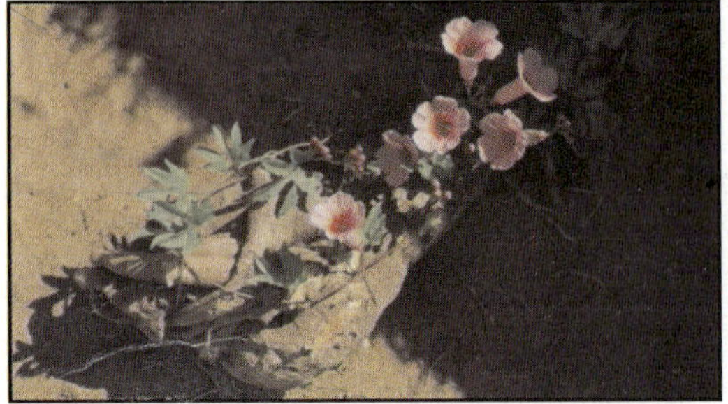

Ipomoea digitata

PLATE : 73

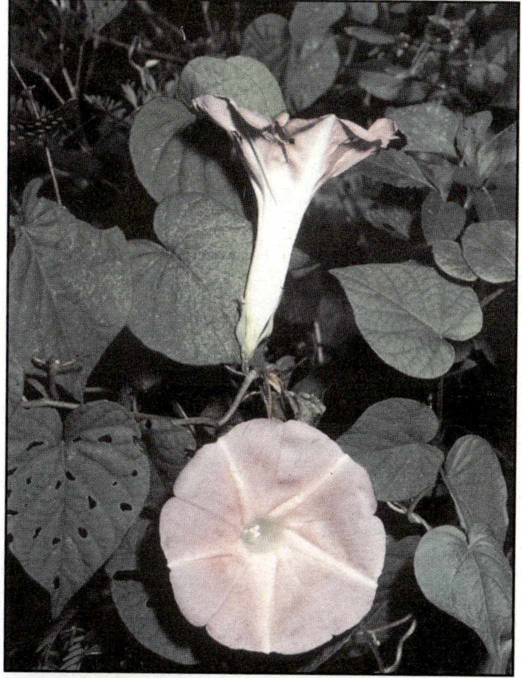

Ipomoea indica

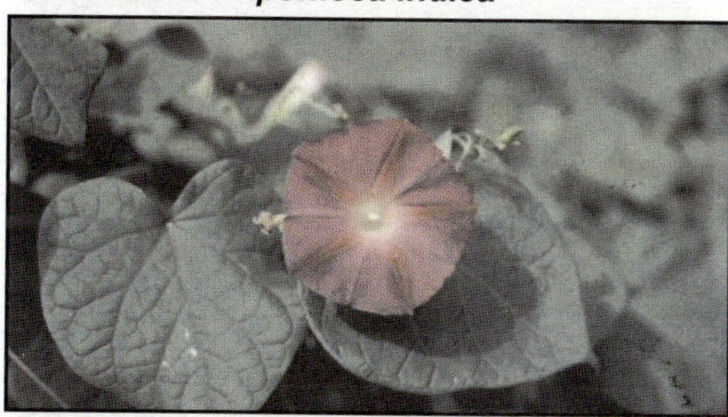

Ipomoea nil

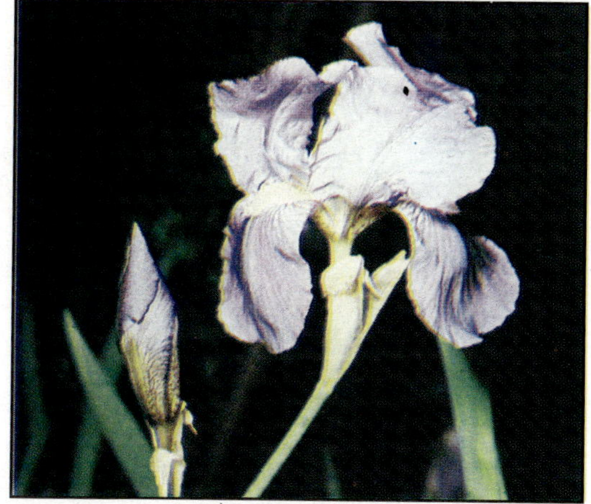

Iris germanica

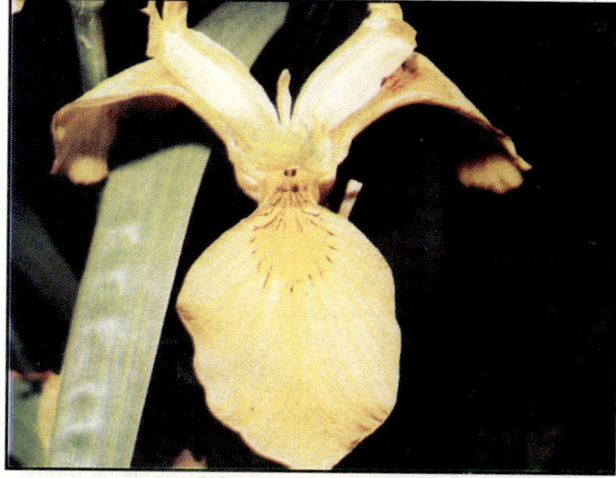

Iris pseudacorus

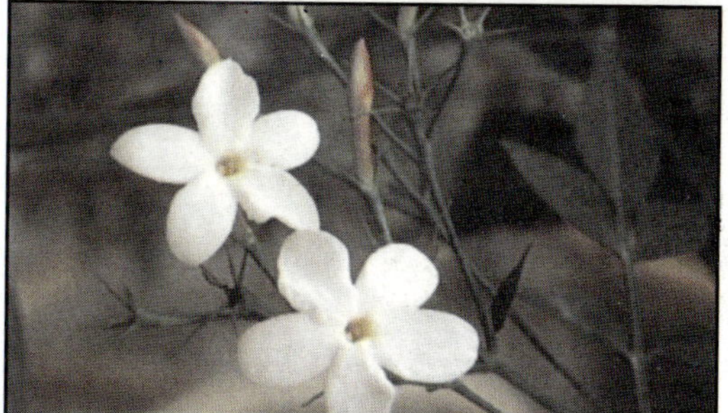

Jasminum grandiflorum

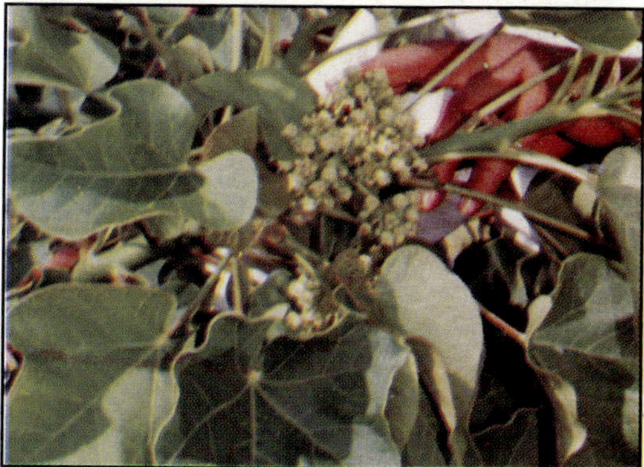

Jatropha curcas

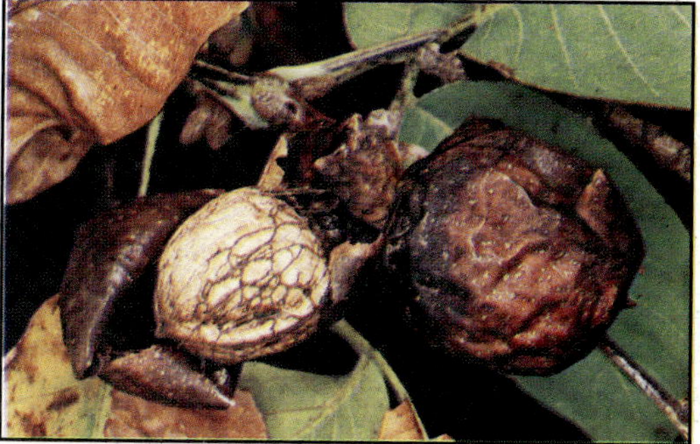

Juglans regia

PLATE : 74

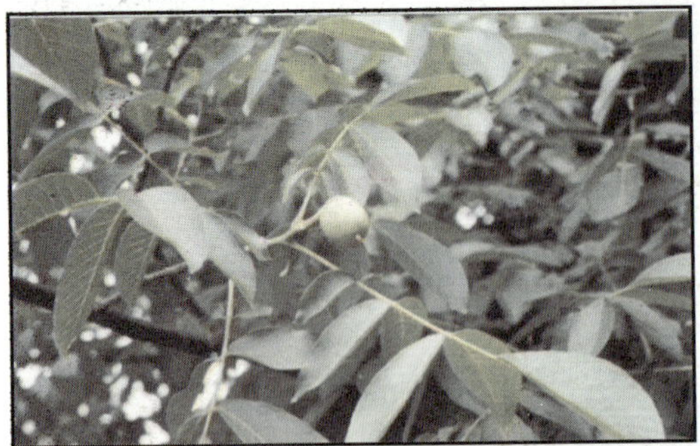

Juglans sinensis

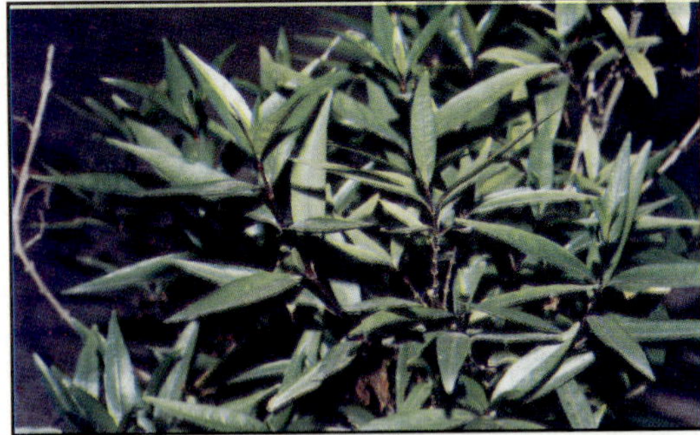

Justicia sendarusse

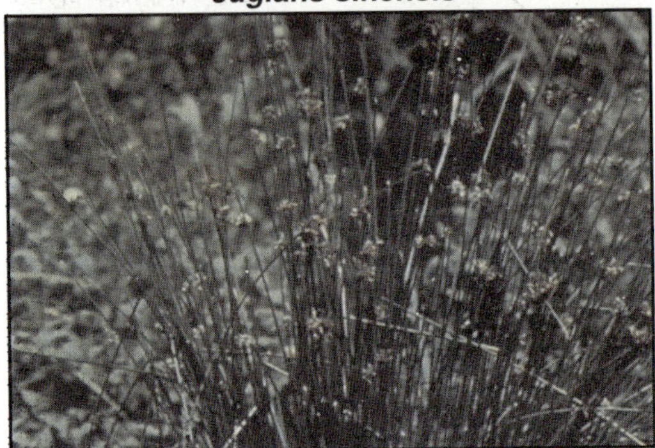

Juncus effusus

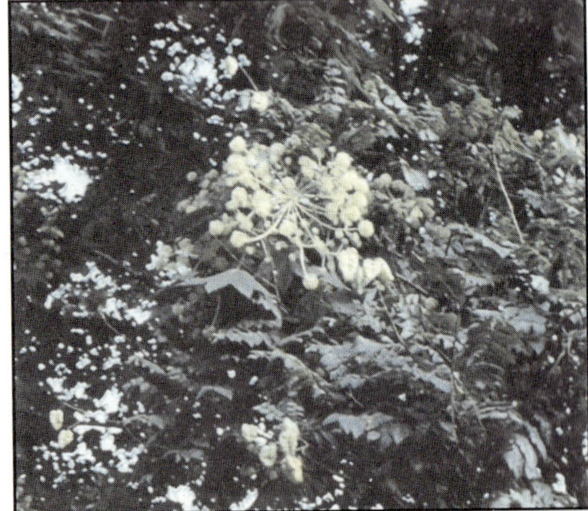

Kalopanax pictus

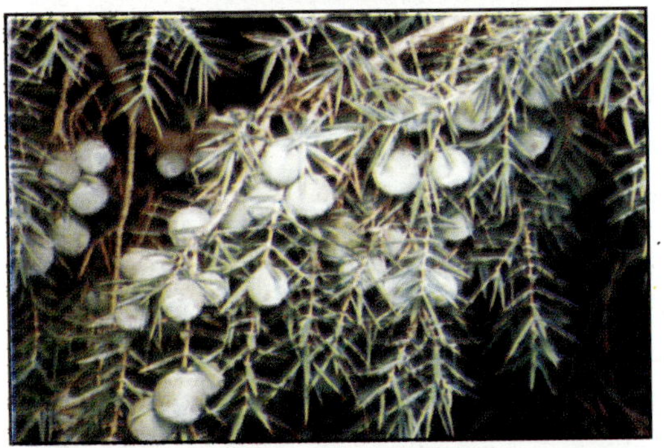

Juniperus communis

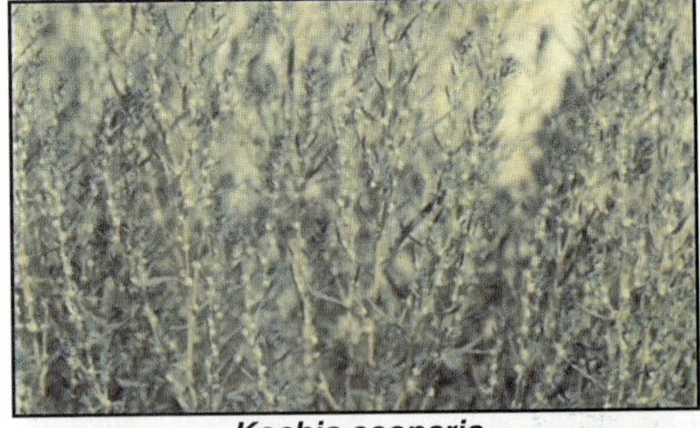

Kochia scoparia

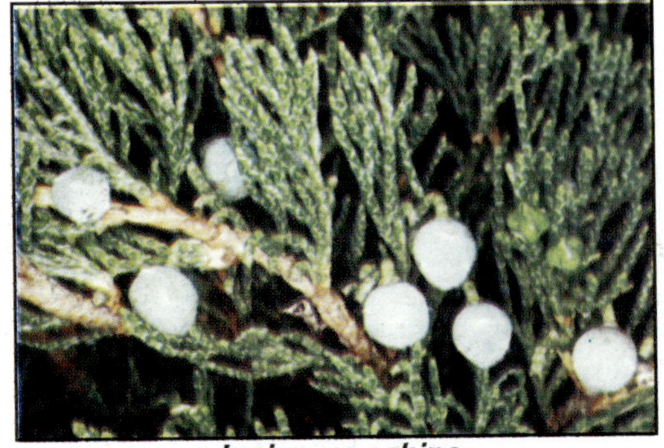

Juniperus sabina

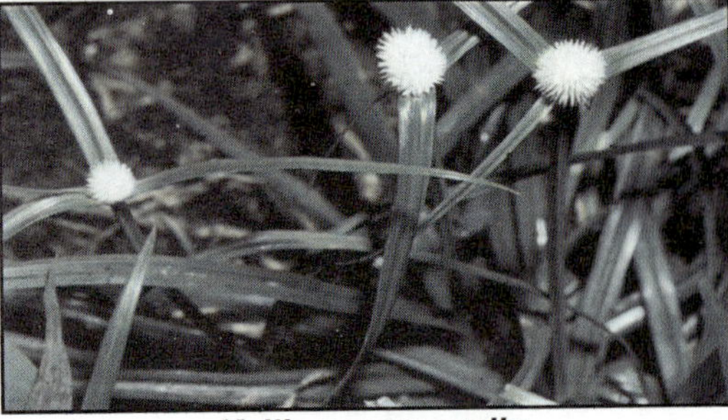

Kyllinga nemoralis

PLATE : 75

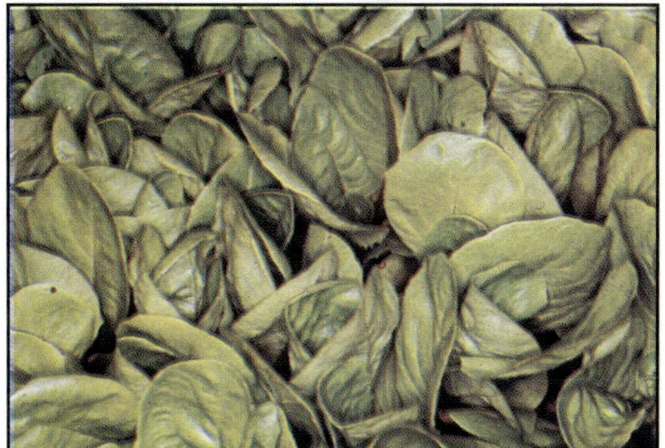

Lactuca sativa

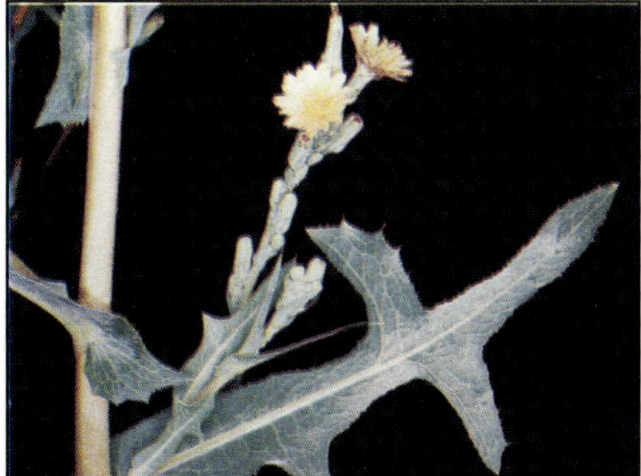

Lactuca virosa

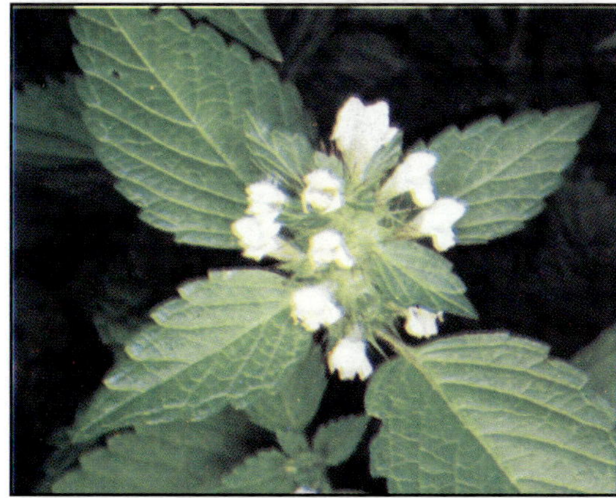

Lamium album

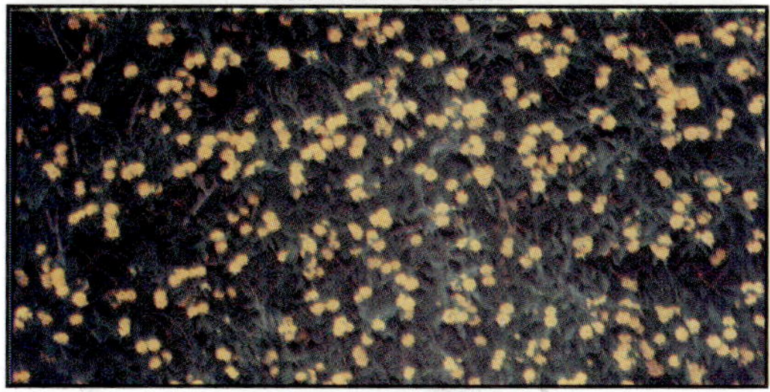

Lantana camara

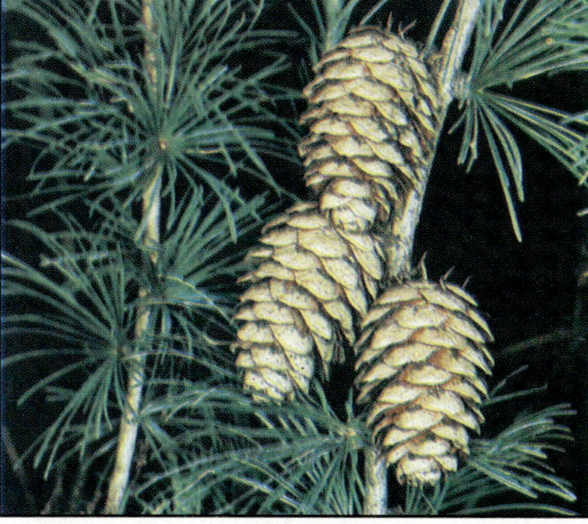

Larix decidua

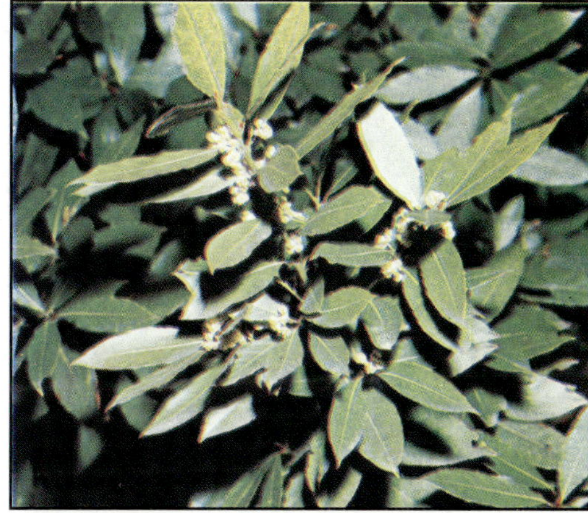

Laurus nobilis

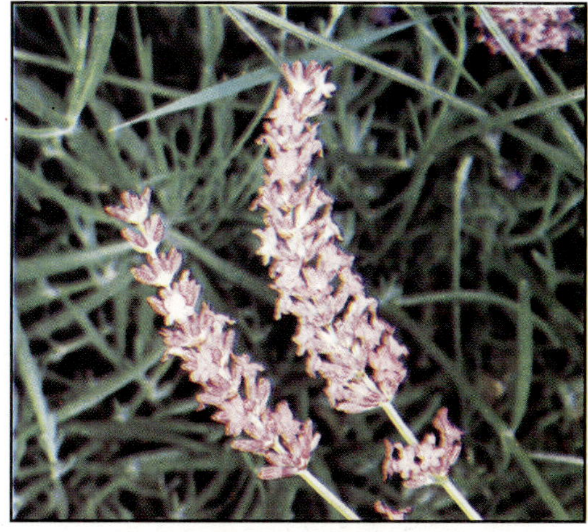

Lavandula angustifolia

PLATE : 76

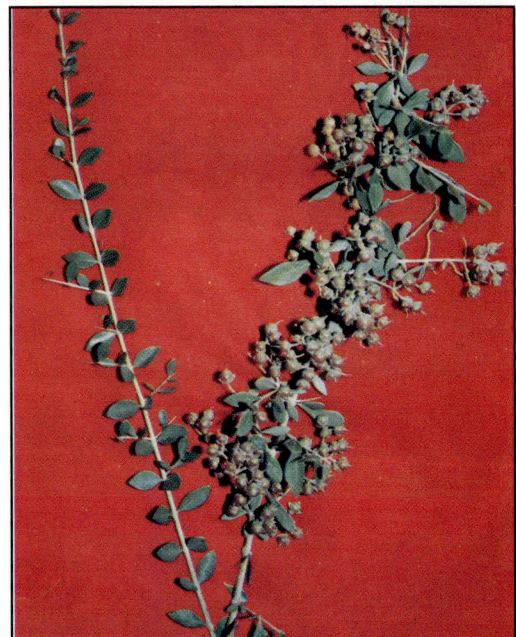

Lawsonia inermis

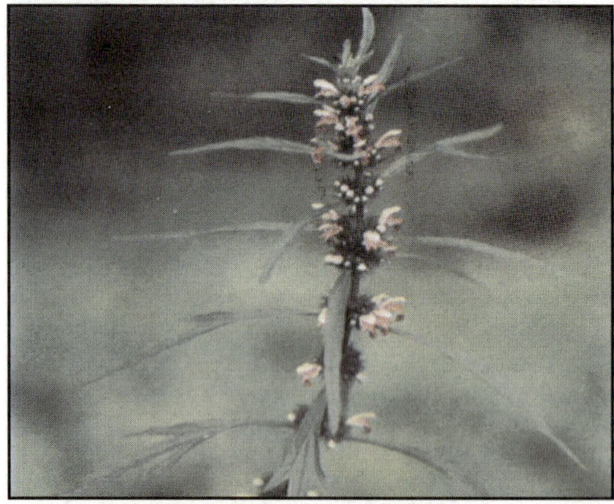

Leonurus japonicus

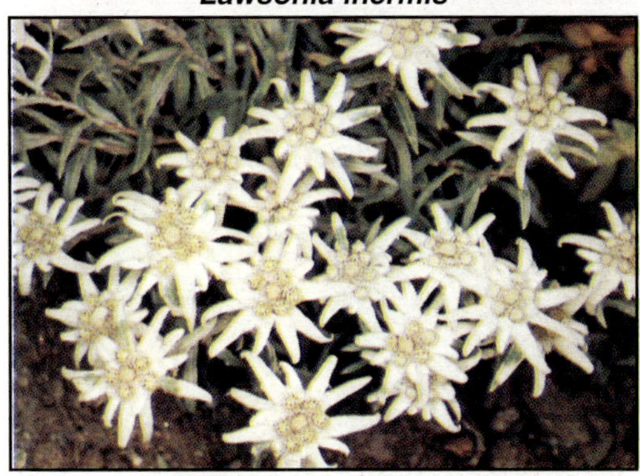

Leontopodium alpinum

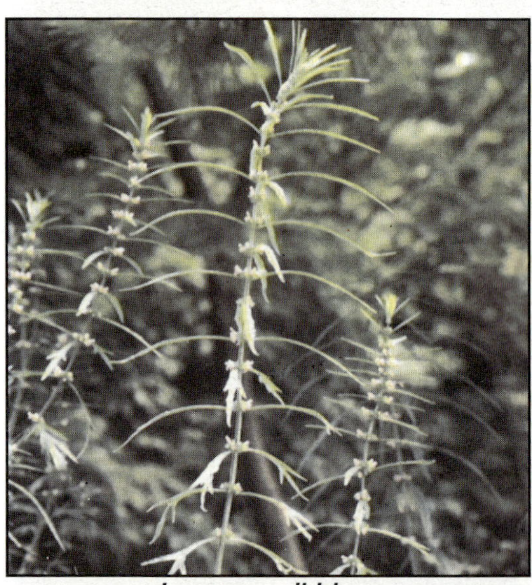

Leonurus sibiricus

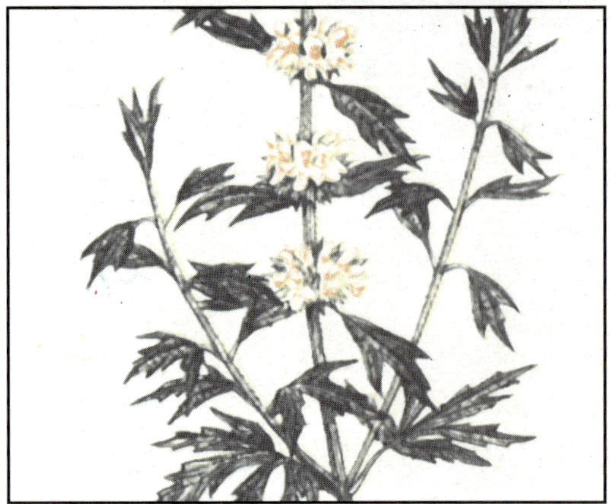

Leonurus cardiaca

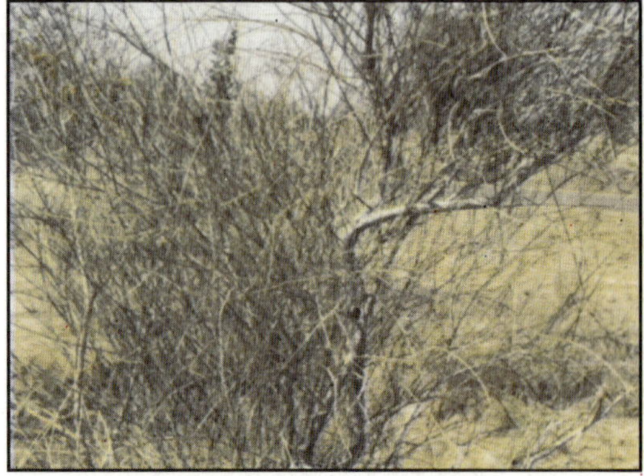

Leptadenia pyrotechnica

PLATE : 77

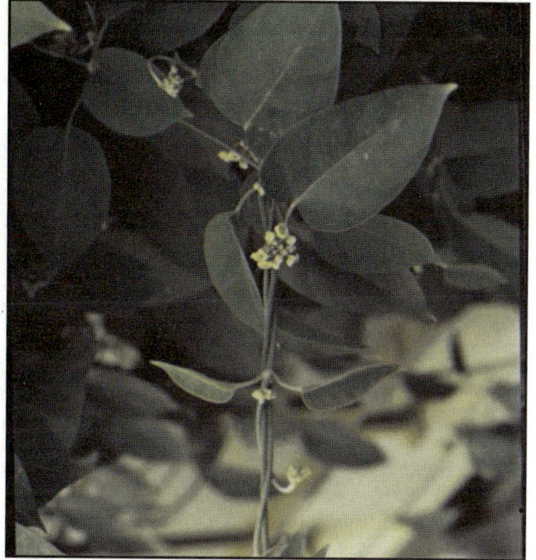

Leptadenia reticulata

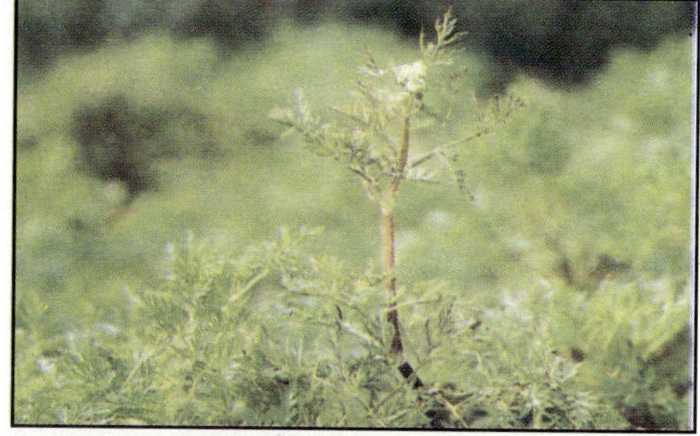

Ligusticum chuanxiong

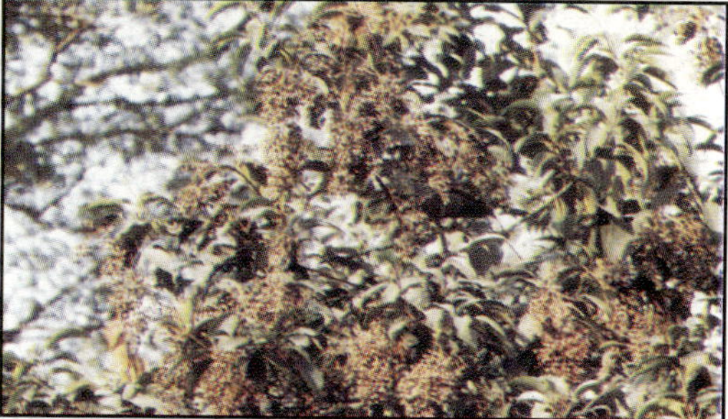

Ligustrum lucidum

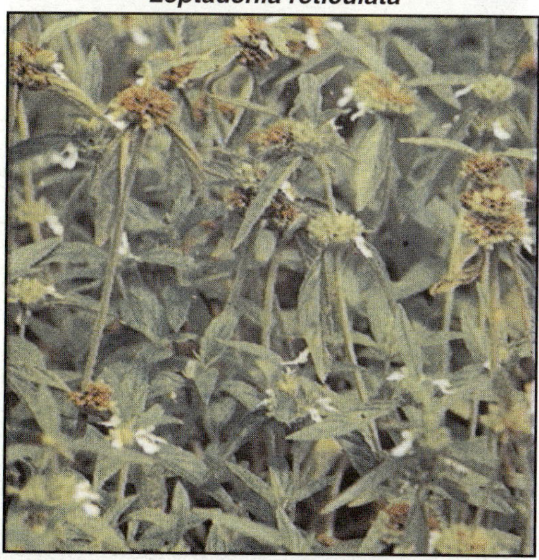

Leucas cephalotes

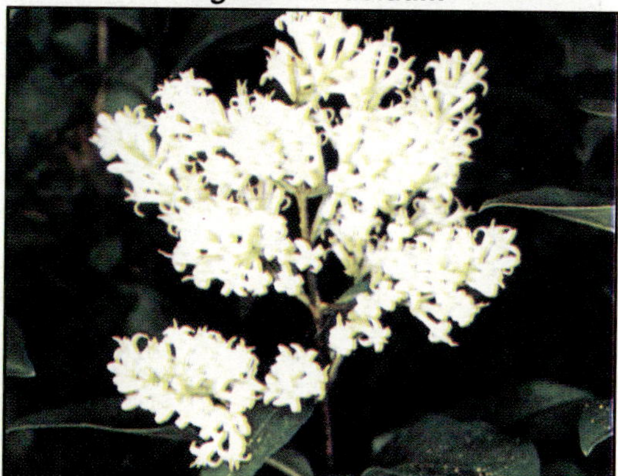

Ligustrum vulgare

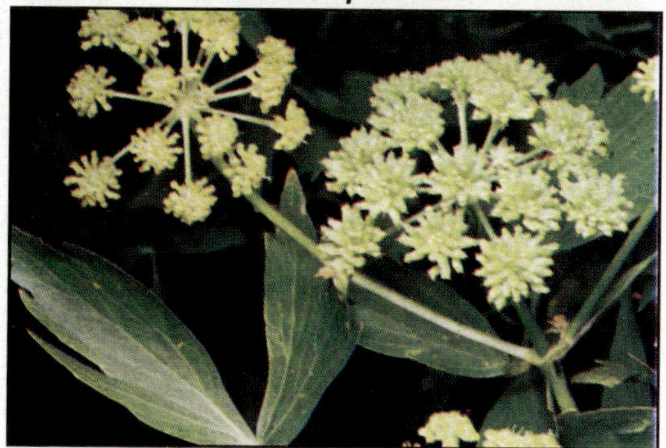

Levisticum officinale

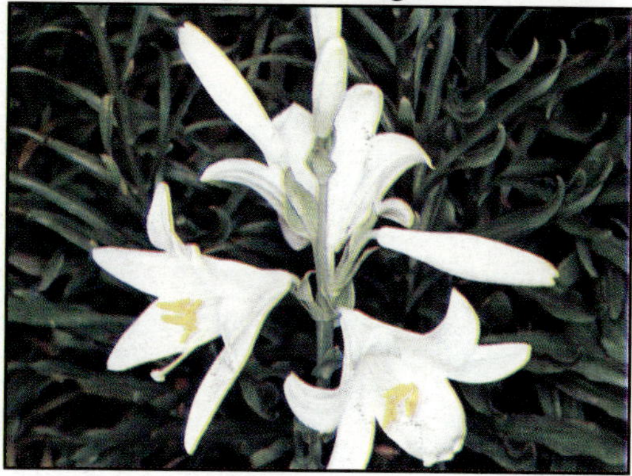

Lilium candidum

PLATE : 78

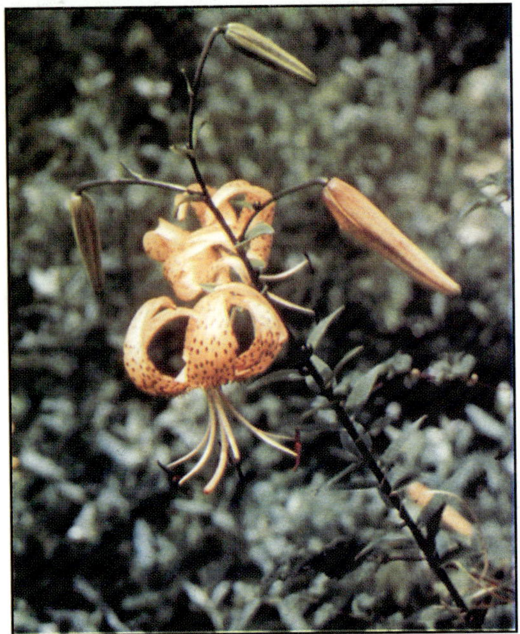

Lilium lancifolium

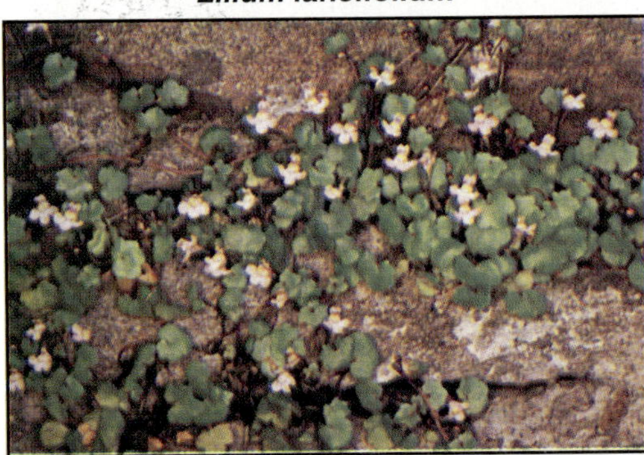

Linaria cymbalaria

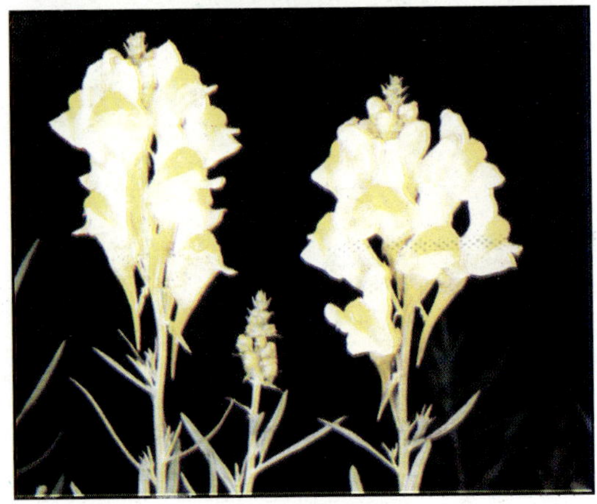

Linaria vulgaris

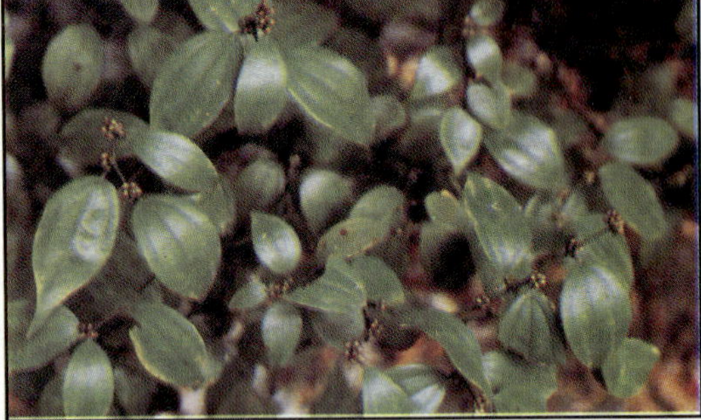

Lindera strychnifolia

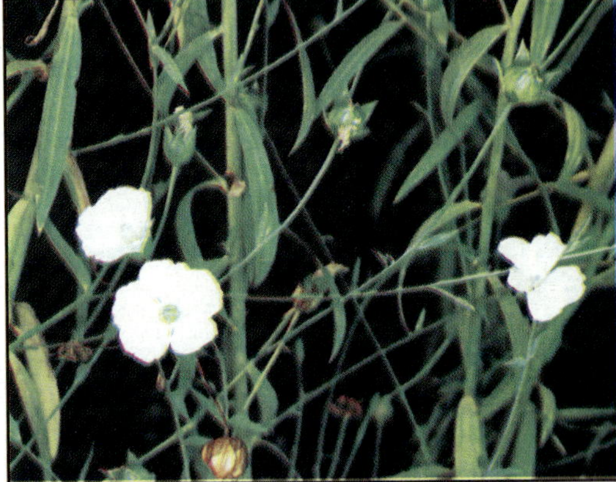

Linum usitatissimum

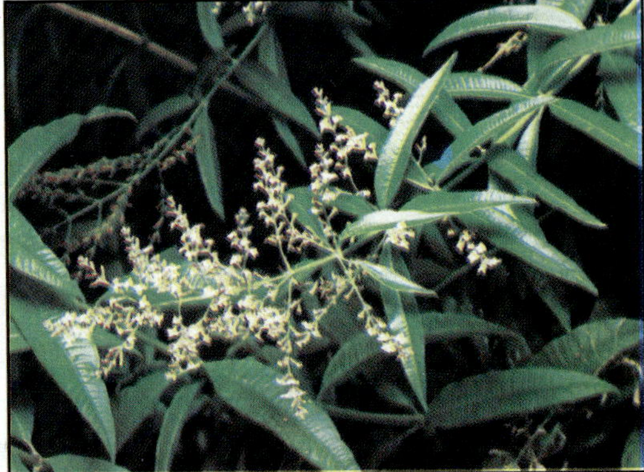

Lippia citridora

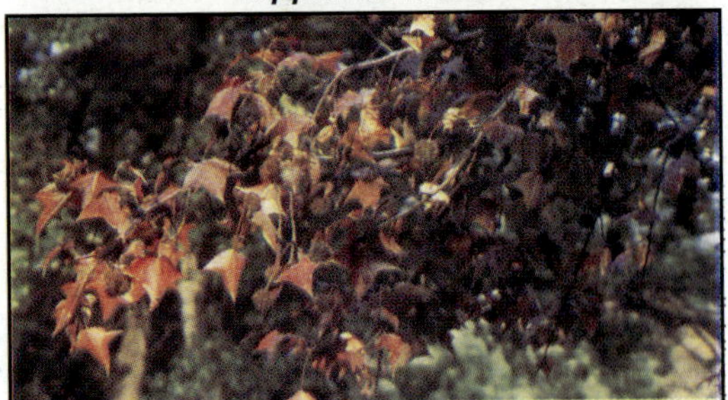

Liquidambar formosana

PLATE : 79

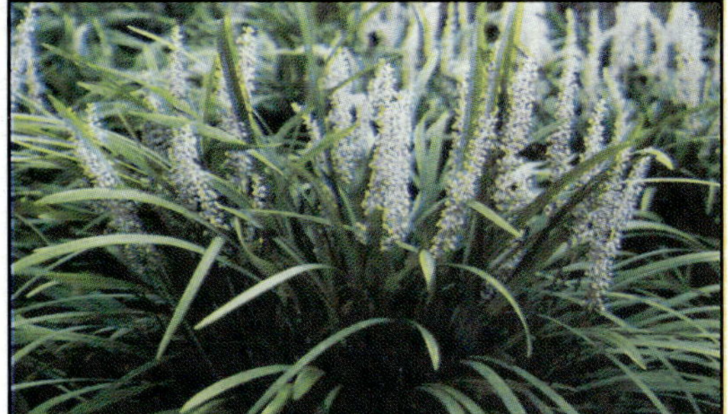

Liriope platyphylla

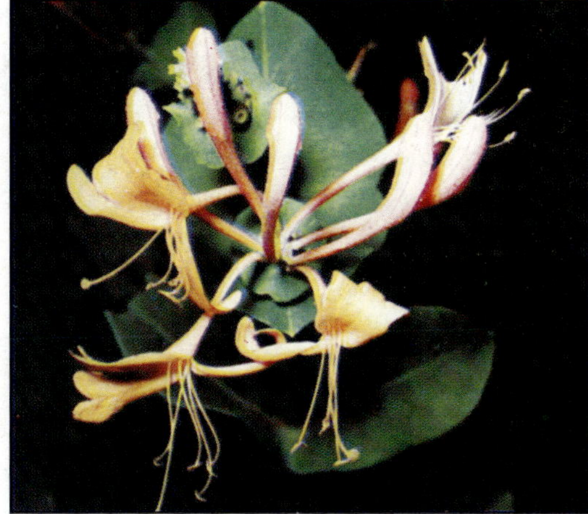

Lonicera caprifolium

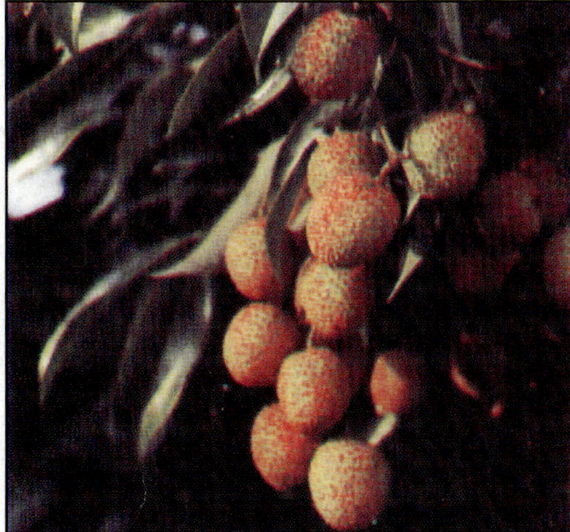

Litchi chinensis

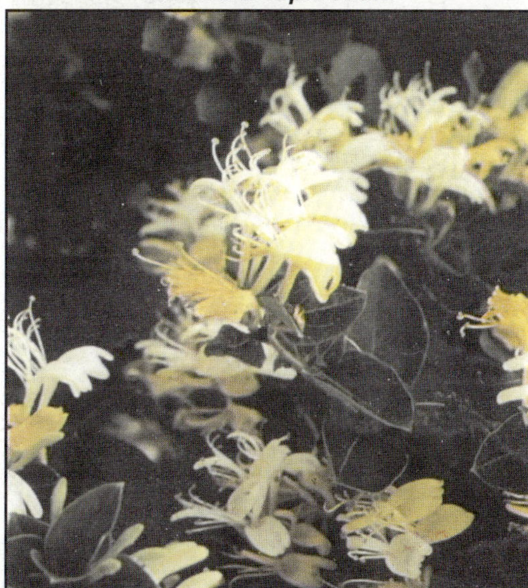

Lonicera Japonica

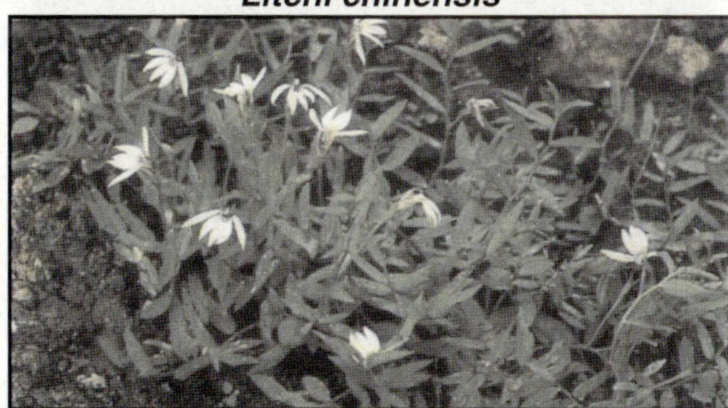

Lobelia chinensis

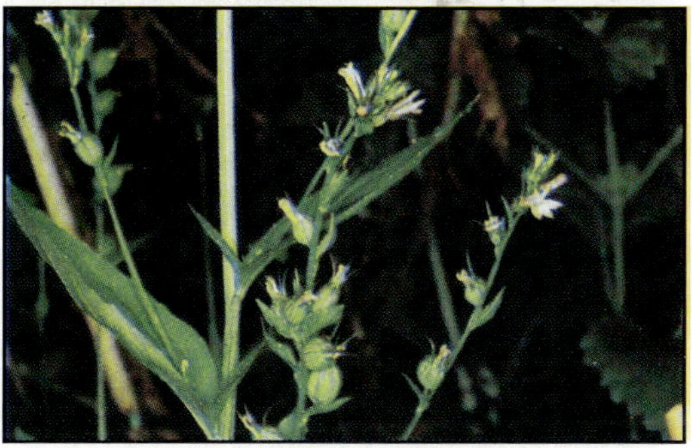

Lobelia inflata

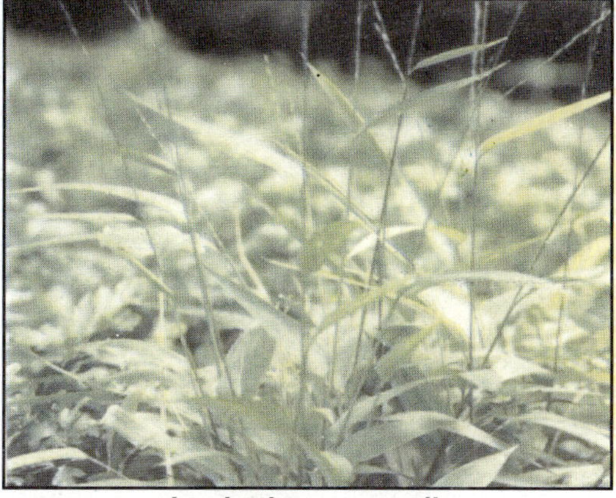

Lophatherum gracile

PLATE : 80

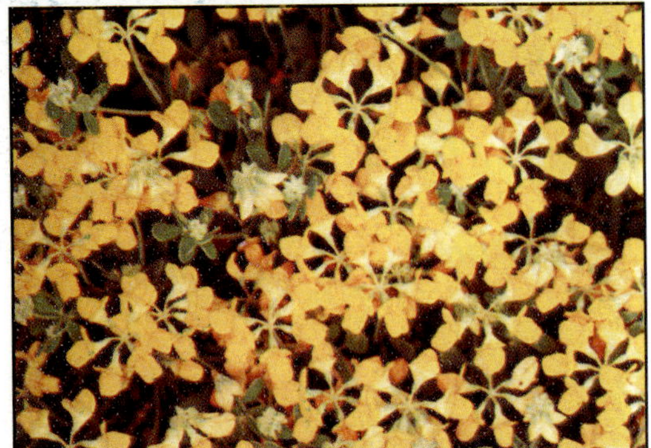

Lotus corniculatus

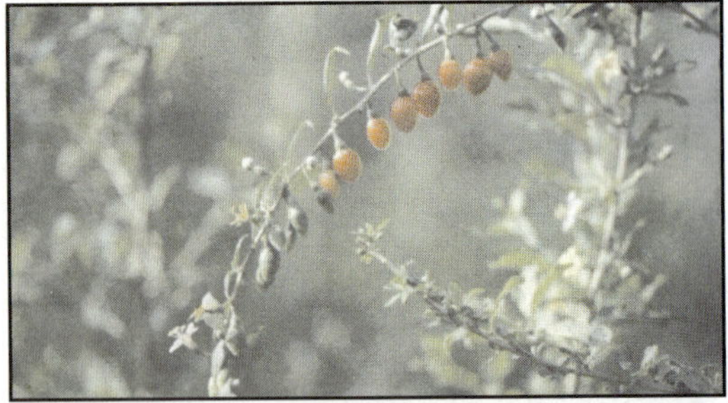

Lycium chinense

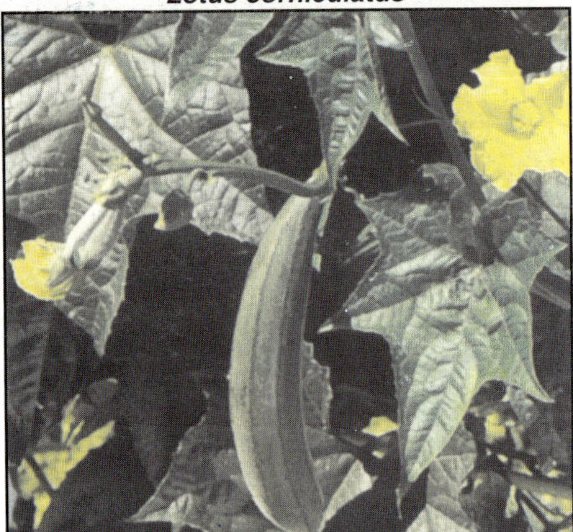

Luffa cylindrica

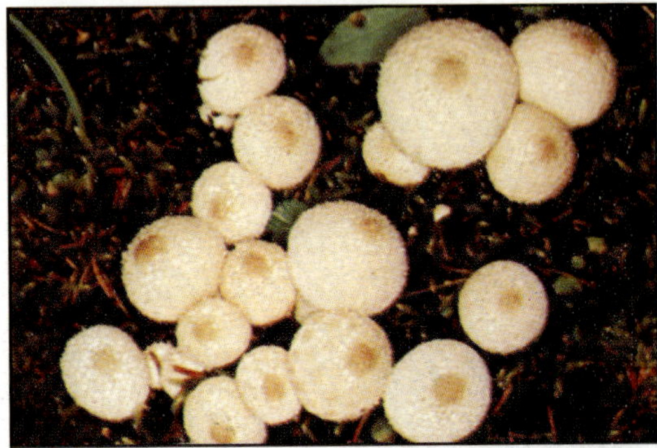

Lycoperdon bovista

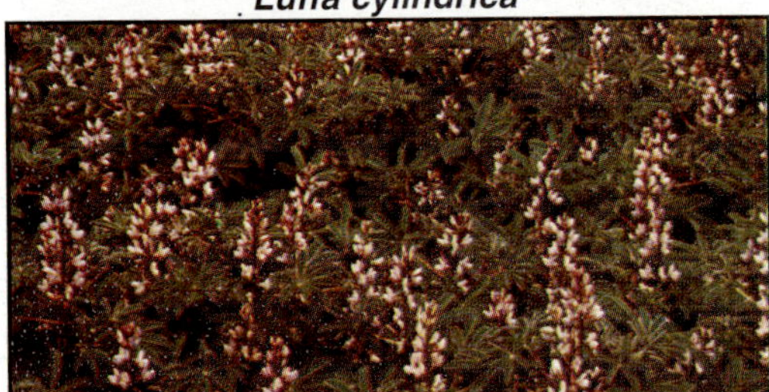

Lupinus albus

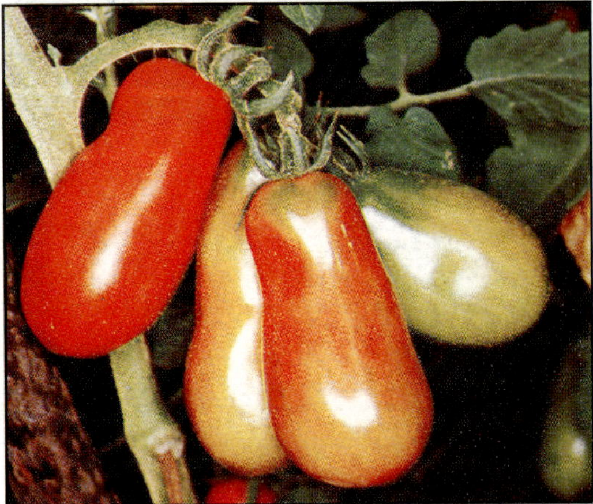

Lycopersicon esculentum

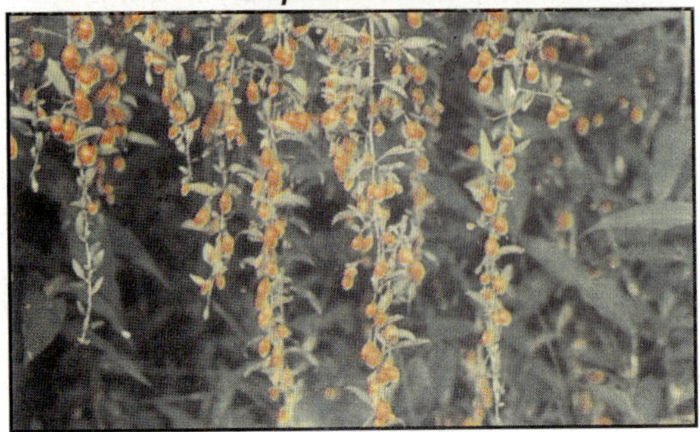

Lycium barbarum

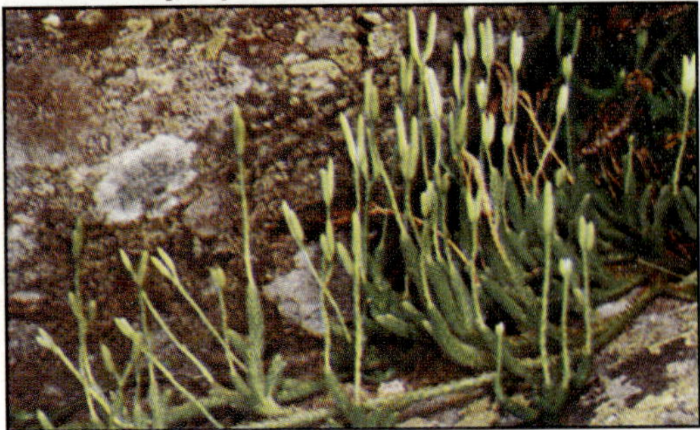

Lycopodium clavatum

PLATE : 81

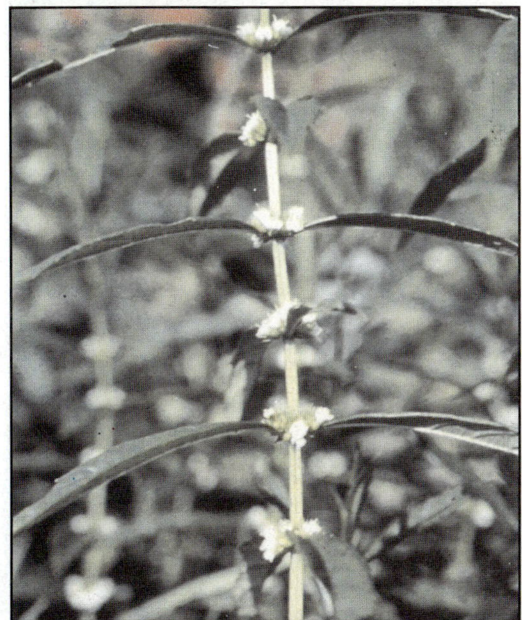

Lycopus lucidus

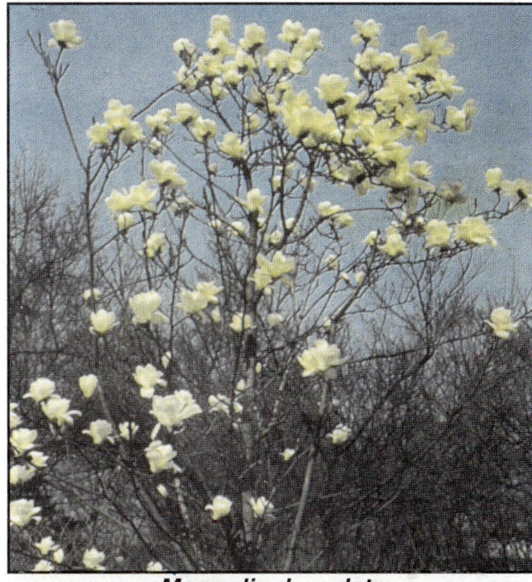

Magnolia denudata

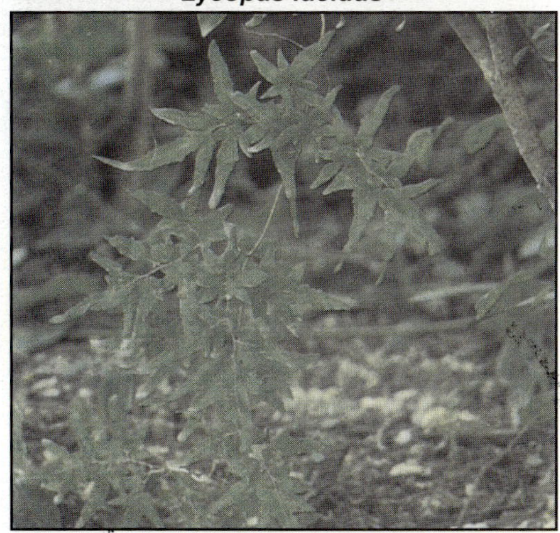

Lygodium japonicum

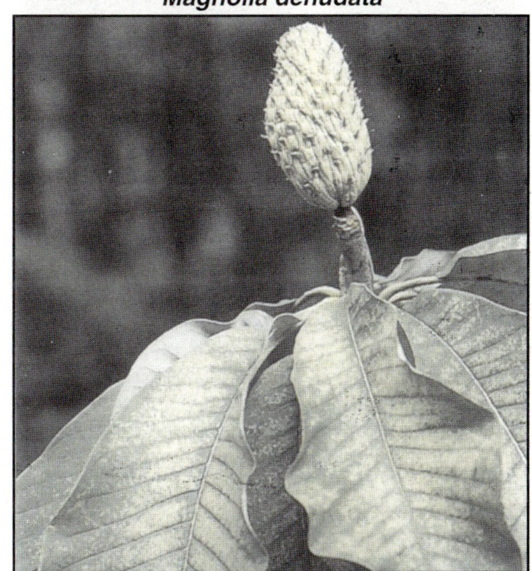

Magnolia officinalis

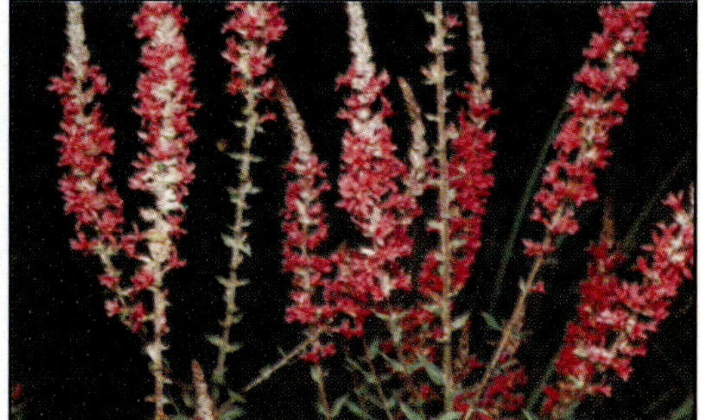

Lythrum salicaria

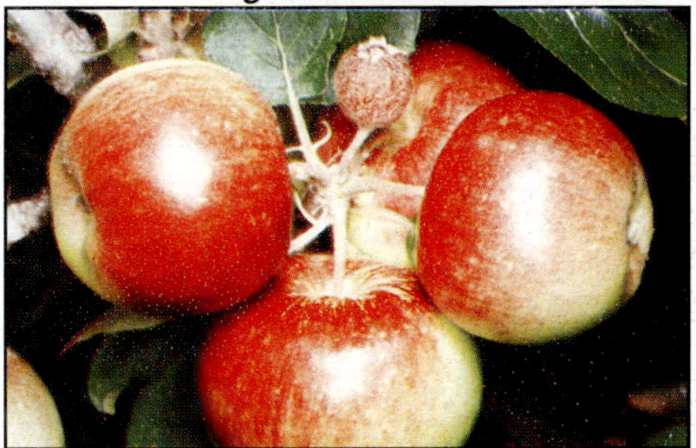

Malus sylvestris

PLATE : 82

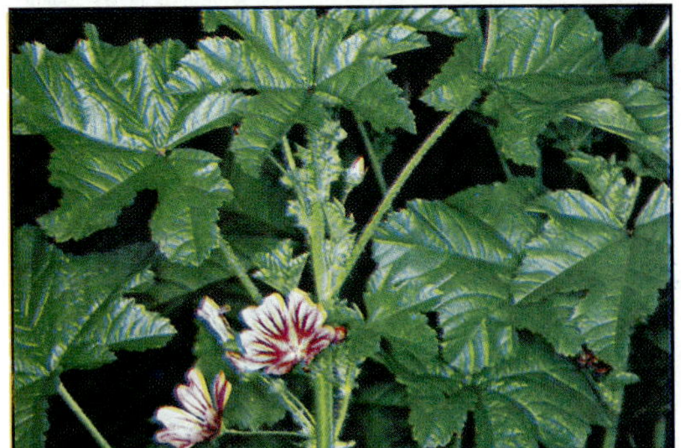
Malva sylvestris

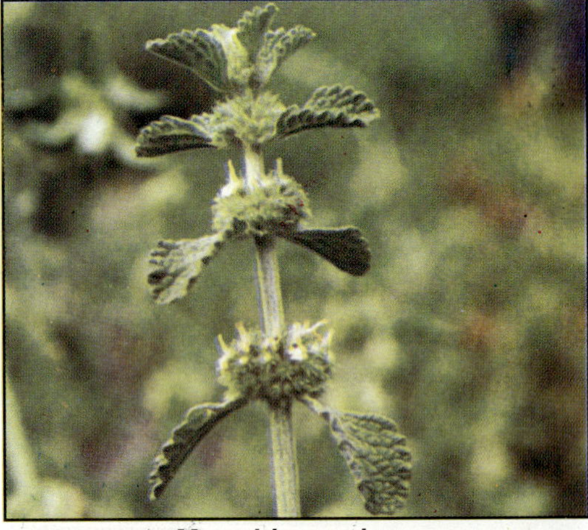
Marrubium vulgare

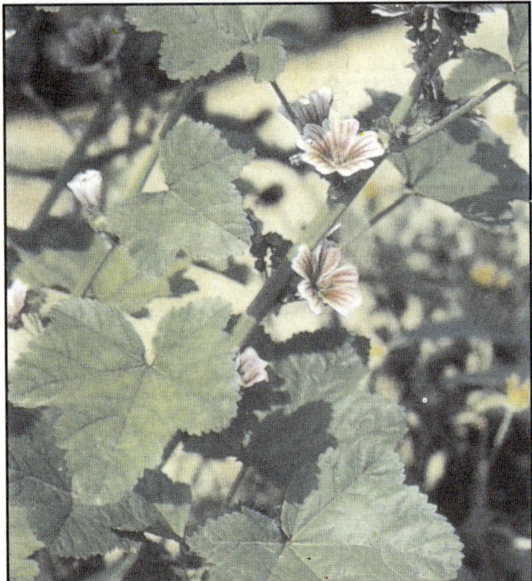
Malva verticillata

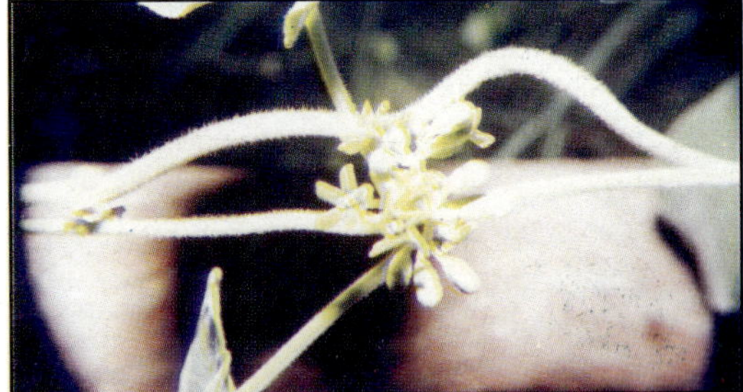
Marsdenia Tenacissima

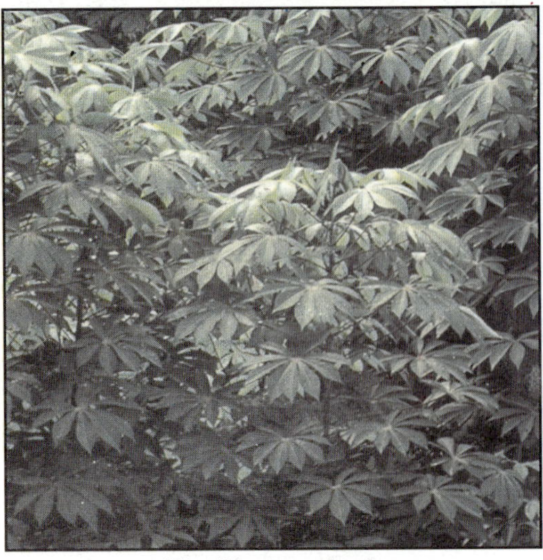
Manihot esculenta

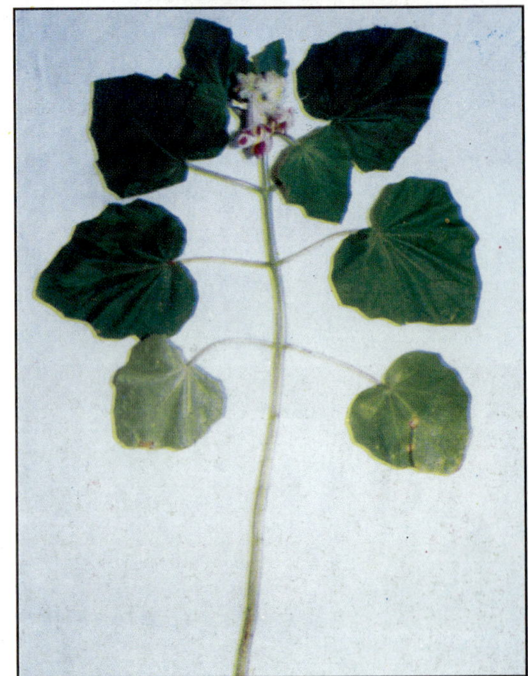
Martynia annua

PLATE : 83

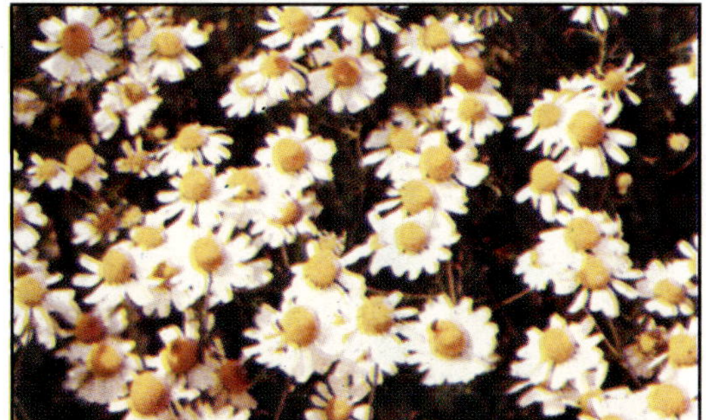

Matricaria chamomillia

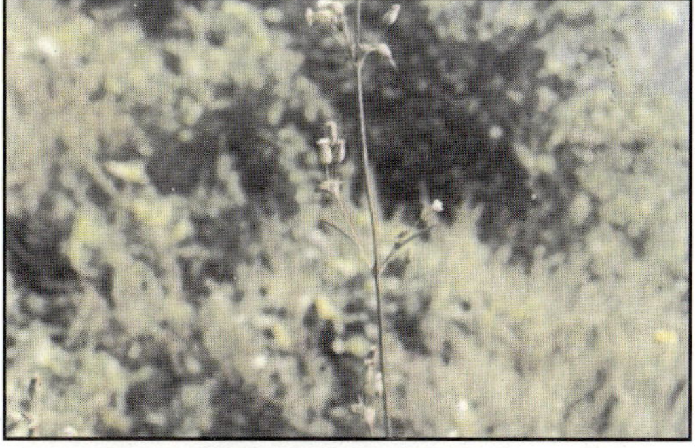

Melandrium firmum

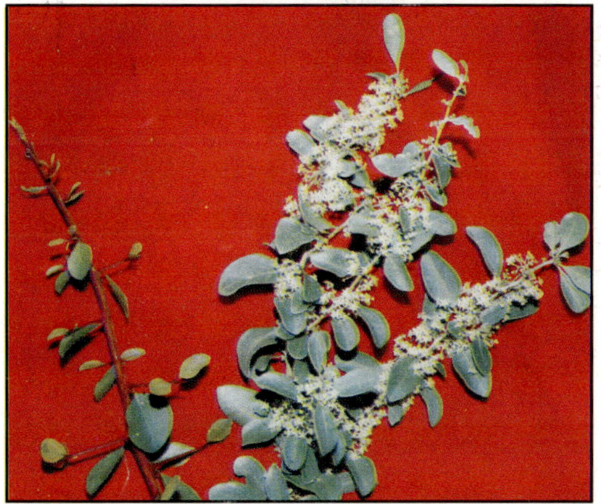

Maytenus emarginata

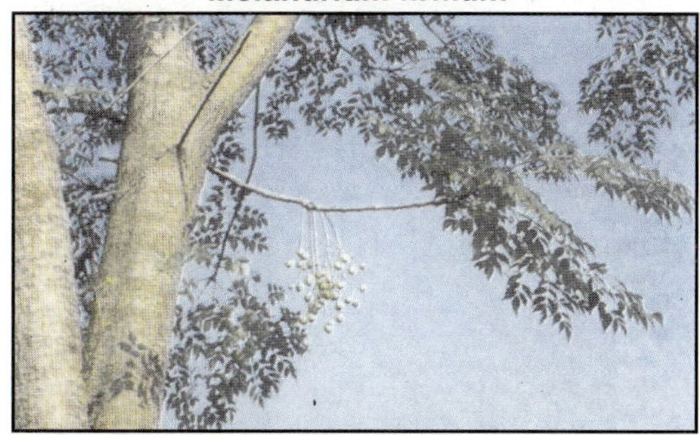

Melia azedarach

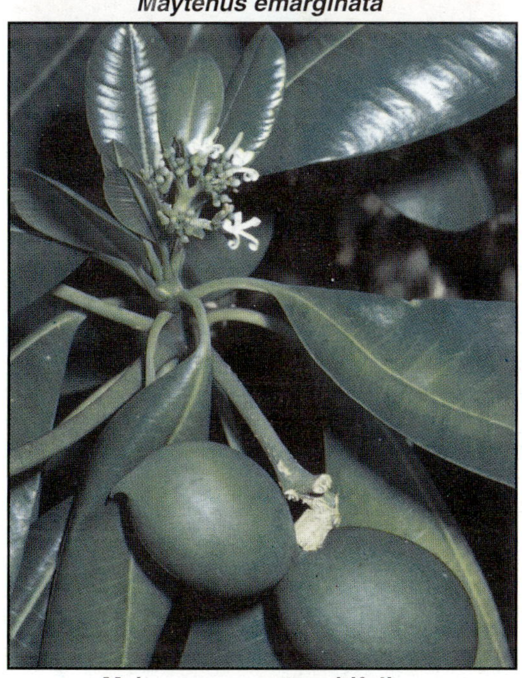

Meisosperma oppositifolium

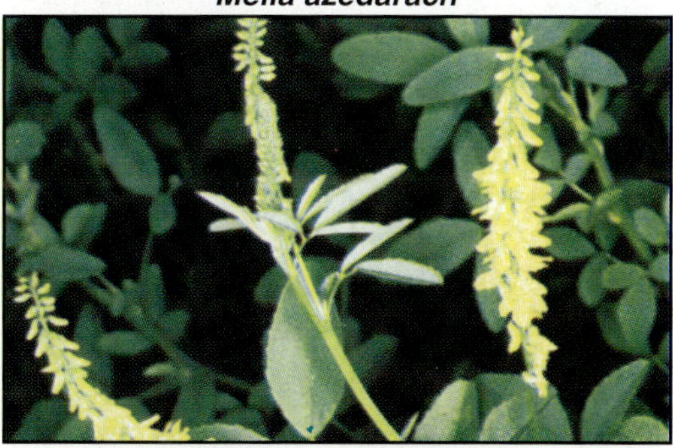

Melilotus officinalis

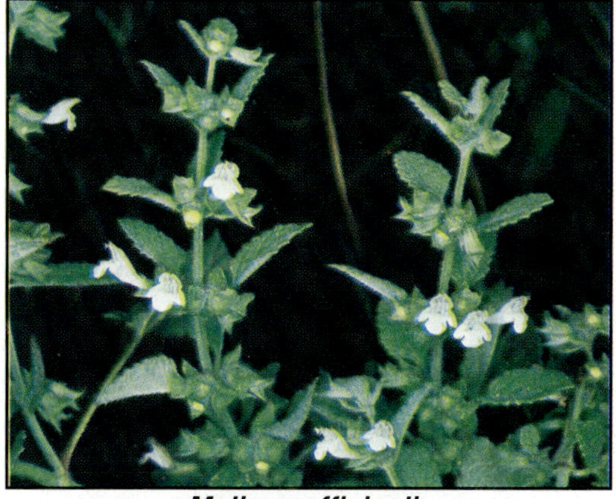

Melissa officinalis

PLATE : 84

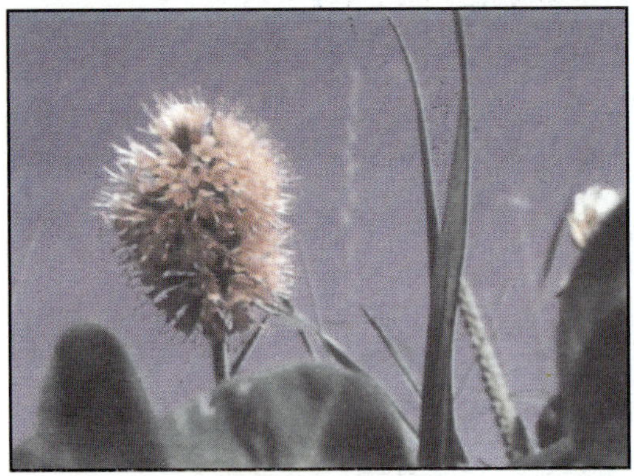
Mentha aquatica

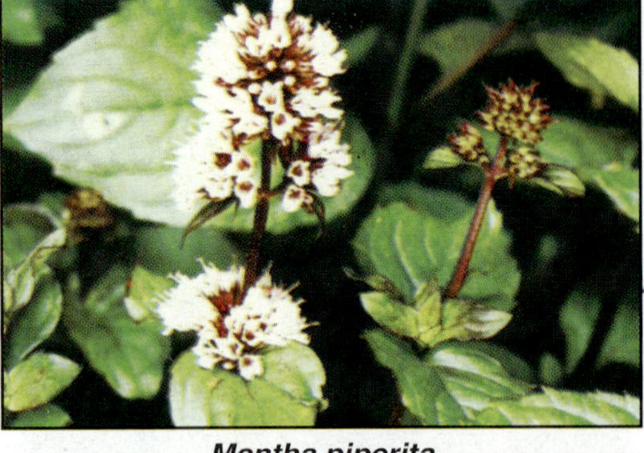
Mentha piperita

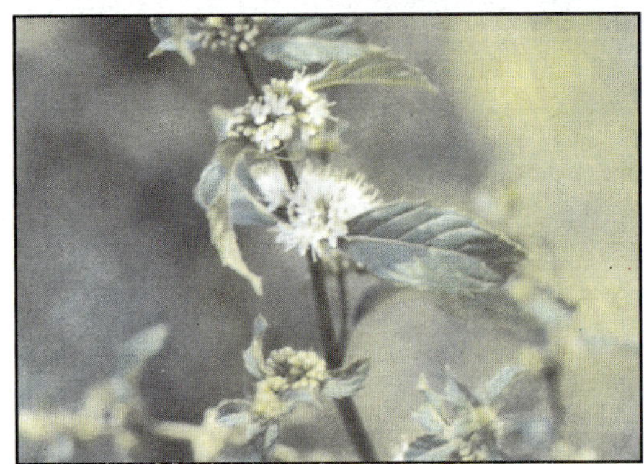
Mentha arvensis

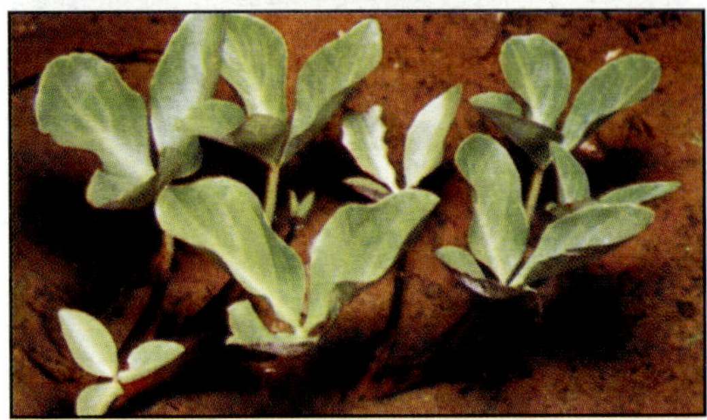
Menyanthes trifoliata

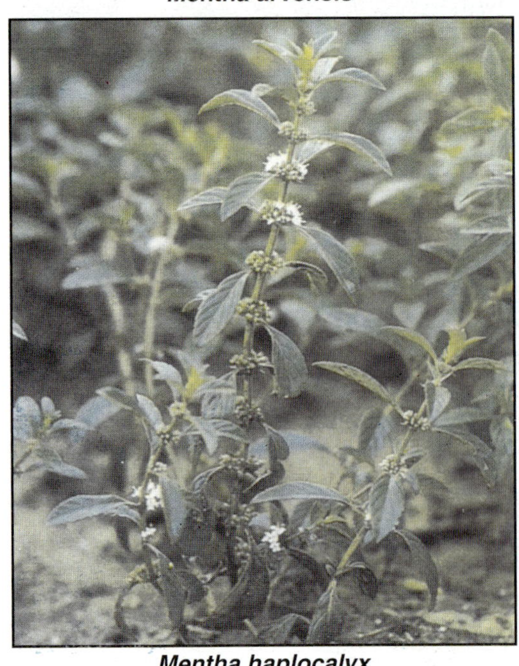
Mentha haplocalyx

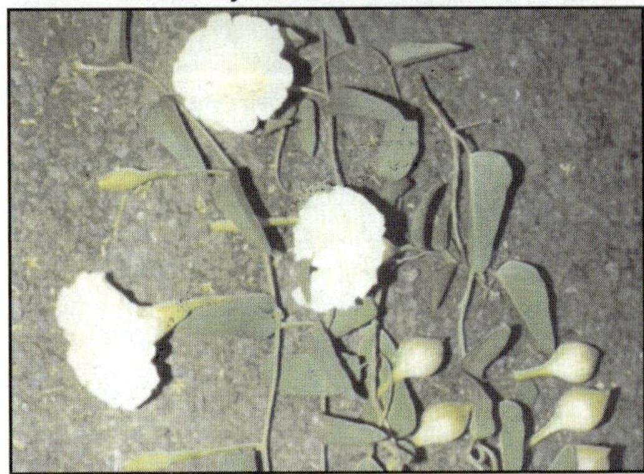
Merremia turpethum

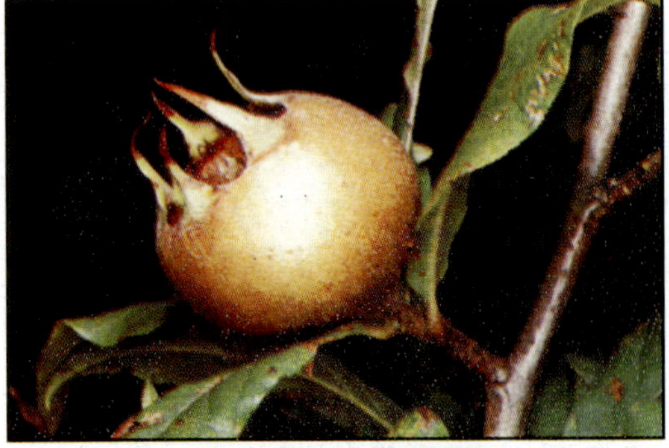
Mespilus germanica

PLATE : 85

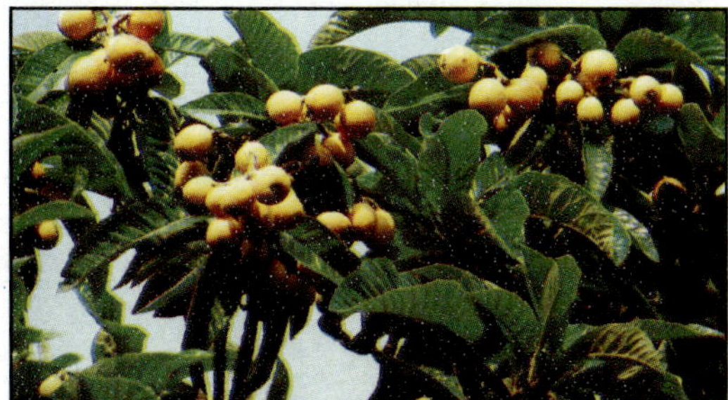

Mespilus japonica

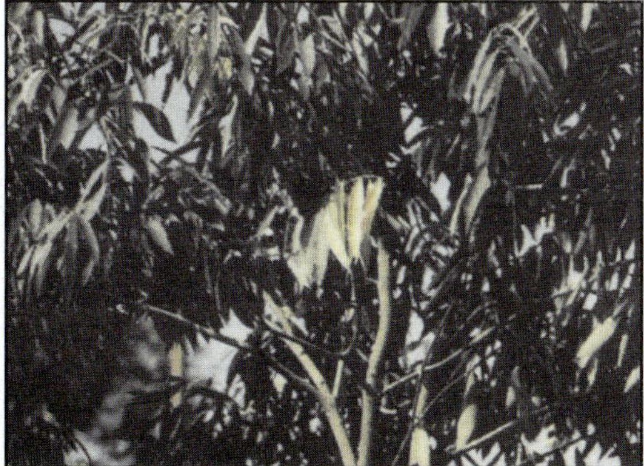

Mesua ferrea

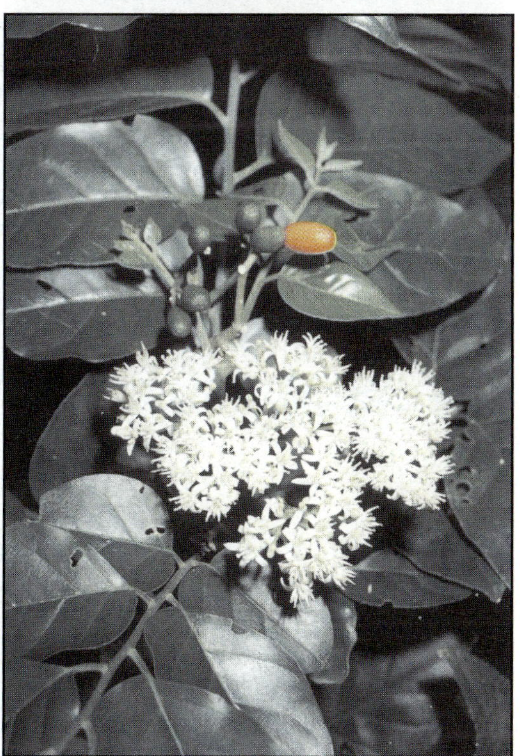

Micromelum minutum

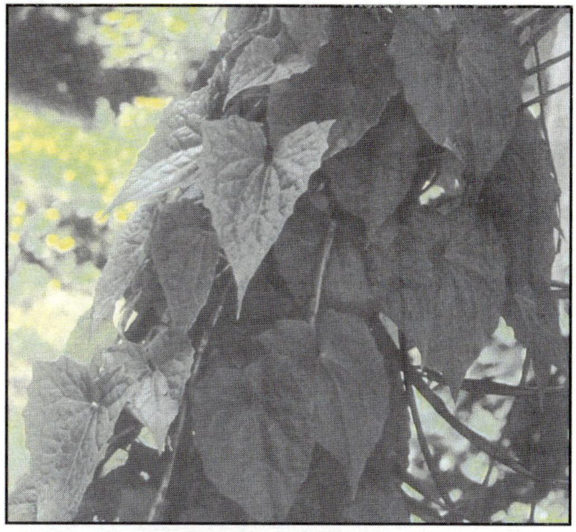

Mikania micrantha

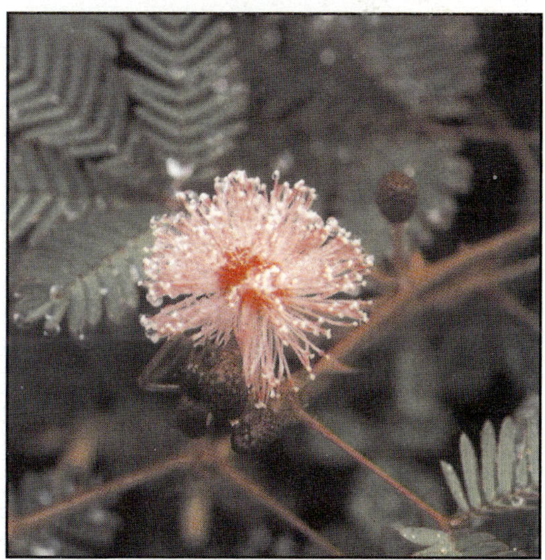

Mimosa pudic Linn

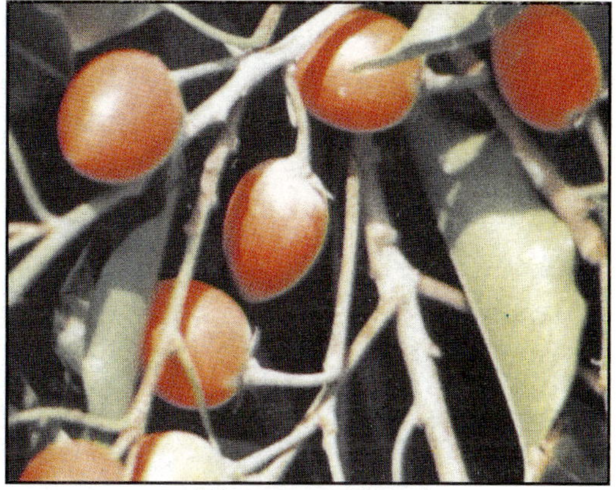

Mimusops elengi

PLATE : 86

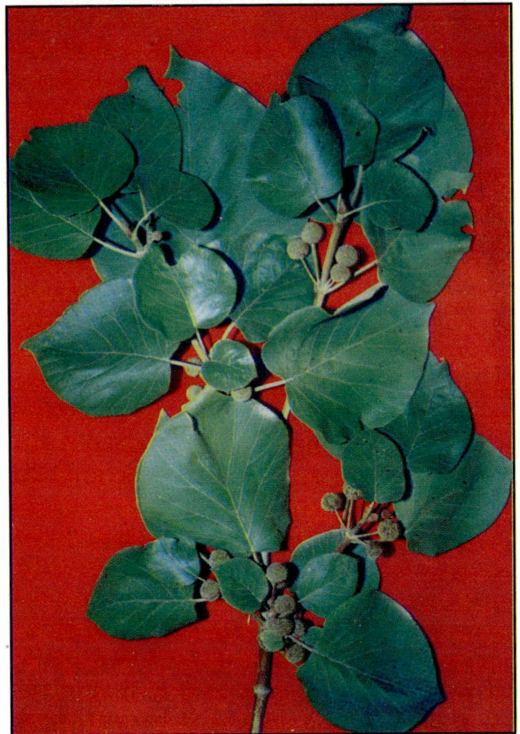

Mitragyna parveflora

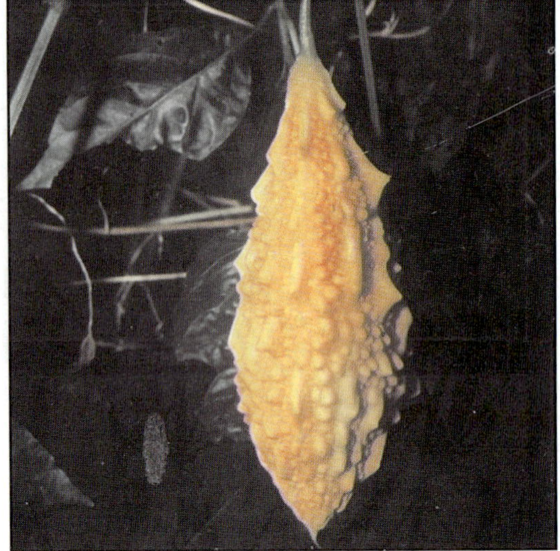

Momordica charantia

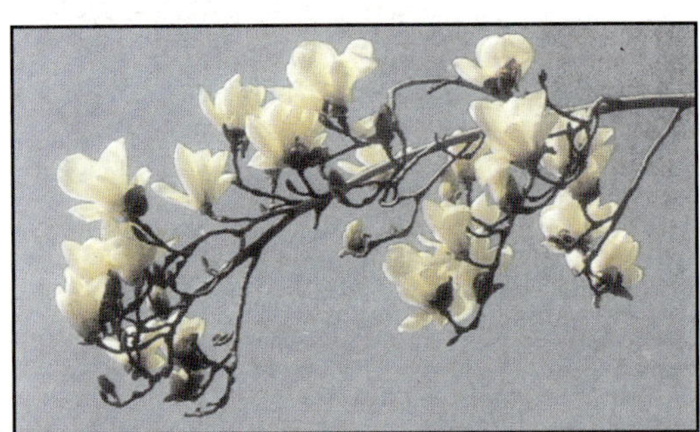

Mognolia denudata

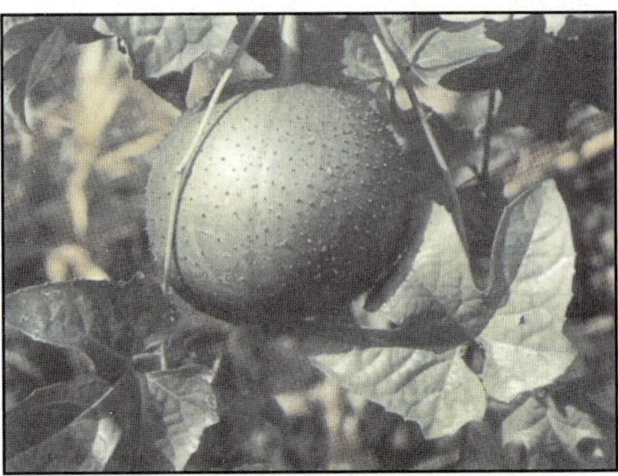

Momordica cochinchinensis

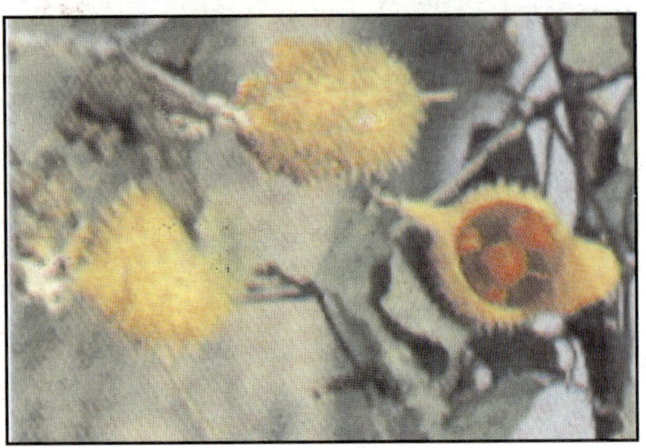

Momordica balsamina

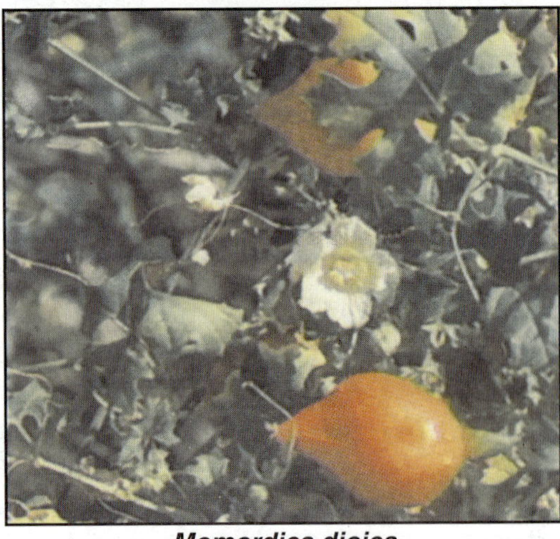

Momordica dioica

PLATE : 87

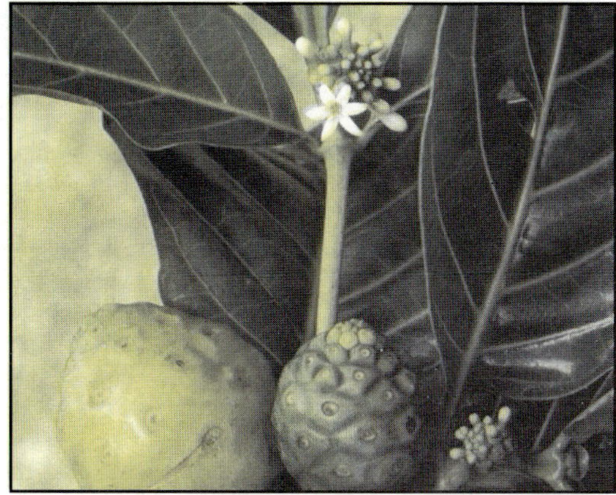

Morinda citrifolia

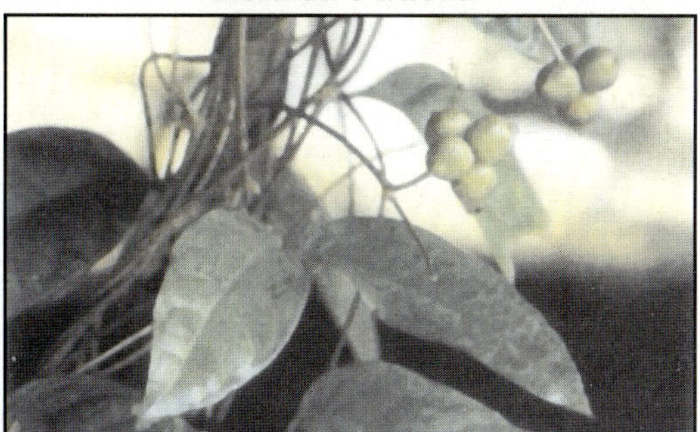

Morinda officinalis

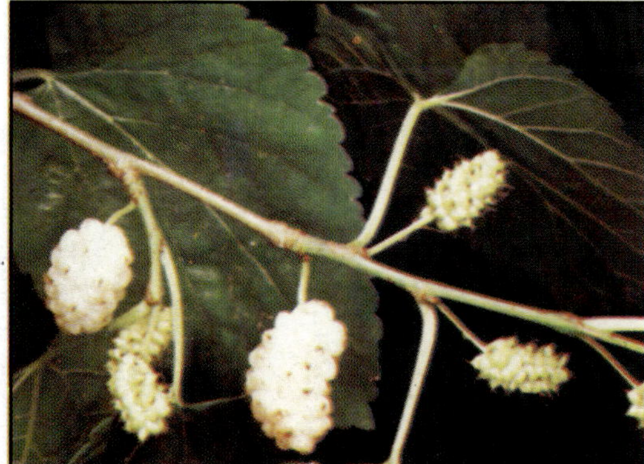

Morus alba

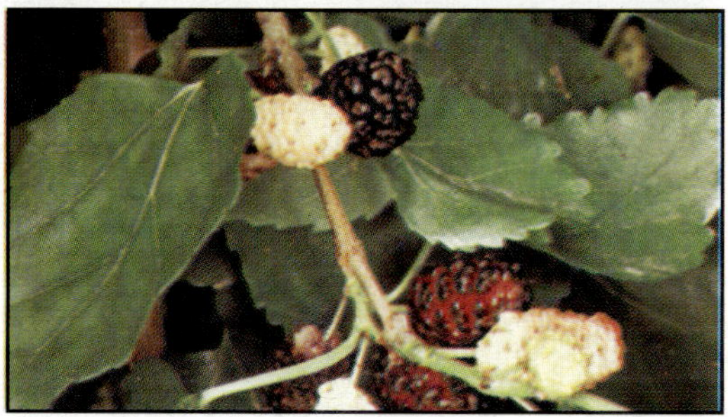

Morus nigra

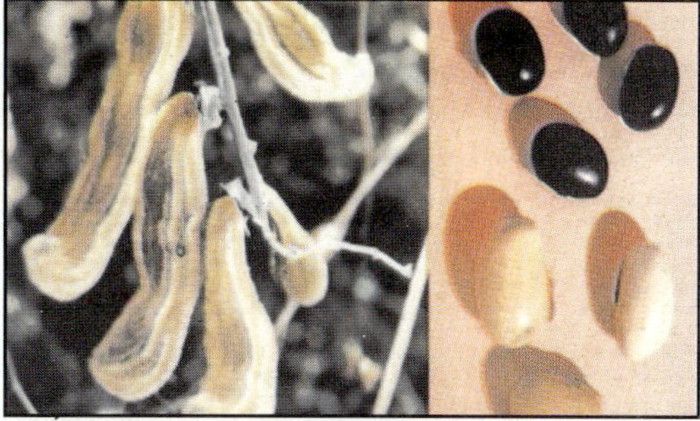

Mucuna pruriens

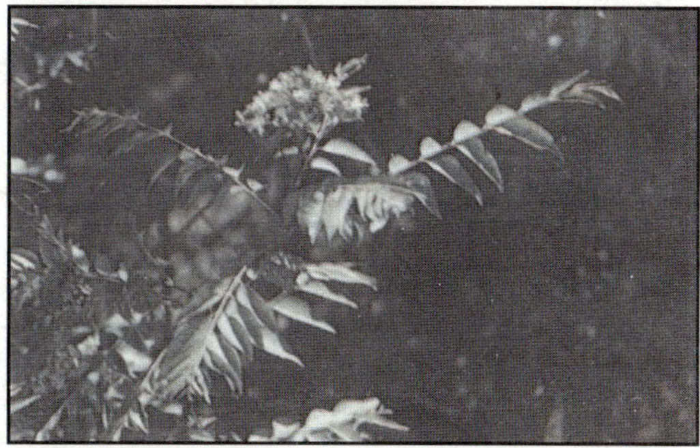

Murraya koenigil

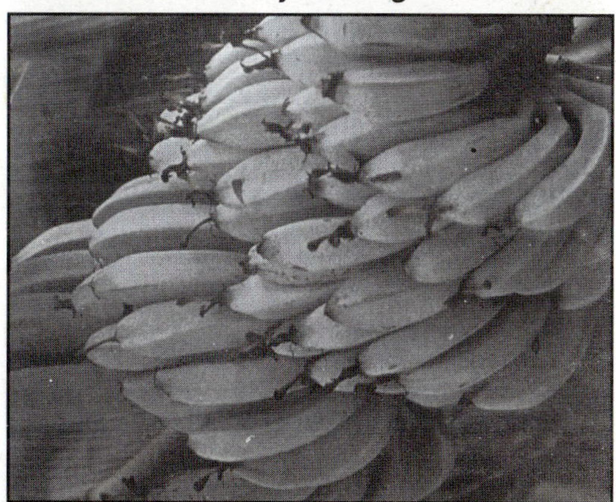

Musa nana

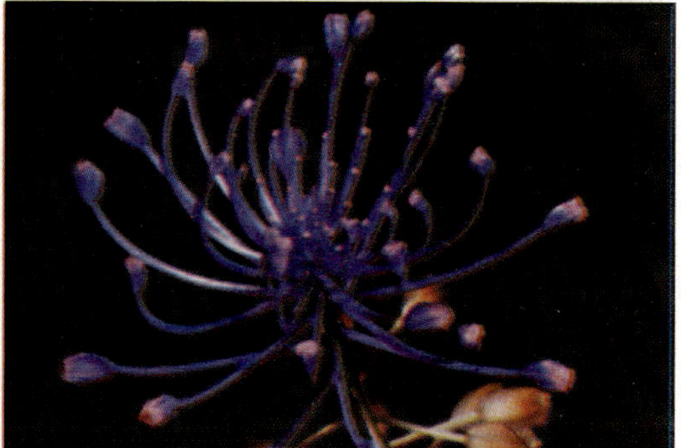

Muscari comosum

PLATE : 88

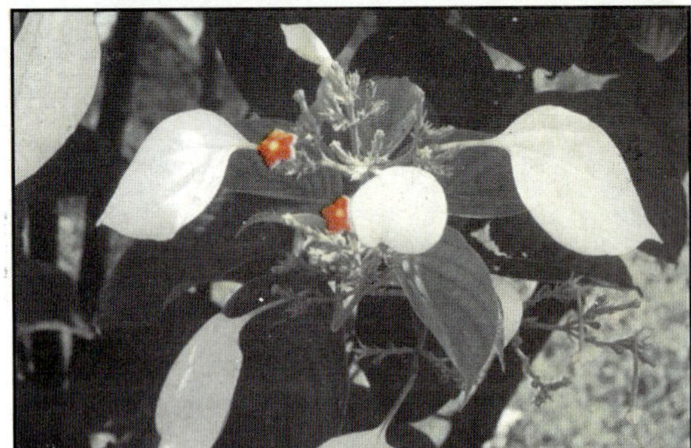
Mussaenda raiateensis

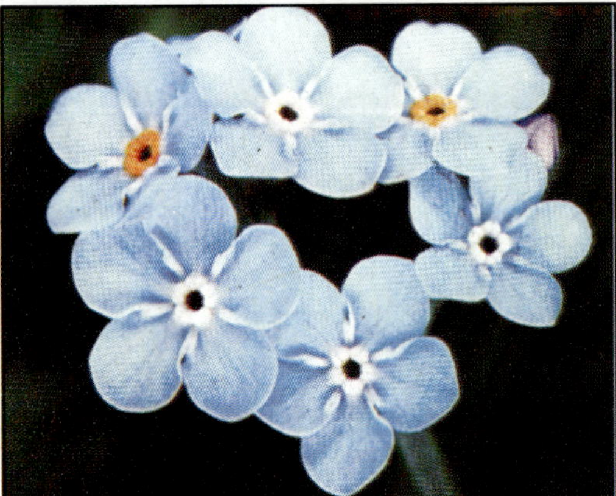
Myosotis alpestris

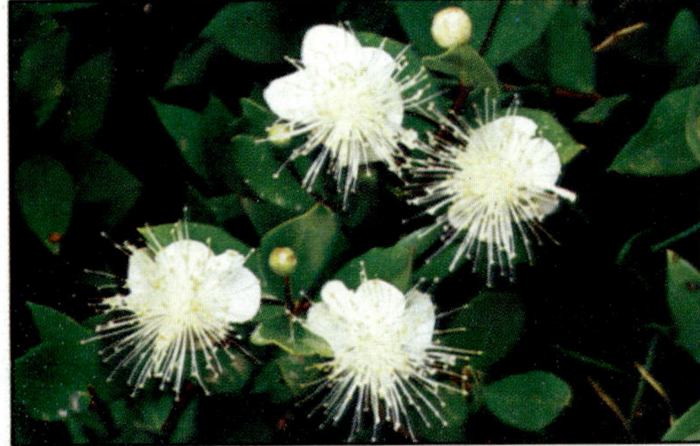
Myrtus communis

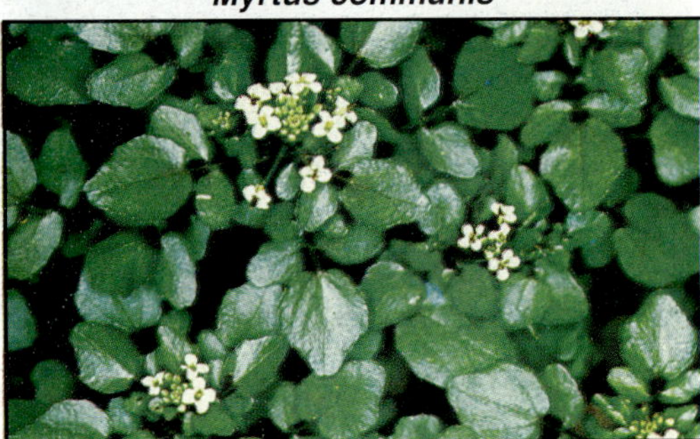
Nasturtium officinale

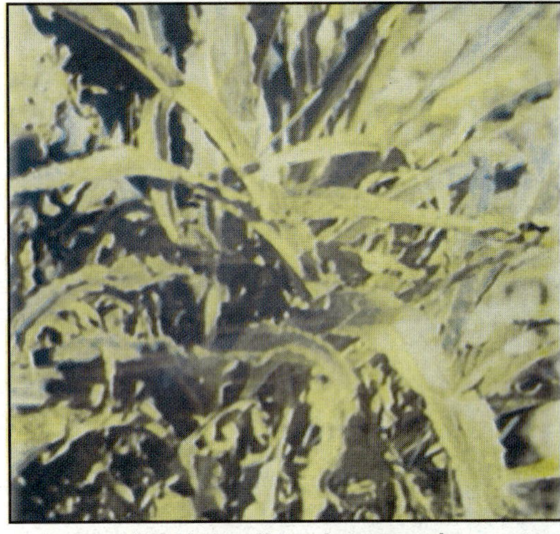
Nardostachys Jatamansi

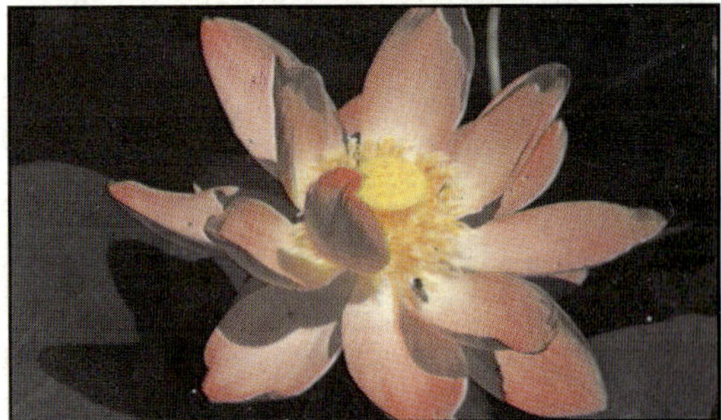
Nelumbo nucifera

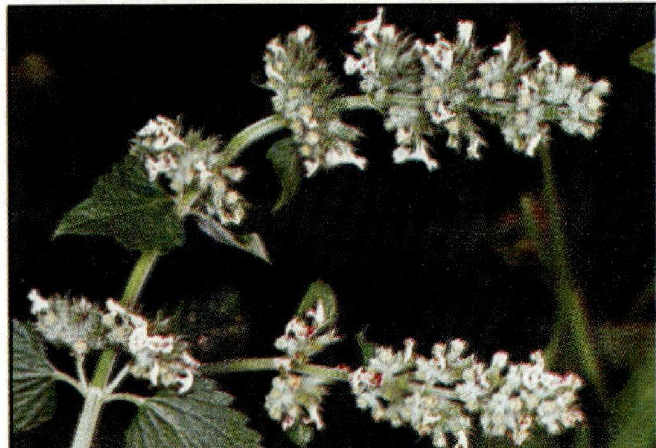
Nepeta cataria

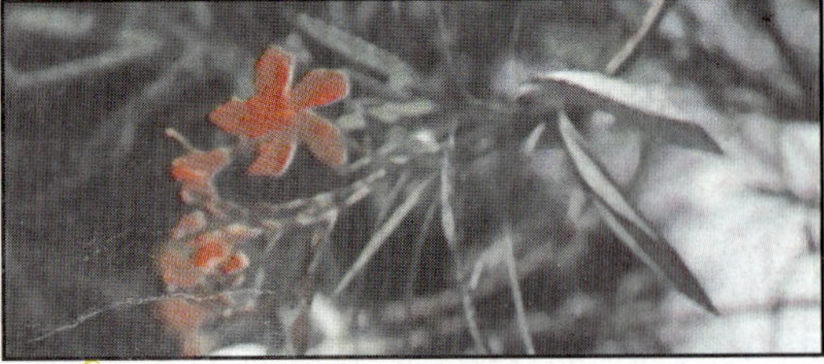
Nerium indicum

PLATE : 89

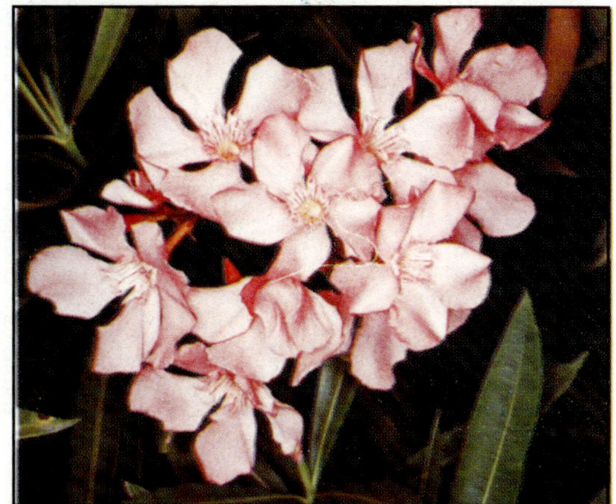

Nerium oleander

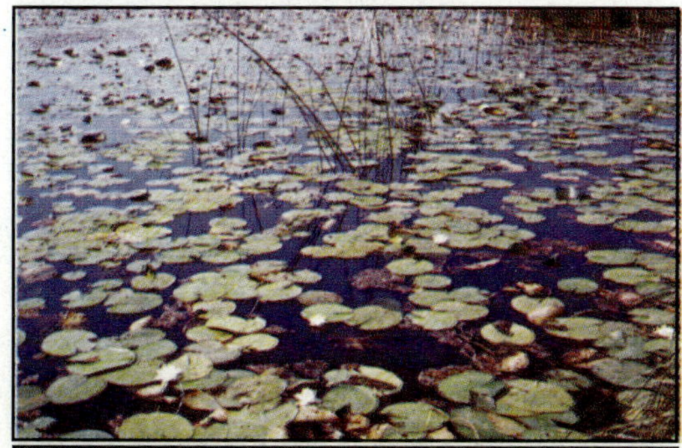

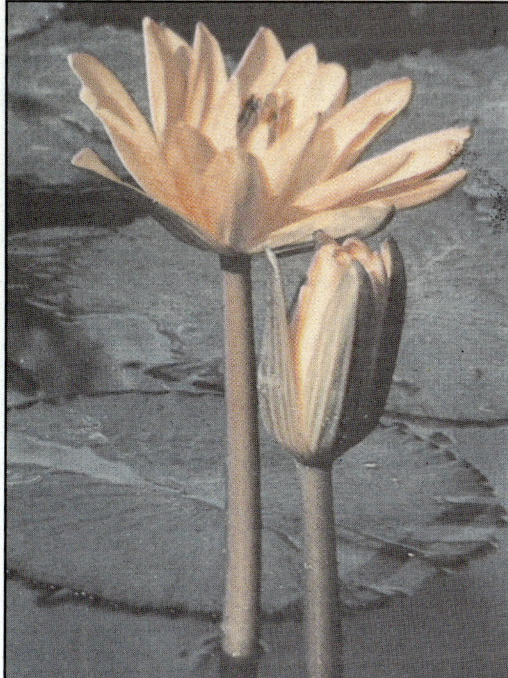

Nymphaea alba

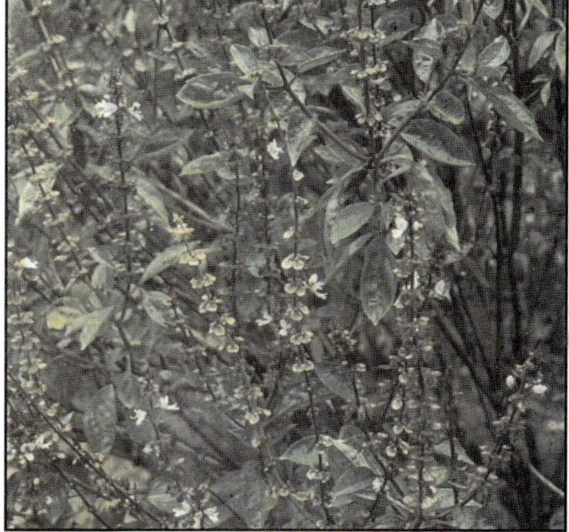

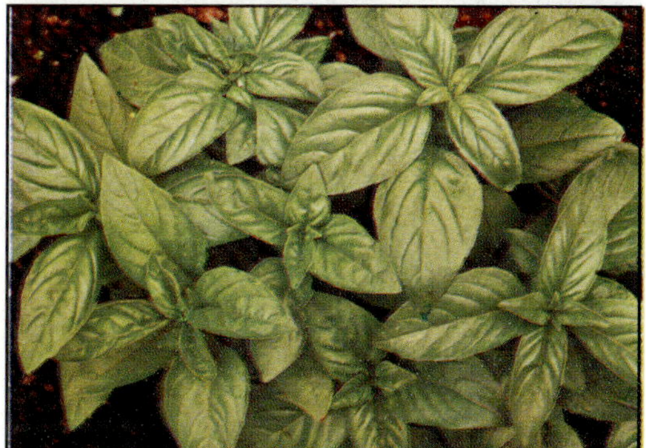

Ocimum basilicum

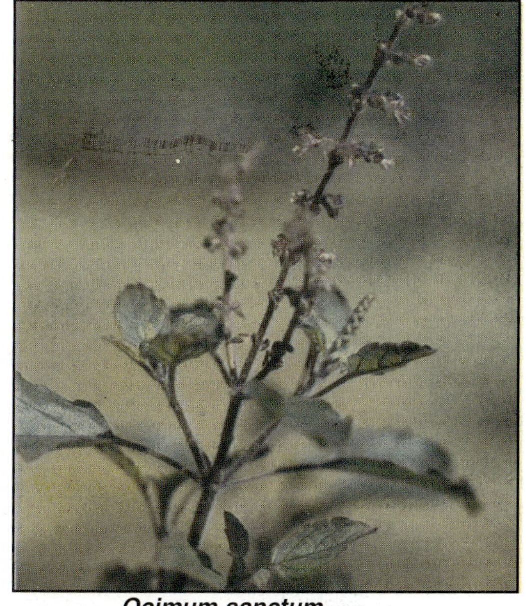

Ocimum sanctum

PLATE : 90

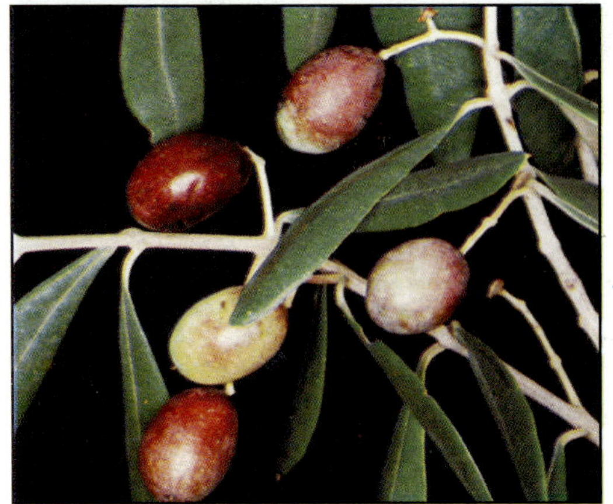

Oela europaea

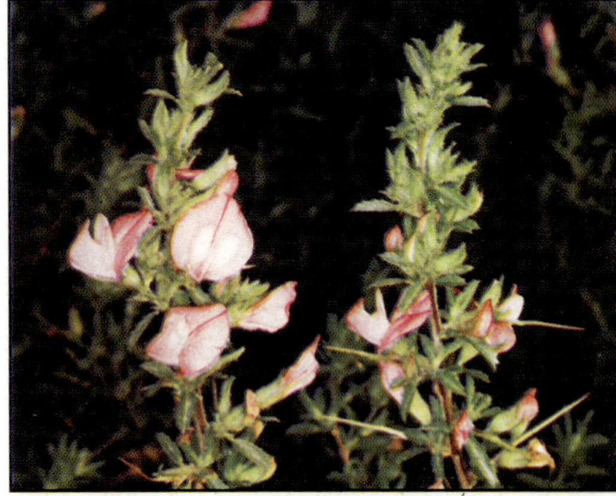

Ononis spinosa

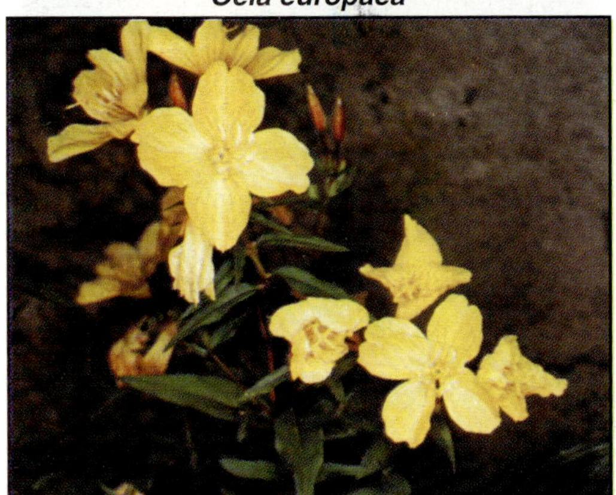

Oenothera biennis

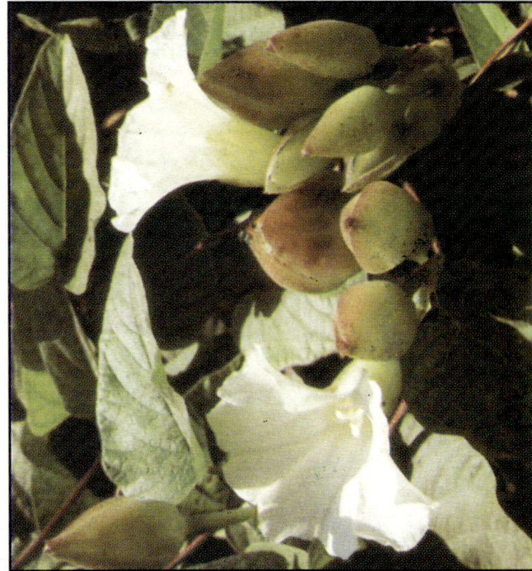

Operculina turpethum

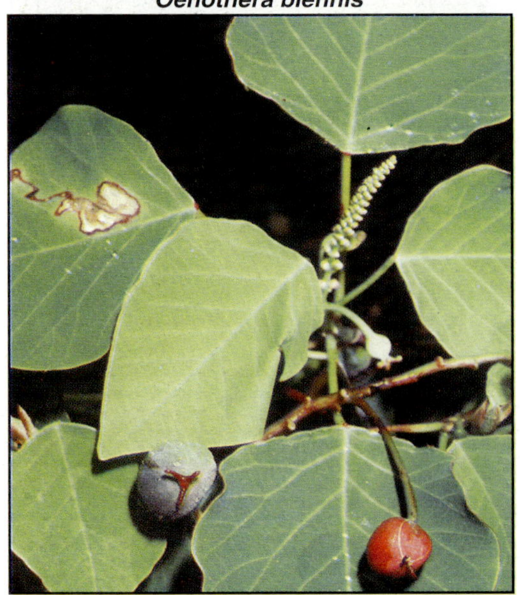

Omalanthus nutans

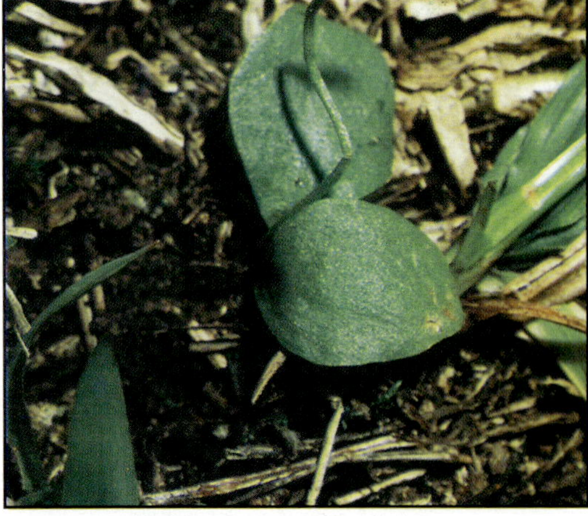

Ophioglossum petiolatum

PLATE : 91

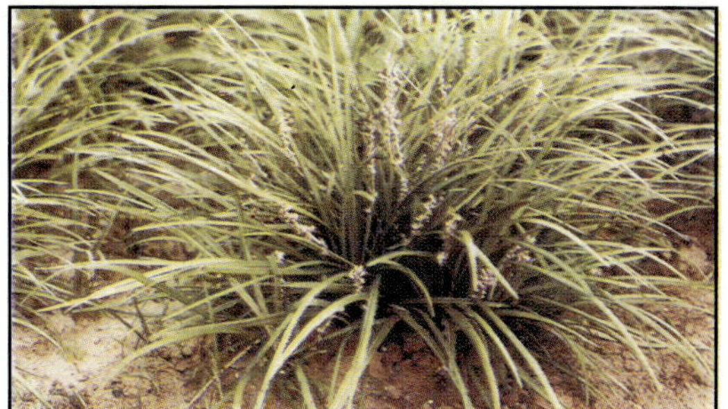

Ophiopogon japonicus

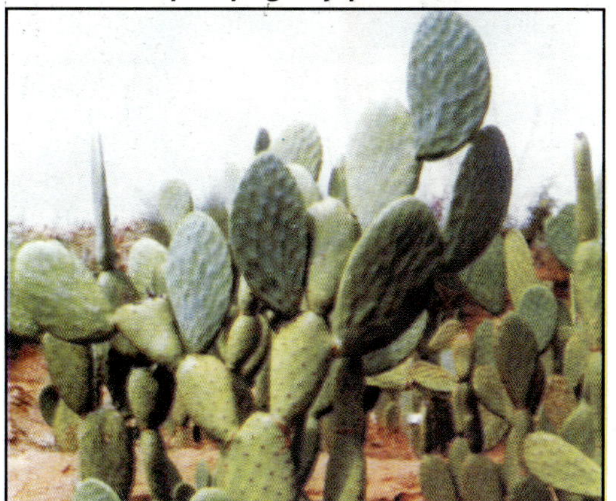

Opuntia ficus-indica

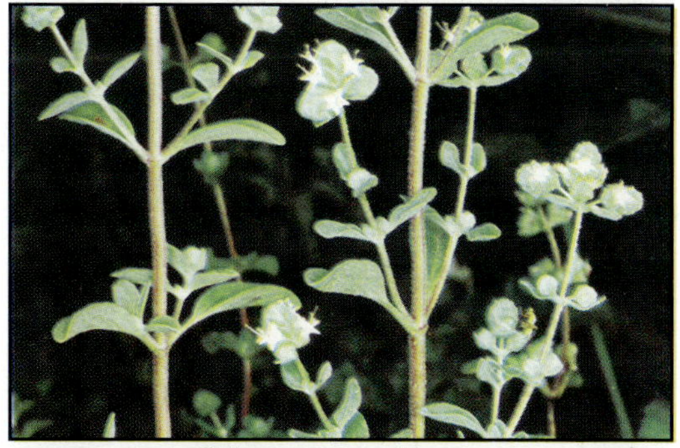

Origanum majorana

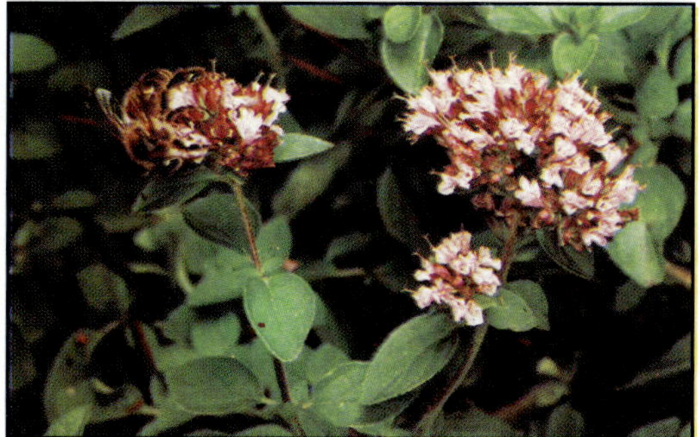

Origanum vulgare

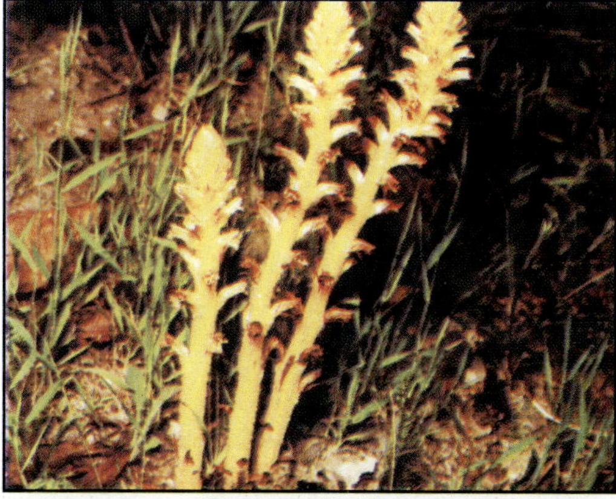

Orobanche flava

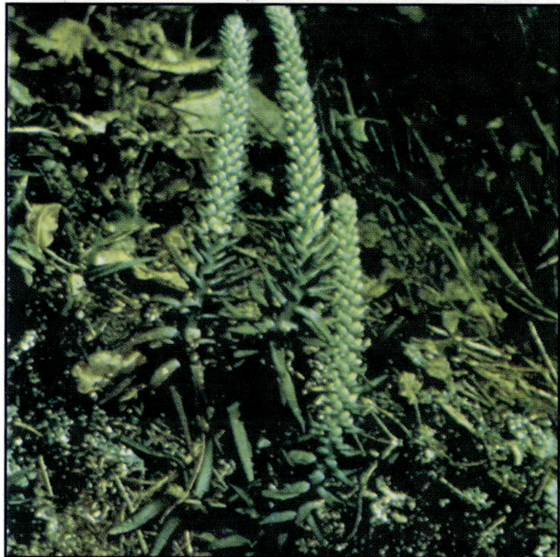

Orostachys japonicus

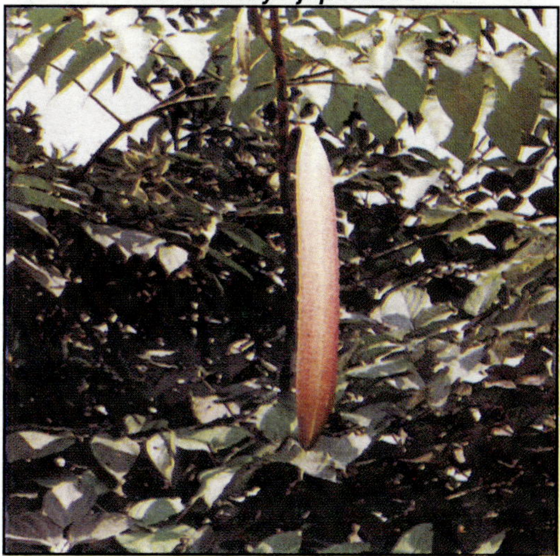

Oroxylum indicum

PLATE : 92

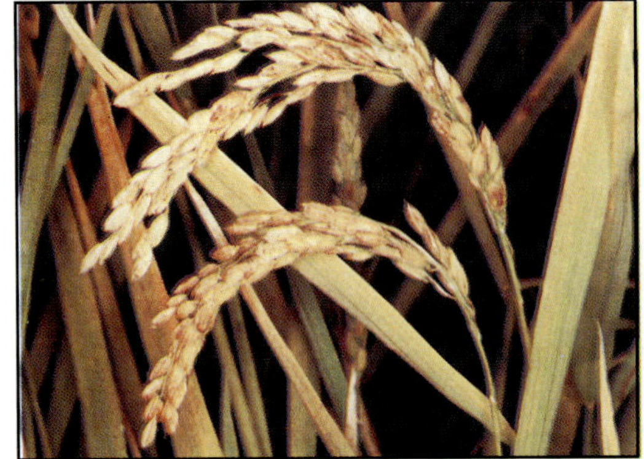

Oryza sativa

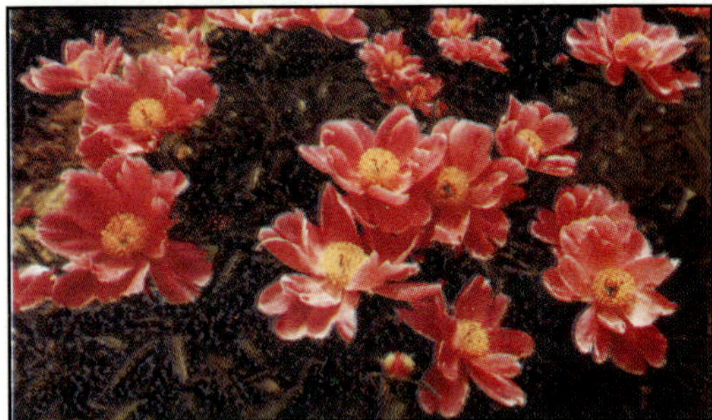

Paeonia lactiflora

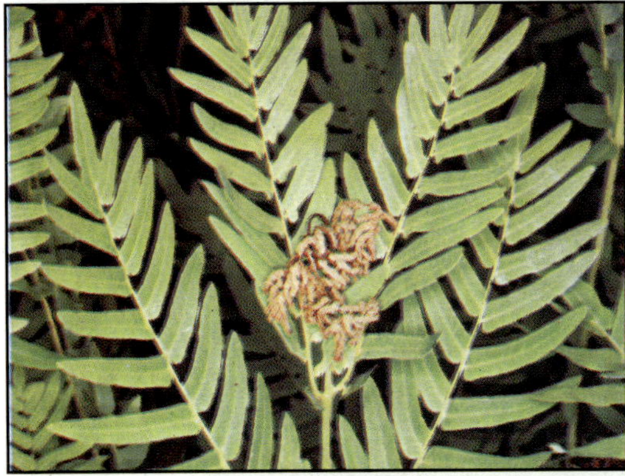

Osmunda regalis

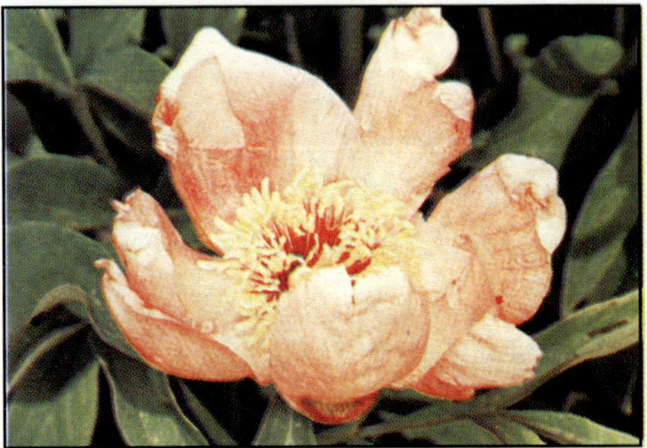

Paeonia officinalis

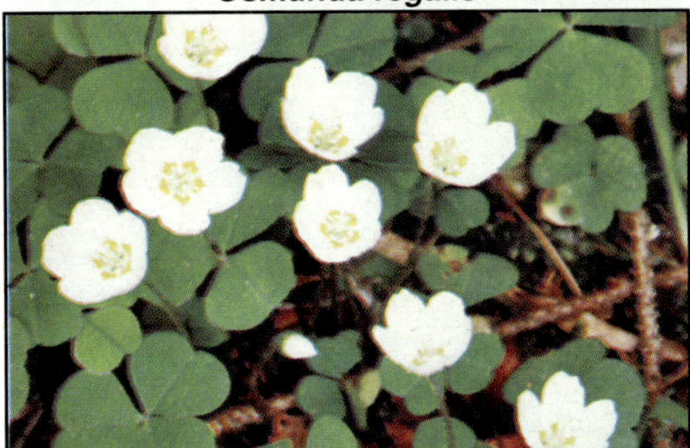

Oxalis acetosella

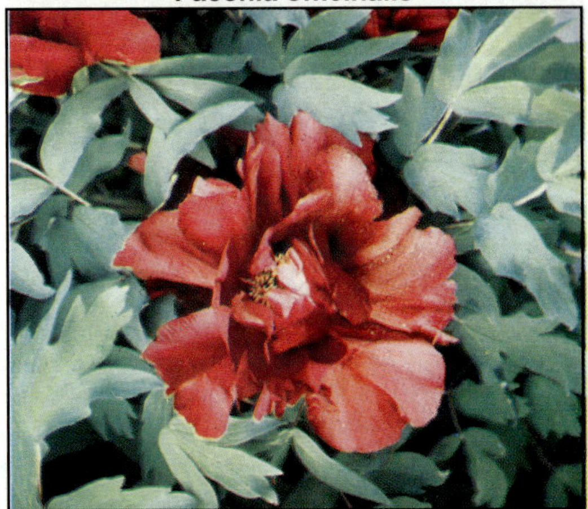

Paeonia suffruticosa

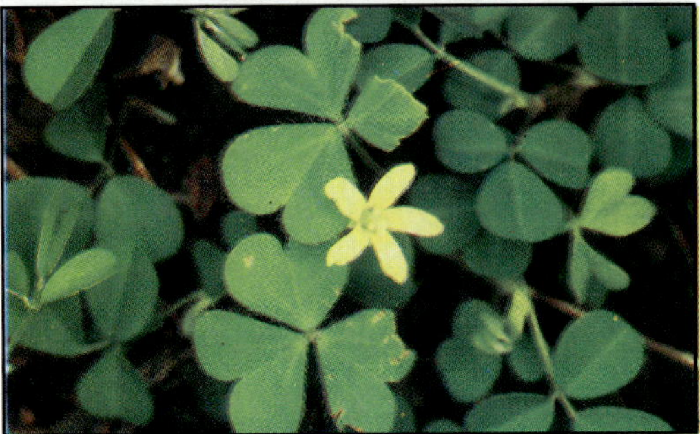

Oxalis corniculata

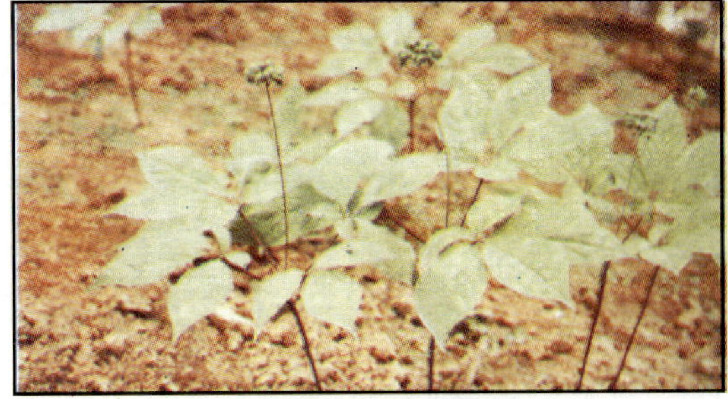

Panax ginseng

PLATE : 93

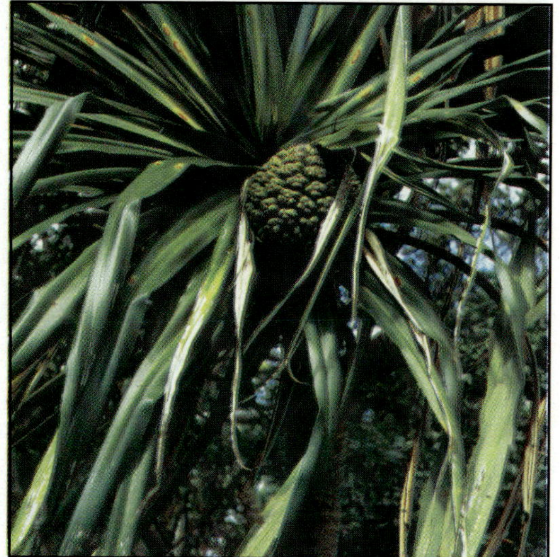

Pandanus pyriformis

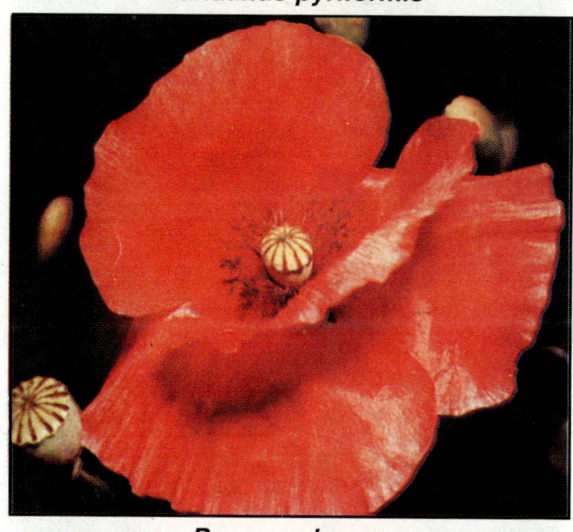

Papaver rhoeas

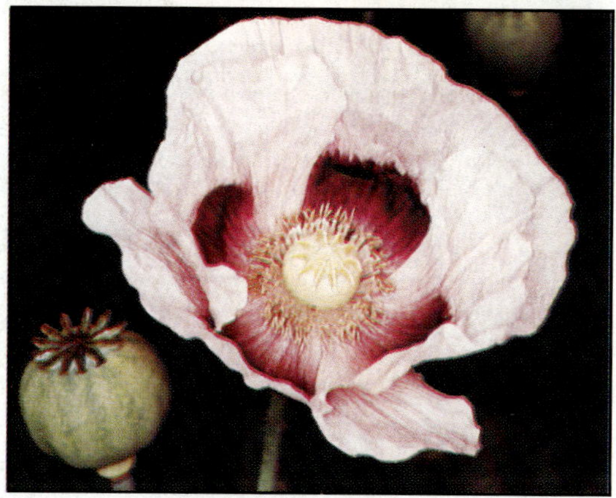

Papaver somniferum

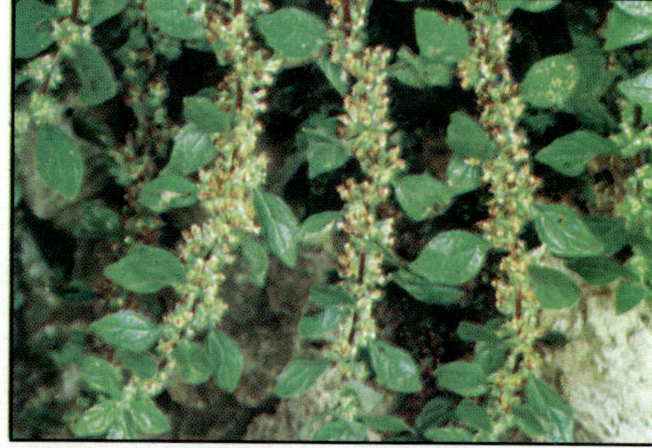

Parietaria officinalis

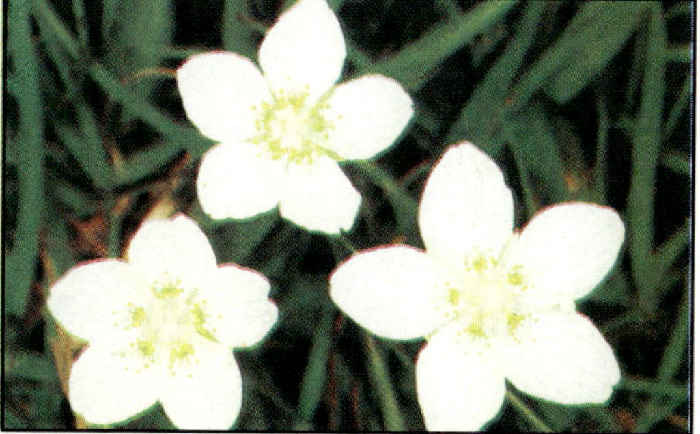

Parnassia palustris

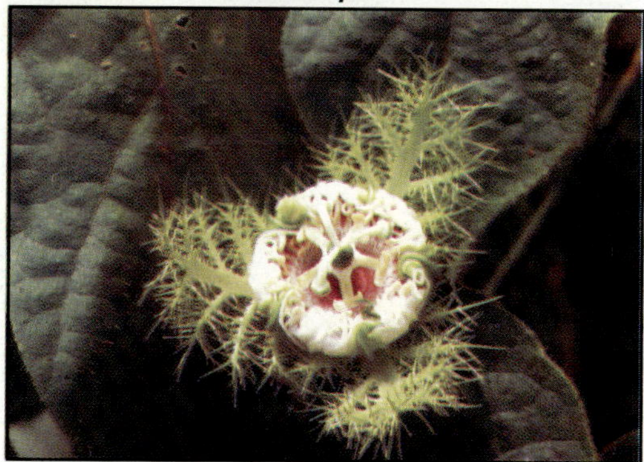

Passiflora foetida

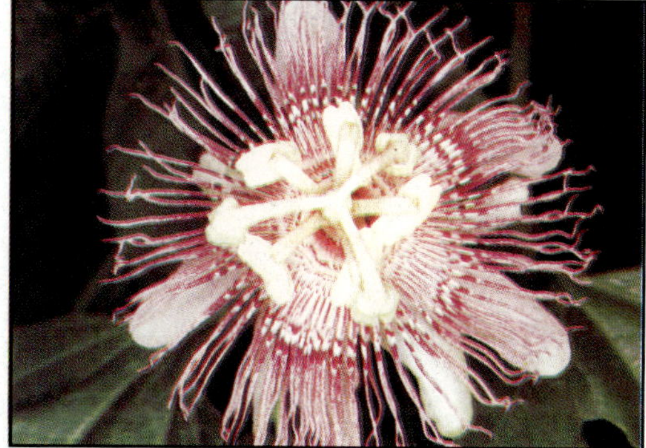

Passiflora incarnata

PLATE : 94

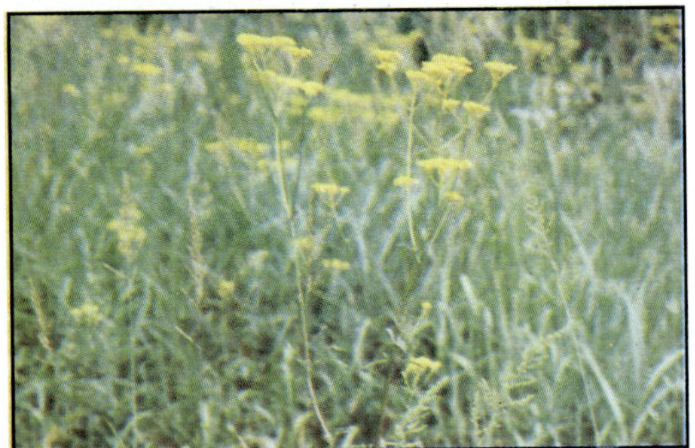

Patrinia scabiosaefolia

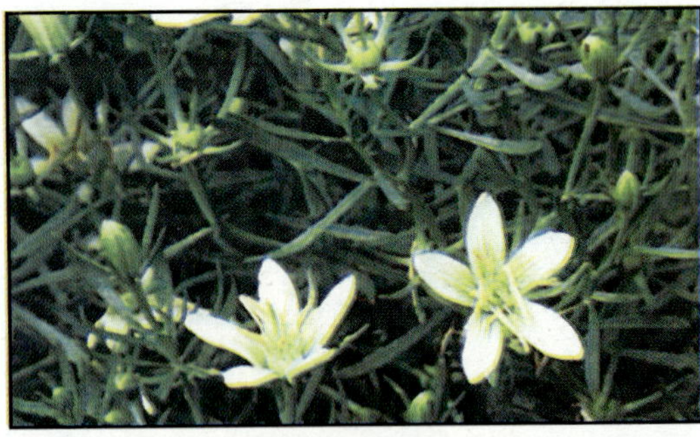

Peganum harmala

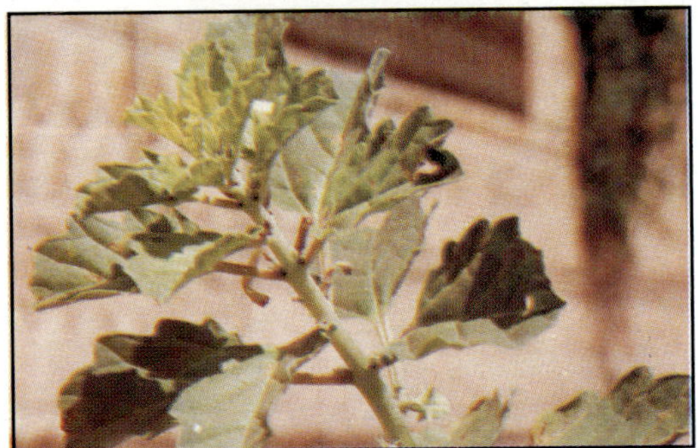

Pedalium murex

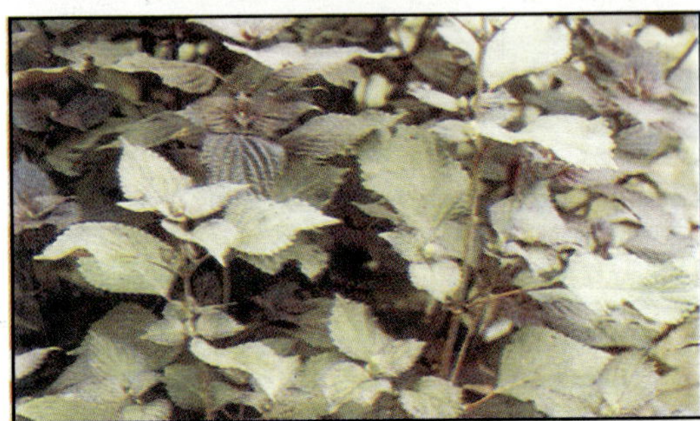

Perilla frutescens

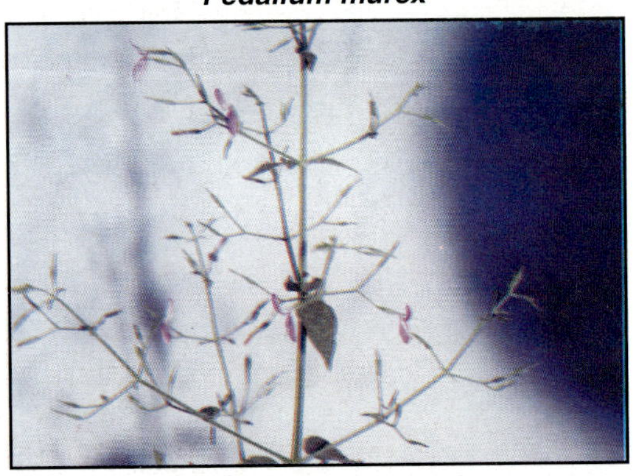

Peristrophis bicalicalcita

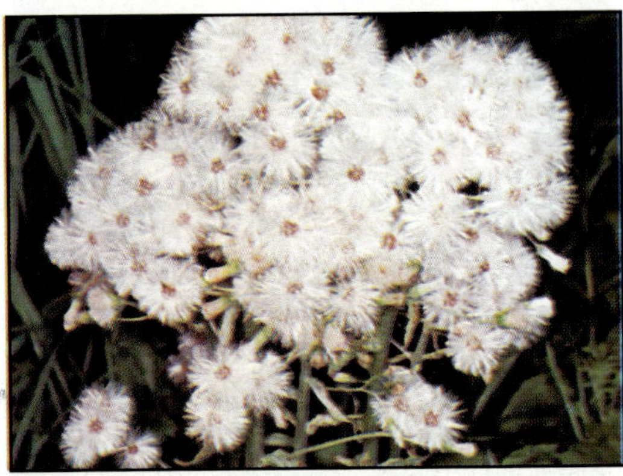

Petasites albus

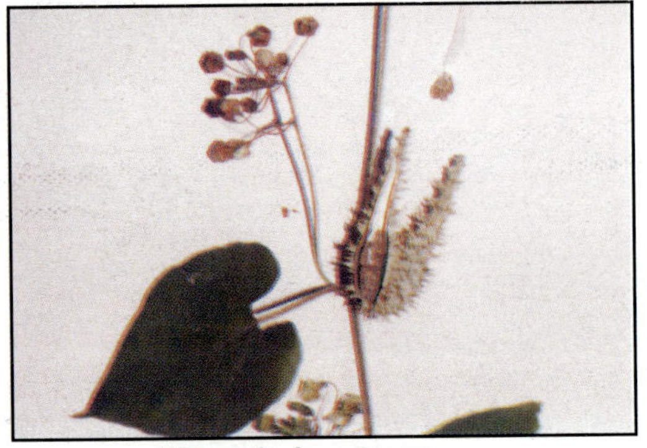

Pergularia extensa

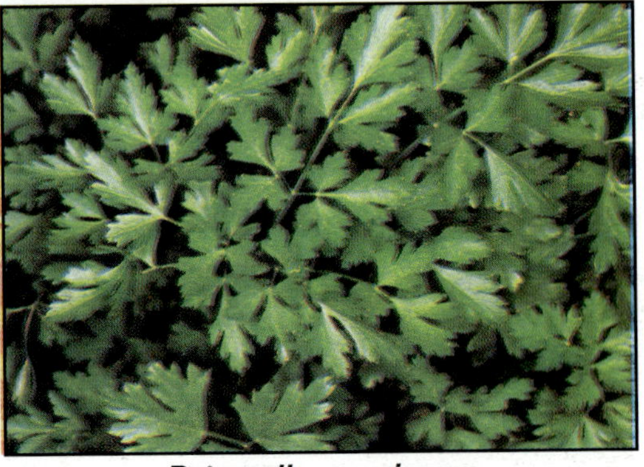

Petroselinum crispum

PLATE : 95

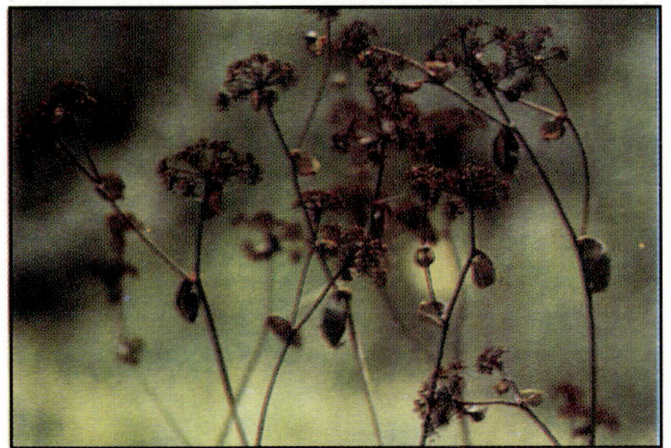
Peucedanum decursivum

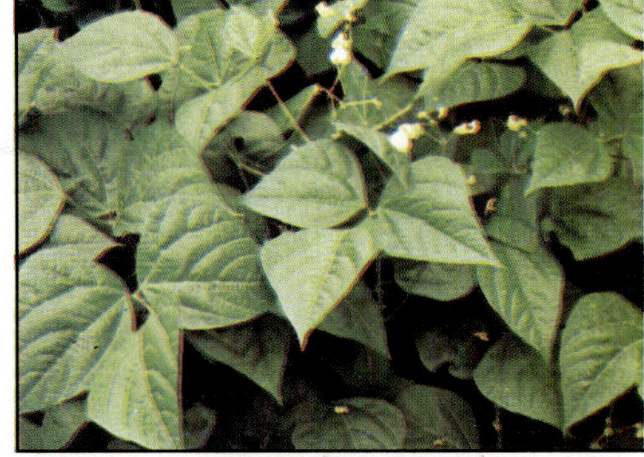
Phaseolus vulgaris

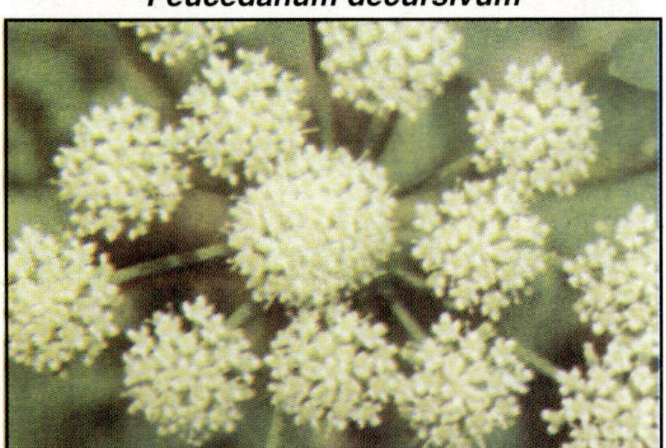
Peucedanum japonicum

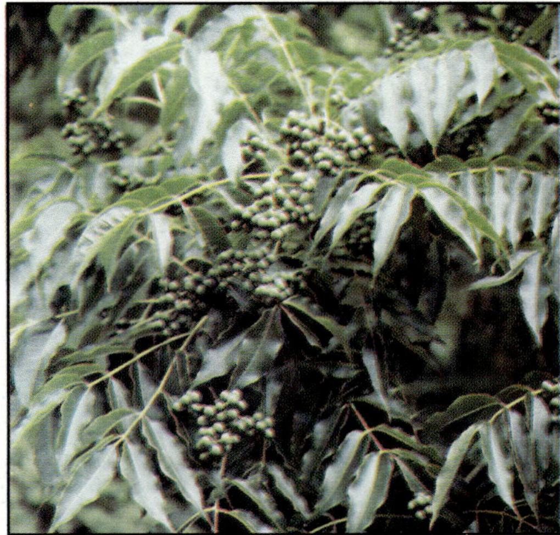
Phellodendron amurense

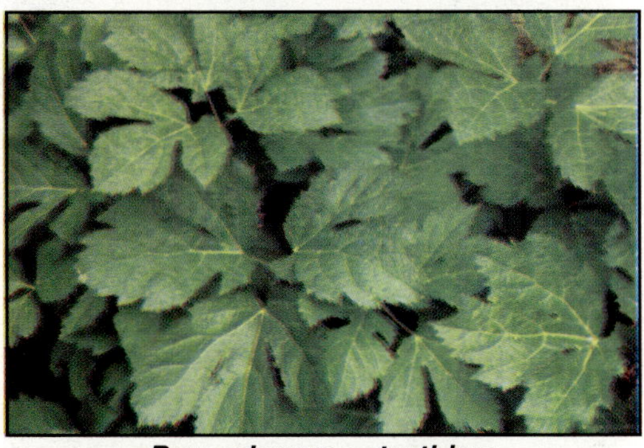
Peucedanum ostruthium

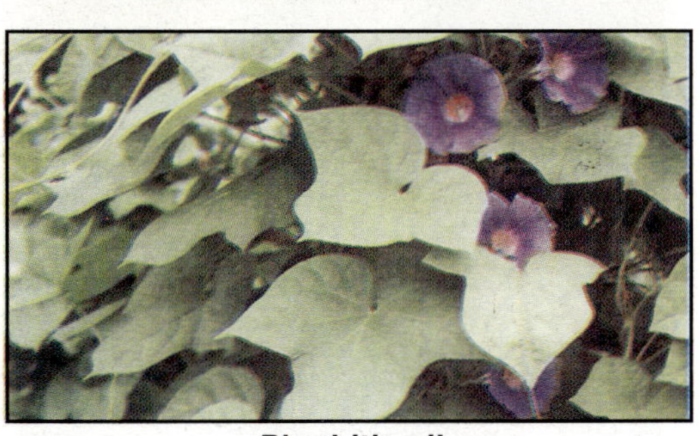
Pharbitis nil

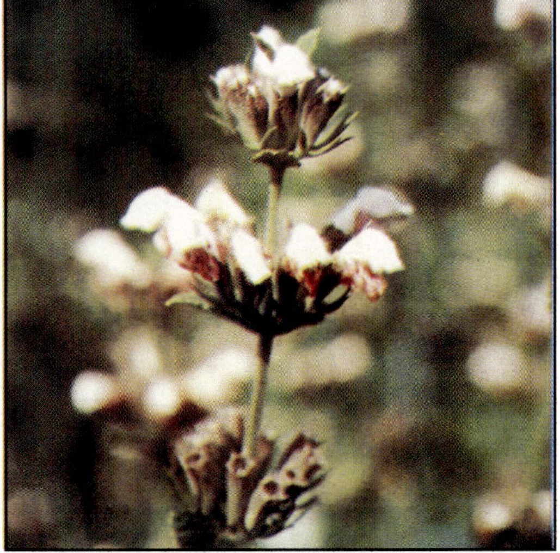
Phlomis umbrosa

PLATE : 96

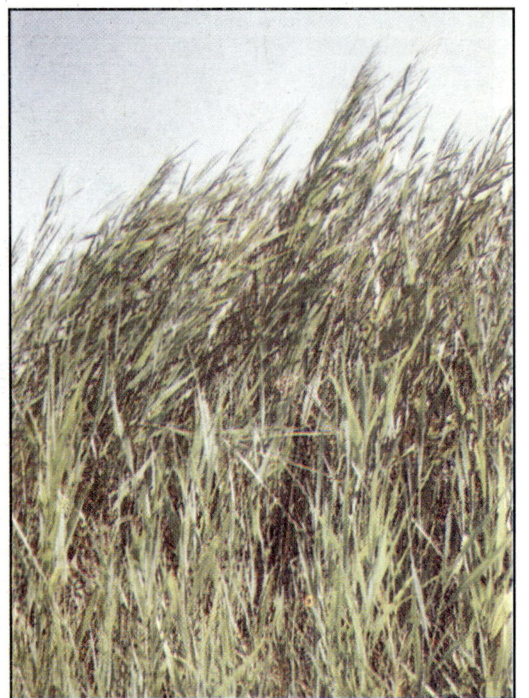

Phragmites communis

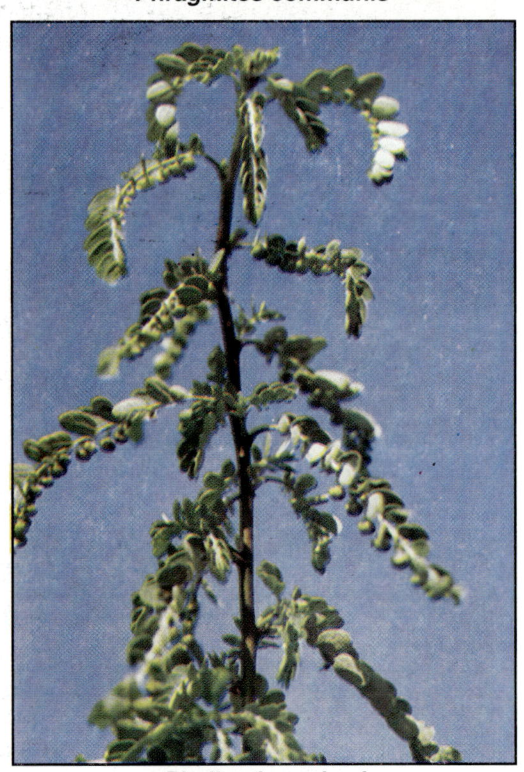

Phyllanthus niruri

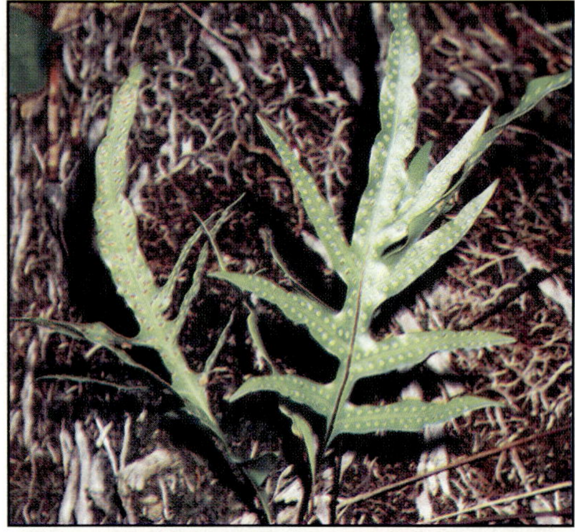

Phymatosorus scolopendeia

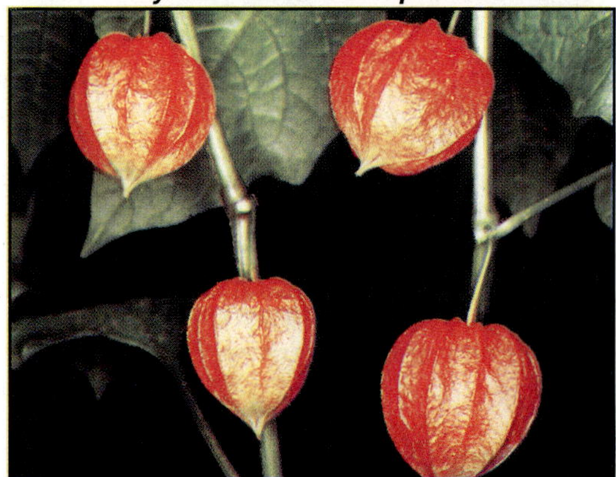

Physalis alkekengi

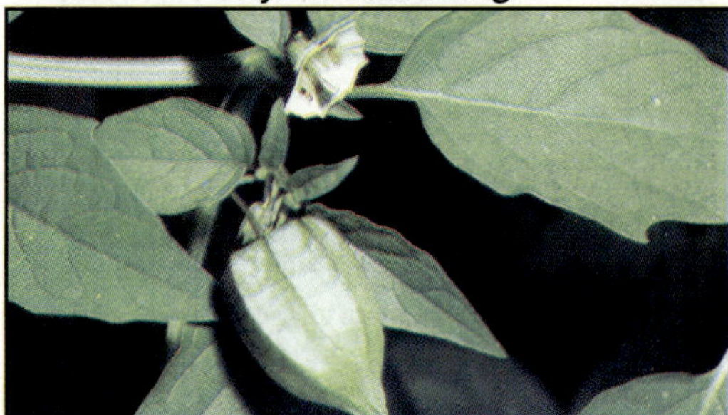

Physalis angulata

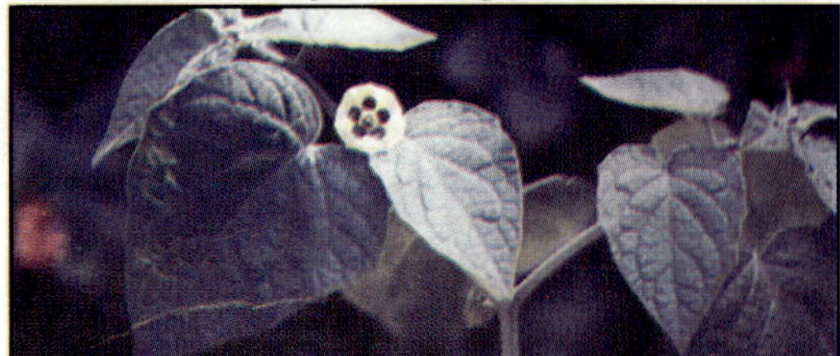

Physalis minima

PLATE : 97

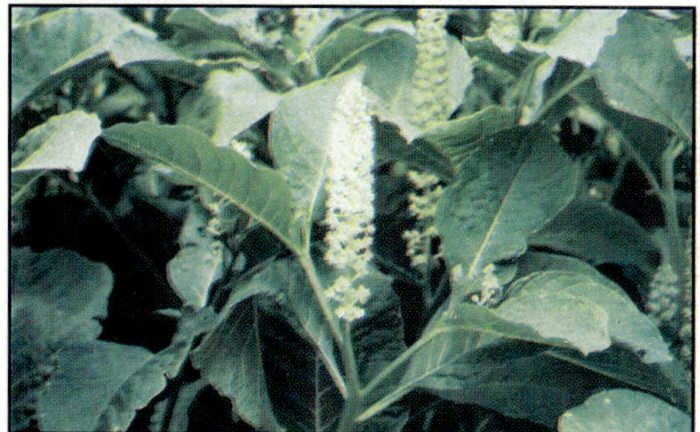

Phytolaca esculenta

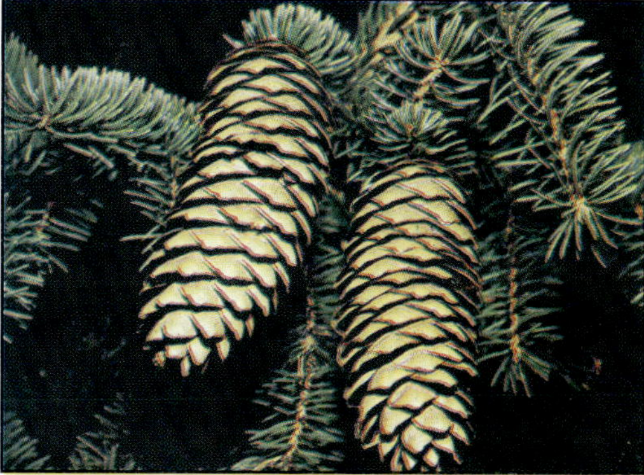

Picea abies

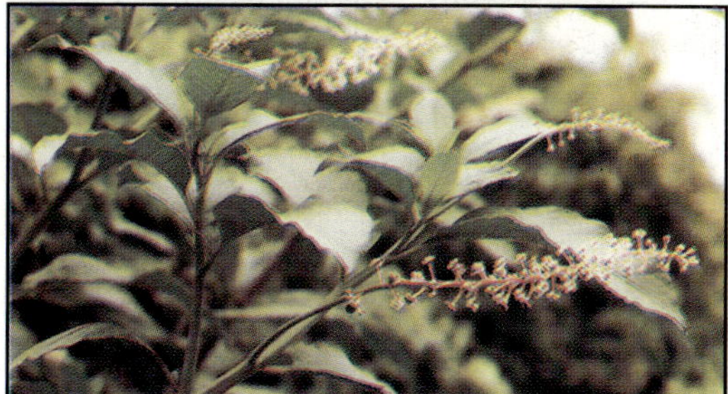

Phytolacca acinosa

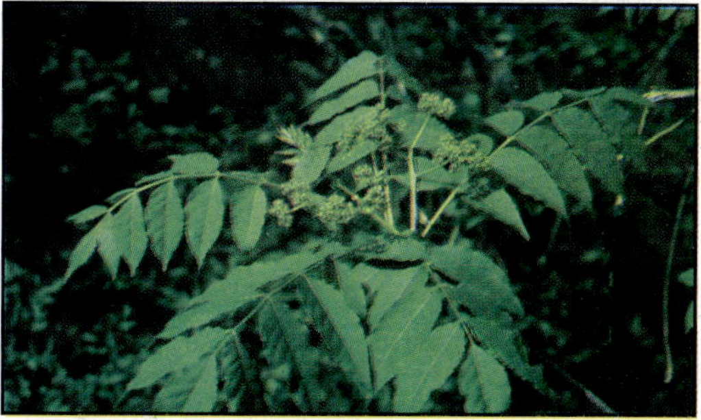

Picrasma quassioides

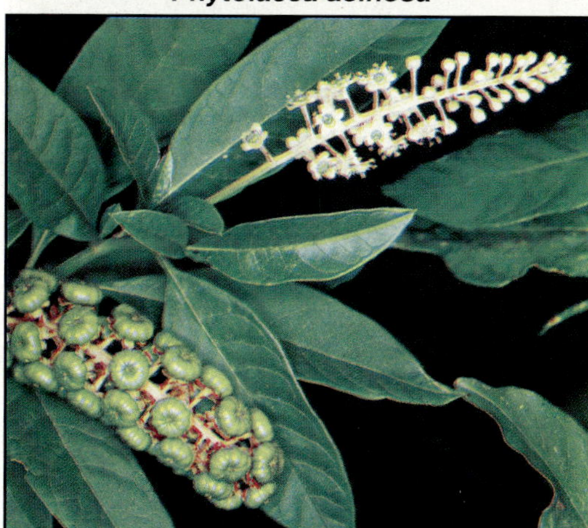

Phytolacca americana

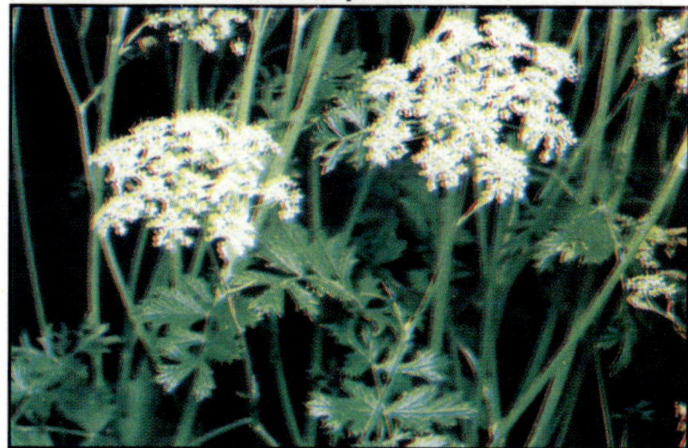

Pimpinella saxifraga

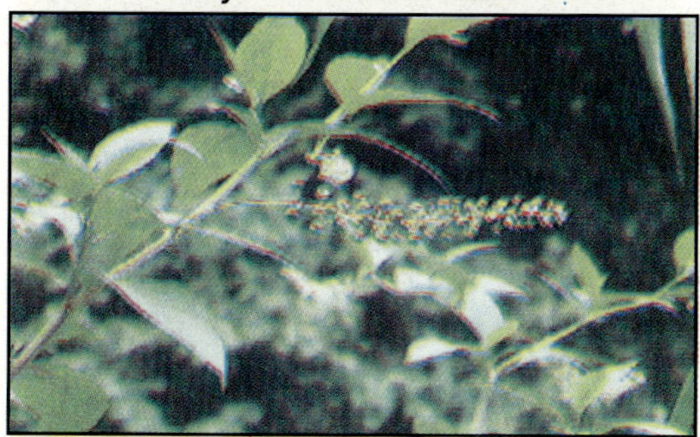

Phytolacca dioica

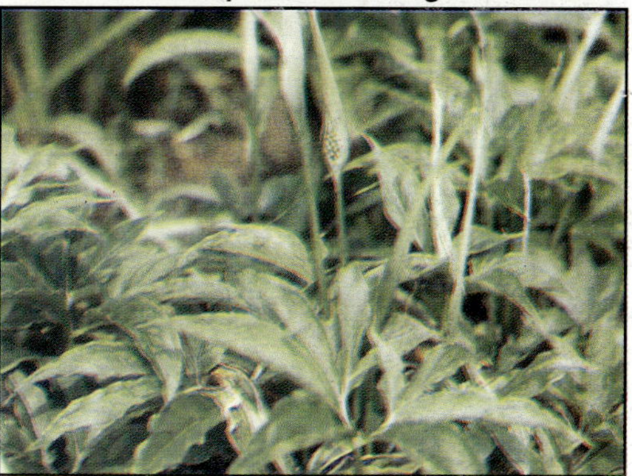

Pinellia pedatisecta

PLATE : 98

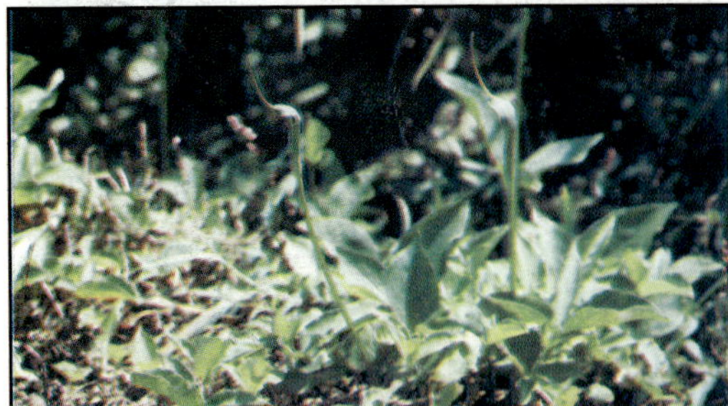

Pinellia ternata

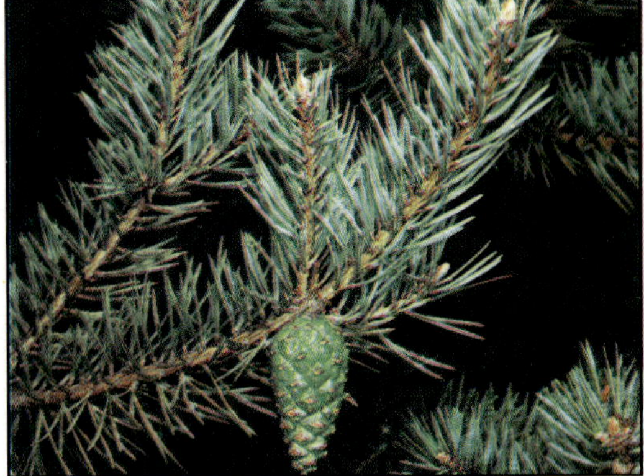

Pinus sylvestris

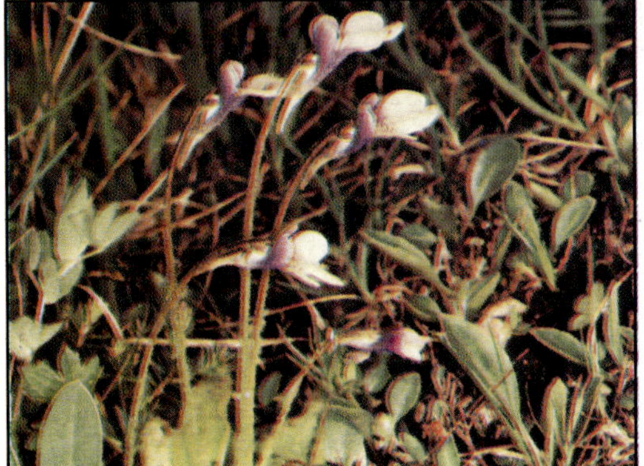

Pinguicula vulgaris

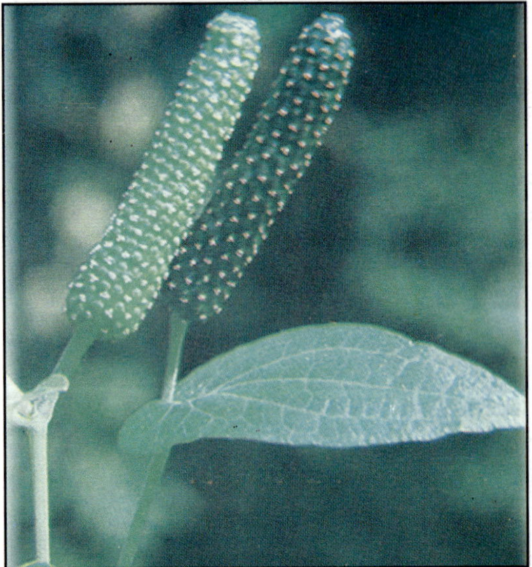

Piper longum

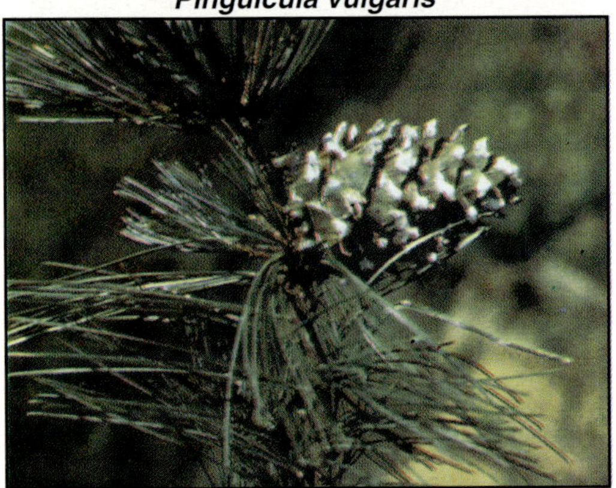

Pinus koraiensis

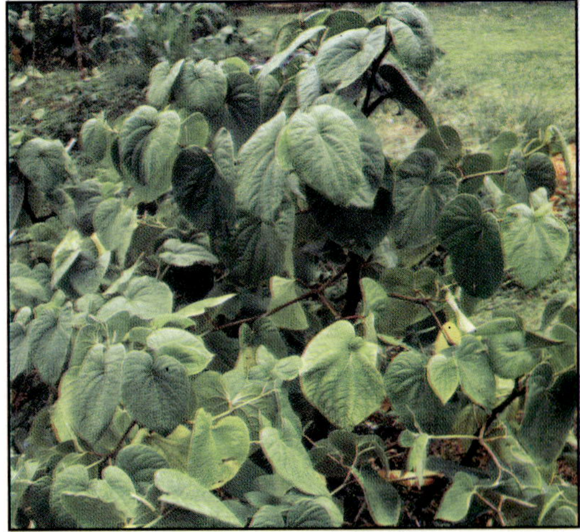

Piper methysticum

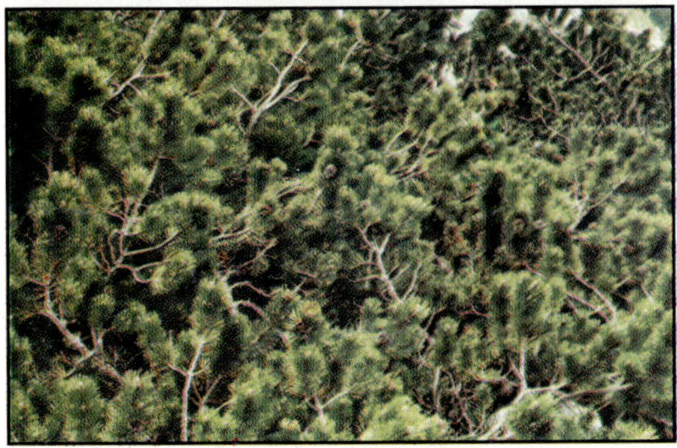

Pinus mugo

PLATE : 99

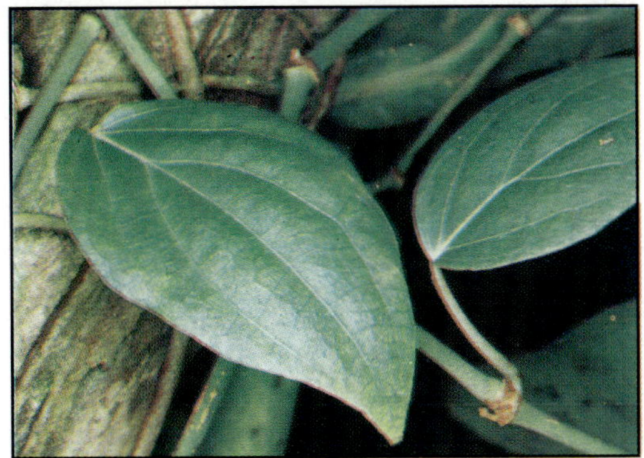
Piper nigrum

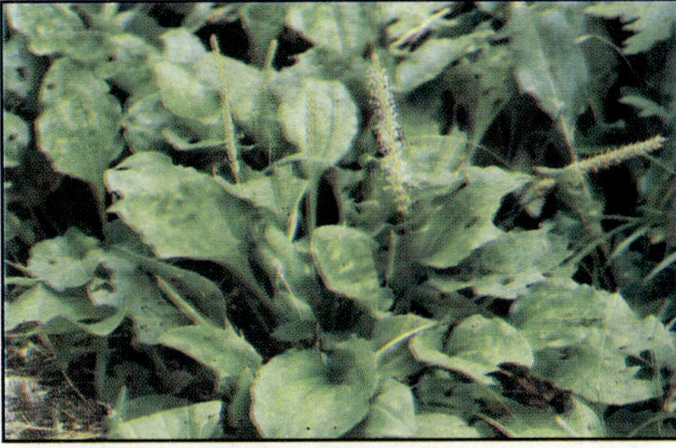
Plantago asiatica

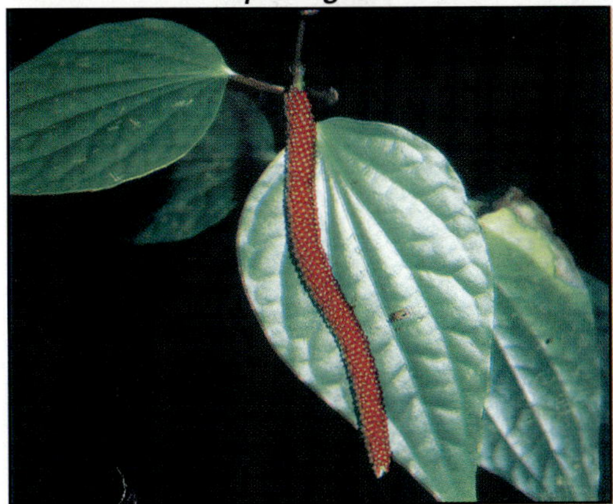
Piper purberulum

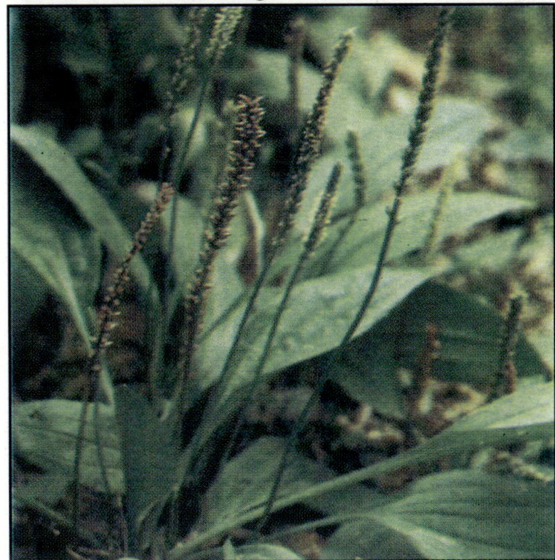
Plantago depressa

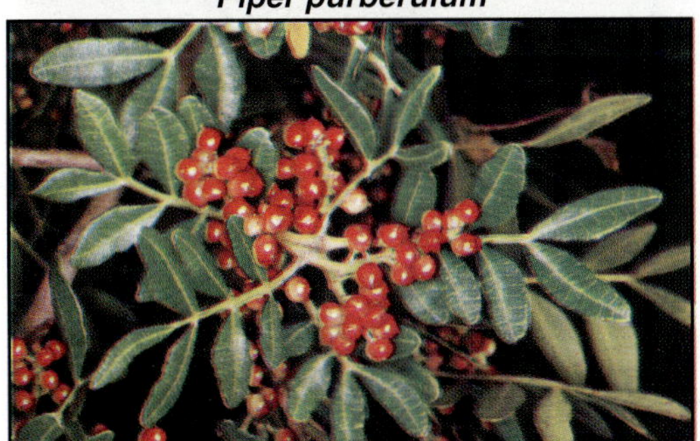
Pistacia lentiscus

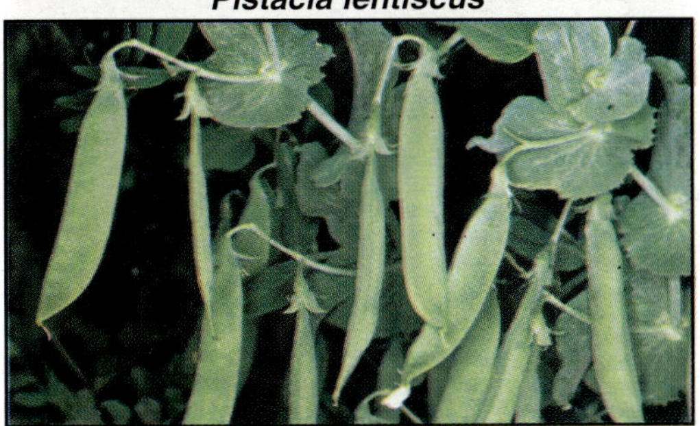
Pisum sativum

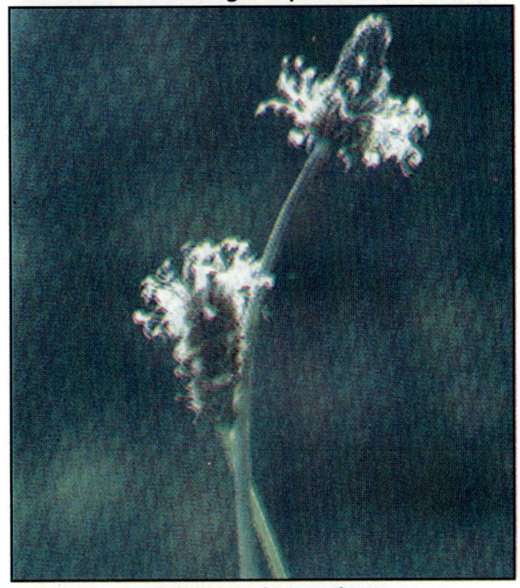
Plantago lanceolata

PLATE : 100

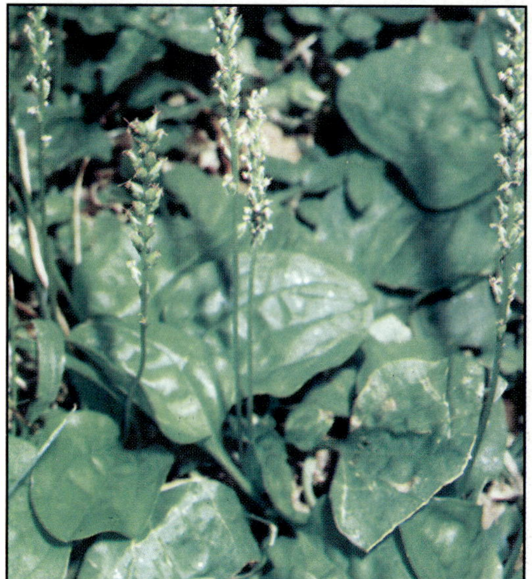
Plantago major

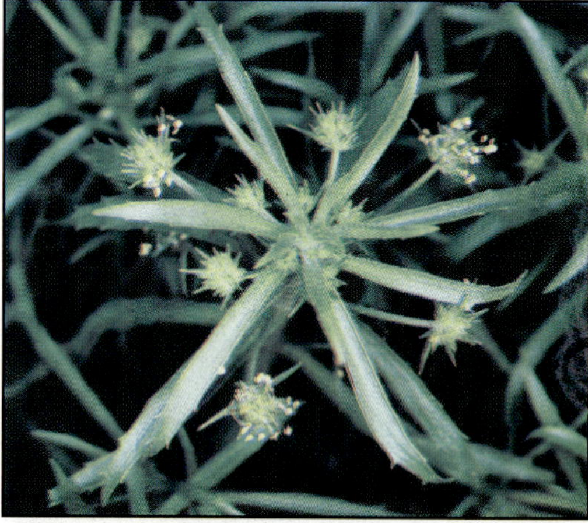
Plantago psyllium

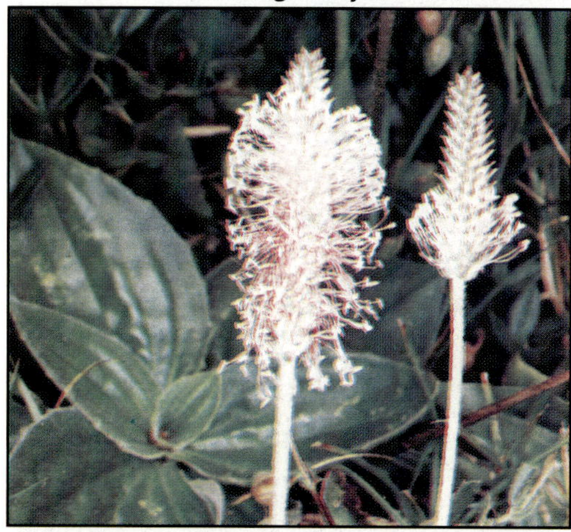
Plantago media

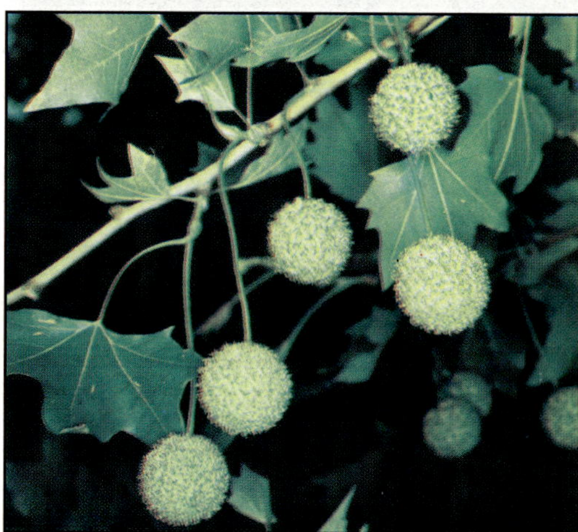
Plantanus orientalis

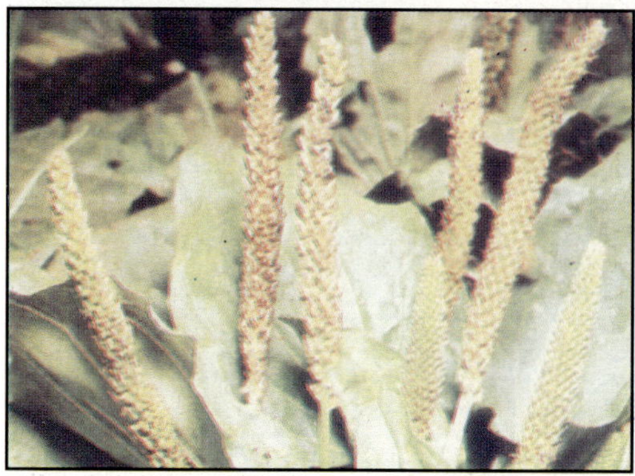
Plantago ovata Forsk

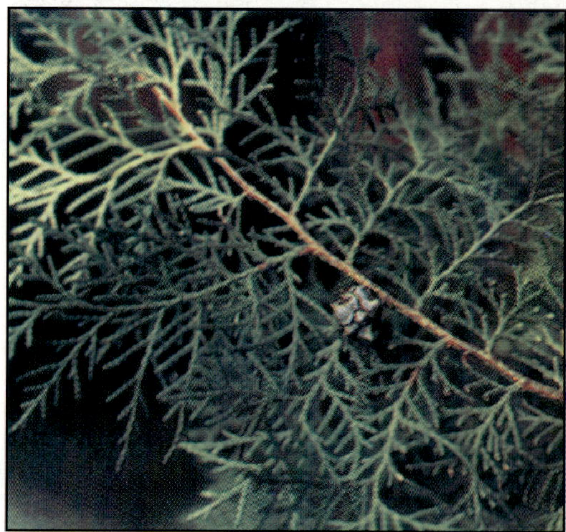
Plantycladus arientalis

PLATE : 101

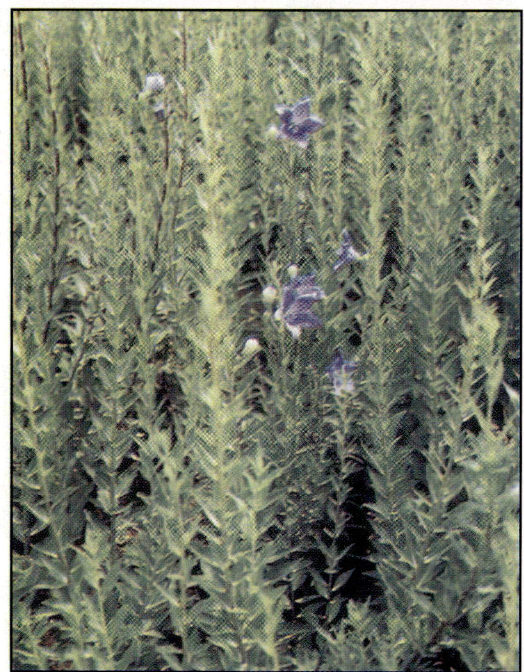

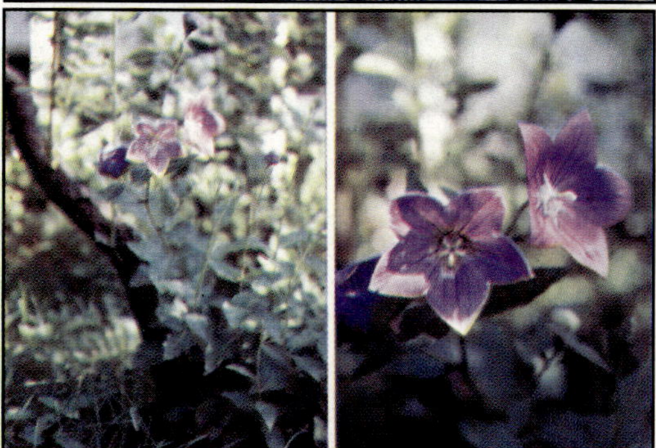

Platycodon grandiflorum

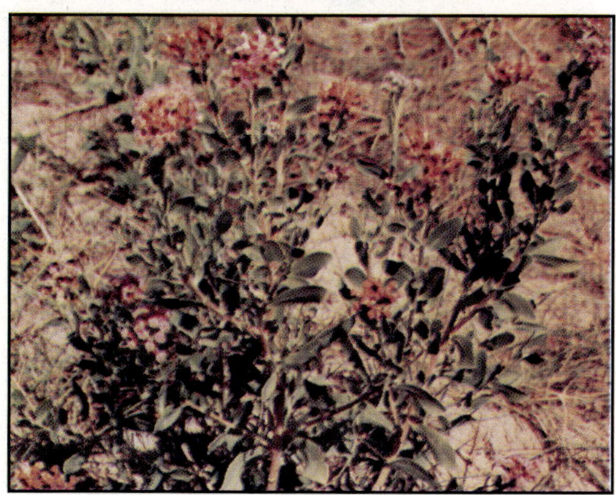

Pluchea lanceolata

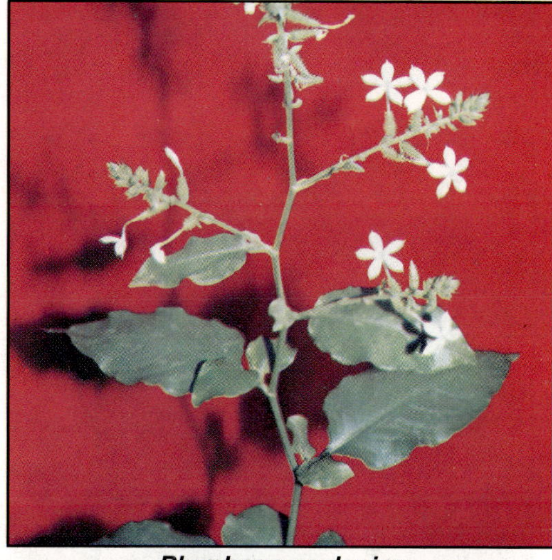

Plumbago zeylanica

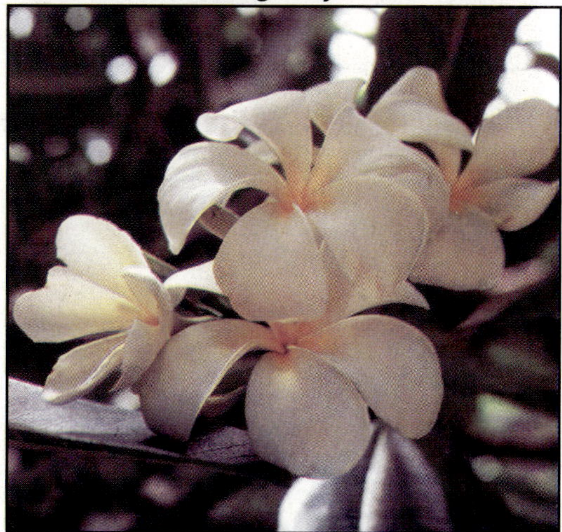

Plumeria rubra

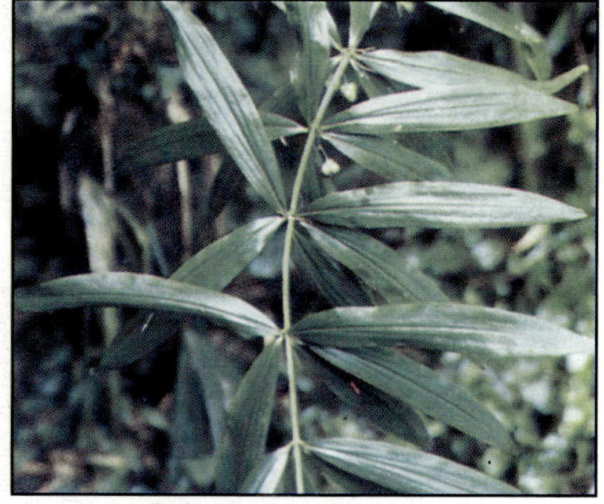

Polygonatum kingianum

PLATE : 102

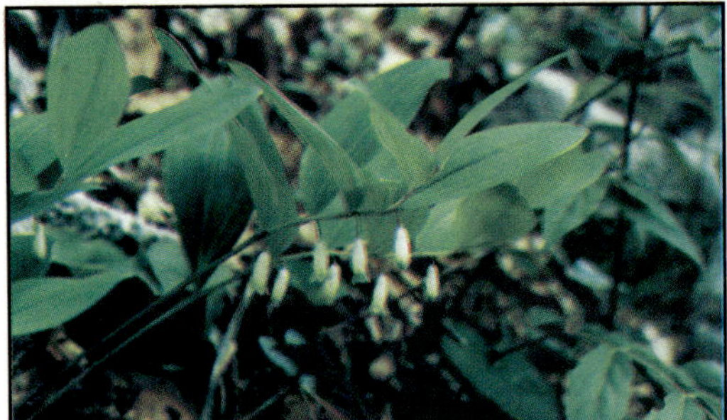

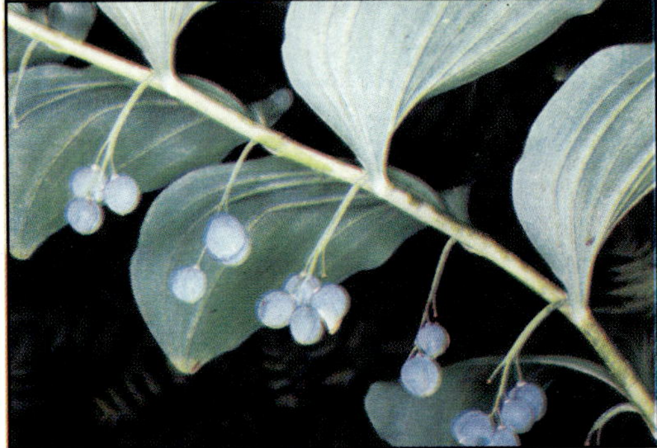

Polygonatum odoratum

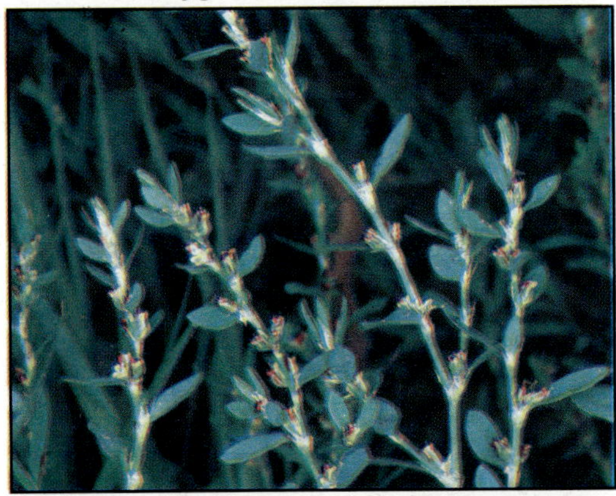

Polygonum aviculare

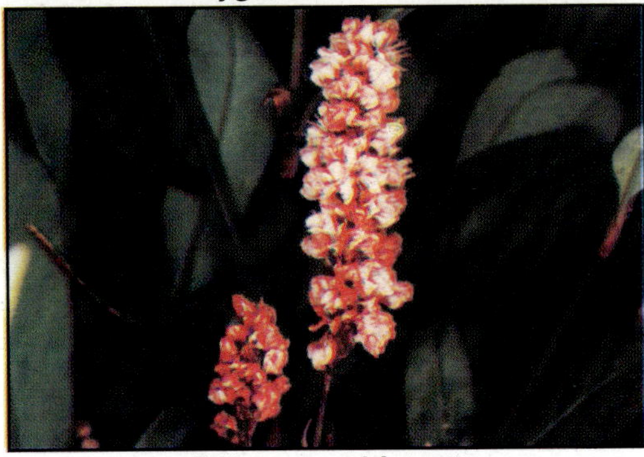

Polygonum bistorta

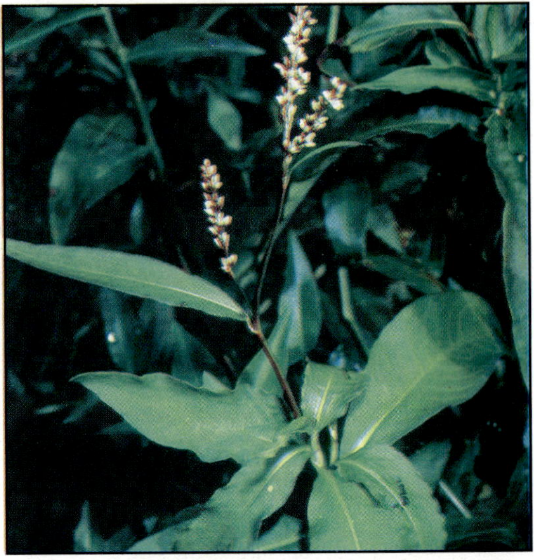

Polygonum dichrotomum

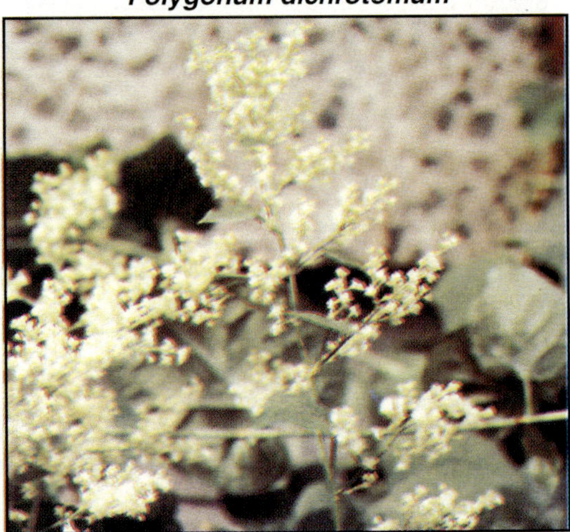

Polygonum multiflorum

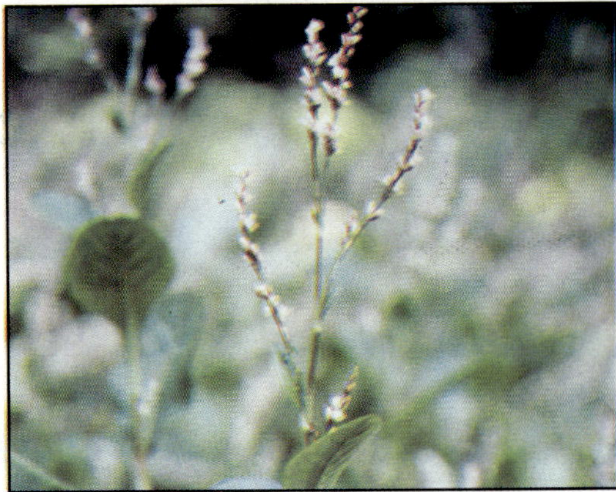

Polygonum tinctorium

PLATE : 103

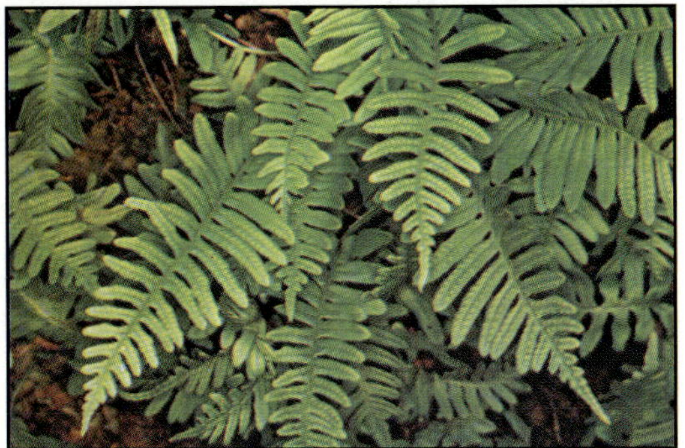

Polypodium vulgare

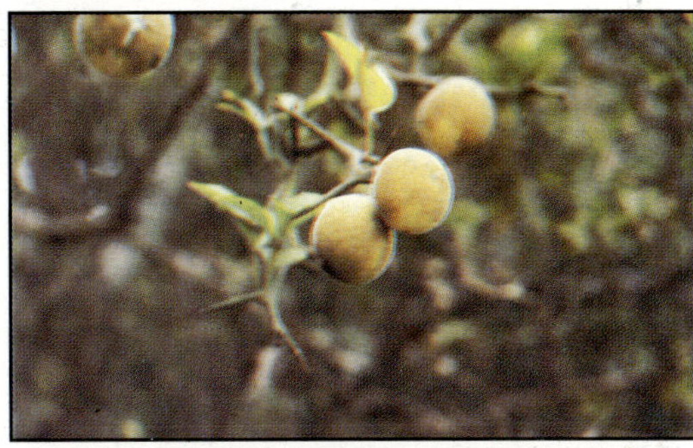

Poncirus trifoliata

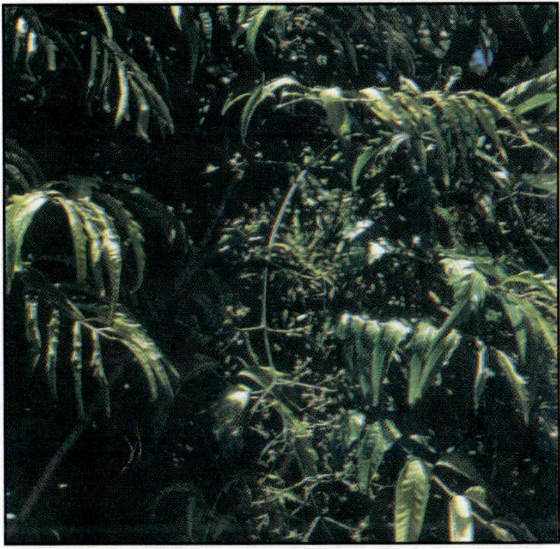

Polyscias fruticosa

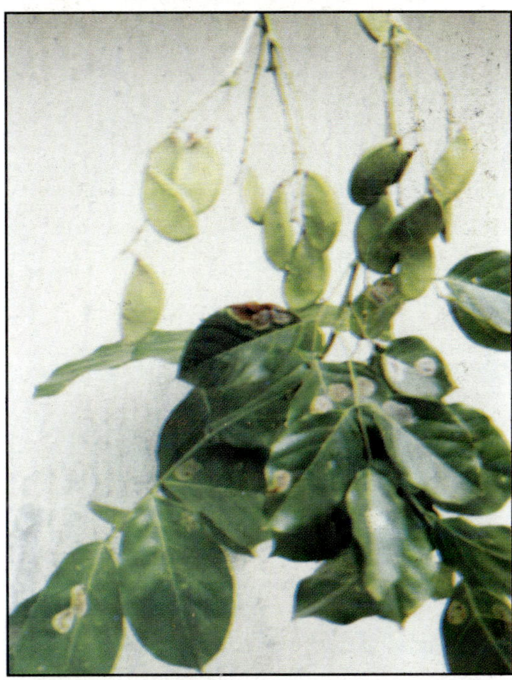

Pongamia pinnata

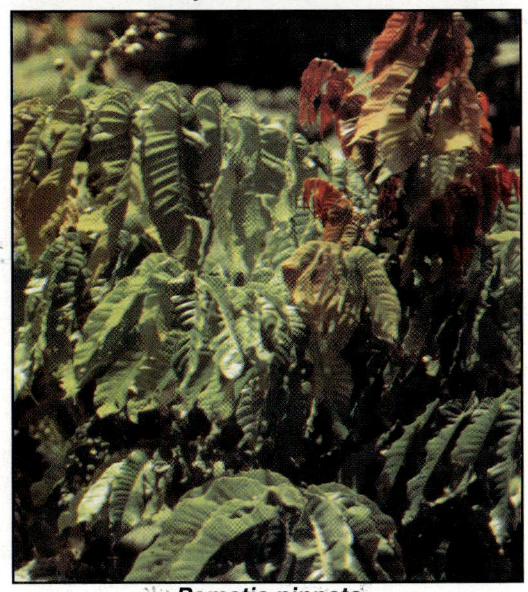

Pometia pinnata

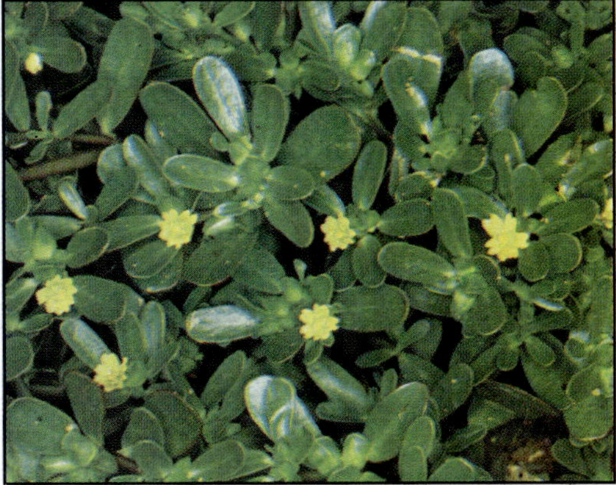

Portulaca oleracea

PLATE : 104

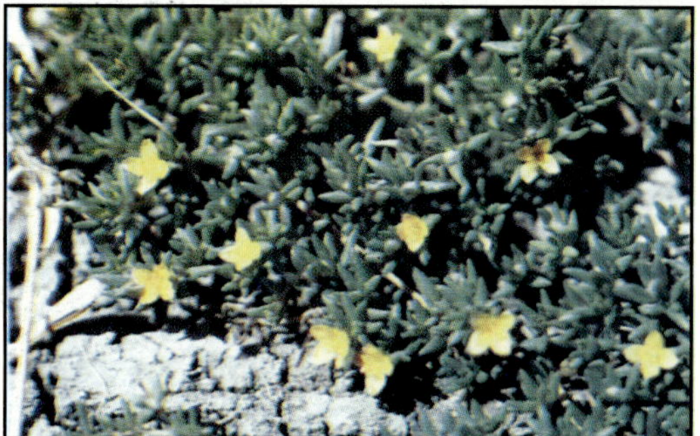
Portulaca quadrifida

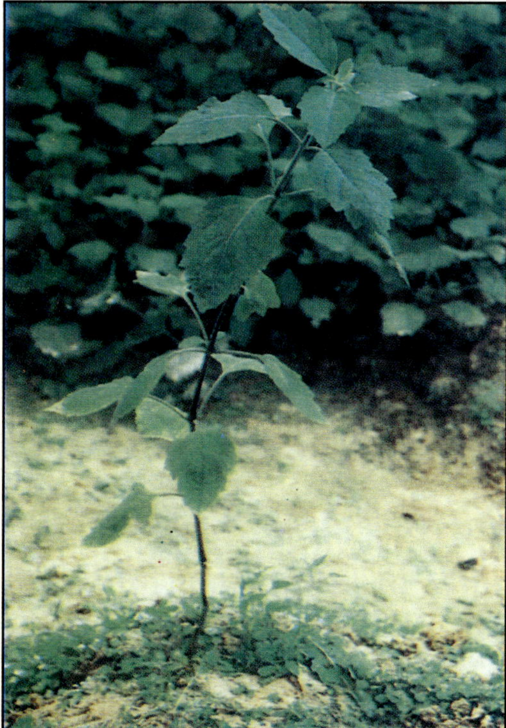
Posostemon cablin

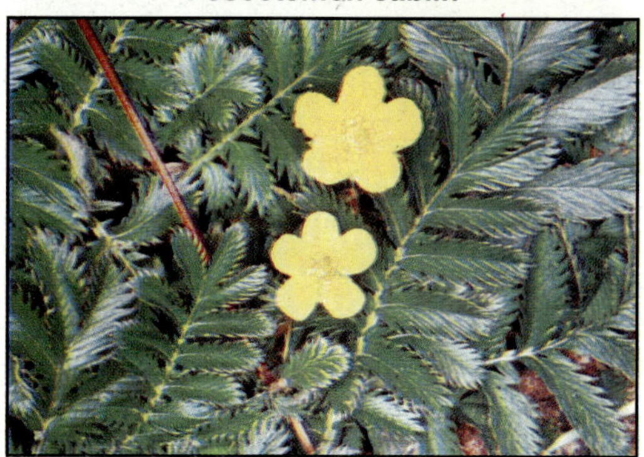
Potentilla anserina

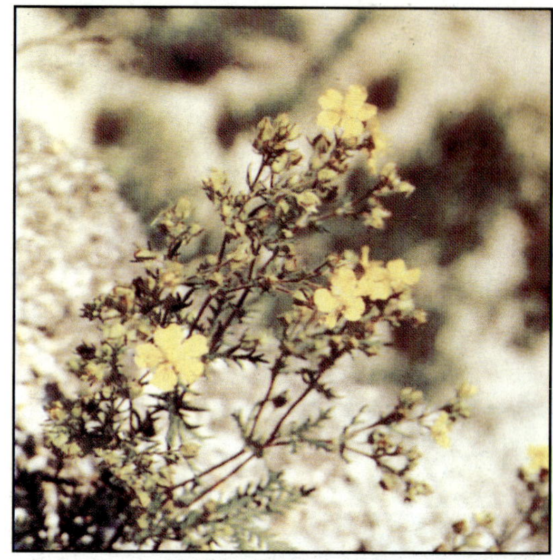
Potentilla chinensis

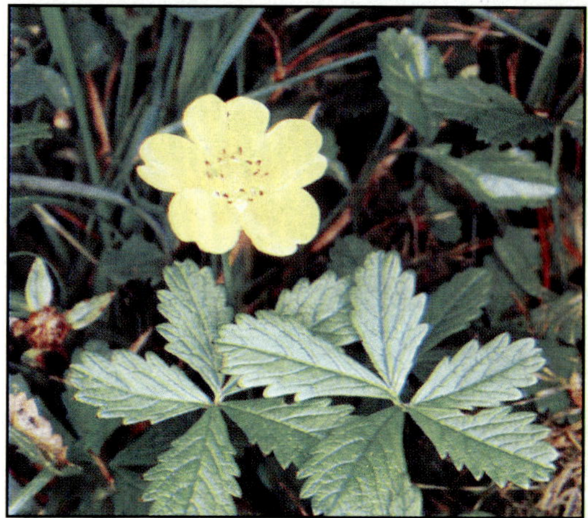
Potentilla reptans

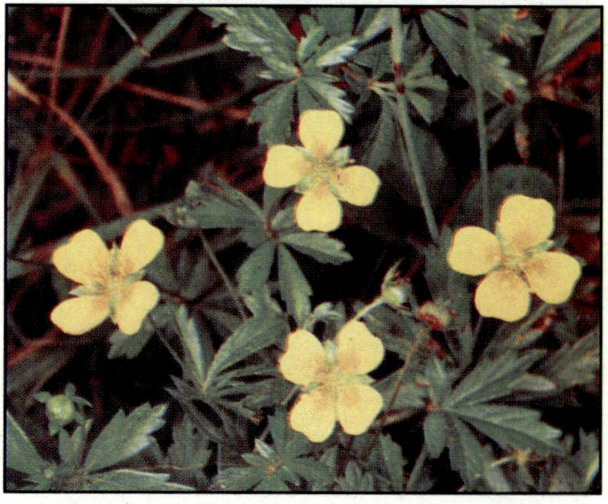
Potentilla tormentilla

PLATE : 105

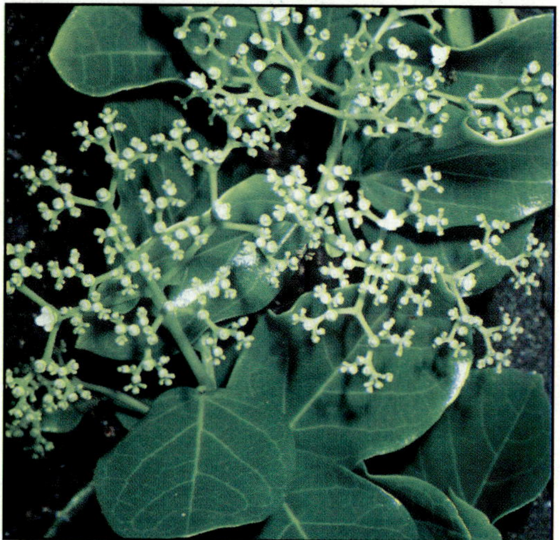

Premna serratifolia

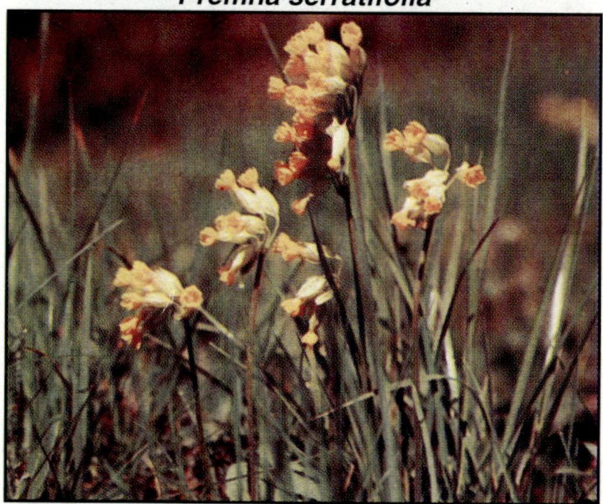

Primula veris

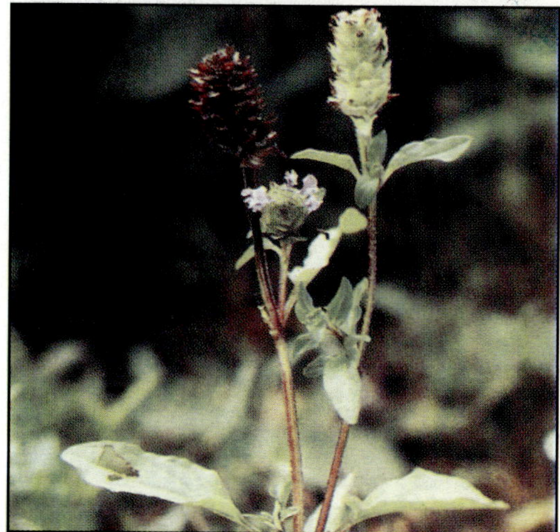

Prunella vulgaris

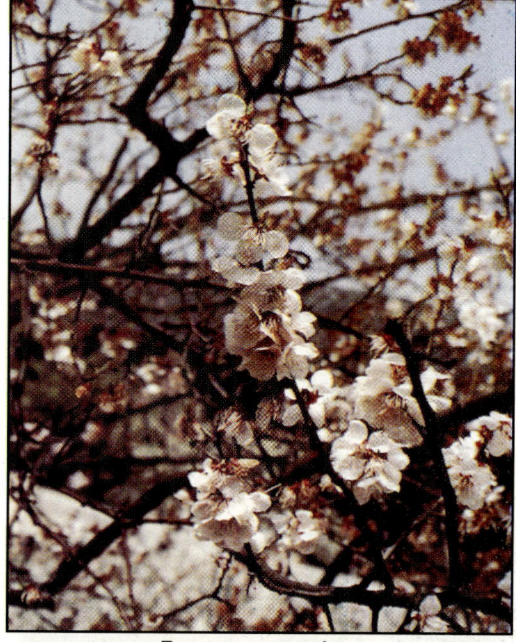

Prunus armeniaca

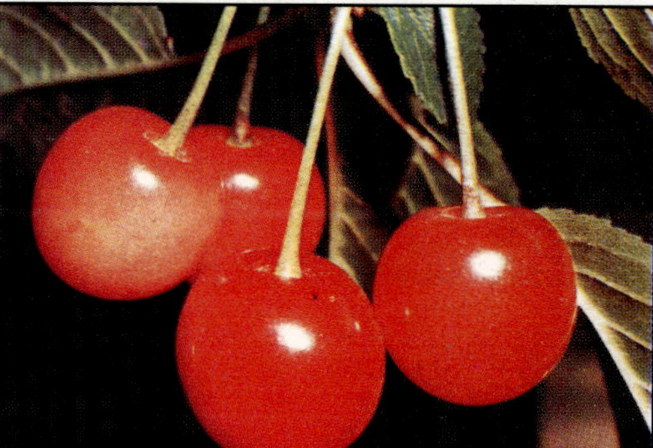

Prunus avium

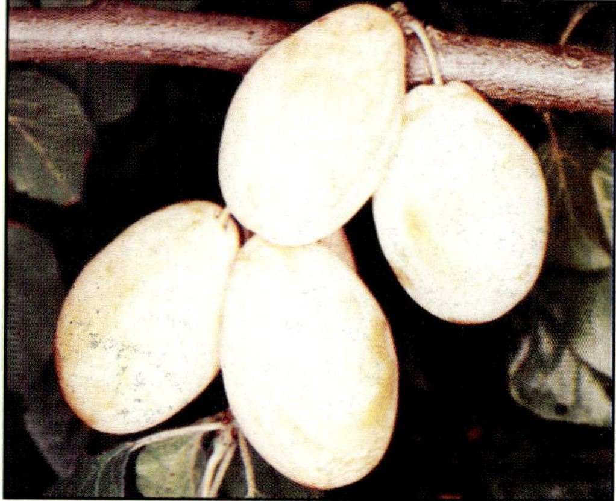

Prunus domestica

PLATE : 106

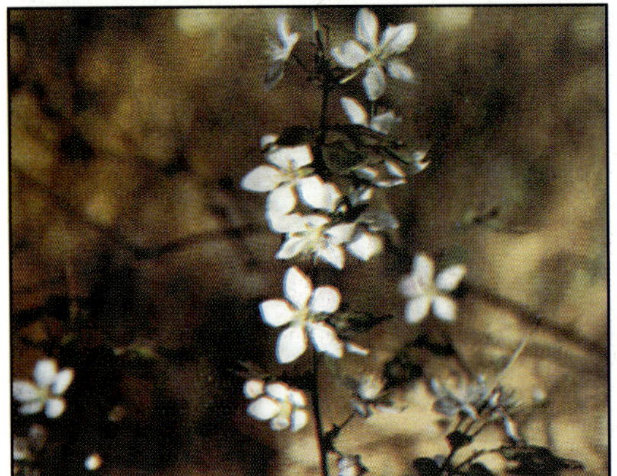

Prunus japonica

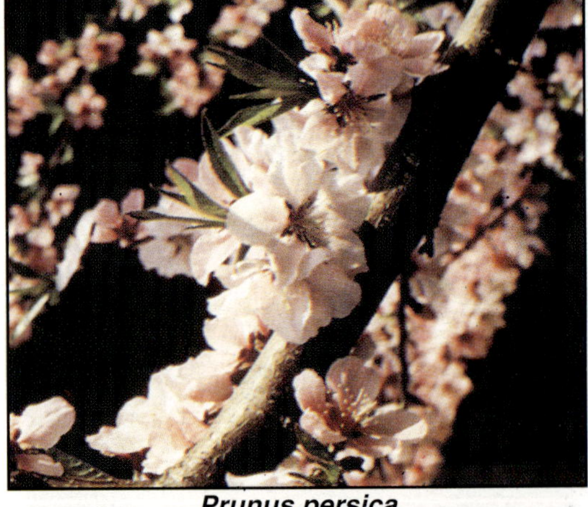

Prunus persica

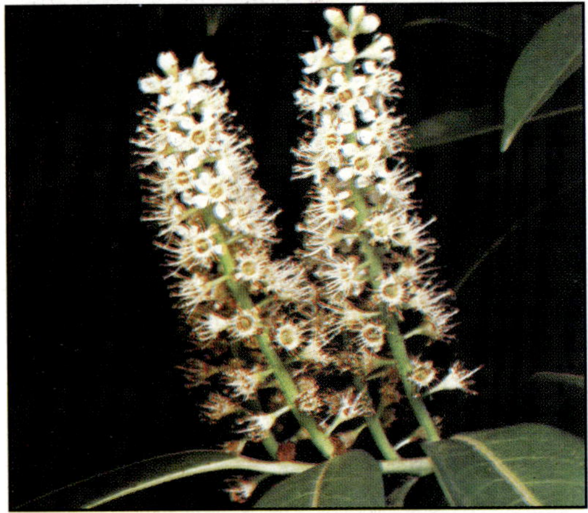

Prunus laurocerasus

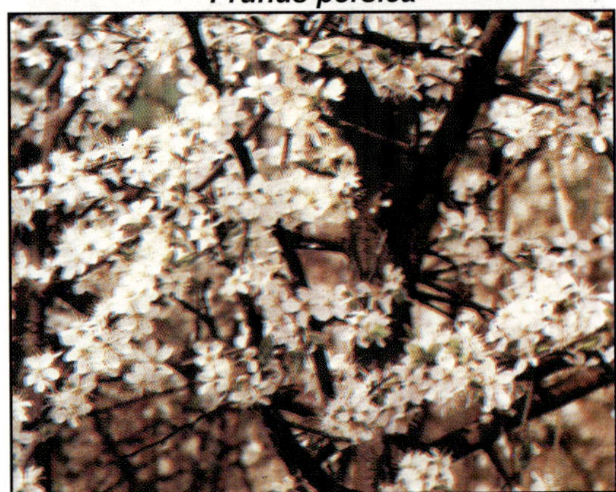

Prunus spinosa

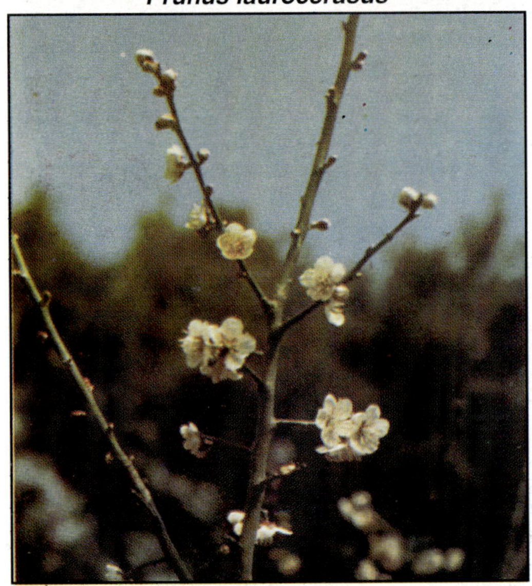

Prunus mume

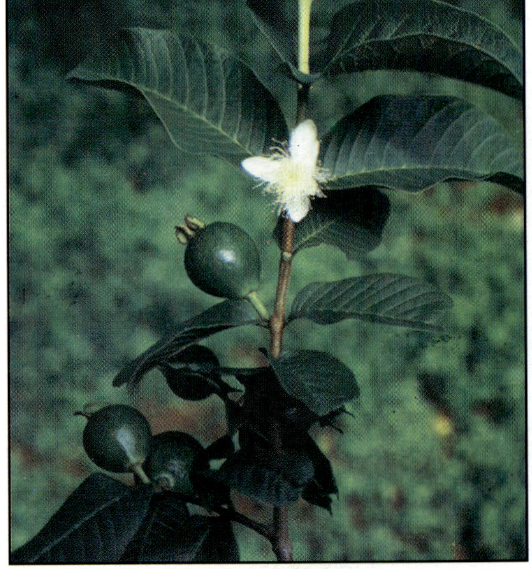

Psidium guajava

PLATE : 107

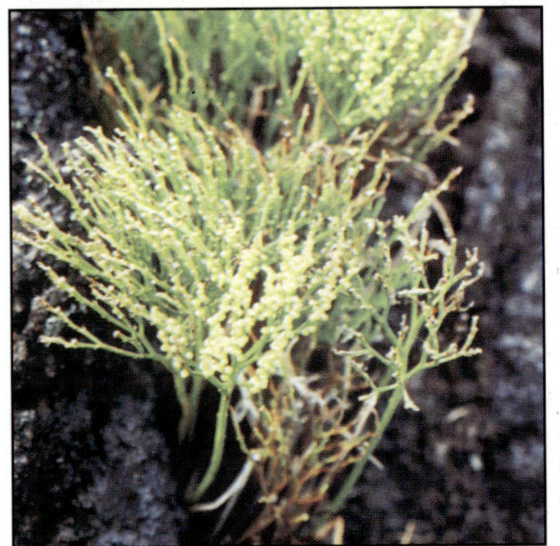

Psilotum nudum

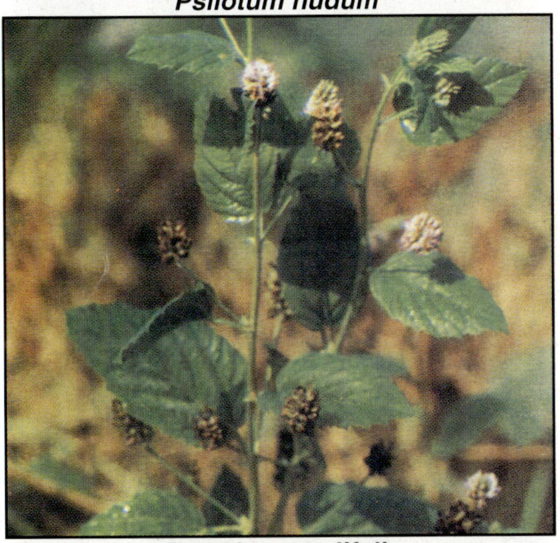

Psoralea corylifolia

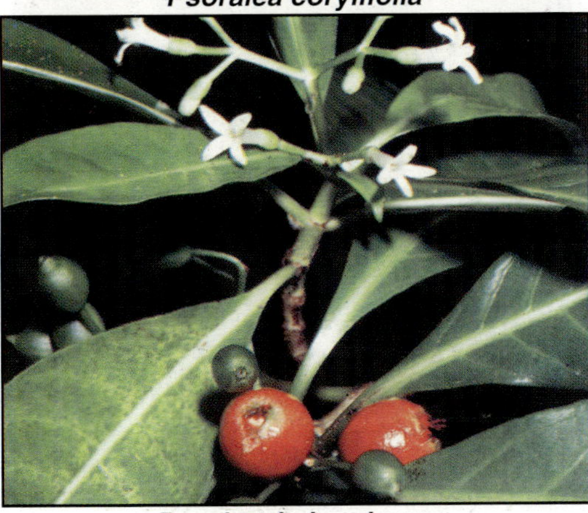

Psychotria insularum

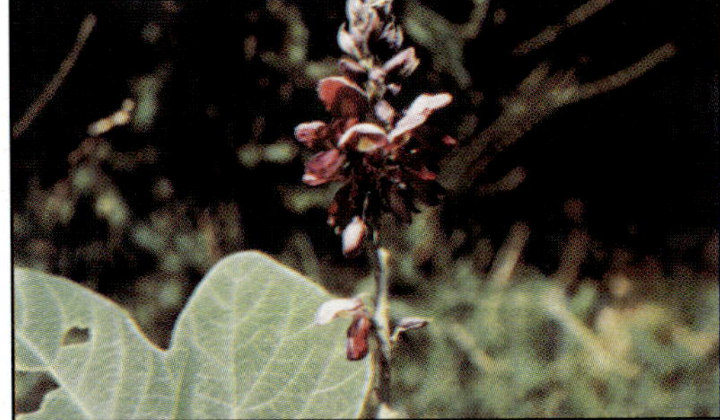

Pueraria lobata

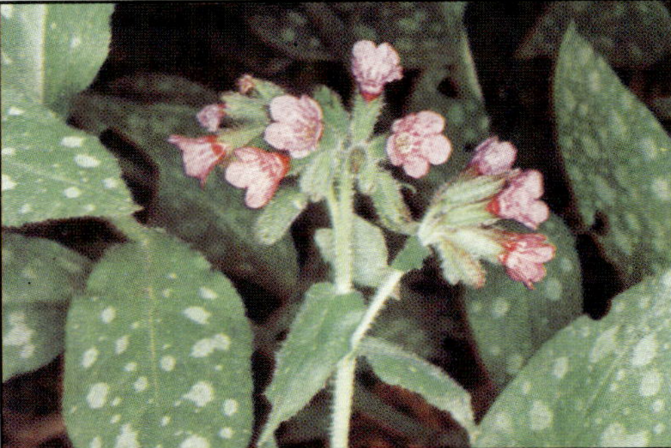

Pulmonaria officinalis

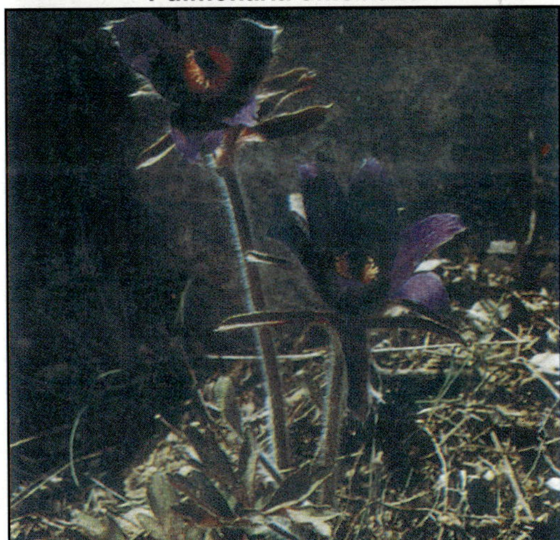

Pulsatilla chinensis

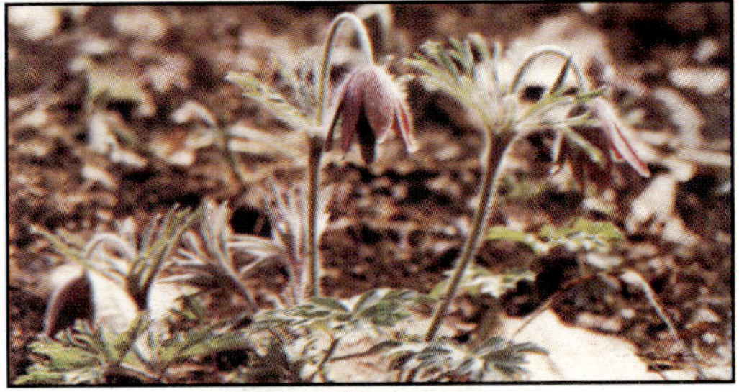

Pulsatilla koreana

PLATE : 108

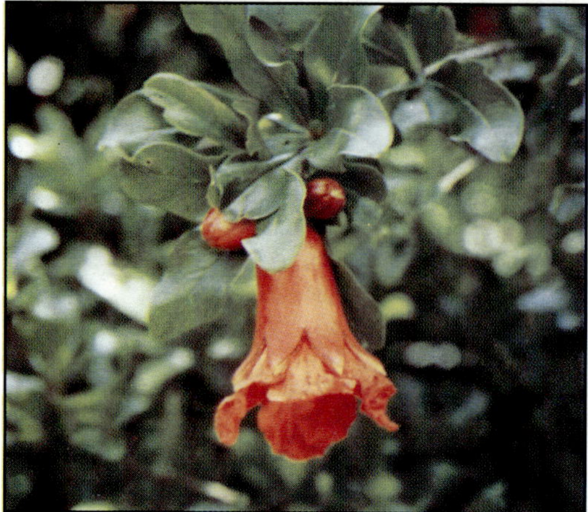

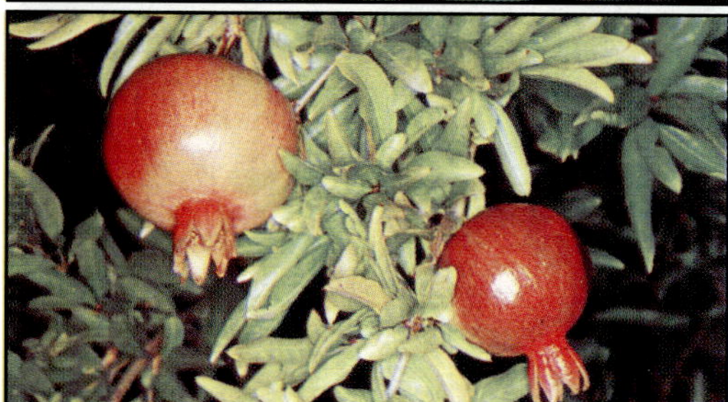

Punica granatum

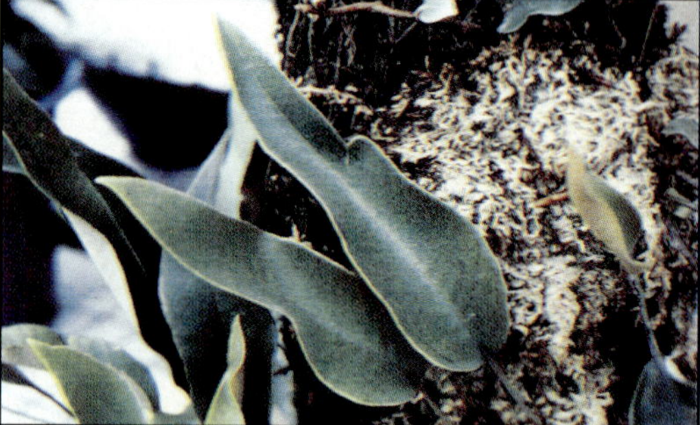

Pyrrosia lingua

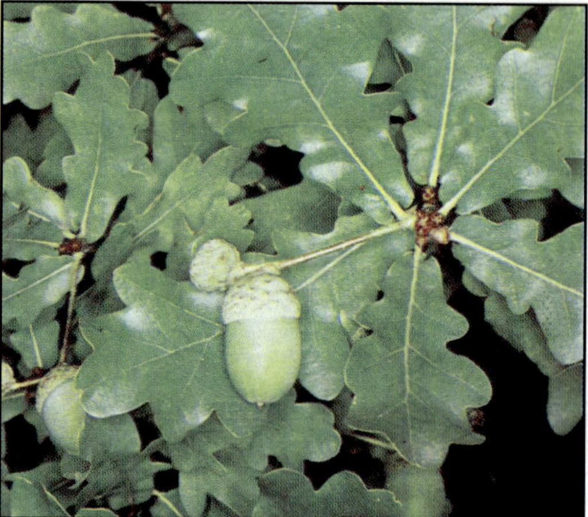

Quercus robur

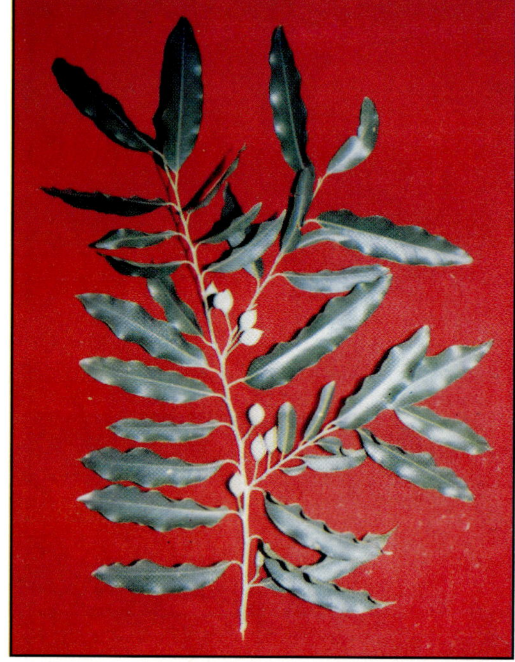

Putranjiva roxburghii

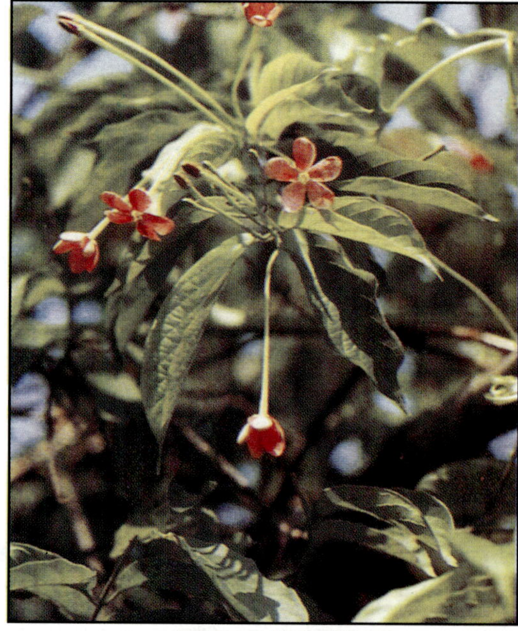

Quisquqlis indica

PLATE : 109

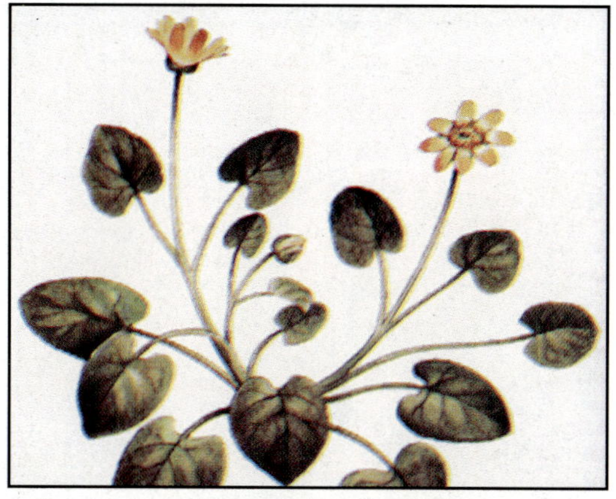

Ranunculus ficaria

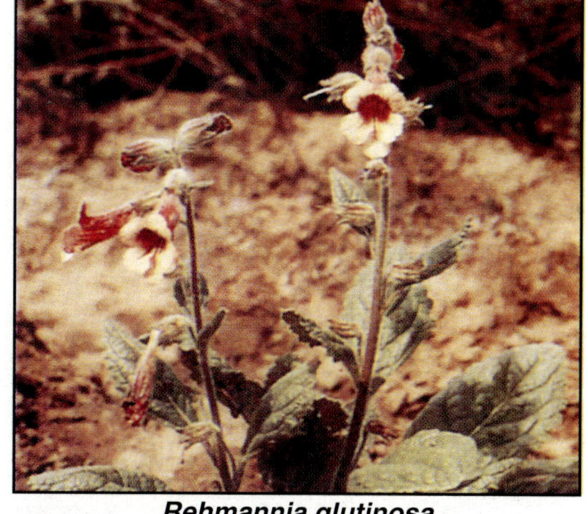

Rehmannia glutinosa

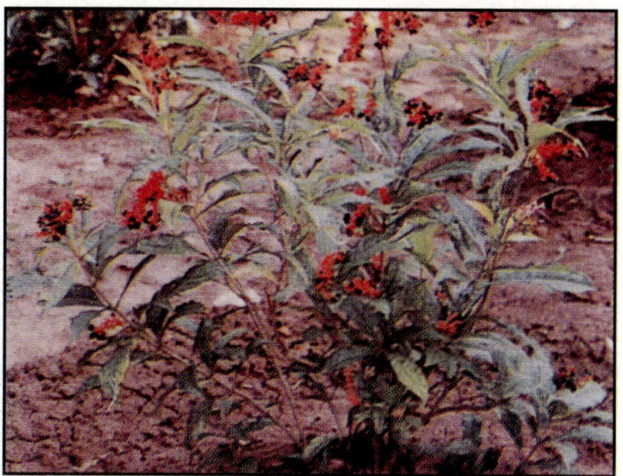

Rauwolfia serpentina Benth

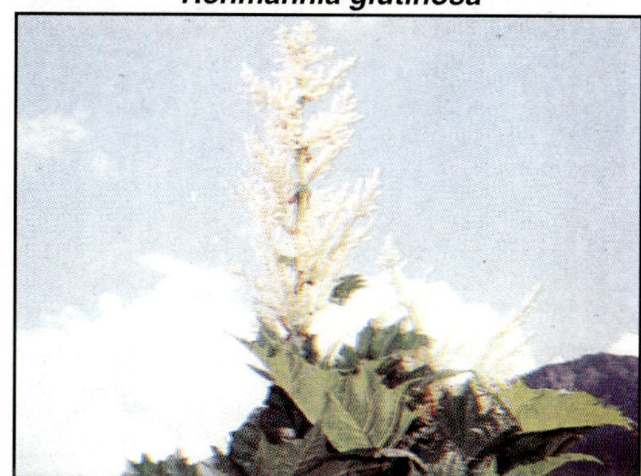

Rheum palmatum

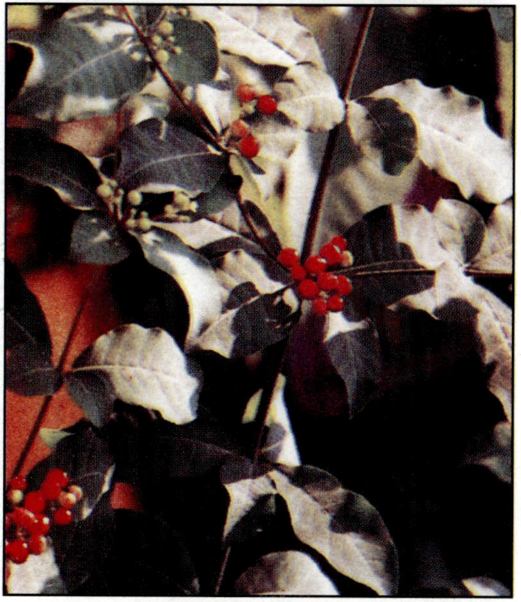

Rauwolfia tetrafela

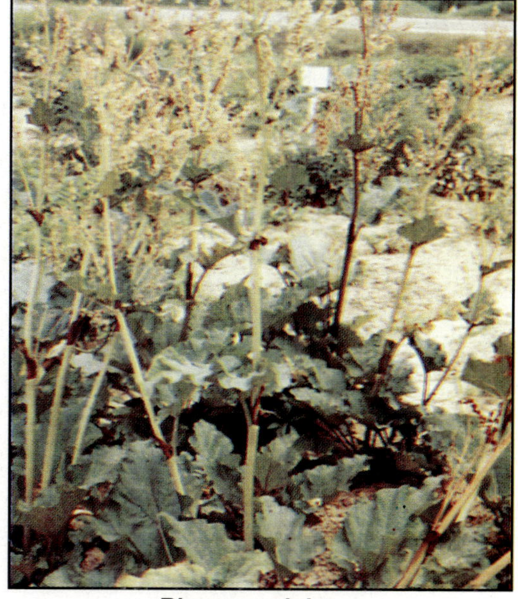

Rheum undulatum

PLATE : 110

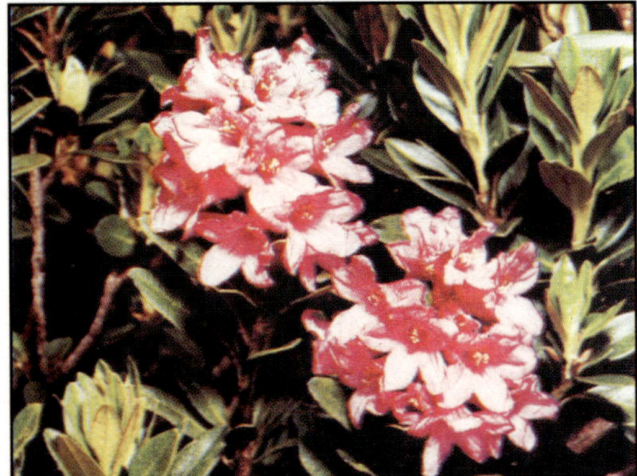

Rhododendron ferrugineum

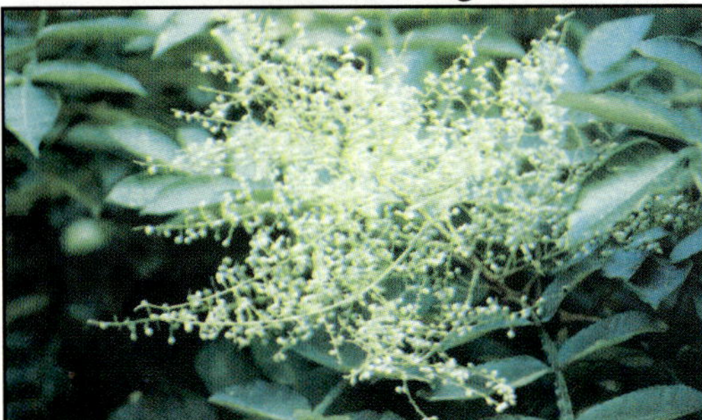

Rhus chinensis

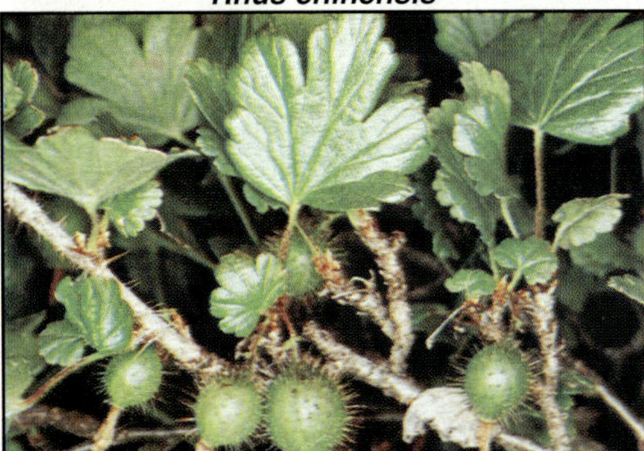

Ribes grossularia

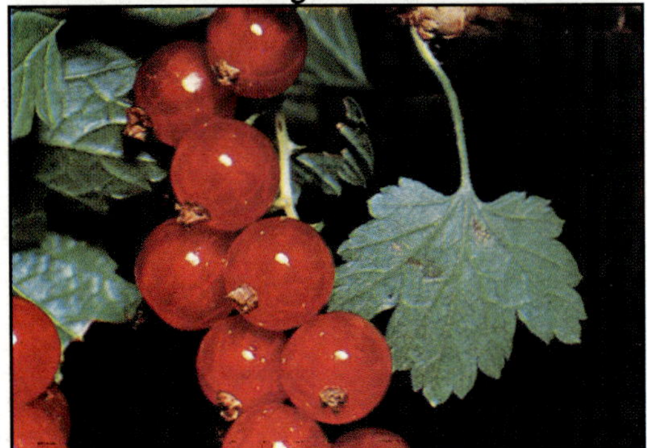

Ribes rubrum

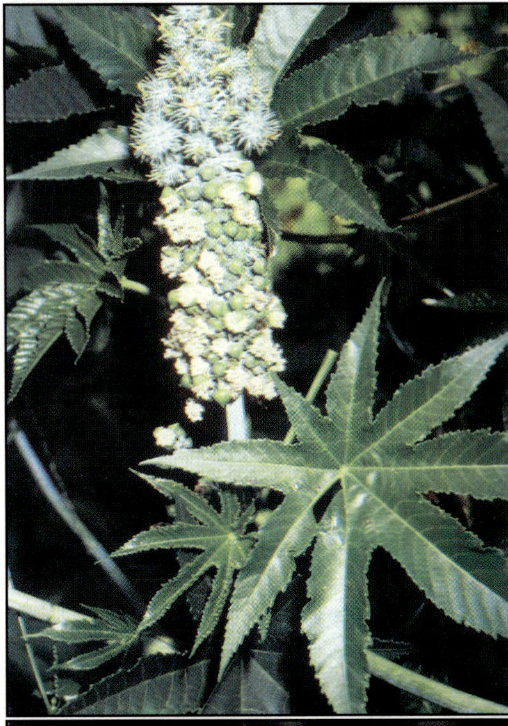

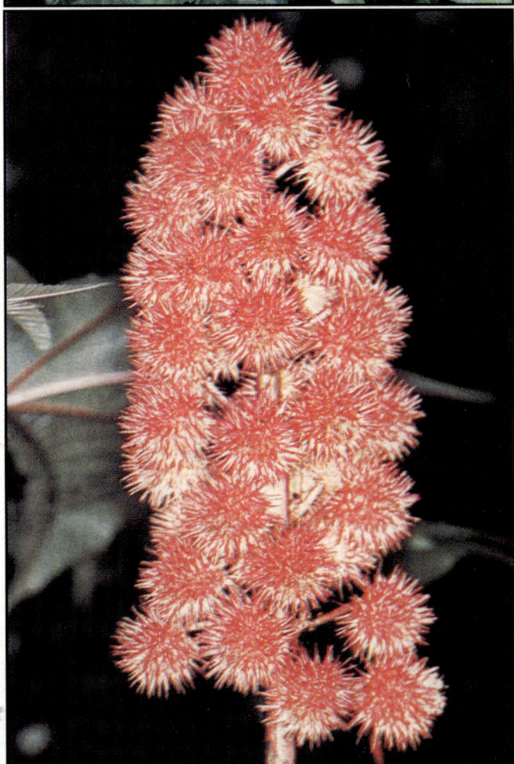

Ricinus communis

PLATE : 111

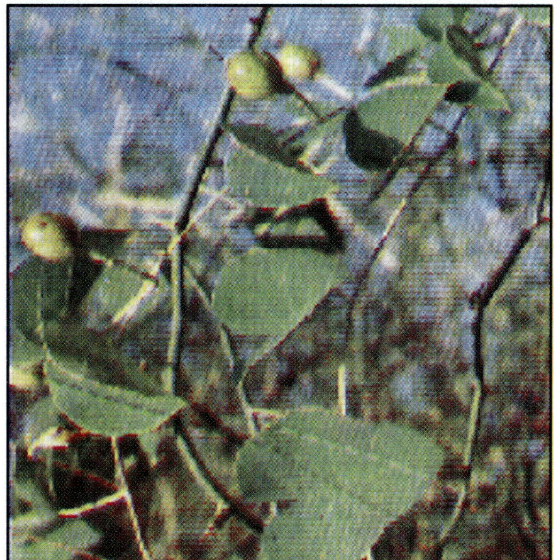
Rivea hypocrateriformis

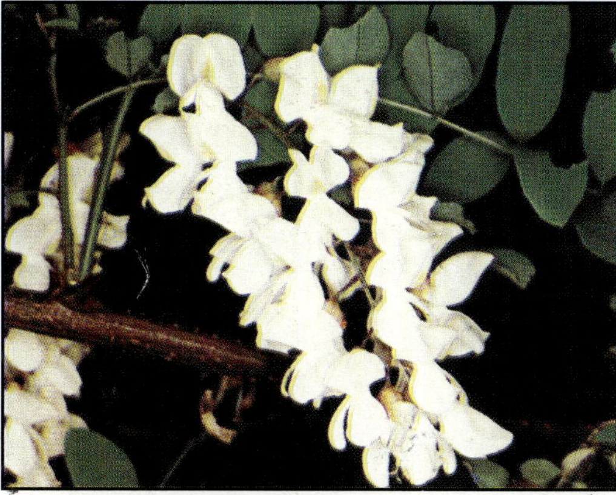
Robinia pseudacacia

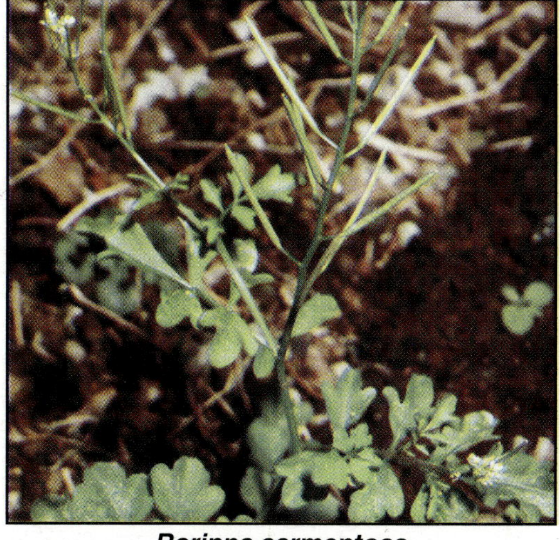
Rorippa sarmentosa

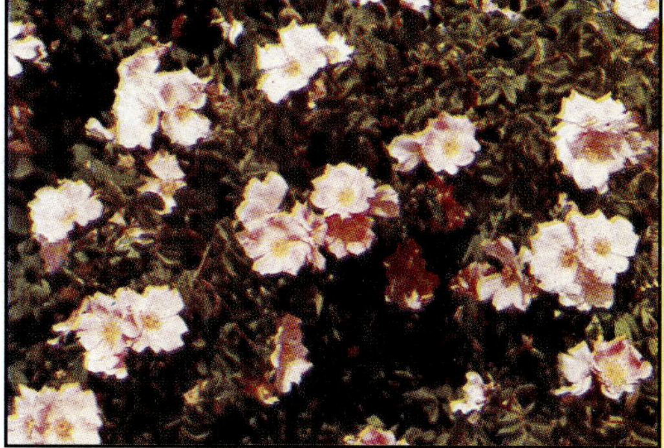
Rosa canina

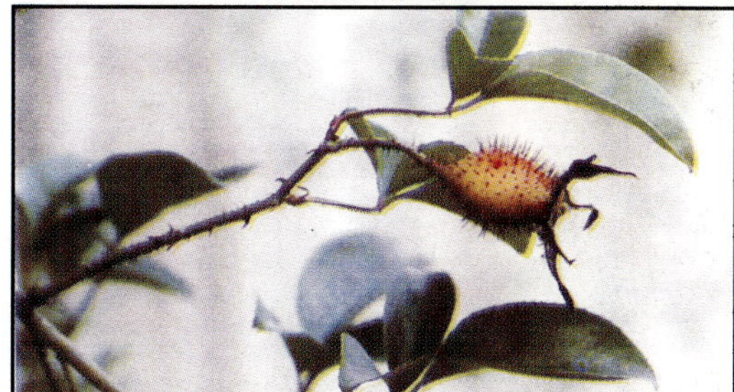
Rosa laevigata

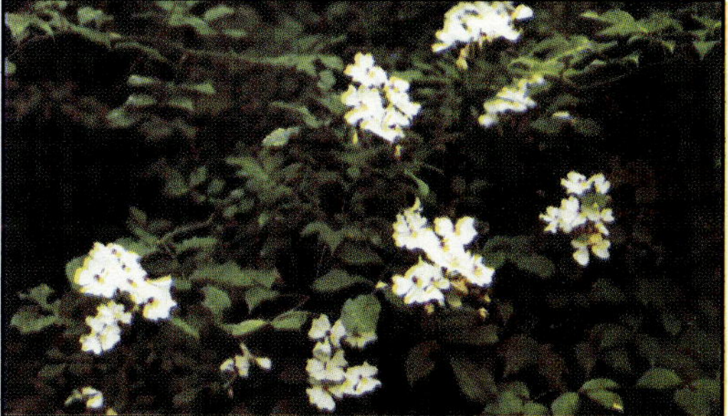
Rosa multiflora

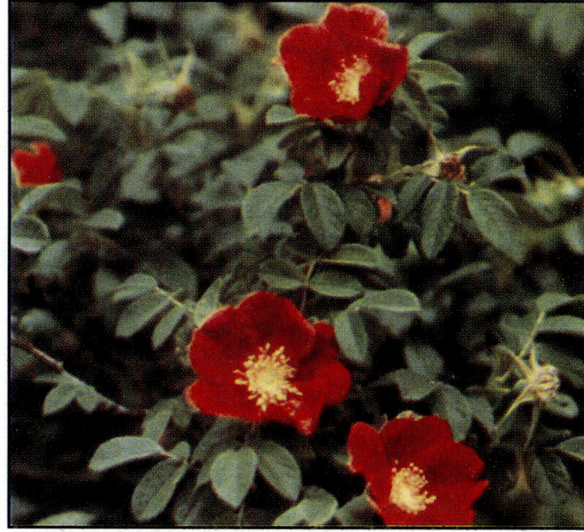
Rosa rugosa

PLATE : 112

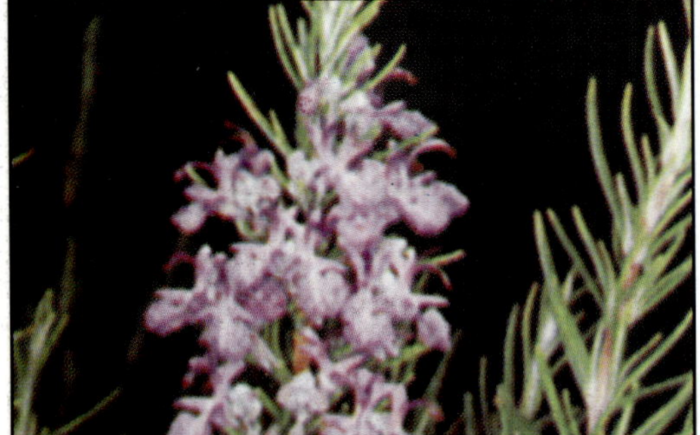

Rosmarinus officinalis

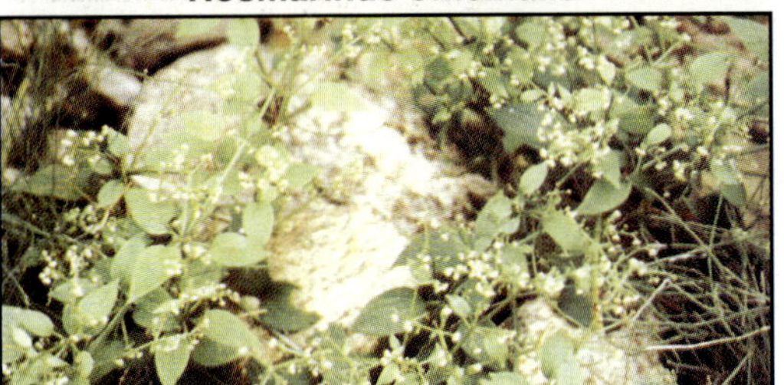

Rubia akane

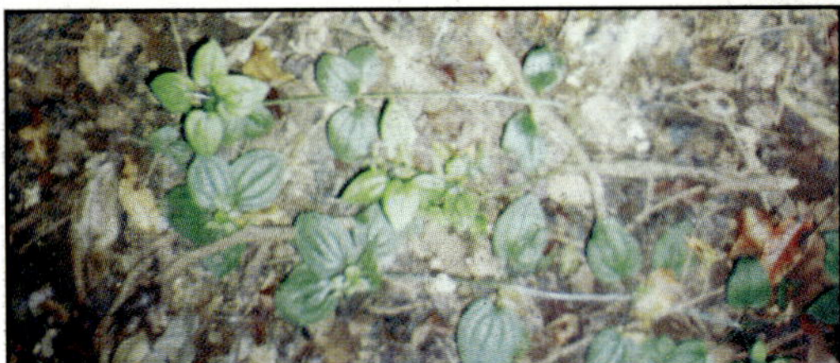

Rubia cordifolia

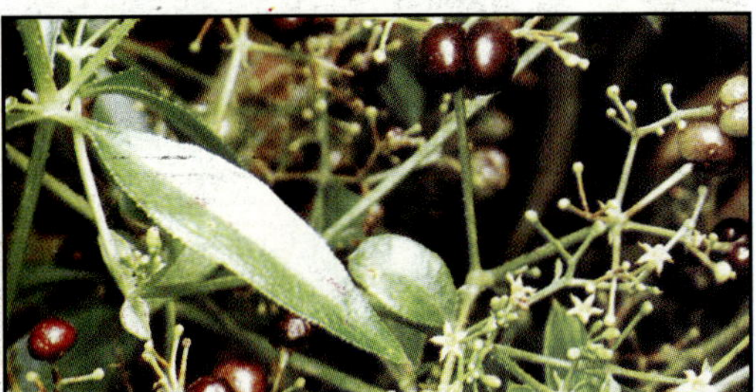

Rubia tinctorum

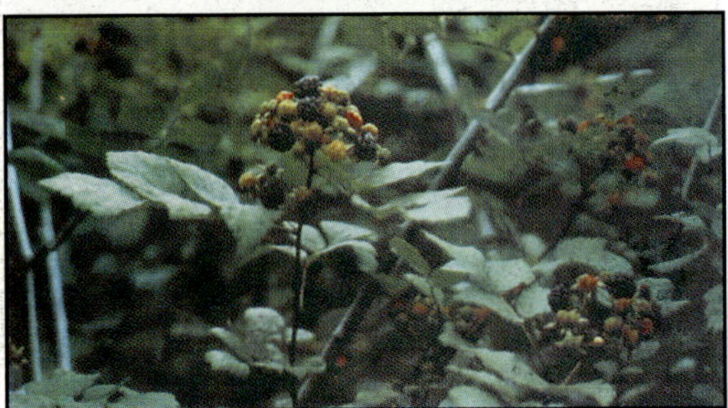

Rubus coreanus

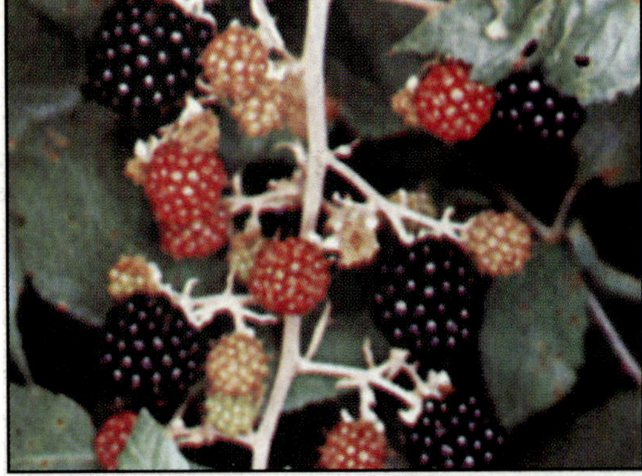

Rubus fruticosus

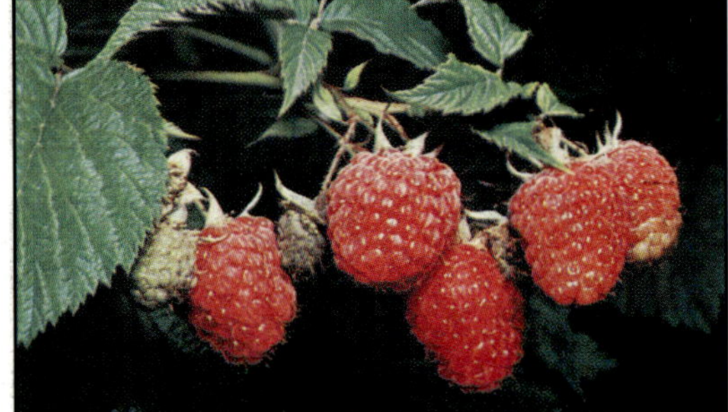

Rubus idaeus

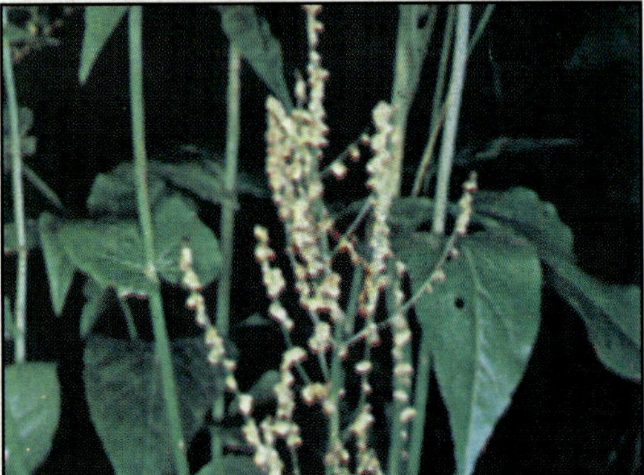

Rumex acetosella

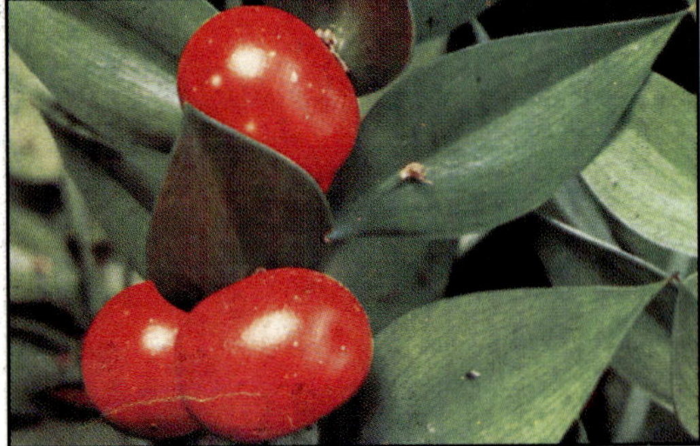

Ruscus actuleatus

PLATE : 113

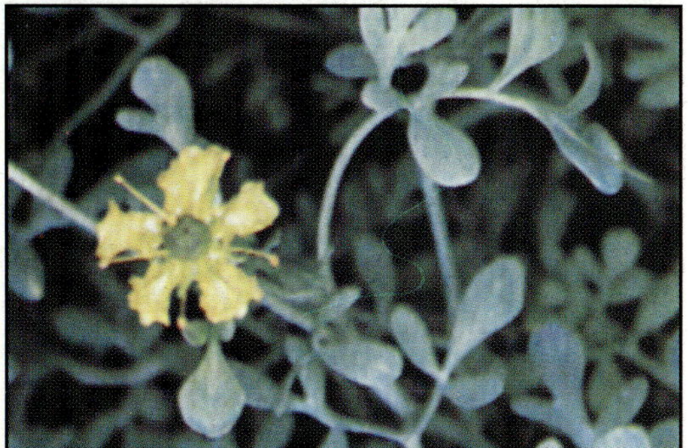
Ruta graveolens

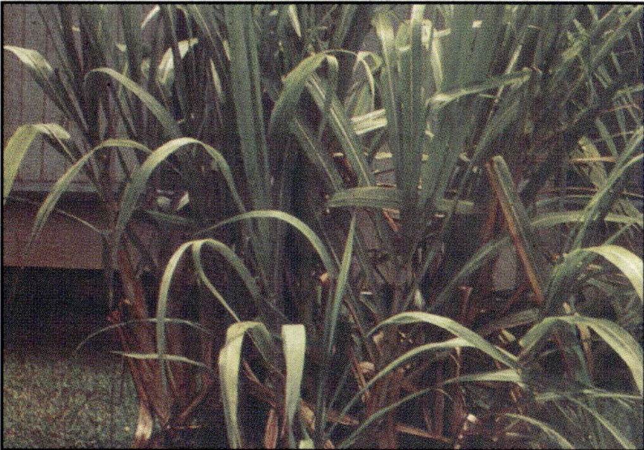
Saccharum officinarum

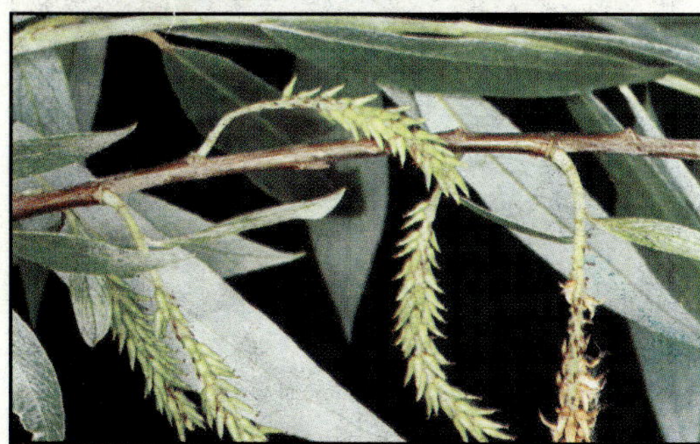
Salix alba

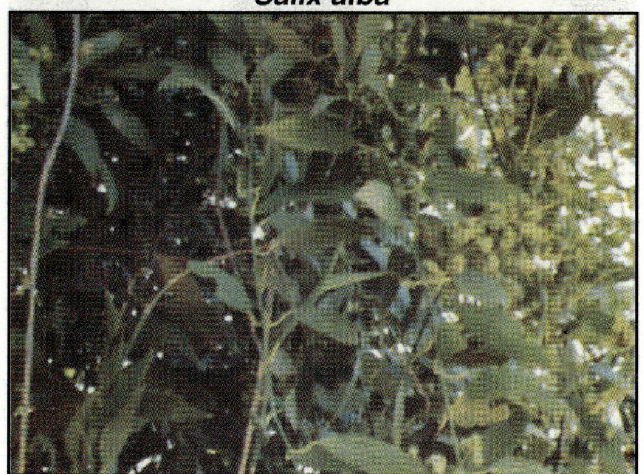
salvadora persica

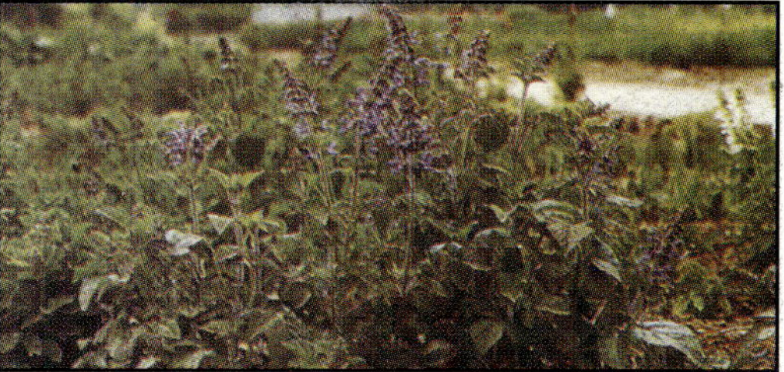
Salvia miltiorrhiza

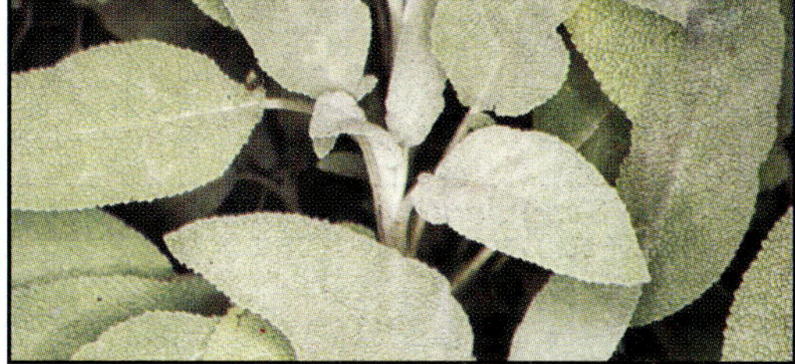
Salvia officinalis

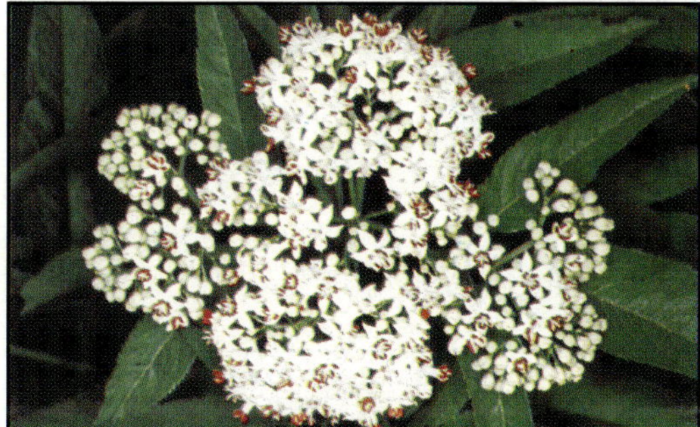
Sambucus ebulus

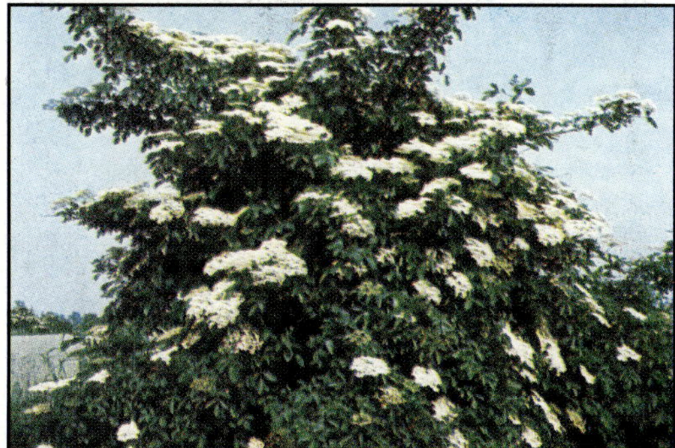
Sambucus nigra

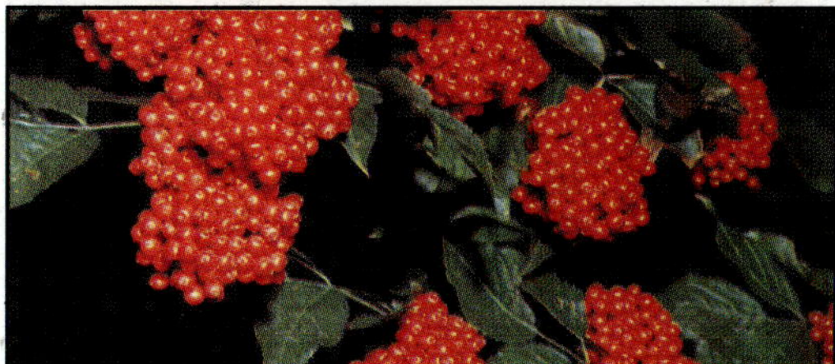
Sambucus racemosa

PLATE : 114

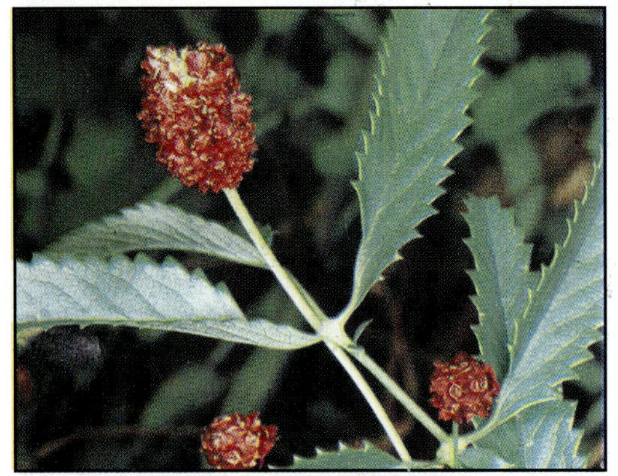
Sanguisorba officinalis

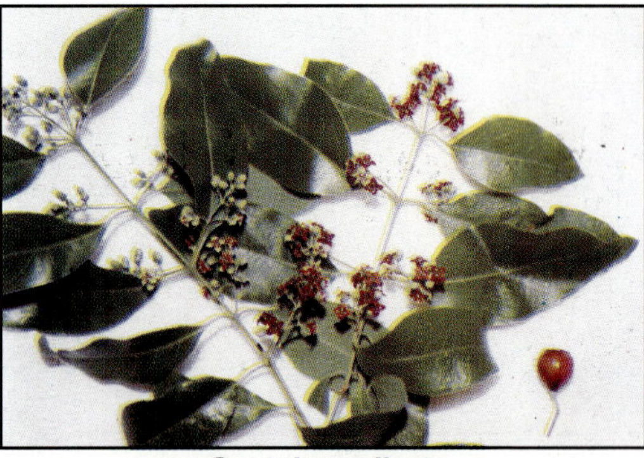
Santalum album

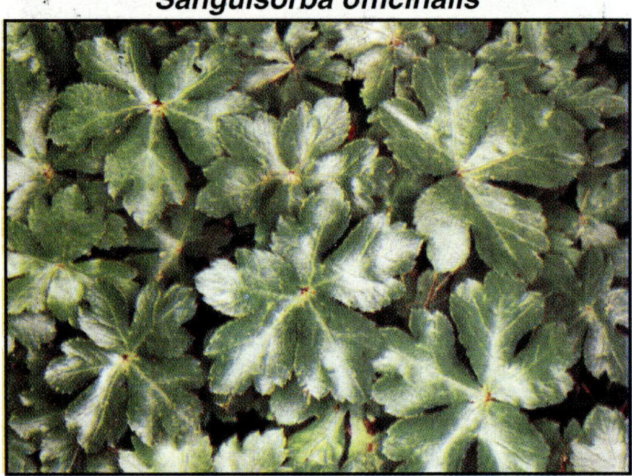
Sanicula europaea

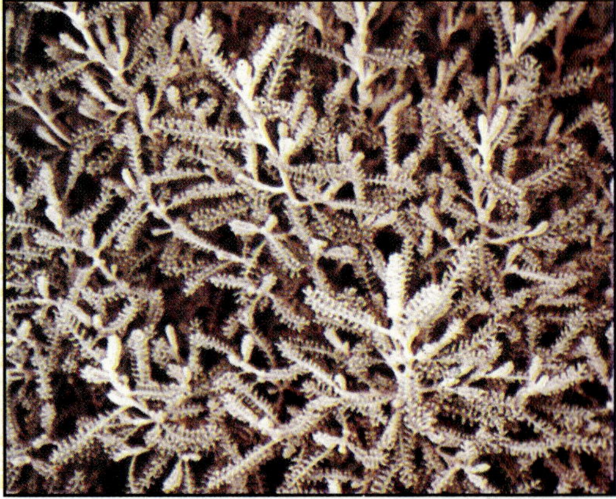
Santolina chamaecyparissus

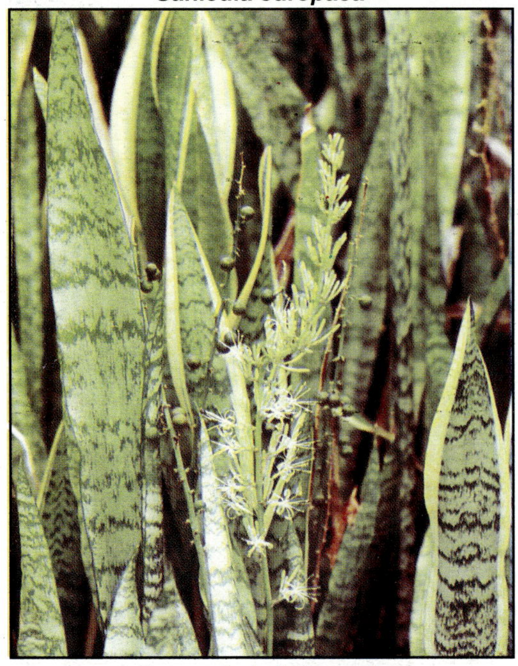
Sansevieria trifasciata

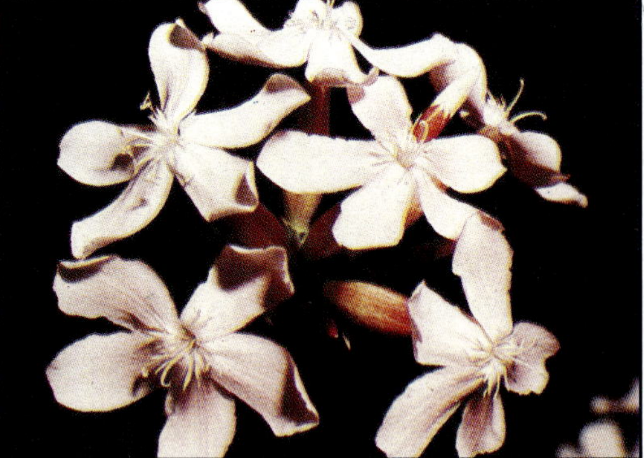
Saponaria officinalis

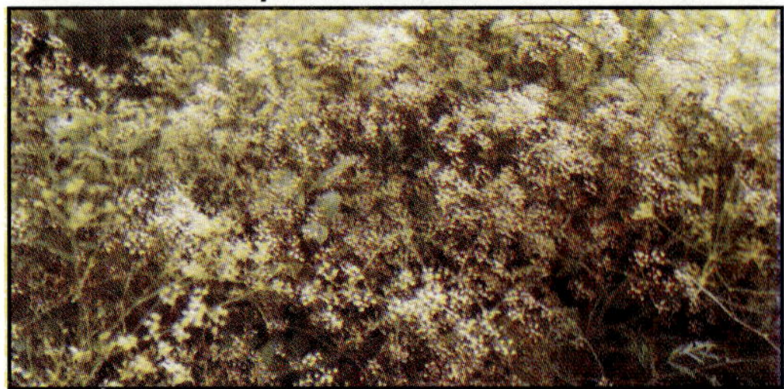
Saposhnikovia divaricata

PLATE : 115

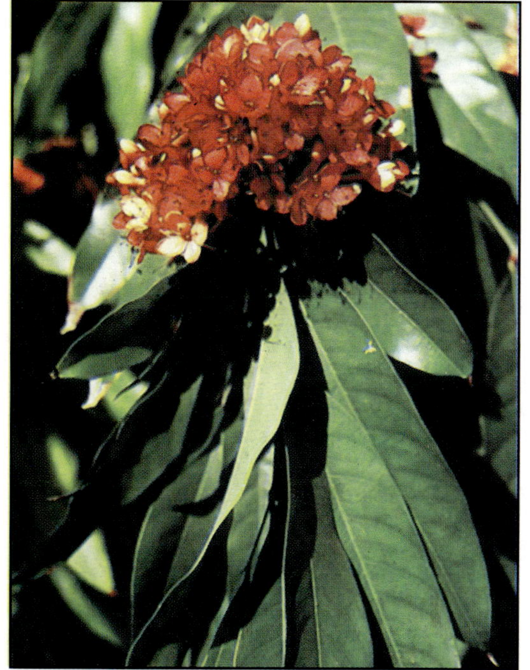

Saraca asoka

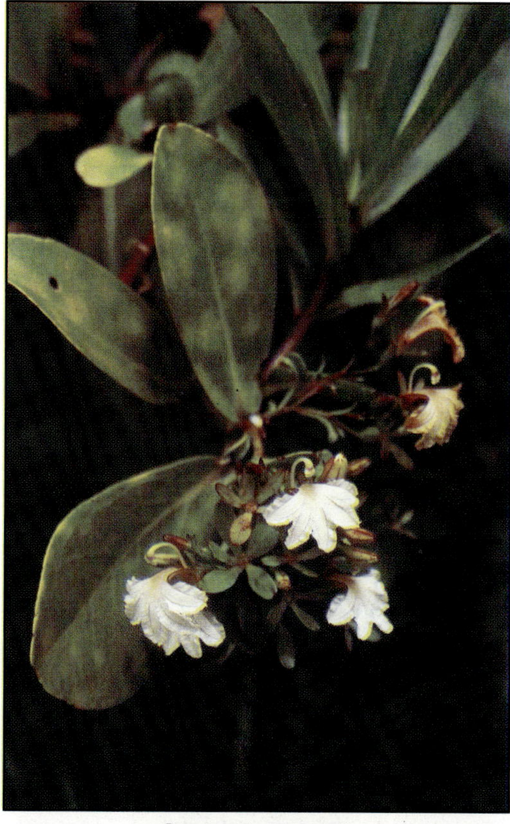

Scaevola taccada

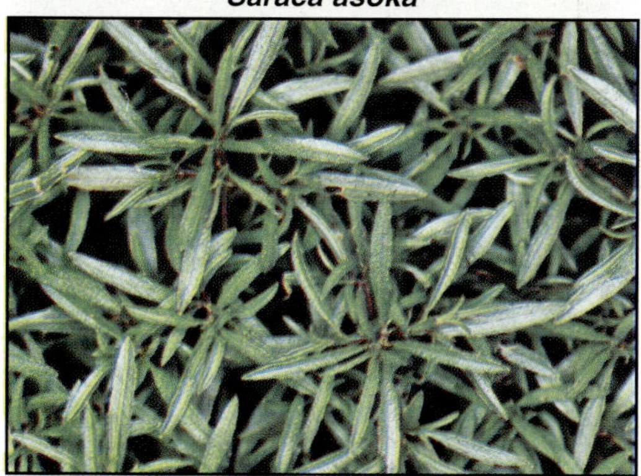

Satureja hortensis

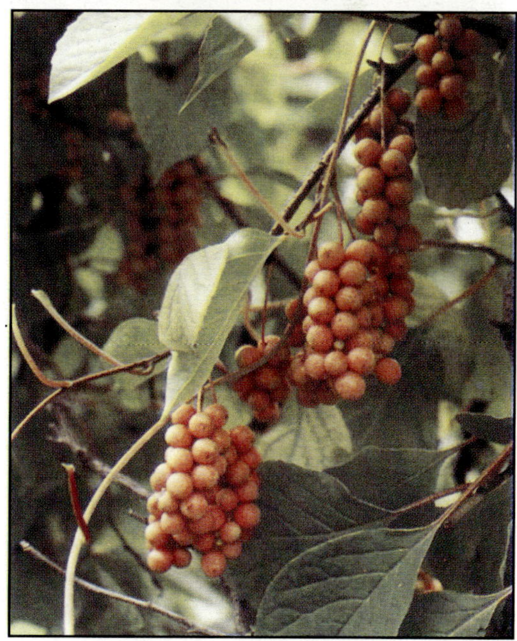

Schisandra chinensis

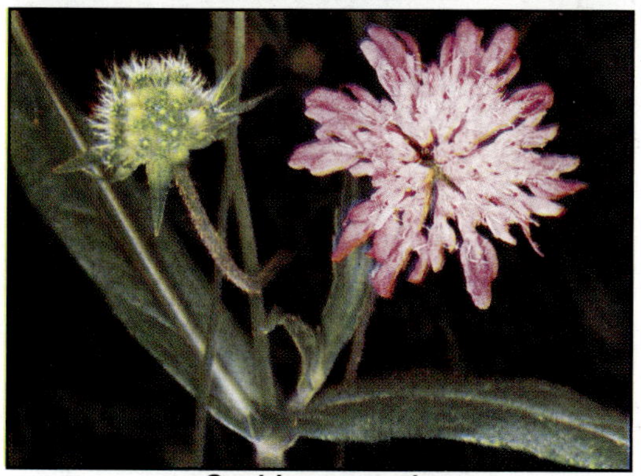

Scabiosa succisa

PLATE : 116

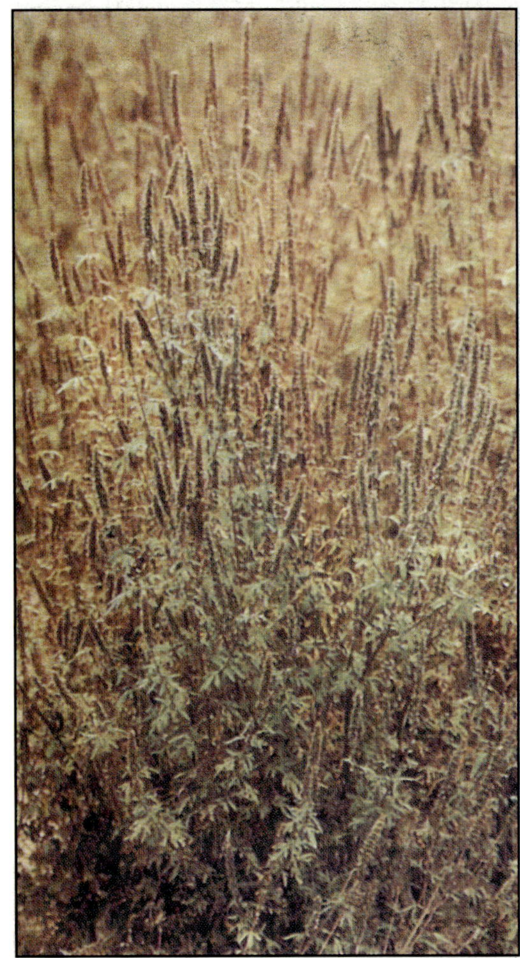

Schizonepeta tenuifolia

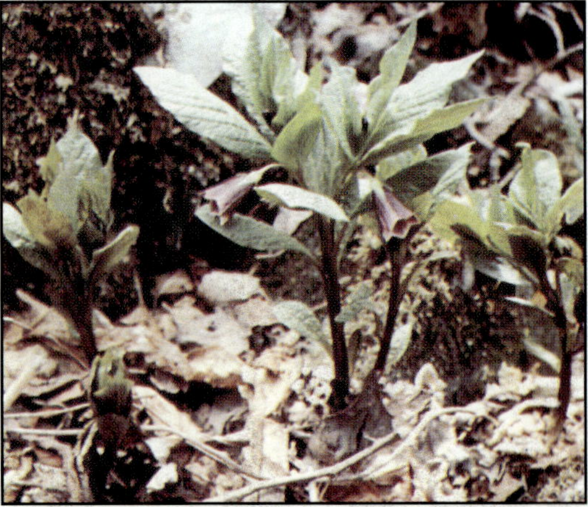

Scopolia japonica

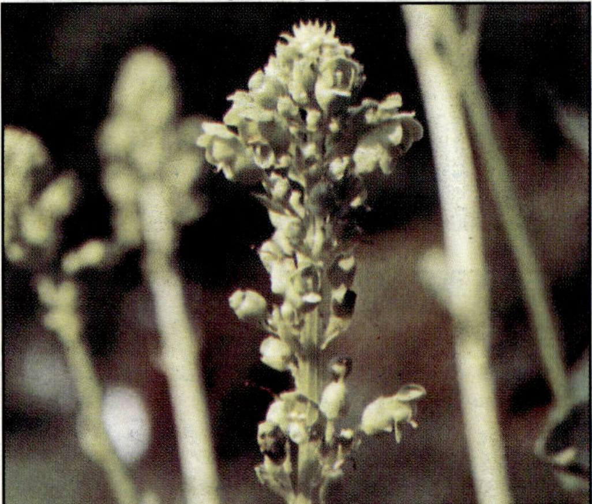

Scrophularia buergeriana

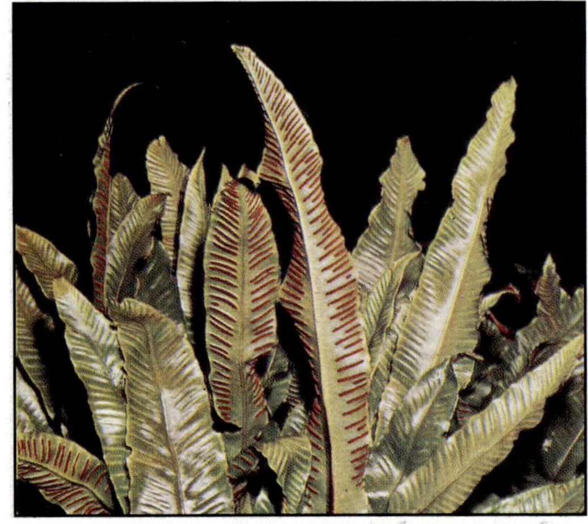

Scolopendrium officinale

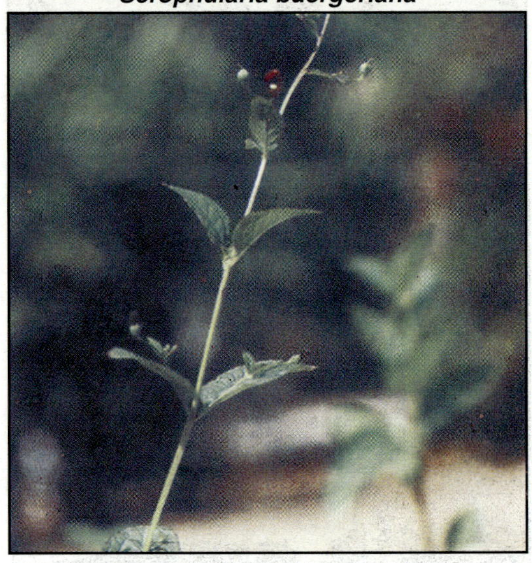

Scrophularia ningpoensis

PLATE : 117

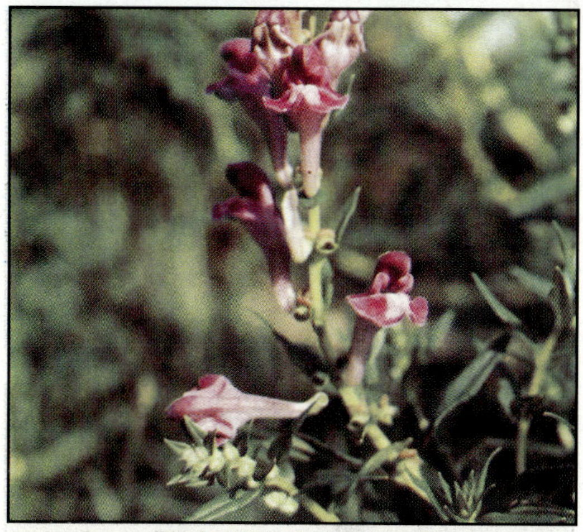

Scutellaria baicalensis

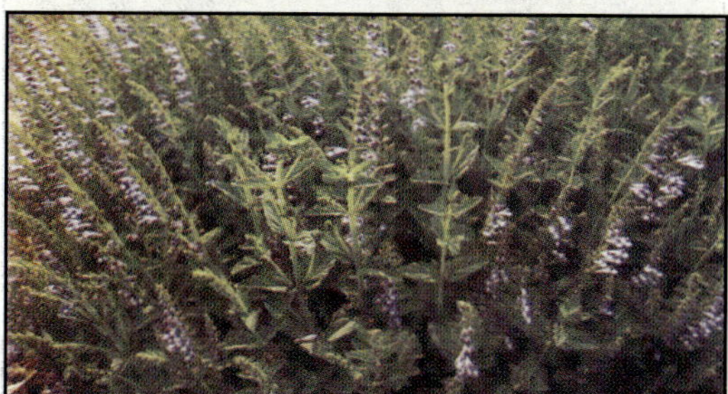

Scutellaria barbata

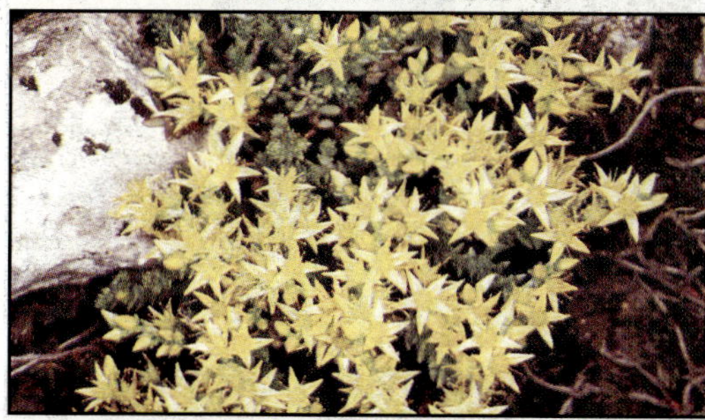

Sedum acre

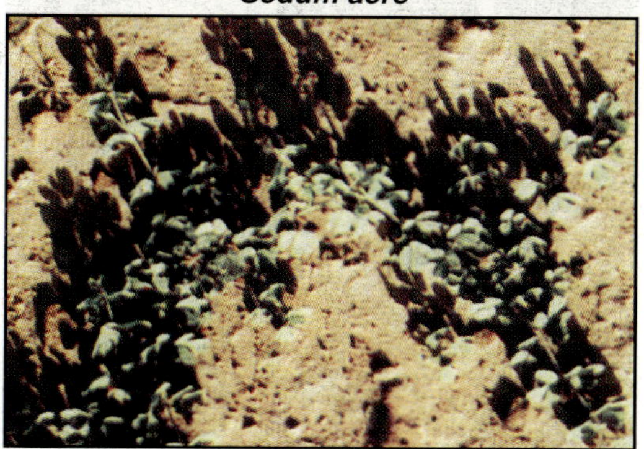

Seetzenia lanata

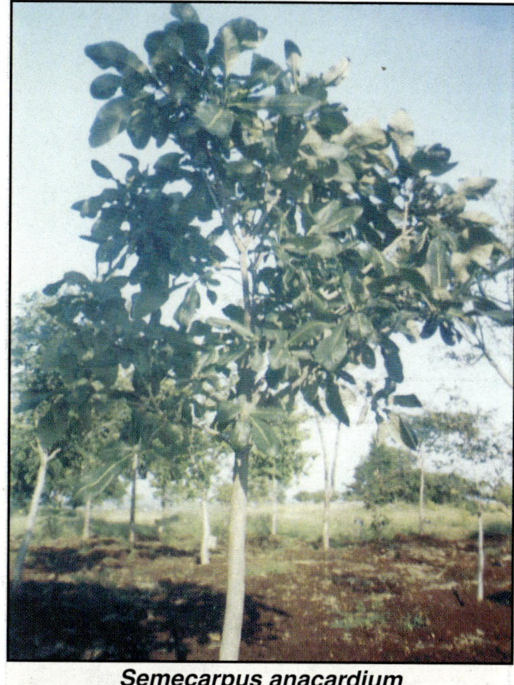

Semecarpus anacardium

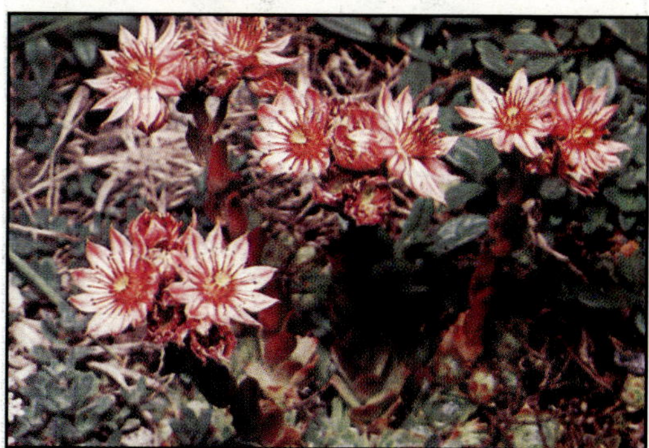

Sempervivum arachnoideum

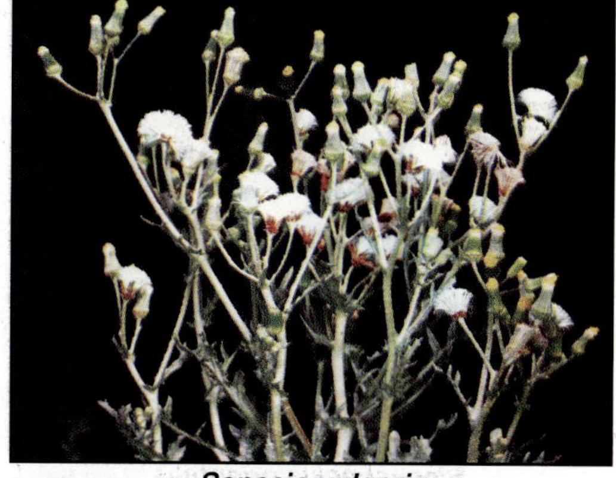

Senecio vulgaris

PLATE : 118

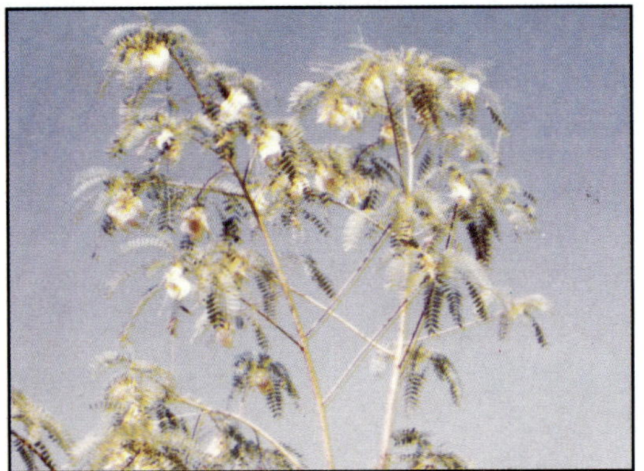

Sesbania grandiflora

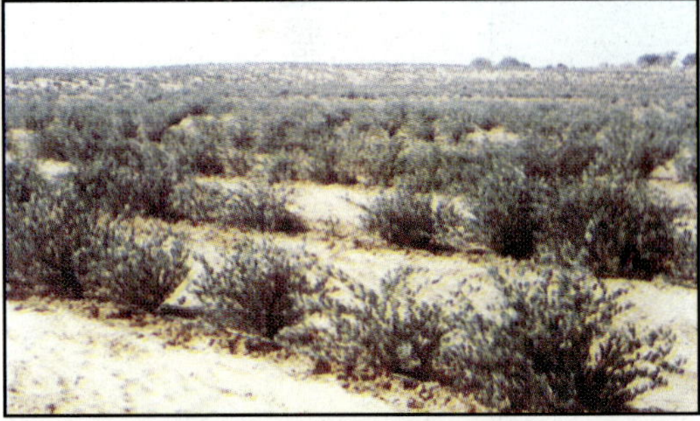

Simmondsia chinensis

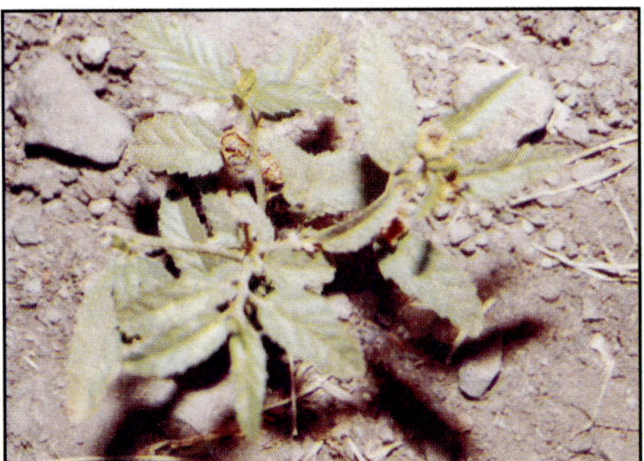

Sida cordifolia

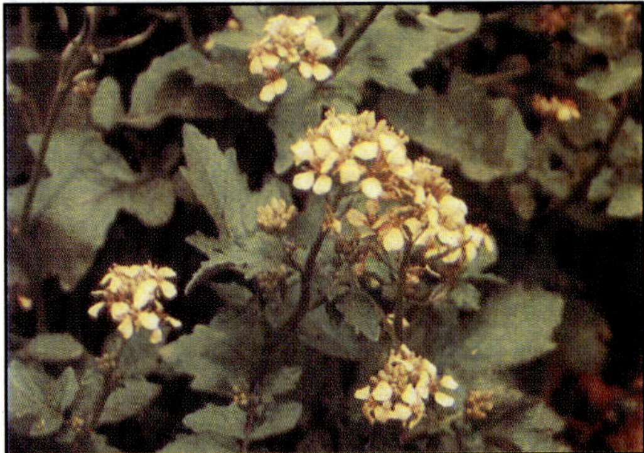

Sinapis alba

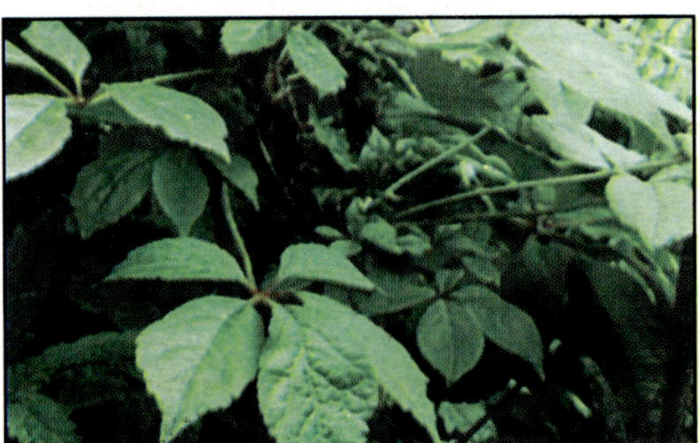

Siberian ginseng

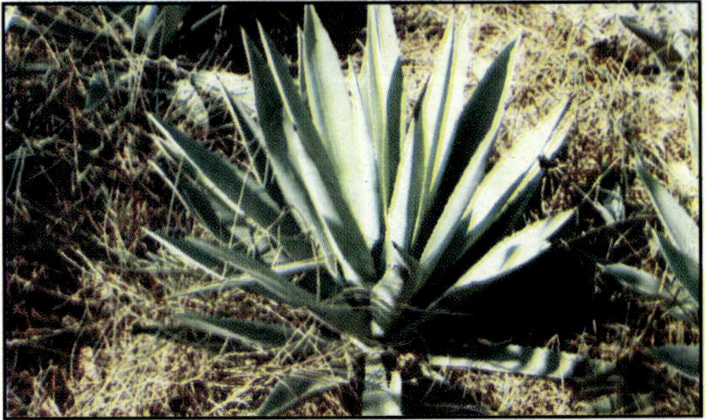

Sisal sislana

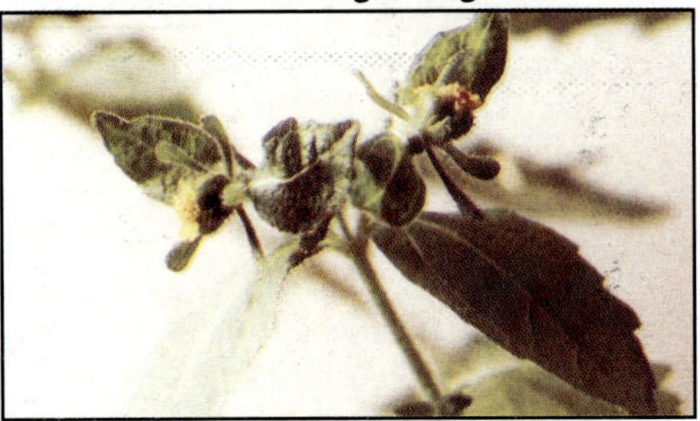

Siegesbeckia orientalis

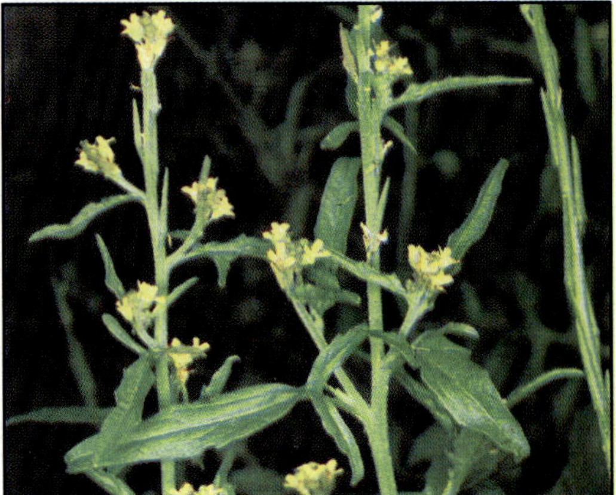

Sisymbrium officinale

PLATE : 119

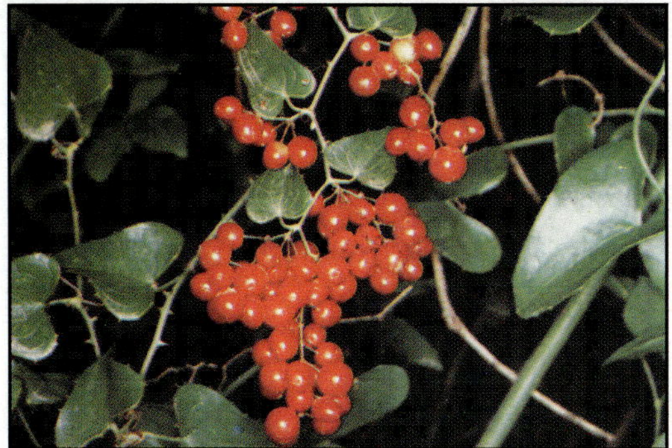
Smilax aspera

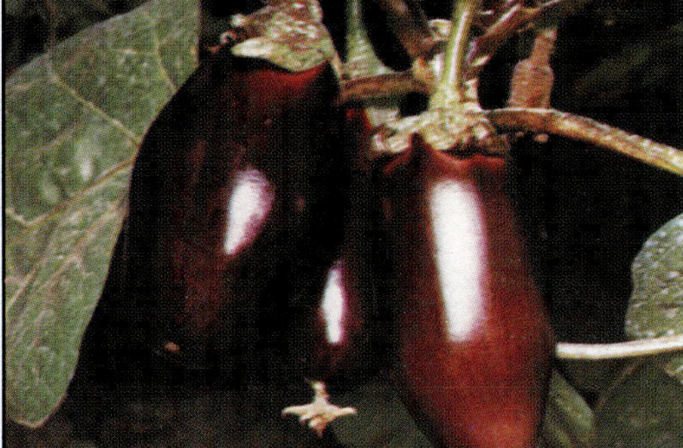
Solanum melongena

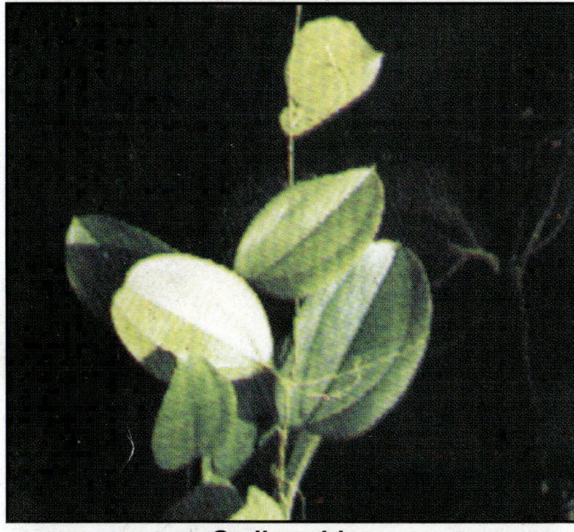
Smilex china

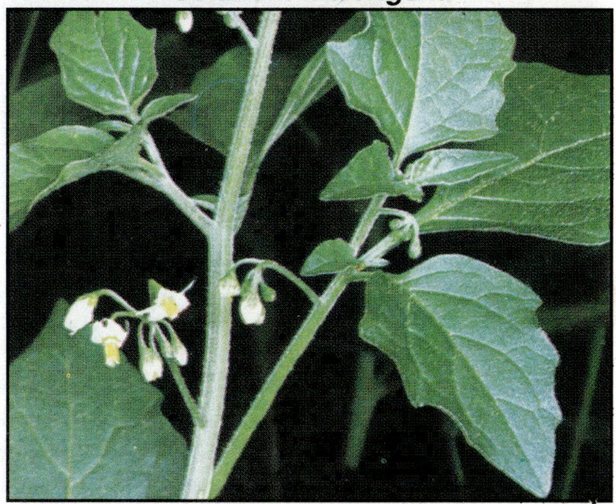
Solanum nigrum

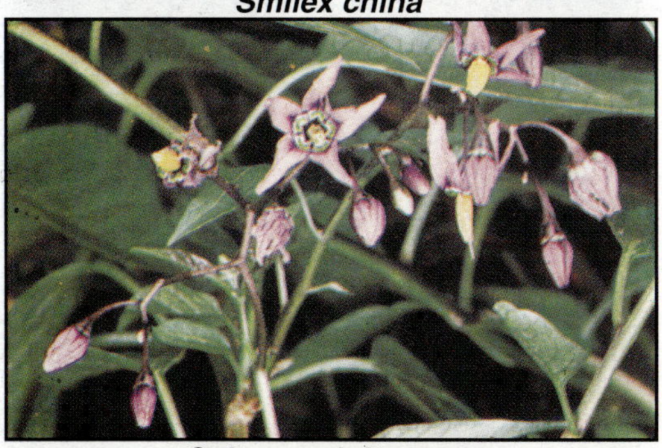
Solanum dulcamara

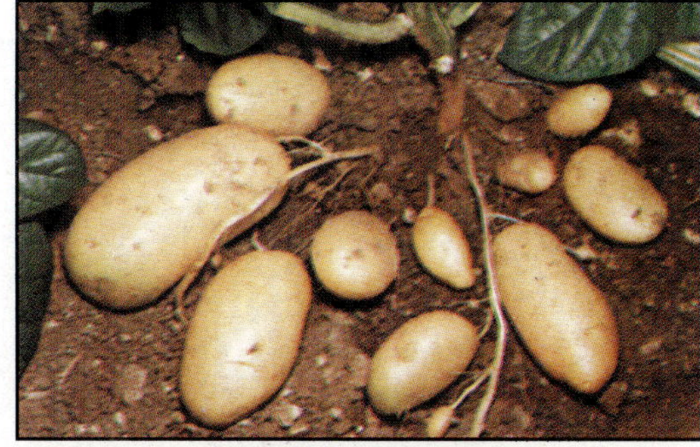
Solanum tuberosum

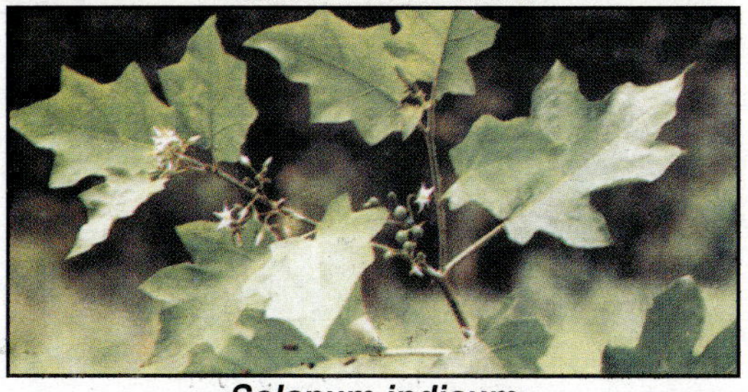
Solanum indicum

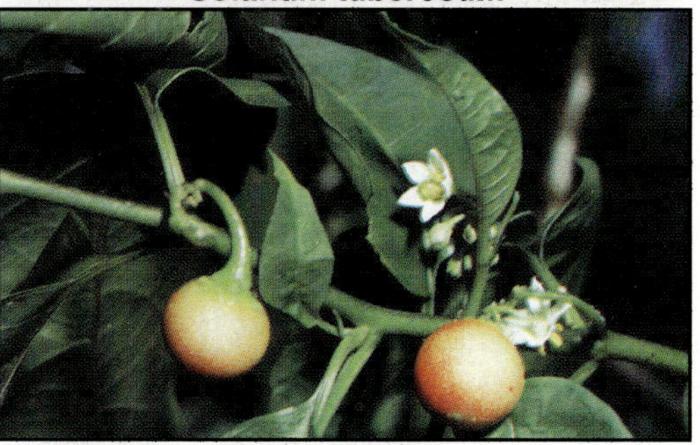
Solanum viride

PLATE : 120

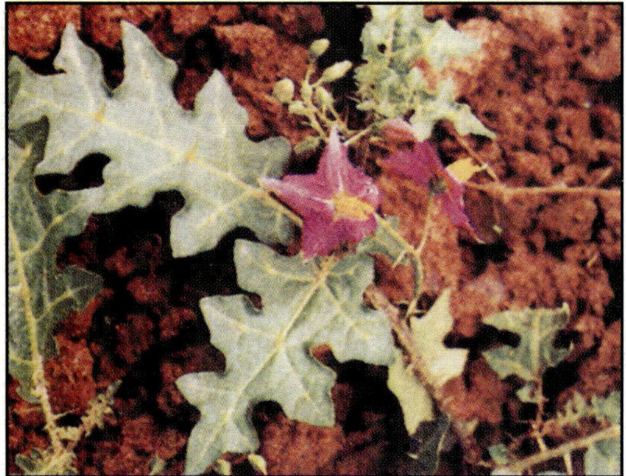

Solanum xanthocarpum

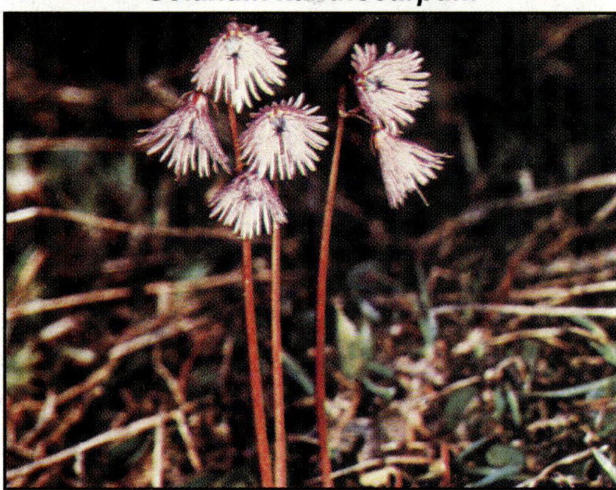

Soldanella alpina

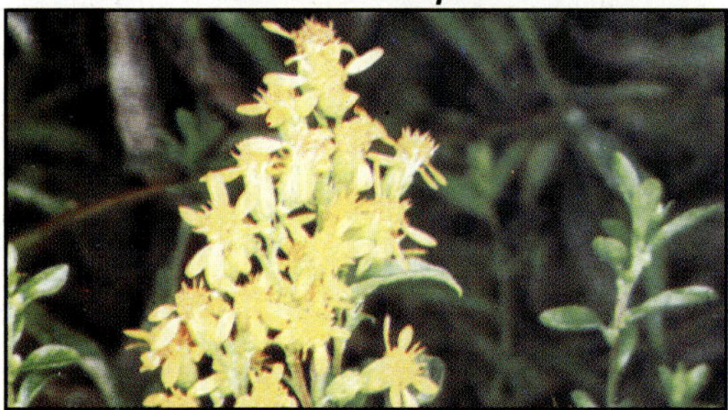

Solidago virgaurea

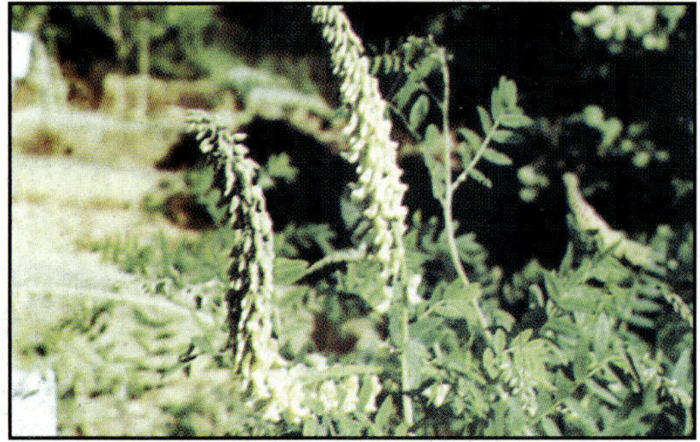

Sophora flavescens

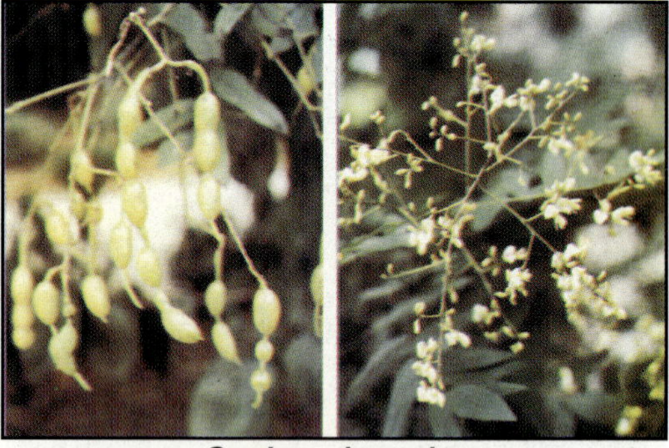

Sophora japonica

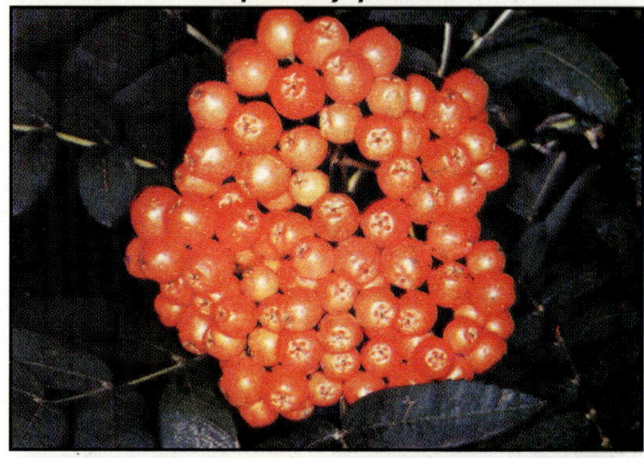

Sorbus aucuparia

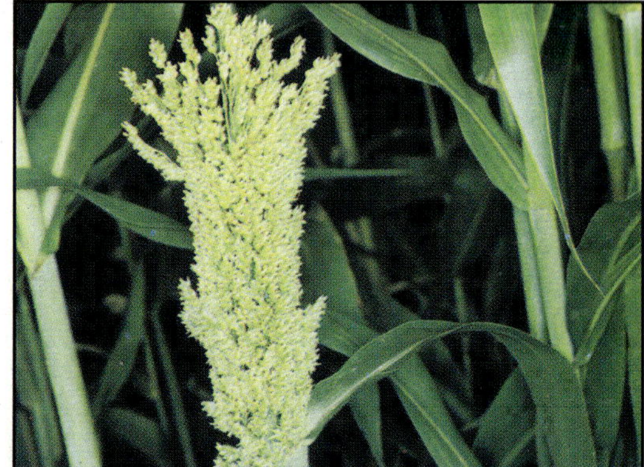

Sorghum bicolor

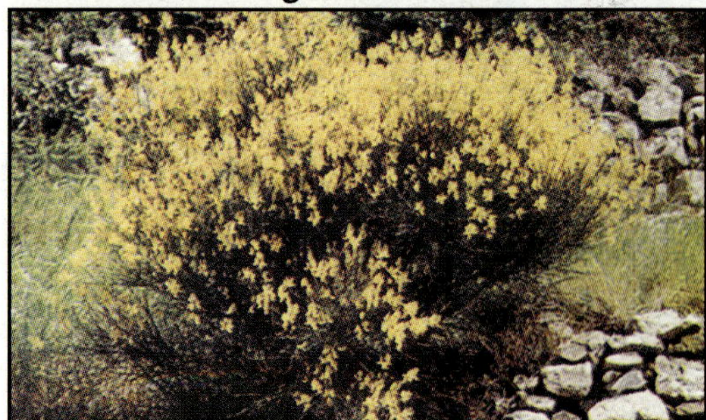

Spartium junceum

PLATE : 121

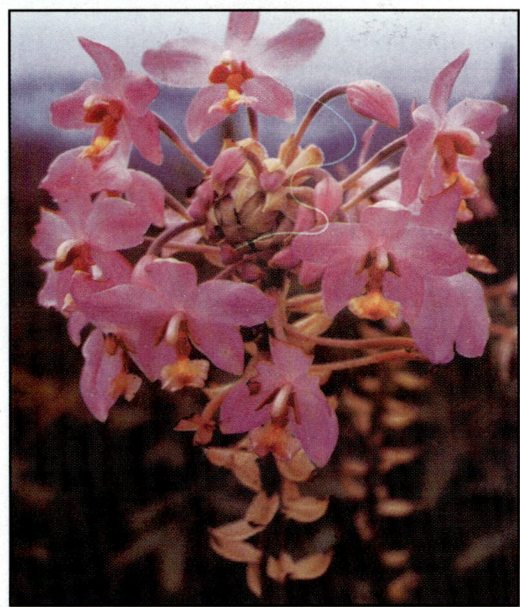

Spathoglottis pacifica

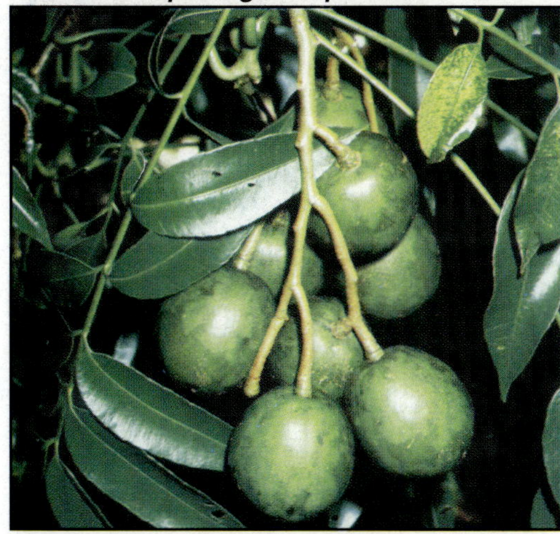

Spondias dulcis

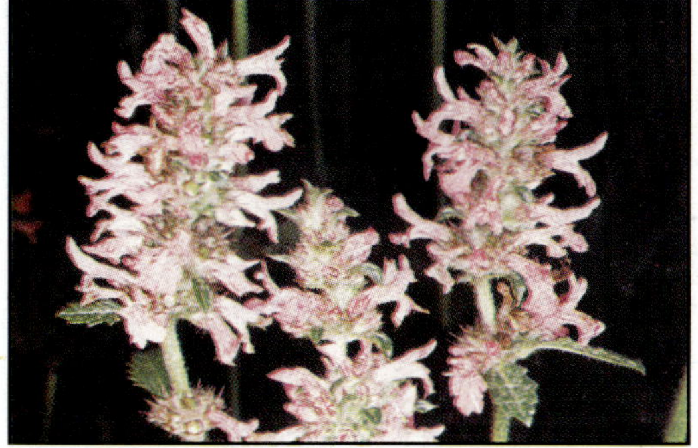

Stachys officinalis

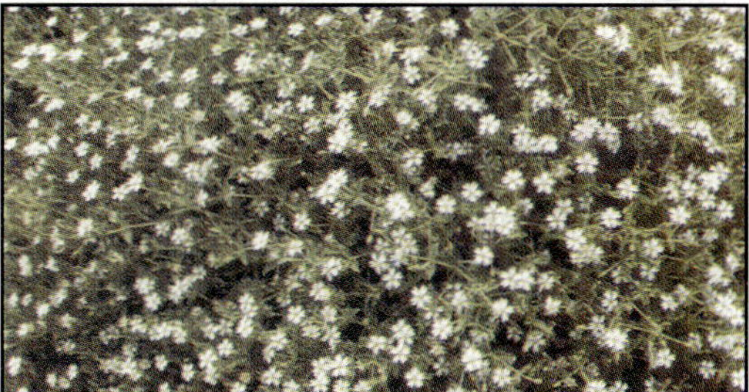

Stellaria dichotoma

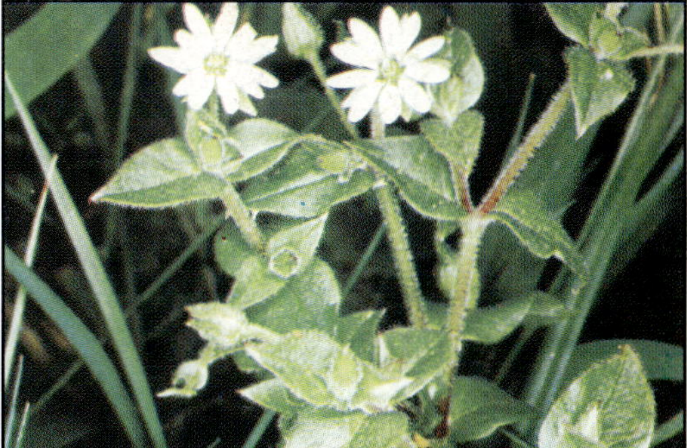

Stellaria media

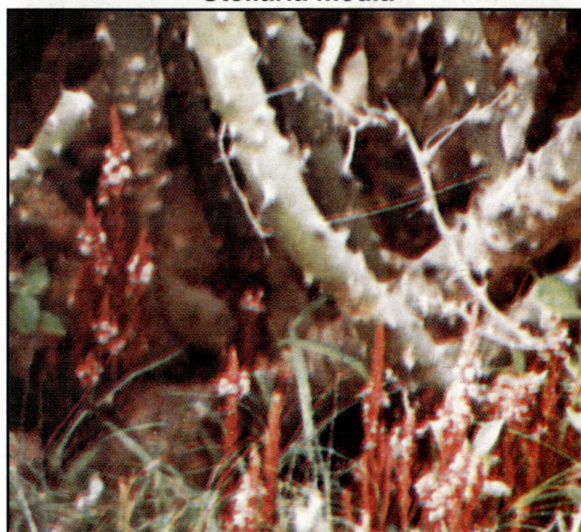

Striga gesnerioides

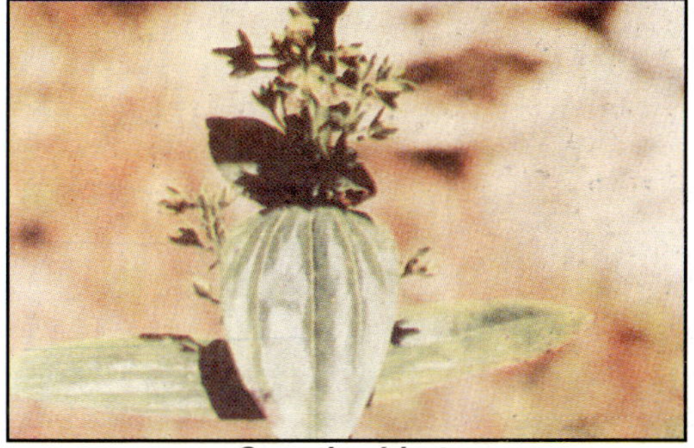

Swertia chirata

PLATE : 122

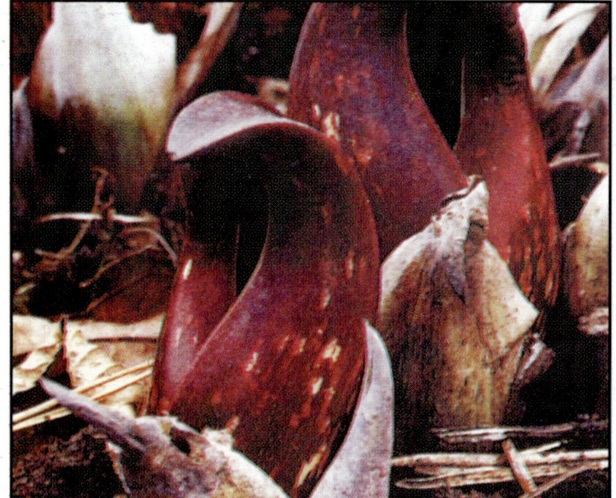

Symplocarpus foetidus

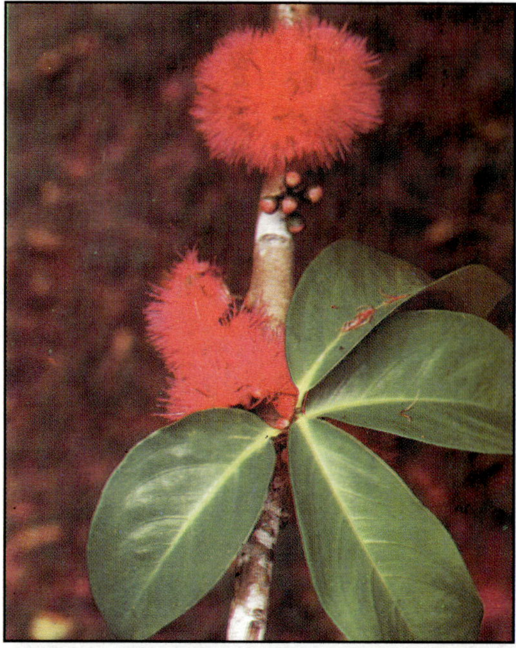

Syzygium malaccense

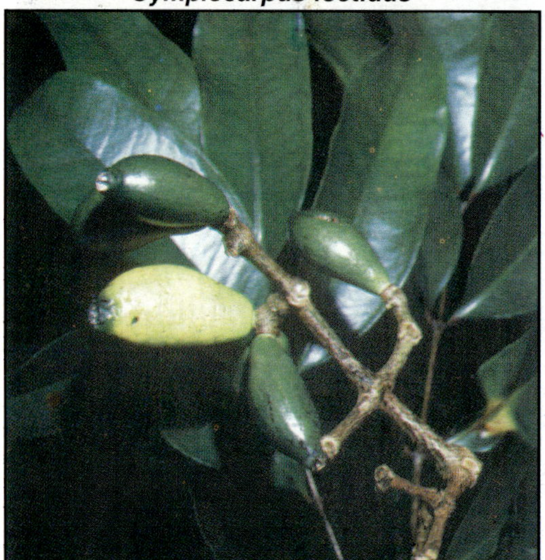

Syzygium cornocarpum

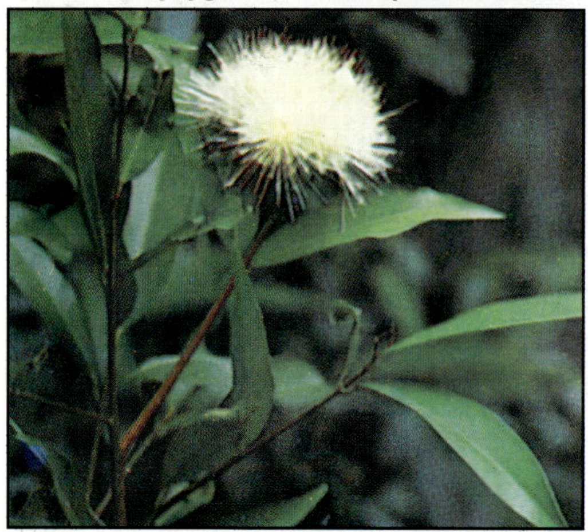

Syzygium cumini

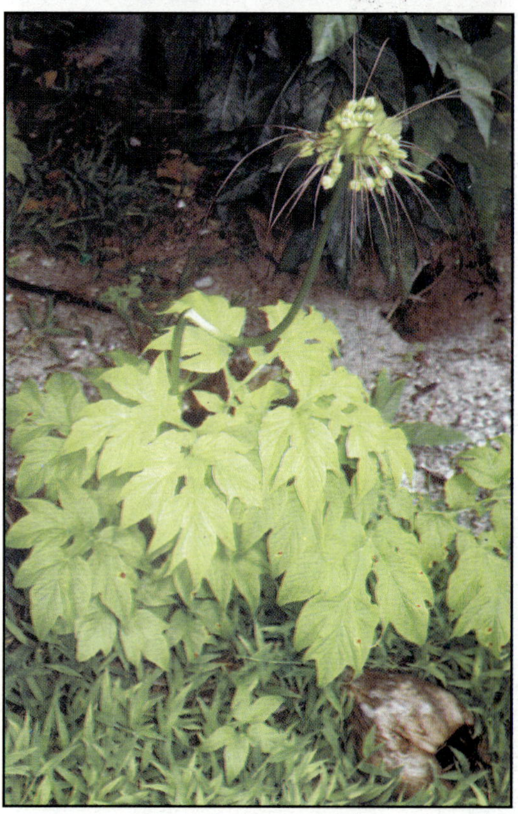

Tacca lentopetaloides

PLATE : 123

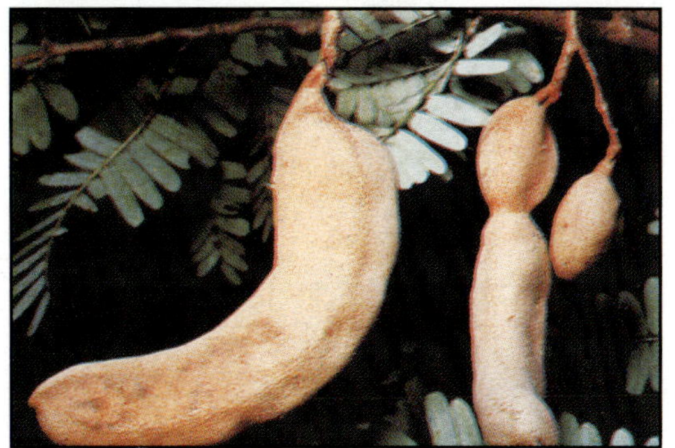

Tamarindus indica

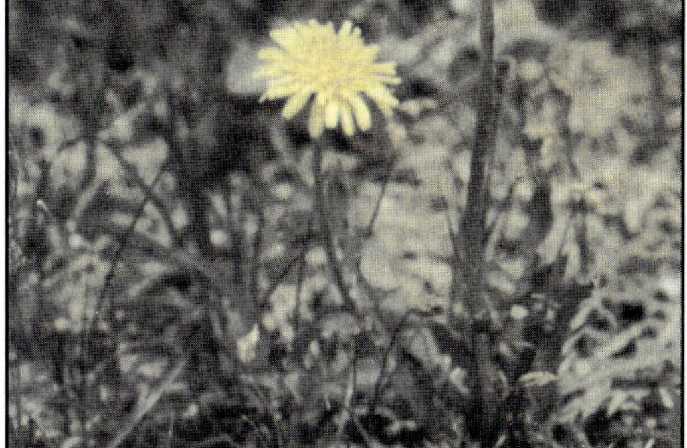

Taraxacum mongolicum

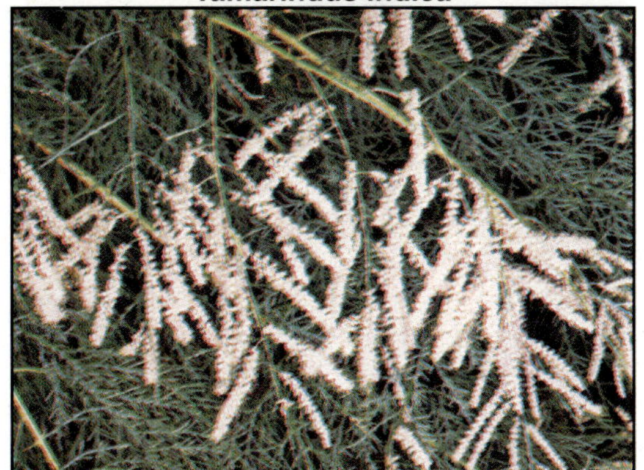

Tamarix gallica

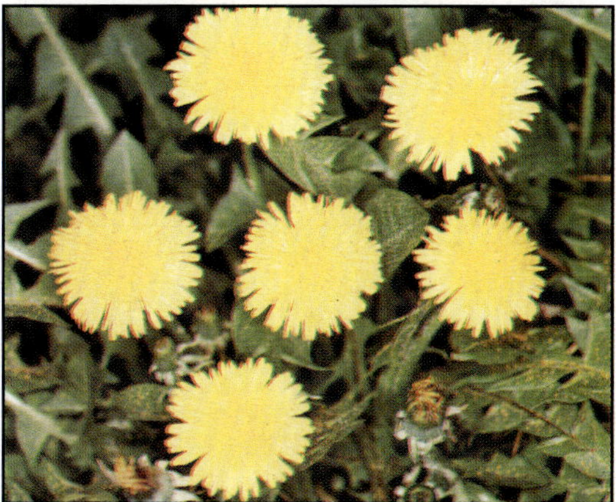

Taraxacum officinale

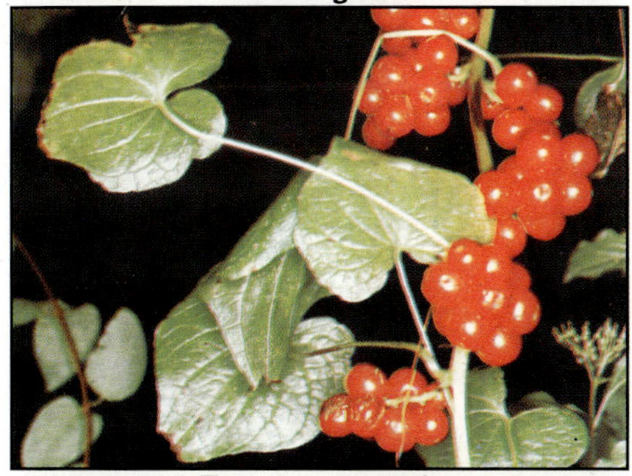

Tamus communis

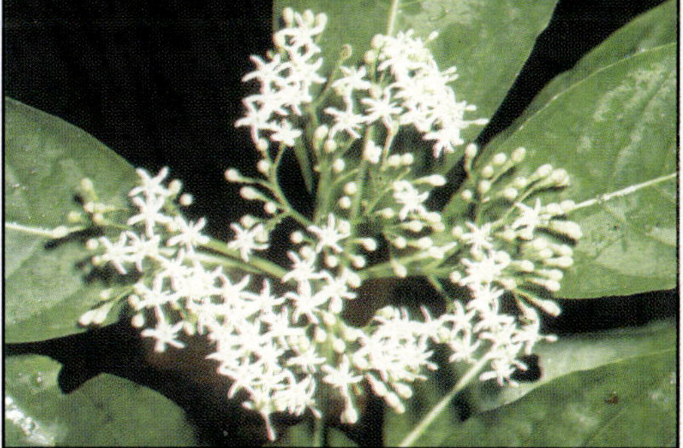

Tarenna sambucina

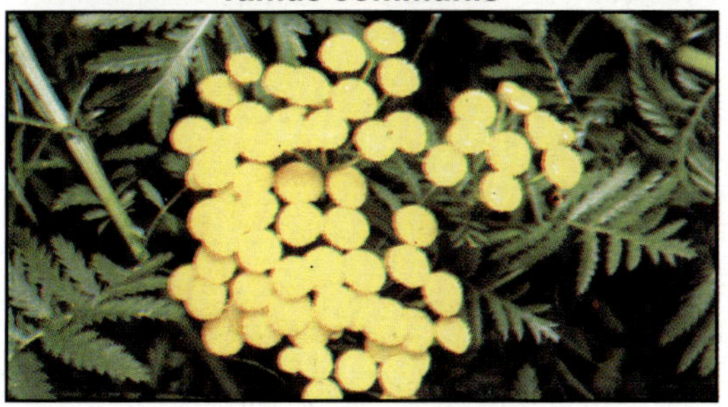

Tanacetum vulgare

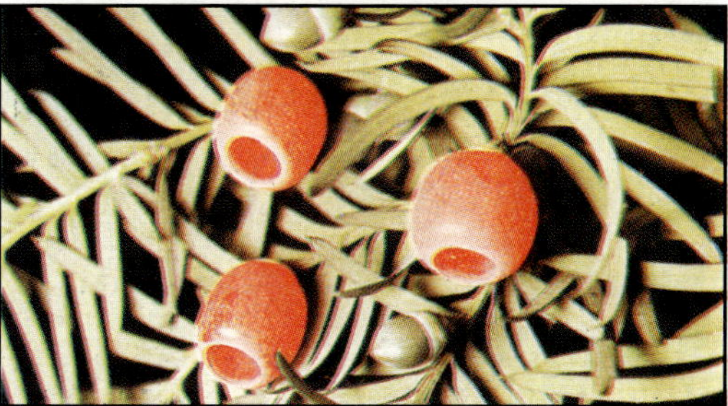

Taxus baccata

PLATE : 124

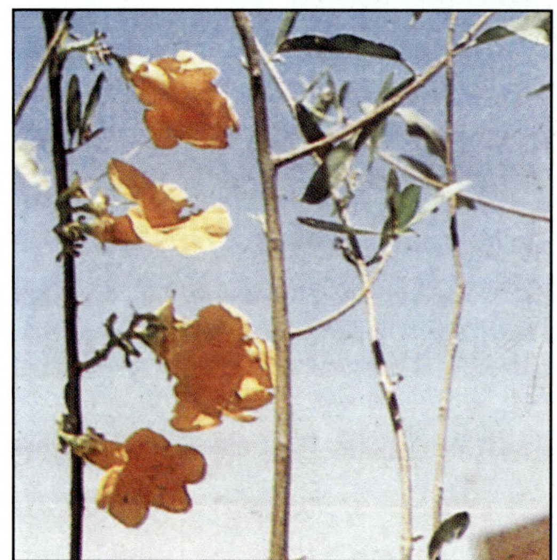

Tecomella undulata

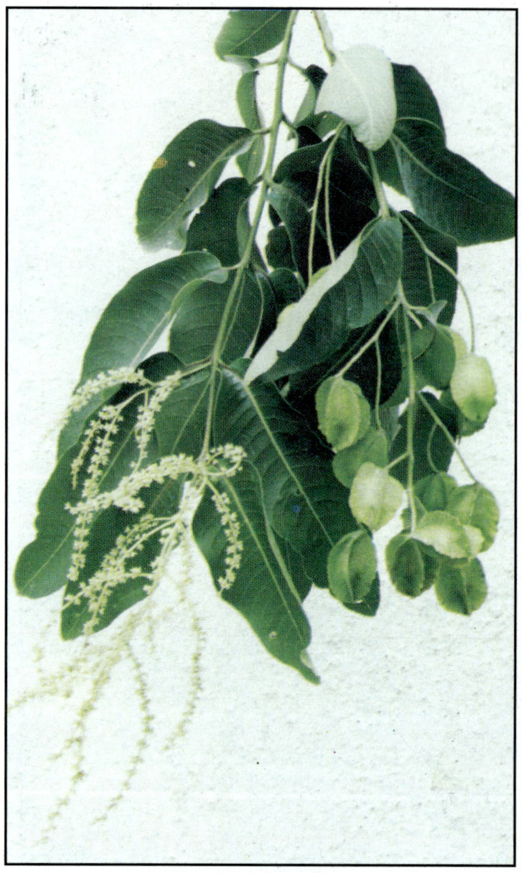

Terminalia arjuna

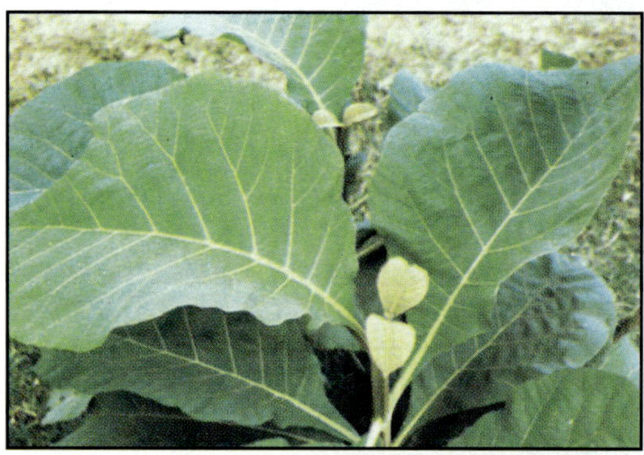

Tectona grandis

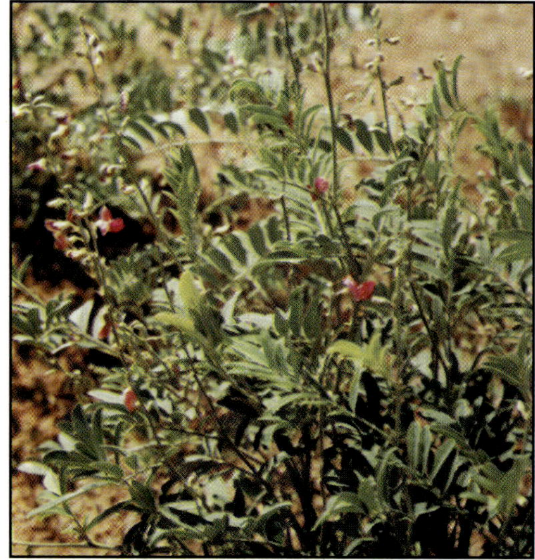

Tephrosea purpurea

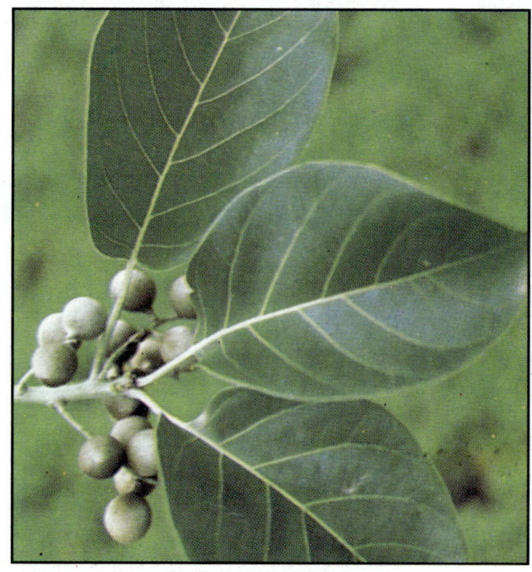

Terminalia bellirica

PLATE : 125

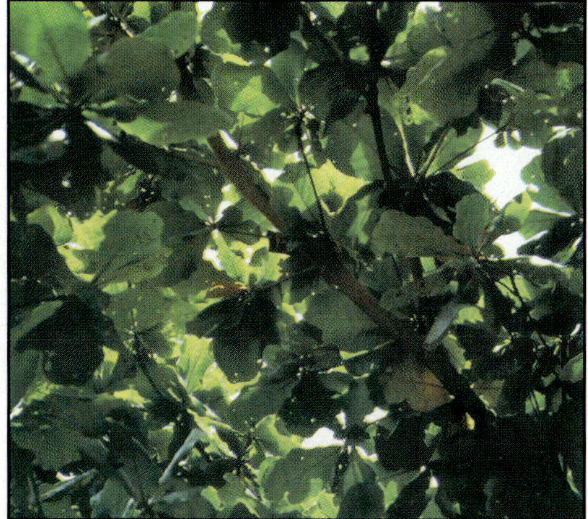

Terminalia catappa

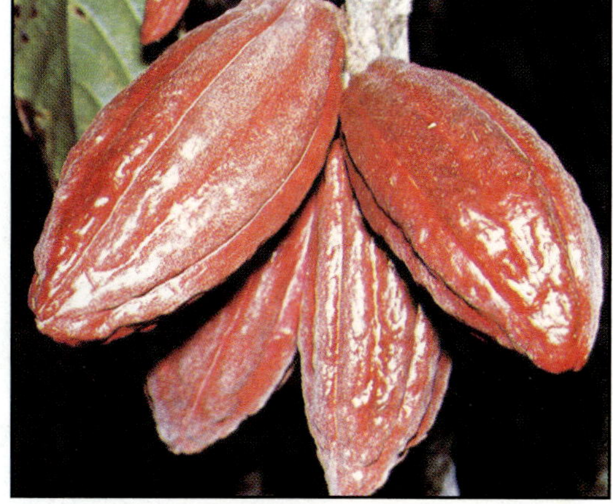

Theobroma cacao

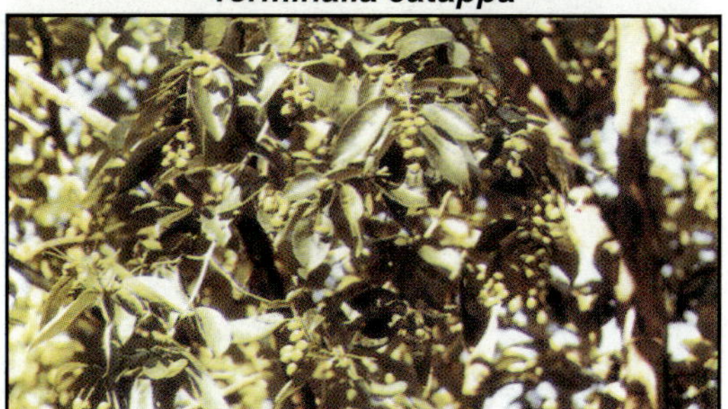

Terminalia chebula

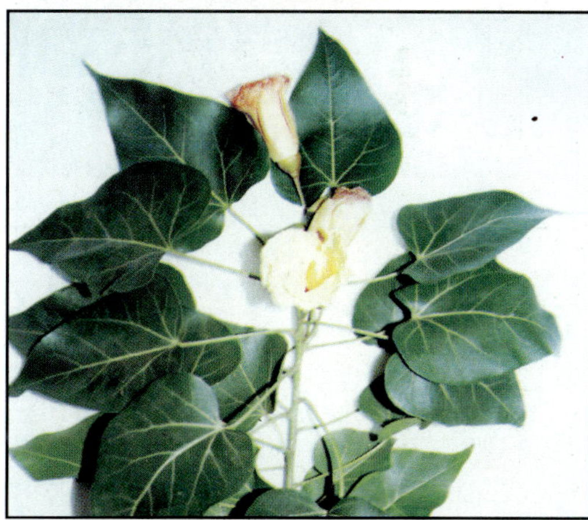

Thespesia populnea

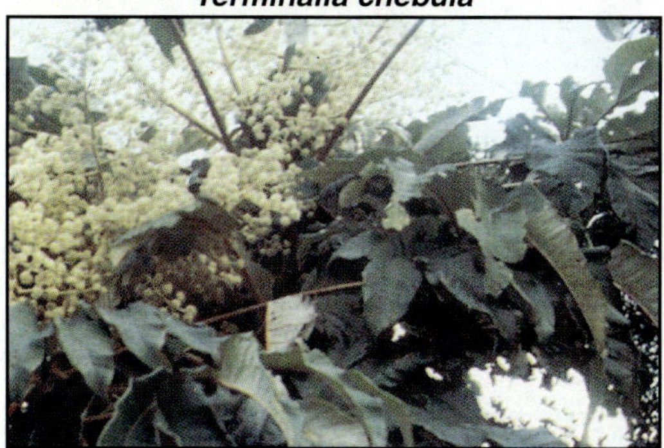

Tetrapanax papyrifer

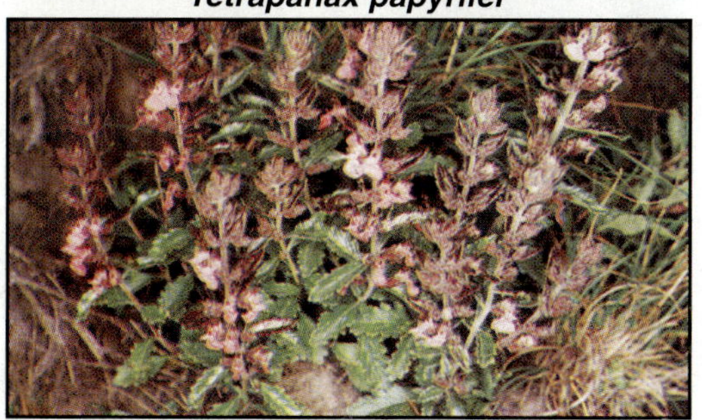

Teucrium chamaedrys

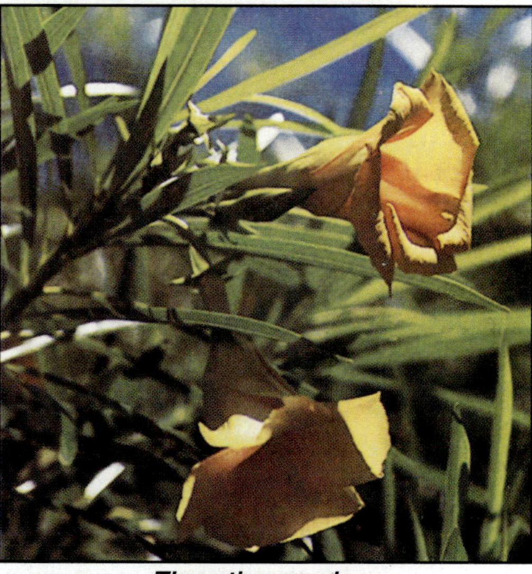

Thevetia peruviana

PLATE : 126

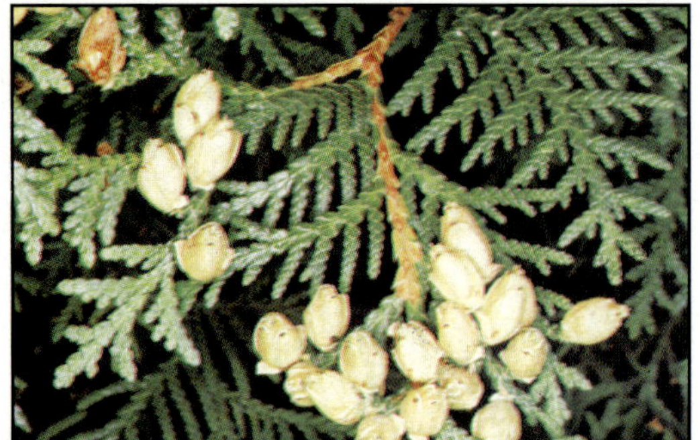

Thuja occidentalis

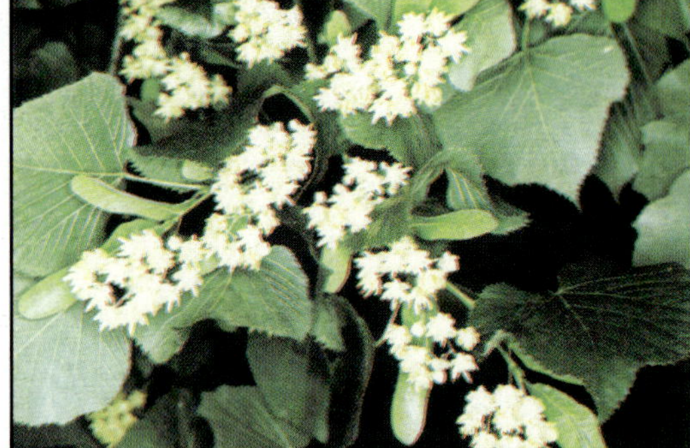

Tilia platyphyllos

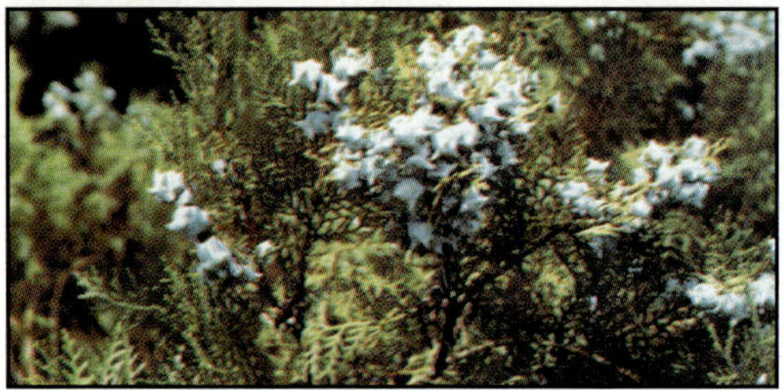

Thuja orientalis

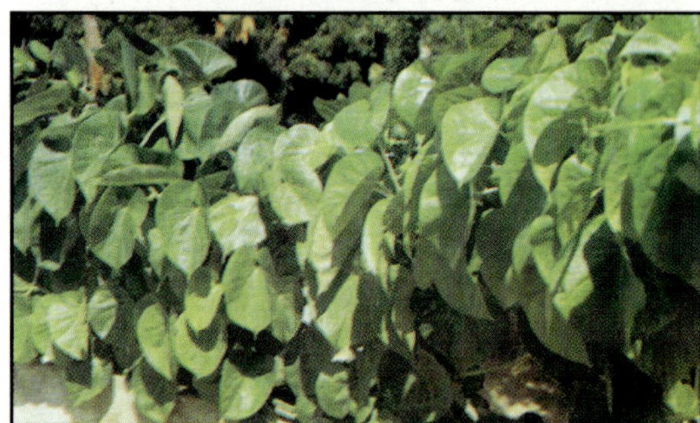

Tinospora Cordifolia

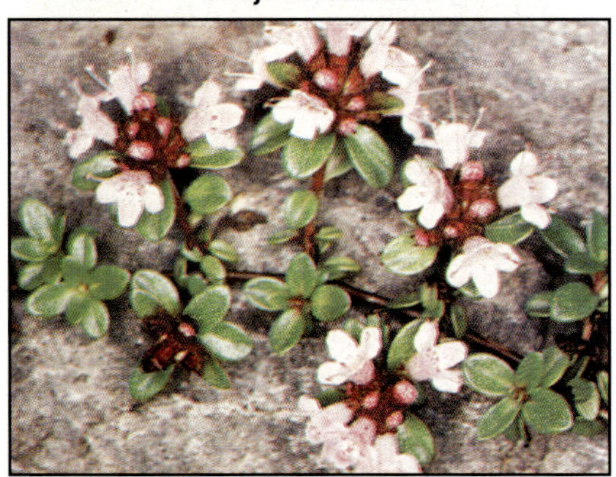

Thymus serpyllum

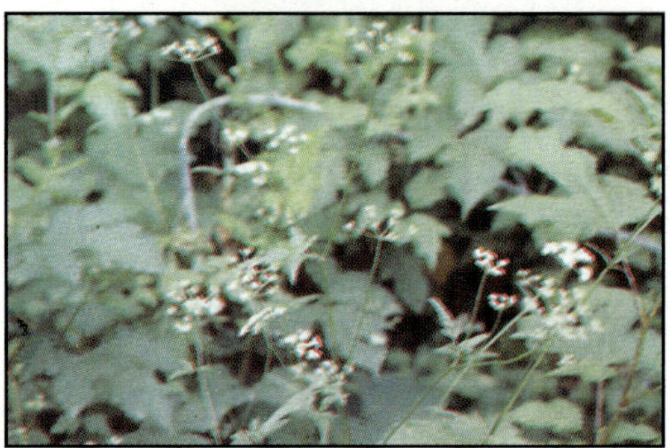

Torilis japonica

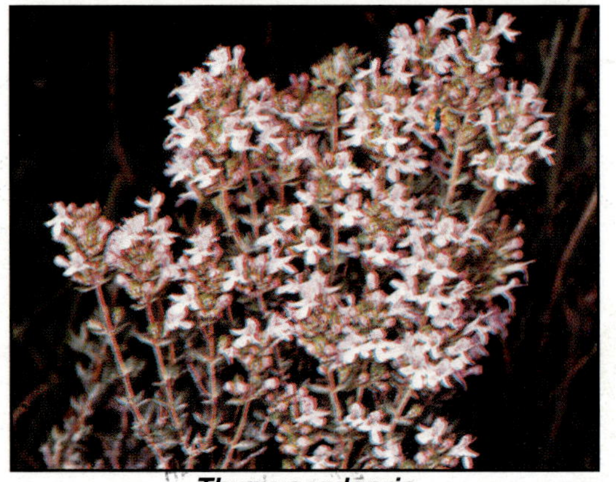

Thymus vulgaris

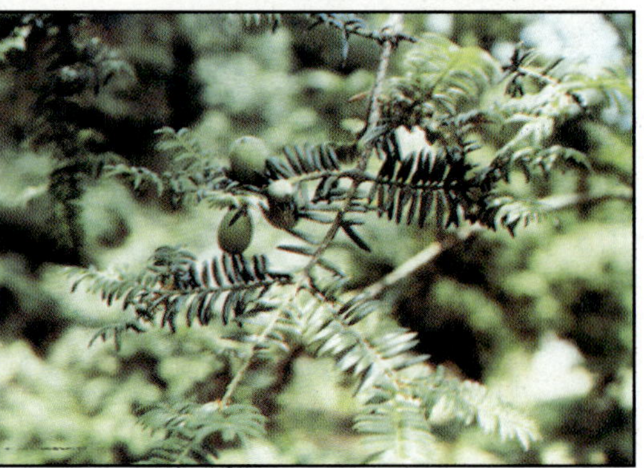

Torreya nucifera

PLATE : 127

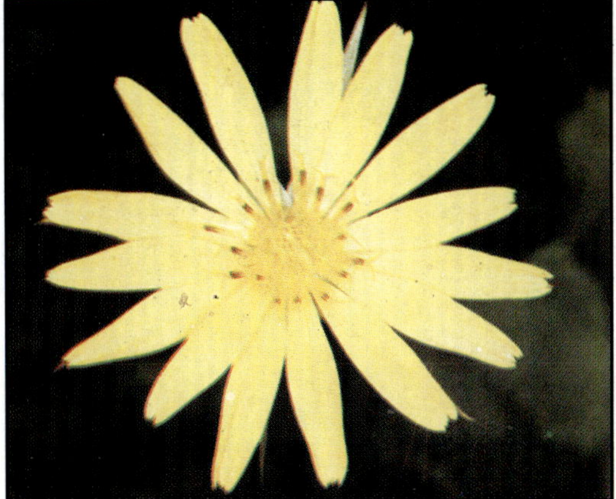

Tragopogon pratensis

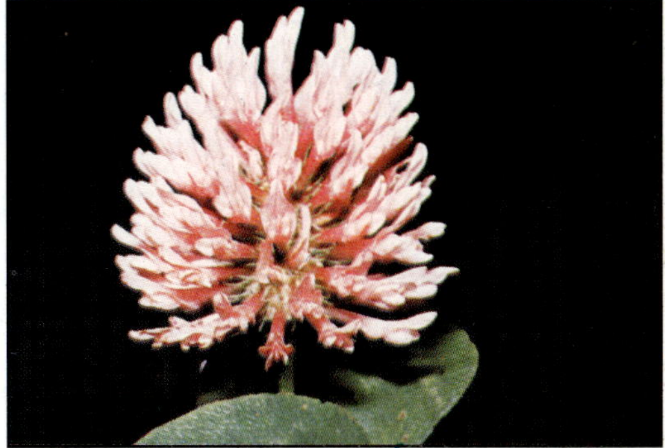

Trifolium arvense

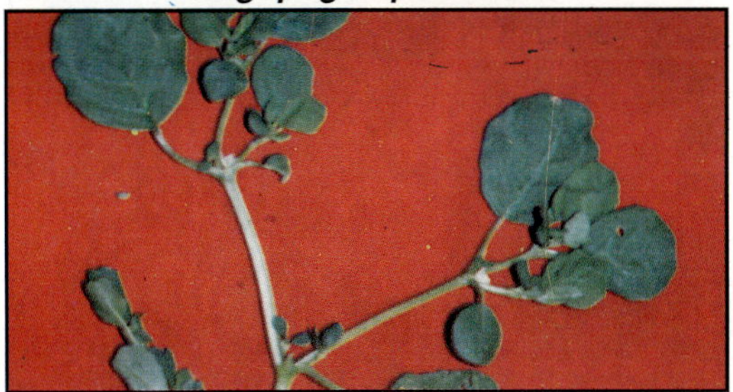

Trianthema portulacastrum

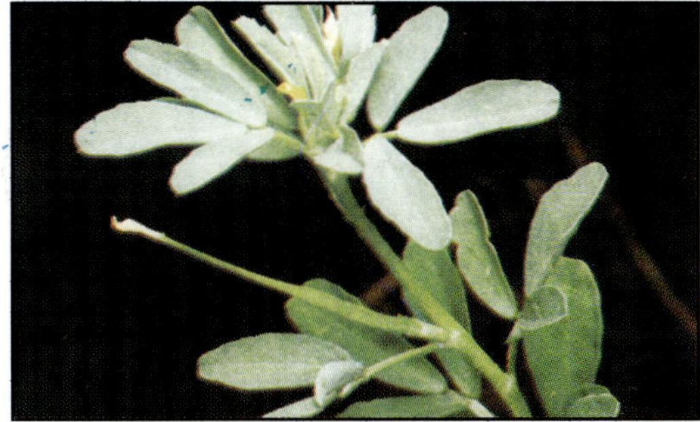

Trigonella foenum-graecum

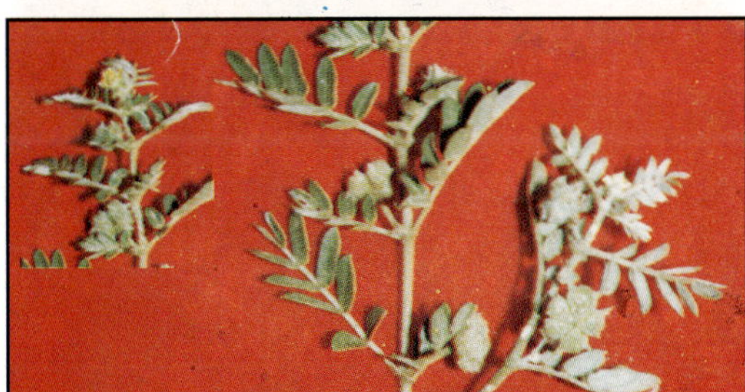

Tribulus terrestris

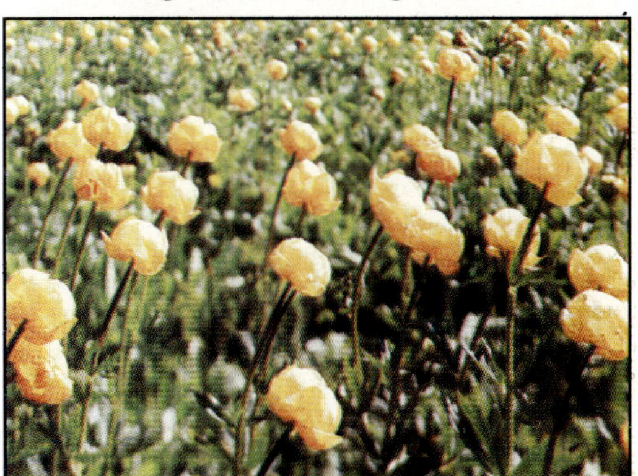

Trollius europaeus

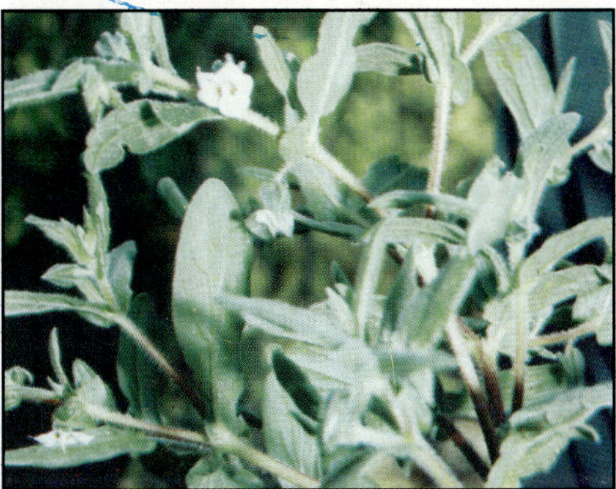

Trichodesma indicum

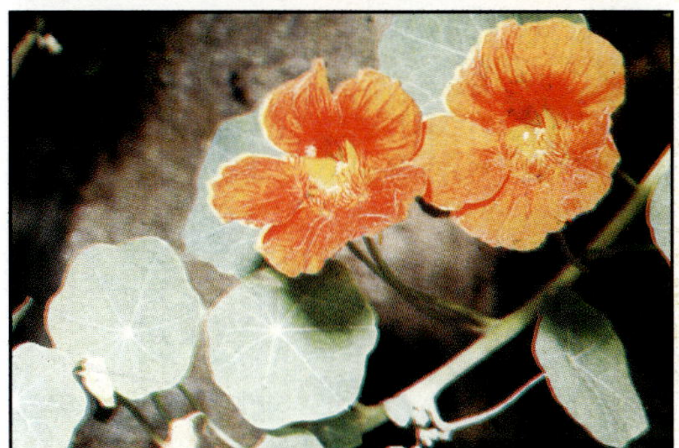

Tropaeolum majus

PLATE : 128

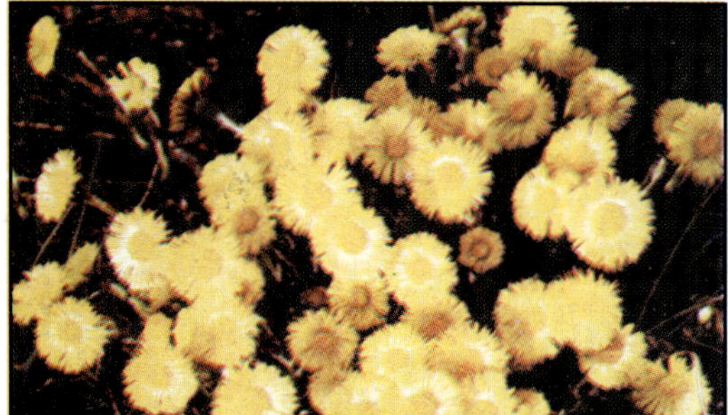

Tussilago farfara

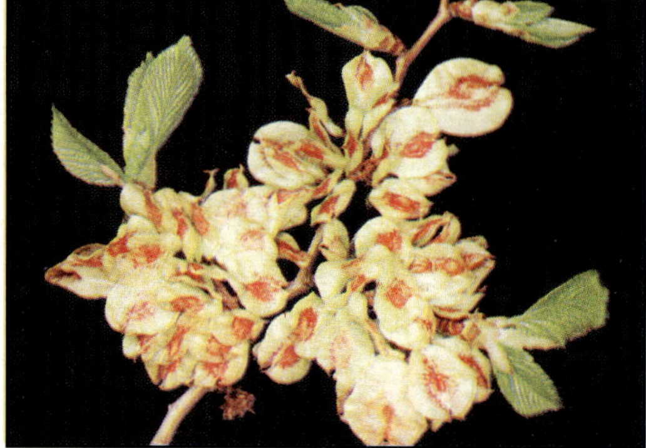

Ulmus procera

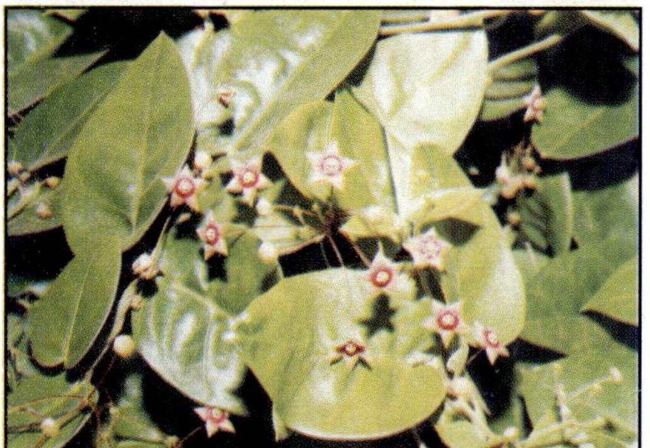

Tylophora indica

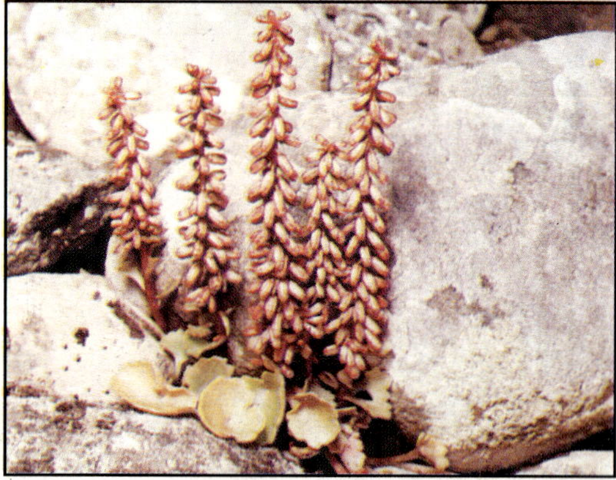

Umbilicus rupestris

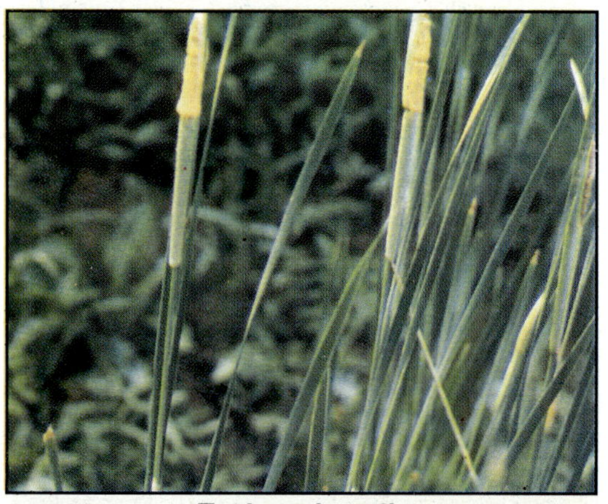

Typha orientalis

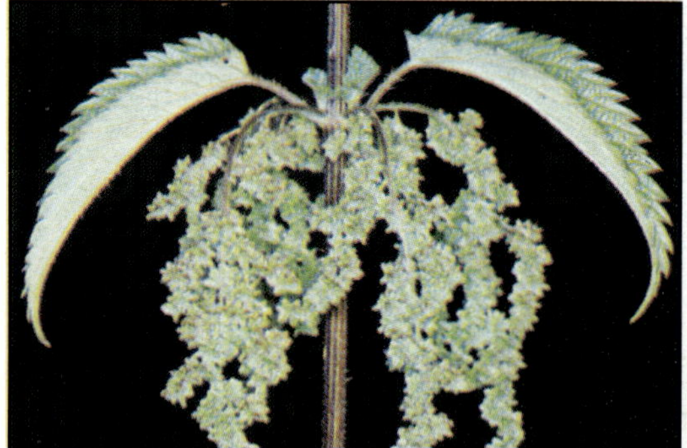

Urtica urens

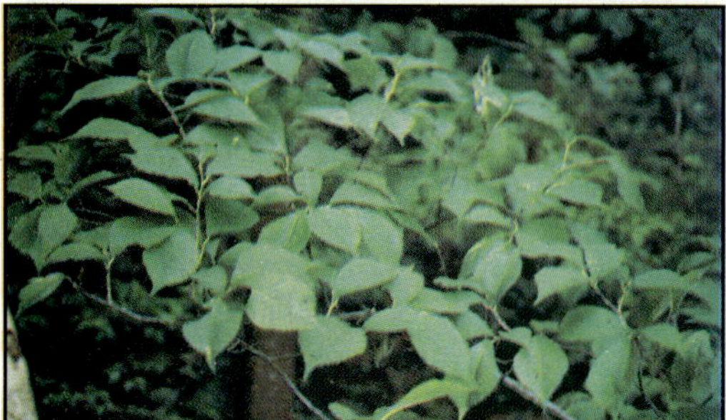

Ulmus macrocarpa

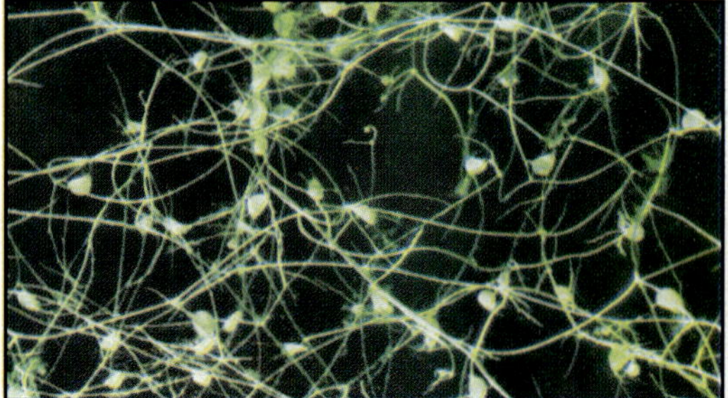

Utricularia vulgaris

PLATE : 129

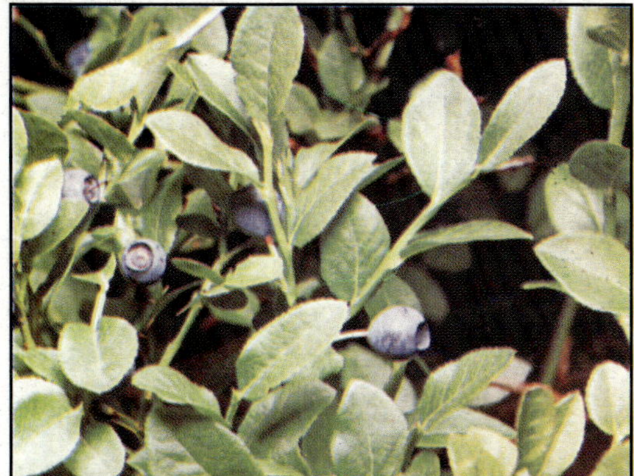
Vaccinium myrtillus

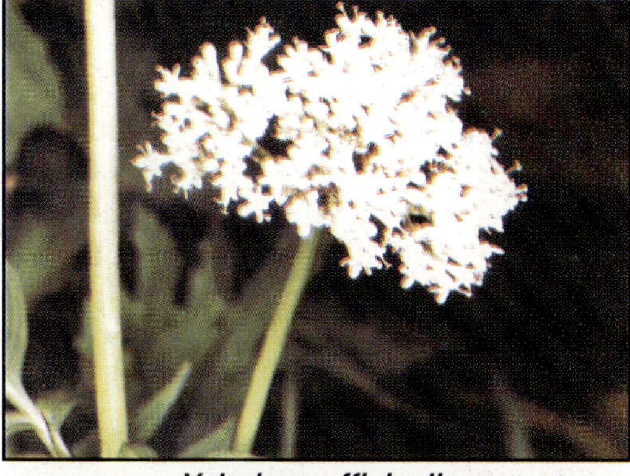
Valeriana officinalis

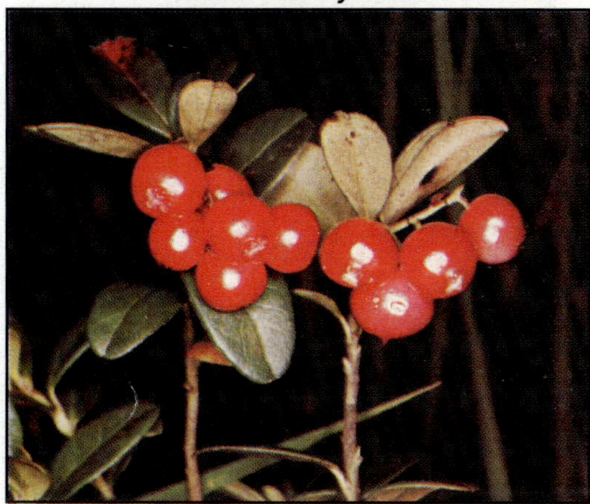
Vaccinium vitis-idaea

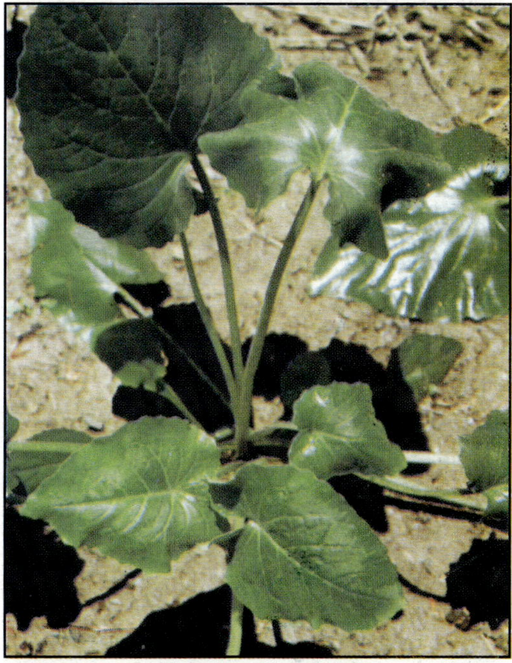
Valeriana wallichii

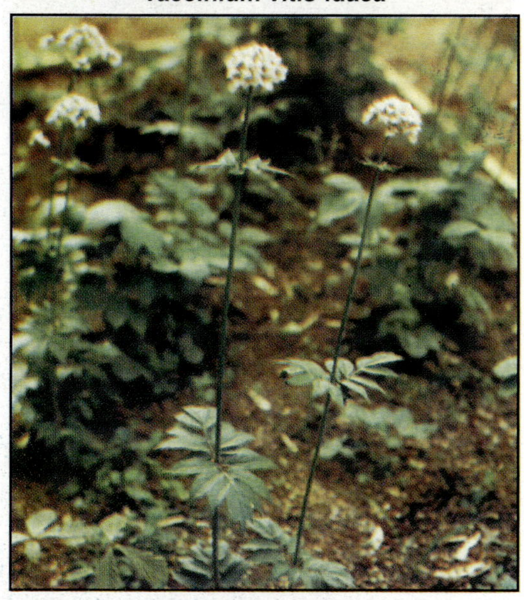
Valeriana fauriei

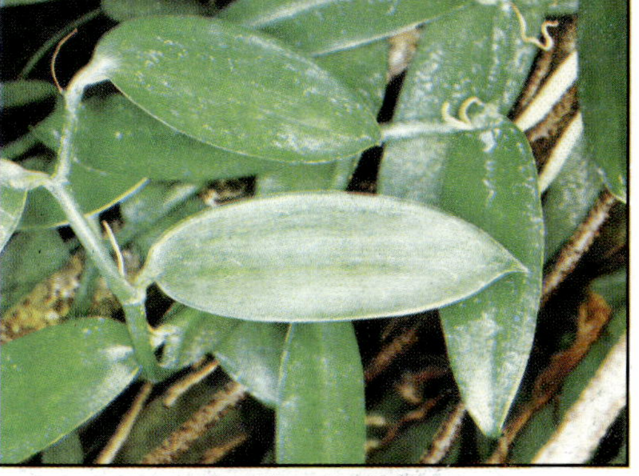
Vanilla planifolia

PLATE : 130

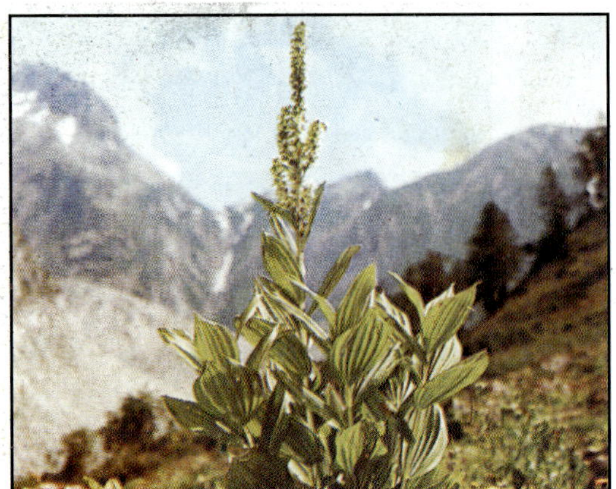

Veratrum album

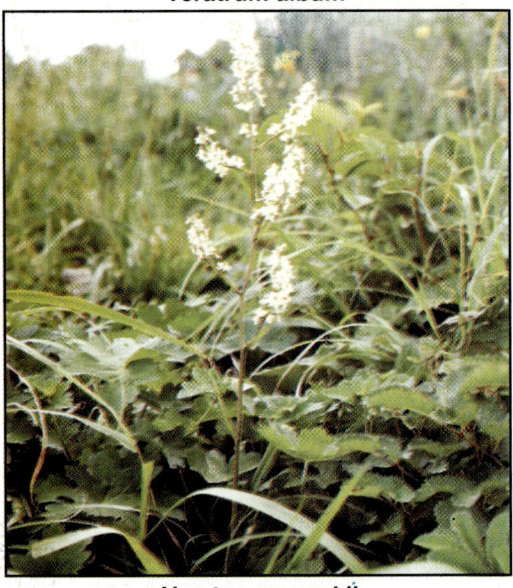

Veratrum maackii

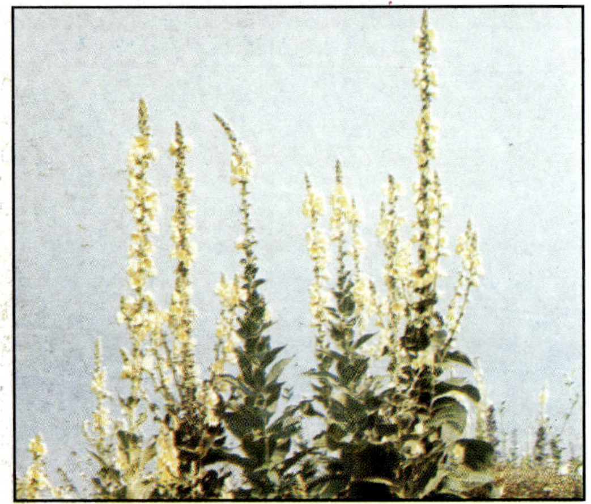

Verbascum thapsus

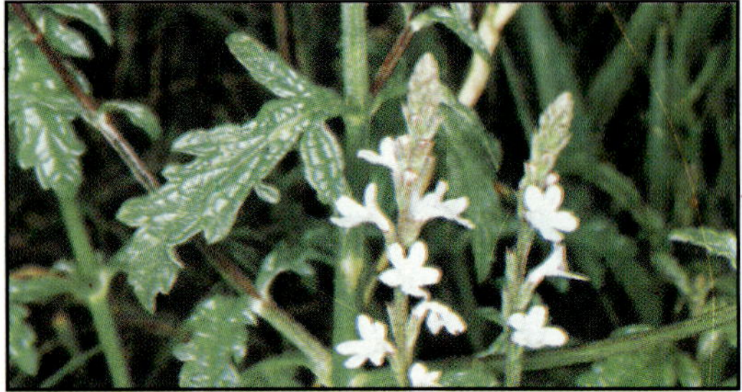

Verbena officinalis

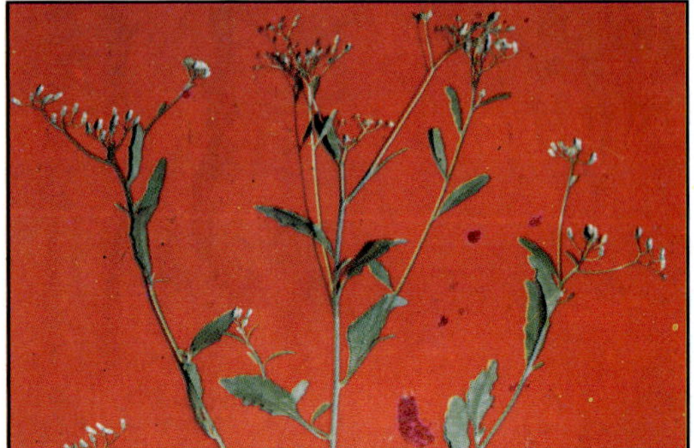

Vernonia cinerea

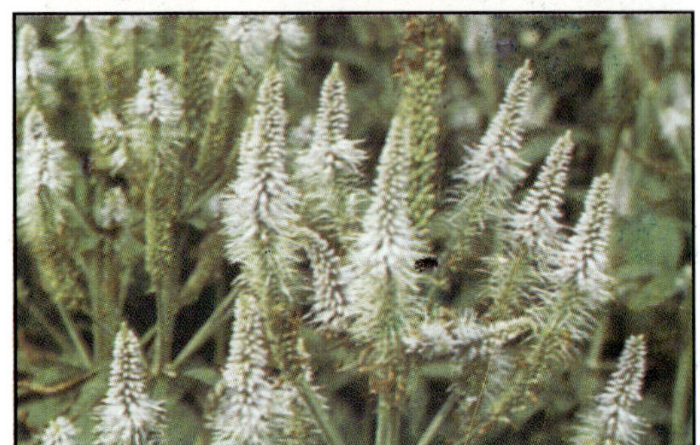

Veronicastrum sibiricum

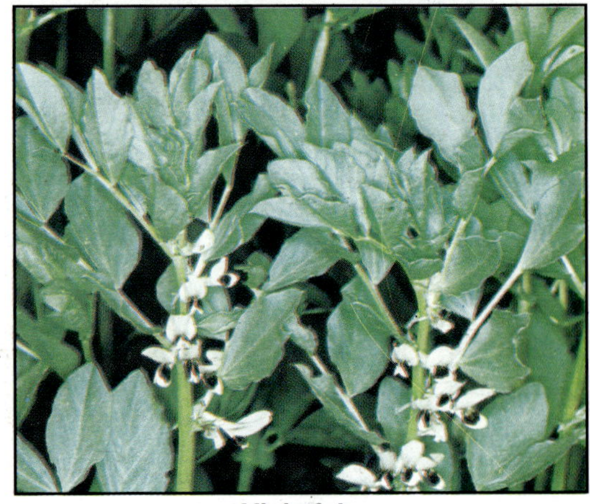

Vicia faba

PLATE : 131

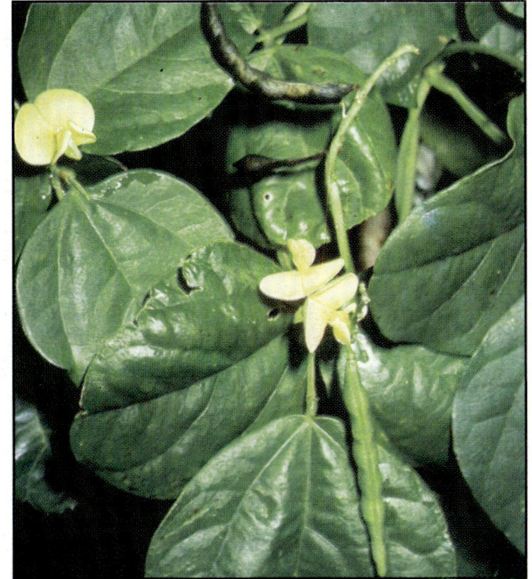

Vigna marina

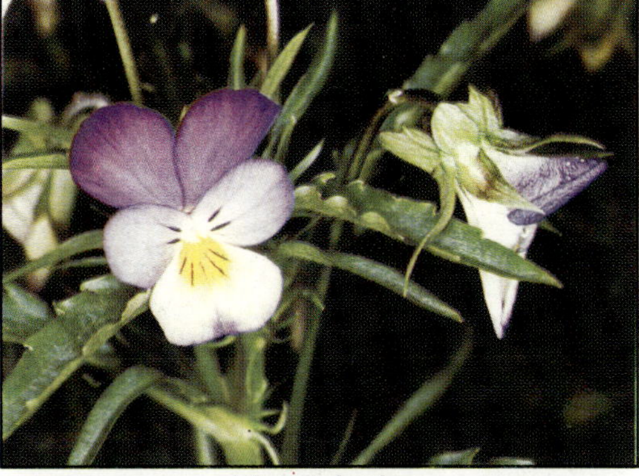

Viola tricolor

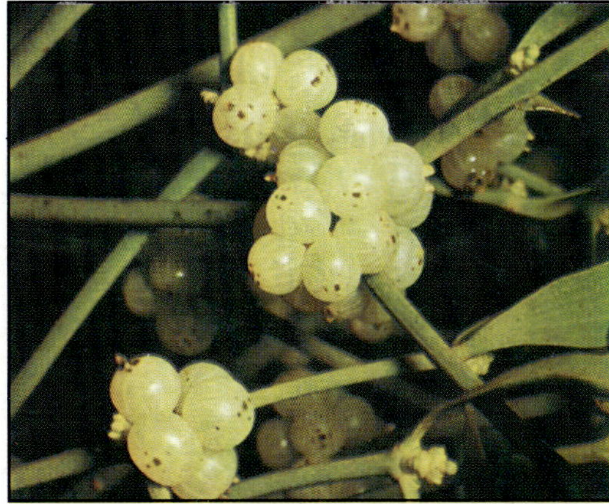

Viscum album

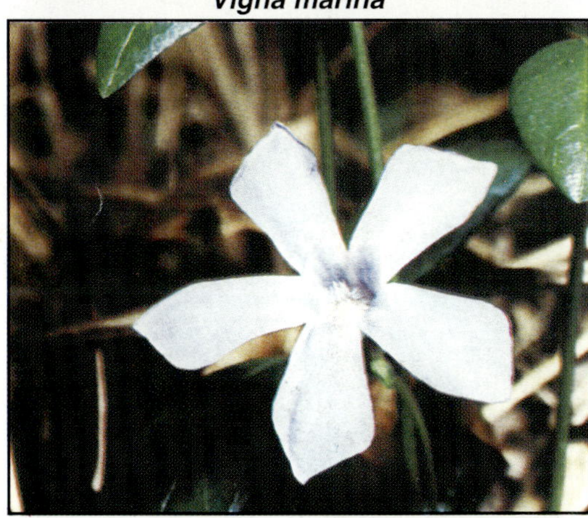

Vinca minor

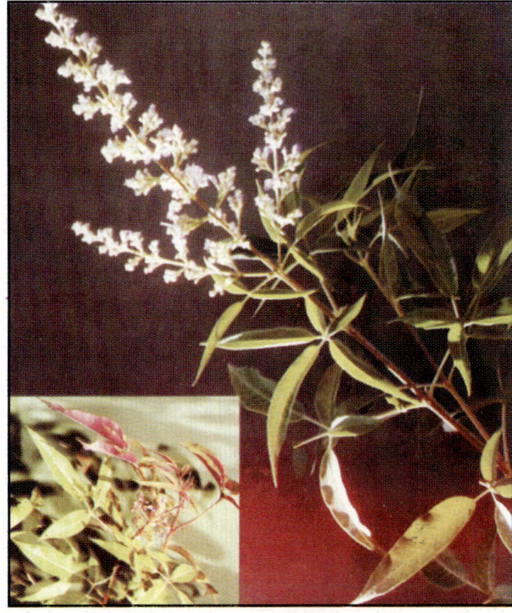

Vitex negundo

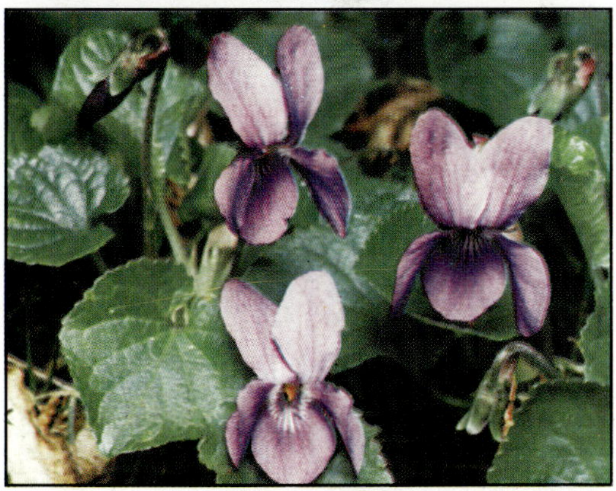

Viola odorata

PLATE : 132

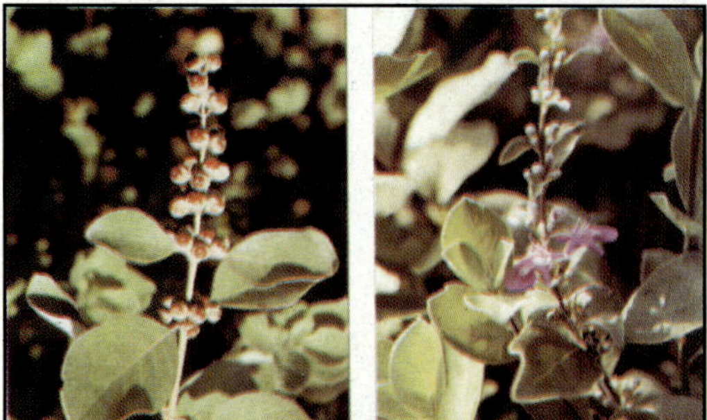

Vitex rotundifolia

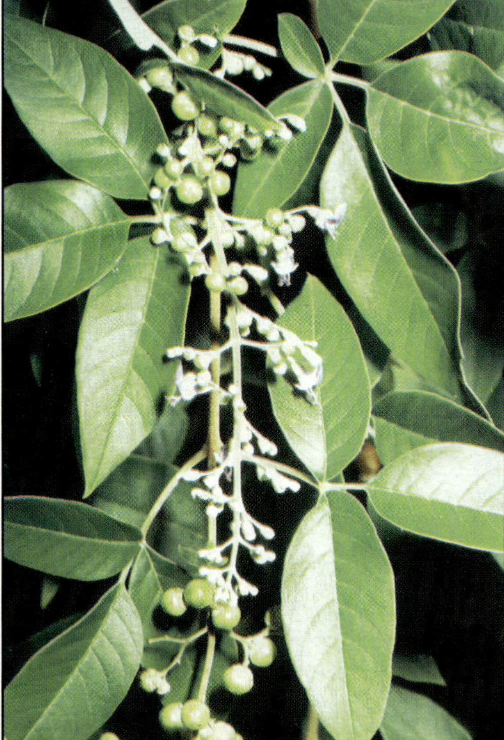

Vitex trifolia

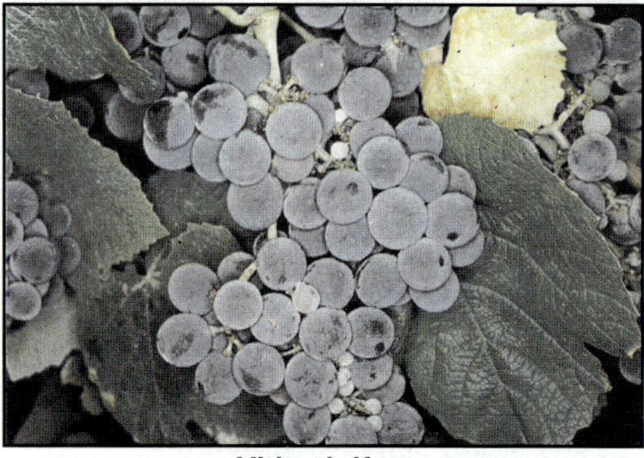

Vitis vinifera

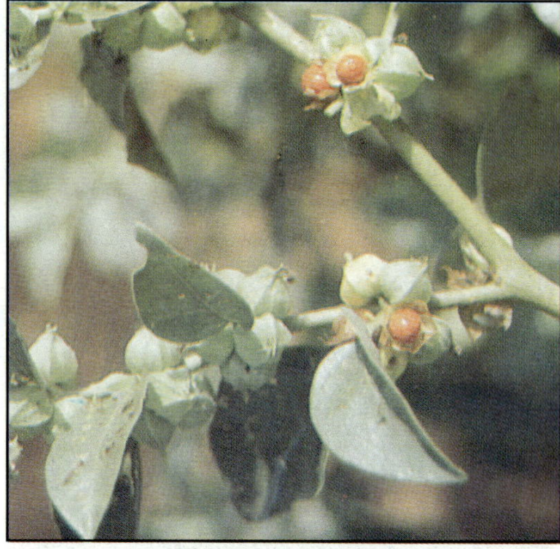

Withania somnifera

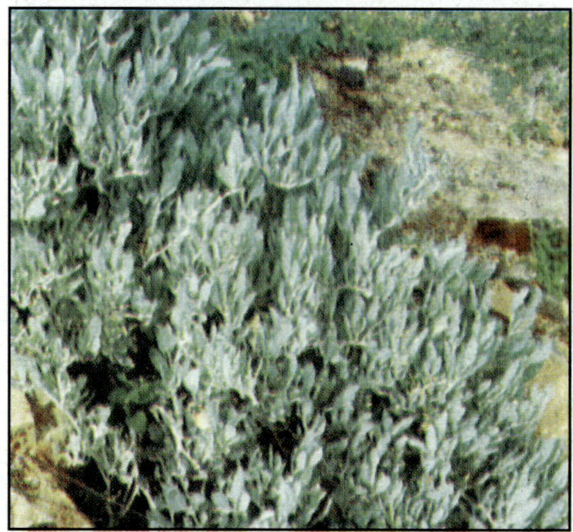

Withinia Coagulans

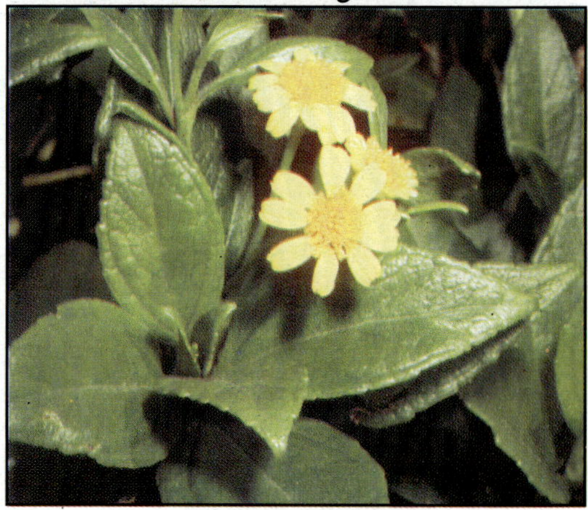

Wollastonia biflora

PLATE : 133

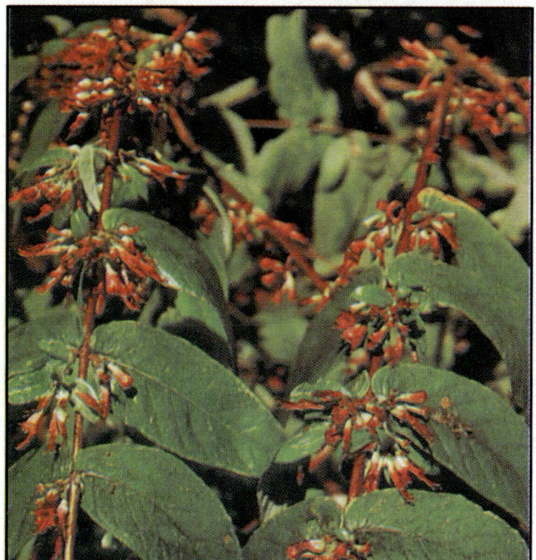

Woodfordia fruticosa

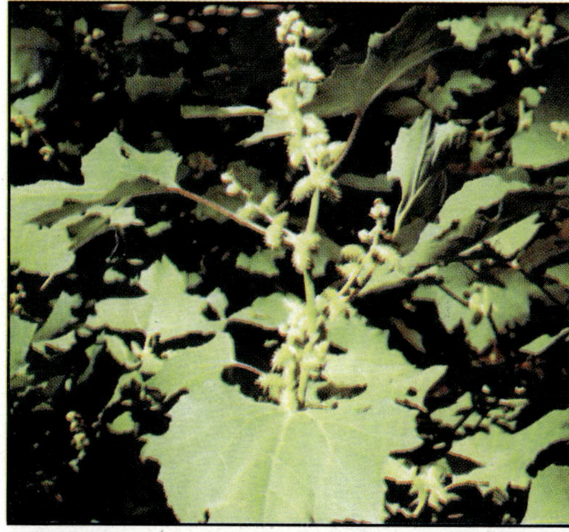

Xanthium strumarium

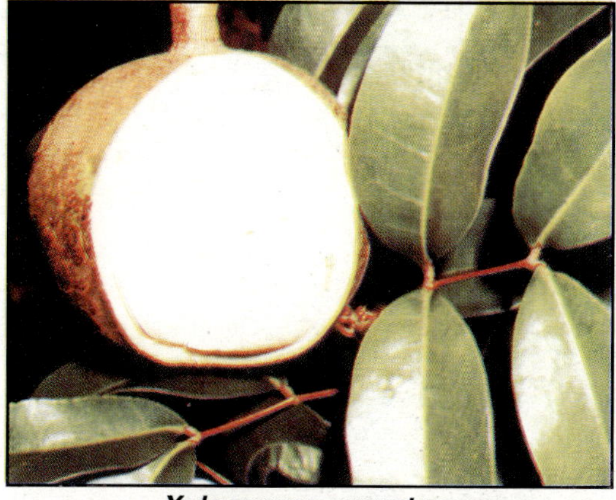

Xylocarpus granatum

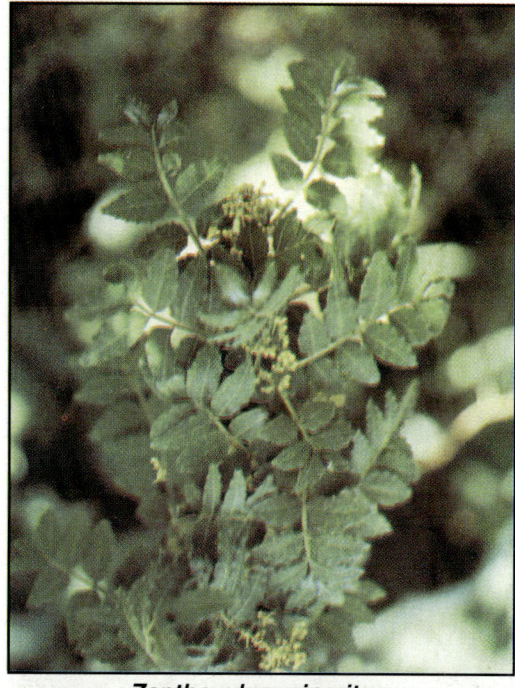

Zanthoxylum piperitum

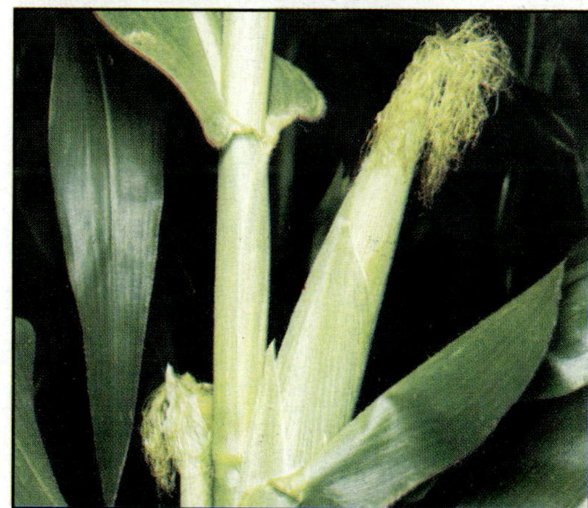

Zea mays

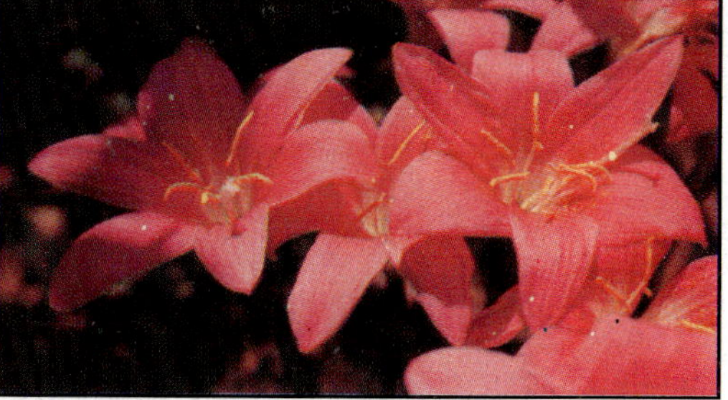

Zephyranthes grandiflora

PLATE : 134

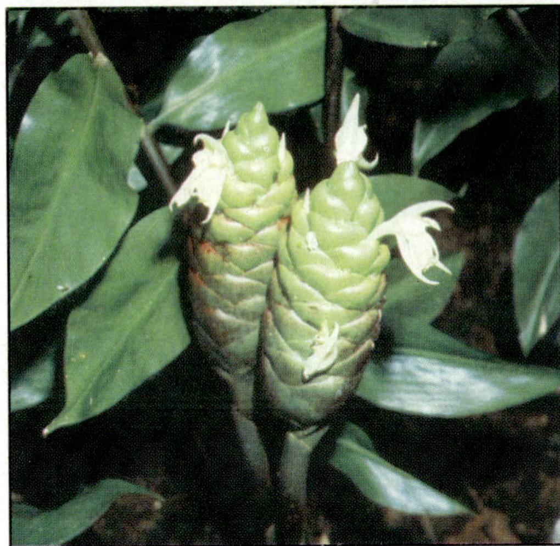

Zingiber zerumbet

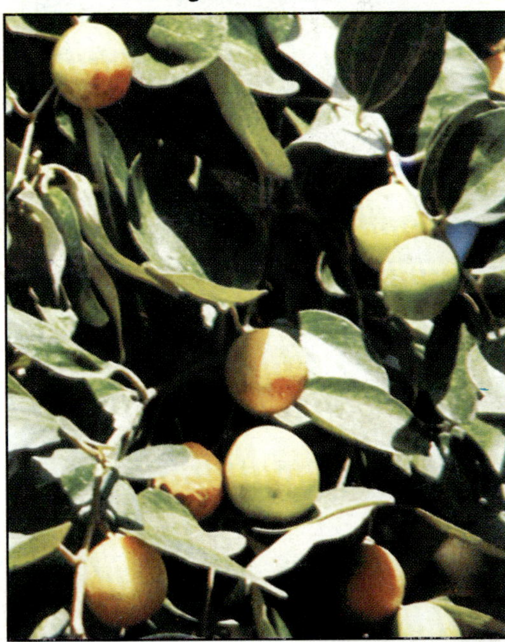

Ziziphus jujuba

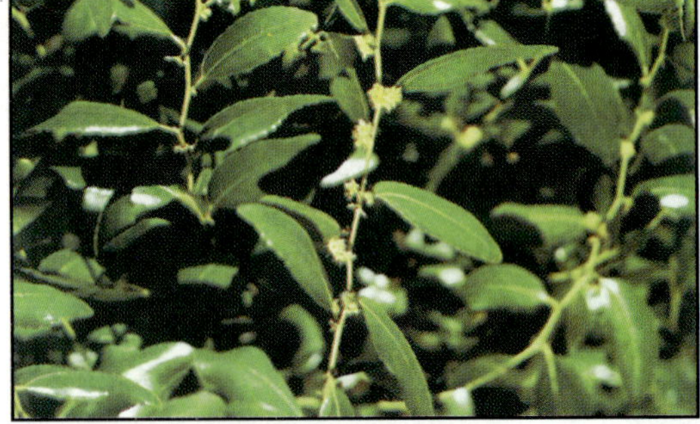

Ziziphus montanum

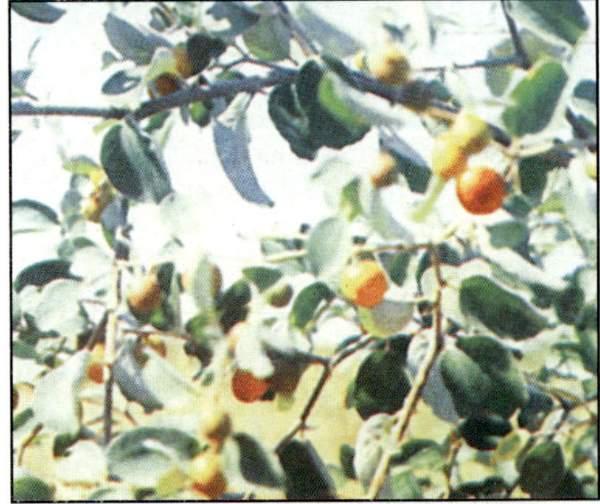

Ziziphus nummularia

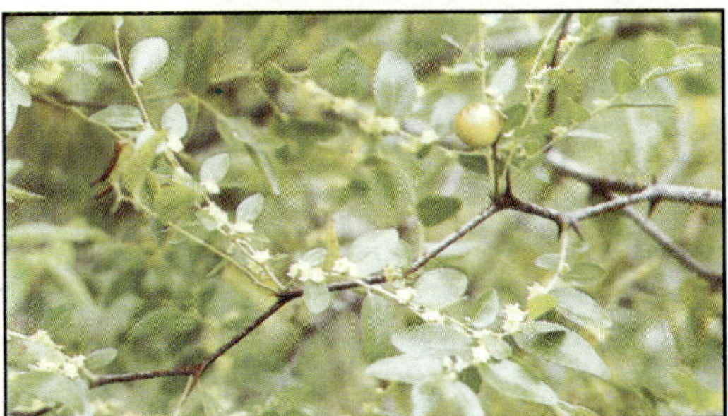

Ziziphus spinosa

SECTION : IV

Medicinal Plants: Resources

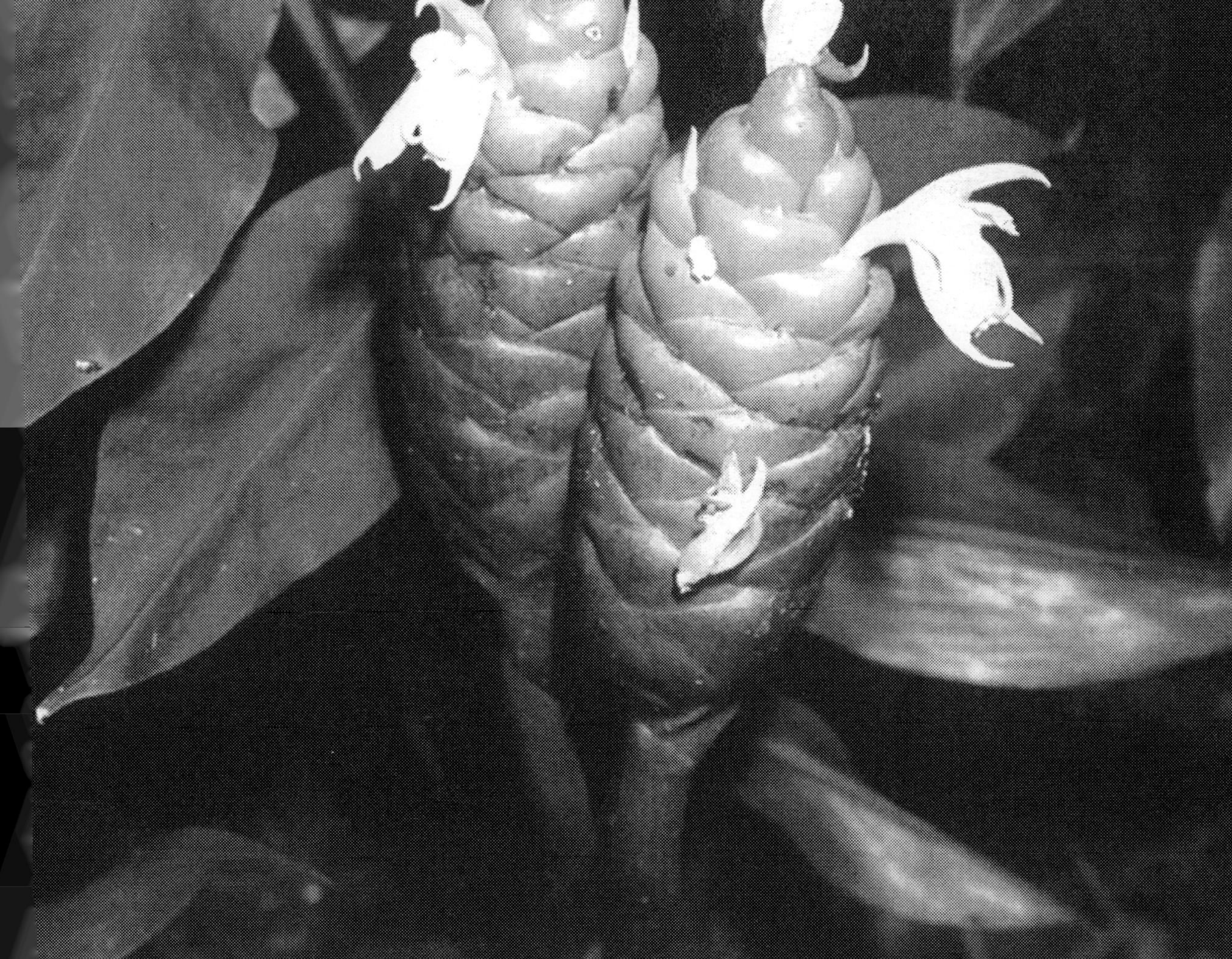

1 EXTRACTORS

1 Alchem International Pvt. Ltd.
5, Empire Estate
Mehrauli – Gurgaon Road
Sultanpur
New Delhi – 110 030

2 Alchem Laboratories
B-21, Industrial Estate
Partapur
Meerut – 250 103 (UP)

3 Alembic Chemical Works
Baroda

4 Alkaloids Corpn.,
8, Bentick Street,
Kolkatta – 700 001

5 Amsar Private Ltd.
47, Laxmibai Nagar Indl. Estate
Indore

6 Ansar Industries
4/3367, H.K. Street
Zampa Bazar
Surat – 395 003

7 Auro Impex Pvt. Ltd.
8, C-1-4936, Dehgam Road,
Industries Township
VAPI – 396 195

8 Ayurchem Products
W-74, MIDC, Phase II
Dombivili (East)
Thane – 421 201

9 Bengal Chemicals & Pharmaceuticals Ltd.
153, Dharamtala Street,
Kolkatta – 700 013

10 Bhavnagar Oil & Chemicals
Industries Pvt. Ltd.,
141, Dalamal Tower,
Nariman Point,
Mumbai – 400 021

11 Bhilware Herbal Extract Co.
H-3, Lane-6, Ibrahimganj,
Bhopal – 1 (M.P.)

12 Bicon India Pvt. Ltd.,
20th K.M. Hosur Road,
Hebbagodi – 562 158
Dist. Bangalore

13 Biological Evans Ltd.,
C-1-4936, Dehgam Road,
Industries Township
VAPI – 396 195

14 Central Institute of Medicinal and
Aromatic Plants,
P.O. CIMAP
Lucknow – 226 016

15 Chemical Industrial & Pharmaceuticals
Laboratories Ltd.,
Vikhroli,
Mumbai – 400 079

16 Chemiloids
40-15-14, Brindavan Colony,
Vijaiwada – 520 010 (AP)

17 CIBA – Giegy of India Ltd.,
Bhandup,
Mumbai – 400 078

18 CIPLA Research Centre & Factory
Vigonagar P & T Office,
Bangalore

19 Concept Pharmaceuticals Ltd.,
167, CST Road,
Santacruz (East), Kalina
Mumbai – 400 098

20 Deccan Phytochemicals
309, Kabra Complex,
61, MG Road,
Secundrabad – 500 003 (AP)

21 Eastern Natural Herb Extracts Ltd.,
53-B, Akurli Industrial Estate,
Akurli Road, Kandivili (East),
Mumbai – 400 101

22 Fortune Biotech Ltd.,
6-6-125, Annam Gardens
Kavadiguda
Secunderabad – 500 380

23 Glaxo Laboratories (P) Ltd.,
Dr. Annie Besant Road,
Worli, Mumbai – 400 018

24 Herbochem,
38, Technocrats Industrial Estate,
Balanagar, Hyderabad – 500 037

25 Hillgreen Company
17, 93th Cross,
Vasanthanagar Extension
Bangalore – 560 052 Karnataka

26 Indo German Alkaloids,
Mahakali Caves Road,
Andheri (East), Mumbai – 400 093

27 Jayant Oil Mills
13, Sitalwadi, Mazgaon,
Mumbai

28 Kaizen Organics (P) Ltd.,
G-17, RIICO Industrial Area
Bagru (Extn) Phase II
Jaipur (Raj.)

29 Kisalaya Pharmaceuticals Pvt. Ltd.
Plot No. 548, Sector – III
Industrial Area, Pithampur
Dist. Dhar (M.P.)

30 Kothari Phytochemicals International
766, Anna Nagar,
Madurai – 625 020

31 Kulu Aromatics
Shamshi – 175 126
Dist. Kullu (H.P.)

32 Kumaon Chemical Products
Village Shivalalpur,
P.O. Ramnagar – 244 715
Nainital

33 Lepro Herbals (P) Ltd.,
5, Empire Estate
Mehrauli – Gurgaon Road
Sultanpur
New Delhi – 110 030

34 Liberty Oil Mills Pvt. Ltd.
302, Dalamal House,
206, Nariman Point,
Mumbai – 400 021

35 Mehta Pharmaceuticals Pvt. Ltd.
G-T Road, Chheharta
Amritsar – 143 105

36 Mumbai Extraction Pvt. Ltd.,
Daya Mandir, 1st Floor
123-25, Mumbadevi Road
Mumbai – 400 003

37 N. B. Laboratories
40, Farm Land,
102 , Ganga,
Ramdas peth
Nagpur (M.S.)

38 Natural Remedies (P) Ltd.,
Manandi Arch
242/29, 2nd Floor, 9th Main,
3rd Block, Jayanagar
Bangalore – 560 011

39 Navyug Pharmaceuticals
48, Industrial Area, Phase II,
Panchkula – 134 113 (Haryana)

40 New India Agro Chemical Ind.
4013, Yawai Road,

41 Organokem Laboratories
xcNear Janata Vidyalaya
Yeola Dist. Nasik

42 Polybond Chemicals
4, Bhaktinagar Station Plot,
Rajkot – 360 002

43 Rathi Papains Pvt. Ltd.
75-76-A, Mittal Court,
Nariman Point,
Mumbai – 400 021

44 Regional Research Laboratory
Canal Road,
Jammu Tawi

45 Rohini Herbals (P) LTd.,
35, Jaora Compound,
M.Y. Hospital Road
Indore – 452 001

46 S. M. Herbals
A-106, Lajpatnagar I,
New Delhi

47 S. M. Organics
30, Hanuman Lane, Canought Place,
New Delhi – 110 001

48 Sami Chemicals & Extracts Ltd.,
19/1, 1st Main, IInd Phase,
Peenya Industrial Area,
Bangalore – 560 058

49 Sandoz India Ltd.,
Sandoz House, Dr. A. B. Road
Worli, Mumbai – 400 018

50 Shashi Phytochemicals Industry,
1, Old Industrial Area,
Alwar (Rajasthan)

51 Sheeba Laboratories Pvt. Ltd.,
B-151, Avas Vikas Colony,
Delhi Road, Saharanpur – 247 001

52 Smith Stanistreet Pharmaceuticals Ltd.
18, Convent Road,
Kolkatta – 700 014

53 Synthozyme Laboratories (P) Ltd.,
G-1, Add1, MIDC,
Jalgaon – 425 003 (MS)

54 Tarani Herbal International
34/3155, Beedanpura
Karol Bagh,
New Delhi

55 Toxicity Research Unit
Maharani Lakshmi Bai Medical College
Pharmacology Department
Jhansi – 284 128 (UP)

56 Toxicology Research Foundation
KUM 2057 Sadashiv, Vijayanagar Colony
Pune – 411030 (MS)

57 Tribal Health Care Research Project
(Siddha)
90-B, Shiva Rajpath,
North Arcot District
Thrupathur (Tamil Nadu)

58 Tribal Health Care Research Project
(Siddha)
Saujanya Nilaya, Main Road,
Chikmagalur District
Kalasa – 577 124 Karnataka

59 Tribal Health Care Research Project
Car Nicobar – 744 301
Andaman & Nicobar Islands

60 Tribal Health Care Research Project
D.N.K. Colony, 1 Dharmapura,
District Bastar
Jagdalpur – 494 005 (CG)

61 Tribal Health Care Research Project
Hospital Campus, Rama Block
Jhabua – 457 661 (MP)

62 Tribal Health Care Research Project
Ranka Block
Palamau District – Bihar

63 Tribal Health Care Research Project
Ziro – 791 120 (AP)

64 Tropical Botanic Garden & Research
Institute
Karimancode, Pacha-Palode P.O.
Thiruvananthapuram – 692562 (Kerala)

65 Tropical Forest Research Institute
Mandla Road
Jabalpur – 482001 (MP)

66 True Food Corporation
17, Kamer Building
38, Cawaji Patel Street,
Mumbai – 400 023

67 Uma Ayurved Bhawan Pvt. Ltd.
Kasganj – 207 123 (U.P)

68 World Coconut Germplasm Centre
Sipighat – Andaman & Nicobar Islands

69 Yogi Herbal Ltd.,
D-28, Industrial Area,
Haridwar – 249 401 (Uttaranchal)

2 EDUCATIONAL INSTITUTES

UNIVERSITY & COLLEGE RESEARCH CENTRE

1 Agricultural Research Station
Bahadari
Mandsaur – 458001 (MP)

2 Ajmal Khan Tibbia College
Aligarh Muslim University
Aligarh – 202001 (UP)

3 Andhra University
Waltair – 530003 (AP)

4 Arid Forest Research Institute
P.O. Krishi Upaz Mandi, New Pali Road
Jodhpur – 342005 Rajasthan

5 Aromatic & Medicinal Plants
Research Station
P.O. Asamanoor, Ernakulam
Dist. Odakkali – 683549
Kerala

6 Ayurvedic & Unani Tibbia College
82 Tibbia College Building, Ajmal Khan
Road,
Karol Bagh
Delhi – 110005

7 Banaras Hindu University
Institute of Medical Sciences
Varanasi – 221005 (UP)

8 Berhampur University
Botany Department
Ecology & Floristcs Laboratory
Berhampur – 760007
Orissa

9 Bhagalpur University
Postgraduate Botany Department
Bhagalpur – 812007
Bihar

10 Bharathidasan University
Chemistry Department
P.O. Khajamalai
Tiruchirapalli – 620024
Tamil Nadu

11 Bharathira University
Coimbatore – 641041
Tamil Nadu

12 Bidhan Chandra Krishi
Viswavidyalaya
Mohanpur – 741252
West Bengal

13 Birla College
Zoology Department
Reproductive Physiology Section
Kalyam – 421361
West Bengal

14 Botanical Survey of India
Andaman & Nicobar Circle
Horticultural Road, Haddo
Port Blair – 744102,
Andaman & Nicobar Islands

15 Botanical Survey of India
Arid Zone Circle
Subhas Nagar
Jodhpur – 342003 Rajasthan

16 Botanical Survey of India
Arunachal Pradesh Circle
Itanagar – 791110
Arunachal Pradesh

17 Botanical Survey of India
Central Circle
10 Chatham Lines
Allahabad – 211002 (UP)

18 Botanical Survey of India
Central National Herbarium
Botanic Garden, Sibpur
Howrah – 711103 West Bengal

19 Botanical Survey of India
Eastern Circle
Woodlands
Shillong – 793003 Meghalaya

20 Botanical Survey of India
Indian Botanic Garden
Sibpur
Howrah – 711103 West Bengal

21 Botanical Survey of India
Indian Museum
Industrial Section
Botanical Museum
1 Sudder Street
Kolkatta – 700016
West Bengal

22 Botanical Survey of India
Northern Circle
192 Kaulagarh Road
Dehra Dun – 248195 (UC)

23 Botanical Survey of India
Sikkim Himalayan Circle
Gangtok – 737101 Sikkim

24 Botanical Survey of India
Southern Circle
P.O. Lawley Road,
Tamil Nadu Agricultural
University Campus
Coimbatore- 641002 Tamil Nadu

25 Botanical Survey of India
Western Circle
7 Koregaon Road
Pune – 411001 Maharashtra

26 Botany Department
Centre of Advanced Study
35 Ballygunge Road, Circular Road
Kolkatta – 700019
West Bengal

27 Kolkatta University
87/1 College Street
Kolkatta – 700073
West Bengal

28 Central Council for Research in
Homoeopathy
JLN Bhartiya Chikitsa Evum Homoeopathy
Anusandhan Bhawan, 61-65
Institutional Area, Opp. D Block
Janakpuri
Delhi – 110058

29 Central Council for Research in Unani
Medicine
Central Herb Garden & Museum
National Botanical Research Institute
Campus
Rana Pratap Marg
Lucknow – 226001 (UP)

30 Central Council for Research in Unani
Medicine
JLN Bhartiya Chikitsa Evum Homoeopathy
Anusandhan Bhawan, 61-65
Institutional Area, Opp. D Block,
Janakpuri
Delhi – 110058

31 Central Council for Research
in Ayurveda & Siddha
JLN Bhartiya Chikitsa Evum
Homoeopathy Anusandhan Bhawan,
61-65 Institutional Area, Opp D.
Block, Janakpuri
Delhi – 110058

32 Central Drug Research Institute
Chattar Manzil Palace
Lucknow – 226001 (UP)

33 Central Institute of Medicinal & Aromatic
Plants
P.O. CIMAP
Lucknow – 226016 (UP)

34 Central Plantation Crops Research Institute
Post Kudlu
Kasaragod – 671124 Kerala

35 Central Plantation Crops Research Institute
Regional Station
Dakshina Kannada Dist.
Vittal – 574273 Karnataka

36 Central Research Institute for Unani
Medicine
11/4/625 Dilkhusha, A.C. Guards
Hyderabad – 500004
Andhra Pradesh

37 College of Agriculture
Indore – Madhya Pradesh

38 College of Science
Botanical Laboratory of Pharmacoanatomy
92 Acharya Prafulla Chandra Road
Kolkatta – 700009
West Bengal]

39 Council of Scientific & Industrial Research
Publications & Information Directorate
Dr. K.S. Krishnan Marg
Delhi – 110012

40 Delhi University
Botany Department
Near Delhi Railway Station
Delhi – 110007

41 Dr. Hari Singh Gour
Vishwavidyalaya
Sagar – 470003
Madhya Pradesh

42 Dr. Y.S. Parmar University of
Horticulture & Forestry
Nauni-Solan – 173230
Himachal Pradesh

43 Forest College & Research Institute
Coimbatore Dist.
Mettuppalayam – 641301
Tamil Nadu

44 Forest Research Institute
Botany Division
P.O. New Forest
Dehra Dun – 248006 ((UC)

45 Forest Research Institute
P.O. New Forest
Dehra Dun – 248006 (UC)

46 Forestry Department
Nauni-Solan – Himachal Pradesh

47 Foundation for Revitalization of Local
Health Traditions
50 MHS Layout, 3rd Main, 2nd Stage,
Anandnagar
Bangalore – 560024 Karnataka

48 G.B. Pant Institute of Himalayan
Environment & Department
Kosi-Katarmal
Almora – 263643 (UC)

49 G.B. Pant University of Agriculture
& Technology
Udham Singh Nagar
Dist. Pantnagar – 263145 (UC)

50 Gandhi Krishi Vigyana Kendra
Bangalore – 5600065 Karnataka

51 Grant Medical College
Department of Medicine
Mumbai – Maharashtra

52 Gujarat Agricultural University
Anand – 388110 Gujarat

53 Gujarat Ayurved University
Dhanwantari Mandir
Jamnagar – 361008 Gujarat

54 Haryana Agricultural University
Plant Breeding Department
Hissar – 125004 Haryana

55 Himachal Pradesh Krishi
Vishva Vidyalaya
Kangra Dist.
Palampur – 176062
Himachal Pradesh

56 HNB Garhwal University
P.B. 38
Srinagar – 246174 (UC)

57 Hoechst India Ltd.
Lal Bahadur Shastri Marg, Mulund
Mumbai – 400080
Maharashtra

58 Homoeopathic Drug Research Institute
B-1433 Indira Nagar
Lucknow – 226016 Uttar Pradesh

59 Horticultural Research Station
Ambalavayal P.O.
Wynad – 673593 Kerala

60 Indian Council of Agricultural Research
Krishi Anusandhan Bhawan, Pusa
Delhi – 110012

61 Indian Council of Forestry Research
& Education
P.O. New Forest
Dehra Dun- 248006 (UC)

62 Indian Council of Medical Research
Ansari Nagar
Delhi – 110029

63 Indian Institute of Ayurveda for Drug
Research
Near Ranikhet
Tarikhet – 263645 (UC)

64 Indian Institute of History of Medicine
Osmania Medical College Buildings,
Putlibowli
Hyderabad – Andhra Pradesh

65 Institute of Forest Genetics & Tree Breeding
Forest College Campus, R.S. Puram
Coimbatore – 641002 Tamil Nadu

66 Institute of Forest Genetics & Tree Breeding Seed Technology Division
Forest College Campus, R.S. Puram
Coimbatore – 641002 Tamil Nadu

67 Institute of Forest Productivity
Ranchi – Bihar

68 Institute of Rain & Moist Deciduous Forest Research
A.T. Road, Tarajan P.O.
Jorhat – 785001 Assam

69 Institute of Wood Science & Technology
18th Cross Road, Malleswaram
Bangalore – 560003 Karnataka

70 Jadavpur University
Kolkatta – 700032 West Bengal

71 Jamia Hamdard
Faculty of Pharmacy
Mehrauli-Badarpur Road,
Hamdard Nagar
Delhi – 110062

72 Jamia Hamdard
Faculty of Science
Botany Department
Mehrauli-Badarpur Road,
Hamdard Nagar
Delhi – 110062

73 Jawaharlal Nehru Ayurvedic Medicinal Plants Garden & Herbarium, Kothrud
Pune – 411029 Maharashtra

74 Jawaharlal Nehru Krishi Vishwa Vidyalaya
(Jawaharlal Nehru Agricultural University)
Krishi Nagar, Adhartal
Jabalpur – 482004 Madhya Pradesh

75 Kasturba Medical College
Manipal – 576119
Karnataka

76 Kerala Agricultural University
Vellanikkara
Thrissur – 680654 Kerala

77 Kerala University
Kariavattom
Thiruvananthapuram – 695034
Kerala

78 Kumaon University
Nainital – 263002 (UC)

79 Lallubhai Motilal College of Pharmacy
P.B. 4011, Navrangpura
Ahmedabad – 380009 Gujarat

80 Lok Swasthya Parampara Samvardhan Samithi
P.B. 7102, Trichy Road, Ramanathapuram
Coimbatore – 641045 Tamil Nadu

81 Lucknow University
Lucknow – 226007 (UC)

82 Madras Medical College
Institute of Pharmacology
Medicinal Chemistry Research Centre
Madras – 600003 Tamil Nadu

83 Marathwada Krishi Vidyapeeth
College of Veterinary & Animal Sciences
Parbhani – 431402 Maharashtra

84 Medical College
Pharmacology Department
Thiruvananthapuram – 695001
Kerala

85 Mohan Lal Sukhadia University
Pratap Nagar
Udaipur – 313001 Rajasthan

86 Nagpur University
Amravati Road
Nagpur – 440010 Maharashtra

87 Narendra Dev University of Agriculture & Technology
Horticulture Department
Faizabad – 224229 (UP)

88 National Botanical Research Institute
Rana Pratap Marg
Lucknow – 226001 (UP)

89 National Bureau of Plant Genetic Resources
Indian Agricultural Research Institute Campus, Pusa
Delhi – 110012

90 North-Eastern Hill University
School of Agricultural Sciences & Rural Development
Medziphema – 797106
Nagaland

91 Orissa University of Agriculture & Technology
Bhubaneswar – 751003 Orissa

92 Osmania University
Hyderabad – 500007 Andhra Pradesh

93 Pepper Research Station
Panniyur, Cannanore
Dist. Taliparamba – 670141 Kerala

94 Plant Systematics & Ethnobotany
Laboratory
Srinagar – 246174 (UC)

95 Poona University
Ganeshkhind
Pune – 411007 Maharashtra

96 Punjab Agricultural University
Ludhiana – 141004 Punjab

97 Punjab University
Sector 14
Chandigarh – 160014

98 Punjabi University
Patiala – 147002 Punjab

99 Punjabrao Krishi Vidyapeeth
P.O. Krishi Nagar
Akola – 444104 Maharashtra

100 Rajasthan University
Jaipur – 302004 Rajasthan

101 Ranchi University
Ranchi – 834008 Jharkhand

102 Regional Research Institute (Ayurveda)
476/6 Sitapur Road
Lucknow – 226007 (UP)

103 Regional Research Institute (Ayurveda)
Rajendra Memorial Research Institute
Building, Kadam Kuan
Patna – 800007 Bihar

104 Regional Research Institute of Unani
Medicine
1 West Mada Chruch Street, Royapuram
Madras – 600013 Tamil Nadu

105 Regional Research Institute of Unani
Medicine
Aligarh Muslim University, Department of
Research in Unani Medicine
Aligarh – 202001 (UP)

106 Regional Research Institute of Unani
Medicine
Dist. Balasore
Bhadrak – 756100 Orissa

107 Regional Research Institute of Unani
Medicine
Nawab Manzil, Guzri
Patna- 800008 Bihar

108 Regional Research Institute of Unani
Medicine
University of Kashmir, University Health
Centre, Hazratbal
Srinagar- 190006 Jammu & Kashmir

109 Regional Research Laboratory,
Canal Road
Jammu Tawi – 180001 Jammu & Kashmir

110 Regional Research Laboratory,
Jorhat- 785006 Assam

111 Reproduction Biology Laboratory
Almora – 263601 (UC)

112 SK University of Agricultural
Science & Technology
Shalimar – 191121 Jammu & Kashmir

113 SKN College of Agriculture
Rajasthan Agricultural University Campus
Jobner – 303328 Rajasthan

114 Spices Board India
Sugandha Bhavan, N.H. Bypass,
Palarivattam
Cochin – 682025 Kerala

115 Sri Venkateswara University
Tirupati – 517502 Andhra Pradesh

116 St. Xavier's College
Botany Department
Palayamkottai – 627002 Tamil Nadu

117 Survey of Medicinal Plants & Collection
Unit
112 Government Arts College Campus
Udhagamandalam – 643002
Tamil Nadu

118 Tamil Nadu Agricultural University
Lawley Road
Coimbatore – 641003 Tamil Nadu

119 Temperate Forest Research Institute
Shimla – Himachal Pradesh

120 Tibetan Medical & Astro Institute
Men-Tsee-Khang Exports
13 Jaipur Estate, Nizamuddin East
Delhi – 110013

121 Tropical Botanic Garden &
Research Institute
Karimancode, Pacha-Palode P.O.
Thiruvananthapuram – 692562
Kerala

122 Tropical Forest Research Institute
Mandla Road
Jabalpur – 482001
Madhya Pradesh

123 University of Agricultural Sciences
Gandhi Krishi Vigyana Kendra Campus
Bangalore – 560065
Karnataka

124 Voluntary Health Association of India
40 Qutab Institutional Area
Delhi – 110016

125 Wildlife Institute of India
Chandrabani, P.B. 18
Dehra dun – 248001 (UP)

126 Zandu Pharmaceutical Ltd.,
70, Gokhale Road South, Dadar
Mumbai – 400025 Maharashtra

AYURVEDIC COLLEGES

1 ALN Rao Memorial Ayurved Medical College
Koppa – 577 126
Dist. Chickmagalore (Karnataka)

2 Anantha Laxmi Govt. Ayurved College
Station Road,
Warangal – 506 002 (A.P.)

3 Aryakanya Shuddha Ayurved Mahavidyalaya
Kereli Bagh
Vadodara – 390 018

4 Ashtang Ayurved Mahavidyalaya
2062, Sadashiv Peth
Vijaynagar Colony
Pune – 411 030 (Maharashtra)

5 AV Samiti's Ayurved Maha Vidaylaya
Bijapur – 586 101 (Karnataka)

6 Ayurved & Unani Tibbia College
Ajmal Khan Road, Karol Bagh
New Delhi – 110 005

7 Ayurved College
Pathanjali puri, Thadgam (Via)
Coimbatore – 641 108 (Tamil Nadu)

8 Ayurved Mahavidyalaya
Ganeshwadi, Panchavati
Nasik – 422 003 (Maharashtra)

9 Ayurved Mahavidyalaya
Gaya – 823 991 (Bihar)

10 Ayurved Mahavidyalaya
Heggeri Extension
Old Hubli – 580 024 (Karnataka)

11 Ayurved Mahavidyalaya
Near Sion Railway Station
Sion
Mumbai – 400 022 (Maharashtra)

12 Ayurved Mahavidyalaya
Shri Shivaji Nagar
Tal: Rahuri, – 413 796
Dist. Ahmednagar (Maharashtra)

13 Bundelkhand Govt. Ayurved College
Jhansi – 294 001 (U.P.)

14 Chaitanya Ayurved Mahavidyalaya
Sakegaon
Bhusawal – 425 201 (Maharashtra)

15 Dayanand Ayurved College
Mahatma Hansraj Marg
Jalandhar City – 144 088 Punjab

16 Dayanand Ayurved Medical College & Hospital
Siwan – 841 221 (Bihar)

17 DMM Ayurved Mahavidyalaya
Aarni Road, Shivaji Nagar
Yeotmal – 445 001 Maharashtra

18 Dr. BRKR Govt. Ayurvedic College
S.R. Nagar, Erragadda
Hyderabad – 500 038 (A.P.)

19 Dr. N.R. Sastry Govt. Ayurved College
Bandar Road
Vijayawada – 520 002 (A.P)

20 Ganga Educational Society's Ayurved Medical College
Kolhapur – 416 012 (Maharashtra)

21 Gaur Brahaman Ayurved College
Rohtak – 124 001 (Haryana)

22 Gopabandhu Ayurved Mahavidyalaya
Puri – 752 002 (Orissa)

23 Government Dharam Samaj Sanskrit Mahavidyalaya
Muzaffarpur (Bihar)

24 Govt. Akhandanand Ayurved College
Opp. Victoria Garden Bhadra
Ahmedabad – 380 001 Gujarat

25 Govt. Ashtang Ayurved Mahavidyalaya & Hospital
Lok Manya Nagar
Indore – 420 009 (M.P)

26 Govt. Ayurved College & Hospital
Balangir – 767 001 Orissa

27 Govt. Ayurved College
Ajwa Road
Baroda – 390 001 Gujarat

28 Govt. Ayurved College
Atarra – 210 201 Dist. Banda, (UP)

29 Govt. Ayurved College
Herbala Road, Ulubari
Guwahati – 781 001 Assam

30 Govt. Ayurved College
Kadam Kuan
Patna – 800 003 Bihar

31 Govt. Ayurved College
Patiala – 147 001 Punjab

32 Govt. Ayurved College
Rewa – 486 001 (M.P)

33 Govt. Ayurved College
Sadar Bagh
Junagarh – 362 001 Gujarat

34 Govt. Ayurved College
Wazirabad
Nanded – 431 601 (Maharashtra)

35 Govt. Ayurved Mahavidyalaya
Raje Raghuji Nagar
Nagpur – 440 001 Maharashtra

36 Govt. Ayurveda College
Dhanwantari Nagar
Tripunithura – 682 301
Dist. Ernakulam, Kerala

37 Govt. Ayurveda College
M.G. Road
Thiruvananthapuram – 695 001
Kerala

38 Govt. Ayurvedic College
Gorakhpur

39 Govt. Ayurvedic College
Gwalior – 473 001 (M.P)

40 Govt. Ayurvedic College
Raipur – 492 001 (M.P)

41 Govt. Ayurvedic College
Tuijapur Road, Madhban
Osmanabad – 413 501 Maharashtra

42 Govt. College of Indian Medicine &
Hospital, Vishweshwariah Circle
Sayau Rao Road
Mysore – 570 021 Karnataka

43 Govt. College of Indian Medicine
Dhanvantari Road
Bangalore – 560 009 Karnataka

44 Govt. Dhanwantri Ayurved College
Mangalnath Road
Ujjain – 456 001 (M.P)

45 Govt. Gurukul Ayurved College
Gurukul Kangari
Haridwar – 249 401 (UC)

46 Govt. Rishikul Ayurved College
Haridwar – 249 401 (UC)

47 Govt. Taranath Ayurved College
Anantapur Road
Bellary – 583 101 Karnataka

48 Hanuman Shikshan Prasark Mandal's
Ayurved Mahavidyalaya
Peth Vadagaon, Tq. Hatkanacgala,
Dist. Kolhapur Maharashtra

49 J.S. Ayurved Mahavidyalaya
College Road
Nadiad – 387 001 Gujarat

50 Karmavir Vyankatrao Tanaji Randhir
Ayurved College
Boradi – 401 701
Tal. Shirpur, (Maharashtra)

51 Karnataka Liberal Education Society
Shri BM Kankanwadi Ayurved
Mahavidyalaya
Shahapur
Belgaum – 590 003 Karnataka

52 Kaviraj Ananta Tripathy Sarma Ayurved
College
Ankushpur – 761 100,
Ganjam (Orissa)

53 Lal Bahadur Shastri Govt.
Ayurved Mahavidyalaya
Handia – 221 503 Allahabad (UP)

54 M.M.M. Govt. Ayurved Mahavidyalaya
Udaipur – 313 001 (Rajasthan)

55 Maharashtra Arogya Mandal
Hadapsar – 411 028
Pune (Maharashtra)

56 Mohta Ayurved Mahavidyalaya
Sadulpur – 331 023
Dist. Churu, (Rajasthan)

57 National Institute of Ayurved
Madhav Vilas Palace, Amer Road
Jaipur – 302 002 (Rajasthan)

58 Nitishwar Bhartiya Chikitsha Vigyan Sansthan & Hospital
Mukherjee Seminar Campus
Harisabha Chowk, Ramna
Muzaffarpur – 842 002 (Bihar)

59 Parsurampuriya Ayurved College
Sikar – 332 001 Rajasthan

60 PBN Institute of Indian Medical Sciences
Ranti Road
Madhubani – 847 211 Bihar

61 RA Podar Medical College (Ayurved)
Worli, Mumbai – 400 018
(Maharashtra)

62 Rajkiya Ayodhya Shivkumari Ayurved Mahavidyalaya
Begusarai – 850 101 Bihar

63 Rajkiya Ayurved Mahavidyalaya
Paprola – 176 115
Dist. Kangra (H.P)

64 Rajkiya Lalit Hari Ayurved College
Pilibhit – 262 001 (UP)

65 Rajkiya Maharani Rameshwari Bhartiya Chikitsa Vigyan Sansthan
Mohanpur – 846 007
Darbhanga (Bihar)

66 Ravindernath Mukherji Ayurved Mahavidyalaya
Dist. Champaran
Motihari – 845 401 Bihar

67 S.S.M.D. Ayurved College & Hospital
G.T. Road
Moga – 142 001 Punjab

68 S.V. Ayurved College
T.T. Devasthanams
Tirupati – 517 501 (A.P.)

69 Sangam Sewabhavi Trust's Ayurved Mahavidyalaya
Sanjivan Hospital, Nasik Poona Road
Sangamner – 422 605 (Maharashtra)

70 Seth Chandanmal Mutha Aryangla Vaidyak Mahavidyalaya
Cendamal
Satara – 415 001 Maharashtra

71 Seth Govindji Raoji Ayurved Mahavidyalaya
21/A/13, Budhwar Peth, Samarat Chowk
Sholapur – 413 002 Maharashtra

72 Seth JP Govt. Ayurved Mahavidyalaya
Opp. Sardar Bagh Bhadra
Bhavnagar – 364 001 Gujarat

73 Sh. DM College of Ayurveda
Udupi – 576 101 (Karnataka)

74 Sh. Gangadhar Shastri Gune Ayurved Mahavidyalaya
Vishrambag
Ahmednagar – 414 001 Maharashtra

75 Shri Ayurved Mahavidyalaya
Dhanwantri Marg, Hanuman Nagar
Nagpur – 440 009 Maharashtra

76 Shri Balahanuman Ayurved Mahavidyalaya
At & Post Lodhra – 382 835
Dist. Mehsana (Gujarat)

77 Shri Bhanwar Lal Dugar Ayurved
Vishwabharati (Gandhi Vidya Mandir)
Sardar Shahar – 331 403
Dist. Churu, (Rajasthan)

78 Shri Dhanwantri Ayurved Mahavidyalaya
Ahiroli, Buxar
Bhojpur – 802 101 (Bihar)

79 Shri Dhanwantry Ayurved College & Pandit
Kedarnath Memorial Ayurved Hospital
Sector 46-B
Chandigarh – 160 017

80 Shri Gulab Kunverba Ayurved Mahavidyalaya
Dhanwantri Mandir
Jamnagar – 361 008 Gujarat

81 Shri Gurudev Ayurved Mahavidyalaya
Gurukul Ashram (Mozari)
Amrawati – 444 601 Maharashtra

82 Shri Krishna Govt. Ayurved College
Kurukshetra – 132 118 Haryana

83 Shri Laxminarayan Ayurved College
Sant Tulsidas Marg
Amritsar – 143 001 Punjab

84 Shri Maru Singh Memorial Mahila Ayurved Degree College
Kanya Gurukul
Khanpur Kalan – 124 301
(Sonepat) Haryana

85 Shri Mastnath Ayurved College
Asthal Bohar
Rohtak – 124 001 (Haryana)

86 Shri Moti Singh Jageshwari Ayurved Mahavidyalaya
Chhapra – 841 301 (Bihar)

87 Shri Nursinghanath Ayurved College & Research Institute
Nrusinghnath P.O., Paikmal
Dist. Sambalpur – 768 029 (Orissa)

88 Shri OH Nazar Ayurved College
Near Railway Station
Shri Swami Atmanand Saraswati Road
Surat – 395 003 (Gujarat)

89 Shri Radha Krishna Toshniwal Ayurved Mahavidyalaya
Station Road
Akola – 444 001 Maharashtra

90 Shri Venkataramana Ayurved College
144, Kutchery Road, Mylapore
Madras – 600 004 Tamil Nadu

91 Smt. KG Mittal Punarvasu Ayurved College
Netaji Subash Road
Mumbai – 400 002 Maharashtra

92 Sri Yatindra Narayan Ashtang
Bhagalpur – 812 006 Bihar

93 SRM Govt. Ayurved College
Bareilly – 243 001 (UP)

94 State Ayurved College
Tulsidas Marg
Lucknow – 226 004 (UP)

95 Swami Kalyandev Govt. Ayurved College
Rampur
Muzaffar Nagar (U.P)

96 Swami Raghavandracharya Ayurved Mahavidyalaya
Karjara Station P.O., Manjholi
Gaya – 823 001 Bihar

97 Tilak Ayurved Mahavidyalaya
583/2, Rasta Peth
Pune – 411 011 Maharashtra

98 Vaidyaratnam Ayurveda College
Ollur – Thikkattussery
Trichur – 680 322 Kerala

99 Vasant Dada Patil Ayurved Medical College
South Shivaji Nagar
Sangli – 416 416 Maharashtra

100 Vasant Kusum's Rural Yog & Ayurved Sanshodhan
Paratishthanam's Sidh Kalan Ayurved Mahavidyalya
Nehru Chowk
Sangamner – 422 605
Dist. Ahmednagar Maharashtra

101 Vidarbha Ayurved Mahavidyalaya
Hanuman Nagar
Amrawati – 444 605 Maharashtra

102 VPS Varier Ayurveda College
Kottakkal, Edarikode P.O. – 675 501
Malappuram Dist. (Kerala)

103 Yashwant Shikshan Prasark Mandal's
Sri Yashwant Ayurved College
At & Post Kedali – 416 114
Tel. Panhala, Dist. Kolhapur (Maharashtra)

104 Yerala Medical Trust & Research Center's
Ayurved Medical College
Mumbai – 400 012 Maharashtra

INSTITUTES OF UNANI MEDICINE

1 Central Herb Garden & Museum
Regional Research Institute of Unani Medicine
163-164, Terhi Pulia
Kursi Road, P.O. Batha Saboli, Aliganj
Lucknow – 226 007 (UP)

2 Central Research Institute of Unani Medicine
Opp. E.S.I. Hospital
A.G. Colony Road, Erragadda
Hyderabad – 500 838 Andhra Pradesh

3 Chemical Research Unit
Department of Research in Unani Medicine
Near Office of Dean, Faculty of Science
Aligarh Muslim University
Aligarh – 202 002 (UP)

4 Drug Standardization Research Unit
Central Research Institute of Unani Medicine
Opp. E.S.I. Hospital
AG Colony Road, Erragadda
Hyderabad – 500 838 Andhra Pradesh

5 Drug Standardization Research Unit
Department of Chemistry, Central College
Bangalore – 560 001 Karnataka

6 Drug Standardization Research Unit
Department of Chemistry, New College
P.B. No. 684, P.O. Rayapatta, 87,
Peters Road
Chennai – 600 014 Tamil Nadu

7 Drug Standardization Research Unit
Jamia Hamdard, Hamdard Nagar
New Delhi – 110 062

8 Drug Standardization Research Unit
Regional Research Institute of Unani
Medicine, 163-164, Terhi Pulia,
Kursi Road P.O. Batha Saboli, Aliganj
Lucknow – 226 007 (UP)

9 Family Welfare Research Unit
Govt. Nizamiah Tibbiya College
Hyderabad – 500 002 Andhra Pradesh

10 Family Welfare Research Unit
Regional Research Institute of Unani
Medicine, J.J. Hospital Compound
Behind Eye Benk, Byculla
Mumbai – 400 008 Maharashtra

11 Information Centre
Central Council for Research in Unani
Medicine, 61-65, Institutional Area
Pankha Road, Janakpuri
New Delhi – 110 058

12 Literary Research Institute of Unani
Medicine
Jamia Hamdard, Hamdard Nagar
New Delhi – 110 062

13 Regional Research Institute of Unani
Medicine
1, West Mada Church Street, Royapuram
Chennai – 600 001 (Tamil Nadu)

14 Regional Research Institute of Unani
Medicine
163-164, Tehri Pulia, Kursi Road
P.O. Batha Saboli, Aliganj
Lucknow – 226 007 (UP)

15 Regional Research Institute of Unani
Medicine
79-B, 1st Floor, Chittaranjan Avenue
Kolkatta – 700 073 West Bengal

16 Regional Research Institute of Unani
Medicine
A.K. Tibbiya College Hospital (New Block)
Aligarh Muslim University
Aligarh – 202 002 (UP)

17 Regional Research Institute of Unani
Medicine
Bhadrak – 756 100 Orissa

18 Regional Research Institute of Unani
Medicine
Nawab Manzil, Guzri
Patna – 800 008 Bihar

19 Regional Research Institute of Unani
Medicine
University of Kashmir, Hazrat Bal
Srinagar – 190 006 Jammu & Kashmir

20 Regional Research Institute of Unani
Medicine, J.J. Hospital Compound
Behind Eye Bank, Byculla
Mumbai – 400 008 Maharashtra

COLLEGES OF UNANI MEDICINE

1 A.K.I. Tibbia College and Hospital
Nagpada, Hasrat Mohani Chowk
Mumbai – 400 001 Maharashtra

2 Ajmal Khan Tibbia College
Aligarh University
Aligarh – 202 002 (UP)

3 Ayurvedic and Unani Tibbia College
Karol Bagh, New Delhi – 110 005

4 Kolkatta Unani Medical College
Maulvi Abdul Haleem Lane
Kolkatta – 700 016

5 Deoband Unani Medical College
Naya Bans, Near Talhavi Chungi
Deoband – 247 554
Dist. Saharanpur (UC)

6 Dr. Abdul Haq Unani Medical College
& Hospital
Park Road, Kurnool – 518 001
Andhra Pradesh

7 Government Nizamiah Tibbi College
Charminar, Hyderabad – 500 001
Andhra Pradesh

8 Government Unani Medical College
Arignar Anna Govt. Hospital of
Indian Medicine, Chennai – 600 106
Tamil Nadu

9 Government Unani Medical College
No. 261 1st Floor, Indian Red Cross
Society Building
Mahadeva Nagar, Race Course Road
Bangalore – 560 039

10 Hamdard Tibbi College
Hamdard Nagar,
New Delhi – 110 062

11 Ibn-e-Sina Tibbia College
Binapara, Dist. Azamgarh (UP)

12 Jamia Tibbia, Deoband – 247 554
Dist. Saharanpur (UC)

13 Mohammedia Tibbia College and
Assayer Hospital
P.O. Box No. 128, Mansoora
Malegaon – 423 203
Dist. Nasik (Maharashtra)

14 Nizamia Unani Medical College
& Hospital
Bari Road, Gaya – 823 001 Bihar

15 Rajasthan Unani Tibbia College
11/4636, Handipura,
Chawkri Ram Chandra Ji,
Jaipur – 302 00

16 Rajputana Unani Tibbia College
Khander ka Rasta, Near Char Darwaza
Jaipur – 302 002

17 Saifia Hamidia Unani Tibbia College
Burhanpur – 450 331
Dist. Khandwa (MP)

18 Salfia Unani Medical College
Laheria Sarai, Darbhanga – 846 001
Bihar

19 Taj Tibbia College
Jamia Arabia, Rasheed Nagar
Nagpur – 440 002 Maharashtra

20 Takmil ut-Tibb College
Jhawai Tola, Hakim Abdul Aziz Road,
Lucknow – 226 003 (UP)

21 Unani Medical College & Hospital
Anglo-Urdu School Campus,
New Modi Khana
K.B. Hidayatullah Road
Pune – 411 001 Maharashtra

22 Unani Medical College and Hospital
Gulshan-e-Masoom Azam Colony
Dargah Road, Parbhani – 431 401
Maharashtra

23 Unani Medical College and Hospital
Muzaffarpur, Kadam Kuan,
Patna – 800 003 Bihar

24 Unani Medical College
Himmatganj, Allahabad – 211 001
(UP)

25 Zulfequar Haider Unani Medical College
& Hospital, P.O. Box No. 12,
Nawalpur, SIWAN – 841 226 Bihar

SIDDHA CENTRES

1 Ayushya Ayurvedic Centre
Kovalam
Thiruvananthapuram

2 Devaki Ayurvedic Health Care Centre
Vazhuthacaud
Thiruvananthapuram

3 Gopals Ayurvedic Beach Resort
Main Beach Kovalam
Thiruvananthapuram – 695527 (Kerala)

4 Hotel Samudra
Kovalam (Kerala)

5 Ideal Ayurvedic Centre
Chowara, Kovalam
Thiruvananthapuram – 693501 (Kerala)

6 Kairali Ayurvedic Health Resort
Olassery Post Kodumbu
Palakkad – 678551 (Kerala)

7 Keraleeya Ayurveda Samajam Hospital and
Nursing Home
Shornur – 679123

8 Nagarjuna Ayurveda Resport
Thannipuzha Okkal P.O.
Kaladi (Kerala)

9 Rajah Healthy Acres
P.B.No.2
Chavakkad – 680506 (Kerala)

10 Santhigiri Health Care Centre
Olasseri Post
Palakkad – 678551 (Kerala)

11 Santhigiri Hospital Complex
Koliacode P.O.
Pothencode
Thiruvananthapuram – 695607 (Kerala)

12 Somatheeram Ayurvedic Beach Resort
Chowara P.O.
South Kovalam
Thiruvananthapuram – 695501 (Kerala)

13 Sree Sankara Gardens
Pambupara P.O.
(Via) Vandanmedu
Ankkara Kumily (Kerala)

14 Sreedhari Ayurvedic Health Resort
Koottala P.O.
Thrissur – 680652 (Kerala)

15 Surya Ayurvedics Ltd.
Kanjany
Thrissur (Kerala)

3 RESEARCH INSTITUTIONS

1 Agricultural & Processed Food Products Export Development Authority (APEDA)
4th Fl., Ansal Chambers 2,
6 Bhikaji Cama Place
Delhi – 110 066

2 All India Ayurvedic Congress (Akhila Bharatiya Ayurveda Mahasammelan)
Dhanwantri bhavan, Road,
66, Punjabi Bagh
Delhi – 110 026

3 All India Ayurvedic Specialists (Post Graduate) Association (Akhil Bhartiya Ayurveda Visheshajan Sammelan)
Secr.: K. Dharam Vir, 320 Narela
Delhi – 110 040

4 All India Institute of Medical Sciences (AIIMS)
Pharmacology Department
Ansari Nagar
Delhi – 110 029

5 All India Unani Tibbia Conference
2077 Qasim Jan Street
Delhi – 110 006

6 Amala Cancer Research Centre (ARRC)
Amala Nagar
Thrissur – 680 553 Kerala

7 Arid Forest Research Institute
P.O. Krishi Upaz Mandi,
New Pali Road
Jodhpur – 342005 Rajasthan

8 Arya Vaidya Sala
Malappuram District
Kottakal – 676 503 (Kerala)

9 Arya Vaidyan Rama Varier Educational Foundation of Ayurveda (AVREFA)
366 Trichy Road
Coimbatore – 641 018 Tamil Nadu

10 Ayurvedic Research Centre
Ayurvedic & Unani Tibbia College Campus
Ajmal Khan Road, Karol Bagh
Delhi – 110 005

11 Ayurvedic Research Unit
National Institute of Mental Health & Neuro-Sciences,
P.B. 2779, Hosur Road
Bangalore – 560 029 (Karnataka

12 Banaras Hindu University,
Varanasi – 221005 (Uttar Pradesh)

13 Basic Chemicals, Pharmaceuticals & Cosmetics Export promotion Council (CHEMEXCIL)
Jhansi Castle, 4th Fl., 7 Cooperage Road
Mumbai – 400 039 (Maharashtra)

14 Bhaba Atomic Research Centre (BARC)
Bio-Organic Division
Trombay
Mumbai – 400 085 (Maharashtra)

15 Bhaba Atomic Research Centre (BARC)
Plant Biotechnology Section
Trombay
Mumbai – 400 085 (Maharashtra)

16 Birla Institute of Scientific Research (BISR)
78 Syed Amir Ali Avenue
Kolkatta – 700 019 (West Bengal)

17 Botanical Survey of India (BSI)
Botanic Garden, Sibpur
Howrah – 711 103 (West Bengal)

18 Botanical Survey of India
Andaman & Nicobar Circle
Horticultural Road, Haddo
Port Blair – 744 102
Andaman & Nicobar Islands

19 Botanical Survey of India
Arid Zone Circle
Subhash Nagar
Jodhpur – 342 003 (Raj.)

20 Botanical Survey of India
Arunachal Pradesh circle
Sankai View
Itanagar – 791 110 (AP)

21 Botanical Survey of India
Central Circle
10 Chatham Lines
Allahabad – 211 001 (UP)

22 Botanical Survey of India
Eastern Circle
Woodlands
Shillong – 793 003 (Meghalaya)

23 Botanical Survey of India
Northern Circle
192, Kaulagarh Road
Dehra Dun – 248 195 (UC)

24 Botanical Survey of India
Sikkim Himalayan Circle
Gangtok – 737 101 Sikkim

25 Botanical Survey of India
Southern Circle
P.O. Lawley Road,
Tamil Nadu Agricultural University Campus
Coimbatore – 641 002 Tamil Nadu

26 Botanical Survey of India
Western Circle
7 Koregaon Road
Pune – 411 001 Maharashtra

27 Captain Srinivasa Murti Drug
Research Institute For Ayurveda (CSMDRIA)
Arignar Anna Government Hospital
Campus, Arumbakkam
Madras – 600 016 Tamil Nadu

28 Cardamom Research Centre
Appangala- Kerala

29 Catholic Hospital Association of India
(CHAI)
Community Health Department
P.B. 2126, 157/6 Staff Road,
Gunrock Enclave
Secunderabad – 500 003 (AP)

30 Central Council For Homoeopathy (CCH)
JLN Bhartiya Chikitsa Evum Homoeopathy
Anusandhan Bhawan, 61-65 Institutional
Area, opp. D Block, Janakpur
Delhi – 110 058

31 Central Council For Indian Medicine (CCIM)
JLN Bhartiya Chikitsa Evum Homoeopathy
Anusandhan Bhawan,
61-65 Institutional Area
opp. D Block, Janakpur
Delhi – 110 058

32 Central Council for Research in
Homoeopathy (CCRH)
JLN Bhartiya Chikitsa Evum Homoeopathy
Anusandhan Bhawan, 61-65 Institutional
Area, opp. D Block, Janakpuri
Delhi – 110 058

33 Central Council for Research in Yoga
& Naturopathy
JLN Bhartiya Chikitsa Evum Homoeopathy
Anusandhan Bhawan,
61-65 International Area,
Opp. D Block, Janakpuri
Delhi – 110058

34 Central Council For Research In
Ayurveda & Siddha (CCRAS)
JLN Bhartiya Chikitsa Evum Homoeopathy
Anusandhan Bhawan,
61-65 Institutional Area,
opp. D Block, Janakpuri
Delhi – 110 058

35 Central Council For Research in
Unani Medicine (CCRUM)
JLN Bhartiya Chikitsa Evum Homoeopathy
Anusandhan Bhawan,
61-65 Institutional Area,
opp. D Block, Janakpuri
Delhi – 110 058

36 Central Drug Research Institute
Chattar Manzil Palace
Lucknow – 226001 (UP)

37 Central Food Technological Research Inst.
Cheluvamba Mansion
Mysore – 570013 Karnataka

38 Central Herb Garden & Museum
National Botanical Research Institute
Campus, Rana Pratap Marg
Lucknow – 226 001 (UP)

39 Central Institute of Medicinal & Aromatic Plants
P.O. CIMAP
Lucknow – 226016 (UP)

40 Central Plantation Crops Research Institute, Post Kudlu
Kasargod – 671124

41 Central Research Institute (Ayurveda)
Dhanwantari Bhawan, Road 66, Punjabi Bagh
Delhi – 110 026

42 Central Research Institute (Ayurveda)
Near Rajdhani College, New Capital, Ashok Nagar
Bhubaneswar – 751 009 Orissa

43 Central Research Institute (Ayurveda)
Raja Ramdeo Anadilal Podar Institute, Worli
Mumbai – 400 018 (MS)

44 Central Research Institute (Siddha)
Arignar Anna Government Hospital Campus, Arumbakkam
Madras – 600 106 (TN)

45 Central Research Institute for Unani Medicine
114/625 Dilkhusha, A.C. Guards
Hyderabad – 500 004 (AP)

46 Central Tuber Crops Research Institute, Sree Kariyam
Thiruvananthapuram – 695017 (Kerala)

47 Centre for Advanced Research on Standardisation, Quality Control & Formulation of Selected Traditional Remedies Punjab University, Pharmaceutical Sciences Department
Chandigarh – 160014

48 Centre for Minor Forest Products for Rural Development & Environmental Conservation
HIG – 2/8 General Mahadev Singh Road, Indirapuram P.O. Kanwali
Dehra Dun – 248001 (UC)

49 Centre for Science & Technology for Rural Development Biotechnology Unit
Kannamangalam North
Mavelikara – 690106 Kerala

50 Centre for Tribal Medicine
North Wayanad
Manantavady – Kerala

51 Council for Traditional Medical Sciences of Assam
Khanikar Puthibharal, Tetelitol
Golaghat P.O. – 785621 Assam

52 Council of Scientific & Industrial Research Complex, Palampur
Mission Road
Palampur – 176061 Himachal Pradesh

53 Council of Scientific & Industrial Research, 2, Rafi Marg
New Delhi – 110001

54 DCOMPWB Research Laboratory
Mungpoo (Darjeeling) – 734313
West Bengal

55 Directorate of Cinchona & Other Medicinal Plants, Govt. of West Bengal
10/1A, Indian Mirror Street
Kolkatta – 700013 West Bengal

56 Dr. A. Lakshmipathi Research Centre in Ayurveda, V.H.S. Medical Centre,
TTTI Post Office
Madras – 600 113 Tamil Nadu

57 Drug Research Scheme (Multidisciplinary) (Siddha)
Central Research Institute,
A.A. Government Hospital Campus
Arumbakkam
Madras – 600 016 Tamil Nadu

58 Drug Standardisation Research Unit (Siddha)
Captain Srinivasa Murti Drug Research Institute for Ayurveda,
A.A. Government Hospital Campus,
Arumbakkam
Madras – 600 106 Tamil Nadu

59 Drug Standardisation Research Unit (Siddha)
Regional Research Centre (Ayurveda),
Government Central Pharmacy Annex,
Ashok Pillar, Jayanagar
Bangalore – 560 011 Karnataka

60 Drug Standardisation Research Unit (Siddha)
Regional Research Institute (Drug Research), Poojapura
Thiruvananthapuram – 695 012 (Kerala)

61 Drug Standardisation Research Unit
Central College, Chemistry Department
Bangalore – 560 001 Karnataka

62 Drug Standardisation Research Unit
Jamia Hamdard, Research Division,
Mehrauli-Badarpur Road, Hamdard Nagar
Delhi – 110062

63 Drug Standardisation Research Unit
National Botanical Research Institute,
Rana Pratap Marg
Lucknow – 226001 (U.P.)

64 Drug Standardisation Research Unit
New College, Chemistry Dept,
87 Peters Road
Madras – 600014 Tamil Nadu

65 Drug Standardisation Research Unit
Osmania University, Chemistry Department
Hyderabad – 500007 Andhra Pradesh

66 Drug Standardisation Research Unit
Regional Research Institute of Unani
Medicine, Aligarh Muslim University,
Department of Research in Unani Medicine
Aligarh – 202 001 (UP)

67 Drug Standardisation Research Unit
University of Kashmir, University Health
Centre, Hazratbal,
Srinagar – 190006 (J&K)

68 Drug Standardisation Unit
Banaras Hindu University,
Institute of Medical Sciences,
Dravyaguna Department
Varanasi – 221 005 (UP)

69 Drug Standardisation Unit
Gujarat Ayurved University, Pharmacy
Department,
Dhanvantari Mandir
Jamnagar – 361 008 Gujarat

70 Drug Standardisation Unit
Homoeopathic Pharmacopoeia Laboratory,
Central Government Offices Complex,
Kamla Nehru Nagar
Ghaziabad – 201 002 (UP)

71 Drug Standardisation Unit
Osmania University Building 32,
Botany Department,
Vikram Puri, Habsigunda
Hyderabad – 500 007 (AP)

72 Drugs Testing Laboratory
Palace Road
Bangalore – 560001 (Karnataka)

73 Food & Drug Toxicology Research
Centre
National Institute of Nutrition,
Jamai-Osmania Campus
Hyderabad – 500007 (AP)

74 Food & Drugs Laboratory
National Highway 8, near Polytechnic Inst.
Vadodara – 390002 Gujarat

75 Forest Research Institute
P.O. New Forest
Dehra Dun – 248006 (UC)

76 Foundation for Revitalization of
Local Health Traditions
50-MHS Layout, 3rd Main,
2nd Stage Anandnagar
Bangalore – 560024 Karnataka

77 G.B. Pant Institute of Himalayan
Environment & Development
(G.B. Pant Himalaya Paryavaran Evam
Vikas Sansthan)
Almora –263643 (UC)

78 Guggulu Herbal Farm
Near Ajmer
Mangaliawas – 303 001 (Raj.)

79 Haffkine Institute for Training,
Research & Testing
Acharya Donde Marg, Parel
Mumbai – 400012 (MS)

80 Hamdard National Foundation
2/3 Asaf Ali Road
Delhi – 110002

81 Herbals Academy
3-D, Sindhu House, Nanabhai Lane,
Flora Fountain, Fort
Mumbai – 400001 (MS)

82 Homoeopathic Drug Research Institute
B-1433 Indira Nagar
Lucknow – 226 016 (UP)

83 Indian Council of Agricultural
Research
Krishi Anusandhan Bhawan, Pusa
Delhi – 110012

84 Indian Council of Forestry
Research & Education
P.O. New Forest
Dehra Dun – 248006 (UC)

85 Indian Council of Medical Research
Ansari Nagar, Medical Enclave,
P.O.B. 4502
Delhi – 110029

86 Indian Drug Manufactures Association
102-B, Poonam Chambers,
Dr. Annie Besant Road, Worli,
Mumbai – 400018 (MS)

87 Indian Drugs Research Association
516-B, Shivjinagar
Pune – 411005 (MS)

88 Indian Institute of Ayurveda for Drug Research
Near Ranikhet
Tarikhet – 263 645 (UC)

89 Indian Institute of Chemical Biology
4 Raja S.C. Mullick Road
Kolkatta – 700032 West Bengal

90 Indian Institute of Chemical Technology
Organic Chemistry Division
Uppal Road
Hyderabad – 500007 (AP)

91 Indian Institute of History of Medicine (IIHM)
Osmani Medical College Buildings,
Putlibowli
Hyderabad (Andhra Pradesh)

92 Indian Institute of Horticultural Research
255 Upper Palace Orchards
Bangalore –560080 Karnataka

93 Indian Institute of Kayachikitsa
Patiala – 147 001 Punjab

94 Indian Institute of Panchakarma
Thrissur District
Cheruthuruthy P. O. – 679 531 Kerala

95 Indian Pharmacological Society
Government Medical College,
Pharmacology
& Therapeutics Department
Jammu – 180001 (J&K)

96 Indian Society for Promotion o
Medicinal & Aromatic Plants
B-221Chittarajan Park
Delhi – 110019

97 Indian Society for Spices
National Research Centre for Spices,
P.O.B. 1701, Mari Kunnu P.O.
Calicut – 673012 Kerala

98 Indian Society of Genetics & Plant Breeding
Indian Agricultural Research Institute,
Genetics Division, NRL Buildings, Pusa
Delhi – 110012

99 Indian Society of Pharmacognosy
Dr. H.S. Gour Vishwavidyalaya,
Pharmaceutical
Sciences Department
Sagar – 470003 (MP)

100 Indian Society of Plant
Genetic Resources
National Bureau of Plant Genetic Resources,
Indian Agricultural Research Institute
Campus, Pusa
Delhi – 110012

101 Institute of Alternative Medicine & Research
Ambala-Shimla Highway
Panchkula – Haryana

102 Institute of Forest Genetics &
Tree Breeding
Forest College Campus, R.S. Puram
Coimbatore – 641002 (TN)

103 Institute of Forest Productivity
Ranchi – Jharkhand

104 Institute of Indian Medicine
36 Kothrud
Pune – 411029 (Maharashtra)

105 Institute of Postgraduate Education
& Research in Ayurveda
249 Acharya Prafulla Chandra Road
Kolkatta – 700009 (West Bengal)

106 Institute of Rain & Moist
Deciduous Forest Research
A.T. Road, Tarajan P.O.
Jorhat – 785001 (Assam)

107 Institute of Research in Indigenous
System of Medicine
Approach Road
Joginder Nagar – 176120 (HP)

108 Institute of Science
15 Madam Cama Road, Fort
Mumbai – 400032 (MS)

109 Institute of Wood Science &
Technology
18th Cross Road, Malleswaram
Bangalore – 560003 Karnataka

110 International Association for the
Study of Traditional Asian Medicine,
Zandu Pharmaceutical Works Ltd.,
Gokhale Road South
Mumbai – 400025 (MS)

111 International Institute of Ayurveda
Ramanathapuram
Coimbatore- 641045 (TN)

112 Jawaharlal Nehru Ayurvedic
Medicinal Plants Garden & Herbarium
Kothrud
Pune – 411 029 (Maharashtra)

113 Kerala Forest Research Institute
Dist. Thrissur
Peechi – 680653 Kerala

114 Literary Research & Documentation
Department (Siddha)
Central Research Institute,
A.A. Government Hospital Campus
Arumbakkam
Madras – 600

115 Lok Swasthya Parampara Samvrdhan
Samithi
P.B.7102, Trichy Road, Ramanathapuram
Coimbatore – 641045 Tamil Nadu

116 M.S. Swaminathan Research Foundation
Community Gene Bank
3rd Cross Road, Taramani Institutional Area
Madras – 600113 Tamil Nadu

117 Maharashtra Association for the
Cultivation of Science
Science & Technology Department
Law College Road
Pune – 411004 Maharashtra

118 Malaria Research Centre
22 Sham Nath Marg
Delhi – 110054

119 Medicinal Plants Garden-Cum-
Demonstration Centre
Regional Research Centre (Ayurveda),
Sankai View
Itanagar – 791 110 Arunachal Pradesh

120 Ministry of Defence Research &
Development Organization Defence
Agrotechnological Research Laboratory
Pithoragarh – 262501 (UC)

121 National Ayurveda Academy
M.G. Road
Thiruvananthapuram – 695012
Kerala

122 National Botanical Research Institute
Rana Pratap Marg
Lucknow – 226001 (UP)

123 National Bureau of Plant
Genetic Resources
Indian Agricultural Research Inst.
Campus, Pusa
Delhi – 110012

124 National Chemical Laboratory
Dr. Homi Bhabha Road
Pune – 411008, Maharashtra

125 National Institute of Ayurveda
Madhav Vilas Palace, Amer Road
Jaipur – 302002 Rajasthan

126 National Institute of Homoeopathy
Block GE, Sector 3, Bhidan Nagar,
Salt Lake City
Kolkatta – 700091 West Bengal

127 National Institute of Immunology
Ayurvedic Drug Testing Project
Jawaharlal Nehru University Complex,
Aruna Asaf Ali Marg
Delhi – 110067

128 National Institute of Nutrition
Jamai-Osmania
Hyderabad – 500007 Andhra Pradesh

129 National Institute of Unani Medicine
Srigandadhakavalu Village,
Bangalore – Karnataka

130 National Integrated Medical
Association
G-2 Mohan Kunj, M.J. Phule Marg,
Naigaun Dadar
Mumbai – 400014 (Maharashtra)

131 National Research Centre for
Spices
Mari Kunnu P.O.
Calicut – 673012 Kerala

132 Niamath Science Acadamy
49 Bharathi Salai
Madras – 600005 Tamil Nadu

133 Perfumes & Flavours Association of India
2-B, Court Chambers, 35 New Maine Lines
Mumbai – 400020 Maharashtra

134 Pharmacognosy Research Unit
Kolkatta University, Botany Department,
35 Ballygunge Circular Road
Kolkatta – 700 019 West Bengal

135 Pharmacognosy Research Unit
Jawaharlal Nehru Ayurvedic Medicinal Plants Garden
& Herbarium, Kothrud
Pune – 411 029 Maharashtra

136 Pharmacological Research Unit
Banaras Hindu University,
Institute of Medical Sciences,
Pharmacology Department
Varnasi – 221 005 (UP)

137 Pharmacological Research Unit
Central Research Institute (Ayurveda)
Road 66, Punjabi Bagh
Delhi – 110 026

138 Pharmacological Research Unit
K.G. Medical College,
Pharmacology Department
Lucknow – 226 003 (UP)

139 Pharmacological Research Unit
Medical College,
Pharmacology Department
Thruvananthapuram – 695 001 (Kerala)

140 Pharmacological Research Unit
SMS Medical College,
Pharmacology Department
CCRAS
Jaipur (Rajasthan)

141 Pharmacological Research Unit
University College of Medicine,
Pharmacology Department,
244-B, J.C. Bose Road
Kolkatta – 700 020 (WB)

142 Pharmacopoeial Laboratory for Indian Medicine
A Wing, 3rd fl., Central Government Office Building, Kamala Nehru Nagar
Ghaziabad – 201002 (UP)

143 Rashtriya Ayurveda Vidyapeeth
(National Academy of Ayurveda)
Dhanwantri Bhawan, Road 66,
Punjabi Bagh
Delhi – 110026

144 Regional Research Centre (Ayurved)
Government Central Pharmacy Annex,
Ashok Pillar, Jayanagar
Bangalore – 560 011 Karnataka

145 Regional Research Centre (Ayurveda)
1093 Gorepeth
Nagpur – 440 010 Maharashtra

146 Regional Research Centre (Ayurveda)
A Block, North Wing,
Indira Gandhi Stadium Complex,
Bandra Road
Vijayawada – 520 010 Andhra Pradesh

147 Regional Research Centre (Ayurveda)
Gandhi Bhawan
Mandi (HP)

148 Regional Research Centre (Ayurveda)
Government Ayurvedic College, Jalukbari
Guwahati – 781 014 Assam

149 Regional Research Centre (Ayurveda)
Gwalior Road
Jhansi – 248 003 (UP)

150 Regional Research Centre (Ayurveda)
Hastinapur – 250 404 (UP)

151 Regional Research Centre (Ayurveda)
Rehari Chowk
Jammu – 180 005 J & K

152 Regional Research Centre (Ayurveda)
Sankai View
Itanagar – 791 110 Arunachal Pradesh

153 Regional Research Centre (Ayurveda)
Tadung
Gangtok – 737 101 (Sikkim)

154 Regional Research Inst. of Unani Medicine
1 West Mada Church Street, Royapuram
Madras – 600013 Tamil Nadu

155 Regional Research Inst. of Unani Medicine
Aligarh Muslim University,
Department of Research in Unani Medicine
Aligarh – 202001 (UP)

156 Regional Research Inst. of Unani Medicine
Bhadrak – 756100
Dist. Balasore (Orissa)

157 Regional Research Inst. of Unani Medicine
J.J. Hospital Compound, Byculla
Mumbai – 400008 Maharashtra

158 Regional Research Inst. of Unani Medicine
University of Kashmir, University Health Centre, Hazratbal
Srinagar – 190006 (J&K)

159 Regional Research Institute (Ayurveda)
14 Jagannath Dutta Lane
Kolkatta – 700 009 West Bengal

160 Regional Research Institute (Ayurveda)
476/6 Sitapu Road
Lucknow – 226 007 (UP)

161 Regional Research Institute (Ayurveda)
Madhav Vilas Palace,
Amer Road
Jaipur – 302 002 (Raj.)

162 Regional Research Institute (Ayurveda)
Poojapura
Thiruvananthapuram – 695 012 (Kerala)

163 Regional Research Institute (Ayurveda)
Rajendra Memorial Research Institute
Building, Kadam Kuan
Patna – 800 007 (Bihar)

164 Regional Research Institute (Ayurveda)
Taj Manzil, Sardar Bagh
Junagadh – 362 001 (Guj.)

165 Regional Research Institute (Ayurveda)
Ullas Bhawan, Kherapathi,
Killa Road, P.B. 3
Gwalior – 474 002 (MP)

166 Regional Research Institute (Siddha)
Government Pharmacy (upstairs),
Indra Nagar, Gorimedu
Pondicherry – 605 006

167 Regional Research Laboratory,
Bhubaneswar
Sachivalya Marg
Bhubaneswar – 751013 Orissa

168 Regional Research Laboratory,
Canal Road
Jammu Tawi – 180001 J & K

169 Regional Research Laboratory,
Jorhat – 785006

170 Regional Research Laboratory,
P.O. Industrial Estate, Pappanamcode
Thiruvananthapuram – 695019 (Kerala)

171 Research Project on Tibetan System of
Medicine
(Amchi Research Unit)
Amchi Association Building
Leh – 194 101 (J & K)

172 School of Tropical Medicine
Chittaranjan Avenue
Kolkatta – 700073 (West Bengal)

173 Society for Health Alternatives
Holistic Health Centre, Bibbewedi
Pune – 411037 (MS)

174 Society for Promotion of Minor
Forest Produce
Tropical Forest Research Institute,
Mandla Road
Jabalpur – 482001 (MP)

175 Society of Economic Botanists &
Phytochemists
18 Ashirvad Enclave, Chakrata Road
Dehra Dun – 248001 (UC)

176 Society of Ethnobotanists
Central Drug Research Inst.
Botany Division
Lucknow – 226001 (UP)

177 Spices Board India
Sugandha Bhawan, N.H. Bypass,
Palarivattam
Cochin – 682025 (Kerala)

178 State Forest Research Institute
Polipathar, Narmada Road
Jabalpur – 482008 (MP)

179 Survey of Medicinal Plants &
Collection Unit
112, Government Arts College Campus
Udhagamandalam – 643 002 (TN)

180 Survey of Medicinal Plants Unit (Siddha)
Government College of Indian Medicine,
Tirunelveli District
Palayamkottai – 627 002 (TN)

181 Survey of Medicinal Plants Unit
Regional Research Inst. of Medicine,
Dist. Balasore
Bhadrak – 756100 (Orissa)

182 Survey of Medicinal Plants Unit
Regional Research Inst. of Unani Medicine,
University of Kashmir,
University Health Centre, Hazratbal
Srinagar – 190006 (J&K)

183 Swamy Prakashananda Ayurveda
Research Centre
13th N.S. Road, Juhu
Mumbai – 400049 (MS)

184 Tamil Nadu Government Cinchona
Department
Nilgiris, P.B 6
Udhagamandalam – 643001 (TN)

185 Temperature Forest Research
Institute
Shimla – Himachal Pradesh

186 Tibetan Medical & Astro Institute
Khara Danda Road, Dist. Kangra
Dharamsala – 176215 (HP)

4 PHARMACEUTICALS

1 Aimil Pharmaceuticals (I) Pvt. Ltd.
2994/4, Street No. 17, Ranjit Nagar
New Delhi – 110008

2 Ajmal Fragrances and Flavours (P) Ltd.
1, Cecil Court, 24, Mahakavi Bhushan Road
Colaba, Mumbai – 400039

3 Ajmera Pharmaceuticals Pvt. Ltd.
B-9, 'A' Industrial Area, Pologround
Indore – 452003

4 Akhand Ayurvedic Rasayansala
276, Sector – E, Sanwer Road
Industrial Area, Indore

5 Alarsin Pharmaceuticals
Alarsin House, A-32, Road No. 3
Opp. ESIS Hospital, MIDC
Andheri (E) Mumbai – 400093

6 Alchem International Private Ltd.
201, Empire Plaza,
Mahrauli-Guragaon Road
Sultanpur, New Delhi – 110030

7 Alchemy Chemicals
302 PI Estate, SC Road No2
Goregaon East, Mumbai 400063

8 Alembic Chemical Works Co. Ltd.
Alembic Road, Vadodara – 390003

9 Alkaloids Corporation
8, Bentick Street, Kolkatta – 700001

10 Alkaloids Pvt. Ltd.
61 M.G. Road, 309 Kabra Complex
Secunderabad – 5000003, AP

11 Allen Laboratories Pvt. Ltd.
Allen House, 224/H, Maniktala Main Road
Kolkatta – 700054

12 Allen Pharmaceuticals
2-3-105 Aberprt, Hyderabad – 500013

13 Alrasin Marketing (P) Ltd.
MIDC, PB9416
Opp: ESIS Hospital
Andheri East
Mumbai 400093

14 American Remedies Limited
No. 14, L.B. Road, Adyar
Chennai – 600020

15 Amrutanjan Limited Research and
Development Laboratory
42/45 Luz Church Road, P.O. Box No. 612
Mylapore
Chennai – 600004

16 Amruth Kesari Depot
364 Avenue Road
Bangalore

17 Amsar Private Limited
47, Lakshmi Nagar, Industrial Estate, Fort
Indore – 452006

18 Anand Medicaids Private Ltd.
4 DLF Industrial Area, Najafgarh Rd.
New Delhi 110015

19 Ancient Herbs Ltd.
1117/2A Varinder Nagar
Ludhiana 141001

20 Ancient Pharma
5 SPG Church Lane, 1st Floor, P.B. 184
Madurai – 625001

21 Anil Ayurpharma
Ladiwala Estate, Hingwala Lane
Ghatgopar (East), Mumbai – 4000077

22 Anu Chem Industries
872/874, Marshall House, 25 Strand Road
Kolkatta 700001

23 Anuja Pharmaceuticals
5 Rajmahal Shopping Centre, 55-E
Mathura Das Vasanji Road, Andheri East
Mumbai – 400069

24 Apar Chem Product
203 Kailash – I Navrangpura Post
Ahmedabad 380009

25 Apothecaries Sundries Mfg. Co.
ASCO House I-30A Kirti Nagar
New Delhi 110015

26 Arochem Silvassa Limited
Scent House, Station Road, Goregaon (West)
Mumbai – 400062

27 Aromatic and Allied Chemicals
B-8, Industrial area, C.B. Gang
Bareilly – 243502

28 Artifacts
577 Sector 9
Faridabad 121006

29 Arvind Inter Trade
3, 2nd Lane, Pantheon Road
Chennai 600008

30 Arya Aushadhi Pharmaceuticals Works
35/A/5 Fort Industrial Estate
Indore – 452006

31 Arya Ayurveda Ashram
P-73 Amritlal Mukherjee Road
Thakurpukur, Kolkatta – 700063

32 Arya Vaidya Pharmacy (Coimbatore) Ltd.
1382 Trichy Road, Coimbatore – 641018

33 Arya Vaidya Pharmacy
9/1 Queens Road,
Opp: Indian Express Bldg.
Bangalore 560001

34 Arya Vaidya Pharmacy
P.O. Palghat, Kanjikode – 678621
Kerala

35 Arya Vaidya Sala
District Malappuram, Kottakal – 676503
Kerala

36 Ascent International
30 Harishkunj International
Ahmedabad 380051

37 Asoj Soft Caps Private Limited
Plot No. G-9, Cross Road, 'A' Marol, MIDC
Andheri (E), Mumbai – 400093

38 Assam Chemical and Pharmaceutical Pvt. Ltd.
A.K. Azad Road, Gopinath Nagar
Guwahati – 781016

39 Atlanta Enterprises
B-46 Chandra Nagar
Indore 452008

40 Atreya Ayurvedic Pharmacy
P.B. 20 Delhi Road, Badot – 250611

41 Auro Impex Pvt. Limited
8, Camac Street, 2nd Floor
Kolkatta – 700017

42 Aurochem (I) Pvt. Ltd.
B-74, 75, Sector 2, Noida – 201301

43 Avo Chem Industries
Jaypica House, Dolatganj,
Gwalior – 474001

44 Ayulabs Pvt. Ltd.
Gondal Road, Vavdi,
Rajkot – 360004

45 Ayur Herbals
7/28 South Patel Nagar
New Delhi 110008

46 Ayurchem Products
31-32 Patil Bhawan, Netaji Sibhash Road
Mulund (W), Mumbai – 400080

47 Ayurgandha Products
28 Bhera Enclave, Paschim Vihar
New Delhi 110087

48 Ayurved Sewa Sangh
Shanti Gali, Ravivan Peth, Nasik

49 Ayurved Sumshodhanalaya Ltd.
1379 Shukravar Peth, Natubaug
Pune 411002

50 Ayurved Vikas Sansthan
C-83 Gandhi Nagar, Moradabad

51 Ayurveda Rasashal
25 Karve Road
Pune 411004

52 Baidyanath Ayurved Bhawan Ltd.
1 Gupta Lane, Kolkatta – 700006

53 Bain Dass Ravi Mohan
1st Floor, Bhawan Majith Mandi
Amritsar

54 Bajaj Sewashram Ltd.
Manduadih, Varanasi – 221003

55 Balsara Herbal Products Pvt. Ltd.
12-A, Jorawal Bhuvan, Second Floor
Maharishi Karve Road, Mumbai – 400021

56 BDH Industries Ltd.
Nair Baug, Akurli Road
Kandivli East, Mumbai – 400101

57 Bevit Pharmaceuticals Ltd.
Mackinnon Mackenzie Blg., 3rd Floor
Ballard Estate, Mumbai – 400038

58 Bhagwat Pharmaceutical Laboratories
18/73, Bhagwat Mension, Kampoo Kothi
Gwalior – 474001

59 Bharathi Impex
44 New Bangaru Naidu Colony
KK Nagar West, Chennai 600078

60 Bharati Rasyanagar
27, Nakukeshwar Bhattacharjee Lane
Kolkatta – 700026

61 Bharatiya Aushdhi Nirman Shala (BAN)
Dr. Vikram Sarabhai Marg, Gondal Road
Rajkot – 360004

62 Bindumadhav Ayurved Pratishthan
8 Nanak Society, 1st Floor, Manmala Tank Road
Mumbai – 400016

63 Biolink Healthcare Ltd.
66 Princess Stree
Mumbai 400 001

64 Bio-Synth India
347, Dawa Bazar, Ist Floor, RNT Marg
Indore – 452002

65 Bio-Ved Pharmaceuticals Pvt. Ltd.
6, Paarth, Prabhat Road 84/1/1
Pune – 411004

66 Biovedic India Ltd.
K-21 Hauz Khas Enclave
New Delhi 110016

67 BKM Indigenous Pharmaceuticals
TC25/3386 Chirakulam Road)
Thiruvanthapurm 695001

68 Blue Star Laboratories
107, Risal Complex, Shiva Market
Pitampura, New Delhi – 110034

69 Mumbai Alkaloides Pvt. Ltd.
194, Samuel Street, Mumbai – 400009

70 Mumbai Drug and Pharma Ltd.
Nair Baug, Akurli Road, Kandivli (E)
Mumbai – 400101

71 C.I. Laboratories
56/1, Biplabi Ras Behari Basu Road
Kolkatta – 700001

72 Cadila Pharmaceuticals Ltd.
IRM House, Off. C.G. Road
Navrangpura, Ahmedabad – 380009

73 Chandrashree Laboratories and Farm Products Pvt. Ltd.
Sanatorium Road, Shri Jaswant Bhawan
Rau, Indore – 453331

74 Charak Pharmaceuticals (India) Ltd.
Evergreen Industrial Estate, Shakti Mills Lane
Dr. E. Moses Road, Mahalaxmi
Mumbai – 400011

75 Chem Pharma Corporation
146, Habibulah Road, T. Nagar
Chennai – 600017

76 Chemiloids
40-15-14
Brindavan Colony
Vijayawada 520010 Andhra Pradesh

77 Chemitech Laboratories
465/4, Vashist Marg, Raja Park
Jaipur – 302004

78 Chimera Gentec Pvt. Ltd.
C-255, Sector-51
Noida 201303

79 Chirayu Pharmaceuticals
14, Din Dayal Market, MLB Road
Gwalior – 474009

80 Cipla Ltd.
Virgo Nagar P.O.
Bangalore 560049
Karnataka

81 Creasons Son Brand Products
Narula Building, CHS Flat No. 9,
Road No. 21, Chambur,
Mumbai – 4000071

82 Crimson Labs. Pvt. Ltd.
7, Kasturba Market, Kampoo
Gwalior – 474009

83 Croford Pharmaceuticals Pvt. Ltd.
B-5/142, Indira Nagar
Lucknow – 226016

84 Crown Pharma Exports
E-74A Gangotri Enclave, Alakananda
New Delhi 110019

85 Crystal India
C-316 Yojana Vihar
New Delhi 110092

86 Dabur Ayurvedic Specialities Ltd.
Harsha Bhawan, Block E
Connaught Place, New Delhi 110001

87 Dabur India Limited
8/3 Asaf Ali Road, Darya Ganj
New Delhi – 110002

88 Dabur India Ltd. (Pharma Division)
3, Factory Road, Near Safdarjung Hospital
New Delhi – 110029

89 Dabur India Ltd.
9, Netaji Subhash Chandra Bose Road
P.O. Narendrapur – 743508
District 24 Pargana

90 Dabur Research Foundation
22, Site IV, Sahibabad,
Ghaziabad – 201010

91 Dacca Ayurvedic Pharmacy Ltd.
26/1 A, Shanagar Road
Kolkatta – 700026

92 Dangi Laboratories
C-1, Shalimar Industrial Estate, Matunga
Mumbai – 400019

93 Deccan Ayuvedashram Pharmacy Ltd.
17-1-204-8 Saidabad
Hyderabad 500059

94 Deccan Phytochemicals
309, Kabra Complex, 61 MG Road
Secundrabad – 500003

95 Deendayal Aushadhi (P) Ltd.,
5, Industrial Area
Gwalior – 474 004 (MP)

96 Dehlvi Remedies Pvt. Ltd.
B-18 Sector – 9
Noida 201301

97 Deshrakshak Aushdhalaya Ltd.
Kankhal, Haridwar – 249408 (UC)

98 Dey's Medical Stores (Mfg.) Ltd.
17, Collin Lane, 2nd Floor
Kolkatta – 700016

99 Dhanvantri Drugs
Laxmi Bhawan, Main Road
E-87, Fondrem Raibandan
Panjim, Goa – 403006

100 Dhanwantari Ayurveda Matam
Station Road
Thiruvananthpuram – 695012
Kerala

101 Dhara Pharmaceuticals
194/2 Nehru Park, Vastrapur
Ahmedabad 380015

102 Dhariwal Industries
F-8, Mandor Industrial Area,
Mandore
Jodhpur (Raj)

103 Dharmani Drugs Research &
Training Institute
1131, Sector IV,
Gurgaon – 122001 Harayana

104 Dhawan International
B-134 G.F. Front, Malaviya Nagar
New Delhi 110017

105 Dhootapapeshwar Limited
135, Nanubhai Desai Road
Opp. Wilson High School
Mumbai – 400004

106 Diamex India Ltd.
S-1/17 Bela Road, Civil Lines
New Delhi 110054

107 Digamber Exports Pvt. Ltd.
A-12 Lajpat Nagar – 1
New Delhi 110025

108 Dindayal Aushadalaya (P) Ltd.
Din Dayal Market, MLB Road
P.O. Box No. 50
Gwalior – 474009

109 Dogra Drugs Pharma
29 Industrial Estate, Bilaspur – 174001

110 The Zandu Pharmaceutical Works Ltd.
70 Gokhale Road
South Dadar
Mumbai 400025 Maharashtra

111 Dr. K.S. and Sons
66, Manikkara Street
Kumbakonam – 612001

112 Sandu Brothers (P) Ltd.
D/124, TTC, MIDC
Shirvane, Nerul
Navi Mumbai 400614 Maharashtra

113 Bio-Ved Pharmaceuticals (P) Ltd.
6 Pradeep Chambers
Bhaadarkar Institute Road
Pune 411005 Maharashtra

114 Dr. Roopas Herbal System (P) Ltd.
75 Usha Chambers
Central Market, Ashok Vihar
New Delhi 110052

115 Gufic Health Care Ltd.
Subhash Road – A
Vile Parle East
Mumbai 400057 Maharashtra

116 East India Pharmaceuticals Works Ltd.
6, Lttle Russell Street
Kolkatta – 700071

117 Eastern Drug
11-A, Earle Street, P.O. Box 10454
Kolkatta – 700026

118 Eisen Pharmaceuticals Co. (P) Ltd.
34/7 Erandwana, Deccan Gymkhana
Pune – 411004

119 Eisenhower International
A-8 East of Kailash
New Delhi 110065

120 Emami Group of Companies
18 R.N. Mukherjee Road
Kolkatta

121 Ensys Nature Products
52, 3rd Marine Street, Marine Lines
Mumbai 400002

122 Envin Bioceuticals Pvt. Ltd.
Sharda Nagar, P.O. Box No. 203
Saharanpur – 247001

123 Ethneco Exports Pvt. Ltd.
C-6-3-4-3, Sector - 4 CBD Belapur
New Mumbai 400614

124 Fair Pharma
T.A. majeed, Broadway, Eranakulam
Cochin – 682031

125 Famay Marketing Services P. Ltd.
D-120 Krishna Park, K.D. Road
New Delhi 110062

126 Fem Care Pharma Ltd.
ASD-36, Ashwin Nagar
CIDCO, Nasik – 422009

127 Fixus Ltd.
4240-D Panna Bhavan, 2 Ansari Road
Darya Ganj, New Delhi 110002

128 Foodaids
D2/33 Rajasthali, Pitampura
New Delhi 110034

129 Franco-Indian Pharmaceuticals Pvt. Ltd.
676-680, Bapurao Jagtap Marg
Mumbai – 400011

130 Gajraj Mehandi Udyog
51, Lunet Building, 3rd Floor, Dr. Ambedkar Road
Dadar (East), Mumbai – 400014

131 Gandhi Vidya Mandir
19 Synagogue Street
Kolkatta 700001

132 Ganga Pharmaceuticals
C/o Ganga Ayurved Bhandar, 5 Dattani Trade
Centre, Chandrawarkar Road, Borivili (West)
Mumbai – 400092

133 Gavit Herbal E.H. Pharma
Jawahar Nagar, 4723/15B
Adhartal, Jabalpur

134 Gemini Drgu Pvt. Ltd.
85 Fifth Street, Mangalapuram
Thanjavur 613007

135 George Herbals Pvt. Ltd.
A-156 Shivalik, Malaviya Nagar
New Delhi 110017

136 Global Exims
366/A Tolichowki
Hyderabad 500008

137 Glyco Remedies
C-73, Okhla Industrial Area, Phase I
New Delhi – 110020

138 Gomtesh Laboratories
25-D, Sector – B, Sanwer Road
Indore – 452003

139 Government Ayurvedic Pharmacy
Bolangir (Orissa)

140 Government Central Pharmacy
Jayanagar, Bangalore

141 Graham Brothers
124-A, North Cotton Road
Tuticorin – 628001

142 Green (India) Labs.
25-B, Besant Road, Madurai – 625002

143 Growel Pharmaceuticals
A-31, Talkatora Industrial Estate
Lucknow – 226011

144 Guapha Remedies Pvt. Ltd.
A-24, Sector 7, Noida – 201301

145 Gufic Health Care Ltd.
Subhash Road A, Vile Parle (E)
Mumbai – 400057

146 Gujarat Ayurveda University Pharmacy
Jamnagar – 3621001

147 Gujarat Ayurveda Vikasa
Mandal Bhawan, Ahmedabad – 380014

148 Gujarat Terce Lab. Ltd.
209 Samir Complex Opp. M. Market
Ahmedabad 380009

149 Gurukul Kangri Pharmacy
P.O. Gurukul Kngri,
Haridwar – 249404 (UC)

150 Hamdard (Waqf) Laboratories
Hamdard Building, 2/3 Asif Ali Road
Darya Ganj, New Delhi – 110002

151 Harsha Pharma Pvt. Ltd.
WZ-49H, 1st Floor, Bodella, Vikas Puri
New Delhi 110018

152 Heal Ayurveda Pharmacy Ltd.
1382 Trichy Road, Coimbatore – 641018

153 Helios Pharmaceuticals
Helios House, 659/1, Gulbai Tekra,
2nd Lane
Panchwati, Ahmedabad – 380006

154 Herbal (APS) Pvt. Ltd.
BM Das Road
Patna – 800004

155 Herbal Indica
351, Industrial Area, Phase II
Chandigarh – 160002

156 Herbal Native Drugs Pvt. Ltd.
30, Vijay Nagar
Amritsar – 143001

157 Herbal Remedies (I) Pvt. Ltd.
F-9/5, MIDC, Chikalthana
Aurangabad – 431210

158 Herbindus
New Industrial Area, Kanjikode East
Palakkad 678621

159 Herbolab
Jay Bhawan, 23 Kazi Sayed Street, Mandvi
Mumbai – 400009

160 Herbo-Med (P) Ltd.
68 Hemachandra Naskar Road
Kolkatta – 700010

161 Herbs & Health Makers (I) Ltd.
61-62, Dawa Bazar RNT Marg
Indore 452001

162 Herbs Era Pharmaceuticals (P) Ltd.
P.O. Udayraipur – 745275
District 24-Parganas (WB)

163 Hering and Cant
Hering and Cant Building, 3rd Floor, 263
Dr. D.N. Road, Fort, Mumbai – 400001

164 Hill Green Company
17, 13th Cross
Vasanth Nagar East
Bangalore 560052
Karnataka

165 Himalaya Drug Co. (P) Ltd.
Shivsagar Estate E, Dr. Annie Besant Road
Worli, Mumbai – 400018

166 Himalaya Drug Co.
Makali
Bangalore 562123 Karnataka

167 Himani Limited
Taher Mansion, 10th Floor
8 Bentink Street, Kolkatta – 700001

168 Hindustan Pharmaceuticals
Kotmit Singh, Taran Taran Road
Amritsar – 143001

169 Hitashi Chemicals
11 Ezra Street
Kolkatta – 700001

170 Hiten Chemicals
45, Cavel Cross Lane, Opp. G.T. High
School
Kalbadevi Road, Mumbai – 400002

171 Honeybee Natural Products Ltd.
193B Sainik Farms
New Delhi 110062

172 ICMC Corporation Ltd.
F-29, 1st Floor, 769 Anna Salai
Chennai 600002

173 IMPCOPS
Dr. Muthulakshmi Road
Tiruvanmipur
Chennai 600041

174 Indfrag (P) Ltd.
5-913 Manipal Centre
Dickenson Road
Bangalore 560042
Karnataka

175 India Herbals
T-55/A, Liots Beach Road, Besant Nagar
Chennai – 600090

176 Indian Herbs Research & Supply Co.
P.B. 5 Sharda Nagar
Sharanpur 247009

177 Indian Herbs
164/3 Vasvi Temple Road,
Vishweshvapuram
Bangalore 560004

178 Indian Medical Practitioner's Cooperative Pharmacy and Stores
Lattice Bridge Road, Adyar,
Chennai – 600041

179 Indian Medicine Industries
"Nagalands", Seetharampuram,
Vijayawada – 520004

180 Indian Medicines Pharmaceutical Corporation Ltd.
A Govt. of India Undertaking
Mohan, District Almora – 244715

181 Indian Remedies
127, Kalyandas Udhyog Bhawan,
Near Century Bazar
Worli, Mumbai – 400025

182 Indira Dinesh Chemicals
131, HSIDC Kundli Industrial Estate
Kundli, Sonepat – 131028

183 Indo Phyto Chemicals Pvt. Ltd.
F2/2 Vasant Vihar
New Delhi 110 057

184 Indo World Trading Corporation
303 Prakash Chambers, 6 N.S. Marg
New Delhi

185 Indo-French Laboratories Pvt. Ltd.
P.O. Box No. 1115, No. 19,
III Main Road Ramnagar,
Nanganallu, Chennai – 600061

186 Indo-German Alkaloids
IGA Complex, Mahakali Road
P.O. Box 7376, Andheri (E)
Mumbai – 400093

187 J. and J. De Chane Laboratories Pvt. Ltd.
4-1-324, Residency Road
Hyderabad – 500001

188 Jain Ayurvedic Pharmacy
15-9-472 Siddiamber Bazar
Hyderabad 500012

189 Jain Ayurvedic Pharmacy
19-2-246/J Royal Lab Compound
Chandulal Baradari Hyderabad – 500264

190 Jainsom Pharma Pvt. Ltd.
238 H. Industrial Estate, Kanjurmarg West
Mumbai 400078

191 Jamna Pharmaceuticals
48-B, Sector-C, Industrial Area
Mandi Deep – 462046, District Raisen

192 JB Chemical and Pharma Ltd.
Plot No., 215-216, GIDC Industrial Area
Panoli – 394116

193 Jiwadaya Netraprabha Karyalaya
55, Gam Devi Road, Ground Floor
Plasa Panch Sheel Estate, Old Victoria Mill
Compound, Mumbai – 400007

194 Jupiter Pharmaceuticals Ltd.
25, Dr. Lalit Banerjee Sarani
Kolkatta – 700073

195 K.V. Health Care Products Pvt. Ltd.
27-F, Kamala Nagar
Delhi – 110007

196 Kamal Pharmacy (Ayurvedic)
1498, Bhagirath Palace, Chandni Chowk
Delhi – 110006

197 Karnataka Antibiotics & Pharmaceuticals Ltd., Nirman Bhawan,
Dr. Rajkumar Road
Ist Block, Rajajinagar
Bangalore – 560010

198 Kisalaya Herbals Ltd.
2-A Ratlam Kothi, AB Road
Indore

199 Knight Queen Chemicals Pvt. Ltd.
A-14 Wazirpur Industrial Area, Ring Road
New Delhi 110052

200 Kothari Laboratories
Arihand, Link Road,
Sagar – 470002

201 Kothari Phytochemicals International
766 Anna Nagar
Mudurai 625020 Tamilnadu

202 Krimson Finechem Pvt. Ltd.
2/34 Nityanand Nagar, 4 SN Street
andheri East, Mumbai 400069

203 Kruzer Herbals
B-20/2, Okhla Industrial Area, Phase II
New Delhi – 110020

204 Kuria Mal & Sons
Mehandi Godown, Delhi Gate
Faridabad Old, Haryana 121002

205 Lenwlls Marketing (P) Ltd.
8-B/17, Samhita Complex
Andheri-Kurla Road, Near Crown Silk Mills
Mumbai – 400072

206 Libra Drugs (India)
145/146/92-B, Mangalwar Peth
Parge Chowk, Pune – 411011

207 Lotus Health Care
"Ashirwad", bangla No. 612,
Post Shelu via Narul
Karjat, District Raigadh – 410101

208 Lotus Herbals Ltd.
B-9 Sector – 58
Noida 201 301

209 Lupin Laboratories Ltd.
159 CST Road, Kalina, Santa Cruz East
Mumbai – 400098

210 Lupin Labs Ltd.
198-202, New Industrial Area No. 2
Mandideep – 462046, District Raisen

211 M.K. Industries
C-44, MP Shah Indl. Estate, SS Road
Ahmedabad 361002

212 M.M. Pharma Remedies
Shahpur Bunglow, Khanpur
Ahmedabad 380001

213 M.P. Pharmaceuticals
121, New Industrial Area II
Mandideep, District Raisen

214 Maan Pharmaceuticals Ltd.
Plot No. 1, Phase 2, GIDC, Modhera Road
Mehsana – 384002 (Gujarat)

215 Madhura Pharma Research Labs.
292, 294 Phase IV, Peenya Industrial Area
Bangalore – 560958

216 Madonna Pharmaceuticals Research Pvt. Ltd.
208/7, Rishi Bankim Chandra Road
Kolkatta – 700073

217 Maharishi Ayurved Products Limited
Plot No. 17-18,
Noida Export Processing Zone
Noida – 201305

218 Maharishi Ayurveda Corporation Ltd.
A-14 Mohan Estate, Mathura Road
New Delhi – 110044

219 Mahesh Pharmaceuticals
Plot No. 94, Sector – H
Govindpura Industrial Area, Govindpura, Bhopal

220 Majeesa Foods (P) Ltd.,
52/54, Old Hanuman Lane
31, 4th Floor, Parvati Bhawan,
Kalbadevi Road,
Mumbai –2 (MS)

221 Mangaldas & Com
109 Masjid Bunder Road
Mumbai – 400003

222 Maxeswell Pharmaceuticals
33/5, SSI area, 5th Block,
3rd Cross Rajaji Nagar
Bangalore – 560010

223 Maxo Laboratories Ltd.
35-E, Kamla Nagar, P.O. Box 2156
Delhi – 110007

224 Meghdoot Gramodhyog Sewa Sansthan
Head Office Meghdoot Building,
Ashok Vihar Aliganj,
Lucknow – 226020

225 Mehta Pharmaceuticals Pvt. Ltd.
G.T. Road, Chhehartta
Amritsar – 143105

226 Mendine Pharmaceuticals Pvt. Ltd.
36 A&B, Alipore Road
Kolkatta – 700027

227 Merpha Laboratories
58-59, Raja Colony, Collector Office Road
Trichy – 620001

228 Miracle Laboratories
1101, OTC Road, Near Pai Vihar Hotel
Bangalore 560002

229 MMC Healthcare Ltd.
23 Gandhi Nagar, Alwarthirunagar
Chennai 6000087

230 Moderna Remedies Corporation
10 Kader Terrace, Deorukha Road, Dadar
Mumbai – 400014

231 Modi Research (P) Ltd.
1796-A, Kotla Mubarakpur,
Delhi – 110003

232 Mohabey Herbal Products Pvt. Ltd.
Factory, Plot No. 76-A, Industrial Area,
Dist. Raisen
Mandi Deep – 462046

233 Mona Pharmachem
3/7010, Navjivan (7th Floor)
Lamington Road, Mumbai – 400108

234 Mount Mettur Pharmaceutical Ltd.
No. 16, North Road, Mandavelipakkam
Chennai – 600028

235 Multani Ayurveda
H-36 Connaught Place
New Delhi 110001

236 Mysore Essential Oils & Naturals
11, 2nd Cross, 5th Main
Gaganahalli Extension
Bangalore 560032
Karnataka

237 N.M. India Cosmetics Co.
J-268 Gali No. 5, 31/1 Pusta
Telecom Block
Karatar Nagar, New Delhi 110053

238 Nagarjuna Herbal Concentration Ltd.
Kalayanthani, Thodupuzha – 685588

239 Narniat Pharmaceuticals and Chemicals
Pvt. Ltd.
Naduvattom P.O. North Beypore
Calicut – 673015

240 Narsanj Pharmaceuticals
22/24, Champa Gali Cross Lane,
Singpuri Building
Room No. 3-A, Second Floor
Mumbai – 400002

241 Natco Parenterals Limited
Natco House, Road No. 2,
Banjara Hills
Hyderabad – 500033

242 National Pharma
P.B. No. 214, Medical College Road
Thanjavur – 613004

243 Natural Drug and Alkaloid Co. Pvt. Ltd.
4127, Naya Bazar (2nd Floor), PB No. 1297
Delhi – 110006

244 Natural Products Company
23 Chitra, Rabodi
Thane 400601

245 Natural Remedies Pvt. Ltd.
164.3 Vasavi Temple Road
V.V. Puram, Bangalore-560004

246 Naturence Research Labs Ltd.
A-91 Malviya Nagar
New Delhi 1100017

247 Natures Lab
45-B, Kewal Industrial Estate, S.B. Road
Lower Parail, Mumbai – 400012

248 Navashakti Ayurvidalaya Pvt. Ltd.
4960, Ashtabhuja, P.B. 8,
Bhusawal – 425201
District Jalgaon Devi Road

249 Navbal Industries
(Mfr of herbal physiotherapy goods)
2959 Gali No. 12 Ranjit Nagar
New Delhi 110008

250 Neeta Enterprises
(Deals in herbal medicines)
A/4, B/4 Avdhut Nagar, C.S. Road
Mumbai 400068

251 Nutrine Confectionary Company Ltd.
B.V. Reddy Colony, P.O. Box 38
Chittoor – 517001

252 Omkar Ayurved Mandir
At and Post Mangaon, District Raigad
Kulata – 402104 (MS)

253 Opal Products
2/9 Three View Bldg. Pradhadevi
Mumbai 400016

254 Orchid (India)
Jyoti Nagar, Guwahati – 781021

255 Oushadhi, The Pharmaceutical Corporation
(IM) Kerala Ltd.
Thrissur – 680001

256 Ozone Pharmaceutical Limited
1, Local Shopping Complex, Block A-3
Janakpuri – New Delhi – 110058

257 P.K. Pharma
16, Third Floor, Dawa Bazar,
Indore (MP)

258 Pal's Herbal Products India Ltd.
21-7-506/2, New No. 1088
Shakkar Kota, Hyderabad – 500002

259 Pans Laboratories
1, Kishanlal Darshan Complex
Navghar Road, Bhyander (East) – 401105
District Thane

260 Parle Pharma
24/147 S.J. Road, Vile Parle East
Mumbai 400057

261 Parle Products Pvt. Ltd.
North Level Crossing, Vila Parle (E)
Mumbai – 400057

262 Penal Herbal and Company
219, Dwarka Nagar,
NB Road, Badhora – 460001,
District Baitul (MP)

263 Penjon Limited
104, Industrial Estate, Penjon House
577 M.G. Road, Indore – 452001 (MP)

264 Pentavox India Ltd.
479 Sangat Road, P.O. Box No. 446
Ludhiana 141001

265 Pett Pharmaceuticals
C/6, Yashomangal Apartments
Near City Post, Dr. Patwardhan Road,
Panwel
District Raigadh – 410206

266 Pfizer Limited,
Express Towers
Nariman Point
Mumbai – 400021

267 Pharm Products Pvt. Ltd.
'Vijai', Medical College Road
PB No. 205, Thanjavur – 613007

268 Pharma Products Pvt. Ltd.
Vijai Medical College Road,
Thanjavur – 613007

269 Pharmaveda
Tejpal Road, Vile Parle East
Mumbai – 400057, Maharashtra

270 Phyto Medical
1/12, Udhyog Nagar, Industrial Estate
SV Road, Goregaon (West)
Mumbai – 400062

271 Phyto-Pharma (Research and Development)
T-4 Neelgiri Apartments
Opp. SNDT College
Karve Road, Pune

272 Planned Pharma Pvt. Ltd.
80 Marine Drive, Neelam, E-road West
Mumbai 400002

273 Poddar Prayogshala
(Mfr. of Ayurvedic health care products)
12 Hathi Khana Azad Market
New Delhi 110006

274 Prabhat Ayurvedic Pharmacy
Katra Sher Singh
Amritsar 143006

275 Pride Pharmaceuticals (P) Ltd.
First Floor, 1-12/B, Gandhi Nagar
Gwalior – 474002

276 Arya Vaidya Sala
Kottakal 676503 Kerala

277 Rajasthan Ayurvedic Research Laboratories
4 Dhamni Market,
Swai Mansingh Highway
Jaipur – 302003

278 Rajvaidya Shital Prasad and Sons
4771, Bharat Ram Road, 23 Darya Ganj
New Delhi – 110002

279 Rallis India Limited (Pharma Division)
Ralli House, P.O. Box 229
21 Damadardas Sukhadvala Marg
Mumbai – 400001

280 Ramkrishn Industries
158, A.B. Prabhu Building, Mogul Lane
Behind Shitladevi, Mahim,
Mumbai – 400016

281 Regal Chemicals
11, Palsikar Colony, Indore – 452004

282 Rovers Marketing Pvt. Ltd.
(Merchant Exporter of Herbal Products)
302 Sarthak Complex, C.G. Road
Ahmedabad 380009

283 Sagar Chemicals & Sagar Pharmacy
59/21, New Rohtak Road
New Delhi – 110005

284 Sagar Pharmaceuticals
"Varada" No. 375, Ist 'B' Main, Phase I
Girinagar, Bangalore – 560085

285 Sai Health Care
216 Dayanand Vihar, VM Extension
New Delhi 110092

286 Saiba Industries Pvt. Ltd.
129/131, Kazi Syed Street
Mumbai – 400003

287 Saini Herbs Pvt. Ltd.
17, 19, 20 KS Complex, Kanishka Hotel
Ashoka Road, New Delhi 110001

288 Sakthi Industries
Unit 2 near Milk Project
Vijayawada 520009

289 Sami chemicals & Extracts (P) Ltd.
1382 South End Main Road
9th Block, Jayanagar East
Bangalore 560069 Karnataka

290 Sandu Brothers
V.N. Purav Marg, Chembur
Mumbai – 400071

291 Sanjivani Herbal Pharma
105 VIP View Kareli Baug
Baroda 390018

292 Sanmar Speciality Chemicals Ltd.
8 Cathedral Road
Chennai 600086 Tamilnadu

293 Sanros Pharma
Jivdani Road, Virar – 401303

294 Santa Products Ltd
Sagar Plaza, Main Vikas Marg
New Delhi 110092

295 Santosh Ayurvedic Drug Supply Co.
33/102 Dariyasthan St. Masjid Bunder
Mumbai 400003

296 Sarabhai Piramal Pharmaceuticals Ltd.
Wadi, Vadodara – 390007

297 Sareen Herbal
E-101 Greater Kailash Enclave 1
New Delhi 110048

298 Shahnaz Herbals
M-84-A, Greater Kailash – I
New Delhi – 110048

299 Shalaks Chemicals
C-3, Puja House,
Karampura Community Centre
Milan Complex,
New Delhi – 110015

300 Shama (Unani and Ayurvedic) Laboratories
3651 Lal Kuan,
Delhi – 110006

301 Sharangdhar Pharmaceuticals Pvt. Ltd.
Vrindavan, 91/1 Parvati
Pune – 411009, Maharashtra

302 Sharda Drug Industries Pvt. Ltd.
Chandrama Banglo, 529 Camp
Parasneesh Colony, Satara – 415001

303 Shashi Phytochemical Industry
1, Old Industrial Area
Alwar

304 Shiv Ayurvedic Pharmacy
Kasganj – 207123, District Etah

305 Shraddha Exports
518 S.C. Centre, Nr. GPO
Salapose Rd, Ahmedabad 3800001

306 Shree Baidyanath Ayurved Bhawan Ltd.
!72-B, Gusainpura, Jhansi – 284002

307 Shree Baidyanath Ayurved Bhawan Ltd.
28, Ishwar Nagar, Mathura Road
New Delhi 110065

308 Shree Baidyanath Ayurved Bhawan Ltd.
28, Ishwar Nagar
New Delhi – 110065

309 Shree Baidyanath Ayurved Bhawan Ltd.
Baidyanath Bhawan Road
Patna – 800001

310 Shree Baidyanath Ayurved Bhawan Ltd.
Naini, Allahabad – 211008

311 Shree Baidynath Ayurved Bhavan Ltd.
Great Nag Road
Nagpur 440009 Maharashtra

312 Shree Dhanwantari Labs (Cal.)
244, Chittranjan Avenue
Kolkatta – 700006

313 Shree Dhootapapeshwar Limited
135, Nanu Bhai Desai Road, Khetwadi
Mumbai – 400004

314 Shri Anand Dharmik Vastu Bhandar
32/5 Rani Bagh Chowk
New Delhi 110034

315 Shri Dhanwantri Ayurvedic Pharmacy
277 East Mohan Nagar
Amritsar – 143006

316 Siddhayu Ayurvedic Research
Foundation Pvt. Ltd.
Great Nag Road
Nagpur (MS)

317 Sidhi Pharmacy Pvt. Ltd.
8 Civil Lines, Lalitpur – 284403

318 Simla Chemicals Pvt. Ltd.
(Mfr./Exporter of herbal products)
A-76 Phase – 1 Naraina Industrial Area
New Delhi 110028

319 Sind Ayurvedic Pharmacy
375 Kalba Devi Road, Mumbai – 400002

320 Sitaram Ayurved Pharmacy
MG 65-5/10, Sidharth Colony, Chambur
Mumbai – 400071

321 SMB Eximtrade Pvt. Ltd.
108 H New Alipore, Block F
Kolkatta 700053

322 SOL Pharmaceutical Ltd.
5-9-98/2, Fateh Maidan, Saphire Building
Hyderabad – 500001

323 Southern Herbals Ltd.
45 Ramraj Mansions
100 Feet Road, Vysya Bank Colony
BTM, IInd State Layout
Bangalore 560076 Karnataka

324 Srikrishn Ausdhylaya
2990, Tilak ali Corner, Behind Congress Bhawan
Ratnagiri – 415612

325 State Government Ayurvedic Pharmacy
Joginder Nagar – 176120
Himachal Pradesh

326 State Government Ayurvedic Pharmacy
Near Paonta, Sirmaur
Himachal Pradesh

327 Supreem Pharma
C-49, Hit Nikatan, Konkan Nagar
Bhandup (West), Mumbai – 400078

328 Surya Herbal Ltd.,
C-33, Sector-59,
Noida – 201 301 (UP)

329 Swami Laxminarain Pharmacy Ltd.
Raiji Ka Ghar, Johri Bazar
Jaipur

330 Swastik Formulations Pvt. Ltd.
CK 36/1-A, Bansphatak
P.B. No. 1022, Varanasi – 221001

331 Synthochem
7-B Shahjahanpur Road,
Bareilly – 243005

332 Taarani Herbals International
33/3155 Beadonpura, Karol Bagh
New Delhi 110005

333 Taniya Herbals
Type III/77, A.G. Colony
Bhadbhada Road, Bhopal

334 The Aroma Shop
C4A/40C Janak Puri
New Delhi 110058

335 The Himalayan Drug Company
Makali, Nelamangala, Bangalore – 562123

336 The Women Palace
Saboo Market, Topi Bazar, Lashkar
Gwalior, Madhya Pradesh 474001

337 Themis Pharmaceuticals
38, Suren Road, Andheri (East)
Mumbai – 400093

338 Tirubal Enterprise
(Dealing in Ayurvedic drugs)
4 VGP Selvanagar Vijayanagar
Velachery, Chennai-600042

339 Trichy Ayurvedic Union (P) Ltd.
31-A Chinnakadai Stret
Tiruchirapalli 620002
Tamilnadu

340 Triguna Ayurvedic Research Laboratory
47 Friends Colony, Mathura Road
New Delhi – 110065

341 TTK Pharma Ltd.
8, Old Trunk Road, Pallavaram
Chennai – 600043

342 Ujjawal Pharmaceuticals
MIDC, Plot No. L-1, Phase III
Shivar-Shibani, Akola

343 Uma Ayurved Bhawan Pvt. Ltd.
Kasganj – 207123,

344 Universal Ayurved
545/C, Shanti Nagar, Nagpur – 440002

345 Universal Exports Pvt. Ltd.
41 Sankari Main Road, Annathapatti
Salem 636005

346 Universal Medicaments Pvt. Ltd.
545 Shanti Nagar, P.O. Box No. 308
Nagpur – 440002

347 Unjha Ayurvedic Pharmacy
Dhanwantary Prasad, Station Road
Unjha 307026

348 Unjha Formulations
State Highway, 8, Khali Char Rasta
Khali, Sidhpur – 384151

349 Unjha Pharmacy
11, Krishanlal Zaveri Road
Bhuleshwar, Mumbai – 400004

350 Urja Pharmaceuticals Pvt. Ltd.
20/B Gokulnagar, Usmanpura,
Ashram Road,
Ahmedabad – 308013

351 Uttam Laboratories
Sadar Bazar,
Karnal (Haryana)

352 V N Sons
985 Sadashiv Peth, Bhupathi Complex
Pune – 411030, Maharashtra

353 V.N. Pharma
Sukh Sadan, 1st Floor, Anand Bawa
Chakala
Jamnagar – 361001

354 Vasu Pharmaceuticals Pvt. Ltd.
967/4, GIDC, Makarpura
Vadodara – 390010

355 Venkateswara Ayurveda Nilayam (P) Ltd.
Chintaluru – 533232, Alamuru Mandal
District East Godawari

356 Vetsfarma Ltd.
Police Lines Road,
Jalandhar – 144001

357 Vicco Laboratories
12, Dharmputra, Dr. Ambedkar Road
Dadar, T.T., Mumbai – 400014

358 Vikas Pharma (I) Pvt. Ltd.
1/3848 Bhagwanpur Khera, Loni Road,
Shahdara
Delhi – 110032

359 Vins Herbs
17 NGO New Colony Palayamkottai
Tirunelveli 627007

360 Vishwa Pharma
K-37/48, Gwaldas Sahu Lane
P.O. Box 1033, Varanasi – 221001

361 Vyas Pharmaceuticals
98-C, Sector-E,
Sanwer Road Industrial Area
(Behind Chautha Sansar),
Indore – 452004

362 Warrier Herbal Product Ltd.
PB No. 826
Visitors Building Complex
M.G. Road
Thrissur 680004 Kerala

363 Warrier Herbal Products Ltd.
P.B. No. 826
Visitors Building Complex
MG Road, Thrissur – 680004
Fax. 0487-427143

364 Welex Laboratories (P) Ltd.
5/46 Tardeo Airconditioned Market
Tardeo
Mumbai 400034 Maharashtra

365 Wings Pharmaceuticals (P) Ltd.
J-13, Udyog Nagar, Peera Garhi Chowk
Delhi – 110041

366 World Wide Connections
185/A GIDC Industrial Estate, Naroda
Ahmedabad 382330

367 Worldveda Enterprises
Krishnakripa
Cochin 682304

368 Wyeth Laboratories Ltd.
Nyloc House, 254-D2
Dr. A.B. Road, Post Box 9109
Mumbai – 400025

369 Yamuna Pharmacy
Yamuna Pharmacy Lane, Jagadhari Road
Yamuna Nagar – 135001
Harayana

370 Yash Pharma Laboratories Pvt. Ltd.
13-B, Navyug Niwas
Dr. Bhadkamdar Marg,
Mumbai – 400007

371 Zandu Pharmaceutical Works Ltd.
70 Gokhale Road South
Mumbai 400025

372 Zandu Pharmaceuticals Ltd.
GIDC, Plot No. 82,
Vapi – 396195
District Valsad (Gujarat)

373 Zylac Pharmaceuticals
914, Arya Samaj Road
Fazilka – 152123, District Ferozepur

5 ANALYTICAL AND TESTING FACILITIES

1 Alembic Limited
Alembic Road
Vadodara – 390 003

2 Anchrom Analytical Pvt. Ltd.,
Anand Bldg., Mithagar Road,
Mulund (East)
Mumbai – 400 081

3 Andhra University
Pharmaceutical Science Department
Waltair – 530003
Andhra Pradesh

4 Arbro Pharmaceutical Ltd.
8/32, Industrial Area
Kirti Nagar
New Delhi – 110 015

5 Bengal Immunity Research Inst.
39 Achraya J.C. Bose Road
Kolkatta – 700017
West Bengal

6 Birla Institute of Scientific Research
78 Syed Amir Ali Avenue
Kolkatta – 700019
West Bengal

7 Cadila Laboratories Pvt. Ltd.
244 Ghodasar, Maninagar
Ahmedabad – Gujarat

8 Central Drug Research Inst.
Chattar Manzil Palace
Lucknow – 226001 (UP)

9 Central Drugs Laboratory
3 Kyd Street
Kolkatta – 700016 West Bengal

10 Central Institute of Medicinal &
Aromatic Plants
P.O. CIMAP
Lucknow – 226016 (UP)

11 Chem-Med Analytical Laboratories
5-6-7 Kakad Estate, Worli, Seaface Road
Mumbai – 400018 Maharashtra

12 Ciba-Geigy Research Centre
Aarey Road, Goregaon East
Mumbai – 400063 Maharashtra

13 Drug Standardization Unit (Ayurveda)
Gujarat Ayurved University, Pharmacy
Dept., Dhanvantari Mandir
Jamnagar – 361008 Gujarat

14 Drug Standardization Unit (Homoeopathy)
Homoeopathic Pharmacopoeia Laboratory,
Central Govt. Offices Complex, Hapur Road
Chungi
Ghaziabad – 201002 Uttar Pradesh

15 Drug Standardization Unit (Homoeopathy)
Osmania University Buildings 32, rm,
4 Botany Department, Vikram Puri,
Habsigunda
Hyderabad – 500007
Andhra Pradesh

16 Drugs Testing Laboratory
Palace Road
Bangalore – 560001
Karnataka

17 Food & Drug Toxicology Research Centre
National Inst. of Nutrition,
Jamai-Osmania Campus
Hyderabad – 500007 Andhra Pradesh

18 Food & Drugs Laboratory
National Highway 8,
Near Polytechnic Inst.
Vadodara – 390002 Gujarat

19 Forest Research Inst.
P.O. New Forest
Dehra Dun – 248006 (UP)

20 Haffkine Inst. for Training Research & Testing
Acharya Donde Marg, Parel
Mumbai – 400012
Maharashtra

21 Homoeopathic Drug Research Inst.
B-1433 Indira Nagar
Lucknow – 226016 Uttar Pradesh

22 Homoeopathic Pharmacopoeia Laboratory
Central Govt. Offices Complex,
Hapur Road Chungi
Ghaziabad – 201002 Uttar Pradesh

23 Indian Drugs & Pharmaceuticals Ltd.
IDPL Complex, Dandahera-Gurgaon Road
Gurgaon – 122001 Haryana

24 Indian Institute of Chemical Biology
4 Raja S.C. Mullick Road
Kolkatta – 700032 West Bengal

25 Indtech Analytical
K-227, Ansa Industrial Estate,
Saki Vihar Road,
Mumbai – 400 072

26 Industrial Perfumes Ltd.
Hay Bunder Road, P.O. Tank Road,
Sewri P.O.
Mumbai – 400033 Maharashtra

27 Jamia Hamdard
Faculty of Medicine
Mehrauli-Badarpur Road,
Hamdard Nagar
Delhi – 110062

28 Jamia Hamdard
Faculty of Pharmacy
Mehrauli-Badarpur Road,
Hamdard Nagar
Delhi – 110062

29 Jamia Hamdard
Faculty of Science
Biochemistry Department
Mehraul-Badarpur Road,
Hamdard Nagar
Delhi – 110062

30 Nagpur University
Pharmaceutical Sciences Dept.
Amravati Road
Nagpur – 440010 Maharashtra

31 National Chemical Laboratory
Dr. Homi Bhabha Road
Pune – 411008 Maharashtra

32 National Institute of Ayurveda
Madhav Vilas Palace, Amer Road
Jaipur – 302002 Rajasthan

33 National Institute of Nutrition
Jamai-Osmania
Hyderabad – 500007
Andhra Pradesh

34 National Research Centre for Spices
Mari Kunnu P.O.
Calicut – 673012 Kerala

35 Oil Technology Research Inst.
Anantapur – 515001 Andhra Pradesh

36 Organon (India) Ltd.
Himalaya House, 38 Chowringhee Road
Kolkatta – 700071 West Bengal

37 Pharmacopoeial Laboratory for Indian Medicine
A Wing, 3rd fl., Central Govt. Office Building
Kamala Nehru Nagar
Ghaziabad – 201002 (UP)

38 Ranbaxy Laboratories Ltd.
A-1, Phase 1, Okhla Industrial Area
Delhi – 110020

39 Regional Research Laboratory,
Canal Road
Jammu Tawi – 180001
Jammu & Kashmir

40 Regional Research Laboratory,
Jorhat – 785006 Assam

41 Regional Research Laboratory,
Sachivalya Marg
Bhubaneswar – 751013 Orissa

42 Regional Research Laboratory,
P.O. Industrial Estate, Pappanamcode
Thiruvananthapuram, 695019
Kerala

43 SAMI Labs Ltd.,
19/1 & 19/2, 1 Main, II Phase,
Peenya Industrial Area
Bangalore – 560 058

44 Sandoz (India) Ltd.
R&D Centre
P.O. Sandoz Baug, Kolshet Road
Thane – 400607 Maharashtra

45 Sgabtga Buitecgbucs Pvt. Ltd.,
3rd Floor, Serene Chambers Road No. 7,
Banjara Hills,
Hyderabad

46 Sonit Aromatic Chemicals Pvt. Ltd.
257/258, IV Phase, Peenya Industrial Area
Bangalore – 560058 Karnataka

47 Wyeth Laboratories Ltd.
Steelcrete House, Dinshaw Wacha Road,
P.O.B. 11056
Mumbai – 400020
Maharashtra

48 Zandu Pharmaceutical Works Ltd.
Gokhale Road South, Dadar
Mumbai – 400025 Maharashtra

6 HERBERIA AND MEDICINAL GARDENS

1 Allahabad University
Botany Department
Allahabad – 211001 UP
India

2 Andhra Pradesh
Botany Department
Waltair – 530003
Andhra Pradesh
India

3 Arid Forest Research Institute
New Pali Road,
Jodhpur – 342 005 (India)

4 Banaras Hindu University
Botany Department
Varanasi – 221005 UP
India

5 Banaras Hindu University
Faculty Agriculture
Mycology & Plant Pathology Dept.
Varanasi – 221005
Uttar Pradesh
India

6 Bangladesh National Herbarium
Zoo Road, Mirpur – 1
Dhaka – 1216
Bangladesh

7 Baroda University
Baroda – Gujarat
India

8 Bhabha Atomic Research Centre
Trombay
Mumbai – 400085
Maharashtra
India

9 Bhagalpur University
Postgraduate Botany Department
Bhagalpur – 812007
Bihar
India

10 Botanical Garden
Pondicherry
India

11 Botanical Garden
Waghai Saputara Road, Dangs
Dist. Waghai-Dangs – 394730
Gujarat
India

12 Botanical Survey of India
Andaman & Nicobar Circle
Horticultural Road, Haddo
Port Blair – 744102
Andaman & Nicobar Islands
India

13 Botanical Survey of India
Arid Zone Circle
Subhash Nagar
Jodhpur – 342003
Rajasthan
India

14 Botanical Survey of India
Arunachal Pradesh Circle
Sankai View
Itanagar – 791110
Arunachal Pradesh
India

15 Botanical Survey of India
Central Botanical Laboratory
Botanic Garden, Sibpur
Howrah – 711103
West Bengal
India

16 Botanical Survey of India
Central Circle
10 Chatham Lines
Allahabad – 211001 (UP)
India

17 Botanical Survey of India
Central National Herbarium
Botanic Garden, Sibpur
Howrah – 711103
India

18 Botanical Survey of India
Eastern Circle
Woodlands
Shillong – 793003
Meghalaya
India

19 Botanical Survey of India
Indian Museum
Industrial Section
Economic Herbarium
1 Sudder Street
Kolkatta – 7000016
West Bengal
India

20 Botanical Survey of India
Northern Circle
192 Kaulagarh Road
Dehra Dun – 248195 (UC)
India

21 Botanical Survey of India
Sikkim Himalayan Circle
Gangtok – 737101
Sikkim
India

22 Botanical Survey of India
Southern Circle
Tamil Nadu Agricultural University Campus
Lawley Road
Coimbatore – 641003
Tamil Nadu
India

23 Botanical Survey of India
Western Circle
7 Koregaon Road
Pune – 411001
Maharashtra
India

24 Burdwan University
Botany Department
Burdwan – West Bengal
India

25 Burma Forest Herbarium
Forest Research Institute
P.O. –650
Yezin, Pyinmana
Myanmar

26 Kolkatta University
Botany Department
35 Ballygunge Circular Road
Kolkatta – 700019 West Bengal
India

27 Calicut University
Botany Department
Calicut – 673635
Kerala
India

28 Central Arid Zone Research Inst.
Light Industrial Area
Jodhpur – 342003 Rajasthan
India

29 Central Council for Research in Unani
Medicine
JLN Bhartiya Chikitsa Evum Homoeopathy
Anusandhan Bhawan, 61-65 Institutional
Area,
Opp. D Block, Janakpuri
Delhi – 110058
India

30 Central Council for Research in
Ayurveda & Siddha
JLN Bhartiya Chikitsa Evum Homoeopathy
Anusandhan Bhawan, 61-65 Institutional
Area
Opp. D Block, Janakpuri
Delhi – 110058
India

31 Central Council for Research in
Ayurveda & Siddha
Research Project on Tibetan System of
Medicine
Amchi Association Building
Leh – 194101 Jammu & Kashmir
India

32 Central Council for Research in
Unani Medicine
Central Herb Garden & Museum
National Botanical Research Inst.
Campus, Rana Pratap Bagh
Lucknow – 226001 (UP)
India

33 Central Council for Research
in Homoeopathy
JLN Bhartiya Chikitsa Evum Homoeopathy
Anusandhan Bhawan, 61-65 Institutional
Area
Opp. D Block, Janakpuri
Delhi – 110058
India

34 Central Drugs Research Inst.
Botany Division
Chattar Manzil Palace
Lucknow – 226001 (UP)
India

35 Central Institute of Medicinal &
Aromatic Plants
P.O. CIMAP
Lucknow – 226016 (UP)
India

36 Central Institute of Medicinal &
Aromatic Plants
Regional Centre
Attuvampatti, P.B. 22
Kodaikanal – 624101 Tamil Nadu
India

37 Central Research Institute (Siddha)
Arignar Anna Govt. Hospital Campus,
Arumbakkam
Madras – 600106
Tamil Nadu
India

38 Central Research Institute for
Unani Medicine
11/4/625 Dilkhusha, A.C. Guards
Hyderabad – 500004
Andhra Pradesh
India

39 Central Research Institute
Near Rajdhani College,
New Capital,
Ashok Nagar
Bhubaneswar – 751009
Orissa
India

40 Central Salt & Marine Chemicals
Research Institute
Bhavnagar – 364002
Gujarat
India

41 Council of Scientific & Industrial Research
Publications & Information Directorate
Raw Materials Herbarium & Museum
Dr. K.S. Krishnan Marg
Delhi – 110012
India

42 Delhi University
Botany Department
Near Delhi Railway Station
Delhi – 110007
India

43 Dr. A. Lakshmipathi Research
Centre in Ayurveda
V.H.S. Medical Centre, TTTI Post Office
Madras – 600113 Tamil Nadu
India

44 Dr. Hari Singh Gour Vishwavidyalaya
Botany Department
Sagar – 470003
Madhya Pradesh
India

45 Drug Standardization Unit (Homoeopathy)
Homoeopathic Pharmacopoeia Laboratory,
Central Govt. Offices Complex, Hapur Road
Chungi
Ghaziabad – 201002 Uttar Pradesh
India

46 Drug Standardization Unit (Homoeopathy)
Osmania University Buildings 32,
32 rm. 4, Botany Dept, Vikram Puri,
Habsigunda
Hyderabad – 500007
Andhra Pradesh
India

47 Eden Gardens
Kolkatta – 700021
West Bengal
India

48 Forest Research Institute
Botany Division
P.O. New Forest
Dehra Dun – 248006 Uttaranchal
India

49 Forest Research Institute
Silviculture Division
P.O. New Forest
Dehra Dun – 248006
Uttaranchal
India

50 Forest Research Institute
Xylarium
P.O. New Forest
Dehra Dun – 248006
Uttaranchal
India

51 Government Botanic Garden
Thiruvananthapuram – 695001
Kerala
India

52 Gujarat Agricultural University
Agricultural Botany Department
Junagadh – 362001
Gujarat
India

53 Gujarat Ayurved University
Jamnagar – 380 008 (India)

54 Gujarat University
School of Sciences
Botany Department
Ahmedabad – 380009
Gujarat
India

55 Guru Nanak Dev University
Biology Department
Amritsar – 143005 Punjab
India

56 Herbarium
Art & Science University
Mandalai
Myanmar

57 Herbarium
Biological Sciences Department
Quaid-e-Azam University
Islamabad
Pakistan

58 Herbarium
Botanical Sciences Division
Pakistan Museum of Natural History
P.O. Box No. 1761 Garden
Avenue, Shakarparian
Islamabad
Pakistan

59 Herbarium
Botany Department
University of Karachi, Sind
Karachi – 75270
Pakistan

60 Herbarium
Botany Department
University of Peshawar
Peshawar
Pakistan

61 Herbarium
Botany Department, Islamia College
University of Peshawar
Peshawar
Pakistan

62 Herbarium
Department of Botany
University of Colombo
Colombo 3
Sri Lanka

63 Herbarium
Department of Botany
University of Jaffna,
Jaffna,
Sri Lanka

64 Herbarium
Department of Botany
University of Ruhuna
Ruhuna
Sri Lanka

65 Herbarium
Hakgala Botanic Garden
Hakgala
Sri Lanka

66 Herbarium
Natural Drug Division
Pakistan Council of Scientific &
Research Laboratories
University of Peshawar
Peshawar
Pakistan

67 Herbarium
Pakistan Forest Institute
Peshawar
Pakistan

68 Herbarium
Pharmaceutical Department
Union of Burma Applied
Research Institute
Yangon
Myanmar

69 Herbarium
Yangon University, Yangon
Myanmar

70 Himachal Pradesh Krishi Vishva Vidyalaya
Near Naranda Railway Station,
Kangra Dist. Palampur – 176062
Himachal Pradesh
India

71 Homoeopathic Drug Research Institute
B-1433 Indira Nagar
Lucknow – 226016
Uttar Pradesh
India

72 Homoeopathic Pharmacopoeia Laboratory
Central Govt. Offices Complex,
Hapur Road
Chungi
Ghaziabad – 201002
India

73 Indian Agricultural Research Institute
Mycology & Plant Pathology Division
Herbarium Cryptogamiae Indiae Orientalis
Pusa
Delhi – 110012
India

74 Indian Agricultural Research Institute
Plant Introduction Division
Pusa
Delhi – 110012
India

75 Indian Drugs Research Association
516-B, Shivajinagar
Pune – 411005
Maharashtra
India

76 Indian Institute of Ayurveda for
Drug Research
Near Ranikhet
Tarikhet – 263645
Uttaranchal
India

77 Institute Français
10 St. Louis Street
Pondicheery – 605001
India

78 Institute of Forest Genetics & Tree
Breeding Seed Technology Division
Seed Harbarium
Forest Campus College, R.S. Puram
Coimbatore – 641002 Tamil Nadu
India

79 Institute of Forest Genetics &
Tree Breeding Fischer Herbarium
Forest Campus College, R.S. Puram
Coimbatore – 641002
Tamil Nadu
India

80 Institute of Research in Indigenous System
of Medicine
Approach Road
Joginder Nagar – 176120
Himachal Pradesh
India

81 Institute of Wood Science & Tech.
18th Cross Road, Malleswaram
Bangalore – 560003 Karnataka
India

82 Jabalpur University
Pachpedi
Jabalpur – Madhya Pradesh
India

83 Jamia Hamdard
Faculty of Science
Botany Department
Mehrauli-Badarpur Road,
Hamdard Nagar
Delhi – 110062
India

84 Jawaharlal Nehru Ayurvedic Medicinal
Plants Garden & Herbarium
Kothrud
Pune – 411029
Maharashtra
India

85 Jai Narain Vyas University
Botany Department
Jodhpur – Rajasthan
India

86 Kashmir University
Botany Department
Srinagar – 190006
Jammu & Kashmir
India

87 Lalbagh Gardens
Bangalore – 560004
Karnataka
India

88 Lalit Narayan Mithila University
Botany Department
Darbhanga – 846004
Bihar
India

89 Lloyd Botanic Garden
Darjeeling – 734101
West Bengal
India

90 Lucknow University
Lucknow – 226007
(UP)
India

91 M.S. Swaminathan Research Foundation
Community Gene Bank
3rd Cross Road, Taramani Institutional Area
Madras – 600113
Tamil Nadu
India

92 Madurai Kamraj University
Plant Sciences Division
Madurai – 622021
Tamil Nadu
India

93 Magadh University
Postgraduate Botany Department
Bodh Gaya – 824234
Bihar
India

94 Maharashtra Association for the
Cultivation of Science
Research Institute
Ajrekar Mycological Herbarium
Law College Road
Pune – 411003
Maharashtra
India

95 Marathwada University
Aurangabad – 431004
Maharashtra
India

96 Nandan Kanan, State Botanical Garden
Dist. Cuttack, Barang
Orissa
India

97 National Botanical Research Institute
Rana Pratap Marg
Lucknow – 226001 (UP)
India

98 National Bureau of Plant Genetic Resources
National Herbarium of Cultivated Plants
FIC Building, Indian Agricultural Research
Institute Campus, Pusa
New Delhi – 110012
India

99 National Herbarium & Plant Laboratories
Department of Plant resources
Ministry of Forests & Soil Conservation
P.O. Box: 3708 KATH.
Godawary, Lalitpur
Kathmandu
Nepal

100 National Herbarium of Bhutan
National Biodiversity
Programme
Ministry of Agriculture,
Serbithang,
P.O. Box : 875, Thimphu,
Bhutan

101 National Herbarium
Department of Agriculture
Royal Botanic Garden
P.O. Box – 15
Peradeniya
Sri Lanka

102 National Herbarium
Pakistan Agricultural Research Centre
Park Road
Islamabad – 45500
Pakistan

103 National Institute of Homoeopathy
Block, GE, Sector 3, Bhidan Nagar,
Salt Lake City
Kolkatta – 700091
West Bengal
India

104 Orchid Research & Development
Centre Botanic Garden
Bhalukpong
Tippi – 790114
Arunachal Pradesh
India

105 Osmania University
Botany Department
Herbarium & Botanical Museum
Hyderabad – 500007
Andhra Pradesh
India

106 Pharmacopoeial Laboratory for
Indian Medicine
A Wing, 3rd floor,
Central Govt. Office Building
Kamala Nehru Nagar
Ghaziabad – 201002 (UP)
India

107 Presidency College
Botany Department
Madras – 600005
Tamil Nadu
India

108 Punjab University Herbarium
Department of Botany
Quaid-e-Azam Campus
Lahore-54590
Pakistan

109 Punjab University
Botany Department
Sector 14
Chandigarh – 160014
India

110 Punjabi University
Botany Department
Patiala – 147002
Punjab
India

111 Rajasthan Agro Forestry Corporation,
Sonamukhi Nagar, Sangaria Phanta
Jodhpur – 342 005 (India)

112 Rajasthan University
Botany Department
Jaipur – 302004
Rajasthan
India

113 Ravi Shankar University
Biosciences Department
Raipur – 492010 Chhatisgarh
India

114 Regional Research Centre (Ayurveda)
1093 Gorepeth
Nagpur – 440010
Maharashtra
India

115 Regional Research Centre (Ayurveda)
A Block, North Wing, Indira Gandhi
Stadium
Complex, Bandra Road
Vijayawada – 520010
Andhra Pradesh
India

116 Regional Research Centre (Ayurveda)
Gandhi Bhawan
Mandi – Himachal Pradesh
India

117 Regional Research Centre (Ayurveda)
Govt. Ayurvedic College, Jalukbari
Guwahati – 781014
Assam
India

118 Regional Research Centre (Ayurveda)
Govt. Central Pharmacy Annex,
Ashok Pillar,
Jayanagar
Bangalore – 560011 Karnataka
India

119 Regional Research Centre (Ayurveda)
Rehari Chowk
Jammu – 180005 Jammu & Kashmir
India

120 Regional Research Centre (Ayurveda)
Sankai View
Itanagar – 791110
Arunachal Pradesh
India

121 Regional Research Centre (Ayurveda)
Tadung
Gangtok – 737101
Sikkim
India

122 Regional Research Centre
Gwalior Road
Jhansi – 248003
(UP)
India

123 Regional Research Institute (Ayurveda)
14 Jagannath Dutta Lane
Kolkatta – 700009
West Bengal
India

124 Regional Research Institute (Ayurveda)
476/6 Sitapur Road
Lucknow – 226007 (UP)
India

125 Regional Research Institute (Ayurveda)
Madhav Vilas Palace, Amer Road
Jaipur – 302002
Rajasthan
India

126 Regional Research Institute (Ayurveda)
Poojapura
Thiruvananthapuram – 695012
Kerala
India

127 Regional Research Institute (Ayurveda)
Rajendra Memorial Research Institute Building
Kadam Kuan
Patna – 800007 Bihar
India

128 Regional Research Institute (Ayurveda)
Taj Manzil, Sardar Bagh
Junagadh – 362001
Gujarat
India

129 Regional Research Institute (Ayurveda)
Ullas Bhawan, Kherapathi,
Killa Road, P.B. 3
Gwalior – 474002 (MP)
India

130 Regional Research Institute of Unani Medicine
1 West Mada Chruch Street, Royapuram
Madras – 600013
Tamil Nadu
India

131 Regional Research Institute of Unani Medicine
Aligarh Muslim University,
Department of Research in Unani Medicine
Aligarh – 202001 (UP)
India

132 Regional Research Institute of Unani Medicine
Dist. Balasore
Bhadrak – 756100
Orissa
India

133 Regional Research Institute of Unani Medicine
Nawab Manzil, Guzri
Patna – 800008
Bihar
India

134 Regional Research Institute of Unani Medicine
University of Kashmir, University Health Centre,
Hazratbal
Srinagar – 190006
Jammu & Kashmir
India

135 Regional Research Laboratory,
Canal Road
Jammu Tawi – 180001 Jammu & Kashmir
India

136 Regional Research Laboratory,
Extension Centre
Palampur – Himachal Pradesh
India

137 Regional Research Laboratory,
Sachivalya Marg
Bhubaneswar – 751013
Orissa India

138 Sarabhai Foundation
Retreat Botanical Garden
Shahibag
Ahmedabad – 380004
Gujarat
India

139 Saurashtra University
Biosciences Department
Rajkot – 360005
Gujarat
India

140 School of Tropical Medicine
Chittaranja Avenue
Kolkatta – 700073
West Bengal
India

141 Sikkim State Forest Department
Gangtok – Sikkim
India

142 South Gujarat University
Biosciences Department
P.B. 49
Surat – 395001
Gujarat
India

143 St. Joseph's College
Centre for Taxonomic Studies
P.B. 5031
Bangalore – 560001
Karnataka
India

144 St. Joseph's College
Rapinat Herbarium
Tiruchirapalli – 620002
Tamil Nadu
India

145 St. Xavier's College
Botany Department
Blatter Herbarium
Mahapalika Marg
Mumbai – 400001
Maharashtra
India

146 Survey of Medicinal Plants &
Collection Unit (Homoeopathy)
112 Govt. Arts College Campus
Udhagamandalam – 643002
Tamil Nadu
India

147 Survey of Medicinal Plants Unit (Siddha)
Govt. College of Indian Medicine,
Tirunelveli
Dist. Palayamkottai – 627002
Tamil Nadu
India

148 Swami Maheshwaranand Ashram
Village post : Jadan
Dist: Pali Marwar Rajasthan (India)

149 The Chittagong University
Herbarium
Department of Botany
Chittagon University
Chittagong – 4331
Bangaldesh

150 Tibetan Medical & Astro
Institute (Men-Tsee-Khang)
Khara Danda Road, Dist. Kangra
Dharamsala – 176215
Himachal Pradesh
India

151 Tropical Botanic Garden &
Research Institute
Karimancode, Pacha-Pacha-Palode P.O.
Thiruvananthapuram – 692562
Kerala
India

152 University of Agricultural Sciences
College of Basic Sciences & Humanities
Gandhi Krishi Vigyana Kendra Campus
Bangalore – 5600065
Karnataka
India

153 Utkal University
Botany Department
Vani Bihar
Bhubaneswar – 751004
Orissa
India

154 Vaidya Gopi Kishan Parihar
Village Post Birai
Teh: Bhopalgarh
Dist. : Jodhpur Rajasthan (India)

155 Vikram University
School of Studies in Botany
Ujjain – 456001
Madhya Pradesh
India

156 Zandu Pharmaceutical Works Ltd.
Gokhale Road South, Dadar
Mumbai – 400025
Maharashtra
India

157 A.A. Enterprise Ltd.
2113 Parakeet Terrace
Maloney, Trinidad
West Indies

158 A.A. Sayia & Co. Inc.
One Newark Street, Hoboken, NJ 11791
USA

159 A.M. Todd Co.
Box 711, Kalamazoo
Michigan 49005
USA

160 Abdul Kaleq Abdullah
P.O. Box 374 Abu Dhabi
U.A.E.

161 Abdulla al Omran Trading Est.
P.O. Box 16720 Dubai
U.A.E.

162 Abdulla Fahad Al Ajlan
P.O. Box 1357 Riyadh
Saudi Arabia

163 Abel Lemon Food Service Pty. Ltd.
2 Railway Parade, Murrumbeena VIC 3163
Australia

164 Abu Dhabi National Food Stuff Co.
P.O. Box 2378 Abu Dhabi
U.A.E.

165 Acana Mercantile Inc.
Sutte 204, 208 Dundas Street East,
Belleville,
Ontario K8N 1E3
Canada

166 Accurate Ingredients Inc.,
60 Eileen Way Syosset NY 11791
USA

167 Adams, Joseph, Corporation
5740 Grafton Road,
P.O. Box 273,Valley City, OH 44280,
USA

168 Adron Inc.
94 Fanny Road,
P.O. Box 270 Boonton, NJ 07005
USA

169 Ahmad Taher Gen Trdg. Est.
P.O. Box 7607 Dubai
U.A.E.

170 Ahmed S Al Hamad Trdg. Est.
P.O. Box 1346 Riyadh
Saudi Arabia

171 Al Bida Enterprises
P.O. Box 7891 Dubai
U.A.E.

172 Al Hamli Trading Est.
P.O. Box 16651 Jeddha
Saudi Arabia

173 Al Inshirah Trading Est.
P.O. Box 16828 AL Raas Dubai
U.A.E.

174 Al Keddah Trading Co.
P.O. Box 13264 Jebel Ali Dubai
U.A.E.

175 Al Khair General Trading
P.O. Box 1466 Jaddah 21431
Saudi Arabia

176 Al Muhwar Trading Est.
P.O. Box 4808 Sharjah
U.A.E.

177 Al Salah Establishment
P.O. Box 16460 Jeddah 21464
Saudi Arabia

178 Al Sawani For Trading and Services Co. Ltd.
P.O. Box 52826 Riyadh 11573
Saudi Arabia

179 Al Sharif and Al Daboos Trdg. Est.
P.O. Box 4173 Dubai
U.A.E.

180 Alfayiz Trading Office
P.O. Box 5960 Jeddah
Saudi Arabia

181 Algerian Coffee Stores Ltd.
52 Old Compton Street
London W1V 6PV
UK

182 Allied Enterprises
P.O. Box 1578 Dubai
U.A.E.

183 Alps Pharmaceutical Ind. Co. Ltd
TSUJI-Koraibashi Bldg., 4-7
Koraibashi 2-Chome, Osaka 541, Japan

184 American Mercantile Corpn.
5690 Summer Avenue
P.O. Box 240654 Memphis, TN 38134
USA

185 Andard Mount Ltd.
West Africa House,
Ashbourne R
GB-London W 5 3QP, England

186 Angelika Duval
Thyme Cottage
87 World's End Lane
Green Street Green
Kent BR6 6AE
UK

187 Ankram Company
30, Abdel Raheim Sabri Street
Dokki, Cairo, Egypt

188 Aoboshi & Co. Ltd.
2-3-5, Ikenohata,
Taito-Ku Tokyo-110
Japan

189 Apex Resources Inc.
(Exporters Herbal Products)
9003 Marksfield Road Suite 3
Lousville 40222, USA

190 Apex Resources Inc.
9003 Marksfield Road
Suite 3, Louisville 40222
USA

191 Aquario Commercio De Electronica
Rua de Alegria 93-A
4000 Porto Portugal

192 Arabian Development Ent. For Trading
P.O. Box 40418 Riyadh
Saudi Arabia

193 Arabian Trading Corporation
P.O. Box 5894 Jeddah
Saudi Arabia

194 Arco Establishment USA
83, Cedar Lane Englewood, NJ 07631
USA

195 Asoka spices Co. Ltd.
2-13-16, Higashi, Sakashita,
Itabashi-Ku Tokyo 174
Japan

196 Aum Commodities PTE Ltd.
101 Cecil Street #19-09 Tong Eng
Building
Singapore 0106

197 Ayurvedic Helse Norge ANS
4003 S. Westshore Blvd. Apt. #2008
Tampa 33611, USA

198 B.E. International Foods Ltd.
Grafton House, Stockings Water Road,
Ensfield, Middlesex, Em3 7JZ
England
UK

199 Bafarat Spices and Herbs Shops
P.O. Box 11652
Jeddah 21463, Saudi Arabia

200 Bahadi Trading Est.
P.O. Box 19738 Jeddah 21445
Saudi Arabia

201 Baharain Pharmacy & Gen. Store
P.O. Box 56, Manama, Baharain
Tel: (973) 253491
Kuwait

7 FOREIGN BUYERS

1 Bahasan Trading Est.
P.O. Box 612 Jeddah
Saudi Arabia

2 Balanced bodies Enterprises
15 Potter Street Sutie 1
Haddonfield 08033
USA

3 Baldwins
173 Walworth Road
London SE17
UK

4 Baltimore spice Co., the
P.O. Box 5858
Baltimore MD 21208
USA

5 Barwinnock Herbs
Barrhill Ayrshire
Scotland KA26 ORB
UK

6 Bashir Al Halees Corp.
P.O. Box 30569 Jeddah 21487
Saudi Arabia

7 Basic American Foods
P.O. Box 599
Bacaville CA 95696-0599
USA

8 Bechara Yordan Obegi
P.O. Box 343, Damascus, Syria

9 Bender and Cassel Blackhorse Road,
Letch Worth, Herts, SG6 1HL England
UK

10 Blessed Herbs
Martha & Michael Volahoh
109 Barre Plains Road
Oakham, Mass USA 01068

11 Bohara Industries Co. Ltd.
P.O. Box 8982 Jeddah 21492
Saudi Arabia

12 Botanicals International
2550 El Presidio Street
Long Beach, CA 90810, U.S.A.

13 BPS Fragrance
20090 Buccinasco (MI)
ITALY

14 Brithish Pepper & Spice Co. Ltd.
Rhosili Road, Brack Mills,
Old Northamptonshire,
Northamption NN4, England
UK

15 Brome & Schimmer
Greatbridge Road Estate
Romsey Hampshire SO5 OHR
(Wholesale only)
UK

16 Buchanan Trading Inc.
4174, Dundas Street West,
Toronot, Ontario M8X, 1X3
Canada

17 Bush Beach Ltd.
Stanley Green Ltd.
GB-Cheadle H.,
Cheadle SK8 6RN, England

18 Bush Boake Allen (NZ) Ltd.
128-130 Stoddard Road,
New Zealand

19 Bush Boake allen Ltd.
Blackhorse Lane, Walthamstow,
London E17 5QP
UK

20 Bush Broake Allen Clinc.
312, St. Patrick Street,
LassalleQuebec H8N 2H2
Canada

21 Cade-Grayson Co.
2445 Cades Way Vista CA 92083
USA

22 Cains coffee Company
13131 Broadway Extn.
P.O. Box 25009 Oklahoma City, OK 73125
USA

23 Cal-compack foods
4906 West first Street
P.O. Box 265 Santa Ana, CA 92702-0265
USA

24 Candlesby Herbs
Cross Keys Candlesby
Spilsby Lincolnshire PE23 5SF
UK

25 Cerebros Gregg's Limited
East Tamaki Road,
P.O. Box 58-095, East Tamaki, Auckland
New Zealand

26 Champon, L.A. & Co., Inc.
1404 OAK Tree Road
P.O. Box 950 ISELIN, NJ 08830
USA

27 Charles Carey
The Oil Merchant
47 Ashchurch Grove
London W12 9BU
UK

28 Chia Shin Trading Co., Ltd.
P.O. Box 22841, Taipei City, Taiwan

29 Chii Yea Trading Co., Ltd.
10, Alley 19, Lane 50, Wu Hsing
Sungshan Dist, Taipei City, Taiwan

30 Chinese-Cheer Trading Co., Ltd.
2F, 2, Lane 107, San Ho Rd, Sec 3
Sahchung City, Taipei Hsien, Taiwan

31 Chun Che Trading Co., Ltd.
55, Ku Shan 1 Rd, Kushan Dist,
Kaohsiung City, Taiwan

32 Chunilal Purushottam & Co.
P.O. Box 2937 Dubai
U.A.E.

33 Clos d' Aguzon
Saint Auban Sur l' Ouvese
26170 Buis –les-Barronies
France

34 Codidex Pharma S.P.R.L.
Rue Josse Impens,
1030 Brussels, Belgium

35 Commercial Markets
P.O. Box 764 Dammam 31441
Saudi Arabia

36 Cordovi, V.A. Inc.
P.O. Box 763 Two Park Avenue, Man-
Hasset N.Y. 11030
USA

37 Cottage Delight Unit
8, Churnetside Industrial Park,
Station Road, Cheddleton,
Staffs, ST13 7EE, England
UK

38 Covent Garden General Store
111 Long Acre
London WC2N 4BA
UK

39 CPC (UK) Ltd.
Food Ingredients Division,
Claygate House, Esher,
Surry Kt 10 9 PN
UK

40 Crew Corp.
10-9-606, Uehommachi, 6-Chome,
Tennoji-Ku, Osaka 543,
Japan

41 CTC Spice Corp.
152 Madison Avenue Suite 300 Newyork,
NY 10016
USA

42 Culpeper Ltd.
Hadstock Road
Linton Cambridgeshire CB1 6NJ
UK

43 Cyclo Products Inc.
P.O. Box 01557, Los Angles,
CA 90001, U.S.A.

44 Daarnhou Wer & Co.
105, Cecil Street, #12-01 The Octagon,
Singapore 0106

45 Daarnihouwer (New York) Inc.
2125 Center Street, Suite 506
P.O. Box 1928 Fort Lee, NJ 07024
USA

46 Daiel Sangyo Kaisha, Ltd.
18, Honjin-Dori 4-Chome,
Nakamuraku, Nagoya 453
Japan

47 Dainan Boeki Kaisha, Ltd.
3-3, Minam-Kyuhoji-Machi,
3-Chome, Chuo-Ku, Osaka 541,
Japan

48 Deep South Blenders
3763 Derbingny Street Metairie, LA 70001
USA

49 Dmt New York, Inc.
20 Exchange Place
32nd Floor New York, NY 10005
USA

50 Docks Des Alcools SA
57 Rue De Villiers, F-92200
Neuilly Sur Seine, France

51 Dolma
19 Royce Avenue
Hucknall
Nottinghamshire NG15 6FU
UK

52 Dooley International Corp.
C.P.O. Box 10696
Seoul, South Korea

53 Du Pont De Nemours (Belgium)
100, Rue De La Fusee, B-1130
Bruxelles, Belgium

54 Dublin Street Service Station
14 Dublin Street, Wanganui,
New Zealand

55 Dunn. G.S. & Co. Limited.
80, Park Street North Hamilton,
Ontario L8R 2m9
Canada

56 Dunningham D.M. Ltd.
2 Hobson Street, Auckland,
New Zealand

57 Durkee Food service corpn.
926 Euclid Avenue Cleveland OH 44115
USA

58 Durkee-French Foods, Inc.
1665 Valley Road
P.O. Box 942 Wayne, NJ 07474-0942
USA

59 E.C. Arnold Ltd.
Boston Road, Heckington,
Lincs NG34 9JE England
UK

60 East Anglican Food Ingredients Ltd.
Gorse Lane Ind Estate,
Wade Road, Clacton, On Sea,
Essex CO15 4LT, England
UK

61 East West Herbs Ltd.
Langston Priory Mews
Kingham
Oxfordshire OX7 6UP
UK

62 Ecom Trading Corporation
120, Dynamic Drive Suite 23,
Scarborough, Ontario Miv 4T5,
Canada

63 Eduardo Caremoli
Vial Casiraghi 508
20099 Sesto S. Giovanni
Milano, ITALY

64 Edwin Trading Co., Ltd.
7F-1, 337, Hsin Yi Rd, Sec 4
Ta-An Dist, Taipei City,
Taiwan

65 Eikoco Co. Ltd.
6-1, Nihonbashi Hon-Cho, 2-Chome,
Chuo-KU Tokyo 174
Japan

66 Ely Lilly Italia SPA
Via Gramsci, 733
I-50019 Sesto Florentino (Fi), Italy

67 Empire Foodstuffs Ltd.
60-66 Kingsford,
Smith Street, Wellington,
New Zealand

68 Equilibrium S.A.
8, Route De Buchillon, Ch-1162
Saint Prex, Switzerland

69 F.R. Benson & Partners Ltd.
Crossroads House, 165,
The Parade Watford, Herts, WD1 Inj.
England
UK

70 Fallowfield Herbs
Morrells Farm Buildings
Vinehall Road Whatlington
Battle East Sussex
UK

71 Famy Enterprises
P.O. Box 6348 Dubai
U.A.E.

72 Fastrade International Est.
P.O. Box 11337 Dubai
U.A.E.

73 Felton Worldwide Ltd.
The Spice Ware house,
Pepperalley, Banbury, Oxon Ox 16 8JB,
England
UK

74 Fiddes Paynes Ltd.
17a-21a Woolton Street,
Liver-pool 1.25 5NR England.
UK

75 Flavorite Labs, Inc.
P.O. Box 1315 Memphis TN 38101
USA

76 Flora Dist. Ltd.
7400 Fraser Park Drive, Burnaby
B C V5J 5B9, Canada

77 Florasynth Canada Inc.
5800 AVE Andover Ave.,
VII Lemonth-Royla Quebec H4T 1H
Canada

78 Florida 734, Piso 1, Off
1005 Buenos Aires, Argentina

79 Fold Garden
26 Fold Lane
Biddulph Staffordshire ST8 7SG
UK

80 Foodingredients Service
Bilton Road, Bletchley,
Milton Keynes, MKI 1HP, England
UK

81 Foodpro National Inc., (Quest)
2610 J.B. Deschamps Blvd. Lachine,
Qoebec H&T 1C9,
Canada

82 Foodstuff Trading
P.O. Box 20561 Riyadh 11465
Saudi Arabia

83 Foreign-Domestic Chemicals
95 Chestnut Ridge Road, Montvale,
NJ 07645, U.S.A.

84 Forever V-Win Corporation
(Exporters Herbal Products)
No.31 Jalan Laksamana 10, Off Sungai Jati
Taman Desa Idaman, Klang 41200,
Malaysia

85 Franklin Trading Co. Inc.
990 Franklin Avenue Garden City NY
11530
USA

86 Frontier Herbs
Box 299
Norway, Iowa 523118, USA
1-800-669-3275

87 Fukunda Ryu Co., Ltd.,
5-11, Nishitemma 1-Chome
Kita-Ku, Osaka 530, Japan

88 Furth, Louis, Inc.
52-15 Flushing avenue
P.O. Box 19 Maspeth, NY 11378
USA

89 G.D. Searle
5200 Old Orchard Rd.
Skokie, IL 60077, U.S.A.

90 Gaban Spice Co. Ltd.
Ginza Maruki Bldg., 8F2-4 Kanda-Jinbo-
CHO,
Chiyoda-KU Tokyo
Japan

91 Gaur Cosmetics
455 Sentinel Unit
Unit 602, Toronto M3J 1V5
Canada

92 Gel Spice co., Inc.
48 Hook Road Bayonne NJ 07002
USA

93 Gelda Scien. & Ind. Dev. Inc.
5466 Gorvan Drive,
Mississauga, Ontario L4w 3E8
Canada

94 General Medicine Sup Ctr, Ltd.
P.O. Box 792, TaipeiCity, Taiwan

95 General Spice, Inc.
238 St. Nichols Avenue,
South Plain Field NJ 07080
USA

96 Gerald McDonald & Co.
1st Andrews Hill London EC4V 5HA
England
UK

97 Giant Medical Corporation
P.O. Box 101-53, Taipei City,
Taiwan

98 Gilroy Foods Inc.
P.O. Box 1088 GIL Roy, CA 95021
USA

99 Glaxo Australia Pty. Ltd.
Mountain Highway,
P.O. Box 168, Boronia 3155, Victroria
Australia

100 Golombeck, Morris J. Inc.
960 Franklin Ave., Brooklyn
NY 11225, U.S.A.

101 Golombeck, Morris J. Inc.
960 Franklin Avenue Brokklyn, NY 11225
USA

102 Great Eurasia Corp
9F, 101, Fu Hsin N Rd,
Chungshan Dist
Taipei City, Taiwan

103 Great Wealth Intern'l Corp
P.O. Box 55-134,
Taipei City, Taiwan

104 Griffith Laboratories USA
1 Griffith Center Alsip, IL 60658
USA

105 Gulf Delta Corp.
P.O. Box 252, Safat 13003, Kuwait

106 H.J. Langdon & Co. Pty. Ltd.
351-336 King Street,
Melbourne VIC 3000,
Australia

107 Hall G.S. & Co. Ltd.
P.O. Box 536/563,
Auckland
New Zealand

108 Harris Freeman & Co.
1380 N. Mccan Street Anaheim, CA 92806
USA

109 Hax Ltd.
306 Archway Road, London N6 5AU
UK

110 Heaven Scent Herbs
Rose Cottage
Heathfield Langford Budville
Somerset TA21 ORP
UK

111 Heller Seasonings & Ingredients, Inc.
P.O. Box 128, Bedford Park II 60499
USA

112 Herbarium Inc., 11016 152nd Ave.
Kenosha, WI 53142, U.S.A.

113 Herbimex
GPO Box 1514, Brisbane QLD 4001,
Australia

114 Herbs Products Company
John W.Du Vall. Jr.
PO Box 898, 11010 Magnolia Bouleward
N.Hollywood, CA 91603-0895, USA

115 Herbs, Minerals & Goods
Don Harouff
21215 Bennington Road
elkhorn, NE 68022, New England

116 Hereford Herbs Ltd.
Ocle Pychard Hereford HRI 3RB England
UK

117 Heron Product (M) Sdn. Bhd.
10-A JL. Jejaka 7, T.Mal Cheras
55100 Kuala Lumpur, Malaysia

118 Hiang Kie (Pvt.) Ltd.
52 Genting Lane #04-05 Hiang Kie
Complex 1, Singapore 1334

119 Hiap Ho Trading Co., Ltd.
2, Al 17, Ln 46, Ti Hua St, Sec 1
Yenping Dist, Taipei City, Taiwan

120 Hiltfields Ltd.
OAK House, Leigh Road, Worsley,
Manchester M28 4LS Engloand
UK

121 Hindustan Importers
48 Dingley Ave,
Dandenong Vic 3175
Australia

122 Hino Pharmaceutical Co., Ltd.,
3-15, Doshomachi 2-Chome
Chuo-Ku, Osaka 541, Japan

123 Hip Shing Tai Co., (Japan) Ltd.
P.O. Box 620, Kobe Port
Kobe 650, Japan

124 Hoel Kogyo Co. Ltd.
Kyugetsu-Kanda Bldg.,
8F 2-4 Kanda-Jinbo-CHO, Hiyoda-KU,
Tokyo
Japan

125 Homviora Arznei Hagdeorn Gmbh
Arabellastrasse 5, D-8000
Munchen 81, Germany

126 Hsiangou Trading Co., Ltd.
P.O. Box 634, Taipei City,
Taiwan

127 Hyades Trading Co., Ltd.
4F-1, 142, Cheng An E Rd, Sec 2
Chungshan Dist, Taipei City, Taiwan

128 Hybritech Europe S.A.
12, All. Des Noiseties, S.A.
B-4900 Angleur, Belgium

129 I Chang Trading Co., Ltd.
66, Ho Chuan St, Kushan Dist,
Kaohsiung City, Taiwan

130 Ibrahim A Al Ajlan Est.
P.O. Box 1356 Riyadh
Saudi Arabia

131 ICC Trading (Taiwan) Ltd
P.O. Box 1369, Taipei City,
Taiwan

132 Ichimaru Co., Ltd. J Bldg., 3-7
Fushimimachi, 2-Chome,
Chuo-Ku, Osaka 541, Japan

133 Iden Croft Herbs Ltd.
Frittenden Road Staplehurst Kent TN12
ODN
UK

134 Ikeda Corporation
Shin Tokyo Bldg. 3-1, Marunouchi 3-
Chome
Chiyoda-KU, Tokyo-100
Japan

135 Indian Emporium.
178B Brunswick Street,
Fitzroy Vix 3065
Australia

136 Industries La Locomotora S.L.
C/Locom., 5 Cabezo De Torres
E-30110 Murcia, Spain

137 International Brokers Inc.,
185, Ridgedale Avenue Cedar knolls, NJ
07927
USA

138 Introplant Tropenpflanzen
Trottstrasse 16, D-3500
Kassel, Germany

139 Istituto Gentili SPA
Via Mazzini, 112
I-56100 Pisa, Italy

140 J.H. Rayner (Mincinglane) Ltd.
Berisford Wing, 1 Prescott Street, London,
E1 8AY UK

141 Jaya International Inc.
34 United Squire,
Scarborough, Ontario M1B 2C2
Canada

142 Jeffreys Miller & Co.Ltd.
Leyland Mill Lane, W Wigan, Lancs WN1
2SB
UK

143 Jin Jin Enterprise Co., Ltd.
P.O. Box 3717, Taipei City,
Taiwan

144 John chambers
15 Westleigh Road
Barton Seagrave
Kettering
Northamptonshire NN15 5AJ
UK

145 John F Seyfried & sons Ltd.
Mickelton, Chipping Campden,
Glocs, GI55 6SS England
UK

146 K.H.L. Flavours, Inc.
59-25 63RD Street Maspeth NY 11378
USA

147 K.Kobayashi & Co. Ltd.
Boeki Building, 4F-123 Higashimachi,
Chou-KU Kobe 651-01
Japan

148 Kaisers Pharm & Medical Corp.
P.O. Box 3717
Taipei City Taiwan

149 Kalsec, Inc. 3711 West main
P.O. Box 511 Kalamazoo, MI 49005
USA

150 Kanegrade Ltd.
9 Bowman Estate, Bessember Drive,
Stevenage, Herts, SGI 2DI, England
UK

151 Kaneka Sunspice Co. Ltd.
Yasuda Seimei-Jso Bldg. 1 10-19,
Jusu-Higashi Yodogawa-Ku, Osaka 532
Japan

152 Kemila – Preparat AB, Box 609
S – 191 26 Solentuna,
Sweden

153 Kharrit Research Centre Press
951 North Main Street
Apartment 56, Sumter 229150
USA

154 Kimoha Enterprises
P.O. Box 16828 Dubai
U.A.E.

155 Kirby Commodity Packers & Suppliers
Park Lane, Abram,
Wigan, WN2 5XJ, England
UK

156 Koshiro Co., Ltd.
5-8, Doshomachi 2-Chome
Chuo-Ku, Osaka 541, Japan

157 Koyaku Company Ltd.
13-1, Shimosone Shinmachi
Kokuram-Ku, Kitakyushu 800-02
Japan

158 Kroger Company, The
Pontiac Foods Division
P.O. Box 25469 Columbia, SC 29224-5469
USA

159 Kushal Trading Co.
P.O. Box 208 Dubai
U.A.E.

160 L. Noel & Sons Ltd.
Stanhill Lane, Oswaldstwistle,
Accrington, Lancs BB5 4PR, England
UK

161 La Champion & Co.
P.O. Box 950
Iselin, New Jersey 08830
USA

162 Laboratorio de applications
Calle Lope de ruedo 46
E – 30220 Madrid Spain

163 Laboratorio Vitafarma Ltd.
P.O. Box 51130, Santiago, Chile

164 Lal's Trading Co. Ltd.
P.O. Box 11096 Dubai
U.A.E.

165 Lawry's Foods, Inc.
570 West Avenue 26 Los Angeles, CA
90065
USA

166 Lee Mckeand & son
80-88, Greville Street,
Prahran Vic 3181
Australia

167 Legg, A,C., Packing Co., Inc.
2319 First Avenue North
P.O. Box 10283 Birmingham AL 35202
USA

168 Leo's Imports
98 Payten Ave,
Punchbowl NSW 2196
Australia

169 Lian Huat & Co. PTE Ltd.
163, Tras Street #11-02/04 Lian Huat
Building
Singapore 0207

170 Liberty Foodstuff Trading Est.
P.O. Box 16746 Dubai
U.A.E.

171 Lion Corporation
3-7, Honjo 1-Chome
Sumida-KU, Tokyo-130
Japan

172 Lion Foods
Faraday Road, Astmoor Industrial Estate,
Runcorn.
Cheshire WA7 1PE, England
UK

173 Litster K.I. Ltd.
251, Bartley Drive Toronto,
Qntario M4A 2N7
Canada

174 Little Herbs
11 Sadlers Way Hertford Hertfordshire
SG14 2DZ
UK

175 Lombard World Trade, Inc.
Third Street Newyork NY 10038
USA

176 Lucas Ingredients Ltd.
Moravian Road, Kingswood,
Bristol, BS 15 2NG, England
UK

177 Lucid Import & Medical Corp
283, Ming Shen W Rd
Yenping Dist. Taipei City,
Taiwan

178 Lucky Traders
P.O. Box 2160 Dubai
U.A.E.

179 M.Duche & Sons (UK) Ltd.
Berisford Wing, 1 Prescot Street,
London B1 8AZ
UK

180 M.O. Azizkhan Trading Est.
P.O. Box 37 Jeddah 21411
Saudi Arabia

181 Mac Andrews & Forbes Co.
Third Street Jefferson Avenue Cameden, NJ 08104
USA

182 Macleod Ross & Co. Ltd.
Broadwall House, 21 Broadwall,
London SE1 9PL
UK

183 Maganlal Nagindas & Co. Ltd.
RM 528, Edomachi Bldg.,
98, Edomachi, Chuo-Ku, Koba 651
Japan

184 Mail Order Herb Shop
5615 Memorial Drive
Stone MTN 30083 USA

185 Malagasy Agencies Inc.
20 Potash Road Oakland, NJ 07436
USA

186 Manage Develop. Fukunaga Co. Ltd
457-8, Tonohara
Chikushino City, 818 Japan

187 Mandalia (U.K.) Ltd.
287/289 Burntoak Broadway, Edgware,
Middlesex, HA8 SED England
UK

188 Manheimer, Inc.
47-22 Pearson Place Long Island City NY 11101-4481
USA

189 Mantab Inc.
115 Hymus Boulevard Ponte Claire
Montreal, Qubec H9R 1E5
Canada

190 Marmorek, Herbert & son
P.O. Box 140036
Brooklyn NY 11214-0005
USA

191 Martin, W.M.E., & Sons Co., Inc.
Suite 215, Colonial Off. Bldg.
P.O. Box 408, 14,
Vander Venter Ave Port Wasthington, NY 11050
USA

192 Master Foods of Australia Pty. Ltd.
26-49 Smith Street,
Matraville, N.S.W. Sydney, 2036
Australia

193 May Trading Est.
P.O. Box 2495 Dammam 31451
Saudi Arabia

194 Mayway Corporation
1338 Cypress St., Mandela Pkwy.
Oakland, CA 94607, U.S.A.

195 MC Clancy Seasoning Co.,
One Spice Road Ft. Mill, SC 29715
USA

196 MC Clement Sales Co. Inc,
1 S. 280 Summit Avenue
Oakbrook Terrace IL, 60181
USA

197 Mc. Cormick Foods
Dormer Road, Thame Park Industrial Estate,
Thame, Oxon, OX9 3SL, England
UK

198 MCC Foods Ltd.
Worcester Road, Evesham,
Worcs WR11 4QU England
UK

199 McCormic Lion Co. Ltd.
1-3-7, Honjo, Sumida-Ku Tokyo 130
Japan

200 Medexport, Import Dept.
31, Korp., 2, Ul Kakhovka
Moscow 113461
Russia

201 Meer Corporation
9500 RailRoad Avenue
P.O. Box 9006 North Bergen, NJ 07047
USA

202 Mehndi Me
15436 SW Foster Lane
No. 296 Beaverton 97007
USA

203 Mercantum (US) Corp.
225 Broadway New York, NY 10007
USA

204 Michans Y Roy Ltd.
Hauser Chemical Research Inc.,
4750 Nautilus Court S.
Boulder, Co 80301, U.S.A.

205 Mikuni & Co. Ltd.
4-10, Doshomachi 2-Chome,
Chuoku, Osaka 541
Japan

206 Mil Waukee Seasoning Inc.
N113 W 18900 Carnegie Dr.,
P.O. Box 339,Germantown WI 53022
USA

207 Milldspice Gmbtt
Camwal Road, Starbeck,
Harrogate HG1 4PY, England
UK

208 Mincing Trading Corp,
528 Ferry Street Newark, NJ 07105
USA

209 Mobarak H Al Dosari
P.O. Box No. 59462
RIYADH – 11532,
Saudi Arabia
F.H. Taussig Inc., 111 Brook St.
Scarsdale, NY 10583, U.S.A.

210 Mohamed and Abdulla Sal Saadi
P.O. Box 59 Dammam 31411
Saudi Arabia

211 Mohammed Thaffen Est for Trading
(Food Supply Division) P.O. Box 4398
Dammam 31491
Saudi Arabia

212 Mohammed Zulfikar Ali
P.O. Box 4402 Abu Dhabi
U.A.E.

213 Mohd. G. Hadban Al Ghambi Est.
P.O. Box 15327 Riyadh 11444
Saudi Arabia

214 Mootah Medical Co.
P.O. Box 17561
Jeddah 21494, Saudi Arabia

215 Morishita Jintan Co., Ltd.
1-30, Tamatsukuri 1-Chome
Chuo-Ku, Osaka 540, Japan

216 Mother Earth Herbs
Kathy Sedler
P.O. Box 1078
Wheatland, California 95692 USA

217 Mr Cormic Stange
Rossmore Road Ellesmere Port,
South Wirral, L65 3DA, England
UK

218 Mr. A.A. Spencer
69 Pine Grove Brookmans Park
GB – Hatfield AL 9 7BL,
England

219 Mueller, Ludwing, Co., Inc.
Two Park, Avenue Newyork NY 10016
USA

220 Multilinks Ltd.
(Mfrs. & Exporter Ayurvedic products)
12 The Broadway
Southall UBI IPS, UK

221 Mumbai Food Stuff Trading LLC
(Deals in Herbal Products)
PO Box No. 29603
Dubai, UAE

222 Musallam Brobaid Trading
P.O. Box 1398 Dubai
U.A.E.

223 N.I. Ibrahim Company (Flavogypt)
8, Falaki Street, Alexandria, Egypt

224 N.V. Sofarex
Van Varenberghstraat 49
B-2600 Berchem

225 Naseem Est. for Trade and Service
P.O. Box 5971 Jeddah 21432
Saudi Arabia

226 Nathalie Lopez
A Touch of Spice Ltd.
21 The Highlands
Bexhill-on-Sea
East Sussex TN39 5HL
UK

227 National Supplies Store
P.O. Box 994 Aub Dhabi
U.A.E.

228 National United Super Markets
P.O. Box 60931 Riyadh 11555
Saudi Arabia

229 Nature's Sunshine Products
95 A Jalan Jejaka Semblian
55100 Kuala Lumpur, Malaysia

230 Natures Herbs Sdn. Bhd.
62, 1/F, Jalan SS 2/66, 47300 Petaling
Jaya, Selangor, Malaysia

231 Natwar and Co.
P.O. Box 2748 Dubai
U.A.E.

232 Neal Street East
5-7 Neal Street
London WC2H 9PU
UK

233 Neal's Yard Apothecary
London WC2
UK

234 Neelkant Trading Co.
P.O. Box 826 Dubai
U.A.E.

235 Net Foods Ltd.
Brookland Farm, Stone Aller-ton Axbridge
Somerest,
BS26 2NU, England
UK

236 New Great Asia Trading Co. Ltd.
P.O. Box 3191, Taipei City,
Taiwan

237 Nihon Kaken Company Ltd.
1-6-6 Yurakucho, Chiyodaku Tokyo 100,
Japan

238 Nihon Sibre Hegner
K.K. Shin-Kokusai Bldg.
7th Floor 4-1 Marunouchi 3-Chome,
Chiyoda-Ku Tokyo 100,
Japan

239 Norfolk Lavender Ltd.
Caley Mill Heacham
King's Lynn
Norfolk PE31 7JE, UK

240 Northern Sales Co. Ltd.
200 Portage Avenue Winnipeg,
Manittoba, Canada R3C 3X2
Canada

241 Olfactory Corporation
P.O. Box 21620, Oxnad,
CA 93034, U.S.A.

242 Om Luik
4 Hols Brook Road IL Ford Essex,
IGI LIF, England
UK

243 Omar K Alesayi and Co. Ltd.
P.O. Box 21592 Jeddah 21492
Saudi Arabia

244 Omer Ben Salem Basaffar
P.O. Box 33 Jeddah
Saudi Arabia

245 Organon Taiwan Ltd.
P.O. Box 39558, Taipei City,
Taiwan

246 Oriental Trading Est.
P.O. Box 17889 Jeddah
Saudi Arabia

247 Ostindo International Pty. Ltd.
10 Abbot Road,
Hallam Vic 3803
Australia

248 Overseas Produce Corpn.
129 Halstead Avenue
P.O. Box 296, Mamaroneck NY 1054
USA

249 Overseas Spice Company
528 Ferry Street Newark NJ 07105
USA

250 Pacific Spice Company Inc.
722 Stanford Avenue
Los Angeles CA 90021
USA

251 Palestine Grocery
P.O. Box 6091 Jeddah 21442
Saudi Arabia

252 Panda United Corp. Ltd.
Riyadh 11471
Saudi Arabia

253 Paramount Trading Corporation
P.O. Box 943 Dubai
U.A.E.

254 PARC Scientifique
Rue Du Bosquet 7
B – 1348 Louvain-La-Neuve,
Belgium

255 Passuto Products
7, Seax Way, Southfields,
Laindon Essex, SS15 66SL, England
UK

256 Paterson Jenks Plc.
Castle House, 71/75, Desborough Road,
Higwycombe, bucks HP11 2HS, England
UK

257 Pelon LLC
163 E, Main Street
Liffle falls 07424-1733
USA

258 Pepper Alley Herbs
The Spice Warehouse
Pepper Alley
Banbury, Oxon, OX16 8JB
UK

259 Petty Wood & Co. Ltd.
15/16, Dufferin Street,
EC1Y 8NU, London
UK

260 Pfannenschmidt
P.O. Box 20224, D-2000
Hamburg 54, Germany

261 Pharma Industries Ltd.
P.O. Box 604, Manila,
Philippines

262 Pharmaton-Korea Co., Ltd.
C.P.O. Box 2533, Seoul,
South Korea

263 Pier 3 Imports
3717 Capps Hill Drive
Charlotte – 28216-2726
USA

264 Pierce A. Arnold & Son Ltd.
12, Park Roadk Hackbridge,
Wallignton, Surry, SM6 7ES England
UK

265 Powell Torma Sales Ltd.
230 Watt Line, Mississauga,
Ontario L4Z IIP4
Canada

266 Premier Distributors Ltd.
5-9 Cleaveland Road,
P.O. Box 4026, Parnell, Auckland
New Zealand

267 Quest int. Canada Inc.
P.O. Box 460, 15 Farmers Avenue,
Vankleek Hill, Ontario KOB 1RO
Canada

268 Quest Intnl Ingredients
1090 Pratt Boulevard Elk Grove Village IL
60007
USA

269 R. Sarant & Co. Ltd.
Priestley Road, Basingstoke,
Hants RG 24 9PU
UK

270 R.M. Jones Foods Ltd.
Threxton Industrial Estate, Threxton Raod
Watton, Norfolk IP25 6BR, England
UK

271 Rashwell Company
P.O. Box 5394 Dubai
Saber Food/ Stuff
P.O. Box 50574 Dubai
U.A.E.

272 Reutter Ltd.
P.O. Box 51130
Santiago, Chile

273 RHM Ingredients Ltd.
OWL Lane, Ossett Wakefield W Yorks,
WF5 9AX England
UK

274 Robert Bryce & Co.
145 Glenlyon Road,
Brunswick Vix, 3056
Australia

275 Rogers Foods/Chili Products
A Divin. Of Universal Foods Corpn. 151,
South Walnut P.O. Drawer R. Turlock CA
95381
USA

276 Rolimpex, P.O. Box 364
PL-00 950 Warszawa, Poland

277 Rosemary Titterington
Iden Crfot Herbs Ltd.
Frittenden Road
Staplehurst
Kdent TN 12 ODH
UK

278 Rucker & Salann Ltd.
7 SEAX Way, Southfields, Laindon,
Essex, SS15 6SL, England
UK

279 S & B Shokuhin Co. Ltd.
18-6 Nihonbashi-Kabutocho,
Chuo-Ku. Tokyo 104
Japan

280 S.L. Borrasosa
C/Locom., 5 Cabezo de Torres
E-30110 Murcia
Spain

281 Saeed Omar Bamousa Est.
P.O. Box 476 Dammam 31411
Saudi Arabia

282 Safeway Stores, Inc.
2643 Prince Street Brookl Yn. Ny. 11201
USA

283 SAG Trading Est.
P.O. Box 3339 Riyadh 11471
Saudi Arabia

284 Said Abdulla Bawazeer Est.
P.O. Box 22033 Riyadh
Saudi Arabia

285 Sakai Spice Mfg. Co. Ltd.
1-29-11, Nakajima Urawa Saitama
Japan

286 Salem A Bin Mahfooz Est.
P.O. Box 755 Jeddah 21421
Saudi Arabia

287 Salem Abdulkader Bajubair Est.
P.O. Box 113 Jeddah 21411
Saudi Arabia

288 Salema Bin Mhfooz Est.
P.O. Box 4288 Riyadh
Saudi Arabia

289 Sanofibio-Induatries Ltd.
Mill REEF House, 9-14 Cheap Street,
Newbury Berks RG14 4DN.
UK

290 Sargold Ltd.
17 Air Street, London WI
UK

291 Saudi Marketing Co. Ltd.
P.O. Box 4605 Dammam 31412
Saudi Arabia

292 Saudi Sachet Services
P.O. Box 15383 Riyadh 11444
Saudi Arabia

293 Saudi Trading Co. Ltd.
P.O. Box 383 Riyadh 11411
Saudi Arabia

294 Sclavo SPA
Via Fiorentina, 1
I-53100 Siena, Italy

295 Scott, E.L., & Company Inc.
One World Trade Center Suite 1313 New York, NY 10048
USA

296 Seishin Trading Co. Ltd.
Sanshine Bldg., 2.1 Sannomiya-cholchome.
Chuo-Ku Kobe 650
Japan

297 Seng Yuang Trading Co., Ltd.
3/F, 14, Lane 185, Nanking W Rd
Yenping Dist., Taipei City, Taiwan

298 Seven Brother trading Inc.
3400 San Fernando Road Los Angeles, CA 90065
USA

299 Shah Trading Company Ltd.
3451 McNicoll Ave. Scarborough,
Ontario Miv 2V3
Canada

300 Sharjah Trading Co.
P.O. Box 2210 Dubai
U.A.E.

301 Shin Ho Shing Company, Ltd.
P.O. Box 1566, Taipei City,
Taiwan

302 Shing Yu Trading Co., Ltd.
4F-1, 42, Chung An E Rd, Sec 2
Chungshan Dist, Taipei City,
Taiwan

303 Shuang Lung Trading Co., Ltd.
2F, 112, Ti Hua St, Sec 1
Yenping Dist, Taipei City,
Taiwan

304 Siber Hegner Ltd.
Mackenzie House, 221-241, Beckenham Road
Kent BR34UF, England
UK

305 Sleryo International NV
Henvelstraat 3-2530
Boechout, Belgium

306 Sokol & Company
5315 Dansher Road Countryside IL 60525
USA

307 Somejant Sa
Rue De Boetendael 147
B-1180 Bruxelles, Belgium

308 Southwick Country Herbs
Southwick Farm
Nomansland Tiverton
Devon EX16 8NW

309 Speciality Seeds, Herbs & Spices
12623 S.W. Green Drive Culver, Or 97734
USA

310 Spice Craft
910 Spruce Craft St. Louis, MO 63102
USA

311 Spicemanns Ltd.
59 Kelvin Avenue, Hillingdon Industrial Estate,
Glasgow G52 4LR England
UK

312 Spices of the Orient Pvt. Ltd.
245 Pandan Loop
Singapore 0512

313 Spices of the Orient
48 Buckingham Drive Wanneroo WA 6163
Australia

314 Spicetec, Ld.
185 Alexandria Way Carol Stream IL 60188
USA

315 Stange Japan K K
3-5-3, Kayaba-CHO, Chuo-KU Tokyo 103
Japan

316 Stewart Foods Pty. Ltd.
47 Neridah Street,
Suite 10, Chats-wood,
Australia

317 Suffolk Herbs
Sawyers Farm
Little Cornard
Sudbury
Suffolk CO10 ONY
UK

318 Sulaiman and Abdul Mohsin
Al Saad al Rossais P.O. Box 44 Riyadh
Saudi Arabia

319 Sun Tsuang Enterprise Co. Ltd.
1F, 29, The Ho Rd
Yungho City, Taipei Shien,
Taiwan

320 Sunrider International
3111 Lomita BL Vd.
Torrance, CA 90505, U.S.A.

321 Swegian Company,
P.O. Box 59269
Taipei City, Taiwan

322 T Choithram and Sons
P.O. Box 5249 Dubai
U.A.E.

323 T.O. Food Co. Ltd. 14-44 Minaminagasaki
2-Chome Toshima-KU, Tokyo 171
Japan

324 Taiwan Excelsior Inc
5F, 141, Jen Ai Rd, Sec 3
Ta-An Dist, Taipei City,
Taiwan

325 Takasago International Corporation
3-19-22 Takanawa Minatoku, Tokyo-108
Japan

326 Takasago Spice Co. Ltd.
tamaru Shoji Co. Ltd.
Taiso-Marine Bldg. Taiso-MarineBldg., 23,
Kaigan-Dori 4-Chome, Naka-Ku, Yokohama
231, Japan

327 Tasmenian Alkaloids Pty. Ltd.
P.O. Box 130,
Westbury Tasmania 7303
Australia

328 Taste Maker. U.S.A.
1 Abercombay Street, Port of Spain,
Trinidad and Tobago

329 The Griffith Laboratories Ltd.
757, Pharmacy Avenue Scarborugh
705 Ontario Mil 3J8
CanadaChief Brand Products Ltd.
Uriah Butler Highway, Charlieville
Chaguanas, Trinidad
West Indies

330 The Herbary
Prickwillow
Wly Cambridgeshire
CB7 4SJ
UK

331 The Lebermuth Co.
P.O. Box 4103, South Bend,
In 46634, U.S.A.

332 The Lion Mark Group
Astmoor, Runcorn,
Cheshire WA7 IPE, England
UK

333 The Rayner Essence Group
4 Bullane London N18 ITQ
UK

334 The Supplement Store
1121 S. Military trail
No. 185 Deer field Beach 33442
USA

335 The Tea Council Ltd.
Sir John Lyon House
5 High Timber Street
London EC4 3NJ
UK

336 The Yuh Trading Co. Ltd.
P.O. Box 68-280, Taipei City, Taiwan

337 Thissen S.A. Laboratories
4-6, Rue De La Papyree
B-1420 Briane L'aleud, Belgium

338 Thulsidas lal Chand and Sons
P.O. Box 430 Dubai
U.A.E.

339 Tochimoto Tenkaido Co. Ltd.
3-21 Subhiro-CHO,
Kita-Ku Osaka 530
Japan

340 Tokyo Kishin Co. Ltd.
13-4 Mishuku, Setagaya-KU
Tokyo 154
Japan

341 Tone Brothers, Inc.
P.O. Box 7004 San Moines IA 503001
USA

342 Tow Star Trading Co., Ltd.
P.O. Box 58052, Taipei City,
Taiwan

343 Toyo Koshin Co. Ltd.
1-12, Mansej-Cho, Minami-Ku Yokahama
232
Japan

344 Trade Links
P.O. Box 72 Dammam 31411
Saudi Arabia

345 Traidcraft Plc.
Kingsway, Teamvalley Trading Estate,
Gateshead, NE11 One, England
UK

346 Transit Trading Corpn.
196-198 West Broadway Newyork, NY
10013
USA

347 Tzu Sheng Company Ltd.
P.O. Box 71, Taipei City, Taiwan

348 UHA Marketing (M) Sdn. Bhd.
8 JL. Mega Mend. 5/M Old Klang
58200 Kuala Lumpur, Malaysia

349 Unbar Rothon Ltd.
Radford way Billericay Essex CM12 OBT
England
UK

350 Union Medical Ent Co., Ltd.
P.O. Box 26-784,Taipei City,
Taiwan

351 United National Commercial Co.
P.O. Box 4428, Ruwi, Oman

352 Universe Food Ltd.
Univese House, 52 Queens Road
Weybridge Surrey KT13 OAN England
UK

353 V. Berg & Sons Ltd.
112, Union Street, London SE1 ONL
UK

354 Van De Vries Tradiing Corpn.
150 Varick Avenue Brooklyn, NY 11237
USA

355 Venus Garden Shop
8644 Concord Street
Tacoma, USA

356 Verhaelen GMBH
Muelheimmer Str. 176, W-4100
Duisburg 1, Germany

357 Villeroy & Boch Tableware Ltd.
203 Regent Street
London W1R 2DE
UK

358 Vioergex,V. Salatas Sons Ltd.
35 Deligiorgi St., GR-104 37
Athens, Greece

359 Voon Ng Tong Trading Co., Bhd
489 Jalan Sungei Rambai
14000 Bukit Mertajam,
Malaysia

360 Wamco
P.O. Box 42946 Riyadh 11551
Saudi Arabia

361 Waters Trading Company
65 Pelham Streem,
Carlton Vic 3053
Australia

362 Weiming Union Trading Co., Ltd.
4F, 11, Lane 125, I Tung St
Chungshan Dist, Taipei City, Taiwan

363 Weng Aun Thye
258 Lebuh Pantai
10300 Penang, Malaysia

364 Whittard of Chelsea Ltd.
73 Northcote Road
London SW11 6PJ
UK

365 Whole Herb Company
P.O. Box 1085
Mill Valley, Ca 94942
USA

366 William Foods, Inc.
13301 W. 99th Street Lenexa, KS 66215
USA

367 Wing Hing Co., Ltd.
8823 E. Cordova St., Vancouver,
B C V6A 1M5, Canada

368 Wixon Industries Inc.
1390 E Bolivar Avenue Mil.,
Waukee, WI 53207
USA

369 Woodhouse, Drake & carey (Trdg), Inc.
127 John Street New York Ny 10038
USA

370 World Commodity Trading, Inc.
90 Cutter Mill Road suttee
333N Great Neck, NY 11021-3003
USA

371 World Spice Inc.
223-225 Highland PKWY Rosselle, NJ
07203
USA

372 Xenia Food Communication
1950 Sawtelle Blvd. #300,
P.O. Box 25919 W. Los Angeles Ca 90025-
9998
USA

373 Yamajirushi Jozo Co. Ltd.
15-1, Komono 3-Chome,
Itabashi-Ku, Tokyo 173
Japan

374 Yamamoto Yakuhin Kogyo Co. Ltd.
7-1, Hihonbashi Hon-Cho 4-Chome,
Chuo-Ku, Tokyo 103
Japan

375 Yasuma Co. Ltd.
5-23-2 Hishigotanda Shi-Nagawaku
Tokyo-141
Japan

376 Yuen Fung Trading Co., Ltd.
P.O. Box 1-52, Kaohsiung City, Taiwan

377 Yukawa Sangyo Co. Ltd.
6-6-14, Togoshi Shinagawa-Ku Tokyo 141
Japan

8 NON GOVERMENT ORGANISATIONS (NGO'S)

1 Agharkar Research Institute
G.C. Agarkar Road,
Pune – 411 004 (Maharashtra)

2 Akhil Bhartiya Vanuoushadi Abhyas Mandal
B-16, Basoya Park Society,
Chandlodia
Ahmedabad – 382 481

3 Aloe Laboratories
RT 1, Box 161
Lyford, Texas 78569
USA

4 Aphrodisia Products Inc.
45 Washington Street
Brooklyn, NY 11201
New York USA

5 Asian Medicinal Plants Trust
Sonamukhi Nagar, Sangaria Phanta
Jodhpur – 342 005 (India)

6 Association for Promotion of Medicinal & Aromatic Crops
B-9, UAS Quarters, Hebbal
Bangalore – 560 024 Karnataka

7 BAIF Development Research Foundation
Dr. Manibhai Desai Nagar Warje,
Pune – 411 039

8 BCR Natural Extracts Processing Co. Inc.
62 N Industry Street
Deer Park
New Yorl 11729, USA

9 Botanicals International Inc.
2550 El. Presidio Street
Long Beach
California 90810 USA

10 British Herb Society
134 Buckingham Palace Road
London SW1W 9SA UK

11 British Herb Trade Association
HFU Building
22 Long Acre, Covent Garden
London WC2E 9LY UK

12 British Herbal Medicine Association
Lane House
Cowling Keighley
West Yorksire BD22 OLX, UK

13 Burlington Bio Medical Corporation
100, Fairchild Avenue
Plain View, NY 11803
New York USA

14 Catholic Health Association of India (CHAI)
157/6, Staff Road, Gunrock Enclave,
Secunderabad – 500 009 (A.P.)

15 Center of Minor Forest Products (COMFORPTS)
HIG-2, No. 8, Indirapuram,
P.O. Majra
Dehradun – 248 171 (UC)

16 Centre for Entrepreneurship Development Madhya Pradesh (CEDMAP)
60, Jail Road, Jahangirabad
Bhopal – 462 008 (India)

17 Charabot & Co. Inc.
83, Cedar Lane
Englewood New Jersey 07631
USA

18 Chart Corporation
519 Broad Street, Glen Roack
New Jersey 07452, USA

19 Chelsea Physic Garden
Friends of the Chelsea Physic Garden
66 Royal Hospital Road
London SW3 4HS
UK

20 Cheshire Herbs
Fourfields
Forest Road
Little Budworth near Tarporley
Cheshire CW6 9ES
UK

21 Chhttisgarh Harbal Sansthan
Ravishankar Stadium, P.O. No. 60,
Durg – 491 001 (UC)

22 Cominso (Canada) Ltd.
351 Place Royale
Montreal, CANADA

23 Dominion Herb Distributors Inc.
1447-51
St. Lawrence Boulevard
Montreal, CANADA

24 Dormar Chemicals Inc.
44 Lewis St. Patterson
New Jersey
7501 New Jersey, USA

25 Dr. Sanwarmal Herbals Academy
Chintamani Apartments
1478, Sadashiv Peth, Tilak Road,
Pune – 411 030 (Maharashtra)

26 E.O. Schaffer Chemicals Co. Ltd.
17 Highland Avenue
P.O. Box 142, West Nayark
New York 10994
New York, USA

27 Farmer Friends Club
D. No. 9/25/15A/1, Janatapet (N)
Kavali – 524 201 Nellore DT
Andhra Pradesh

28 Flai Herb & Co.
831 Almar Avenue
Santa Cruz, California
95060, USA

29 Foundation for Revitalisation of Local
Health Tradition (FRLHT)
50 MSH Layout, 2nd Stage,
3rd Main, 2nd Cross, Anandnagar
Bangalore – 560 024

30 General Council and Register of Consultant
herbalists Ltd.
Marlborough House
Swanpool, Falmouth
Cornwall TR11 4HW
UK

31 Green Mountain Herbs Inc.
PO Box 2369, Boulder Colorado
80302 USA

32 Guild of Herbalists
35-37 Grosvenor Gardens
London SW1W OBY
UK

33 Hambledon Herbs Court Farm
Milverton
Somerset TA4 1NF
UK

34 Henry Doubleday Association
148 Forest Road
Tunbridge Wells
Kent TN2 5EY
UK

35 Herb Society
P.O. Box 415
London SW1P 2HE
UK

36 Hollington Nurseries
Woolton Hill
Newbury
Berkshire RG15 9XT
UK

37 INRA
28 Rue de Herrlisheim bte 384
F-68021 Colmar
France

38 Jagram Jan Vikas Samiti
Bedla Road,
Udaipur – 313 011 (Raj.)

39 Jekka's Herbs Farm
Rose Cottage
Shellards Lane
Alveston
Bristol BS12 2SY
UK

40 John Ronaldson & Co. Ltd.
354 Crooked Lane
Cannon Street, London
United Kingdom

41 Kumarappa Gram Swarajya Sansthan
B-190, University Road,
Bapu Nagar,
Jaipur – 302 015 (Raj)

42 L.A. Champson & Co. Inc.
70 Hudson Street
Hoboken N.J. 07030
New Jersey, USA

43 Longley Boxwood Nursery
National collection – Buxus
Rake near Liss
Hampshire GU33 7JL
UK

44 Lupin Herbal Research Centre
Village – Tapovan, P. O. Shivanand
Nagar, Dist. Tehri Garhwal, Uttaranchal

45 M.S. Swaminathan Research Foundation
3rd Cross Road,
Taramani Institutional Area,
Chennai – 600 113 (TN)

46 Meer Corporation
318 West 46th Street
New York 36
USA

47 Mewar Vanaushadi Vikas Sansthan
Chetana Nagar, P.O. Kamlighat,
Via-Deogarh, Raj Samand,
Rajasthan – 313 331

48 National Institute of Medical Herbalists
41 Hatherley Road
Winchester
Hampshire SO22 6RR
UK

49 Natures Herb Company
345 O' Farrel Street
San Francisco 2
California, USA

50 Neal's Yard Remedies
14-15 Neal's Yard
Covent Garden
London WC2 9DP
UK

51 Neem Foundation
67-A, Vithal Nagar, Road No. 12,
Juhu Scheme,
Mumbai – 400 059

52 Neer Corporation
Milly Valley
CA 94941
USA

53 ORFOLK lavender Caley Mill
Heacham Kings Lynn
Norlfolk PE31 7JE
UK

54 Pan Horti Consultants (P) Ltd.,
172-A, Arumuga Nagar,
Ramanathapuram,
Coimbatore – 641 045 (India)

55 Parker Trading Corporation
P.O. Box No. 190
Staten Island, New York 10314
USA

56 Paul Muggenburg
Wandelenwag 24
D2000 Hmburg 1
Germrny

57 Penick Corporation
1050 Wall Street, W Lyndhurst
New Jersey 07071
USA

58 Rajasthan Agro Forestry Corporation
Sonamukhi Nagar, Salawas Road,
Sangaria Phanta,
Jodhpur – 342 005 (Raj)

59 Rober Meyskens
B 7380 Quievrian Belgique
Belgium, Europe

60 S.B. Penick & Co.
50 Church Street
New York, USA

61 Santal Pargana Vikas and Seva Sansthan
Karnibag Road,
B. Deoghar – 814 112 (Bihar)

62 School of Herbal Medicine Physiotherapy
Bucksteep Manor
Bodle St. Green
Hailsham
East Sussex BN27 4RJ
UK

63 Society for Research & Initiatives for
Sustainable Technologies & Institutions
(SRISTI)
C/o Prof. Anil K. Gupta,
Indian Institute of Management,
Vastrapur
Ahmedabad – 380 015

64 Tata Energy Research Institute (TERI)
Seth Darbari Block,
India Habital Centre
Lodi Estate,
New Delhi – 110 003

65 The British Herb Trade Association
Agriculture House
Knightsbridge
London SWIX 7NJ
UK

66 The British Herbal Medicine Association
Lan House Cowling
Keighley
West Yorkshire DB22 01K
UK

67 The Soil Association
86 Colston Street
Bristol BS1 5BB
UK

68 The Tradescant Trust
Friends of the Museum of Garden History
Lambeth Palace Road
London SE1 7LB
UK

69 Triarco Inc.
200 Market Street
Elmwood Park
New Jersey 07407
USA

70 UK Herbal Infusions Association
Central House
High Street
London E15 2PS
UK

71 UTTHAN
102, 6/3 Beniganj,
Allahabad – 211 002 (UP)

72 Verbond van Coopoeratives
Tuinbouwveijlingen
Tiensevest 136
3000 Leuven
BELGIUM
UK

73 Volanteer Health Association of India
Tong Swasthya Bhawan,
15, Tara Present,
Qutub Institutional Area,
New Delhi

74 Wilcox Drug Co. Inc.
P.O. Box 391, Boone
North Carolina 28607
USA

75 Willon Laboratories
P.O. Box No. 85 Green Village, New Jersey
07935 USA

76 World Herb Co. Inc.
459, 18th Avenue
New York 3
USA

77 Zandu Foundation for Health Care
70, Gokhale Road, South Dadar
Mumbai – 400 025 (Maharashtra)

9 GROWERS / SEEDS / PLANTING MATERIAL SUPPIERS

1 Aaradhya Group
1967/1, Right Town
Jabalpur (MP)

2 Aashif Ali (Lat)
Golana, Khambhat, Dist. Anand (Guj)

3 Aayu Trust
303, Harekrisha Complex
Opp. Kothawela Flats,
Ellise Bridge,
Ahmedabad – 380 006

4 Acharya Narendra Dev University
of Agriculture Science & Technology
Narendra Nagar, Kumarganj
Faizabad – 224 229 (UP)

5 Acharya NG Ranga Agricultural Univ.,
Hyderabad – 500 030 (AP)

6 Agarwal Agricultural Farm Res. Centre,
Bed, Kalkhat, Rawatbnata
Chittoregarh (Raj)

7 Agharkar Research Institute
G.C. Agarkar Road
Pune – 411 004 (MS)

8 Akhil Bhartiya Vanousadhi Abhyas Mandal
B-16, Basoya Park Society,
Chandlodia,
Ahmedabad – 382 481 (Gujarat)

9 Akhil Maheshwari
Chandra Shekhar Azad Road
Post Jhora, District Mureina (MP)

10 Andhra Pradesh Forest Department
R & D Circle, Aranya Bhawan,
Saifabad
Hyderabad – 500 004 (AP)

11 Anil Kumar
C/o Durg Sales
109-110, Lower Ground,
Dawa Bazar, RNT Marg,
Indore – 1 (MP)

12 Anrori Agro Herbo Medica (I) P. Ltd.,
Post Box 30,
Nainital – 263 001 (UC)

13 Anthyodhaya Sangh MPCP
P.B. No. 216,
7-A Mission Hospital Road, Woraiyur
Tiruchirapalli – 620 003 (TN)

14 Arvind Kumar Pandey,
Near Sarswati Vidhya Mandir
Birsa – Dahar Road,
Rourkela – 12 (Orissa)

15 Asha Trading Company
P.O. New Forest
Dehra Dun (UC)

16 Ashok Jain
A-8, Navlakha Complex,
Snehnagar, Main Road
Indore – 452 001 (MP)

17 Assam Agricultural University
Jorhat – 785 013 (Assam)

18 Assam Ayurvedic Products (AAP)
Mandakota Manikpur
Dist Kamrup (Assam)

19 Auroville Action Group
Shakti, Auroville
District Viluppuram
pondicherry – 655 101

20 Ayurveda Rasashala
25, Karve Road
Pune – 411 004 (MS)

21 B. K. Chawla
Chawla Nursing Home
Hanumangarh – 335 512 (Raj)

22 BAIF Development Research Foundation
Dr. Manibhai Desai Nagar
National Highway No. 4, Warje
pune – 411 029 (MS)

23 Bajrang Semra
Village – Moibharu
The. Buhana,
Dist. Jhunjhunun (Raj)

24 Balaji Herbal Farms
Ghodadongri
District Baitul – 460 443 (MP)

25 Balram Eangla
Nayan Stores, Sanawad
District Khargon (MP)

26 Balvinder Singh Sandhu
H. No. B-12, 165/15,
New Harjinder Nagar
Faridkot –151 203 (PB)

27 Belgaum Integrated Rural Development Society
BIRDS MPCP, Naganur, Gokak
District Belgaum, Karnataka

28 BGPIHEAD, North East Unit
Vivek Vihar, Itanagar – 791 113 (AP)

29 Bhanwar Lal Pareek
43, Dwarika, Tal Katora, Jaipur (Raj)

30 Bharat Bhushan Chaturvedi
D-86, Koushal Kishore Marg,
Ambawadi
Jaipur (Raj)

31 Bhuralal Narayan Sirsaliya
Dungergaon,
The. : Manawar
Dist Dhar (MP)

32 Bhushan Nandia
7, Dr. Ambedkar Commercial Complex,
G. E. Road,
Durg – 491 001 (CG)

33 Botanical Survey of India (BSI)
Botanic Garden, Sibpur
Howrah – 711 103 (WB)

34 C.M. Kethkar
Neem Mission, 471 Saniwar Peth
Pune – 411 030 (MS)

35 Kolkatta University
Botany Deparment, 35 Bellyganj
Circular Road,
Kolkatta – 700 019 (WB)

36 Capital Project Administration
(Forest Division)
CPA Building, Bittan Market,
E-5 Arera colony,
Bhopal – 462 016 (MP)

37 Catholic Health Associaiton of India (CHAI)
157/5 Staff Road, Post Bag No. 2126
Gunrock Enclave
Secunderabad – 500 009 (AP)

38 CCS Haryana Agricultural University
Plant Breeding Department
Hissar – 125 004 (Haryana)

39 Central Arid Zone Research Institute
Division of Natural Resources and Env.,
Light Industrial Area,
Jodhpur – 342 003 (Raj)

40 Central Institue of Medicinal and Aromatic Plants (CIMAP)
Kukrail Picnic Spot, P.O. CIMAP
Lucknow – 226 015 (UP)

41 Centre for Social Service and Research
Hanumantharayan Kottai,
Dindigul – 624 054
District Dindigulanna, (TN)

42 Charak Herbal and Plantations Service
29, 1st Floor, A.B. Complex
Near Shri Krishna Theatre
Jabalpur – 482 002 (MP)

43 Chouhan Brothers
H. No. 812, Janta Dairy,
Hathital
Jabalpur (MP)

44 CIMAP Field Station
Allasandra (Near Yelahanka)
GKVK Post
Bangalore – 560 065 (Karnataka)

45 CIMAP Field Station
Boduppal, Uppal Road Post
Hyderabad – 500 039 (AP)

46 CIMAP Field Station
P.O. Nagla Dairy Farm
District Udham Singh Nagar – 263 149 (UP

47 College of Agriculture
Department of Horticulture
Rajendra Nagar
Hyderabad – 500 030 (AP)

48 College of Agriculture
Department of Plantation Crops and Spice
Post Vellayani,
Thiruvananthapuram – 695 522 (Kerala)

49 College of Agriculture
Horticulture Department
Shivaji Nagar
Pune – 411 005 (MS)

50 D. R. Prasad
403, Prremasai,
Srinagar Colony,
Hyderabad – 500 073 (AP)

51 D. S. Manesar Farm
1-62, Sector-9,
Noida – 201 301 (UP)

52 Dabur Research Foundation
22, Site-IV,
Sahibabad – 201 010 (UP)

53 Danaram Choudhary
C/o Anraj Krishi Farm, Manai
Jodhpur (Rajasthan)

54 Darshan Shankar Academy of Development Sciences
Kashale, Karzat,
Raigarh – 410 201 (MP)

55 Deputy Conservator of Forest & CEO
Chetak Circle,
(Arawali Green Project)
Udaipur (Raj)

56 Dera Sacha Souda Ashram
Sankhala Phanta
Kolayat (Bikaner)

57 Dera Sacha Souda, Ashram
Sirsa (Haryana)

58 Desert Medicine Research Centre (DMRC)
Post Box 122, New Pali Road
Jodhpur – 342 005 (Raj)

59 Devratan Rathi
E-7/152, Lala Lajpat Rai Society, Arera Colony
Bhopal – 462 004 (MP)

60 Dhanna Singh
V. P. Kukarkheda
Via – Bhim (Rajsamad) Raj

61 Dhanna Singh
Village Post – Kukar Khera,
Via – Bhim, Rajsamand, (Raj)

62 Diamond Herbal Farm
7/2 Civil Centre, Madhatal
Jabalpur (MP)

63 Directorate of Cinchona and Other Medicinal Plants,
10/1A, Indian Mirror Street,
Kolkatta – 700 013 (WB)

64 Directorate of Forest
Silvicultre Division, Lower Lachumere,
Shillong – 793 001 (Meghalaya)

65 Directorate of Horticulture
PWD Shed No. 5, Jawahar Chowk
Bhopal – 462 003 (MP)

66 Divisional Forest Officer
Banswara (Rajasthan)

67 Divisional Forest Officer
Hisar (Haryana)

68 Dr. A. A. Farooqi
B-17, UAS Staff Quarters
Habble
Bangalore – 560 065

69 Dr. N. Radhakrishna Murthy
21/6, Velayutham Colony,
Saligramam
Chennai – 600 093

70 Dr. Sanwarmal Herbals Academy
Chintamani Apartments,
1478 Sadashiv Peth,
Tilak Road
Pune – 411 030 (MS)

71 Dr. Y.S. Parmar University of Horticulture & Forestry
Forest Products Utilisation Department
Nauni
Solan – 173 230 (HP)

72 ENBEE Plantations Ltd.
236, Zone II, MP Nagar
Bhopal – 462 011 (MP)

73 Forest Department of Sikkim Government
Non Timber Forest Produce Division
Forest Annexe, Deorali
Gangtok – 737 101

74 Forest Research Institute
Silviculture Division & Non Wood Forest Products, Division, P.O. New Forest
Dehra Dun – 248 006 (UP)

75 Fragrance and Flavours Dev. Centre
Industrial Area, Makrand Nagar
Kannouj – 209 726 Farrukhabad (UP)

76 G.B. Pant Institute of Himalayan
Environment and Development
(GBPIHNEAD)
Kosi-Katarmal – 263 643 District Almora
UC

77 G.B. Pant University of Agriculture and
Technology, Hill Campus,
Rainchauri – 249 199 (UC)

78 G.D. Mittal
Mittal Musli Farm
Jalgaon Jamod
Dist – Buldhana (MS)

79 Gajraj Singh
Vill – Isepur
P.O. Bilaspur Dist.
Goutam Budhnagar – 203 202 (UP)

80 Gandharv Ayurved Research Institue
4th Mile, Mandla Road, Bilhari
Jabalpur – 482 020 (MP)

81 GBPIHEAD, Garhwal Unit
Post Box 92, Upper Bhaktiyana
Srinagar Garhwal – 246 174 (UC)

82 GBPIHEAD, Himachal Unit
Mohal, Kullu – 175 126 (HP)

83 GBPIHEAD, Sikkim Unit
Tadong, District East Sikkim
Gangtok – 737 102 (Sikkim)

84 Ghanshyam Meena,
Village – Titam Salouna,
Via-Gangapur City,
Dist. – Sawai Madhopur (Raj)

85 Gireesh Sharma
Kamlesh Niketan, Pipli Bazar,
Badi Gali,
Khilchipur – 465 679 (MP)

86 Global Extract Plus
Shakti Niwas, Dharmgarh
Kalahandi – 766 015 (Orissa)

87 Gopal Dass
3/61, Old Rajendra Nagar
New Delhi

88 Gopesh Taparia
Bhallabh Nagar, Ring Road Number 1,
Taparia Compound
Raipur (MP)

89 Gram Bharti
Village Anrori, P.O. Bel
Patwadangar – 263 128
Nainital (UC)

90 Green Future
2nd Floor, 144, Zone-1
M.P. Nagar,
Bhopal (MP)

91 Green Gold Enterprises
Sawarker Colony,
Shivpuri – 473 551 (MP)

92 Gujarat Agricultural University
Sardar Krishi Nagar
District Banaskantha – 385 506 (Guj)

93 Gujrat Agriculture University
Anand – 388 001 (Guj)

94 Harjap Singh Saini
6-C-29, South Extension
Pawanpuri
Bikaner (Raj)

95 Hemaram Okhaji Choudhary
Near Police Chowki, Ranawas
(Via Marwar Jn), Pali, Rajasthan

96 Herbal Garden and Herbarium
Department of ISM&H
Joginder Nagar – 176 120
District Mandi (HP)

97 Hetram Godara
Dhani Sukhera Khede,
P. O. Aboobshahar
Dist Sirsa (Haryana)

98 High Altitude Plant Physiology Research
Centre,
Post Box 14, HNB Garhwal University
Srinagar Garhwal – 246 174 (UC)

99 Himalayan Consortium For Himalaya
Conservation (HIMCON)
Post Box 5,
Ranichauri – 249 199
District Tehri Garhwal (UC)

100 Horti Nursery Networks
30, 2nd Floor, Raji Medical Building, 1128,
EVN Road,
Opp. Govt. H.Q. Hospital
Erode – 638 009 (TN)

101 Horticulture and Food Processing
Department
2 Sapru Marg, Udhyan Bhawan
Lucknow – 226 001 (UP)

102 Human Resource Development and
Research Institute (HRDRI)
Tampha Bazar,
Canchipur (Kyamgei) – 795 003
Imphal (Manipur)

103 Indian Institue of Horticultural Research
255, Upper Palace Orchards
Bangalore – 560 080 Karnataka

104 Indian Institute of Ayurveda for Drug
Research
Tarikhet – 263 663 Ranikhet UC

105 Institute of Public Enterprise (IPE)
Biotechnology Unit
Osamania University Campus
Hyderabad – 500 007 (AP)

106 Institute of Wood Science & Technology
18th Cross Road, Malleswaram
Bangalore – 560 003 (Karnataka)

107 J.S. Industries
Industrial Area, Pratappura Orcha
District Tikamgarh, MP

108 Jagaran Jan Vikas Samiti
Bedla Road
Udaipur – 313 001 (Raj)

109 Jai Narayana Vyas University
Botany Department
Jodhpur – 342 001 (Raj)

110 Jamia Millia Islamia
Dept. of Bioscience (Plant Physiology and
Biochemistry Laboratory),
Jamia Nagar, Okhla
New Delhi – 110 025

111 Jari Booti Sodh Sansthan Kendra
Gopeshwar – 246 401
District Chamoli Garhwal (UC)

112 Jasvinder Pal Singh
577, Gali No. 7, Udaimarg
Raja park,
Jaipur (Raj)

113 Jawaharlal Nehru Ayurvedic Medicinal
Plants Garden and Herbarium
Kothrud,
Pune – 411 029 (Maharashtra)

114 Jawaharlal Nehru Krishi Viswa Vidyalaya
Agricultural Research Station
Mandsaur – 458 001 (MP)

115 Jawaharlal Nehru Krishi Viswa Vidyalaya
Department of Agricultural Botany and
CropPhysiology, Krishi Nagar, Adhartal
Jabalpur – 482 004 (MP)

116 Jaykishan Agarwal
Shivnanda Rice Mills (P) Ltd.,
P.O. Dharamgarh
Dist. Kalahandi – 766 015 (Orissa)

117 Jeevan Herbs
178, Keshavganj
Sagar – 470 002 (MP)

118 Jeevaniya Society
E-III/249, Sector H, Aliganj
Lucknow – 226 024 (UP)

119 Jelmi Herbal Agro Farm
12, Hyotirmaya Complex
Near Hotel Atithi, Jalna Road
Aurangabad – 431 003 (MS)

120 Jonson Enterprises Pvt. Ltd.,
34, New Thanderbalsia Street,
Post Box 905
Washerman Street
Chennai – 21 (TN)

121 K. A. Prasad
52-1/8-5B, NTR Colony,
Gunadala
Vijaiwada – 520 008 (AP)

122 K. Chokal Eangam
25, Parthsarathi, Naykar Street
Tuticorin – 628 001 (TN)

123 K. K. Yadav
N-12, Lowyers Colony
By-pass Road
Agra (UP)

124 Kalyani Samudayik Vikas Kendra
Kawcha, Kathiwada
Dist Jhabua (MP)

125 Kansal Agrotech Pvt. Ltd.,
Kansal Bhawan, Duptyganj
Bulandsahar (UP)

126 Karan Singh
Narayan Bagh, Dabla, Jaisalmer (Raj)

127 Karnataka Forest Department
Aranya Bhawan
Bangalore – 560 003 Karnataka

128 Kedia Nursery
83, Chilbilla, Pratapgarh
Uttar Pradesh

129 Kerala Agricultural University
Aromatic and Medicinal Plants Research Station, P.O. Asamanoor,
District Ernakulam
Odakkali – 683 549 (Kerala)

130 Kerala Agricultural University
Horticltural Research Station,
P.O. Ambalavayal
Wynad – 673 593 (Kerala)

131 Kerala Agricultural University
Vellanikkara, Trichur Kerala

132 Keshra Ram Bishnoi
Vilalge Post Dholia
Via-Lathi,
Jaisalmer

133 Kiran Aroma & Herbs
44, Venkteswar Colony,
Sodala
Jaipur – 19 (Raj)

134 Kisan Sewa Kendra
150-151, Main Market
Padampur – 335 041
Sri Ganganagar (Raj)

135 Krishan Kumar Bhartiya
HIG-3, Indira Nagar
Banga (UP)

136 Krishi Vigyan Kendra
Abusar
Jhunjhunu (Raj)

137 Kriti Agrocom Ltd.
Post Pipriakalan, Via Barahi
District Jabalpur – 483 770 (MP)

138 Kuparam Gurjar
Dadawat, Asind, Bhilwara (Raj)

139 Lalit Narain
C/o Khem Vastralaya,
P. O. Sasamusa
Dist Gopalganj (Bihar)

140 Laxman Singh Panwar
Joshiyana Mohalla, Ghas Mandi
Kila Gate
Gwalior (MP)

141 Laxmi Narain Prajapati
Village & Post Ramsara, Churu (Raj)

142 Laxmikant Sharma
Subhash Nagar
Nenwa Road
Bundi (Raj)

143 Lokendra Singh
110, Vallabh Bari, Gumanpura
Kota – 324 007 (Raj)

144 Loonchand Sinawaria
51F, Narsingh Colony, Ratanada
Jodhpur – 342 001 (Raj)

145 M. Y. Khan
191, Khirjabad Colony,
Dargan Main Road
Khajrana
Indore (MP)

146 M.S. Swaminathan Research Foundation
Community Gene Bank
3rd Cross Road, Taramani Institutional Area
Chennai – 600 113 (TN)

147 Maa Danteshwari Herbal Farm,
DNK Colony, Konda Gaon,
Bastar (CG)

148 Madan Lal Ranzi
Warden, Ward No. 66, Nawibagh
Bairsia Road,
Bhopal (MP)

149 Maharishi Ayurveda Products
Plot 17-18, Noida Export Processing Zone
Noida – 201 305 (UP)

150 Mahatma Phule Krishi Vidhyapeeth
Botany Deparment
Rahuri, District Ahmednagar – 413 733(MS

151 Mahaveer Choudhary
Ward No. 16, Near 132
GSS Power Station
Anoopgarh, Sriganganagar (Raj)

152 Mahaveer Zari Booti Ayurveda Bhawan
Rajeswari Road
Shivpuri – 473 551 (MP)

153 Major Avtar Singh
Farm Chandan
Jaisalmer (Raj)

154 Man Agrotech
Jay Vijai Sadar Society,
Opp. Jyoti Hospital
Visnagar – 384 315 (Gujarat)

155 Manohar Chaudhary
Chaudhar Mohalla, Ashok Nagar
District Guna (MP)

156 Medplan Conservatory Society (MCS)
No. 8, Ist Floor IV Main, II Stage
MSH Colony, Anandnagar
Bangalore – 560 024 (Karnataka)

157 Mewar Vanoushadhi Vikas Sansthan
Kamlighat (Rajmamad) Raj

158 Mittal Musli Farm and Research Centre
Post Jalgaon Jamod
District Buldana – 443 402 (MS)

159 Modi Medicinal Plants and Aromatic Oil Distilleries
Modi Bhawan, Katra Bazar
Panna – 488 001 (MP)

160 Moolchand Golecha
P.O. Khichan,
Phalodi (Raj)

161 MP Council of Science and Technology
26, Kisan Bhawan, Jail Road,
Arera Hills
Bhopal – 462 004 (MP)

162 MP Rajya Van Vikas Nigam
5th Floor, Panchanan Building
Malviya Nagar, Bhopal – 462 003 (MP)

163 Mukesh Chandra Harit
132, Sanjaynagar B Kalwad Road,
Jontwada
Jaipur (Raj)

164 Mukesh Chaurasia
Neelhanth Lodge, Kothi Bazar
Baitul (MP)

165 Mukesh Nathani
555 D/2, Pancholi Chouraha
Ram Nagar,
Ajmer – 305 004 (Raj)

166 Mukesh Seeds
Opposite Old Saifia College
Talkies Road,
Bhopal – 462 001 (MP)

167 N. Kumar Enterprises
84-D, First Floor, Rajguru Market
Hissar – 125 001 (Haryana)

168 Narayan Das Prajapati
Sonamukhi Nagar
Sagaria Phanta, Salawas Road,
Jodhpur – 342 005 (Raj)

169 Narendra Dev University of Agriculture and Technology
Horticulture Department
Narendra Nagar, Kumarganj
Faizabad – 224 229 (UP)

170 Narmada Velly Greenland Pvt. Ltd.,
1, Narmada Club, Cantt.
Jabalpur – 482 008 (MP)

171 National Botanical Research institute
Rana Pratap Marg
Lucknow – 226 001 (UP)

172 National Bureau of Plant Genetic Resources (NBPGR)
National Gene Bank,
Indian Agricultural Research Institute Campus, Pusa
New Delhi – 110 012

173 National Chemical Laboratory (NCL)
Dr. Homi Bhabha Road
Pune – 411 008 (MS)

174 National Institute of Homoeopathy
Block GE, Sector 3, Salt Lake City
Kolkatta – 700 091 (WB)

175 National Institute of Pharmaceutical Education and Research (NIPER)
Sector 67, Phase X, SAS Nagar
Mohali – 160 062 Chandigarh

176 National Research Centre for Medicinal and Aromatic Plants
Boriavi – 387 310, Anand, Gujarat

177 Natural Drugs & Botanicals
C-49, Shyam Park Extn.
Sahibabad (Ghaziabad) UP

178 Natural Remedies Pvt. Ltd.,
Plot No. 5B, Veerasandra Industrial Area
19th KM Stone, Hosur Road
Bangalore – 561 229 (Karnataka)

179 NBPGR, Regional Centre
CAZRI Campus,
Jodhpur – 342 003 (Raj)

180 NBPGR, Regional Centre
Mendre Appa Garden Road
Amrawati Campus
Maharashtra

181 NBPGR, Regional Centre
PKV Campus
Akola – 444 104 (MS)

182 NBPGR, Regional Station
Nagalhat
Bhowali – 263 132
District Nainital, Uttaranchal

183 NBPGR, Regional Station
Phagli
Shimla – 171 004 (HP)

184 NBPGR, Regional Station
Umroi Road
Barapani – 793 103
District Ribhoi, Meghalaya

185 NBPGR, Regional Station
Vellanikkara
Trichur – 680 654 (Kerala)

186 Neem Foundation
67-A, Vithal Nagar, Road No. 12
Juhu Scheme
Mumbai – 400 059

187 Nopa Ram S/o Kishna Ram
Village – Post – Paniwala Mota
Dist. Sirsa, Haryana

188 North Eastern Regional Institute of Science and Technology (NERIST)
Nirjuli, District Papum Pare
Itanagar – 791 109 (AP)

189 Nu Tech Farm
Village Rayan, District Kutch
Gujarat – 370 465

190 O. P. Sharma
5/27, ITI Road,
Aligarh – 202 001 (UP)

191 Orrisa University of Agriculture and Technology
Bhubaneshwar – 751 003 (Orissa)

192 P. J. Agrotech Ltd.,
Flat No. 501A,
SVS Classic Residency,
D.N. 6-3-853/2, Ameerpet,
Hyderabad – 500 016 (AP)

193 Patidar Musli Farm and Research Centre
Vill and P.O. Jotpur,
Tehsil Manavar
District Dhar – 454 446 (MP)

194 Pawan Jariwal
Village – IG Choti,
Dhaka Wali Dhani,
Shri Ganganagar (Raj)

195 Peermade Development Society
Peermade MPCP, P.B. No. 11
Peermade
District Idukki – 685 531 (Kerala)

196 Pitambara Farm,
72, Gosaipura
Jhansi (UP)

197 Prabhudayal Yadav
Vilalge – Biloda
Dist Dhar (MP)

198 Prachi Agro
Station Road, Station Chowk, Aakot,
District Akola Maharashtra

199 Prakash Chand Jain
188, Shastri Nagar
Bhilwara (Raj)

200 Prakash Gursahani
114, Indrapuri
Indore – 452 017 (MP)

201 Prakash Sharma
Kamlesh Niketan, Pipli Bazar
Khilchipur (Dist Raigarh) MP

202 Pratap Seeds Company
Pratap Bhawan, P.O. Panditwari
Dehra Dun – 248 007 (UP)

203 Punjab Agricultural University
Department of Agronomy
Ludhiana – 141 004 (Punjab)

204 R. C. Bhakar
Village – Billowda, Dist. Dhar (M.P.)

205 R. K. Kudesia
B-94, IFFCO Township
Barelly – 243 403 (UP)

206 R.A. Poddar Medical (Ayurvedic) College
Dr. Annie Besant Road, Worli
Mumbai – 400 018 (MS)

207 Rachna Herbal Farm
2/146, Padbazar,
Rajkot – 360 001 (Guj)

208 Radhey Shyam Patidar
Main Gaon, P.O. Piprata
Dist Khargaon (MP)

209 Raghu Nandan Sharma
Chuli Gate, Gangapur City – 322 221
Sawai Madhopur (Raj)

210 Raj and Company
Dashera Maidan
Neemach – 458 441 (MP)

211 Rajasthan Agro Forestry Corporation
Sonamukhi Nagar
Sangaria Phanta, Salawas Road
Jodhpur – 342 005 (Raj)

212 Rajasthan Gau Sewa Sangh
Durga Pura
Jaipur (Raj)

213 Rajeev Ratan Leela
Leela Agricultural Farm
Hanumangarh (Raj)

214 Rajeev Sodhi
29, Samvid Nagar
Kanadia Road
Indore (MP)

215 Rajendra Singh Ranawat
Village & Post Gendaliya
Via – Hamirgarh – 311 025
Dist. – Bhilwara (raj)

216 Rajneesh Gupta
Vandna Bhawan,
P.O. Mohanpur
Jaipur – 303 104 (Raj)

217 Rakesh Shirmal
5, Baikunth Dham Colony,
Khajrana Road,
indore – 452 001 (MP)

218 Raksham Herbals
492, Nehru Nagar, Nandanvan Road,
Nagpur (MS)

219 Ramlal Rupaji Mukati
Sirvi Mohalla, Barwani (MP)

220 Range Forest Officer
Agumbe Range, Agumbe MPCA
Megaravalli – 577 411
District Shimoga, Kerala

221 Range Forest Officer
Alagarkovil Forest Range,
Alagarkovil MPCA
Alagarkovil – 624 007 District Madurai
Tamil Nadu

222 Range Forest Officer
B.R.T. MPCA
Yelandur – 571414,
District Mysore, Karnataka

223 Range Forest Officer
Barijam Forest Range,
Kodaikanal MPCA Berijam
Via Kodaikanal, District Dindigulanna
Tamil Nadu

224 Range Forest Officer
Belthangady Range, Charmadi MPCA
Post Belthangady – 574 214 Karnataka

225 Range Forest Officer
Bhagamandala Forest Range
Talacauvery MPCA,
Madikeri Taluk – 571 247
District Kodagu, Karnataka

226 Range Forest Officer
Bidar Sub Division
Karpakapalli MPCA Humnabad
District Bidar, Kerala

227 Range Forest Officer
Charpa Range, Athirapalli MPCA
Vazhachal via Chalakudy,
P.O. Poringalkutlu, Kerala

228 Range Forest Officer
Charpa Range, Athirapalli MPCA
Vazhachal Via Chalakudy,
P.O. Poringalkutlu, Kerala

229 Range Forest Officer
Chengam Range, Thenmalai MPCA
P.O. Chengam – 606 701
District Tiruvannamalai Sambuvarayar (TN

230 Range Forest Officer
Courtallam Range, Courtallam (Kuttalam)
MPCA, Shencottah, Tamil Nadu

231 Range Forest Officer
Goodrical Range, Triveni MPCA
P.O. Angamoozhy – 689 643
District Pattanamthitta, Kerala

232 Range Forest Officer
Idukki Wildlife Division,
Eravikulam MPCA
District IDUkki – 685 603, Kerala

233 Range Forest Officer
Kulasekaram Range, Main Road
Pechiparai, MPCA
Kulasekaram – 629 163
District Kanyakumari, Tamil Nadu

234 Range Forest Officer
Kumuta Taluk, Devimane MPCA
Kathgal – 581 444
District Uttarakannada, Kerala

235 Range Forest Officer
Magadi Range, Savanadurga MPCA
Magadi – 562 120, District Bangalore
Rural

236 Range Forest Officer
Mertacity (Jodhpur)

237 Range Forest Officer
Minor Forest Range, No. 5,
Kalima Manson, Kurumbaram
(Marakkanam) MPCA, Pudhupalayam Main
road, Cuddalore NT – 670 001
District Viluppuram Ramasamy,
Padayatchiyar (Tamil Nadu)

238 Range Forest Officer
Namakkal Forest Range, Kolli Hills MPCA
Namakkal – 637 001 (TN)

239 Range Forest Officer
Papanasam Project,
Mundanthurai MPCA
P.O. Ambasamudram Taluk (V.K. Puram)
District Tirunelvli Kattabomman, TN

240 Range Forest Officer
Peechi Range, Peechi MPCA
District Thrissur – 680 003, Kerala

241 Range Forest Officer
Peria Range, Wayanadu MPCA
P.O. Mananthavady,
Wayanandu – 670 643 Kerala

242 Range Forest Officer
Sandur Range, Sandur MPCA
Sandur – 583 119, District Bellary,
Kerala

243 Range Forest Officer
Subramanya Range, Subramanya MPCA
Post Subramanya – 574 029, Sullia Taluk
District Dakshina Kannada, Karnataka

244 Range Forest Officer
Tarikere Range,
Kemmangundi MPCA
Tarikere, Kerala

245 Range Forest Officer
Tumkur Range, Kunigal Road
Near Banashankari Temple,
Tumkur – 572 102 (Karnataka)

246 Range Forest Officer
Ulandy Range, Topslip MPCA
Topslip – 642 141
District Coimbatore (TN)

247 Range Forest Officer
Vedaranyam Range Kodikkarai MPCA
Vedaranyam – 614 810 District
Nagappattinam, Qaid-E-Millath (TN)

248 Range Forest Officer
Watrap Range, Thaniparai MPCA
Watrap Srivilliputhur Taluk,
District Kamarajar, Tamil Nadu

249 Range Forest Officer
Wildlife Unit, Kuduremukha MPCA
Karkala – 577 142
District Chikkamagalur, Kerala

250 Ravi Agro Tech and Essential Oil
Distillaries
Village Khajuri Kalan, Post Piplani,
Bhopal (MP)

251 Regional Plant Resource Centre
(Ekamra Kanan)
Adjacent to Chandaka Reserve Forest,
N-2/20 Nayapalli,
Bhubaneswar – 751 015 (Orissa)

252 Regional Research Institute (Ayurveda)
1093 Gorepeth
Nagpur – 440 010 (MS)

253 Regional Research Institute (Ayurveda)
Pharmacognosy Unit,
Ayurvedic College, Poojappura
Thiruvananthapuram – 695 012 (Kerala)

254 Regional Research Institute (Ayurveda)
Post Box 118, Mithun Gate
Itanagar – 791 111 (AP)

255 Regional Research Institute (Ayurveda)
Tadong, District East Sikkim
Gangtok – 737 102 Sikkim

256 Regional Research Laboraotry
Jorhat – 785 006 (Assam)

257 Regional Research Laboratory (Sub Station)
Lamphelpat
Imphal – 795 004 (Manipur)

258 Regional Research Laboratory Branch
Post Box 212, Naharlagun
Itanagar – 791 110 (AP)

259 Regional Research Laboratory
Canal Road,
Jammu Tawi – 180 001 (J&K)

260 Regional Research Laboratory
Sachivalya Marg,
Bhubaneswar – 751 013 (Orissa)

261 Rizwana Attarwala
7-A, United Flats,
Near EME Circle, Shama Road
Baroda – 2

262 Royal Herbs & Musli Farm
Usha Colony, Dabra,
Dwalior (MP)

263 Rupesh Gupta
Parasram Radhey Shyam,
Bhagatsing Chowk,
Sirsa (Haryana)

264 S. D. Mehta
E-8/23, Basantkunj,
Arera Colony,
Bhopal – 462 039

265 S. J. Wanjari
D-18, Tapowan Complex,
Somalwada
Nagpur – 25 (MS)

266 S. N. Gupta
B-8, Sector – 3,
Noida (UP)

267 Sahiram Rao
Village – Samrau
Post – Palli (Osian)
Jodhpur (Raj)

268 Sandeep Bhargawa
761, Sector-8B,
Chandigarh (UT)

269 Sandu Brothers Pvt. Ltd.
D.K. Sandu Marg, Sandu Nagar,
Sandu Wadi, Chembur
Mumbai – 400 071 (Maharashtra)

270 Sanjay Dhoopar
18/46, Penti Naka, Queens Road
Cantt,
Jabalpur (MP)

271 Sanjay Khuswaha
Village Khirki Wala, Post Undha
District Harda (MP)

272 Sansar Nursery and Gardens
Jalkal Campus, Gondey,
Pawan Cinema Road
Pratapgarh – 230 143 (UP)

273 School of Agricultural Sciences and
Rural Development (SASRD)
Medziphema – 797 106

274 Shankar Lal Khatik
Village – Kansedi, Post – Boodh
Vhittorgarh (Raj)

275 Shanker Lal Sharma
V.P.O. Chudi Ajitgarh
Jhunjhunun (Raj)

276 Shanthimalai Trust
Shiva Nagar, P.O. Sri Ramanashramam
Post Bag No. 7,
Thiruvannamalai – 606 603 (TN)

277 Sharda Herbal and Essentials Oils
Block No. 2, Bhaskar,
Sweet Seven Apartments
Opp. Gujral Petrol Pump,
Jalgaon (Maharashtra)

278 Shashank Parulkar
Gangadhar Roo ki Haveli
28/278, Kaithuni Pole
Kota – 324 006 (Raj)

279 Shivnath Singh Lamba
C/o Lamba Book Store,
Bhadra,
Dist. Hanumangarh (Raj)

280 Shrimal Agro Products
284-85, Saket Nagar,
Indore (MP)

281 Shyam Singh
Village – Aakodia, The. : Jaitaran,
Pali (Raj)

282 Society for Himalayan Environment Res.,
Dakpathar Road,
Vikas Nagar – 248 198
District Dehra Dun (UC)

283 Society for Research and Initiative for
Sustainable Technology & Instt. (SRISTI)
B-4, Ravi Niketan Apartments
Near Vastrapuram Gountain
Ahmedabad – 380 015 (Gujarat)

284 Sohanlal Sharma
21, Sachivalaya Colony, Tonk Fatak
Jaipur – 302 015 (Raj)

285 State Forest Research Institute
Polipathar, Narmada Road
Jabalpur – 482 008 (MP)

286 State Forest Research Institute
Post Box 159, Van Vihar
Itanagar – 791 111 (AP)

287 Subhah Agro Products
18/46, Penty Naka, Queens Road Cantt.,
Jabalpur – 482 001 (MP)

288 Subham Aushadhi Ropani
Aamanala, Project Tank, Khamriya
Jabalpur (MP)

289 Subhas GOdara,
2E8, Pawanpuri
Bikaner (Raj)

290 Subhash Khanna
C/o Prakash Medicals,
Rampura Bazar
Kota (Raj)

291 Surendra Pungalia
12, Technocrate Society, Bedla Road,
Udaipur – 313 011 (Raj)

292 Surendra Singh
H-40, Khaturia Colony,
Bikaner (Raj)

293 Synthozyem Laboratories
169, Johri Bazar, Jalgaon (MS)

294 T. P. Shinde
At Post Kusumba
Dist Dhule – 424 302 (MS)

295 Taj Services Ltd.,
33, Nathalal Parekh Marg, Colaba
Mumbai – 400 001 (MS)

296 Tamil Nadu Agriculltural University
College of Horticultural, Lawley Road
Coimbatore – 641 003 (TN)

297 Thanasingh S/o Arjun Singh
Village – Garabadeshar
P. O. Kallu, Bikaner

298 Tibetan Medical and Astro Institute
(Men-Tsee-Khang)
Khara Danda Road,
Dharamshala – 176 215
District Kangra (HP)

299 Tongpang Changri Co-operative Society
Longnak,
District Mokokchung – 789 601 (Nagaland)

300 Trivendra Singh Benda
Village Post Garda,
Tehsil – Kishanganj
Barram (Raj)

301 Tropical Botanical Garden and Research
Institute (TBGRI)
Karimancode, P.O. Pacha-Palode
Thiruvananthapuram – 695 562 (Kerala)

302 Tropical Forest Research Institute (TFRI)
Mandla Road, P.O. RFRC,
Jabalpur – 482 001 (MP)

303 University of Agricultural Sciences (UAS)
Department of Horticulture
GKVK post, Bangalore – 560 065
(Karnataka)

304 UTTHAN-Centre for Sustainable
Development and Poverty Alleviation
102 G/3, Beniganj,
Allahabad – 211 002 (UP)

305 Vidhya Sagar Farms and Plantations Ltd.
Subhash Colony, Guna, Madhya Pradesh

306 Vijay Solvent Ltd.,
Bhagwati Sadan,
Near Rly Station
Alwar (Raj)

307 Vikram Singh Godara
2E8, Pawan Puri
Bikaner (Raj)

308 Vishwanath Nayar
L-3, Anupam Nagar
Raipur – 492 007 (CG)

309 Vivek Khandelwal
Khandelwal Brothers,
Agar Malva (MP)

310 Wimco Limited
5E, Local Shopping Centre
Masjid Moth, Greater Kailash-II
New Delhi – 110 048

311 Y. Anilkumar Reddy
3/52 A, IInd Road, New Town,
Anantpur – 515 001 (AP)

312 Y. Kishore Babu
311/2 RT, P. S. Nagar,
Vijay Nagar Colony,
Hyderabad – 500 457 (AP)

313 Y. Sashirekha
311/2nd, P.S. Nagar
Vijai Nagar Colony,
Hyderabad – 500 547 (AP)

314 Zandu Foundation for Health Care
70, Gokhale Road South, Dadar
Mumbai – 400 025 (MS)

10 TRADERS AND COMMISSION AGENTS

1 A. Govindaraja Mudaliar,
27, Rasappa Chetty Street,
Chennai – 600003

2 A. Kaderali & Company
189 Samuel Street, Khoja Gali
Mumbai – 400009

3 A. Perumal & Co.,
29, Audiappa Naicken Street
Sowcarpet, Chennai – 600079

4 A. S. R. Company
Punalur
Kerala(India)-691305

5 A.G. Singaravel & Co.,
14, Swamy Sannidhi Lane,
East Masti Street,
Madurai – 625001

6 A.M.K. Mohammed Ibrahim
Rowther,
No. 95, Deverpuram Road
Tuticorin – 628003

7 A.M.K. Mohammed
Ibrahim Rowther 95
Davapuram Road
Tuticorin – 628003
Tamil Nadu

8 A.N.S. Enterprises,
No. B-7, Thirumalai Colony
IIIrd Street, Madurai – 625016

9 A.S. Jagadeesan & Firm
2, West Car St.,
Virudhu Nagar – 628001

10 A.S.A. Narayan & Co.,
5, Somasundara Mudali Street
Chennai – 600001

11 A.T. Rathinum Chetty & Co.,
Country Drug Merchants,
261, East Masi Street,
Madurai – 625001

12 A.T. Verma
35, Examiner Press Building
Second Floor, Dalal Street
Mumbai – 400023

13 A.V. Traders
Country Drug Merchants,
218, East Masi Street,
Madurai – 625001

14 A.V.V. Satyanarayana
A.P. Residential School, District
Visakhapatnam
Pedabayalu – 531040

15 Abdul Jaleel,
Green Gunger Merchant,
Kusmi – 577423, Shimoga District

16 Abhudary Industries
27 Market Yard
Sidhpur-384151 Gujarat

17 Abirami Botanical Corporation
55 P.S.S. Nadar Street
Senna & Crude Merchant
Tuticorin-628001 Tamil Nadu

18 Absa Herbals India
82, Buddi Sahib Street, M.K. Garden
Chennai – 600001

19 Adcco Ltd.
District Hoogli
Adcconagar-712121 West Bangal

20 Adco Corporation
67-69 Mohammedan Road
2nd Floor, Dada Manzil
Mumbai -400003

21 Agarwal Trading Company
Tanakpur – 262309 (Champawat)

22 Ahmedali Jafferjee Gandhi
24 Pollock Street
Kolkatta-700001 West Bangal

23 Ajanta Pharma Limited
98, Charkop Industrial Estate,
Hindustan Naka Link Road,
Kanidivili (West)
Mumbai – 400067

24 Ajay Kumar Gandhi
Smita Towers, Shop No. 1, Padamnabh Nagar
Bhopal – 462008

25 Ajmal Fragrances and Flavours P. Ltd.
1, Cecil Court, 24
Mahakavi Bhushan Marg, Colaba
Mumbai – 400030

26 Akhand Aushadhi Bhandar
13, Shitalamata Bazar, Indore – 452003

27 Akhand Ayurvedic Rasayan Sala
276, Sector E, Sanwer Road,
Indore – 452003

28 Akshat Udhyog, Bhanpur Industrial Area
Raipur – 493001

29 Aldrich International
216/2 – A, Aacharya J.B. Road
Kolkatta – 700017

30 All India Drug Supply Company
11 Dariyasthan Street,
Masjid, Bunder Road
Mumbai -400003

31 Aman Impex Pvt. Ltd.
14 Roop Chand Roy Street
Kolkatta-700007

32 Aman Impex Pvt. Ltd.
14, Roop Chand Rai Road
Kolkatta – 700007

33 Amar Chemicals
Annu Talkies, Raipur Road,
Dhamtari – 492145

34 Amar International
330, Katra Hussain Bux
Khari Baoli,
Delhi – 110006

35 Amrutha Kesari
364 Avenue Road
Bangalore-560002

36 Anant Industries / Anant Drug House
Anant House, Shawa Road,
Dhamtari – 492145

37 Andaman & Nicobar Forest Dev. Corp. Ltd.
P. O. Haddo
Port Blair-744103
Andaman & Nicobar

38 Anil Ayurpharma
Ladiwala Estate, Hingwala Lane
Ghatkopar (E),
Mumbai – 400077

39 Anil Goel
JKH Exports, B/62, APMC Complex
Phase II, Market I, Sector – 19, Vashi
New Mumbai – 400705

40 Anrori Agro Herbo Medica (I) Pvt. Ltd.
P.O. Box No. 15, Nainital – 263001

41 Anthyodaya Sangh
PB No. 216, 7-A, Mission Hospital Road, Woraiyur
Thiruchirapalli – 620003 (Tamilnadu)

42 Anu Chem Industries
N-11, Kailash Colony
New Delhi – 110048

43 Aren Exports Pvt. Ltd.
3/25 Steelyard House
67-F, Sant Tukaram Marg
Mumbai – 400009

44 Arjun Das Narayan Das
Gole Bazar, Katni – 482005

45 Aromatic & Allied Chemicals
B-8, Industrial Estate, C.B. Ganj
Bareilly – 243502

46 Arul Jothi Traders
Country Drug Merchants
21, Swamy Sannidhi Lane,
Keela Masi Veethi
Madurai – 625001

47 Arun & Company
Arun Chamber,
P-38 Indian Exchange Place
Kolkatta-700001

48 Arun Chaurasia
53/7 Naya Ganj,
Kanpur – 208001

49 Aruna Brothers
J-27 A, Jangpura Extension
P.B. 352
New Delhi-110001

50 Arunachal Pradesh Forest Co. Ltd.
P.O. Box No. 123, District Papum Pare
Itanagar – 791111

51 Arunachal Pradesh Forest Development Corporation
District Tripa
Deomali-786629
Arunachal Pradesh

52 Arunachal Pradesh Forest Development Corporation Ltd.,
Dist. Tirpa
Deomali – 786629
Arunachal Pradesh

53 Arvind Laboratories
No. 7, Chakrapani Street, Mambalam
Chennai – 600033

54 Arya Vaidya sala
Kottakkal,
District Mallapuram – 676503

55 Arya Vastu Bandar
46 Dispensary Road,
Dehra Dun – 248001 (UC)

56 Arya Vastu Bhandar (Delhi)
2308/203 Sapna Kaushik,
Market Gali, Hinga Beg, Tilak Bazar
Delhi-110006

57 Ashish Overseas Corporation
34 Sarvodaya Industrial Estate,
Mahakali Road
Andheri East,
Mumbai – 400093

58 Ashok Industries
Bhandu Highway, Bhandu
District Mehsana (Gujarat)

59 Ashok Oil Producers,
No. 2/137-A, Perumbadi Road,
Nellorepet,
Gudiyattam 632602 Tamil Nadu

60 Ashok Pathak
114, South Toda,
Juni Indore – 452001

61 Ashok Trading Company
Old Industrial Area, Dhamtari – 492145

62 Asian Drug Company
1244 Chah Rahat
Delhi – 110006

63 Asoj Soft Caps Pvt. Ltd.
Krishna Bai Building
Kahinath Dhuru Road, Agar Bazar
Dadar,
Mumbai – 400028

64 Assam Physiochemical Industries
R.K. Bose Road,
Dhubri – 793301 (Assam)

65 Atul R. Shah
Swastic Medical Store
177-178 Laxmi Road
Pune-411002 (MS)

66 Aurora Export Trading Agency
6-A 3rd Floor,
Saklat Place
Kolkatta-700072

67 Ayurved Samshodhanlaya (ASUM)
1379, Shukrawar Peth, Natu Beg
Pune – 411002

68 Ayurvedic Vikas Sansthan
C-83, Gandhi Nagar
Moradabad – 244001

69 B.D.H. Industries Limited
Nair Baug, Akurli Road, Kandivli (East)
Mumbai – 400016

70 B.K. Industries
G.I.D.C. Estate,
Palanpur – 385002

71 Babu Ram Harish Chand
2114 Khari Baoli,
Delhi – 110006

72 Babulal & Brothers
Premnagar
Dehra Dun (Uttaranchal)

73 Babulal Bhagat
Village Kanawadi, Tehsil Ghodadongri
District Baitul

74 Babulal Sarabhi & Company
Khariar Road
Khariar – 766104

75 Back Impexs International Pvt. Ltd.
Back House, DDA Commercial Complex
13 Masjid Moth,
New Delhi – 110048

76 Bahubali Udhyog
21-A, Tifara Industrial Area
Bilaspur – 495223

77 Balaji Drug House
Country Drug Merchants
14, Swamy Sannidhi Lane,
Keela Mase Veethi,
Madurai – 625001

78 Balaji Enterprises,
491 – B 2nd Floor,
Maduravayal,
Chennai – 102

79 Balisana Isabgol
G.I.D.C. Industrial Estate
Mehsana
Balisana-384110 (Gujarat)

80 BAN MARC
Kamdar Mansion
Dhedar Road
Rajkot-360001 (Gujarat)

81 Banoushadi Jari-Buti Bhandar
S-19 Budh Vihar,
Delhi – 110041

82 Banwari Lal Shree Ram
545 Katra Ishwar Bhawan, Khari Baoli
Delhi – 110006

83 Bardoli Agro Pvt. Ltd.
Sri Ram Industrial Estate
Near Company Kale Marg
Kurla (West)
Mumbai

84 Baskar Benjoin & Co.,
No. 115, T.H. Road
Chennai – 600081

85 Baskar Company
34 New Thandavaraya Frammi Street
Washrmenpet
Chennai-600021

86 Beharilal Hemraj
176 Jamuna Lal Bajaj Street
Kolkatta-700007

87 Beshaj Bhawan
6668 Khari Baoli
Delhi – 110006

88 Bhagwati Trading Company
Satkar Hotel Gali, Station Road, Raipur

89 Bhaleswari Ayurvedic Co.,
62/4, Govindappa Naicken Street
Chennai – 600079

90 Bharat Crude Drug Supply Company
Ravji Mansion
Kazi Syed Street
Mumbai-400009

91 Bharat Drug & Extracts
13 Jail Road Dewas City – 455001
Madhya Pradesh

92 Bharat Drug Company
50, Moti Bazar,
Dehra Dun – 248001 (UC)

93 Bharat Trading Co.,
155, Govindappa Naicken Street
Chennai – 600001

94 Bharat Vastu Bhandar
47, Dhamwala Bazar,
Dehra Dun – 248001 (UC)

95 Bhartia Sons Ltd.,
12 Government Place East
Kolkatta – 700069 (WB)

96 Bhawani Traders
Raipur Road, Dhamtari – 492145

97 Bhilwaray Herbal Extracts Company
H-3, Lane-6, Ebrahimganj,
Bhopal – 462011

98 Bhogilal C. Shah & Company
8/1 South Tukoganj
Nabhodip
Indore-452001

99 Biddle Sawyer & Co. (India) Pvt. Ltd.
25, Dalal Street, Fort
Mumbai-400001

100 Bioveda Herbs Pvt. Ltd.
A-436 B.D.A. Colony Shahpura,
Bhopal – 462011

101 Bisco Company
P.B. 50002, 12/14 Kazi Sayed Street
Mumbai – 400009

102 Biyanis
25 Ganesh Chandra Avenue
Kolkatta (West Bangal)

103 Brij & Company
567-A, Katra Ishwar Bhawan
Khari Baoli
Delhi-110006

104 Brij Bhushan Lal Gupta
Sarafa Bazar
Saharanpur (UC)

105 C. Palaniappan & Son,
2, Reddy Raman Street
Chennai – 600079

106 C. Sundaresan Nair
Drugs Merchant
Kothuval Street,
Chalai, Trivandrum

107 C.M. Jain
1 Carter Road,
9-A- Dhavalgauga Bandra West
Mumbai

108 C.M. Ponnuswamy Nadar & Sons
No. 266, East Masi Street,
Madurai – 625001

109 C.M. Subbaiah Nadar Firm
30 Swamy Sannidhi Lane,
East Masi Street,
Madurai – 625001

110 C.M.N. Annamalai & Co.,
Country Drug Merchants,
30/1-A, Swami Sannidhi Lane,
Madurai – 625001

111 Catholic Hospital Association of
India Community Health Dept.
P.B. 2126, 157/6 Staff Road,
Gunrock Enclave
Secunderabad – 500003 (AP)

112 Chandni and Company
14-1-62 and 63th
Main Road,
Mattupalayam – 641301

113 Chaurasia Agency
53/20 Naya Ganj,
Kanpur – 208001

114 Chengalrayan & Co.,
24, Ebrahim Sait Street,
Chennai – 600079

115 Chhotelal Rajendra Prasad Tiwari
Ghantaghar,
Katni – 482005

116 Chindiya Diyawar (Shahu)
Amla, Near Ram Mandir, District Baitul

117 Chothmall Joshi
"Joshi Kunj" 2nd Mile
Sevoke Road,
Silliguri – 734401

118 Chranji Lal Raut
12th Mile, Sadiya,
P.O. Kukramara District Dibrugarh

119 Classic Medi herbs
323, 3rd Main, JP Nagar, 3rd Phase
Bangalore – 560078

120 Corbet Herbs
Penth Road (Behind SBI), Ram Nagar
District Nainital – 263001

121 Cottage Industries
Shree Arvindo Ashram
3, Rangpillay Street, Pondicherry –
605001

122 Crown Herbal Products
78, Ashtabhujam Road, Choolai
Chennai – 600112

123 D & M Naturals and Fragrances
No. 12, 11th "A" Main Road
11 Stage, West of Chord Road
Bangalore – 560086

124 D. Jamnadas & Company
207 Samuel Street,
Vadgadi
Mumbai-400003

125 Das and Sons
North Lakhimpur, Assam

126 Das Trading Company
Old Bus Stand,
Dhamtari – 492145

127 Dasakarma Bhandar
Barpeta Road, Assam

128 Dashrathlal Ramjibhai Patel
Hari Cotton Mills Compound
Sidhpur-384151 (Gujarat)

129 Deccan Phytochemicals
309, Kabra complex, 61, M.G. Road
Sikandrabad – 500003

130 Deepak Bawa & Company
Majith Mandi
Amritsar-143001 (Punjab)

131 Deepak K. Sharda
Sharda Brothers
Ward No. 1,
Tanakpur – 262309

132 Deepan Trading Corporation
A-47 Maskati Market, Ist fl.,
Ahmedabad – 380002 (Gujarat)

133 Demode and Company
201, Narayana Peth, Laxmi Road
Pune – 411030

134 Devi Enterprises
25 Anjakara Street,
Dharmapuri – 636702

135 Devi Prasad Ashish Kumar
2772 Gali, Arya Samaj Bazar
New Delhi – 110001

136 Devi Sahai Banwari Lal & Sons
20-89-90 Katra Tambacco,
Khari Baoli
Delhi – 110006

137 Devi Sahai Mohan Lal
2210-1 Aggarwal Market
Katra, Tambacoo, Khari Baoli
Delhi-110006

138 Devi ShahaiMohan Lal
2210-1 Aggarwal Market, Katra
Tambacco, Khari Baoli,
Delhi-110006

139 Dhani Ram Ratan Chand
Ghantaghar, Katni – 482005

140 Diamond Exporters
Krishnapadamam Buildings
Anayara P.O.
Thiruvananthapuram – 695012

141 Dinesh Gurbase Bawa Sons
Majith Mandi,
Amritsar – 143001

142 Dogra Drugs Pharma
29 Industrial Estate
Bilaspur – 174001 (HP)

143 Doon Trading Company
Panetitari, Premnagar P.O.
Dehra Dun-248007 (UC)

144 Doshi Enterprises
Ratanbandha,
Dhamtari – 492145

145 Doulat ram Arora
Girdikot
Jodhpur – 342 001

146 Dr. Jain's Special Hearbs
A-10 Raj Complex 2nd fl.,
Miltary Road,
Marol Abdheri East
Mumbai – 400059 (MS)

147 Drug & Alkaloid Company
4127 Naya Bazar
P.B. 1297
Delhi-110006

148 Duncans Agro Industries Ltd.
31 Netaji Subhash Road
Kolkatta (WB)

149 Durga Prasad & Company
2080/81 Katra Tambacco
Khari Baoli
Delhi – 110006

150 Durga Prasad & Company, 2080,
Katra Tobacco Khari Baoli,
Delhi – 110006

151 Durga Singh Martolia
Village Bala (Magar), Post Madlakya
Pithoragarh – 262501 (UC)

152 Eastman & Company
3 Southern Avenue
Kolkatta-700026

153 Elango Traders,
158, Govindappa Naicken Street
Chennai – 600001

154 Enbee Plantations
236, Zone II MP Nagar,
Bhopal – 462011

155 Excel Drug House
18-B Sukeas Lane, Kolkatta – 700001

156 Excelar Trading Company
29/31, Israil Mohalla, Bhagwan Bhawan
Mumbai – 400009

157 Exotic Naturals
401, Sunderwan Complex
A-4, Andheri (W),
Mumbai – 400053

158 Expo International Exporters & Suppliers
20 Old Court House Street
Kolkatta-700001

159 Export Enterpriese
34 Bhagwan Bhawan, 196/198
Samuel Street
Mumbai – 400009

160 Fairdeal Corporation Pvt. Ltd.
66 Lakshmi Building, Sir P.M. Road
Fort, Mumbai – 400001

161 Fakirchand Jagdish Chand Mistry
Village Kahari-Kalam
District Ambala
Bhambhol
Haryana

162 Faqir Chand & Sons
6704 Khari Baoli, Near Fatepuri
Delhi – 110006

163 Farukh Impex
C-3, Dalal Estate, Mumbai Central
Mumbai – 400008

164 Fedelity Flavours
344/18, Main Road
Jaya Nagar, 7th Block,
West Bangalore – 560082

165 Foreign Trade Company of India
12 Walkashwar Road
Mumbai – 400006

166 G. Dass & Company Pvt. Ltd.,
27 W Great Cotton Road
Tuticorin – 628002
Tamilnadu

167 G.B. Viswanatha Chattier,
Big Bazaar,
Palakkad – 678014

168 G.K. Pharma
2725, Chelam Street, Daryaganj
New Delhi – 110002

169 Gadodia Kirana Company
2084 Katra Tambacco, Khari Baoli
Delhi – 110006

170 Gaindamal Babulal & Company
Block B Pocket, W Flat, 74
Shalimar Bagh
Delhi – 110052

171 Gajraj Mehandi Udyog
28, Pali Road
Gajraj House
Sojat City-306104 (Raj)

172 GANDEEPA Kurunchi Bhavanam
Kilavayal – 630410
Ulagampatti via
Sivagangai dist.
Tamilnadu

173 Gandharv Ayurved Research Institute
4th Mile, Mandla Road,
Jabalpur – 482020

174 Ganesh Drugs House,
No. 72, Veerapathiran Street,
Virudhunagar – 626001

175 Ganga Exports
12, Bhaweshwar Vihar
383-A, SVP Road,
Mumbai – 400054

176 Gangaram Mohanlal
54, South Raj Mohalla,
Indore – 452001

177 Gauri Shankar & Company
532 Katra Ishwar Bhawan,
Khari Baoli
Delhi – 110006

178 Gautam Export Corporation
506 Surat Sadan, 5th Floor,
Surat Street
Mumbai – 400009

179 Gayathry & Co.,
Swamy Sannitthi Lane,
Keela Masi Veethi, Madurai – 1

180 Gayatri Enterprises,
32, Arumugam Street,
Chennai – 600001

181 General Mercantila Overseas Corporation
314 Mint Street, P.B. 7401,
Chennai – 600079

182 Genex Corporation
29 New Colony
Tuticorin-628001 (Tamil Nadu)

183 Girdharilal Vithaldas Patel
S.T. Road, Sidhpur – 384151

184 Girijan Corporation Ltd.
East Point Colony
Visakhapatanam
Andra Pradesh-530017

185 Giriraj Enterprises
Highway Unjha
Gujarat

186 Giya Exports
60 Sir Hari Ram Goenka Street
Kolkatta-700007

187 Global Export Pvt. Ltd.
55 Stephen House
4B B-D, Bagh East
Kolkatta-700001

188 Global Link Exports
Dada Manzil No. 1
4th Floor, 67/69 Muhmmad Ali Road
Mumbai – 400003

189 Golden Sat Isabgol Factory
Highway, Kakosi, Chaurasta
Sidhpur – 384151

190 Gopal Brothers
180/82, Samuel Street
Mumbai – 400009

191 Gopal Brothers
578 Katra Ishwar Bhawan
Khari Baoli
Delhi – 110006

192 Govind Prasad Raut
8th Mile Dist. Dibrugarh
Mandi Sadiya
Assam

193 Gulab Chand Laduram Attar,
Naya Bazaar
Ajmer, Rajasthan

194 Guni Gopachal Ayurved Niketan
Chowk Bazar, Gwalior

195 Gutti Ram Sukhanand
290/2 Katra Pedan, Khari Baoli
Delhi – 110006

196 Gwalior Forest Products Ltd.
P.O. Katha Mill, Shivpuri – 473551

197 H.S. Bajaj and Sons
391, Mahesh Chamber, 2nd Floor
Nursi Natha Street,
Mumbai – 400009

198 Hari Ram & Company
2045 Aggarwal Market, Katra Tambacco
Khari Baoli,
Delhi – 110006

199 Hari Ram & Sons
412 Katra Medgran Khari Baoli
Delhi – 110006

200 Haridas Aggarwal & Sons
312 Central Facility Building
APMC Market – I, Phase – II, Vashi
Navi Mumbai – 400703

201 Health Aids
24-25th Cross, Bharti Park Road
Coimbatore – 641043

202 Healthcare Pharmaceuticals
4, Vasant Vilas, St. Andrews Road
Santacruz (West), Mumbai – 400054

203 Hemant and Company
509 Goridia House, 100-102
Kazi Syed Street
Mumbai – 400003

204 Herb & Drug India
29 Nattukottai Chetty Street
Tuticorin
Tamil Nadu-628001

205 Herbal Stores
P.B. 5047, 23 Khadak Street
Mumbai – 400009
Maharashtra

206 Herbs Exporters
D-49 Defence Colony
New Delhi-110024

207 Herbs Indica
351 Industrial Area II
Chandigarh – 160002

208 Hill Green Co.,
No. 17, 13th Cross,
Vasanthanagar Extension,
Bangalore – 560052

209 Himalaya Drug Company
Saharanpur Road
Clement Town
Dehra Dun
Uttaranchal(India)

210 Himalaya Herb Stores
Madho Nagar, P.B. 130
Saharanpur – 247001

211 Himalayan Drug Company
20, Najafgarh,
New Delhi – 110015

212 Himalayan Traders
Katra Dulo,
Amritsar – 143001

213 Himalyan Drugs
Herbs & Alkaloids Syndicate
C-4/33-A, Lawrence Road
Delhi-110035

214 Hindustan Pharmaceuticals
Kot Mit Singh, Taran Taran Road
Amritsar – 143001

215 Hindustan Trading Corporation
Sidhpur – 384151 Gujarat

216 Hiralal Gajdharlal
24 Maktaram Babu Street
Kolkatta – 700007 West Bengal

217 Indian Drug House
6669 Khari Baoli,
Delhi – 110006

218 Indian Drug Merchants,
Chalai, Trivandrum

219 Indian Drugs and Botanical Herbs
Company
103, Ram Nagar, Krishna Nagar
P.O. Box 9416,
Delhi – 110051

220 Indian Herbs Research & Supply Company
Sharda Nagar,
Saharanpur
Uttar Pradesh

221 Indian Herbs Traders
R. No. 6654/2, New Gadodia Market
Khari Baoli,
Delhi – 110006

222 Indo Drugs Hybrid Seeds
218/5 Gali No. Than Singh Nagar
Anand Parbat,
New Delhi – 110005

223 Indo Exports
Bindu Sarover Road
Sidhpur – 384151 Gujarat

224 Indo World Trading Company Ltd.
10 Armanian Street
Kolkatta-700001

225 Indo World Trading Corporation
303 Prakash Chambers
6 Netaji Subhash Marg, Daryaganj
New Delhi-110002

226 Innovations Pharma International
62/12 Old Rajinder Nagar
Delhi – 110050

227 Institute of Alternative
Medicine & Research
Ambala-Shimla Highway panchkula
Haryana

228 Inter Continental Traders,
Hill Produce Merchants
No. 30/637, Big Bazaar Road,
Palakkad – 678014

229 International Traders
Gopinath Building
Gali Batashan, Khari Baoli
Delhi-110006

230 International Traders
Ramesh Chambers, 2nd Floor
14 Garibdat Street, Vadgadi
Mumbai -400003

231 Intra Catholic Centre,
Armenian Street,
Chennai – 600001

232 Ishan Marketing Pvt. Ltd.
901, Nirmal Tower, 22, Barakhamba Road
New Delhi – 110001

233 J.J. Herbals Products
915, Lordganj, Jabalpur – 482002

234 J.K. Drug Stores
163 Nainiappa Naik Street,
Chennai – 600013

235 J.K. Exports
52 K.K. Nagar, C.I.D. Office Corner
Madurai – 625020

236 J.P. Mills
Sighpur – 384151
Gujarat

237 J.R. Pandian
North Cotton Road
Tuticorin – 628001
Tamilnadu

238 Jadavaji Lallubhai and Company
247 Kalbadevi Road, P.O. Box 2034
Mumbai – 400002

239 Jagannath Kashi Prasad Agarwal
Hanumanganj,
Katni – 482005

240 Jagdish Kumar Hari Om and Company
485/2, Katra Ishwar Bhawan, Khari Baoli
Delhi – 110006

241 Jagdish Narayan Hari Mohan
Tanakpur – 262309, District Pithora garh

242 Jaggi Enterprises
8, Lajpath Kunj, Napier Town,
Jabalpur – 482001

243 Jai Hind Trading Corporation
28 New Rohtak Road
Delhi – 110005

244 Jai Industries
Highway
Khali
Sidhpur-384151 (Gujarat)

245 Jai Trading Corporation
11 Barbourne Road
Kolkatta – 700001 (WB)

246 Jailaxmi Exports
2-34-14, Gandhi Nagar, Gundibandi Street
Tenali, Guntur – 522201

247 Jain Herbs Enterprises
Rajeshwari Road, Shivpuri – 493551

248 Jairamdas Khushiram,
P.O. Box No. 37,
No. CC/V/166, Bazaar Road,
Mattanchery,
Cochin – 682002

249 Jairamdas Khusiram
B/48, APMC, Market – I, Phase – II
Turbhe, Navi Mumbai – 400703

250 Jawahar Industries
46 North Cotton Road
Tuticorin
Tamil Nadu

251 Jay Kay & Company
8 Goplnath Building
Khari Baoli
Delhi-110006

252 Jeganath Raj & Sons
Kottampatty Road, Natham,
Dindigul Dist.

253 Jenson Enterprises
34 New Thandavaraya Street
P.B. 905
Chennai-600021 (TN)

254 Jiwanram Sheoduttrai
Block D, Chowringhee Mansion
30 Jawaharlal Nehru Road
Kolkatta-700016
West Bangal

255 Jonson Enterprises Pvt. Ltd.
34 New Thandarvalsia Street, P.B. 905
Washerman Street,
Chennai – 600021

256 Juna Gandhi
515-517 Maulana Azad Road,
Nuli Bazar
Mumbai – 400004

257 K. Akkaretty Nadar & Sons
East Masi Street,
Madurai – 1

258 K. Perumal Pillai
M.G. Road, Trivandrum

259 K. Ramasamy Chetty
177, Rasappa Chetty Street
Chennai – 600003

260 K. Uttam Lal (Exports) Ltd.
Bhagwan Bhawan, 1st Floor
196-198 Samuel Street,
Mumbai – 400009

261 K.D. Shah Enterprises
49/15 Sir C.V. Raman Road,
P.B. 1457 Alwarpet
Chennai – 600013

262 K.M. Abdul Kadhar
145/2 Ettayapuram Road,
Tuticorin – 628002

263 K.P. Esthapanose and Sons
Exporters and Importers
P.O. Box 9, Alwaye – 683101

264 K.V. Patel and Company
S.T. Road, Sidhpur – 384151

265 Kadmi International
Kashi House, 7-A Connaught Place
Delhi – 110001

266 Kalidas Gandhi
Centre Street Camp,
Pune – 411001 (MS

267 Kamal Chand
Bade Pasari, Near City Kotwali
Jabalpur – 482001

268 Kamalkant Chotalal and Company
106 Bhandari street, Narainarao Koli Marg
Mumbai – 400003

269 Kandasmy Chetty,
163, Rasappa Chetty Street,
Chennai – 600003

270 Kanilal Ram Kumar
178 Harrison Road
Kolkatta-700007 (WB)

271 Kannadiyar & Co.,
Country Drug Merchants
260, East Mast Street,
Madurai – 625001

272 Kannappa Chetty & Sons,
No. 83/1, I Main Road,
New Tharagupet,
Bangalore – 560002

273 Kantilal Joitaram Patel
Kakosi Road,
Sidhpur – 384151

274 Kapur International
A-228, Derawala Nagar
New Delhi – 110009

275 Karan Enterprises
4066, Khari Baoli,
Delhi – 110006

276 Karnataka Soaps and Detergent Ltd.
Bangalore – Pune Highway
P.O. Box 5931, Rajaji Nagar
Bangalore – 560055

277 Kashmir Ayurvedic Works
Azad Nagar, Putlighar
Amritsar – 143001 Punjab

278 Kayakalp Herbal Industries
Thuwakheda, Kollar Road, Ginnauri
Bhopal – 462042

279 Kepee Sons,
No. 9/42, Gopra Bazaar,
Calicut – 673001

280 Keshavlal Vithaldas Patel
Gulab Park,
S.T. Road
Sidhpur-384151 (Gujarat)

281 Keshavlal Vithaldas Patel
Gulab Prak, S.T. Road,
Sidhpur – 384151

282 Keshrimal Kastoorchand
Naya Para, Raipur

283 Kirana Trading Company
Raipur Road, Sihawa Chowk,
Dhamtari – 492145

284 Kishalaya Herbals Ltd.
303, Alankar Chambers, 2-A, Ratlam Kothi
A-B Road, Indore – 452001

285 Kishan Chand Vaishno Das
P.O. Box No. 119, Majith Mandi
Amritsar – 143001

286 Kitij Patukala
A-3/8 Chintamani Nagar, Bibnewadi
Pune – 411037

287 Kolaba Business Centre
C 25/5, Middle Circle
Cannaught Place
New Delhi-110001

288 Kothari Phytochemicals (International)
766 Annanagar Madurai – 625020
Tamilnadu

289 Krihivala Herbal and Plant Products
Opp. NGO's House, SBI Road
Sattenapalli – 522403, District Guntur

290 Krishna Ayurvedics,
Pulimood, M.G. Road,
Trivandrum

291 Krishna Kapoor and Company
Woodlands, The Mall, Amritsar – 143001

292 Krishna Pharmacy
Haridwar Road, Kankhal
Haridwar – 249404 (UC)

293 Krishna Traders
20 Harichandra Mullick Street
Kolkatta – 700005

294 Kuria Mal and Sons
Kiran Mansion, 4834/24 Ansari Road
Darya Ganj,
New Delhi – 110002

295 L. Nanalal Bros.
New Anand Bhawan,
Room No. 303, 3rd Floor,
257 Narshi Natha Street, P.B. 5022
Mumbai -400009

296 Lakshmi Syndicate
56, Thatha Muthiappan Street
Chennai – 600081

297 Lala Mata Deen Bhagwan Das
548/49 Katra Ishwar Bhawan, Khari Baoli
Delhi – 110006

298 Laxmi Exports
Laxmi Villa, 20 Pretam Nagar
Sulem Sarai, Allahabad – 211001

299 Laxmidas Haridas Tanna & Company
Gulabi House 3rd Floor
111/115 Kazi Sayeed Street
Mumbai-400009

300 Lehri Mal Anoop Kumar and Company
576 Katra Ishwar Bhawan, Khari Baoli
Delhi – 110006

301 Lupin Laboratories Limited
159, CST Road, Santacruz (East)
Mumbai – 400098

302 M. Ramaswamy & Co.,
No. 80, Thalaiappan St. P.B. No. 9,
Virudhunagar – 626001

303 M. Veerappa & Co.,
APMC Yard,
Batawadi – 572103 (Tumkur)

304 M.K. Industries
No. 1, First Cross Street,
United India Colony,
Chennai – 600024

305 M.K. Nataraja Pillai
No. 49, Emperor Street,
Tuticorin – 628001

306 M.K.M.M. Murugesan & Co.,
259, Keela Masi Veethi,
Madurai 625001

307 M.L. Ramnarayan
Kothi Lala Ramnarayan, M.G. Road
Kannauj – 209726

308 M.M. Abdul Hameed & Sons
P.O. Box No. 12,
Alwaye – 683101 (Kerala)

309 M.P. Rathinam & Co.,
260, Keela Masi Veethi,
Madurai – 625001

310 M.S. Hoda
Piska Farm
Piska Nagri
Ranchi-835303 (Bihar)

311 M.S. Vawda & Company
67 B.R.B.B. Road Canning Street
Kolkatta – 700001 (WB)

312 M.S.M. Ganesan & Co.,
1/L Makkan Compound
Soundamman Koil Street
Dindigul – 1

313 M.S.M. Srinivasan & Co.,
P.O. Box No. 45
1/O, Makkan Compound,
Soundamman Koli Street, Dindigul

314 M.S.P.M. Sanghu Nadar & Sons
Indian Drug Merchants
Dindigul – 624001

315 Madhura Industries
107 Rippon Street
Kolkatta-700016

316 Madhya Pradesh State Minor Forest Product
(T&D) Cooperative Federation Ltd.
38-B Vikas Bhawan, 4th Floor
Bhopal-462011 (MP)

317 Magan Lal & Company
Palton Bazar
Dehra Dun (Uttaranchal)

318 Mahaveer Gothi
C/o Dhan shree Jewelers,
Kothi Bazar
Baitul

319 Mahaveer Jari Booti Ayurved Bhawan
Rajeshwari Road,
Shivpuri – 473551

320 Mahesh Kumar Arun Kumar
P.O. Box No. 64, Hanumanganj,
Katni – 482005

321 Mahesh Trading Company
360/127, Mata Din Road, Sahadat Ganj
Lucknow – 226001

322 Majumdar Consultants
21 Shiv Mandir Shopping Complex
Chittaranjan Park
New Delhi(India)-110019

323 Makkar Pillai,
Alwaye, Kerala

324 Malwa Herbal Collection and Industries
Village Kamorda, Hosangabad Road,
Berkheda
Tehsil Goharganj, District Raisen – 464551

325 Mangal Commercial Corporation
215/88 Panjrenpole Road
Mumbai-400004

326 Manilal & Lallu Bhai Company
P.B. 2008 Kalbadevi Road
Near Narain Mandir
Mumbai-400002 (MS)

327 Manshuji Traders
485/1, Jawahar Marg,
Indore – 452001

328 Marriammal Mooligai Shop
Sunday Market, Thilakar Thidal,
Madurai

329 Matadin Bhagwam Dass
548 Katra Ishwar Bhawan
Khari Baoli
Delhi – 110006

330 Maxo Laboratories Pvt. Ltd.
35-E, Kamla Nagar, P.O. Box 2156
Delhi – 110007

331 Medha Herbal Products
197/1, Ceyon West, Mumbai – 400022

332 Meghalaya Forest Development
Corporation Ltd.
Laohumiera,
Shillong – 703001

333 Meghdoot Gramodhyog Seva Sansthan
E-7/132 Area Colony,
Bhopal – 462016 (MP)

334 Meghdoot Gramoudhyog Sewa Sansthan
Meghdoot Building, Chandan Ganj
Lucknow – 226001

335 Mehta Ove Chem,
No. 12, Kashyap Lane,
Off. BVK Lyengar Road,
Bangalore – 560053

336 Mehta Pharmaceuticals (P) Ltd.
Chheharata
Amritsar-143001

337 Merchants & Traders Pvt. Ltd.
32 Armencences Street
Kolkatta-700001

338 Merchants and Traders Pvt. Ltd.
32 Armencences Street
Kolkatta – 700001

339 Miller & Co. Pvt. Ltd.
24 Netaji Subhash Road
G.P.O. Box 2567
Kolkatta-700001

340 Minex Agencies
71 Ganesh Chandra Avenue
Kolkatta-700013

341 Mishree Lal Ueakay
Sankar Ward, Behind Excise Office
Ganj, Baitul (MP)

342 Modern Agricultural Services
Opp. Plot 60 Jai Hind Colony Deopur
Dhule – 424002 (Maharashtra)

343 Modi Industries
Sidhpur
Gujarat

344 Mohaideen Bai Raw Drug Dealer
Natham, Dindigul Dt.

345 Mohammad Ali Gulam Ali
45, Siyaganj, Indore – 452001

346 Mohammed Hussain Ajmal Hussain
6681/82 Khari Baoli, Delhi – 110006

347 Mohan Kumar & Company
158-187 Samuel Street
Mumbai-400009

348 Mohan Lal Laxmikant
Safdarganj
Northern Railway
Barabanki
Uttar Pradesh

349 Mohanraj Enterprises
151, Chetak Marg
Udaipur – 313001

350 Mohbe herbal Products (P) Ltd.
E-2/333, Area Colony,
Bhopal – 462016

351 Mohd. Hassan / Maqbool Hassan
6681-82, Khari Baoli,
Delhi – 110006

352 Mohhamad Hussain Ajmal Hussain
668/82 Khari Baoli
Delhi – 110006

353 Money Corporation,
T.C. 29/1095, Sreekanteshwaram,
East Road,
Thiruvananthpuram – 695023

354 Mookan Mooligai Shop
1660, Sunday Market
Thilakar Thidal,
Madurai

355 Mr. A. Stalin
Society for Rural Development
Regd. Office No. 1 5th Street
Bharatipuram, Dharmapuri – 636705
Tamilnadu

356 Mukhtyar Husain Gulam Abbas
46, Zumairat Bazar, Bhopal – 462001

357 Mukt Prasad Rameshwar Dayal
Ramnagar – 244714, District Nainital

358 Murari Lal Tek Chand
Katra Ishwar Bhawan
Shop No. 2, Om Market, 40 Khari Baoli
Delhi – 110006

359 Murugan & Bros
78, South Raja Street,
Tuticorin – 628001 (Tamil Nadu)

360 Muthuswam, S.P.
Great Cotton Road
Tuticorin-628001 (TN)

361 Mutual Trader,
49, Badrian Street,
Chennai – 600001

362 Mutual Traders
449 Naya Bans Khari Baoli
Delhi – 110006

363 Mutual Traders
49 Badrian Street,
Chennai – 600001

364 Mutual Traders,
No. 49, Badrian Street,
Chennai – 600024

365 Mysore Agencies
No. 34/1, III Cross, Lalbagh Road,
Bangalore – 560052

366 Mysore Sales International Ltd.
MSIL House
36 Cunningham Road
Bangalore-560052

367 N. Nandagopal Chetty,
41, Rasappa Chetty Street,
Chennai – 600003

368 N. Shobakant & Co.,
59, Govindappa Naicken Street
Chennai – 600001

369 N.L. Satyanarayana Shetty & Sons,
No. 142, Tharagupet,
Bangalore – 560053

370 Nadar P.P.M. Thangayaiah
972/2 North Third Street
Pudukottai

371 Narco Exports
A-340, New Sabzi Mandi
Azadpur, Delhi – 110033

372 Narmada Herbals and Medicinal Plants
Kairobbs Building, Civil Lines,
Near Railway Station,
Jabalpur – 482001

373 Nathi Mal Rugan Mal
6689, Khari Baoli,
Delhi – 110006

374 Nathubhai Kunverji & Company
Arna Bhawan
87-C Broach Street
Mumbai-400009

375 National Drug House
94-A, Ist Floor, Gandhi Gali,
Tilak Bazar, Khari Baoli,
Delhi – 110006

376 National Trading Company
Darshni Gate,
Dehra Dun – 248001 (UC)

377 Natural Bonanza
23, Model Basti
New Delhi – 110005

378 Natural Remedies Pvt. Ltd.
P.O. Box 456, 164/3 Basawi Mandir Road
Bangalore – 560004

379 Navin Bharat Manufacturers
D-373 Deence Colony
New Delhi-110024

380 Navneeth Lal Savilal
64 Mudi Bazar, Mandavi
Mumbai-400003

381 Nemchand Jain & Sons
Naya Bazar, Silliguri – 734405

382 New Kiryana Store
2565 Tilak Bazar, Khari Baoli
Delhi – 110006

383 New Udaya Pharmacy &
Ayurvedic Laboratories
Kadavanthara
Cochin – 682020
Kerala

384 Niharica International
105, Prakash Chambers
6, Netaji Subhash Marg, Daryaganj
New Delhi – 110002

385 Nirmesh
42, Jawara Compound
Mittal Chambers, Second Floor
Indore – 452001

386 Niyogi & Company
352-354 Samuel Street
Vadgadi
Mumbai-400003

387 North Gujarat State Isabgol Industries
Highway
Unjha
Gujarat

388 Om Prakash Madan Lal Pvt. Ltd.
2190-95, Gali Hinga Beg, Tilak Bazar
Delhi – 110006

389 Om Trading Company
330, Katra Hussain Bux
Khari Baoli, Delhi – 110006

390 Organon India Ltd.
Himalya House,
38 Chowringhee Road
Kolkatta-700016 (WB)

391 Orient Traders
615/VI, Bagh Jhanda Singh
Amritsar – 143001 Punjab

392 Oriental Herbs
E-26 Saket
New Delhi-110017

393 Orissa Forest Development
Corporation Ltd.
Bhubaneswar – 750002 Orissa

394 Orissa Overseas
606, Sixth Floor, Ashoka Estate
Barakhamba Road,
New Delhi – 110001

395 P. Rajendran
4/10, Varadaraja Perumal Koil St.
Tondiarpet, Chennai – 600001

396 P. Rajinder Kumar
Exporters and Importers
21-2-156, Gulzar Hauz
Hyderabad – 500002

397 P. Shanti Lal and Company
Raipur Road, Dhamtari – 492145

398 P.A.V. Sundaram
166 New Colony
Tuticorin – 628001 (Tamilnadu)

399 P.G. Money,
Pijoy School Building
Near Bank of Cochin
Munnar – 685612 (Kerala)

400 P.L. Associates
Botwala Building, Top Floor, 8
Horniman Circle
Fort, Mumbai – 400001

401 P.P.M. Nadar Thangayaiah
972/2 North Third Street Pudukottai
Tamil Nadu

402 P.P.M. Thangayaiah Nadar
South Cotton Road
Tuticorin – 628001 (TN)

403 P.S. Jammal & Sons
Street 16
430 Patel Nagar
Talab Tillo, Jammu
Jammu & Kashmir

404 P.S. Nathan & Company
48 Auna Nagar
Tuticorin-628008 (TN)

405 P.S. Sankaralinga Nadar
50 P.S.S. Nadar Street
Tuticorin – 628001 (Tamilnadu)

406 P.S.S. Exports
52, PSS Nadar Street,
Tuticoirn – 628001

407 P.S.S. Exports
No. 523, PSS Nadar Street,
Tuticorin – 628001

408 P.S.S. Gansshan
P.S.S. Nadar Street
North Cotton Road
Tuticorin-628001 (Tamil Nadu)

409 P.S.S.J. Mathan Sankar
P.S.S.J. Suthanthira Enterprises
121, North Cotton Road,
Tuticorin – 628001

410 Padam Prakash Anil Kumar
Kawari Bazar, Saharanpur – 247001

411 Palanichamy V.M.P.K.
T.R. Naidu Street Tuticorin
Tamilnadu

412 Panchsheel Trading Company
G-28, APMC Market – I, Phase – II
Turbhe, Navi Mumbai – 400703

413 Pandit & Company
D-49, Street 11, MIDC
Nasik – 422007
Maharashtra

414 Pannalal Brijlal
Tehri House, Haridwar – 249404

415 Parvatiya Sahkari Bhesaj
Vikas Evam Karya Vikraya Sangh
Pithoragarh – 262501 (UC)

416 Patel Corporation
Highway, Khali Sidhpur – 384151
Gujarat

417 Pearl & Company
Dr. Babasaheb Ambedkar Road
Byculla
Mumbai-400027

418 Penol Herbal and Company
219, Dwarka Nagar, N.B. Road
Badera – 460001, District Betul

419 People's Agricultural Farm
No. 34, S.S. Nagar
Pudukottai – 622001
Tamilnadu

420 Perfumes (India) Pvt. Ltd.
Nanpara House, B.N. Road
Lucknow – 226001

421 Pfimex International Ltd.
4-1-1240 King Kothi Road
Hyderabad – 500001

422 Pharma Impex
10 Middleton Road
Kolkatta-700071

423 Pharmaceutical Crude Drugs Enterprises
Kosi Road, Opposite State Bank
District Nainital
Ram Nagar-244715 (UP)

424 Pharmachem Internatinoal
361 Maulana Azad Road
Mumbai-400004

425 Pharmachem International
8 Camac street, Shantiniketan
Kolkatta – 700017

426 Phulchand Attar
Near Surya Narayan Mandir, Dollatganj
Lakshar, Gwalior

427 Phyto – Biotech International
GNB Road, Ambari
Guwahati – 781001 (Assam)

428 Pillay S.P.M. Pirama Nayagam
South Raja Street
Tuticorin – 628001 Tamilnadu

429 Plaster India
117, 118, S-1/8
Scheme No. 78
Indore – 452001

430 Poneselvan Traders
312 South cotton Road
Tuticorin – 628001 Tamilnadu

431 Prabhat Agri Biotech Pvt. Ltd.
3/6/168/7, First Floor
Haidurguda, Hyderabad – 500029

432 Prabhat Herbs
Latowali, Kankhal,
Haridwar – 249404 (UC)

433 Prasad & Sons
4771 Bharat Ram Road
23 Daryaganj
New Delhi-110002

434 Prashant Traders
Kankhal, Haridwar – 249404

435 Premji Haridas & Company
Bhanushali Chambers
166-170 Sant Tukaram Road
Mumbai
Mumbai (MS)(India)-400001

436 Presus Exports Corporation
Zoriwala Building
Chandi Bazar, Jam Nagar – 361001

437 Puneet Trading Company
10, Ist Floor, Humera Arcade
2/4 Issrail Mohalla, Samuel Street
Mumbai – 400009

438 Punj Traders
2087 Aggarwal Market,
Katra Tambacco,
Khari Baoli
Delhi – 110006

439 Quality Seeds Producer &
Marketer
Shivaji Chowk Parabhani – 431401
Maharashtra

440 Quest Marketing Company
Flat No. 101, 6-3-1112/7, Snowdrop
Apartments
Street No. 3, Green Landa, Begam Peth
Hyderabad – 500016

441 R.G. Herbal Pvt. Ltd.,
M-53 Palika Bhawan, Opp. Hotel
Hyatt Regency, R.K. Puram
Delhi – 110066

442 R.J. Anantharajaiah & Sons
APMC Yard, Batawadi – 572103,
Tumkur

443 R.M.K. Industries
1 First Cross Street, United India Colony
Chennai – 600004

444 R.N. Rajan & Co.,
1, Kumarappa Maistry Street
Chennai – 600001

445 R.S. Rathi
Station Road, Dhamtari – 492145

446 Radharam Sohan Lal
3 Malik Street
Kolkatta-700007 (WB)

447 Radhe Shyam Agarwal
Jaistambh Chowk, Umaria – 484661

448 Radhey Shayam Arvind Kumar Agarwal
2179, Right Town, Jabalpur – 482001

449 Radhey Shyam Rajinder Kumar &
Company
532 Katra Ishwar Bhawan
Khari baoli
Delhi-110006

450 Radhey Sons
367/3 Katra Hussain Baksh
Khari Baoli
Delhi-110006

451 Radhika Enterprise
536, Katra Ishwar Bhawan, Khari Baoli
Delhi – 110006

452 Raj & Company
Dasshera Maidan
Neemuch
Madhya Pradesh(India)-458441

453 Raj Kumar Gupta
Village Bikaman Khurd, Indaura Bagh
Lucknow – 226001

454 Raja Pachailai Shop
24-127, Sunday Market
Thilakar Thidal
Madurai

455 Raja Trading Company
Majith Mandi, Amritsar – 143006

456 Rajan Trading Co.,
28, Govindappa Naicken Street
Chennai – 600001

457 Rajasthan Choorna Bhandar
11/1, Teli Bakhal Malharganj
Indore – 452001

458 Rajendra Brothers
Highway, Khali Sidhpur – 384151
Gujarat

459 Ram Narayan Raj Narayan
Makaran Nagar
Kannauj
Uttar Pradesh-209725

460 Rameshwar Das Chottey Lal
2091 Katra Tambacoo, Khari Baoli
Delhi – 110006

461 Rameshwar Kisan Gopal
Naya Ganj, Kanpur – 208001

462 Ratan Lal & Sons
G.B. Pant Marg (Udham Singh Nagar)
Tanakpur – 262309

463 Robinsomar & Company
2 Mission Row Extension
Kolkatta – 700001 (WB)

464 Rokammal Mooligai Shop
25, Sunday Market
Thilakar Thidal, Madurai

465 Rokaria Agencies
Ampara, Dhamtari – 492145

466 Roli Health Centre
63, Mayur Market, Thatipur, Gwalior

467 Roshan Lal Sham Sunder
50-51 Akali Market Amritsar
Punjab

468 Rosma Overseas Pvt. Ltd.
4-6 Vandhana, 11 Tolstoy Marg
New Delhi – 110001

469 Rural Education and Development
Service (Reads), No. 32-A,
Denkanikottai road
PO Balathotanapalli – 07
Tamilnadu

470 S. Lalchman Singh & Sons
Katra Hari Singh
Amritsar
Punjab-143001

471 S. P. Muthuswami,
Great Cotton Road
Tuticorin – 628001 (TN)

472 S. Sangyong Corporation
206 Arunachal Building
19 Barakhamba Road
New Delhi-110001

473 S. Sattara & Company
1399, Tilak Bazaar, Khari Baoli
Delhi – 110006

474 S.B. Shah
23, Iya Mudali Street
Chentacnpet, Chennai – 600002

475 S.G.A. Kulandaivel Nadar & Sons
No. 223, East Masi Street,
Madurai – 625001

476 S.K. Dutta & Company
215 Old Dalanwala
Dehra Dun-248001 (UC)

477 S.K. Mundra
48, First Floor, Netaji Subhash Road
Kolkatta – 700001

478 S.K. Trading Co.,
195, Govindappa Naicken Street
Chennai – 600001

479 S.P. Muthuswami,
Great Cotton Road,
Tuticorin – 628001

480 S.P.K. Rajamani
56, Strotten Muthiah Mudali Street
Chennai – 600079

481 S.P.M. Pillay
Pirama Nayagam, South Raja Street
Tuticorin – 628001

482 S.S. Trading Company
M.G. Road
P.B. No. 21
Bijapur-586101 (Karnataka)

483 Sadala Herbal Remedies
131, Thapar Chambers-II,
Kalindi Colony, Ring Road,
New Delhi – 110014

484 Sahkari Vikas Sangh Ltd.
Gopeshwar – 246401
District Chamoli Garhwal (UC)

485 Saiba Industries Pvt. Ltd.
129-131, 4th Floor,
Kazi Sayeed Street
Mumbai-400003

486 Sakthi Selvam & Co.,
4, Sankaran Kinatru Street,
Virudhunagar

487 Sanjay Kumar Shailendra Kumar Jain
Sawarkar Colony, Near Sankar Mandir
Shivpuri – 473551

488 Sanjay Kumar Shankar Lal & Company
208 Surat Sadan
88/89 Surat Street
Mumbai-400009

489 Sanjay Traders
Highway, Khali Sidhpur – 384151
Gujarat

490 Santosh Ayurvedic Drug Supply Company
33 Daryansthan Street
Majit Bhandar
Mumbai-400003

491 Santosh Kumar Jar
Lalchand Shrichand Market
Hanumanganj,
Katni – 482005

492 Saraffin International
Kamadhenu No. 57, Bazullah Road
T. Nagar,
Chennai – 600017

493 Saraswati Trading Company
Satkar Hotel Gali, Station Road,
Raipur – 493001

494 Sardar Mal Bachmal Nahar
Zumairati Bazar,
Bhopal – 462001

495 Satpal Kamal & Sons
Bindu Sarover Road
Sidhpur – 384151 Gujarat

496 Satya Narayana Chandra Prakash
Ghandi
P.O. No. 32, Naya Bazar,
Ajmer – 305001

497 Satya Tara and Company
Continental Chambers, 1st Floor,
Room No. 2 142
Nungambakkam High Road
Chennai – 600034

498 Satyam Herbs and Spices
Sihawa, Raipur Road, Dhamtari – 492145

499 Selective Fragrances India Ltd.
Ganganagar Estate
F-126, 127 Malviya Industrial Area
Jaipur – 302017

500 Senthil Trading Co.,
13, Ponnappa Chetty Street
Chennai – 600004

501 Shah Khazi Punsi and Sons
Baitul ganj, Baitul (MP)

502 Shah Phulchand Deepak Kumar Jain
Zumairati Bazar, Bhopal – 462001

503 Shalaks Chemicals
C-3, Puja House, Karampura Community
Centre, Main Complex, New Delhi

504 Shankar & Company
519 Katra Ishwar Bhawan
Khari Baoli
Delhi – 110006

505 Shanthimalai Trust
P.B. No. 7, Shiva Nagar
Sri Ramanashraman PO
Tiruvannamalai – 606603
Tamilnadu

506 Sheetal Prasad Jain
Peeli Kothi, Kamala Ganj,
Shivpuri – 473551

507 Sheetal Traders
Naya Para, Raipur – 495223

508 Sheikh Nazir Ahmed
15 New Iddgha Building
Park Road
Baramula
Jammu & Kashmir

509 Shekherco
P.B. 256,
Muzaffarnagar – 251001 (UP)

510 Shell India
P.B. 1, Sheratallay, P.O. Thayakal
Ernakulam – 688530

511 Shiba Pada Kundu & Sons
168-B, Cotton Street
Kolkatta-700023 (WB)

512 Shiv Trading Company
Satkar Hotel Gali, Station Road,
Raipur – 493001

513 Shivalik Jadi Booti Bhandar
Purani Mandi Chowk, Near Miglani Building
Saharanpur – 247001

514 Shivan Dittamal and Company
Majeet Mandi
Amritsar – 143001

515 Shivnath Khairatilal
Morganj, Saharanpur – 247001

516 Shree Ganesh Aushadhi Bhandar
229 Kalbadevi Road
Mumbai – 400002 (MS)

517 Shree Ram agro Forestry Estate
New Block, 5, First Floor, Farishta Complex
Raipur – 493001

518 Shree Ramajayam Corporation
50 P.S.S. Nadar Street, North Cotton Road
Tuticorin – 628001

519 Shree Suvas Industries
Highway
Chaurasta
Palanpur-385002 (Guj)

520 Shree Swastik Export Corporation
Highway
Chaurasta
Palanpur-385002 (Guj)

521 Shree Swastik Industries (Raipur)
Manasnun
Raipur-492001 (MP)

522 Shree Swastik Industries
Deesa Highway, Chaurasta
Palampur – 385002 (Gujarat)

523 Shreeya Overseas
1701, Nirmal Tower, 26 Barakhamba Road
New Delhi – 110001

524 Shrengi Ayurved Bhandar
Subhash Sadan, Chandrawarkar Road
Behind Dang Kang Chowk, Worli,
Mumbai – 400092

525 Shri Ram Trading Company
Station Road,
Neemach – 458441

526 Shroff Channabasappa & Sons
No. 174-175, Avenue Road,
Bangalore – 560002

527 Shyam Sunder Gupta
2032 Aggarwal Market
Tambacoo Khari Baoli
Delhi-110006

528 Shyam Sunder Gupta
2032 Aggarwal Market, Katra Tambacco
Khari Baoli,
Delhi – 110006

529 Sidhayu Ayurvedic Research
Foundation Pvt. Ltd.
Baidynath House, 20 Great Nag Road
Nagpur – 460009, Maharashtra

530 Sidhpur Isabgol Processing Company
Bindu Sarover Road
Sidhpur-384151 (Guj)

531 Sierra Enterprises
163 Atlanta, 16th Floor, Nariman Point
Mumbai – 400021

532 Sigma Trading Company
Nafees Chambers, 3rd Floor
Lokmanya Tilak Marg
Mumbai-400001

533 Simple Herbs Enterprises
A-216 Somdutt Chambers,
Bhikaji Cama Place
New Delhi – 110066

534 Singapore Bharath Benjamin Co.,
116, T.H. Road,
Chennai – 600081

535 Singhal Trading Company
Satkar Hotel Gali, Station Road
Raipur – 493001

536 Siva Nattu Marundagam,
Bazaar Street, Mylapore,
Chennai – 600004

537 Solai Program
Christianpet, N.A.
Dist. Katpadi – 630027 (TN)

538 Sri Gopalakrishnan & Co.,
78, Varada Muthiappan Street
Chennai – 600001

539 Sri Parasakthi Traders,
219, Govindappa Naicken Street
Chennai – 600001

540 Sri Venkateswara Traders,
224, Govindappa Naicken Street,
Chennai – 600001

541 Sri Venkateswara Trading & Co.,
44, Andiappa Naicken Street
Choolai, Chennai – 600112

542 Sri Vinayagar & Co.,
Plot No. 103-3, Hoodwhart,
4th Lane, Waltax Road,
Chennai – 600079

543 Subhah Agro Products
18/46, Penty Naka, Queens Road, Cantt.
Jabalpur – 482001

544 Suman Trading Company
10-2/32/1 Pamuvair Street, Ramaraopeta
Kakinada – 533004 (AP)

545 Suresh Kapoor
Iswar Bhawan, Khari Baoli
Delhi – 110006

546 Suresh Trading Co.,
No. 432, Bio Bazaar,
Palakkad – 678012

547 Surya Pharmaceuticals
N-1/69, B. Krishna Bagh, Nagwa
Varanasi – 821005

548 Swami Corporation
4 Hari Niwas
C. Road Church Gate
Mumbai-400020

549 Swaroop & Company
330 Katra Hussain Baksh
Khari Baoli
Delhi-110006

550 Swasti Medical Store (Atul R. Shah)
177 – 178 Laxmi Road
Pune – 411002 (MS)

551 Swastic Traders
394 Kuth Bazar Mamaya Chambers
Mumbai-400009

552 Swastik Traders
394 Kuth Bazar, Mamaya Chambers
Mumbai – 400009

553 Syed Noor Ahmed
Santhepet,
Hassan – 573201

554 T.K. Rajan,
189, Govindappa Naicken Street
Chennai – 600001

555 T.S. Vijaya & Co.,
No. 159, Pullakottal Road,
Virudhunagar – 626001

556 Taj Trading & Company
6681 Khari Baoli Delhi – 110006

557 Thenammal & Company
54 P.S.S. Nadar Street
Tuticorin – 628001
Tamilnadu

558 Tibetan Medical & Astro
Institute (Men-Tsee-Khang)
Khara Danda Road,
Dist. Kangra
Dharamsala – 176215
Himachal Pradesh

559 Timex Agencies
9/48 Punjabi Bagh
Delhi – 110026

560 Tirkha Ram Om Prakash
585 Katra Ishwar Bhawan
Khari Baoli
Delhi – 110006

561 Tola Ram India Ltd.
68 Nalini Sett Road
Kolkatta-700070

562 Tribal Cooperative Marketing Development
Federation of India Ltd.
Savitri Sadan 2,
Preet Vihar Community Centre,
Vikas Marg, Delhi – 110092

563 Trimurti Enterprises
3 Satya Niketan, 1st Floor, Moti Bagh-II
New Delhi – 110021

564 Tripura Forest Development & Plantation
Corporatio
Kunjaban
Agartala-799001 (Tripura)

565 Tropical Trading Company
Tuticorin – 628001 Tamilnadu

566 Udayakumar Trading Co.,
60, Venkatesan Ali Street
Chennai – 600001

567 Union Trading Co.,
153/5, Govindappa Naicken Street
Chennai – 600001

568 Universal Carbon Company
46 Ezra Street
Kolkatta-700001 (WB)

569 Urmila Traders
502, Ishwar Bhawan, Khari Baoli
Delhi – 110006

570 Uttam Corporation
194 Khetwadi Main Road
Mumbai – 400004

571 V. Nathan Herbal & Cosmetics Pvt. Ltd.
Shed No. 72, SIDCO Industrial Estate
Kappalur
Madurai-625008 (TN)

572 V.S. Arulangadam & Sons
35 Ginfactory Road P.O. B. 47
Tuticorin – 628002 (TN)

573 V.V. General Traders
1 Sutharashahi Kundanpura
Muzaffar Nagar-251002 (UP)

574 Vadilal Vithaldas Patel
S.T. Road,
Sidhpur – 384151 (Gujarat)

575 Vardman Oushdhi Bhandar
Near employment Office, Ajadpur
Lalitpur – 284403

576 Vasavi Trading Co.,
122, Varadamuthiappan Street
Chennai – 600001

577 Ved Mahila Mandal
Near Gurudwara, Ranjit,
Jabalpur – 482001

578 Venus Herbo Aromatics Pvt. Ltd.
Muhavoor Road, Seithur
Rajapalayam Taluk,
Kamarajar – 626121

579 Vijay Agencies
C-14, APMC, Market – I, Phase – II
Turbhe, Navi Mumbai – 400703

580 Vijay Enterprieses
13, Ponnappa Chetty Street,
Chennai – 600081

581 Vijay Laboratories Pvt. Ltd.
First Floor, Raj Hotel Building
Aminabad Park,
Lucknow – 226015

582 Vijay Lakshmi Industries
Gol Bazar,
Dhamtari – 492145

583 Vinay Aggarwal
Ratanlal and Sons
GB Pant Marg,
Tanakpur – 262309

584 Vishal Traders
Sahadat Ganj
Lucknow – 226003 Uttar Pradesh

585 Vishram
306 Shaikh Menon Street
Mumbai – 400002

586 Warrier Herbal Products Ltd.
P.O. Box. 826, Visitors Buildings Complex
M.G. Road,
Thrissur – 680004

587 Wild Herbs Co.,
P.B. No. 78
Tuticorin – 628001

588 World Trading Corporation
Opposite Parda Bagh, Daryaganj
New Delhi – 110002

589 Yamuna Pharmacy
Yamuna Pharmacy Lane,
Jagadhri Road
Yamuna Nagar – 135001

590 Yan Exporters Pvt. Ltd.
210, Sampann Complex
Navrangpura,
Ahmedabad – 380009

591 Yogi Pharmacy Ltd.
Laskar Road, P.O. Gurukul Kungri
Haridwar – 249404 (UC)

11 IMPORTANT WORLD WIDE WEBSITES

1 **www.7song.com/common.**
Informations on *Common Medicinal Plants of The Northeast*

2 **www.aab.org.uk/meetings/mtgs2003/medplant.htm**
Medicinal Plants and Their Uses
In Association with the Institute of Horticulture. Imperial College, London

3 **www.actahort.org**
II International Symposium On Spices and Medicinal Plants
Convener, P. Tétényi.
Problems Of The Tolerance Of Medicinal Plants.

4 **www.actahort.org/books/73**
I International Symposium On Spices and Medicinal Plants
Convener, CH. Franz. Editor, CH.
Breeding Programme Of Medicinal Plants In Czechoslovakia (J. Luzný).

5 **www.afghan-web.com/fauna/medicinal.html**
Afghanistan Online: Medicinal Plants Found in Afghanistan
Anise Seed The Oil is used to flavor bad tasting medicines. Asafoetida An antispasmodic:

6 **www.ag.arizona.edu/classes/pls480/medicinalplants.html**
Medicinal Plants: Plant Sciences 480/580; Arid Lands Resource
Historical Medicinal Plants Information Guide to Resources in the Science and Engineering Library. Major Lecture Topics. Introduction

7 **www.ag.arizona.edu/classes/pls480/outline2002.html**
Medicinal Plants: Course Outline
Encyclopedia of Medicinal Plants by Chevallier.

8 **www.agnic.org/mtg/1998/medplant.html**
Medicinal Plants for Survival
An International Conference on Medicinal Plants Conservation, Utilisation, Trade and Intellectual and Cultural Property Rights.

9 **www.agric.gov.ab.ca/crops/special/medconf/kulow.html**
Pmapc - Marketing of Medicinal Plants
What is the Opportunity in Medicinal Plants?

10 **www.agric.gov.ab.ca/crops/special/medconf/mirza.html**
Greenhouse Production of Medicinal Plants
Most of the medicinal plants will grow in normally used greenhouse growing media.

11 **www.aircav.com/survival/appb/asappbtoc.html**
Survival - Table of Edible and Medicinal Plants

12 **www.allafrica.com/stories/200209231004.html**
Medicinal Plants; What Hope for the Future? Whenever possible, special gardens should be established for the cultivation of medicinal plants.

13 **www.allayurveda.com/research_medplants.htm**
Allayurveda.Com : Research Findings-Medicinal Plants in oral health care in India. Farooqi, AHA; Jain, SP; Shukla, YN; Ansari, SR; Sushil Kumar (Central Institute of Medicinal Plants)

14 **www.allconferences.net/conferences/20020702022643/ - 18k**
All Conferences. net, GLOBAL SUMMIT ON MEDICINAL PLANTS : Recent trends in Phytomedicine and other alternative therapies for human welfare.

15 **www.all-natural.com/chevbook.html**
The Encyclopedia of Medicinal Plants
This practical reference is the first comprehensive, fully illustrated guide to medicinal plants and their therapeutic properties.

16 **www.aloveria.com/english/plants.htm**
Medicinal Plants - Aloveria®
Canary Medicinal Plants Aloveria ®. Aloe Vera Aloe barbadensis, Orobal Wythania aristata, Hypericum Hypericum canariesis, Canary Sage

17 **www.altnature.com/library/identifying**
Wild, Herbal, Plants, Wildflower, Poisonous Plants, Photos,
Learning to identify and use herbal medicinal plants can be a rewarding hobby as will as a way to offset the high price of herbal extracts from the health food

18 **www.altnature.com/links/wild_herb.htm**
Wild Herb, Medicinal Plants, and Wildflower Conservations Links
Wild Herb, Medicinal Plants, and Wildflower Conservations Links. Maidenhair Fern. Tennessee Wildlife Resources Agency Endangered/Threatened Species.

19 **www.anbg.gov.au/library/medplant.html**
Australian Native Medicinal Plants Bibliography
EV & McCarthy, T. (1983) Australian medicinal plants. Methuen Australia, North Ryde, NSW.

20 **www.ansci.cornell.edu/plants/medicinal/**
Medicinal Plants for Livestock
Answer some basic questions about the safety and efficacy of some medicinal plants Benefits and toxicities of medicinal plants for livestock.

21 **www.ansci.cornell.edu/plants/medicinal/medpl.html**
Medicinal Plants for Livestock
Introduction to Medicinal Plants for Livestock. The idea of using medicinal plants to treat livestock is not new. Many of the active

22 **www.arbec.com.my/endangered%20plants.htm**
Over Extraction Poses Threat To Medicinal Plants, Herbs in
We should not expect rare and endangered plants to be attractive or spectacular. They may have medicinal qualities that cannot be underestimated.

23 **www.arizonacactus.com/medicine.htm**
Medicine
News , Garden , On The Desert , Tortilla Press, Medicinal Plants , Garden Pictures I , , Garden Pictures II , Membership Info , Food and Lodging

24 **www.ars.usda.gov/is/AR/archive/apr98/drug0498.htm**
Harvesting Drugs From Medicinal Plants

25 **www.ars-grin.gov/duke**
Phytochemical and Ethnobotanical Databases
FoodplantDB--Native American food plants. MPNADB—medicinal plants of Native America, Medicinal and Poisonous Plants. Description: Search plants by chemical, activity or ethnobotanical use. Includes list of browsable databases

26 **www.aun.eun.eg/community/cultivation_of_indigenous_medici1.htm**
Cultivation of Indigenous Medicinal Plants
An existing and projected demand for the cultivation of medicinal plants briefly summarized

27 **www.aun.eun.eg/distance/pharmacy/producti/**
Production of Medicinal Plants
Course description. Upon completion of this program, the student should be able to: Understand the sources of Medicinal plants.

28 **www.avro.co.za/africanherb.avro.co.za/keywords.html**
Traditional African medicinal plants, herbs and mutis.

29 **www.ayuherbal.com/medplantcatalogue**
Catalogue of Indian Medicinal Plants
Ayurvedic, herbal medicinal plants, consulting doctors on ayurveda and Pharmacognosy, ayurveda books, education, workshops, literature Search, new herbal recipe

30 **www.ayurvediclife.com/medicinal.htm**
Medicinal Plants. Which as receptacles of light were born three ages

31 **www.barwinnock.com**
Barwinnock herb nursery grows culinary herbs, medicinal plants, fragrant leaf plants and wildflowers using organic gardening principles.
Scottish nursery providing culinary, medicinal and fragrant herb plants that have been organically.

32 **www.bastar.nic.in/mplants.htm**
Informations on Medicinal Plants of the *District Bastar Chhattisgarh - Medicinal Plants*

33 **www.bbc.co.uk/worldservice/sci_tech/highlights/000907_arnold.shtml**
Medicinal Plants of Kenya , Science and Technology , BBC World
Medicinal Plants of Kenya for centuries plants have been used in the treatment of illness.

34 **www.bgci.org.uk/congress_rio_1992/hamilton.html**
International trade in medicinal plants: conservation issues and potential roles for botanic gardens. Alan Hamilton. International trade in medicinal plants.

35 **www.bigchalk.com/cgi-bin/WebObjects/**WOPortal.woa/wa/BCPageDA/sec~GA~7367~~ - 21k
Bigchalk: Homeworkcentral: Medicinal Plants
Informations on Middle School/ Science/ Life Sciences (Biology)/ Plant Sciences (Botany)/ Reference/ Images/ General Botany on Medicinal Plants

36 **www.bio.davidson.edu/Biology/kabernd/seminar/studfold/MedPl/MedPl.html**
This for hundreds of years, indigenous cultures have been using plants for medicinal and spiritual purposes.

37 **www.biopark.org/Plants-Amazon.html**
Ecology, plants, animals, indigenous people, and cultures of the Amazon by noted medical ethnobotanist Dr. Ethan Russo Medicinal Plants of the Peruvian Amazon.

38 **www.botanicadventures.com/resources**
Medicinal Plants Resources. Books. NHBS list of Economic Botany & Ethnobotany books Tibetan Medicinal Plants Companies, Products. Medicinal Plant Products, Inc.

39 **www.cabi-publishing.org/JOURNALS/Abstract/RAMP/Index.asp**
Review of Aromatic and Medicinal Plants - An Online Abstracts
Information on research on medicinal plants, aromatic plants, essential oils, natural products, herbal drugs, herbs and spices.

40 **www.cadefarms.org/herbs.htm**
Medicinal Plants and Herbs
During 1999, the pilot year of our Medicinal Herbs & Plants Project fifteen trial plots were planted in medicinal plants that will be tested for potency.

41 **www.cambiumgardening.com/books/herbs/**
Herbs, Medicinal Plants, Seasonings and Other Specialties
Herbs and medicinal plants come down to us from ancient times, they are interesting and fun to grow, plus they enhance the salad and your family's good health.

42 **www.chili.rt66.com/hrbmoore**
Michael Moore - Sw School of Botanical Medicine
Research, Resources, FAQs, Regional plant checklists Plant Constituents Taken from a variety of sources
Description: Medicinal plant photographs, illustrations, maps, abstracts, constituents, monographs, major papers

43 **www.cieer.org/symposia/presentation**
International Symposium: Ethnobotany, Medicinal Plants, Folk
Informations on Medicinal Plants. Ethnobotany, Medicinal Plants, Folk Traditions. History, Pharmacology. Botany, Muqologia, Istoria, Farmakologia, Eqnoiatria.

44 **www.cimap.org**
Cimap Central Institute of Medicinal & Aromatic Plants Lucknow (UP)
Informations on Medicinal Plants

45 **www.conserveafrica.org/medicinal_plants.rtf**
Overview on Medicinal Plants and. Traditional Medicine in Africa. The Importance of Traditional Medicine in Africa. Status of the medicinal plants base resource.

46 **www.dantewada.nic.in/medi.htm**
Informations on Medicinal Plants.of *Distrct Dantewada Chhattisgarh - Medicinal Plants*
After through survey he was awarded PhD for documenting the Eight Area of the medicinal plants of the world.

47 **www.dittmar.dusnet.de/english/esamoa**
Samoa: Traditional Medicinal Plants
Traditional Medicinal Plants of Samoa. Samoan Medicinal Plants in vrml (3 D).

48 **www.ecouncil.ac.cr/rio/focus/report/english/worldcon.htm**
Andar 'S Experience With Medicinal Plants
Indigenous Peoples and Global Governance: Special Report for Rio+5 Process The World Council of Indigenous Peoples - Conrado Jorge Valiente [Español].

49 **www.edwardrhamilton.com/subject2/hgm.html**
Herb Growing & Medicinal Plants
Catalog, Herb Growing & Medicinal Plants. Current titles are current titles at special prices Botany and Healing: Medicinal Plants of New Jersey and the Region.

50 **www.espace-nature.com/English/herb_store.htm**
Espace Nature - Herbalist Herbal Medicine Aromatic and Medicinal
Since the dawn of time, have been a source of health for man, we offer you a whole range of organically grown aromatic and medicinal plants.

51 **www.export-forum.com/eng/africa_agro_3.htm**
Spices, Condiments, Aromatic and Medicinal Plants From Africa
Africa export offers for spices, condiments, tropical plants and medicinal herbs. Spices,

52 **www.fao.org/docrep/W9195E/w9195e07.htm**
The Supply of Medicinal Plants in Kwazulu-Natal
Percentage of healers reporting changes in the sales of medicinal plants.

53 **www.fao.org/docrep/X5335e/x5335e05**
Non-Wood Forest Products of Bhutan - Medicinal Plants
Trade in medicinal plants in the past. In Bhutan's past, medicinal plants.

54 **www.farmersmarketonline.com/EONS.htm**
Medicinal Seeds Available Direct From Eden Organic Nursery
Now Available: Seed for Medicinal plants, Tobaccos, Specialty vegetables, indoor plants, vines and Organics.

55 **www.fcmsdocs.org/Conference/7th/7anewclassofantihiv.html**
A New Class of Anti-HIV Agents from Medicinal Plants.

56 **www.floraeeb.uconn.edu/collections/medicinal.html**
Medicinal Plants
Special Listing: Medicinal Plants. More importantly, many of the plants in our collections have reputed medicinal properties according to some sources.

57 **www.floridaplants.com/medicinal.htm**
Medicinal Plants. The Order. Atlas of Microscopy of Medicinal Plants, Culinary Herbs, & Spices Betty P. Jackson Derek W. Snowdon; Pub.

58 **www.floridaplants.com/mpharm.htm**
Pharmacology of Medicinal Plants
Poisonous Plants Reference Research. Pharmacology: Anthroposophical Approach to Medicinal Plants; Medicines That Changed the World;

59 **www.forestryimages.org/browse/catsubject.cfm?cat**
Medicinal Plants: Your query produced: records. Subject Name, Order, Family, Scientific Name. medicinal plants, USDA

60 **www.frim.gov.my/tu/ppframe.htm**
Medicinal Plants Division
Forest Research Institute Malaysia Medicinal Plants Division "Natural Healthcare for the Public" Seminar On Medicinal and Aromatic Plants 2001.

61 **www.fs.fed.us/ipnf/eco/yourforest/edibleplants/**
Edible and Medicinal Plants of North Idaho - a guide to common edible and medicinal plants on the Idaho Panhandle National Forests.

62 **www.gajma.com/forums/Table_Talk/posts/15.htm**
Uses of Medicinal Plants in Haiti.

63 **www.generalvitamin.com/product/**
Encyclopedia of Medicinal Plants - General Vitamin
A practical reference guide to more than 550 key medicinal plants and their uses. Encyclopedia of Medicinal Plants

64 **www.geocities.com/littleflowers_2000/medmain.html**
Littleflower's Medicinal Plants of North America
California Herbal Remedies : The History and Uses of Native Medicinal Plants by Lolo Westrich.

65 **www.geocities.com/RodeoDrive/Mall/4992/generalindex3.html**
Littleflower's Medicinal Plants - Jkl Index
Edible and Medicinal Plants of the West, Tom Brown's Guide to Wild Edible and Medicinal Plants, The Encyclopedia of Popular Herbs: From the Herb Research.

66 **www.giga.com/~nacondor/**
Herbs, Nutritional and Medicinal Plants
Exports, Imports and Marketing of Medicinal Plants

67 **www.gisdevelopment.net/application/environment/overview/frcf0001.htm**
Eco-Distribution Mapping of Medicinal Plants of Conservation
GIS Application: Forestry, Ecology & Biodiversity: Eco-distribution mapping of medicinal plants of conservation concern of Southern India.

68 **www.godsremedy.com/qualities.htm**
Gods Remedy - Medicinal Plants and Their Properties
Listing of medicinal plants and their properties including bacteria, microscopic algae, mushrooms, ferns, brushes and trees.

69 **www.grand-bahama.com/plants.htm**
Grand Bahama Island -- Medicinal Plants
Ashrubs (Medicinal Plants) of Grand Bahama Island's. From a botanical viewpoint, perhaps the most interesting plant found on.

70 **www.growinglifestyle.com/h/garden/plants/herb/**
Growing Herbs, Spices and Medicinal Plants
Informations on Medicinal Plants

71 **www.haworthpressinc.com/store/product.asp?sku**
The Haworth Press Online Catalog: Product:
Journal of Herbs, Spices & Medicinal Plants. Levels of Interest and Knowledge in Herbs, Spices, and Medicinal Plants.

72 **www.hellbenderpress.com**
Medicinal Plants
Native Americans have used these medicinal plants for centuries to treat a number of ailments.

73 **www.herbalgram.org/herbalgram/articleview.asp**
Thai Medicinal Plants Recommended for Primary Health Care System
Free Samples Advertise Submit Articles Order Issues Reprint Articles Issue: Thai Medicinal Plants Recommended for Primary Health Care System.

74 **www.herbalgram.org/herbalgram/articleview.asp?a**
Modern Medicinals: Herbs, Spices and Medicinal Plants; Recent Advances in Botany, Horticulture, and Pharmacology.

75 **www.holistic-online.com/Herbal-Med/hol_herb-forms.htm**
Forms of Herbs. The goal of the herbalist is to release the volatile oils, antibiotics, aromatics, and other healing chemicals contained by the herb.

76 **www.hort.cabweb.org/Aromatic/Ramp_cov.htm**
Review of Aromatic and Medicinal Plants covers the literature on cultivated.

77 **www.hort.cabweb.org/Aromatic/ramphome.htm**
Review of Aromatic and Medicinal Plants
The world literature on cultivated and wild species of culinary herbs, spices, essential oil plants and medicinal plants.

78 **www.hort.purdue.edu/newcrop/med-aro/default.html**
A Guide To Medicinal and Aromatic Plants
Aromatic, Spice, and Medicinal Plants, General information about this site, instruction for use, acknowledgments, a comment/suggestion form, and information

79 **www.hort.purdue.edu/newcrop/med-aro/toc.html**
Aromatic and Medicinal Plants Index. A to Z. Abelmoschus moschatus. Achillea millefolium. Aconite. Acorus calamus

80 **www.ics.trieste.it/environment/medicinalplants/ medicinalplants.htm**
Industrial Utilization of Medicinal and Aromatic Plants. Most developing countries are endowed with vast resources of medicinal

81 **www.ics.trieste.it/webservices/databases/mapsdb.htm**
MPNADB (Medicinal Plants of Native America Database). The database includes standardized information on all plants and not specifically on medicinal plants.

82 **www.idrc.ca/reports/read_article_english.cfm?article_num**
IDRC Reports: Global Information Network On Medicinal Plants
MEDPLANT the Global Information Network on Medicinal Plants was created in 1999 as a support to the existing medicinal plant networks.

83 **www.indianmedicine.nic.in/html/plants/plants.htm**
Ayurveda - Indian Systems of Medicine & Homoepathy
Complete Report of the Task Force on Conservation and Sustainable use of Medicinal Plants

84 **www.indmedplants-kr.org**
Indian Medicinal Plants
Full text of book "Database of Medicinal Plants" by Dr. C. Kameswara Rao of Bangalore University.

85 **www.indmedplants-kr.org/Biodiversity_And_Conservati_1.Htm**
Biodiversity and Conservation of Medicinal Plants
Genetic Diversity. Taxonomy and Diversity Of Medicinal Plants. Loss Of Biodiversity.

86 **www.infodienst-mlr.bwl.de/la/lap/pflqual/analymet/Trocknung_E_kurz.htm**
Quality of Microwave Dried Medicinal Plants and Herbs
WD Koller, Th. Drying, especially of medicinal plants and herbs or mushrooms is another application.

87 **www.inforamp.net/~jwhitley/amindmed.htm**
'American Medicinal Plants' and draw on the accumulated wisdom and folklore of years! NEW! ... AMERICAN MEDICINAL PLANTS" by Charles F. Millspaugh.

88 **www.inforamp.net/~jwhitley/harvplnt.htm**
"Identifying and Harvesting Edible and Medicinal Plants"
In Wild (And Not So Wild) Places" by "Wildman" Steve Brill.

89 **www.intracen.org/mns/medplants.html**
Medicinal Plants and Extracts. Market News Service for Medicinal Plants and Extracts presents prices and market intelligence

90 **www.intracen.org/tdc/pmr/t_324.htm**
Trade Documentation Centre - Published Market Research
Descriptors: Medicinal plants, Europe, Marketing research. Language: English.

91 **www.iracambi.com/english/medicinal_plants.htm**
The Iracambi Medicinal Plants Project (IMP) was established with the aim of developing commercially viable and sustainable methods of cultivating the medicinal.

92 **www.islamset.com/sc/plants/pana.html**
Used in the Traditional Arabic Medicine> Inventory of Medicinal Plants

93 **www.kit.nl/about_kit/html**
Domestication of and Trade in Medicinal Plants - Kit Rural Change
KIT Rural Change examines possibilities for domestication of and trade in aromatic and medicinal plants. Enhancing both biodiversity.

94 **www.kol.to/health3.htm**
Kerala - Health
Medicinal Plants Common Name, Malayalam Name, Botonical Name, Family. Black cutch, Karingali, Acacia catachu, Mimosaceae. Asparagus, Sathavari, Asparagus race-mosus

95 **www.kreisels.com/ittm/ayurNET/subject01.htm**
The Ayurnet - Pharmacognosy, Biodynamic Cultivation of Medicinal
Biodynamic Cultivation of Medicinal Plants, Ethno-Botany, Pharmacognosy. Field of Research: Pharmacognosy, Cultivation of Medicinal Plants and Ethno-Botany.

96 **www.kreisels.com/ittm/medicinalPlant/BiodynamicCultivation.htm**
Biodynamic Cultivation of Medicinal Plants At Ittm, Kalimpong
Biodynamic Cultivation Medicinal Plants. at ITTM, Kalimpong ITTM steers New Dimensions in Cultivation Medicinal Plants, Part I. New Dimensions

97 **www.lavoisier.fr/notice/fr2743000280.html**
Livre Pharmacognosy, Phytochemistry, Medicinal Plants, ...
Focussing on medicinal plants, pharmacognosy, phytochemistry, medicinal plants extends to plants that provide additives for pharmaceutical or food technology.

98 **www.lib.umt.edu/guide/ig-mediplants.htm**
Medicinal Plants Information Resources. Prepared by: Barry Brown, Science Librarian

99 **www.library.arizona.edu/library/teams/set/medplant.html**
Medicinal Plants Information Resource Guide
This guide is designed to encourage and facilitate research pertaining to medicinal plants

100 **www.life.umd.edu/classroom/bsci124/lec29.html**
Bsci 124 Lecture Notes - Medicinal Plants
Ask Dr. James A. Duke, noted ethnobotanist and leading authority on medicinal plants.

101 **www.lunerouge.com/produits/prod01_e.htm**
Lune Rouge : Cd-Rom : Medicinal Plants of Madagascar.

102 **www.magdalin.com/herbal**
An Illustrated Herbal - 500 Medicinal Plants and Their Properties
Holistic Medicine, holistic medicine, Traditional Chinese medicine, TCM, Indian Ayurveda, health maintenance, herbal medicine, medicinal plants, herbal remedies

103 **www.mail.ics.trieste.it**
Standardization Techniques for medicinal plants and their products. Description: Herbal medicines in recent period have gained enormous popularity.

104 **www.mda.state.mn.us/esap/greenbook2002/105mig**
Informations on Medicinal Plants*: Potential of Medicinal Plants for Rotational Grazing*

105 **www.mfpfederation.com/content/med_plants.asp**
Minor Forest Produce Federation - Medicinal Plants
Resource Map Tendu Patta Chebulic Myrobolan Sal Seed Gums Other MFPs

106 **www.mind.net/app/planthom.htm**
Medicinal Plants of The Applegate
This sampling provides a brief discussion of some of the plants found in the Applegate Valley of Southwestern Oregon that may be of some medicinal

107 **www.mountainvalleygrowers.com/books/theencyclopediaofmedicinalplants.htm**
They are using is the correct one, and that it is fresh and organically grown.
The Encyclopedia of Medicinal Plants

108 **www.mtnforum.org/calendar/events/0005mpta.htm**
"Medicinal Plants, Traditional Medicines and Local Communities in
Traditional Medicines and Local Communities in Africa: Challenges and Opportunities of the new Millennium" Nairobi, Kenya

109 **www.mtnforum.org/resources/library/impn97a.htm**
"IMPN Newsletter - A special Newsletter of the IDRC Medicinal Plants Network" -Mtn-Forum On-Line Library Document. IMPN Newsletter

110 **www.naturalhealthholistic.com/chevbook.html**
Articles News Nutrition Links Books Find related books at Amazon.com. The Encyclopedia of Medicinal Plants. by and rew Chevallier.

111 **www.naturallist.com/plantme2.htm**
Medicinal Plants 2
Over 100 bioactive ingredients used for hypertension, stop bleeding.

112 **www.naturallist.com/plantmed.htm**
Medicinal Plants
The Petterson Field Guides on Medicinal Plants by Foster and Duke on medicinal applications on plants

113 **www.ncl-india.org/barea/biotech/area07.html**
Medicinal Plants
India is known to be the richest natural resource of medicinal plants. Basic and applied research concerning thorough...

114 **www.nepalicongress.org.np/nepal/medicinal_plants.html**
Medicinal Plants Of Nepal and Their Availability. Medicinal plants of Nepal (1968) enumarated 393 species along with their therapeutio uses.

115 **www.niam.com/corp-web/mediplnt.htm**
Ayurveda: National Institute of Ayurvedic Medicine
Complete and updated profiles on many of these plants from the Ayurvedic

116 **www.nimh.btinternet.co.uk/ejhm/2_2_mm1.htm**
Medicinal Plants of the Pacific North West. back to materia medica Chanchal Cabrera MNIMH, AHG, CAHP.

117 **www.nps.gov/plants/medicinal**
Pca Medicinal Plant Working Group's Website: Green Medicine
Medicinal plants are used commercially, thanks to contributions of traditional cultures worldwide, modern medicine, and pharmacognosy.

118 **www.nps.gov/plants/medicinal/plants.htm**
Mpwg: Medicinal Plants
Green Medicine > Medicinal Plants

119 **www.owc.org.mn/think-3/health/english/emiin%20urgamal.html.**
Medicinal plants are great chemist in nature. There 99 percent of this is produced from medicinal plants.

120 **www.paddleasia.com/tropical_plant_edible.htm**
Thailand tropical plants: edible plants and medicinal plants of southern Thailand. All PaddleAsia tours are educational.

121 **www.pakpost.gov.pk/philately/stamps2002/ medicinal_plants_of_pakistan.html**
Medicinal Plants of Pakistan
Zufa Hyssop was known to the early Greeks, Romans

122 **www.pc4.sisc.ucl.ac.be/prelude.html**
Medicinal Veterinary Plants in Sub Saharan Africa
Data bank resulting from traditional medicinal plants harvests in sub saharan Africa.

123 **www.permacult.com.au/herb/herb09.html**
Medicinal Plants: Herbal Remedy, Natural Remedies
The presentation of "key" medicinal plants features 100 of the best known

124 **www.pharmabiz.com/newsfeat/alter241.asp**
Pharmabiz.Com: Icmr Funded Survey of Medicinal Plants of Western
A detailed multi-centric survey of medicinal plants. By Nandita Vijay, Bangalore

125 **www.phytochemistry.freeserve.co.uk/frames/commerce.htm**
Commercial Research in Medicinal Plants
Commercial research services in the phytochemistry and pharmacognosy of medicinal plants and natural products.

126 **www.phytochemistry.freeserve.co.uk/frames/analysis.htm**
Analysis of Medicinal Plants and Herbs
The analysis of herbal products and medicinal plants are carried out in our laboratories under the supervision of Dr John Wilkinson, Head of the Phytochemistry.

127 **www.planningcommission.nic.in/aboutus/taskforce/tsk_medi**
Task Force On Medicinal Plants
Report of the Task Force on Conservation & Sustainable use of Medicinal Plants
Government of India Planning Commission
March - 2000

128 **www.plantbioassay.com/publications.asp**
Medicinal Plants From Buenavista De Cuellar
Computerized Ethnomedical Database Of Medicinal Plants From Buenavista De Cuellar, Guerrero, Mexico. Medicinal Plants Of Vilcabamba.
A study to generate a computerized ethnomedical database of local indigenous medicinal flora from.

129 **www.plantsavers.org**
Welcome To United Plant Savers
Our Mission: United Plant Savers' mission is to protect native medicinal plants of the United States and Canada and their native habitat
Network of business, government and nonprofit groups trying to stop plant extinction and save native

130 **www.pomegranatecommunications.com**
Herbs and Medicinal Plants Knowledge Card Deck
Informations on Medicinal Plants

131 **www.publications.worldbank.org/ecommerce/ catalog/product?item_id**
World Bank Publications: Medicinal Plants Details
Medicinal Plants: Rescuing a Global Heritage by John Lambert , Noe Vietmeyer

132 **www.rain-tree.com**
Wealth of The Rainforest - Pharmacy To The World From Raintree
Many organizations have demonstrated that if the medicinal plants, fruits, nuts, oils and other resources like rubber, chocolate and chicle, were harvested.
Company and product information and data on the Amazon Rainforest from a USA pharmaceutical company.

133 **www.rain-tree.com/bulkprod.htm**
Rainforest Medicinal Plants From Raintree Nutrition
Brokering medicinal plants into the US market from South and Central America is a growing profitable industry with many participants of varying experience

134 **www.rbgkew.org.uk/peopleplants/wp/wp1/africa1.htm**
People and Plants Online - Working Paper 1: African Medicinal
Throughout Africa, the gathering of medicinal plants was traditionally restricted
to TMPs or to their trainees (Photo 1).
Knowledge of many species was limited
People and Plants Online

135 **www.rhino.org.za/flora_medicinal.htm**
Home Medicinal Plants
Most medicinal plants are presently harvested from wild stocks. Species are harvested

136 **www.rosneath.com.au/ipc6/ch02/brooks2**
Revitalisation of The Indigenous Flora (Particularly Medicinal
Revitalisation Of The Indigenous Flora (Particularly Medicinal Plants) and Traditional Knowledge Of The Coromandel Coastal Region Of South India.

137 **www.rrlbhu.res.in/aromatic.htm**
Aromatic and Medicinal Plants
Facilities: Herbarium of plants of the State of Orissa; Research Garden of Aromatic & Medicinal Plants;

138 **www.ru.ac.za/affiliates/herbarium/leaf2b.html**
Medicinal Plants in The Eastern Cape
The products that they sell range from patent medicines to traditional medicines, which invariably include medicinal plants still in their natural form.

139 **www.sahealthinfo.org/traditionalmeds/antimalarialproject.htm**
Anti-malarial medicines from the medicinal plants of southern Africa project.

140 **www.saps.plantsci.cam.ac.uk/articles/curall.html**
To discover more about the history of plants used in medicine, have a look at the web site of the Royal College of Physicians of Edinburgh

141 **www.seps.org/oracle/oracle.archive/Life_Science.Ecology/2001.03/000983495098.7573.html**
Student's there. Also, many libraries have good books on Medicinal plants. Good luck. Sincerely,. Steven E. Carpenter, Ph.D.

142 **www.siddhacongress.net/dis_med_plants.htm**
Gandeepam.Org Welcomes You
Display of Medicinal Plants Around 500 species of Siddha Medicine. A make shift herbarium will form part of the Medicinal Plants display.

143 **www.somagardens.com/nsps/**
Nova Scotia Plant Savers Saving Wild Medicinal Plants.
United Plant Savers' mission is to protect native medicinal plants of the United States and Canada and their native habitat while ensuring an abundant.
NSPS' mission is to protect native medicinal plants and their habitat. They encourage land stewardship

144 **www.stevenfoster.com/photography/cd/**
Medicinal Plants Volume I - Royalty Free Cd
This royalty free CD ROM contains 102 photos of some of the most popular medicinal plants

145 **www.stuartxchange.com/Collection.html**
How To Collect Medicinal Plants: Philippine Alternative Medicine
Storage Many medicinal plants are seasonal, some not easily accessible, available only in deep forests or mountain peaks.

146 **www.stuartxchange.com/OtherHerbals.html**
List of Other Herbal Medicinal Plants in The Philippines
The voluminous compilation and its regional nomenclatures reflect the widespread cultivation and use of medicinal plants in the Philippines

147 **www.suite101.com/subjectheadings/contents.cfm**
Medicinal Plants Links, Articles and Topics At Suite101.Com
start with. or. contains the word(s). Subject Heading: Medicinal plants, Topics, Articles, Best-Of-Web Recommendations. Topics.

148 **www.sweetsunnah.com**
Sweet Sunnah - Black Seed Derived From Nigella Sativa (Medicinal)
Black seed, a natural herb recommended by the Prophet Muhammad that Sweet Sunnah is proud to carry along with lots of other medicinal plants herbal products.

149 **www.swsbm.com/Ephemera/Ginseng-Harding-1**
Ginseng and Other Medicinal Plants
A Book of Valuable Information for Growers as Well as Collectors of Medicinal Roots, Barks, Leaves,

150 **www.telecom.net.et/~ibcr/Medicinal%20Plants.htm**
Medicinal Plants Genetic
Introduction. Medicinal plants in Ethiopia comprises more than 800 species of flowering plants.

151 **www.teriin.org/biodiv/medicine.htm**
Sustainable Harvest of Medicinal Plants: A Case Study of Biligiri
Case studies. Biodiversity. Sustainable harvest of medicinal plants: a case study of Biligiri Rangaswamy Temple Wildlife Sanctuary, Karnataka, India

152 **www.thinknatural.com/superstore/dept.asp?dept_id**
Think Natural - Natural Living in The Modern World
Vitamins & Minerals Herbs & Medicinal Plants Natural Bodycare Aromatherapy Homeopathy Books & CDs Flower Remedies Pet Health Natural Lifestyle

153 **www.tibetanmedical.com/serv04.htm**
Tibetanmedical.Com Service 4
Medicinal plants from Qingzang plateau.

154 **www.tlahui.com/educai7.htm**
The Mexican Traditional Medicine and its Medicinal Plants. ... Name of the Graduate. The Mexican Traditional Medicine and its Medicinal Plants.

155 **www.tlahui.com/medic/medic7/**
Medicinal Plants Used in Ethnogastroenterology. Fennel. Tlahui-
Medicinal plants used in Ethnogastroenterology, including: Common names, scientific names, habitat, botanical characteristics, properties, uses in traditional.

156 **www.tnhealth.org/imtmp.htm**
Links - Health & Family Welfare Department, Govt. of Tamil Nadu
Introduction to Medicinal Plants: There has been a resurgence in the consumption and demand for medicinal plants.

157 **www.tpwd.state.tx.us/expltx/jrnat/medplants.htm**
Texas Junior Naturalists-Medicinal Plants
Make a Plant Press , Make Seed Balls. Medicinal Plants. Many potential medicinal plants have toxic compounds.

158 **www.tradeforum.org/news/fullstory.php/aid/301/Medicinal_Plants.html**
International Trade Forum - The Quarterly Magazine
It is, therefore, not possible to assess global trade in all medicinal plants.

159 **www.traffic.org/dispatches/archives/june2000/samerica3.html**
Traffic Dispatches Number 14 June 2000
Medicinal plants in trade Medicinal plants as well as their derivative products, such as potions, pills and creams, are sold daily in the local markets

160 **www.tropilab.com/tropicalrainforest.html**
Tropilab Inc, The Tropical Rainforest and Medicinal Plants
The tropical rainforest of Suriname has numerous medicinal plants & herbs used in traditional- and alternative medicine.

161 **www.unani.com/medicinal_plants.htm**
Medicinal Plants/Ethnobotany.
Role of Some common Unani medicinal plants of South India, An appraisal. Germplasm assessment.

162 **www.undp.org.in/Programme/Environment/ mplants/default.htm**
Medicinal Plants Conservation and Sustainable Utilization
Environment Programme Support Sub-Programme for Medicinal Plants Conservation and Sustainable Utilization

163 **www.undp.org.in/Programme/Environment/mplants/toc.htm**
Medicinal Plants Conservation and Sustainable Utilization
Environment Programme Support Sub-Programme for Medicinal Plants Conservation and Sustainable Utilization: CONTEXT 1. Brief Description of Programme Support

164 **www.unep-wcmc.org/species/plants/ghana/aburi.htm**
Medicinal Plants in Ghana
Conservation and sustainable use of medicinal plants in Ghana 1999-2002. Aburi Botanic Gardens. The magnificent central avenue at Aburi.

165 **www.users.argonet.co.uk/users/quilljar/nznat.html**
New Zealand Native Medicinal Plants
It is important to be careful about dose when trying medicinal plants as some can be toxic in the wrong quantity or preparation.

166 **www.vedamsbooks.com/medicina.htm**
Medicinal Plants & Ethnobotany of India
Books on Medicinal
Plants and Ethnobotany. ... Dictionary of Medicinal Plants/RG Brown.
Comprehensive annotated catalogue of books including complete table of contents and jacket excerpts.

167 **www.virtualseeds.com/chinamed-main.html**
Oriental Medicinal Plants
For pictures of many of these plants, visit the University of Washington Medicinal Herb Garden. Additional information.

168 **www.vitex.f9.co.uk/world.htm**
Sara Hamer, Medicinal Plants Are At Risk All Over The World. I
The largest users by far of medicinal plants are commercial companies making over-the-counter remedies. Medicinal Plants are at Risk all over the World.

169 **www.webpages.charter.net/czar207196/120medi.htm**
120 Medicinal Plants
Herbs in the garden: Medicinal plants include every life form (annual, biennial and perennial herbs, deciduous and evergreen trees shrubs, and woody.

170 **www.who.int/medicines/library/trm/medicinalplants/ medplantsdocs.shtml**
Who/Edm/Traditional Medicine/Medicinal Plants
Herbal medicines. Medicinal plants. WHO monographs on selected medicinal plants WHO Geneva, 1999 (92 Swiss Francs).

171 **www.who.int/medicines/library/trm/medicinalplants/medplantspacific.shtml**
Who/Edm/Traditional Medicine/Medicinal Plants in The South
Medicinal Plants in the South Pacific, WHO Regional Publications, Western Pacific Series

172 **www.world.std.com/~krahe**
Herbs and Aromas: Uses, Properties
Herbs and medicinal plants properties and uses. Description and knowledge of Medicinal Plants and Herbs.

173 **www.world.std.com/~krahe/html1.html**
Medicinal Plants List
Medicinal plants and their properties
List of some commonly used medicinal plants

174 **www.wwf.org.uk/core/wildlife**
WWF-Uk: Medicinal Plants
The market for medicinal plants is rapidly expanding, placing great pressure on natural resources.

175 **www.xs4all.nl/~rainmed/bulletin/india1-e.html**
Medicinal Plants In India's Computer City Bangalore. FRLHT's International

12 GLOSSARY

Abdominal tumour: Localized undesirable generally morbid growth of tissue in the abdomen

Abortifacient: An agent that promotes abortion

Abrupt: Ending suddenly

Abscensses: Painful inflammation leading to a localized collection of pus in a cavity formed.

Acaulescent: Having no stem or almost none.

Accrescent: Increasing in size with age

Accumbent: Lying against and face to face

Achene: Single seeded, dry, indehiscent fruit of Asteraceae

Acicular: Shape of a narrow, cylindrical leaf; needle-like.

Acorn: An achene that grows in a cup.

Actinomorphic: Symmetrical in several planes

Aculeate: Bearing prickles.

Acuminate: Gradually tapering to a prolonged point

Acute: Tapering to a sharp point

Adaptogenic: Helps the body adapt to stress and supports normal function

Adhmana: Flatulence

Adnate: Attached by the whole length

Adpressed: Pressed flat to the axis.

Adventitious: Arising irregularly and not in the normal order

Aerial part: Any part of a plant that grows above ground.

Aestivation: The manner in which the part sof the flower are arranged and folded before expansion (in bud)

Agglomerate: Collected or gathered in a mass.

Air-layering: A method of vegetative reproduction.

Albumen: The nutritive tissue stored within the seed outside the embryo

Albumin: A nutritive substance of the embryo of a seed.

Alburnum: The lightest coloured wood immediately beneath the bark; sapwood;

Alcoholate: The product obtained from the alcoholic distillation of medicinal herbs.

Algiform: Resembling an alga

Alluvial: Stream or river-laid soil deposit

Alterative: An drug which corrects disordered process of nutrition and restores the normal function of an organ or of the system

Alveola: A surface cavity

Amavata: Rheumatic diseases

Amenorrhoea: The absence of menstruation during the time of life when it should occur.

Amentia: A last stage of degenerative dementia (a mental syndrome)

Amla: Sour

Amlpitta: Acird peptic disease

Amphitropous: Said of an ovule curved to bring its two ends near together

Amplexicaul: Stem clasping as the bases of some leaves for petioles

Anabolic: Promotes tissue growth

Anaemia: Any condition wherein the number at red blood cells, and the amount of haemoglobin are less than normal

Anaesthetic: Produces insensibility to external sensations.

Anaha: Constipation

Analgesic: That which relieves pain without causing loss of consiousness

Anaphrodisiac: Inhibits libido and sexual activity

Anasarca: Oedema or swelling, due to the fluid, filling the space at subcutaneous connective tissue level

Anastomosing: When veins meet and join to form a net

Anatropous: Said of an ovule inverted on its funicle so that the opening is close to the hilum and the chalaza at the other end

Androecium: The entire male reproductive part of a flower

Androgynous: Male and female flower in the same inflorescence

Angiosperm: Plant with seed in a closed ovary

Anisomerus: When the different series of a flower are unequal in number

Annual: Plants that complete their life-cycle in one year or a season.

Annular: In the form of a ring

Anodyne: A drug that relieves pain

Anorexia: Lack or loss of appetite for food

Anthelmintic: A drug that kills intestinal worms

Anther: That part of the stamen containing pollen

Anthocarp: A false fruit formed by the fusion of the whole or a part of the flower with the fruit itself

Anthraquinones: Irritate the intestinal wall causing a bowel movement

Anti aging agent: An agent that is effective against aging

Anti inflammatory: An agent that suppresses inflammation

Anti pyretic: An agent that reduces/ relieves fever

Anti septic: An agent that destroys the pathogenic micro-organisms or their toxins in blood or other tissues

Anti spasmodic: An agent that prevents/relieves spasms (a sudden repetitive violent muscular contraction)

Anti-aphonic: Restores the voice.

Anti-atonic: Soothes tired muscles.

Antibiotic: Destroys or inhibits micro-organisms

Anticholesterolemic: Prevents the build up of abnormal cholesterol levels in the blood.

Anticoagulant: Prevents blood clotting

Anticous: The fore part that most remote or turned away from the axis

Antidermatosic: Acts to prevent or cure skin complaints.

Antidiarrhoeic: Controls diarrhoea.

Antidropsical: Prevents water retention (dropsy).

Anti-ecchymotic: Prevents bruising.

Anti-enuretic: Prevents bed-wetting and incontinence.

Antifungal: Combats fungal infections

Anti-glycosuric: Reduces level of sugar in the urine; used to treat diabetes.

Anti-icteric: Combats jaundice.

Anti-inflammatory: Reduces inflammation

Antileucorrhoeic: Reduces vaginal discharge sometimes known as 'whites'.

Antimicrobial: Destroys or inhibits micro-organisms

Anti-oedematous: Reduces swelling.

Antioxidant: Prevents oxidation and breakdown of tissues

Antiphlogistic: Reduces inflammation.

Antiplethoric: Acts against high blood pressure and circulatory disturbances.

Antipruritic: Relieves itching.

Antipyretic: Prevents or reduces high temperatures.

Antipyretic: A drug which reduces fever

Antisaturnismic: An antidepressant.

Antisclerotic: Softens unnaturally hard skin.

Antiscorbutic: Prevents or cures scurvy by providing vitamin C.

Antiseptic: Destroys or inhibits micro-organisms that cause infection

Antispasmodic: A drug which counteracts spasmodic disorders

Antitussive: Soothes and relieves coughing

Anti-uricaemic: Prevents build up of abnormal levels of uric acid in the blood (gout).

Anuloma: Mild laxative

Aperient: Mild laxative

Aperitif: Encourages the appetite.

Apex: Tip or upper part

Aphrodisiac: A drug which promotes sexual desire

Apical: Forming a point.

Apicula: A short, sharp, but not rigid point

Apiculate: Ending in a short, sharp point.

Apocarpus: When the carpels are free and separate

Apressed: Pressed closely and flat against another organ

Aquatic: Plants growing in water

Areole: A space marked out in anyway; a small cell or cavity

Arid: Dry locality

Aril: A secondary covering over the seeds of some plants.

Aril: Secondary covering over the seed in certain plants

Arillate: Having aril

Arishta: Medicated wine

Arista: A bristle like appendage, common in grasses

Aristate: Tipped with a beard or awn (e.g. Barley).

Arka: Distillate

Armed: Provided with spines or thorns

Aromatherapy: A method of treatment using essential oils.

Aromatic: Plant with high levels of volatile oil

Aromatic/distilled water: A secondary product of the distillation of medicinal herb essences.

Arsha: Haemorrhoids

Artavajanana: That which promotes ovulation/menstrual flow.

Arthritis: Painful inflammation of the joint

Articulate: Jointed, provided with nodes or joints

Asava: Medicated wine

Ascending: Curving upwards

Aseptic: Free from germs and microorganisms.

Aseptic: Free from contamination by harmful bacteria, viruses or other micro-organisms

Ashmari: Calculus/stone

Asthma: Chromic disease of respiration with attacks of breathlessness, wheezing and tightening of the chest

Astringent: That which causes contraction and hence healing

Atisara: Diarrhoea

Attenuate: Narrowed, tapered

Auricle: A small lobe; an ear-shaped appendage

Autonomic nervous system: Part of the nervous system responsible for the control of bodily dunction that are not consciously directed, e.g. Sweating, beating of the heart

Avaleha: Medicine in a thick viscous from to be licked

Awn: The apical bristle on the bracts that envelop the inflorescences of the Gramineae (grasses). Also called arista or beard.

Axil: The angle formed between the main stem and a branch, leaf stalk or flowering stem.

Axil: Upper angle formed by leaf stem and supporting stem or branch

Axile: Belonging to the axis

Axillary: Situated in an axil

Axis: An imaginary line around which organs are developed; any member which bears lateral subsidiary members

Ayurveda: Traditional Indian system of medicine

Balsamic: Heals or soothes inflammation.

Balya: Beneficial to physical strength, increasing resistance to disease, immunity.

Barbellate: Provided with short, stiff hairs, especially if retrorse

Bark: Outer sheath of tree trunk

Basal: Placed at the base

Basal leaves: Leaves growing from the base of the stem

Basti: Urinary bladder

Basti roga: Disease of bladder

Basti shodhana: Said to cleanse the bladder

Beak: A narrowed, usually solid prolonged tip; not used for leaves

Bearded: Equipped with an awn, beard or arista.

Berry: A fruit with an inner layer to the fruit wall, a fleshy central tissue area and a number of seeds.

Bhedana: Purgation

Bhedaniya: Purgative

Bhrimhana: Having doby-weight increasing effect

Biennial: A plant that completes its life cycle from seed to maturity and death over two growing seasons. Flowering and fruiting often occur in the second year.

Bifid: Two-lobed

Bilabiate: Formed into two lips.

Biliary deobstruent: Promotes the flow of bile.

Biliousness: A complex symptom due to excessive bile secretion leading to nausea (vomiting sensation), discomfort in abdomen and constipation

Bipinnate: Having lobes that themselves having lobes

Biternate: (Of leaves) formed into two sets of three.

Bitter: A bitter principle which acts on the mucous membrance of the mouth and stomach to increase appetite and promote digestion.

Black water fever: Malarial fever

Blade: Expanded part of a leaf, lamina

Blepharitis: Inflammation of the eyelids.

Bole: Stem or trunk of tree

Bract: Reduced leaf subtending flowers

Bracteole: A small bract, often on the petiole or immediately below or on the calyx

Bradycardia: Abnormally slow heartbeat.

Bristle: Stiff hair

Bronchial asthma: An asthmatic condition wherein there is sudden recurrence of attacks of breathlessness affecting one or more larger passages of the lungs

Bronchitis: Inflammation of one or more larger passages of the lungs

Broncho dilator: An agent that expands the air passages of the lungs

Bud: A protruberance on a plant, from which a leaf, shoot or flower develops.

Buddhi smruti prada: Beneficial to intellect and memory

Bulb: A modified bud, usually underground and with fleshy scales or coats

Bulbil: A small, usually aillary bulb in leaf axils

Bullate: Blistered or puckered as the leaf of a savoy cabbage

Caduceus: Dropping off very early; deciduous.

Calamus: The hollow stem of a plant with few articulations.

Calculus: Formation of stones, usually composed of mineral salts in a natural cavity in the body

Caliune, caulinary: Growing from the stem.

Calyptra: The apical part of a root. Also known as the pileorhiza, root-cap.

Calyx: A collective name for the outer whorl of the flower formed by leaf-like parts known as sepals and which are usually green.

Cancer: A disease wherein there is abnormal multiplication of cells

Caphal-algia: Headache

Capitulum, head: An inflorescence consisting of a head of densely-packed stalkless flowers.

Capsule: Dry, many-sectioned fruit which generally splits open to release its numerous seeds.

Carcinogenic: Causes cancer

Cardiac debility: Weakness of heart

Cardiac diseases: Diseases of heart

Cardiokinetic: Strengthens the heart.

Cardiotonic: Improves heart function

Carina: A longitudinal ridge; part of the flowers of legumes.

Carminative: A drug which relieves flatulence

Carpel: One of the modified fertile leaves, a component of the gynaecium that encloses the ovules and bears the stigma.

Carpels: Parts composing the ovule-bearing part of a flower

Carrier oil: Oil such as wheatgerm, to which essential oils are added in order to dilute them for use

Caruncle: Protuberence or peculiar growth near the attachment of seed

Caryopsis: Single seeded, dry, indehiscent fruit of Poaceae

Cataplasm: Or poultice – a hot or warm application of specially prepared medicinal herbs.

Catarrh: Inflammation of a mucous membrane (particularly of the head and throat), with discharge of running nose

Catarrhal bronchitis: Inflammation of mucous membrane of the larger air passages of lungs, with catarrhal discharge

Cathartic: Having a gentle purgative action.

Catkin: A pendulous slender spike of unisexual flowers.

Caustic: Corrosive or burning.

Chakshushya: Beneficial to eyes

Chhardi: Vomiting

Chhedaniya: Lierally, chhedan-cutting asunder, having similar properties on body tissues.

Cholagogue: Amedicament that increases the flow of bile.

Cholera: An acute infectious disease wherein there is severe diarrhoea and vomiting

Choorna: Powder

Chronic Laryngitis: Inflammation of the organ of voice persisting for a long time

Chronic stomachalgia: Pain in the stomach persisting for a long time

Chronic ulceration: Formation/development of ulcer persisting for a long time

Cicatrizer: A medicament which accelerates the formation of scar tissue.

Ciliate: Sort hairs on the margin of an organ

Cinereous: Grey of wood ashes

Circulatory stimulant: Increases blood flow, usually to a given area, e.g. Hands and feet

Cladode: A modified stem resembling a leaf.

Clasping: Sessile leaf whose base partly or wholly surrounds the stem

Clavata: Club shaped

Clay: Stiff tenacious earth

Colic: Abdominal pain produced by strong contractions of intestines or bladder

Colitis: Inflammation of a part of large intestine

Collodion: A yellowish fluid used for sealing wounds or burns.

Collutory: A mouthwash or gargle.

Collyrium: A lotion for eye disorders, an eyewash.

Composite flowers: Flowers of plant of the *Compositae* family, typically having ray or disc flowers, or both

Compound: Leaves or flowers made up of many individual small

Compound leaf: Leaf divided at its midrib into leaflets

Compress: A cloth pad soaked in a hot or cold herbal extract and applied to the skin

Condenser: That part of the distilling apparatus where the vapour condenses.

Cones, strobilus: Bracts forming an inflorescence in a cylindrical-conical shape; characteristic of conifers.

Congestive heart failure: Failure of heart to pump the blood to the body

Conjunctivitis: Inflammation of the delicate membrane lining the eyelids and covering the eye ball

Connate: Joined or attached to ; used with similar parts fused during formation (e.g. Petals).

Consumption: Tuberculosis of the lungs

Convex: Curved outward

Convulsions: Seizure (series of contractions of the muscles)

Coppices: Small wood of undergrowth, grown for periodical cutting

Cordate: Having heart-shaped leaves

Coriaceous: Leather-like.

Corm: An underground stem with sufficient starch

Corn: A horny thickening of a skin layer caused by friction and pressure, which forms a conical mass, producing pain and irritation

Corolla: Collective name of the petals of a flowers

Cortex: The covering of the trunk or main stem and branches of a bush, shrub or tree (bark).

Corymb: Racemose inflorescence with flowers at nearly same height

Coryzide: Relieves the symptoms of the common cold.

Cotyledons: Seed leaves, usually emerging on germination

Counter-irritant: Superficial irritant used to relieve more deep-seated pain or discomfort

Cramps: A painful spasmodic muscular contraction

Cream: A mixture of water and fat or oil that blends with the skin

Creeping: Spreading over or below ground and producing roots

Cremocarp: A type of fruit which breaks up into two individual seeds which hang from the plant (diachaenium).

Crenate: Having round toothed margin

Crown: Corona, also that part of the stem at the surface of the ground

Crustaceous: Having hard and brittle texture

Cryptogamic: Without true flowers and seeds

Culm: Stem of grasses and sedges

Cuneate: Wedge-shaped, tapering gradually towards the base

Cuspidate: Tapering to a long point

Cutting: A method of vegetative reproduction.

Cyathium: Type of inflorescence of the genus euphorbia

Cyme: Inflorescence with the oldest flowers terminating the growth and younger flowers below

Cystitis: Inflammation of the urinary bladder

Cytostatic: Slows down the growth process of tumours.

Daha: Burning sensation

Danta-shoola: Toothache

Dechlorurant: Removes excess salt from the system.

Deciduous: Plant that sheds leaves each year

Decoction: A preparation made by boiling a medicinal herb.

Decongestant: Relieves congestion.

Decorticated: Bark or husk that has been removed.

Decumbent: Spreading horizontally on the ground with the apex finally rising up

Decurrent: A leaf that narrows down into the petiole and main stem.

Decussate: Said of pairs of opposite leaves when they are at a 90° angle to those above and below.

Deepan: Promoting digestive functions

Dehiscent: Fruits, that open at maturity

Delirium: A mental disturbance of sort duration with characteristic overtones in speech

Deltoid: Shaped like an equilateral triangle

Demulcent: An agent having a soothing effect on the skin and mucous membrances

Density: The relationship between the mass of a body and the mass of water occupying an equal volume at 39.2° F. (4°C).

Dentate: Sharpely toothed

Dentifrice: A preparation for condition wherein there is morbid sadness

Depurative: Detoxifying agent

Dermatopathy: Any skin disorder

Detergent: A clearnsing agent that can be used directly on wounds.

Detoxification: The process of aiding removal of toxins and waste products from the body

Diabetes: Any disorder characterized by excessive urine excretion

Diabetes mellitus: A kind of diabetes with increased sugar in the blood

Diachaenium: Cremocarp.

Diaphoretic: An agent that promotes perspiration

Diarrhoea: Abnormal frequent evacuation of watery stools

Dichasial cymes: A cymose inflrescence in which all axes end in flowers

Digestive: Aiding the digestive process.

Digitate: Compound leaf, with leaflets arising from one point; fingered

Dioecious: Plants with male and of female flowers in different plants

Diphteria: An acute infectious bacterial disease affecting the throat

Disc flower: Usually inner flowers in the flower head of the Asteraceae, usually hermaphrodite

Distichous: (Of leaves) having the organs arranged in two vertical rows.

Diuretic: A drug which increases the secretion and discharge of urine

Doctrine of signatures: Theory that the appearance of a plant reveals its medicinal properties

Dormancy: A condition of not growing or germinating

Double-locular: Having two chambers or compartments.

Drastic: Has a violent purgative action.

Dropsy: An abnormal accumulation of fluid in spaces in between the cells of the body. (An old term for oedema)

Drupe: A fruit with a thin outer layer, a fleshy inner layer and a stone consisting of a hard casing and a seed.

Durgandhyanashana: Deodorant

Dynamis: A process in the preparation of homoeopathic medicines.

Dysentry: A condition wherein there is excretion of stools frequently containing blood and mucus etc.

Dysmenorrhoea: Painful menstruation

Dyspepsia: Impairment of functioning in digestion

Dysuria: Painful or difficult urination

Ecchymosis: Causes bruising.

Ecuelle process: A process for extracting the essential oil from citrus fruit.

Electuary: A preparation made from powdered medicinal herbs mixed to a soft paste with honey or sugar.

Elephantiasis: A chronic filarial disease, usually seen in the tropics, due to infection

Elixir: A liquid herbal preparation with a pleasant taste, due to the addition of honey or sugar

Ellipsoidal: Having the nature or shape of an ellipse.

Elliptical: Tapering at both ends with the broadest part across the middle.

Emarginated: Deeply notched at the apex

Emetic: An agent that causes vomiting

Emmenagogue: An agent that promotes menstruation

Emollient: Softens or soothes the skin

Endermic: Acting through the skin.

Endocarp: Inner layer of fertilized ovary or fruit

Endosperm: Reserve food outside embryo but close to it in seed

Enfleurage: A method of extracting essential oils.

Ensiform: (Of leaves) sword-shaped.

Entire: Even margin (leaves)

Epicalyx: Bracts subtending the calyx closely

Epicarp: The outermost layer of the fruit.

Epicotly: Part of the stem between cotyledons and the node of the frits true leaf.

Epilepsy: A diseased condition wherein there is recurrent convulsive attacks

Epiphyte: Plant growing on another

Epispastic: Having a blistering action.

Epistaxis: Nose bleed; blleding at the nose

Erect: Arising upright; perpendicularly

Erytherma: Inflammation of the skin in rose-coloured patches.

Essential oil: Distillation of volatile oils derived from aromatic plants

Ethereal compound: An ether-based medicine.

Eupeptic: A digestive aid.

Euphoric: Gives a general sense of well-being.

Evergreen: Having leaves all round the year

Exalbuminous: Without albumen

Expectorant: A drug that promotes the removal of catorrhal matter and phlegm from the bronchial tubes.

Expectorant: Stimulates coughing and helps clear phlegm from the throat and chest

Extract: A product resulting from a transformation of the simples; it can be dry, semi-fluid or fluid.

Fascicled: Close cluster or bundle (closely aggregated)

Fasciculate: Growing in bundles.

Febrifuge: Reduces fever

Fibrous: Thread-like

Fimbriate: Long hairs on the margins of an organ

Fistular: The hollw, cylindrical stem of a herbaceous plant (e.g. Reed, grass).

Fistulous sores: Fistula is an abnormal passage in the body with lesion of the skin or mucous membrane

Fixed oil: A non-volatile oil (plant constituent). An oil produced by hot or cold infusion (preparation)

Flask: A balloon-shaped glass vessel with a long, narrow neck and usually, a flat bottom; it forms part of a distillation apparatus.

Flatulence: Excessive formation of gases in stomach or intestine

Fleshy: Thick and soft

Flexuous: Full of bends and curves.

Florentine flask: A glass recipient with an outlet to one side, for the distillate.

Floret: A small flower, part of a head or cluster.

Follicles: Dry dehiscent fruit opening by ventral suture

Freckles: A pigmented spot on the skin resulting from exposure to sunlight

Fulvous: Brownish yellow

Galactofuge: A medicine to reduce the flow of milk in nursing mothers.

Galactogogue: A medicine to increases the flower of milk in nursing mothers.

Galanical: A medicine, in a standard formula, prepared from plants

Gall: An excrescence on some part of a plant caused by an insect or disease organism.

Gamopetalous: Having petals that are joined.

Garbhada: Promoting fertility/conception (in females)

Garbhakaraka: See garbhada

Garbhashayya sankochaka: Oxytocic

Garbhashayyottejaka: Uterotropic

Gastric irritability: Irritation in the stomch

Gastropathy: Any disease of the stomach

General debility: General weakness

Geniculate: Bent like a knee

Ghana: Dried aqueous extract

Ghrita: Literally-ghee; (medicated ghee)

Gingivitis: Inflammation of the gums

Glabrous: Hairless.

Glabrous: Not hairy

Glabrous: Without hairs

Gland: Small, usually globose secretory structure, containing liquid; either iside organs (vesicle), or wartlike on the surface, or fixed upon a stalk (glandular hairy).

Glandular tumours: A new growth of tissue of glands

Glaucoma: A disease of the eye characterized by increased intra ocular pressure

Glaucous: Covered with blue green powdery bloom

Glomerule: A cluster of flowers.

Glume: Bracts on the base of a spikelet, usually in pairs (grasses)

Gnarled: Covered with protuberances

Gonorrhoea: Infectius veneral disease

Gout: It is a type of acute inflammatory arthritis

Grahi: That which binds the stools

Granular cell tumour: A new growth like lesion of soft tissue

Granular-conjunctivitis: A granular inflammation of conjunctiva of the eye

Green-manuring: The planting of clover and other nitrogen-fixing plants to enrich the soil.

Guna: Property/ies

Guru: Heavy/that which is digested slowly

Gutika: Pill

Gymnosperm: With unprotected (naked) seeds

Gynaecium: The female part of the flower formed by the carpels.

Haemoppietic: Promotes the formation of blood.

Haemoptysis: Spitting of blood or blood stained sputum

Haemorrhoid: Painful sweeling of veins of the anus

Haemostatic: An agent that stops bleeding

Hair: Uni- or multicellular outgrowth of the epidermis arrow-shaped (leaves)

Hallucination: A case of perception that has no basis in external stimulation

Hallucinogen: An agent that leads to experience false perceptions

Hallucinogenic: Causes visions or hallucinations

Hastate: Basal leaf lobes pointing outwards

Haustorium: Organ of parasites through which they penetrate and tap their host for nutrients and water

Head: Compact inflorescence of essile flowers; racemose type

Heamolytic: Breaks down the red blood corpuscles to separate the harmoglobin.

Heamorrhages: Bleeding

Heartwood: Denser inner part of tree trunk yielding hardest timber

Helminthiasis: The condition at having intestinal vermiform parasites

Hemostatic: Stops or reduces bleeding

Hepatic: Affects the liver

Hepatoprotective: Protects the liver.

Herb: A plant or part of a plant that is valued for its medicinal, culinary or aromatic properties.

Herbaceous: A plant that is not woody and has leafy growth which dies down in winter.

Herbalism: Subject relating the the study of medicinal (officinal) plants.

Herbalist: A person who is knowledgeable about medicinal plants.

Hermophrodite: With bisexual flowers

Herpes: Any inflammatory skin disease marked by the formation of small vesicles in clusters

Hesperidium: A fruit of which the endocarp is divided into chambers.

Hikka: Hiccough

Hikkanigrahaka: That which controls hiccough

Hilum: Scar left on seed at the point of attachment to the fruit

Hirsute: Densely and softly hairy

Hispid: Covered with long stiff hairs.

Homoeopathy: Therapy based on the concept of a close similarity between disease and remedy.

Humour: An important body fluid in traditional European or Indian medicine

Hyaline: Thin and transparent

Hydragogue: An agent producing watery discharge, especially from the bowels

Hyperdipsia: Excessive thirst

Hypertension: High blood pressure

Hypnotic: Induces sleep

Hypocarp: Enlarged pedicel below the fruit

Hypocholesterolic: Excessive cholesterol in the blood.

Hypochondriasis: Morbid anxiety about one's health

Hypocotyls: Part of the stem between root and cotyledons

Hypoglycaemic: Reduces the level of sugar in the blood.

Hypoglycaemic: Lowers blood glucose levels

Hypogynous: Free from but inserted below the ovary

Hypotension: Low blood pressure

Hypotensive: Reduces high blood-pressure.

Hysteria: Psychiatric disorder with delirious speech

Imbricate: Overlapping, like tiles on a roof.

Immune stimulant: Stimulates the body's immune defences to counter infection

Immuno- modulators: An agent that adjusts the immune response to a desired level

Imparipinnate: Leafltets arranged on either side of axis ending with terminal one

Impotency: Lack of reproductive power

In origin: Procumbent trailing loosely on the ground, without rooting

Incised: Deeply cut

Incumbent: Resting or leaning upon

Indehiscent: Not splitting naturally when ripe (fruit)

Indented: With an indented margin.

Indumentum: A covering of hairs

Inflammation: A pathological process where there is pain, heat, redness and swelling

Inflexed: Bent

Inflorescence: A group of flowers that grow on the same stem.

Influenza: An acute viral infection of the respiratory tract

Infusion: Water-based preparation in which flowers, leaves or stems are brewed in a similar way to tea

Inhalation: Breathing of medicinally infused steam or liquid through the nasal pasges

Insectivorous: Traps and digest insects and other small animals

Insomnia: Inability to sleep or sleeplessness

Intercostals neuralgia: Pain extending along the course of one or ore nerves in between the ribs

Intermittent fever: A fever that recurs regularly, e.g. Malaria

Internode: Part of the stem between two nodes

Intrinsic calculi: Stones within urinary tract

Involucre: A collection or rosette of bracts subtending a flower cluster.

Jwara: Pyrexia

Kamala: Jundice

Kanthya: Demulcent beneficial to voice, larynx, throat

Kapha: One of the three Doshas

Karma: Drug Action/Biodynamic effect of drug

Kasa: Cough

Kashaya: Astringent taste, and also, decoction

Keeled: Ridged and folded along the middle

Keshya: Promoting healthy hair

Krimi: Parasites (including microorganisms)

Kshara: Alkaline extract of plant

Kshaya: Pthisis

Kushtha: Dermatoses

Kwatha: Decoction

Labiate: Lipped

Lacerate: With a jagged, irregular margin.

Laciniae: Deep, narrow incisions in the margin of a leaf or petal.

Laciniate: With a margin cut into deep, narrow and irregular strips.

Lactiferous: Yielding milky fluid

Laghu: Light/Easy to digest

Lamina: Leaf-blade

Lanceolate: Lance-shaped, tapering to a pointed apex.

Lateral: On the side

Latex: Milky fluid found in various plants and trees

Lavage: A cleansing of the stomach using emetics in large quantities of water.

Lavan: Salt and salty taste

Laxative: Relaxes the bowels and has a gentle evacuant action.

Layering: A vegetative method of reproduction.

Leaflet: A segment of a compound leaf.

Legume: Or pod, a fruit that opens into two on ripening.

Lekhana: Weight/reducing

Lemma: The inner of two bracts enclosing the flower of a spikelet (grasses); inner to the glumes

Lenitive: Has a mildly analgesic action.

Lenticel: A pore through young bark which allows for gaseous exchange.

Lenticel: Biconvex shaped corky spots on young bark

Lepa: Medicinal paste for topical use

Leucoderma: A condition wherein there is a localized loss of pigmentation of the skin

Leucorrhoea: A whitish, viscid discharge from vagina and uterine cavity

Ligulate: With ligule, which is an appendage at base of leaf

Ligule: A thin appendage at the base of the blade of a leaf.

Linear: Several times as long as broad, with more or less parallel edges, narrow

Liniment: External medication applied by rubbing

Lipid: A preparation with a fatty excipient as a base, greasy to the touch and insoluble in water.

Lithontriptic: A preparation for the elimination of small stones from the body.

Loam: Fertile soil of sand and clay with admisture of decayed organic matter

Lobate: Divided into lobes.

Lobe: A rounded segment of a leaf.

Lobed: Organ deeply divided, with the division not reaching the middle; cleft (leaves, perianth)

Locule: The chamber or cavity of an ovary.

Loculicidal capsule: Dehiscence of capsule where each opens by separate slit

Lomentum: Legume fruit with contractions between seeds which break at maturity

Longevity: Length of duration of life

Lumbago: Pain in the lumbar region

Lunate: Half-moon shaped

Lyrate: Lyre-shaped, the terminal lobe being large than the lateral ones.

Maceration: A simple method of extracting the active principles of a plant, where the ingredients are steeped in liquid.

Madakaraka: Soporific

Madhura: Sweet taste (in context to vipaka-having anabolic effect)

Male potency: Capacity in males to reproduce

Medhya: Beneficial to/ promoting intellect

Medicinal wine: A medicine with a wine base.

Meha: Urnary disease/s

Melancholia: A depressed and unhappy emotional state with abnormal inhibition of mental and bodily activity

Membranous: Skinlike, thin, soft and transparent

Menorrhoea: Excessive menstruation

Mesocarp: The middle layer of pericarp

Metrisis: Inflammation of the uterus.

Metrorrhagia: A uterine haemorrhage.

Midrib: Central or main vein (leaves)

Moniliform: Like string of beads

Monoecius: With flowers of both sexes in the same plant

Mridu: Soft, delicate, mild, gentle

Mucilage: Sticky substance occurring in many plants that relieves irritations and inflammation.

Mucous: Silmy

Mucronate: Divided into several lobes for more than half its length.

Mucronate: With sharp point at apex

Mukha dosha: Mouth lesions

Mukha vairasya: Distaste or loss of taste

Mutra: Urine

Mutra janana: That which increases formation of urine

Mutra samgrahaniya: That which reduce urine output (antidiuretic)

Mutrala: Diuretic

Mydriatic: A preparation that dilates the pupil of the eyes.

Narcotic: A drug that induces sleep with addictive properties

Nausea: An unpleasant sensation with a tendency to comit

Nephritis: Inflammation of the kidneys especially in Bright's Disease.

Nephropathy: Diseases of the kidney

Nervine: Restores the nerves; relaxes the nervous system

Netrahita: Beneficial to eyes

Neuralgia: Pain resulting from irritation or inflammation of a nerve

Neuralgic disorders: Painful disorders of nerves

Neuritis: Inflammation of a nerve

Neuropathy: A functional disturbance or pathological change in peripheral nervous system

Neuters: Neither female or male

Nidra: Sleep

Nidrakara: Sedative/ hypnotic

Node: Joint of a stem, where leaves, branches or secondary roots arise.

Nodose: With knot-like protruberances.

Nut: Dry, indehiscent fruit; usually single-seeded

Obesity: Over weight due to excessive accumulation of body fat

Oblanceolate: Lanceolate, with broadest part towards the apex

Oblique: Non-symmetrically sided (leaves)

Oblong: Longer than broad, with more or less parallel edges

Obovate: Having an oval shape with the narrowest part at the base.

Obtuse: More or less rounded at the apex

Ochrea: Membranous sheath around a node, formed through the fusion of stipules

Odontalgia: Toothache

Odontalgic: Used for the treatment of toothache.

Odontopathy: Any disease of the teeth

Oedema: An abnormal accumulation of fluid in the spaces in between or outside the cells leading to swelling

Oestrogenic: With a similar action to oestrogen in the body, supporting and maintaining the female reproductive organs.

Ointment: A blend of fats or oils that form a protective layer over the skin

Oleolite: A medicine with an oily base.

Ophthalamitis: Inflammation of the eyeball

Ophthalmia: Severe inflammation of the eye

Ophthalmic: Relative to eye diseases.

Ophthalmopathy: Any disease of the eye

Opposite: Arising in pairs on either side from the same node (leaves)

Oral carcinoma: Cancerous growth in the mouth/cancer at the mouth

Oral ulcers: Ulcers in the mouth

Orbicular: More or less circular rounded

Oval: Broadly elliptical

Ovary: Part of a flower that bears the ovules

Ovate: Broadest near the base, tapering towards the obtuse apex; egg-shaped

Ovoid: Egg-shaped; having the solid shape of an egg.

Oxytocic: A medicinal drug used to hasten parturition or stimulate uterine contractions.

Pagina: The surface of a leaf.

Palea: The outer of two bracts enclosing the flower of a spikelet (grasses); inner to the glumes

Palmate: Like outspread fingers of palm

Palmate-lobate: Applied to a palmate leaf with lobes cut more than half-way.

Palmatifid: Applied to a palmate leaf in which the incisions only reach half-way down the pagina.

Palmatiscet: Applied to a palmate leaf with deep divisions forming segments joined at the base.

Pandu: Anaemia

Panicle: A brached cluster of flowers on stalks in a pyramid-shaped arrangement

Pappus: Series of hairs or scales at the apex of achenes; commonly a modification of the calyx

Parasite: Organism which obtains nutrients from another organism by penetrating the host with a haustorium. Hemiparasites still contain chalorophyll, holoparasites are entirely depending on their host; the site of the haustorium in the host defines root-or stemparasites

Parasiticide: Kills parasites

Parasympathetic nervous system: Part of the nervous system involved in vegetative functions, especially digestion

Paregoric: A smoothing remedy for coughs.

Parenchyma: A tissue of undifferentiated cells.

Paripinnate: With equal number of members on either side of rachis

Parshwashula: Lateral chest pain

Parted: (Of leaves) cleft almost to the mid-rib.

Pectoral: Acts on the lungs

Pedicel: Stalk of flowers

Peduncle: Stalk of an inflorescence

Peltate: Petiole attached to lower leaf surface instead of margin

Pendulous: Somewhat hanging

Peptic ulcer: An ulceration of the mucous membrane of the esophagus, stomach or duodenum, due to action of the acid gastric juice

Perennial: Living for many years

Perfoliate: A leaf base which envelops its stem.

Perianth: A collective term for both the calyx and corolla.

Pericarp: Wall of ovary ripened into fruit

Persistent: Remaining naturally attached

Petal: One part of the corolla

Petiole: A leaf-stalk.

Pharmacopeia: A catalogue of officially-recoginized drugs.

Pharyngodynia: Pain in the pharynx

Photosensitive: Heightened sensitivity to sunlight

Phthisis: Tuberculosis

Phyllotaxis: The system of leaf insertion on the stem.

Phytotherapy: Therapy by means of medicinal (officinal) plnts.

Pichchila: Sticky or viscous

Pileorhiza: See calyptra.

Pilose: Thinly sprinkled with long, simple, soft hairs

Pinnate: Compound leaf with leaflets arranged in pairs along a common axis, feathered

Pinnate-parted: Cut almost to the mid-rib.

Pistil: The female part of a flower.

Pitta: One of the three humours (doshas) of body

Placenta: The part of the ovary that bears the ovule

Plethoric: A turgid condition due to an excess number of red blood cells.

Pod: A dry dehiscing fruit

Polygamous: With both besexual and unisexual flowers in the same or on different plants

Poultice: Herbal preparation usually applied hot to affected area to alleviate pain and reduce swelling

Powder: A preparation obtained by the fine powdering of medicinal plants.

Pradarahara: Useful in menstrual and vaginal disorders

Prajasthapana: That which promoters conception

Prakinson's disease: A neurological disorder characterized by tremors, stiffness and slowness

Pravahikahara: Useful in dysentery

Prickle: A small spine

Procumbent: Lying along the ground

Prostaglandins: Chemicals in plants and the human body that have a hormounal action affecting a wide range of conditions including pain and inflammation

Prostrate: Laying flat on the ground

Pruritus: Itching

Pseudocarp: Fruit formed from other than overy

Psoriasis: A chronic, exfoliative skin disease

Pteiole: Stalk of leaf

Puberulous: Slightly hairy with very short haris

Pubescent: Covered with short and soft hairs

Pulvinus: Swollen base of petiole

Punctate: Marked with dots, depressions or glands

Purgative: A very strong laxative

Purulent: Discharging pus.

Pustulate: Like blisters

Pyrenes: A nutlet or one of the small stones of a drupe or similar fruit

Pyriform: Pear shaped

Qi: Vital energy force in Chinese philosophy

Racelcitrant: Seeds, not amenable for storage

Raceme: Inflorescence with acropetal arrangement of pedicelled flowers on main axis

Rachis: Asix of inflorescence or compound leaf

Rakta: Blood

Rakta pitta: Bleeding diathesis

Rakta rodhaka: Haemostatic

Rakta samgrahaka: Haemostatic

Rakta shodhaka: That which purifies 'Rakta'

Rakta vardhana: That which increases blood

Rakta vikara: Diseases of blood

Raktadosha: Diseases of blood

Ralta stambhaka: That which controls bleeding

Rasa: Taste, absorbed elements of food

Rasayana: Rejuvenating body tissues

Ray florest: Outer flowers in the inflorescence of Asteraceae; usually sterile and strap-shaped

Rechana: Purgation

Rectinerved: Describes a leaf with reticulated venation.

Reflexed: Bent dow-or backwards

Remittent fever: Fever wherein the temperature increases varying from 2°F or more in 24 hours, but without return to normal temperaure

Renal calculi: Kindry/renal stones

Reniform: Kidney shaped

Resin: Adhesive insoluble (in water) substance secreted by plant

Resolvent: A preparation to soothe inflammatory conditions.

Retrigerant: A drug which relieves feverishness or produces a feeling of collness

Retuse: A shallow notch in a rounded apex

Revulsive: A preparation that produces revulsion.

Rhachis: Main axis of a compound leaf or an inflorascence

Rheumatism: Any disorder marked by inflammation, degeneration of joints (especially) etc.

Rheumatoid arthritis: A chronic systemic disease primarily of the joints

Rhizome: Non-green underground horizontally growing stem, bearing buds and scale leaves and producing new plants asexually

Rhomboid: Quadrilateral with only opposite sides and angles equal

Rhomboidal: Having shape of rhomboid

Rochana: Stimulating appetite

Rochana: Stimulating appetite

Root: The part of a plant that anchors it in the soil and absorbs nutriment and moisture necessary for growth.

Rootstock: A short, thick rhizome, especially one that is not horizontally but more or less erect.

Roseola: Rose-coloured rash.

Rosette: Basal cluster of radiating leaves

Rosulate: Clustered leaves collected into a rosette

Rubefacient: An agent that reddens the skin

Ruchya: That which stimulates taste

Rugose: Wrinkled

Ruksha: Rough

Runcinate: Applied to a pinnatifid leaf in which the sharply curved cuts between the lobes are directed towards the base.

Runner: A trailing stem that grows along the ground and produces roots.

Sacral fistula: Backache of the lower back.

Sagittate: Arrow shaped.

Samara: An indehiscent winged fruit

Sandhaniya: Uniting

Sangya sthapana: Restoring consciousness

Sara: Fluid, liquid, cathartic

Saraka: Possessing 'sara' property

Sarmentose: Producing long and lithe flexuous runners

Scabies: A contagious skin disease due to itch mite

Scabrid: Covered with small hard hairs or points

Scabrous: Rough to the touch

Scald: To burn with hot liquid or steam

Scale: Small, dry structure; usually a modified leaf

Scaly skin erriuptions: A skin disorder with pealing of the dead skin over it

Scandent: Climbing without aid of tendrils

Scape: A flower stalk which grows from the centre of rosette of leaves.

Scarification: Aterm used for seeds with hard seed coat to hasten germination, aberration of seed coat or soils

Scurvy: A disease due to deficiency of Vitamin C

Sect: (Of leaves) a cut in the surface which reaches the mid-rib or the base.

Sedative: Reduces activity and nervous excitement

Seed: The ripened ovule of a plant containing the embryo; the means by which a plan may propogate sexually.

Semievergreen: Partially evergreen

Seminal weakness: Weakness in ejaculating semen

Semiparasite: Incompletely or partially parasitic

Sepal: A leaf-like part, usually green, that sheathes a flower before it opens.

Serous ulcer: Ulcer secreting serum.

Serrate: Margin regularly sharp, dentate, with teeth pointing towards the apex; saw-toothed (leaves)

Sessile: Without stem or stalk

Seta: Stiff bristle

Setose: Bearing stiff, erect hairs

Sharbata: Syryp

Sheath: Tubular lower part of a leaf enclosing the stem; characteristic for grasses

Sheeta: Cold

Shonitasthapana: That which promotes clotting

Shool: Pain

Shotha: Oedema

Shukrala: Promoting semen

Shukravridhikara: That which increases semen

Shwitra: Vitiligo

Siddha dugdha: Milk boiled with medicines

Siliqua: A fruit that opens on ripening to disclose a diaphragm with seeds.

Silky coma: Tuft of hairs at the end of seed that is silky

Simple: A herb used on its own

Sinuate: Regular wavy margin (leaves)

Sipne: A needle-like modification of the epidermis.

Small pox: Highly contagious, fatal infectious disease marked by fever and distinctive progressive skin eruptions

Smooth: Surface with no outgrowth whatsoever, glabrous

Snehana: Having unctuous properties/ promoting unctuousness in body (see Snigdha)

Snigdha: Unctuous

Sookshma: Minute, subtle

Soporific: Induces sleep.

Sorus: A group of sporangia, which contain the reproductive cells of the plant, on the fronds of a fern.

Spadix: An inflorescence on a single axis surrounded by a type of bract known as a spathe.

Spadiz: Spike inflorescence with fleshy axis

Spasmolytic: Relaxes muscles

Spathe: Large bract enclosing a group of flowers

Spathulate: Spoon-shaped.

Spike: Inflorescence in which sessile, usually unisexual flowers are arranged along a more or less expanded peduncle

Spikelet: Inflorescence of grasses, usually consisting of glumes, lemma, palea and floret

Spine: Sharp pointed, woody outgrowth

Spirit solution: The product obtained from alcoholic maceration of medicinal herbs. Known also as tincture.

Splenobiliary: Bile from the spleen.

Splenomegaly: Enlarged spleen

Stale: The core of the stem (of plants).

Stambhana: To bind, retain

Stamen: The male, pollen-bearing part of a flower.

Stanya: Breast milk

Stellate: Star-like branched hairs

Stem: Main axis of a plant

Sternutatory: An agent that causes sneezing

Steroids: Active chemicals, of animal and plant origin, with powerful hormonal actions

Stigma: Female organ of a flower

Stimulant: Increases rate of activity and nervous excitement

Stipe: Stalk or support for an ovary or carpel

Stipitate: Stalked

Stipule: Leafy or scale-like appendage at the base of a petiole

Stolon: A creeping root that puts out adventitious roots.

Stomachalgia: Pain in the stomach

Stomachic: An agent that improves appetite and digestion

Stomatic: A medicine for complaints of the mouth.

Straggling: Plants, that do not grow erect but spreads or climb over other plant

Stranguary: Slow and painful discharge of urine

Striate: Marked with longitudinal, parralel fine lines

Strigose: Beset with pointed, straight, stiff hairs

Strobilus: See cone.

Stupefacient: Stupefying causing drowsiness.

Style: Zone between the ovary and stigma of a pistil

Styptic: Stops bleeding when applied topically

Subopposite: Nearly opposite

Subsessible: Nearly sessile (without stalk)

Subterete: More or less cylindrical or circular in cross section

Succulent: Thick, soft and juicy

Sucker: A shoot thrown up by an emergent root.

Suffruticose, suffrutescent: Or subshrubby, applied to a small plant with woody branches but a herbaceous apex.

Suppositors: An easily miscible medicated mass to be introduced into a body orifice, as the rectum, urethra or vagina

Swaras: Juice of plant

Swarya: Beneficial for voice

Swedajanana: Promoting diaphoresis, diaphoretic

Swedana: Diaphoretic

Sycoium, syconus: A fleshy, false fruit that contains achenes.

Sympathetic nervous system: Part of the nervous system involved in maintaining arousal, alertness and muscle tone

Synergic: The combined effect of certain substances that exceeds the sum of their individual effects.

Syphilis: A veneral disease

Systemic: Affecting the body as a whole rather than individual organs

Taenifuge: Combats tapeworms (taeniae).

Tail: Extended outgrowth of leaves

Taila (Tailam): Oil

Tapering: Narrowing to an acute point

Taproot: The main anchoring root which grows much larger than the secondary roots.

Tendril: Slender, flexible, spirally coiling leafless organ; supports a climbing plant

Terminal: Growing at the top.

Terpense: Plant medicine prepared by macerating herb in water and alcohol

Tessellate: Chequered

Testa: Outer coat of seed

Tikshna: Acute, irritant

Tikta: Bitter

Tiller: Offshoot from an axillary bud

Tincture: A spirit solution.

Tomentose: Densely, soft and of very short hairs; cottony

Tonic: A medicine to improve the general health of a person.

Tonify: Strengthens and restores body systems

Topical: Application of herbal remedy to body surface

Toxifuge: Dispels poisons.

Triboliate: Compound leaf of three leaflets

Tridosha: Body humours (three in nos.)

Trifoliate: Three leaflets

Trigeminal: Pertaining to trigeminal nerve (deals with chewing, etc).

Trigonal: Triangular in cross section.

Trilocular: Having three chambers or cells.

Tripinnate: Thrice pinnate

Tripinnatisect: A leaf in which the pinnately divided leaflets are themselves pinnately divided.

Trituration: Reduction to a fine powder by grinding.

Truncate: End cut off more or less square

Tuber: A swollen, underground stem containing a store of nutritive materials.

Ture leaves: Leaves other than the cotyledons

Turion: A fleshy, underground bud shooting up from the root.

Twacha: Skin

Twagdosha: Dermatoses (see Tawacha)

Twining: Climbing with the stem

Udarada: Urticaria

Umbel: Umbrella-like arrangement of flowers with all flower stems arising from the same point

Umbilicate: Having a navel-like depression.

Umbrageous: Giving shade

Undulate: More or less irregular wavy margin

Urethrorrhoea: Abnormal discharge from the urethra

Urinary calculi: Stones in urinary tract

Urocolitic: An inflammation of the urinary ducts.

Urogentital: Pertaining to the urinary and genital organs.

Uropathy: Any disease of the urinary tract

Ushna: Hot, heating

Vaginopathy: Any disease at the vagina

Varnya: Beneficial to complexion (varna-complexion)

Vascoconstrictive: Cases dilation of the blood vessels.

Vascular tissue: Plant tissue consisting of ducts or vessels that, in the higher plants, forms the tissue.

Vasoconstrictor: Contracts and narrows blood vessels

Vasodilator: Relaxes and widens blood vessels

Vasodilatory: Causing relaxation of the blood vessels.

Vata: One of the three doshas

Vati: Pill

Vayasthapana: Promotes longevity/anti-aging

Vedana: Pain, discomfort

Vedanasthapana: Analgesic

Veerya: That which brings about action of a drug

Venation: The arrangement of the veins in a leaf.

Veneral disease: Sexually transmitted disease

Vermifuge: A drug which expels intestinal worms.

Verminosis: Infestation by worms

Verrucose: Warty

Vesical calculi: Stones in bladder

Vesicant: Blistering agent.

Vesicle: Gland inside an organ

Vexillum: The large, upper petal of a papilionaceous.

Villous: Bearing long, soft, shaggy, hairs

Vipaka: Ultimate effect of the pharmacologic agent or food on body

Visha: Poison

Vitamin supplement: A preparation to combat vitamin deficiency (avitaminosis).

Volatile oil: Plant constituent distilled to produce essential oil

Vrana: Ulcer/wound

Vranaropana: That which promotes healing of ulcers or wounds

Vranashotha: Inflammation

Vranavisha: Toxins from the wound

Vrishya: That which promotes virility

Vulnerary: A preparation for healing wounds.

Vulnerary: Heals wounds

Vyatha: See vedana

Warts: A skin disorder with a horny surface and finger like shape

Warty: Covered with small, hard excrescence

Whooping cough: An infection disease marked by inflammation of mucous membrane of the respiratory tract and peculiar type of cough etc

Whorl: A circular arrangement, at the same level on a stem, of three or more leaves or flowers.

Wildcrafting: Harvesting herbs from the wild

Xerophilus: Plant adapted to dry climatic conditions

Yakrit: Liver

Yakritottejaka: Liver stimulant

Yield: The percentage of the final product obtained after the transformation of the materials used.

Yin and yang: Complementary opposites in Chinese philosophy

Yonidosha: Diseases of female reproductive system

13 LIST OF BOOKS AND PERIODICALS

BOOKS

1 **100 Red Listed Medicinal Plants**
D. K. Ved
2000
FRLHT, Bangalore

2 **A Handbook of Cacti & Succulents**
Clive Innes
1988
Ward Leck Ltd, London

3 **A Handbook of Organic Farming**
A.K. Sharma
2002
Agrobios (India), Jodhpur

4 **Abstract Bibliography on Senna**
M. Mohan Rao
1975
Indian Drugs Research Association, Pune

5 **Aconites of India: a Monograph**
Stapf. Otto
1904
Today & Tomorrow's Printers & Publishers, Delhi

6 **Adhabhut Zari Butiya**
M. K. Roy
1997
Bishen Singh Mahendra Pal Singh, Dehradun

7 **Advances in Research in Indian Medicine**
K.N. Udupa
1970
Banaras Hindu University, Varanasi

8 **Agrotechniques of Medicinal and Aromatic Crops (Hindi)**
Dr. Ravindra Sharma
2002
Daya Publications, Delhi

9 **Amalaka and Baumi Amalaka**
Krishnamurthy
1992
Books for All, Delhi

10 **Ancient Indian Medicine**
P. Kutumbiah
1962
Orient Longman Ltd., Bombay

11 **Arid Legumes**
N.D. Yadava
1994
Agrobios (India), Jodhpur

12 **Assessment of Threatened Plants of India**
S.K. Jain
1983
Botanical Survey of India, Calcutta

13 **Astanghridyam (Hindi)**
Lal Chandra Vaidya
1963
Motilal Banrsidas, Delhi

14 **Ayurveda & Aromatherapy**
Light Miller
1998
Motilal Banarasidas, New Delhi

15 **Ayurveda & Modern Medicine**
Dr.Lele
2001
Bhartiya Vidya Bhavan, Mumbai

16 **Ayurveda for Health and Long Life**
R.K. Garde
1993
D.B. Taraporevala Sons. & Co. (P) Ltd., Bombay

17 **Ayurveda for Healthy Living**
T.L. Devaraj
1992
UBS Publishers, Delhi

18 **Ayurveda for Mother and Child**
Bhagwan Dash
1975
Delhi Diary Publishers, Delhi

19 **Ayurveda, the Science of Self-Healing**
Vasant Lad
1994
Motilal Banarsidass Publishers Pvt. Ltd., Delhi

20 **Ayurvedic Cure for Common Diseases**
N. Murthy
1982
Orient Paperbacks, Delhi

21 **Ayurvedic Cures for Common Diseases**
Bhagwan Dash
1993
Hind Pocket Books, Delhi

22 **Ayurvedic Drugs and Their Plant Sources**
V.V. Sivarajan
1994
Oxford & IBH Publishing Co. Pvt. Ltd., Delhi

23 **Ayurvedic Flora Medica**
N.S. Moss
1978
Vaidyasarathy Press, Kottayam

24 **Ayurvedic Healing for Women**
Atreya
2000
Motilal Banarasidas, New Delhi

25 **Ayurvedic Healing, a Comprehensive Guide**
David Frawley
1994
Motilal Banarsidass Publishers Pvt. Ltd., Delhi

26 **Ayurvedic Medicinal Flora of Gujarat State**
Maltiben Chouhan
2000
Gujarat Ayurved University, Jamnagar

27 **Ayurvedic Medicine Past and Present**
Shiv Sharma
1987
Krishnadas Academy, Varanasi

28 **Ayurvedic Pharmacology & Therapeutic Uses of Medicinal Plants**
Vaidya V.M. Gogte
2000
Bhartiya Vidya Bhavan, Mumbai

29 **Ayurvedic Treatments of Kerala**
N.S. Moss
1946
Vaidyasarathy Press, Kottayam

30 **A-Z Encyclopedia of Gardening Plants**
Dorling Kindersley
1996
Dorling Kindersley, London

31 **Bael Cultivation and Processing**
R.N. Singh
1984
Indian Council of Agricultural Research, Delhi

32 **Bael, Wood apple, Lemons, Castor**
Krishnamurthy
1992
Books for All, New Delhi

33 **Banana**
Indian Council of Agricultural Research, New Delhi

34 **Banyan and Peepul**
Krishnamurthy
1992
Books for All, Delhi

35 **Beshaja Kalpana: Pharmacology in Traditional Medicine**
V.O. Saji
1991
Lok Swasthya Parampara Samvardhan Samithi, Coimbatore

36 **Bibliography on Pharmacognosy of Medicinal Plants**
Roma Mitra
1985
National Botanical Research Institute, Lucknow

37 **Bihar Ke Adivasi Avom Zari Butiya (Hindi)**
Dr. Mayaram Uniyal
Baidya Nath Ayurvedic Sansthan, Patna

38 **Biofertilizers for Sustainable Agriculture**
A.K. Sharma
2002
Agrobios (India), Jodhpur

39 **Bombay Materia Medica and Their Therapeutics**
Khory
1887
Peridical Expert Book Agency, Delhi

40 **British Pharmaceutical Codex**
K.S. Ahluwalia
1962
Manager of Publications, Delhi

41 **CACTI**
Marcus Schneck
1992
New Burlington Books, London

42 Cashew: Production and Processing Technology
R.C. Mandal
2000
Agrobios (India), Jodhpur

43 **Catalogue of Medicinal Plants Exhibits**
S. N. Bal
1984
Bisensingh Mahendra Pal Singh, Dehradun

44 **Charak Sahita Vol. & II (Hindi)**
Dr. Tripati
1996
Choukambha Surbharti Prakashan, Varanashi

45 **Charak Samhita**
Priyadaranjan Ray
1980
Indian National Science Academy, Delhi

46 **Chemistry of Medicinal Plants Part 1**
1993
Central Council for Research in Unani Medicine, Delhi

47 **Chinese Medicine & Ayurveda**
Robert Svoboda
1998
Motilal Banarasidas, New Delhi

48 **Citrus in India**
NISCOM
NISCOM, New Delhi

49 **Coconut: Production and Protection Technology**
R.C. Mandal
2000
Agrobios (India), Jodhpur

50 **Colour's From Nature Vol 1 & 2**
SERI
2000
Oxford & IBH Publishers Pvt. Ltd., New Delhi

51 **Commercial Drugs of India**
N.B. Dutt
1928
Bishen Singh Mahendra Pal Singh, Dehra Dun

52 **Commercial Guide to the Forest Economic Products of Mysore**
G. Krishnamurti Naidu
1917
Government Press, Bangalore

53 **Common Healing Herbs**
Prem Kishore
1983
ICCRAS, New Delhi

54 **Common Medicinal Plants of Darjeeling and the Sikkim Himalayas**
K. Biswas & R.N. Chopra
1982
Periodical Expert Book Agency, Delhi

55 **Common Trees**
H. Santapu
1966
National Book Trust India, New Delhi

56 **Common Weeds of Central Sudan**
M. Braun
1991
Scientific Books, Weikersheim, Germany

57 **Companion to Chopra's Glossary of Indian Medicinal Plants**
B. N. Mehrotra
1987
Bishen Singh Mahendra Pal Singh, Dehra Dun

58 **Comparative Hindu Materia Medica**
Chandra Chakraberty
1923
Neeraj Publishing House, Delhi

59 **Compendium of Indian Medicinal Plants**
P. Ram Rastogi
1990
Central Drug Research Institute and Publications & Information Directorate (CSIR), Lucknow and Delhi

60 **Compendium of Indian Medicinal Plants Vol-1, 2,3,4,5, & 6**
NISCOM
NISCOM, New Delhi

61 **Complete Book of Home Remedies**
H. Abdul Hameed
1982,
Orient Paperbacks, Delhi

62 **Contribution of Indian Ethnobotany**
S.K. Jain
1997
Scientific Publishers. Jodhpur

63 **Creative Planting with Climbers**
Jane Taylor
1991
Ward Lock Ltd., London

64 **Cultivation and Utilization of Aromatic Plant**
C.K. Atal
1982
Regional Research Laboratory (CSIR), Jammu Tawi

65 **Cultivation and Utilization of Medicinal Plants**
C.K. Atal
1982
Regional Research Laboratory (CSIR), Jammu Tawi

66 **Cultivation of Medicinal & Aromatic crops**
A.A. Farooqi
2001
University Press, Hyderabad

67 **Cultivation of Medicinal Plants**
K. Biswas
1959
Director of Publicity, Calcutta

68 **Cultivation of Medicinal Plants in Jammu and Kashmir**
J.C. Luthra
1956
Indian Council of Agricultural Research, Delhi

69 **Cultivation Practices Some Commercially Important Medicinal Plants**
R. B. S. Rawat
2002
National Medicinal Plants Board, New Delhi

70 **Current Research on Medicinal Plants**
B.N. Dhawan
1986
Indian National Science Academy, Delhi

71 **Damask Rose for Rose Oil and Rose Water**
V. Chandra
1979
National Botanical Research Institute, Lucknow

72 Development of Cardiovascular Drugs from Herbal Sources
R.B. Arora
1965
Handard National Foundation, Delhi

73 **Dictionary of Economic and Medicinal Plants**
A.C. Dutta
1985

74 **Dictionary of Economic Plants in India**
Umrao Singh
1996
Indian Council of Agricultural Research. Delhi

75 Dictionary of Flowering Plants in India
H. Santapu
1998
NISCOM, New Delhi

76 Dictionary of Indian Folk Medicine and Ethnobotany
S.K. Jain
1991
Deep Publications, Delhi

77 **Dictionary of Indian Medicinal Plants**
Akhtar Husain
1992
Central Institute of Medicinal & Aromatic Plants, Lucknow

78 **Dictionary of the Economic Products of Indian**
George Watt
1889
Periodical Expert Book Agency, Delhi

79 **Dictionary of the Flowering Plants in Indian**
H. Santapau
1983
Council of Scientific & Industrial Research, New Delhi

80 **Directory of Spice Suppliers**
Edited
1992
Spices Board Indian, Cochin

81 Domestication of Medicinal Plants in the Arid zone of Rajasthan
Padma Prajapati (Ph.D.)
2001
Unpublished

82 Domestication, Production and Utilization of New Crops
J. Smartt & N. Hag
1997
ICUC, Dhaka

83 **Drug Plants of India Vol – 1 & 2**
V.S. Agarwal
1997
Kalyani Publishers, Delhi

84 **Drug Plants of Indian: Root Drugs**
V.S. Agarwal
1985
Kalyani Publishers, Delhi

85 **Drug-Plant Resources of Central Indian**
R.C. Srivastava
1989
Today & Tomorrow's Printers & Publishers, Delhi

86 **Dry Culinary Herbs**
Edited
1991
International Trade Centre, Geneva

87 **Easy Growing**
Kevin Heinze
1986
South Down Press, Melbourne

88 **Economic Plants of India**
M.P. Nayar
1989
Botanical Survey of India, Calcutta

89 **Economic Plants of India**
V.S. Agarwal
1986
Bishen Singh Mahendra Pal Singh, Dehra Dun

90 **Economic Plants of North East India**
Sudhir Kumar
1999
Scientific Publishers, Jodhpur

91 **Edible Nuts**
G. E. Wickens
1995
FAO, Rome

92 **Encyclopedia of Indian Medicine**
S.K. Rao
1985
Popular Prakashan Pvt. Ltd., Bombay

93 **Encyclopedia of Organic Garding**
HDRA
2001
Dorling Kindersley, London

94 **Ethnobotany and Medicinal Plants of Indian Subcontinent**
J.K.Maheshwari
2000
Scientific Publishers, Jodhpur

95 **Ethnobotany in South Asia**
J.K.Maheshwari
1996
Scientific Publishers, Jodhpur

96 **Ethnobotany of Rajasthan, India**
V.Singh
1998
Scientific Publishers, Jodhpur

97 **Everybody's Guide to Ayurvedic Medicine**
J.F. Dastur
1978
D.B. Taraporevala Sons & Co. (P) Ltd., Bombay

98 **Facts and Fallacies about Coconut oil**
P. K. Thampan
1994
Peekay Tree Crops Dev. Crop., Cochin

99 **Fifty Useful Herbs**
A. Gardiner
1995
Promotional Reprint Co. London

100 **Flavours and Fragrances of Plant Origin**
J. J. W. Coppen
1995
FAO, Rome

101 **Flora of Indian Desert**
M. M. Bhandari
1978
M.P.S. Reports, Jodhpur

102 **Flora of Rajasthan Vol. I to III**
B.V. Shetty & V. Singh
1987
Botanical Survey of India, Kolkatta

103 **Flowering Trees and Shrubs in India**
D.V. Cowen
1970
Thacker & Co. Ltd., Bombay

104 **Folk and Modern Medicine**
Kakar
Lok Swasthya Parmpara Samvardhan Samithi

105 **Food For Thought**
Bertus Haverkort
1999
Zeel Books Ltd., The Netherlands

106 **Foods that Heal**
H.K. Bakhru
Orient Paperbacks, Delhi

107 **Fruits and Vegetables in Ancient India**
P.V. Sharma
1979
Chaukhambha Orientalia, Delhi

108 **Fundamentals of Ayurvedic Medicine**
Bhagwan Dash
1989
Konark Publishers (P) Ltd. And Bansal & Co., Delhi

109 **Garden Plants**
Peter Mchoy
1994
Marshall Cavendish Books, London

110 **Garden Trees**
Francis Ritter
1996
Dorling Kindersley, London

111 **Ginger and Turmeric**
Krishnamurthy
1992
Books for All, Delhi

112 **Glimpses of Indian Ethnobotany**
S.K. Jain
1981
Oxford & IBH Publishing Co. Pvt. Ltd., Delhi

113 **Glimpses of Indian Medicinal Plant Drug Development Research**
R.B. Arora
Indian Institute of History of Medicine, Delhi

114 **Glossary of Indian Medicinal Plants**
R.N. Chopra
1956
Council of Scientific & Industrial Research, Delhi

115 **Glossary of Indian Medicinal Plants with Active Principles, Second Supplement**
L.V. Asolkar
1992
Council of Scientific & Industrial Research Publications & Information directorate, Delhi

116 **Glossary of Indian Medicinal Plants With Supp. & Second Supp. (Set of 3 Books)**
NISCOM
NISCOM, New Delhi

117 **Glossary of vegetable Drugs in Brhattrayi**
K.C. Chunckar
1972
Chowkhamba Sanskrit Series Office. Varanasi

118 **Glossary of Vegetable Drugs in Vagbhata**
S.R. Godbole
1966
Indian Drugs Research Association. Pune

119 Good Manufacturing Practices and Requirements of Premises, Plant and Equipment for Pharmaceutical Products
Govt. of India
2001
Govt. of India, New Delhi

120 **Gourds and Pumpkins**
Krishnamurthy
1992
Books for All, Delhi

121 **Gragrant Herbs**
Krishnamurthy
1979
Books for All, Delhi

122 Guide to Natural Remedies for Health & Well Being
Enrique Garza
1998
Orvit Publishing, Maxico

123 **Guide to the Economic Plants of South India**
D. Sundararaj
1959
Periodical Expert Book Agency, Delhi

124 Gums, resins and Latexes of Plant Origin
J. J. W. Coppen
1995
FAO, Rome

125 **Hand Book of Agriculture**
ICAR
2001
ICAR, Delhi

126 **Hand Book of Horticulture**
Dr.R.L.Chadha
2002
ICAR, Delhi

127 **Handbook of Ayurveda**
Bahgwan Dash
1983
Concept Publishing Company, Delhi

128 **Handbook of Ayurveda Medicinal Plants**
L.D. Kapoor
1990
CRC Press, Boca Raton, USA

129 **Handbook of Common Ayurvedic Remedies**
Edited
1974
Central Council for Research in Ayurveda & Siddha, Delhi

130 **Handbook of Common Ayurvedic Remedies in Siddha System of Medicine**
G. Veluchamy
1991
Central Council for Research in Ayurveda & Siddha, Delhi

131 **Handbook of Common Remedies in Unani System of Medicine**
Ummal Fazal
1976
Central Council for Research in Indian Medicine & Homoeopathy, Delhi

132 **Handbook of Domestic Medicine and Common Ayurvedic Remedies**
Edited
1978
Central Council for Research in Indian Medicine & Homoeopathy, Delhi

133 **Harad and Baheda**
Krishnamurthy
1992
Books for All, Delhi

134 **Heal with Herbs**
Avijit Hazra
1995
NISCOM, Delhi

135 **Healing Forests, HealingPeople**
Manjul Bajaj
1995
IDRC, New Delhi

136 **Healing Herbs**
Prem Kishore
1979
Central Research Institute, Bhubaneswar

137 **Herbal Beauty & Hair Care**
Suman Mahendru
Manoj Publications, Delhi

138 Herbal Cosmetics & Ayurvedic Medicines
P. K. Chattopadhyay
NIIR, Delhi

139 **Herbal Cure Series**
Bhagwan Dash
B. Jain Publishers (P) Ltd., Delhi

140 **Herbal Cures**
C. Thakkur
1975
Ancient Wisdom Publications, Bombay

141 **Herbal Drugs in Indian Pharmaceutical Industry**
S.L. Kapoor
1979
National Botanical Research Institute, Lucknow

142 **Herbal Foods**
N. Ramaswami Pillai
1985
Nature Cure Publishing House, Pudukkottai

143 **Herbal Medicine for Human Health**
R. Roy Chaudhury
1992
World Health Organization, Delhi

144 **Herbal Spices-Domestic Survey**
Edited
Spices Board India, Cochin

145 **Herbs & Spices**
J. Kybal
1995
Harveys Book Shop Ltd., Wingston U.K.

146 **Herbs that Heal: Natural Remedies for Good Health**
H.K. Bakhru
1992
Orient Paperbacks, Delhi

147 **History and Natural History of Ephedra as Soma**
S. Mahdihassan
1987
Pakistan Science foundation, Islamabad, Pakistan

148 **History of Indian Medicine**
Girindranath Mukhopadhyaya
1992
Munshiram Manoharlal Publishers Pvt. Ltd. Delhi

149 **Home Remedies: a Handbook of Folk Medicine**
Girija Khanna
1982
Tarang Paperbacks, Delhi

150 **Horticultural and Economic Plants of the Nilgiris**
S. Krishnamurthy
1953
Government Botanic Gardens Centenary Committee, Udhagamandalam

151 **How to Grow Medicinal Plants for Primary Health Care**
D.K. Ved
1995
Foundation for Revitalization of Local Health Traditions, Bangalore

152 **Illustrated Materia Medica of Indo-Tibetan Medicine**
Bhagwan Dash
1987
Classics India Publications, Delhi

153 **India Herbal Therapies**
C. P. Khare
2000
Visha Vijai Pvt. Ltd., New Delhi

154 **Indian Medicinal Plants**
Dr.Paranjpe
2001
Chaukhambha Sanskrit Pratisthan

155 **Indian Medicinal Plants**
Kirtikar & Basu
1918
Periodical Expert Book Agency, Delhi

156 **Indian Medicinal plants Used in Ayurvedic Preparations**
A.C. Dey
1980
Bishen Singh Mahendra Pal Singh, Dehra Dun

157 **Indian Medicinal Plants Vol 1,2,3,4,5**
P.K.Warrier
2002
Orient Longman, Hyderabad

158 Indian Medicinal Plants, a Compendium of 500 Species
Vaidya Sala Arya
1996
Orient Longman Ltd., Delhi

159 **Indian Therapeutics**
D.V. Sandu
1987
Sir Satguru Publications, Delhi

160 **Indigenous Drugs of India**
J.C. Ghosh
1940
P.K. Ghosh School of Chemical Technology, Calcutta

161 **Indigenous Drugs of India**
R.N. Chopra
1958
Academic Publishers, Delhi

162 **International Expert Consultation on NWFP**
Edited
1995
FAO, Rome

163 **Introduction to Ayurveda**
C. Thakkur
1975
Shri Gulabkunverba Ayurvedic Society, Jamnagar

164 **Introduction to Dravyaguna**
P.V. Sharma
1976
Chaukhambha Orientalia, Varanasi

165 **Ipecac Cultivation in India**
K. Biswas
Indian council of Agricultural Research, Delhi

166 **Ipomoea**
S.C. Datta
1959
National Botanical Garden, Lucknow

167 **Isabgol, Cultivation in India**
D. Gopani
1969
Ministry of Food & Agriculture, Government of India, Delhi

168 **Isabgol, Gokhru and Bhahmi**
Krishnamurthy
1992
Books For All, Delhi

169 **Jadi Bution ki Saral Kheti**
N. D. Prajapati
2002
Rajasthan Agroforestry Corpn., Jodhpur

170 **Jivanopayogi Zari Butiya (Hindi)**
C. M. Srivastava
1999
Manoj Publications, Delhi

171 **Jojoba New Crop for Arid Lands**
Edited
1985
National Academy Press, Washington D.C.

172 **Kashyapiyakrishisukti**
Kashyapa
2002
Asian Agri History Foundation, Secunderabad

173 **Kew: A World of Plants**
Heather Angel
1993
Royal Botanical Gardens, Kew, UK

174 **Khas, Kesar, Nagakesar, Khaskhas**
Krishnamurthy
1992
Books for All, Delhi

175 **Lillies: Their Care & Cultivation**
Michael Juffrson-Brown
1990
Cassel Publishers Ltd., London

176 **Mahua; The Tree of the Poor**
Ram Prasad
1993
International Book Distributors, Dehra Dun

177 **Major Essential Oil-Bearing Plants of India**
Akhtar Husain
1988
Central Institute of Medicinal & Aromatic Plants, Lucknow

178 **Major Medicinal Plants of India**
R.S. Thakur
1989
Central Institute of Medicinal & Aromatic Plants, Lucknow

179 **Major Spices of India**
P.S. Prithu
1993
Indian Council of Agricultural Research, New Delhi

180 **Manual of Ethnobotany**
S.K. Jain
1987
Scientific Publishers, Jodhpur

181 **Manual of Indian Spices**
S.N. Mahindru
1994
Academic Foundation, Delhi

182 Marketing Directory of Medicinal and Aromatic Crops (Hindi)
CEDMAP
2002
CEDMAP, Bhopal

183 Marketing Directory of Medicinal Plants
Sushil Kumar
1979
CIMAP Lucknow

184 **Materia Indica**
Whitelwa Ainslie
1926
Neeraj Publishing House, Delhi

185 **Materia Medica**
John Martin Honigberger
1952
B.R. Publishing Corporation, Delhi

186 **Materia Medica (Reprint)**
Henry G. Greenish
1999
Scintific Publishers, Jodhpur

187 **Materia Medica of Ayurveda**
Bhagwan Dash
1980
Concept Publishing Company, Delhi

188 **Materia Medica of Ayurveda Based on Madapala's Nighantu**
Bhagwan Dash
1991
B. Jain Publishers (P) Ltd., Delhi

189 **Materia Medica of Indian and Their Therapeutics**
Nanabhai Nvrosji Katark
1903
Neeraj Publishing House, Delhi

190 **Materia Medica of the Hindus, with a Glossary of Indian Plants**
U.C. Dutt
1877
Mittal Publications, Delhi

191 **Materia Medica of Tibetan Medicine**
Bhagwan Dash
1994
Sri Satguru Publications. Delhi

192 **Matricaria for Blue Oil**
V. Chandra
1979
National Botanical Research Institute, Lucknow

193 Medical and Economic Aspects of Some Indian Medicinal Plants
R.N. Chopra
1932
Patna University, Patna

194 **Medical and Economical Botany**
John Lindley
1849
Bishen Singh Mahendra Pal Singh, Dehra Dun

195 **Medical Systems with a Holistic Approach**
S.N. Tripathi & Y.B. Tripathi
1994

196 **Medicinal & Aromatic Plants of Himachal Pradesh**
Dr. Narain Singh
1999
Indus Publishing Company, Delhi

197 **Medicinal and Poisonous Legumes of India**
Jean F. Caius
1989
Scientific Publishers, Jodhpur

198 **Medicinal and Poisonous Plants of India**
Jean F. Caius
1986
Scientific Publishers, Jodhpur

199 **Medicinal Chemistry Research in Indian**
Harkishan Singh
1985
Central Drug Research Institute, Lucknow

200 **Medicinal Flora of Garhwal Himalayas**
M.R. Uniyal
1989
Baidyanath Ayurved Bhawan Ltd., Nagpur

201 **Medicinal Flora of India**
James Duke
1981
Economic Botany Laboratory, USA

202 **Medicinal Flowers**
G. Pandey
1992
Sri Satguru Publications, Delhi

203 **Medicinal Herbs and Essential Oils**
A. Gardiner
1995
Promotional Reprint Co. London

204 **Medicinal Pants of Patalkot**
H.O. Sexena
1971
State Forest Research Institute, Jabalpur

205 **Medicinal Plants**
Edited
1986
Indo-German Chamber of Commerce, Bombay

206 **Medicinal Plants**
S.G. Joshi
2000
Oxford & IBH Publishers, New Delhi

207 **Medicinal Plants**
S.K. Jain
1979
National Book Trust, Delhi

208 **Medicinal Plants & Minerals of Uttarankhan Himalaya**
Dr. Mayaram Uniyal
1997
Baidyanath Ayurvedic Research Centre, Patna

209 **Medicinal Plants and Herbs for Health**
Gunaram Khanikar
1993
Khanikar Puthibharal, Golaghat

210 **Medicinal Plants for Forest Conservation and Health Care**
Gerard Bodeker
1997
FAO, Rome

211 **Medicinal Plants Growing in the Districts of Andhra Pradesh through Which the River Krishna Flows**
K. Raghunathan
1976
Central Council for Research in Indian Medicine & Homoeopathy, Delhi

212 **Medicinal Plants in China**
Edited
1990
World Health Organization (WHO)

213 **Medicinal Plants in Skin Care**
S. Kumar
1994
Central Institute of Medicinal & Aromatic Plants, Lucknow

214 **Medicinal Plants in the Republic of Korea**
Edited
1990
World Health Organization (WHO)

215 **Medicinal Plants in the South Pacific**
Edited
1990
World Health Organization (WHO)

216 **Medicinal Plants in Viet Nam**
Edited
1990
World Health Organization (WHO)

217 **Medicinal Plants of Andhra Pradesh**
Edited
1999
CCRUM, New Delhi

218 **Medicinal Plants of Bombay Presidency**
S.P. Agharkar
1991
Scintific Publishers, Jodhpur

219 **Medicinal Plants of Conservation Concern in Southern India**
D.K. Ved
2000
FRLHT, Bangalore

220 **Medicinal Plants of Gwalior Forest Division, Madhya Pradesh**
V.K. Singh
1984
Central council for Research in Unani Medicine, Delhi

221 **Medicinal Plants of India**
C.K.N. Nair
1998
Nag Publishers, Delhi

222 **Medicinal Plants of India**
S.K. Jain
1991
Reference Publications Inc., Algonac, Michigan (USA)

223 **Medicinal Plants of Indian and Pakistan**
J.F. Dastur
1977
D.B. Taraporevala Sons & Co. (P) Ltd., Bombay

224 **Medicinal Plants of Indian Vol. I & II**
G.V. Satyavati
1976
Indian Council of Medicinal Research, New Delhi

225 Medicinal Plants of Kachchh (Gujarat)
H. R. Goyal
1998
CCRAS, New Delhi

226 **Medicinal Plants of Kerala Forests**
Edited
1981
Kerala Forest Research Institute, Peechi, Kerala

227 Medicinal Plants of Madhya Pradesh Distribution, Cultivation & Trade
K. P. Tiwari
1998
SFRI Jabalpur

228 **Medicinal Plants of Saharanpur**
B.S. Ahuja
1965
Gurukul Kangri Vishwavidyalaya, Hardwar

229 **Medicinal Plants of the Arid Zone**
I.C. Chopra
1960
Today & Tomorrow's Printers & Publishers, Delhi

230 **Medicinal Plants of the Sikkim Himalaya: Status, Usage and Potential**
Lalitkumar Rai
1994
Bishen Singh Mahendra Pal Singh, Dehra Dun

231 **Medicinal Plants Used in Homoeopathy Vol-1&2**
Vikramaditya
1997
Homoeopathic Pharmacopeia Laboratory, Ghaziabad (UP)

232 **Medicinal Plants Useful in Mother and Child Health**
S. N. Venugopal
1992
Lok Swasthya Parampara Samvardhan Samithi, Coimbatore

233 **Medicinal Plants Useful in Primary Health Care**
S. N. Venugopal
Lok Swashya Parampara Samvardhan Samithi, Coimbatore

234 **Medicinal Plants: New Vistas of Research**
J.N. Govil
1993
Today & Tomorrow's Printers & Publishers, Delhi

235 **Melia**
C.R. Mitra
1962
National Botanic Gardens, Lucknow

236 **Minor Forest Product of India**
S.S. Negi
1993
Periodical Expert Book Agency, Delhi

237 **Minor Forest Products (Medicinal Plants)**
Edited
1989
Tropical Forest Research Institute, Jabalpur

238 **Minor Forest Products in Mysore: A Survey**
M.N. Ramaswamy
1945
Superintendent, Government press, Bangalore

239 **Minor Species of India**
P.S. Prithu
2001
ICAR, New Delhi

240 **Miracles of Indian Herbs**
G.S. Verma
1982
Rasayan Pharmacy, Delhi

241 **Miracles of Neem Tree**
G.S. Verma
Rasayan Pharmacy, Delhi

242 **Monograph on Eucalyptus**
D.N. Tewari
1992
Suraya Publications, Dehra Dun

243 **Monograph on Neem**
D.N. Tewari
1992
International Book Distributors, Dehra Dun

244 **Monograph on Teak**
D.N. Tewari
1992
International Book Distributors, Dehra Dun

245 **Narcotic Drugs**
Anil Aggarawal
1995
National Book Trust, New Delhi

246 **Nardostachys, Jatamansi: a Chemical, Pharmacological and Clinical Appraisal**
R.B. Arora
1965
Indian council of Medical Research, Delhi

247 **Natural Colourants and Dyestuffs**
C. L. Green
1995
FAO, Rome

248 **Natural Medicines**
Edited
1999
Eastern Publisers, New Delhi

249 **Natural Pesticides from the Neem Tree**
(IInd International Neem Conference)
1984
Eschbon, Germany

250 **Natural Pesticides from the Neem Tree**
(IIIrd International Neem Conference)
1987
Eschbon, Keniya

251 **Natural Plant Products: a Practical Guide**
R.D. Chaudhury
1989
Amsar Private Limited, Indore

252 **Natural Plant Products: Classification for End Use**
R.D. Chaudhury
1983
Amsar Private Limited, Indore

253 **Neem**
C.R. Mitra
1963
Indian Central Oilseeds Committee, Hyderabad

254 **Neem**
N. S. Ranghawa
1993
Society of Pesticide Science, India

255 **Neem and It's Relatives**
Krishnamurthy
1992
Books for All, Delhi

256 **Neem, Research and Development**
N.S. Randhawa
Indian Agriculture Research Institute, Delhi

257 **Neem: Free No More**
Foundation for Revitalization of Local Health Traditions, Bangalore

258 **New Manual of Homeopathic Materia Medica and Repertory**
Boericke
2001
B. Jain Publishers, New Delhi

259 **Nidaana: Diagnosis in Traditional Medicine**
R. Aruna
1991
Lok Swasthya Parampara Samvardhan Samithi, Coimbatore

260 Notable Plants in Ethnomedicine of India
S.K. Jain
1991
Deep Publications, Delhi

261 **Observations on Medico-Botany of Andaman and Nicobar Islands**
Edited
1988
Central council for Research in Ayurveda & Siddha, Delhi

262 **One Hundred Beautiful Trees of India, a Descriptive and Pictorial Handbook**
Charles McCann
1959
D.B. Taraporevala Sons & Co. (P) Ltd., Bombay

263 **Onion and Garlic**
Krishnamurthy
1992
Books For All, Delhi

264 **Opium Poppy**
Akhtar Husain & J.R. Sharma
1983
Central Institute of Medicinal & Aromatic Plants, Lucknow

265 **Organic Agriculture**
P. K. Thampan
1995
Peekay Tree Crops Dev. Crop., Cochin

266 **Organic Food and Beverages**
Edited
1999
International Trade Centre, Geneva

267 **Organics in Soil Health & Crop Production**
P. K. Thampan
1993
Peekay Tree Crops Dev. Crop., Cochin

268 **Our Trees**
RPN Sinha
1968
Publication Division, Govt. of India New Delhi

269 Outline of Pharmacopoeial Drugs of Vegetable Origin
S.N. Bal
1940
P. Ghosh & Co., Calcutta

270 **Pharmacognosy**
C.K. Kokate
1990
Nirali Prakashan, Pune

271 **Pharmacognosy**
Varro E. Tyler
1981
K.M. Varghese Company, Bombay

272 **Pharmacognosy of Ayurvedic Drugs-Kerala**
K. Narayana Aiyar
Kerala University, Pharmacognosy Department, Thiruvanthapuram

273 **Pharmacognosy of Indian Leaf Drugs**
S.C. Datta & B. Mukerji
1952
Government of India Press, Calcutta

274 **Pharmacognosy of Indian Root and Rhizome Drugs**
S.C. Datta
1949
Manager of Publications, Calcutta

275 **Pharmacognosy of Indigenous Drugs Vol. I, II & III**
K. Raghunathan & Roma Mitra
1982
Central Council for Research in Ayurveda & Siddha,

276 **Pharmacological Investigation on Certain Ayurvedic and Siddha Plants**
Edited
Central Council or Research in Ayurveda & Siddha, New Delhi

277 **Pharmacopoeia Indica, Being a Collection of Vegetable, Mineral and Animal Drugs in Common Use in India**
Kartick C. Bose
1932
Bishen Singh Mahendra pal Singh, Dehra Dun

278 **Pharmacopoeia of India**
Edited
1955
Controller of Publications, Delhi

279 **Pharmacopoeia of Siddha Medicine**
Edited
1956
Indian Medical Practitioners' co-operative Pharmacy & Stores Ltd., Madras

280 **Pharmacopoeia of Tibetan Medicine**
Bhagwan Dash
1995
Sri Satguru Publications, Delhi

281 **Pharmacopoeial Standards for Ayurvedic Formulations**
Edited
1987
Central Council or Research in Ayurveda & Siddha, Delhi

282 **Physico-Chemical Standards of Unani Formulations**
Edited
1986
Central Council for Research in Unani Medicine Delhi

283 Phytochemical Investigations of Certain Medicinal Plants Used in Ayurveda
V.N. Pandey
1990
Central Council for Research in Ayurveda & Siddha, Delhi

284 **Plant Families: How to Know Them**
H.E. Jacques
1999
Agro Bios India, Jodhpur

285 **Plant Food Flavours**
Santosh Mehtani
1999
NISCOM, New Delhi

286 **Plant Genetic Resources: Conversation and Management, Concepts and Approaches**
R.S. Paroda & R.K. Arora
1991
International Board for Plant Genetic Resources, Regional Office for South & South-East Asia, Delhi

287 Plant Geography of Western Rajasthan
Padma Prajapati
1998
Unpublished

288 **Plants and Drugs of Sind**
James A. Murray
1881
Ajay book Service, Delhi

289 Plants for Reclamation of Wastelands
NISCOM
1990
NISCOM, New Delhi

290 Plants in the Indian Puranas: an Ethnobotanical Investigation
P. Sensarma
1989
Naya Prokash, Calcutta

291 **Plants of the Quran**
M.I.H. Farooqi
1989
Sidrah Publishers, Lucknow

292 **Poisonous Plants of India**
R.N. Chopra
1965
Indian council of Agricultural Research, Delhi

293 **Poppies of Indian Region**
H.S. Debnath
1986
Botanical Survey of India, Calcutta

294 **Practical Bazaar Medicines**
G.T. Birdwood
1936
Asian Educational Services, Delhi

295 **Prayogatmak Abinav Daryagum Vigyan (Hindi)**
Dr. Mayaram Uniyal
1991
Shri Baidyanath Ayurveda Bhawan Ltd., Patna

296 **Production Technology of Medicinal & Aromatic Crops**
A. A. Farooqi
1993
Natural Remedies Pvt. Ltd., Bangalore

297 **Promotion of Non-Wood Forestry Produce Through Social Forestry**
N.C. Hegde & J.N. Daniel
1993
Bharatiya Agro-Industry Foundation (BAIF), Development Research Foundation, Pune

298 **Propagation of Tropical and Sub-Tropical Horticultural Crops**
T.K. Bose
1986
Naya Prokash, Calcutta

299 **Psyllium Production and Marketing in India**
D.P. Mathur
1990
Oxford & IBH Publishing Co. Pvt. Ltd., Delhi

300 **Pyrethrum**
S.C. Datta & O.P. Virmani
National Botanic Gardens, Lucknow

301 **Rastaringini (Hindi)**
Kashinath Sastina
1979
Motilal Banarsidas, Delhi

302 **Rauvolfia Serpentina**
R.L. Badhwar
1955
Manager of Publications, Delhi

303 **Rauvolfia Serpentina**
S.C. Datta & O.P. Virmani
1964
National Botanical Gardens, Lucknow

304 **Recent Advances in Medicinal, Aromatic and Spice Crops**
S.P. Raychaudhuri
1991
Today & Tomorrow's Printers & Publishers, Delhi

305 **Red Data Book of Indian Plants**
M.P. Nayar & A.P.K. Sastry
1987
Botanical Survey of India, Calcutta

306 **Regulation of Collection, Transit and Trade of Medicinal Plants**
Ashok K. Jain
2000
WWF India, New Delhi

307 **Report on Propagation methods of Medicinal Plants of India**
Edited
Tropical Botanic Garden & Research Institute and Lok Swasthya Parampara Samvardhan Samithi, Thiruvananthapuram and Coimbatore

308 **Resource Assessment of Non-Wood Forest Products**
Jennifer L. G. Wong
2001
FAO Rome

309 **Review of Research on spices and Cashewnut in India**
S.G. Aiyadurai
1966
Indian Council of Agricultural Research, Regional Office-Spices & Cashewnut, Ernakulum

310 **Review of Work on Indian Medicinal Plants (Including Indigenous Drugs and Poisonous Plants)**
R.N. Chopra & I.C. Chopra
1955
Indian Council of Medicinal Research, Delhi

311 **Role of Traditional Asian Medicine in Primary Health Care**
I. Wolffers
1990
Free University press, Amsterdam

312 **Romance of Empire Drugs**
1946
Stafford Allen & Sons, London

313 **Root Crops**
Daisy E. Kay
1973
Tropical Development & Research Institute, London

314 **Rose and Rose Oil Industry in India**
Regional Research Laboratory (CSIR), Jammu Tawi

315 **Seed Spices in Rajasthan**
Edited
1994
Agricultural Marketing Board Jaipur

316 Selected Medicinal Plants of India
Ramus Deora
1992
Chemexcil, Mumbai

317 Selected Poisonous Plants from the Tribal Areas of India
K. Thothathri
1985
Botanical Survey of India, Calcutta

318 **Siddha Formulary**
Edited
1988
Controller of Publications, Delhi

319 **Silviculture in the Tropics**
Hans Lamprecht
1989
GTZ, Germany

320 **Single Drug Remedies with Illustrations**
N.S. Mooss
1976
Vaidyasarathy Press (P) Ltd., Kottayam

321 **Sodasangahrdayam: Essentials of Ayurveda**
Priya V. Sharma
1993
Motilal Banarsidass Publishers Pvt. Ltd., Delhi

322 **Some Beautiful Indian Trees**
Ethelbert Blatter
1954
Bombay Natural History Society, Bombay

323 **Some Controversial Drugs in Indian Medicine**
Bapalal (Vaidya)
1982
Chaukhambha Orientalia, Varanasi

324 **Some Medicinal Plants of Kashmir**
S.N. Bal
Botanical Survey of India, Calcutta

325 Some Promising Plants Drugs of Ayurveda
Edited
CCRAS, New Delhi

326 **Some Useful Aromatic Plants**
R.I. Badhwar
1964
Manager of Publications,

327 Delhi

328 **Source Book of Indian Medicine: an Anthology**
Krishnamurthy
1991
B.R. Publishing Corporation, Delhi

329 **Speaking of Ayurvedic Remedies for Common Diseases**
T.L. Devaraj
1985
Sterling Publishers (P) Ltd., Delhi

330 **Spices**
Krishnamurthy
1992
Books for All, Delhi

331 **Spices and Condiments**
J.S. Pruthi
1987
National Book Trust, Delhi

332 Spices, Plantation Crops, Medicinal & Aromatic Crops
N. Kumar
2000
Oxford & Ibh Publications

333 **Standardization of Single Drugs in Unani Medicine**
Edited
1987
Central Council for Research in Unani Medicine, Delhi

334 **Status Report on Aromatic & Essential Oil**
NISCOM
NISCOM

335 **Status Report on Medicinal Plants**
NISCOM
NISCOM

336 **Status Report on Medicinal Plants for NAM Countries**
Akhtar Husain
1993
Centre for Science & Technology of the Non-Aligned & Other Developing Countries

337 **Studies in Indian Medicinal Plants Used in Ayurveda: Cathartics**
G.S. Pendse
1961
Indian Drugs Research Association, Pune

338 **Studies on Guggulu: Clinical and Experimental Trial Guggulu in Medo-Roga**
1989
Central Council for Research in Ayurveda & Siddha, Delhi

339 **Studies on Medicinal Plants in Dhanvantri Nighantu**
D.K. Kamat
1972
D.K. Kamat, 18 Rasta Peth, Pune

340 **Studies on the Medicinal Plants of Kerala Forests**
V.P. Nambiar
1985
Kerala Forest Research Institute, Peechi

341 **Substitute and Adulterant Plant**
Sunit Garg
1992
Periodical Expert Book Agency, Delhi

342 **Supplement of Cultivation & Utilization of Aromatic Plants**
Edited
1982
R.R.L., Jammu

343 **Supplement to Cultivation & Utilization of Medicinal Plants**
Edited
1982
R.R.L., Jammu

344 **Survey of Arecanut Crop in Indian Union**
K.K. Nambiar
1949
Indian Central Arecanut Committee, Ernakulum

345 **Sushruta Samhita**
Edited
1974
Motilal Banrasidas, Delhi

346 **Susruta Samhita, a Scientific Synopsis**
Priyadaranjan Ray
1980
Indian National Science Academy, Delhi

347 **Susurat Sahita (Hindi)**
Dr. Danetar
1974
Motilal Banarsidas, Delhi

348 **Textbook of Pharmacognosy**
C.S. Shah & J.S. Qadry
1989
B.S. Shah Prakashan, Ahmedabad

349 **The Ayurvedic Formulary of India Part-2**
Govt. of India
The Controller of Publication, Delhi

350 The Ayurvedic Pharmacopoeia of India Part-1 Vol 1, 2 & 3
Govt. of India
The Controller of Publication, Delhi

351 **The Economic Plants of North East India**
Sudhir Kumar
1999
Scientific Publishers, Jodhpur

352 **The Encyclopedia of Herbs, Spices & Flavourings**
Elisabeth Lambert Ortiz
1992
Dorling Kindersley, London

353 **The Encyclopedia of Medicinal Plants**
Andrew Chevallier MNIMH
1996
Dorling Kindersley, London

354 **The Forest Types of India**
S. K. Seth
1968
Govt. of India Press Nasik

355 **The Green Pharmacy(Reprint)**
James A. Duke
2002
Scientific Publishers, Jodhpur

356 **The illustrated herbs Endypedia**
Kathi keville
1991
Grange books, London

357 **The Medicinal and Poisonous Legumes of India**
J.F.Caius
1989
Scientific Publishers, Jodhpur

358 **The Medicinal and Poisonous Plants of India**
J.F. Caius
1998
Scientific Publishers, Jodhpur

359 **The Medicinal Plants of North East India**
Sudhir Kumar
2002
Scientific Publishers, Jodhpur

360 **The Role of Bamboo, Rattan & Medicinal Plants in Mountain Development**
Madhav Karki
1996
INBAR, Jorbagh, New Dehi

361 **The Small Garden**
John Brookes
1989
Tiger Books International, London

362 **The Treatise of Indian Medicinal Plants Vol. 1,2,3,4,5 & 6**
Edited
2001
NISCOM, New Delhi

363 **The Unani Pharmacocoeia of India**
Govt. of India
1999
Govt. of India (ISM&H) New Delhi

364 **The Wealth of India**
NISCOM
NISCOM, New Delhi

365 **Therapeutic Guide to Ayurvedic Medicine**
Ram R. Pathak
1970
Baidyanath Ayurveda Bhawan Ltd., Patna

366 **Threatened Plants of India**
S.K. Jain (Editor)
1983
BSI, Kolkotta

367 **Tibetan Medicinal Plants**
T.J. Tsarong
1994
Tibetan Medical Publications, Kalimpong

368 **Tibetan Medicine and Other Holistic Health-Care Systems**
Tom Dummer
1988
Paljor Publications, Delhi

369 **Tibetan Medicine Series 1-13**
Edited
1980
Library of Tibetan Works & Archives, Dharmsala

370 **Traditional Medicinal Plants in Skin Care**
1994
Central Institute of Medicinal & Aromatic Plants, Lucknow

371 **Traditional Medicine**
Biswapali Mukherjee
1993
Oxford & IBH Publishing Co. Pvt. Ltd., Delhi

372 **Treatise on Tropical Therapeutics**
R.N. Chopra
1954
U.N. Dhur & Sons Ltd., Calcutta

373 **Trees**
Allen J. Coombes
1992
Dorling Kindersley, London

374 **Trees & Shrubs**
John Kelly
1995
David & Charles UK

375 **Trees and Tree Farming**
P. K. Thampan
1994
Peekay Tree Crops Dev. Crop., Cochin

376 **Trees For Dry Lands**
Drake Hocking
1993
Oxford & IBH Publishing Co., New Delhi

377 **Tribal Medicine**
Maire D'Souza
1993
Society for Promotion of Wastelands Development, Delhi

378 **Tribal Medicine**
Dr. S. Vedavathy
1997
Herbal Folklore Research Centre, Tirupati

379 **Tropical Garden Plants**
T. K. Bose
1991
Horticulture & Allied Publishers, Kolkata

380 **Tropical Indian Medicinal Plants Propagation Methods**
D.K. Ved
2000
FRLHT, Bangalore

381 **Ultraviolet and Visible Spectra of herbal Drugs**
Asif M. Shafiullah
1992
Aligarh Muslim University Press, Aligarh

382 **Unani System of Medicine in India, a Profile**
Edited
1991
Central Council for Research in Unani Medicine, Delhi

383 Unique Medicinal Plant: Holy Basil, Tulsi
Yash Rai
Gala Publishers, Bombay

384 **Use of Traditional Medicine in Primary Health Care, a Manual or Health Workers in South East Asia**
Edited
1990
World Health Organisation, South-East Asia Regional Office, Delhi

385 Useful Cosmetic Herbs for Skin Care, Hair Care, Beauty Care & Toiletries
Edited
2000
Institute of Natural & Modern Cosmetech Faridabad

386 **Useful Plants of India**
Edited
NISCOM, Delhi

387 **Useful Plants of India: with Notices of Their Chief Value in Commerce, Medicine and the Arts**
Heber Drury
1873
International Book Distributors and Periodical Expert Book Agency, Dehra Dun and Delhi

388 **Using Herbs in the Home**
A. Gardiner
1995
Promotional Reprint Co. London

389 **Utilisation of Neem and Its By-products**
C.M. Ketkar
1976
Directorate of Non-edible Oils & Soap Industry, Khadi & Village Industries Commission, Bombay

390 Value Addition of Indian Essential Oils
S. C. Varshney
2001
Som Extracts, Delhi

391 **Vanoshadhi Chandrodaya Vol. & II (Hindi)**
Chandra Raj Bhandari
1998
Choukambha Sanskrit Sansthan, Varanashi

392 **Vegetable Drugs of India**
Devaprasad Sanyal
1924
Bishen Singh Mahendra Pal Singh, Dehra Dun

393 **Vegetable Materia Medica of India**
Emmanuel Roberts
1931
Bishen Singh Mahendra Pal Singh, Dehra Dun

394 **Vegetable Materia Medica of Western India**
William Dymock
1883
Educational Society Press, Bombay

395 **Vetiver Grass**
National Research Council
1993
National Academy Press, Washington

396 **Vetiver Grass**
P. K. Yoon
1993
The World Bank

397 **Wealth of Susruta**
Krishnamurthy
International institute of Ayurveda, Coimbatore

398 **Western Epitomes of Indian Medicine**
D.V. Subba Reddy
1966
Osmania Medical College, Upgraded Department of history of Medicine, Hyderabad

399 **What Trees is That?**
Stirling Macoboy
1979
Weldon Publishing, Sydney

400 **Wild Edible Plants of India**
R. K. Arora
1996
NBPGR, New Delhi

401 **Wild Fruits of the Sub-Himalayan Region**
Chiranjit Parmar
1982
Kalyani Publisher, Delhi

402 **Workshop on Drug Research in Ayurveda**
Edited
1993
Central Council for Research in Ayurveda & Siddha, Delhi

403 **Workshop on Information Management for the Medicinal & Aromatic Plants Industry**
H.C. Jain
1994
Council of Scientific & Industrial Research Publications & Information directorate, Delhi

404 **Workshop on Literary Research in Ayurveda & Rasashstra**
Edited
Indian Institute of History of Medicine, Hyderabad

405 **Workshop on Medicinal & Aromatic Plants**
Edited
1985
Indian Institute of Horticultural Research Coimbatore

406 **Workshop on Traditional Systems of Medicine & Primary Health Care**
Edited
1984
Arya Vaidyan Rama Varier Education Foundation of Ayurveda, Coimbatore

407 **World Directory of Ethnobotanists**
S.K. Jain
1986
Society of Ethnotanists, Lucknow

408 **Yoga of Herbs, an Ayurvedic Guide to Herbal Medicine**
David Frawley
1994
Motilal Banarasidass Publisher Pvt. Ltd., Delhi

409 **Zari Buti Chikitsa (Hindi)**
Dr. Saxena
1998
Rajasthan Patrika, Jaipur

PERIODICALS

1 **Agricultural Today**
G-30, Lajpat Nagar-II,
New Delhi-110024
Phone: 6910927-28, 6316747
Fax: 6849107
E-mail: agritoday@card.org.in
website: http://www.card.org.in

2 **Agriculture & Industry Survey**
Vadamlai Media Private Limited
Vadamlai Media Group No. 25,
17th Main, HAL, II Stage,
Bangalore 560008

3 **Agrobios New Letter**
Dr. Updesh Purohit
Behind Nasrani Cinema,
Chopasani Road, Jodhpur-342 003
Phone: 0291-643993
E-mail: agrobios@sify.com

4 **Amruth**
Medplan Conservatory Society
No. 8, 1" floor, 4th main,
MSH Layout, Anandnagar
Bangalore 560024, India
Phone: +91 80 3434464/65
Fax: +91 80 3334167
E-mail: medplan@eth.net
website: www.frlht.india.org

5 **Ancient Science of Life**
A.V.R. Educational Foundation of Ayurveda
P.B. No. 7102, Ramanathapura,
Coimbatore – 641045. India

6 **Arogya (Hindi)**
Arogya Mandir Gorkhpur-273003 (UP)
Phone: 0551-310469/310805
E-mail: arogya_mandir@indiatimes.com & info@arogyamandir.com
website: www.argyamandir.com

7 **Arogya, a Journal of Health Sciences**
Kasturba medical College,
Biochemistry Department
Manipal-576119 Karnataka

8 **Arogyadham (Hindi)**
Arya Samaj Road,
Muzaffarnagar – 251 001 (UP)
www.arogyadham.com

9 **Arunachal Forest News**
Orchidologist,
Orchid Research & Development Centre
Tippi
Bhalukpong-790114
Arunachal Pradesh

10 **Aryavaidyan**
Arya Vaidya Sala
malappuram District
Kottakal-676503 Kerala

11 **Ayu**
Gujarat Ayurved University
Dhanwantri Mandir, P.B. 511
Jamnagar-361008 Gujarat

12 **Ayurveda Mahasamelan Patrika (Hindi)**
Dhanvantri Bhavan
Road No. 66 Punjabi Bagh
New Delhi – 110026

13 **Ayurwave**
Dr. Giridhara Kaje
Prashanthi Ayurvedic Centre
#51,7th Cross, Bet. Sampige & Margosa Road,
Malleshwaram, Bangalore-560003
Phone: 91-80-3341105, 3361105
E-mail: info@kajeayurveda.com
website: www.kajeayurveda.com

14 **Baliraja (Marathi)**
Krishi Vigyan Prakashan Pune –411002
Phone/Fax: 020-4473225/4452540
E-mail: balirajaa@vsnl.net
website: www.biliraja.com

15 **Bharatiya Bouddhik Sampada**
Dr. V.K. Didolkar
Kedar 26, Cement Road,
Shivajinagar
Nagpur – 440010.
Phone: 525163

16 **Bhartiya Nariyal Patrika (Hindi)**
Nariyal Vikash Board
Kera Bhavan Kochi-682011
Phone: 0484-376265, 377266, 377267
Fax: 91-484-377902
E-mail: enk_cdbkochi@sancharnet.in
website: www.coconutboard.nic.in

17 **BSI Newsletter**
Botanical Survey of India
P.O. Botanic Garden
Howrah – 711103 West Bengal

18 **CCRAS Newsletter**
Central Council for Research in Ayurveda & siddha
JLN Bhartiya Chikitsa Evum Homoeopathy
Anusandhan Bhawan, 61-65
Omstotiteopma; Area.
Opposite D Block, Janakpuri
Delhi – 110058

19 **CCRH News Letter**
Central Council for Research in Homoeopathy
JLN Bhartiya Chikitsa Evum Homoeopathy
Anusandhan Bhawan, 61-65
Omstotiteopma; Area.
Opposite D Block, Janakpuri
Delhi – 110058

20 **CCRH Quarterly Bulletin**
Central Council for Research in Homoeopathy
JLN Bhartiya Chikitsa Evum Homoeopathy
Anusandhan Bhawan, 61-65
Omstotiteopma; Area.
Opposite D Block, Janakpuri
Delhi – 110058

21 **CCRUM Newsletter**
Central Council for Research in Homoeopathy
JLN Bhartiya Chikitsa Evum Homoeopathy
Anusandhan Bhawan, 61-65
Omstotiteopma; Area.
Opposite D Block, Janakpuri
Delhi – 110058

22 **CDRI Newsletter**
Central Drug Research Institute, National Information
Centre for Drugs & Pharmaceuticals
Chattar Manzil Palace, P.B. 173
Lucknow-226001 Uttar Pradesh

23 **Central Plantation Crops Research Institute, Newsletter**
Central Plantation Crops Research Institute
Post Kudlu
Kosaragoda – 671124 Kerala

24 **Central Tuber Crops Research Institute, Annual Research Highlights**
Central Tuber Crops Research Institute
Sree Kariyam,
Thiruvananthapuram – 695017 Kerala

25 **Chikitsa Pallav (Hindi)**
P. O. Pangara – 210 129
Dist. Banda (UP)

26 **CIMAP Newsletter**
Central Institute of Medicinal & aromatic Plants
P.O. CIMAP,
Lucknow (UP)
www.cimap.org

27 **CSIR Complex, Newsletter**
Council of Scientific & Industrial Research Complex,
Palampur Mission Road
Palampur – 176061 Himachal Pradesh

28 **CSIR News**
Council of Scientific & Industrial Research
Publications & Information Directorate
Dr. K.S. Krishnan Marg, Delhi-110012

29 **Current Research on Medicinal and Aromatic Plants (CROMAP)**
Central Institute of Medicinal & Aromatic Plants
P.O. CIMAP
Lucknow-226016 Uttar Pradesh
www.cimap.org

30 **Dhanvantri (Hindi)**
Harish Pharma, Vijaygrah, Aligarh (UP)
Phone: 0571-862219

31 **Down to Earth**
Centre for Science and Environment
41, Tughlakabad Institutional Area,
New Delhi –110062 India
Phone: 91-11-608 1110, Fax: 91-11608 0870, 608 5879
E-mail: sales@csenidia.org
website: www.cseindia.org

32 **Drugs and Pharmaceuticals: Current Highlights**
Central Drug Research Institute, National Information
Centre for Drugs & Pharmaceuticals
P.B. 173 Chattar Manzil Palace,
Lucknow-226001 Uttar Pradesh

33 **Drugs and Pharmaceuticals: Industry Highlights**
Central Drug Research Institute, National Information
Centre for Drugs & Pharmaceuticals
P.B. 173 Chattar Manzil Palace,
Lucknow-226001 Uttar Pradesh

34 **Eco News Africa**
P.O. Box No. 10332
00100, Nairobi, Kenya
www. Econewsafrica.org

35 **Environment (Hindi)**
Ministry of Environment & Forest 'B' Block
Environment House Room No. 904
C.G.O., Complex Lodhi Road New Delhi – 110003
Phone: 4363961

36 **Farming Japan**
Farming Japan Co. Ltd.,
7th Floor, Kojima Building,
4-2, Uchikanda 1-chome, Chiyoda-Ku
Tokyo-101-0047 Japan

37 **Food Technology Abstracts (FTA)**
Central Food Technological Research Institute,
National Information Centre for Food Science & Technology
Cheluvamba Mansion
Mysore-570013Karnataka

38 **Footsteps**
Tear fund, 100 Church Rd,
Teddington, TW11, 8QE UK

39 **Forests, Trees & People Newsletter**
GPO Box 11321,
Maitidevi Battishputali
Kathmandu, Nepal

40 **Gaun ka Guni (Hindi)**
Jagran Jan Vikash Samiti, Sapetiya Road
Bedla, Udiapur (Rajasthan)
Phone: 0294-441322

41 **Green News**
C/o Aruna Traders,
Babu Gram, IDPL,
Rishikesh – 249 202 (U.C.)

42 **Hamdard Medicus**
Hamdard Foundation Pakistan
Nazimabad, Karachi – 74600, Pakistan

43 **Health & Environment**
Centre for Science and Environment
41, Tughlakabad Institutional Area,
New Delhi –110062 India
Phone: 91-11-6081110, 3394, 608 6399
Fax: 91-11608 0870, 608 5879
E-mail: sales@csenidia.org
website: www.cseindia.org

44 **Herbal Cure**
Dr. Ahmad Rasool
10-4-41 Humayun Nagar
Hyderabad-500028 Andhra Pradesh

45 **Herbal Gram**
P.O. Box – 144345,
Austin, Texas 78714-4345
Phone – 512/926-4900
Fax – 512/926-2345
Email – abc@herbalgrow.org
Web – www.herbalgram.org

46 **Heritage Healing**
Healthcare Communication (P) Ltd.,
#8, 5th Cross Extn,
Bakthavatchalam Nagar
Adyar, Chennai 600020 India.
Phone : 91-44-4422780, 4422781 Fax :
91-44-4404070
E-mail : himal@md2.vsnl.net.in &
heritagehealing@yahoo.com

47 **Honey Bee**
Honey Bee, Indian Institute of
Management,
Vastrapur Ahmedabad – 380015 India
Phone: 91-79-6324927 Fax: 91-79-
6307341
E-mail: honeybee@sristi.org

48 **IIHR Newsletter**
Indian Institute of Horticultural Research
255 Upper Place Orchards
Bangaore – 560080 Karnataka

49 **Indian Chemical Society, Journal**
Indian Chemical Society
92 Acharya Prafulla Chandra Road
Calcutta-700009 West Bengal

50 **Indian Cocoa, Arecanut and Spices Journal**
Directorate o Cocoa, Arecanut & Spices
Development
c/o Ministry of Agriculture, Horticulture
Division
Calcutt-63005 Kerala

51 **Indian Coconut Journal**
Coconut Development Board
Kera Bhavan Kochi – 682011, India
Phone: 0484 – 377266 Fax: 91-0484-
377902
E-mail: cdbkochi@vsnl.com &
enk_cdrkochi@sancharnet.nic.in
Website: www.coconutboard.nic.in

52 **Indian Drugs**
Indian Drug Manufacturers Association
102-B Poonam Chambers, Dr. Annie
Besant Road, Wori
Bombay-400018 Maharashtra

53 **Indian Farming**
ICAR, Krishi Anusandhan Bhavan, Pusa
New Delhi 110012

54 **Indian Forest Bulletins**
Forest Research Institute
P.O. New Forest
Dehra Dun-248006 Uttar Pradesh

55 **Indian Forester**
Forest Research Institute (S.K. Aggarwal)
P.O. New Forest
Dehra Dun – 248006 Uttar Pradesh

56 **Indian Horticulture**
ICAR, Krishi Anusandhan Bhavan,
Pusa, New Delhi 110012

57 **Indian Journal of Arecanut, Spices & Medicinal Plants**
Directorate of Arecanut & Spices
Development
Ministry of Agriculture Department
of Agriculture & Co-operation
West Hill P.O., Calicut – 673005 Kerala

58 **Indian Journal of Chemistry**
Council of Scientific & Industrial Research,
Publications & Information Directorate
Dr. K.S. Krishnan Marg, Delhi-110012

59 **Indian Journal of Indigenous Medicine**
Society of Indigenous Medicine
Sharda Nagar
Saharanpur-247001 Uttar Pradesh

60 **Indian Journal of Minor Forest Produce**
Society for promotion of Minor Forest Produce
Tropical Forest Research Institute, Mandla Road
Hablpur-482001 Madhya Pradesh

61 **Indian Journal of Natural Products**
Indian Society of Pharmacognosy
c/o Dr. H.S. Gour Vishwavidyalaya, Pharmaceutical
Sciences Department
Sagar Department
Sagar-470003 Madhya Pradesh

62 **Indian Journal of Pharmaceutical Sciences**
Indian Pharmaceutical Association
Kalina, Santa Cruz East
Bombay-400098 Maharashtra

63 **Indian Journal of Soil conservation**
Indian Association of Soil & Water Conservationists
218, Kaulagarh Road, Dehradun – 248195
Uttarancahl, India

64 **Indian Journal of Unani Medicine**
Central Council for Research in Unani Medicine
JLN Bhartiya Chikitsa Evum Homoeopathy
Anusandhan Bhawan 61-65 Institutional Area,
opposite D Block , Janakpuri
Delhi – 110058

65 **Indian Journal of Veterinary Medicine**
Indian Society for Veterinary Medicine
c/o Orissa Veterinry College, Department of Medicine
Bhubaneswar- Orissa

66 **Indian Medicine**
Indian Medicine Industries
Dubagunta Nivas
Vijaywada-520002 Andhra Pradesh

67 **Indian Perfumer**
Essential Oil Association of India
Dua Complex, 24 Veer Savarkar Block, Shakarpur,
Viks Marg
Delhi-110092

68 **Indian Spices**
Spices Board India
Sugandha Bhavan, N.H. Bypass, Palarivattam
Cochin-682025 Kerala

69 **Intensive Agriculture**
Editor, Intensive Agriculture, Krishi Vistar Bhavan
Directorate of Extension, Ministry of Agriculture
IARI Campus, Pusa, New Delhi – 110012
E-mail: patanga_editor@rediffmail.com

70 **International Trade Forum**
ITC, 54-56, Rue De Montbrillant,
1202 Geneva, Switzerland,
Phone: +41 22 7300111
Fax: +41 22 733 4439
E-mail: itcreg@intracen.org
website: http://www.intracen.org

71 **Journal Naturaceuticals, Functional & Medical Foods**
The Haworth Herbal Press
10, Alice Street, Binghamton,
New York 13904 – 1580 USA
Email – getinfo@haworthpressinc.com
www.haworthpress.com

72 **Journal of Herbal Pharmacotherapy**
The Haworth Herbal Press
10, Alice Street, Binghamton,
New York 13904 – 1580 USA
Email – getinfo@haworthpressinc.com
www.haworthpress.com

73 **Journal of Herbs, Spices and Meditional Plants**
The Haworth Herbal Press
10, Alice Street, Binghamton,
New York 13904 – 1580 USA
Email – getinfo@haworthpressinc.com
www.haworthpress.com

74 **Journal of Scientific Research in Plants and Medicines**
Yogi Pharmacy Ltd.
Laksar Road, P.O. Gurukul Kangri
Hardwar-249404 Uttar Pradesh

75 **Journal of Spices and Aromatic Crops**
Indian Society for Spices
c/o National Research Centre for spices,
P.O.B. 1701,
Mari Kunnu P.O.
Calicut-673012 Kerala

76 **Kheti (Hindi)**
ICAR Krishi Anusandhan Bhavan, Pusa
New Delhi – 110012

77 **Kheti Dunyia (Hindi New Paper)**
K.D. Complex, Gaushala Road Patiala-147001, Punjab
Phone : 214575/700386 Fax : 0175-217098

78 **Kisan Bharti (Hindi)**
Govind Vallabha Panth Krishi avom Prodhogiki Vishvavidhalaya
Panth Nagar-263145,
Udhyam Singh Nagar (Uttaranchal)

79 **Kisan World**
101, Mount Road, Guindy
Chennai – 600 032

80 **Krishak Bharati (Hindi)**
Directorate of Extension,
Chandrashekhar Azad Agriculture & Technology University,
Kanpur – 208 002 (UP)

81 **Krishak Jagat (Hindi New Paper)**
Krishak Jagat P.O. Box-37, Bhopal-462011 (MP)

82 **Krishak Vandana (Hindi)**
Nanda Kishore Patel M.N. 6, Matri Nagar,
Maharajpur Jabalpur-482004 (MP)
Phone : 353692, 344024

83 **Krishi Chayanika (Hindi)**
ICAR Krishi Anusandhan Bhavan, Pusa
New Delhi – 110012

84 **Krishi Jeevan (Gujarati)**
Gujrat State fertilizer & Chemicals Ltd.,
P.O. Fertilizer Nagar
Baroda – 391 750 (Gujarat)

85 **Market News Services For Medicinal Plants**
International Trade Centre
Palais des Nations
CH-1211, Genewa-10
Switzerland

86 **Maru Krishi Chyanika (Hindi)**
Central Arid Zone Research Institute
(CAZRI), Jodhpur – 342 003

87 **Medicinal and Aromatic Plants Abstracts (MAPA)**
NISCOM
Dr. K.S. Krishnan Marg
Delhi-110012

88 **MFP News**
Centre of Minor Forest Products for Rural Development & Environmental Conservation
HIG-2/8 General Mahadev Singh Road,
Indirapuram P.O. Kanwali
Dehra Dun-248001 Uttar Pradesh

89 **My Forest**
My Forest, Silviculturist, Central Zone
1st Cross, Arekere, Mico Layout,
Near Forest Complex Boresanipalya,
Bannerghatta Road, Bangalore 560076

90 **Namah**
Sri Aurobinodo Society
Pondicherry 605001
Phone: 91 –0413-336396/7/8

91 **Namaths Herbal Unani Med**
136, Jani Jehan Khan Road, Royapettah
Chennai – 6000014

92 **Natural Product Radiance**
The Sales and Distribution Officer,
National Institute of Science Communication (NISCOM)
Dr. K.S. Krishnan Marg, New Delhi 110012
Phone: 5786301-7 Fax: 5787062
E-mail: sales@niscom.res.in

93 **Naturopathy**
Bapu Nature Cure Hospital, Gandhi Nidhi
Patparganj, New Delhi-110091
Phone: 2795205, 2795247 Fax: 2795254
E-mail: natucure@nda.vsnl.net.in
website:
www.naturopathyinternational.8k.com
www.naturopathyacademy.org

94 **NBPGR newsletter**
National Bureau of Plant Genetic Resources
Indian agricultural Research Institute Campus, Pusa
Delhi-110012

95 **NBPGR Research Highlights**
National Bureau of Plant Genetic Resources
Indian Agricultural Research Institute Campus, Pusa
Delhi-110012

96 **Neem: News Letter of International Neem Network**
Indian Council of Forestry Research & Education
P.O. New Forest
Dehra Deun-248006 Uttar Pradesh

97 **Non-Wood News**
Non-Wood News-FOPW
FAO, Viale delle terme di Caracalla
00100 Rome, Italy
E-Mail: non-wood-news@fao.org
website:
www.fao/foreshtry/nwfp/nonwood.htm

98 **PAFAI Journal**
Perfumes & Flavours Association of India
2-B, Court Chambers, 35 New Mrine Lines
Bombay-208002 Uttar Pradesh

99 **Perma Culture**
Permanent Publications,
Hyden House Ltd.,
The Sustainability Centre,
East Meon, Hampshire, GU32, IHR,
England
www.permaculture.co.uk

100 **Phal-Phul (Hindi)**
Indian Council of Agricultural Research
Krishi Anusandhan Bhavan, Pusa Gate,
New Delhi – 110012
Phone: 5854649

101 **Pharma Research**
Express Pharma Pulse, Business
Publications Division, Indian Express
Newspapers (Bombay) Ltd., 1st Floor,
Express Towers, Nariman Point, Mumbai-
400021. India
Phone: 2301020 Fax : 022-2301007

102 **Plant Science**
Association for Advancement of Plant
Sciences
c/o Agricultural Refinance & Development
Corporation
Calcutta-700001 West Bengal

103 **Planta Medica**
Georg Thieme Verlag
P.O. Box 301120, D-7045
Stuttgart, Germany

104 **Regional Health Forum**
World Health Organization
Regional Office for South-East Asia
Indraprastha Estate
New Delhi 110002, India
Email: Dixitr@whosea.org

105 **Review of Aromatic and Medicinal Plants**
CAB International
Wallingford, Oxon, OX10, 8DE
UK

106 **Richters Herb letter**
357, Hwy 47, Goodwood,
Ontario LOC IAO Canada
www.richters.com
Email – orderdesk@richters.com

107 **RRL-Jammu, Newsletter**
Regional Research Laboratory, Jammu
Canal Road
Jammu Tawi-18001 Jammu & Kashmir

108 **RRL-Jorhat, News Letter**
Regional Research Laboratory, Jorhat
Jorhat-785006 Assam

109 **RRL-Thiruvananthapuram, Newsletter**
Regional Research Laboratory,
Thiruvananthapuram
P.O. Industrial State, Pappanamcode
Thiruvananthapuram-695019 Kerala

110 **Sachitra Ayurveda (Hindi)**
Shri Baidyanath Ayurveda Bhavan Ltd.
Baidyanath Bhavan Road, Patna –800001

111 **Sayama Kon (Hindi New Paper)**
Chiranjilal Mathur
13, Viradvila, Tejaji Marg, New Sanganer
Road, Sodala, Jaipur-302019
Phone: 0141-294556

112 **Science Reporter**
Publisher
257, Driba Kalan, Delhi 110006

113 **Science Tech Entrepreneur**
Centre for Entrepreneurship Development
Madhya Pradesh (CEDMAP)
60, Jail Road, Jehangirabad,
Bhopal – 462008. India
Phone: 91-0755-766437 Fax: 91-0755-
763401
E-mail: cedmap@vsnl.com
website: www.cedmapindia.com

114 **Suchi (Hindi)**
Shri Trimurthi Pharmacy Compound
47A Industrial Area Bikaner-334001
Phone: 542290

115 **Sudhanidhi (Hindi)**
Sudhanidhi Office Vijaygrah, Aligarh (UP)

116 **Sujh-Bujh (Hindi)**
Bhartiya Praband Sansthan, Vastrapur,
Ahmedabad-15
Phone: 6324927
Fax : 6307341
E-mail : honeybee@sristi.org
website : http://www.sristi.org.

117 **Swasthya**
Krishna Gopal Ayurved Bhawan
Post Kaleda-Krishna Gopal
Dist – Ajmer – 305 408 (Raj.)

118 **Traffic Bulletin**
TRAFFIC International,
219c, Huntingdon Road,
Cambridge, Cambs
CB3 0267 4297 – UK

119 **Udhyamita (Hindi)**
Centre for Entrepreneurship Development
Madhya Pradesh
60, Jail Road, Jehangirabad, Bhopal – 462008. India
Phone: 91-0755-766437 Fax: 763401
E-mail: cedmap@vsnl.com website: www.cedmapindia.com

120 **Unnat Krishi (Hindi)**
Krishi Vistar Bhavan, Directorate of Extension,
Ministry of Agriculture, IARI Campus, Pusa,
New Delhi – 110 012
E-mail : patanga_editor@rediffmail.com

121 **Vaniki Sandesh**
State Forest Research Institute
Polipathar, Narmada Road
Jabalpur-482008 Madhya Pradesh

122 **Vanoshadhi (Marathi)**
Vaidya Sunil B. Patil
Ayurveda Punchkarm Centre, 1449/C,
Laxmipuri, Kolhapur
Phone: 0231-642725

123 **Vishva Krishi Sanchar (Hindi)**
Vishva Agro Marketing & Communication
Mohasin Manzil, 252, Shopping Centre
Kota-7, Rajasthan
Phone: 0744-363066, 364571
Fax: 0744-422219

124 **Wood Energy News**
Regional Wood Energy Development Programme in Asia,
FAO Regional Office,
Maliwan Mansion, Phra Atit Road,
Bangkok – 10200 (Thailand)
www.rwedp.org

COMMON NAMES OF MEDICINAL PLANTS IN DIFFERENT LANGUAGES